T0318871

Veterinary Anaesthesia

Content Strategist: Robert Edwards
Content Development Specialists: Nicola Lally and Alison McMurdo
Project Manager: Julie Taylor
Designer/Design Direction: Miles Hitchen
Illustration Manager: Jennifer Rose
Illustrator: Antbits Ltd

Veterinary Anaesthesia

Eleventh Edition

K. W. Clarke MA, VetMB, DVA, DVetMed, DipECVAA, FHEA, MRCA, FRCVS

Hon Professor of Veterinary Anaesthesia, Royal Veterinary College, University of London, UK

C. M. Trim BVSc, DVA, DipACVAA, DipECVAA, MRCVS

Professor Emeritus of Anesthesiology, Josiah Meigs Distinguished Teaching Professor, College of Veterinary Medicine, University of Georgia, Athens, Georgia, USA

L. W. Hall MA, BSc, PhD, DVA, Dr (Hons Causa) Utrecht, DipECVAA, DipACVA (Hon), FRCA, FRCVS (deceased)

Reader in Comparative Anaesthesia, University of Cambridge, UK

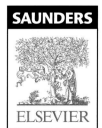

Edinburgh London New York Oxford Philadelphia St Louis Sydney Toronto 2014

SAUNDERS
ELSEVIER

First edition 1941
Second edition 1947
Third edition 1948
Fourth edition 1957
Fifth edition 1961
Sixth edition 1966
Seventh edition 1971
Eight edition 1983
Ninth edition 1991
Tenth edition 2001
Eleventh edition 2014

ISBN: 9780702027932
E-ISBN: 9780702054235

British Library Cataloguing in Publication Data
A catalogue record for this book is available from the British Library

Library of Congress Cataloging in Publication Data
A catalog record for this book is available from the Library of Congress

Notices
Knowledge and best practice in this field are constantly changing. As new research and experience broaden our understanding, changes in research methods, professional practices, or medical treatment may become necessary.

Practitioners and researchers must always rely on their own experience and knowledge in evaluating and using any information, methods, compounds, or experiments described herein. In using such information or methods they should be mindful of their own safety and the safety of others, including parties for whom they have a professional responsibility.

With respect to any drug or pharmaceutical products identified, readers are advised to check the most current information provided (i) on procedures featured or (ii) by the manufacturer of each product to be administered, to verify the recommended dose or formula, the method and duration of administration, and contraindications. It is the responsibility of practitioners, relying on their own experience and knowledge of their patients, to make diagnoses, to determine dosages and the best treatment for each individual patient, and to take all appropriate safety precautions.

To the fullest extent of the law, neither the Publisher nor the authors, contributors, or editors, assume any liability for any injury and/or damage to persons or property as a matter of products liability, negligence or otherwise, or from any use or operation of any methods, products, instructions, or ideas contained in the material herein.

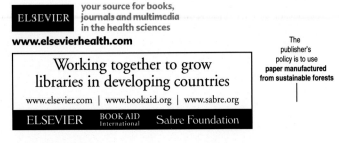

ELSEVIER your source for books, journals and multimedia in the health sciences
www.elsevierhealth.com

Working together to grow libraries in developing countries
www.elsevier.com | www.bookaid.org | www.sabre.org

ELSEVIER   BOOK AID International   Sabre Foundation

The publisher's policy is to use paper manufactured from sustainable forests

Printed in China

Contents

Contributors

Jennifer G. Adams DVM, DipACVIM, DipACVAA
Hull, Georgia, USA

Kate Borer-Weir BVSc, PhD, DVA, DipECVAA, FHEA, MRCVS
Lecturer in Anaesthesia
Royal Veterinary College
Hatfield, Hertfordshire, UK

K. W. Clarke MA, VetMB, DVA, DVetMed, DipECVAA, FHEA, MRCA, FRCVS
Hon Professor of Veterinary Anaesthesia
Royal Veterinary College
University of London, UK

Stephen J. Divers BVetMed, DZooMed, DipACZM, DipECZM (Herpetology), MRCVS
Professor of Zoological Medicine
Department of Small Animal Medicine & Surgery
College of Veterinary Medicine
University of Georgia
Athens, Georgia, USA

Leslie W. Hall MA, BSc, PhD, DVA, Dr (Hons Causa) Utrecht, DipECVAA, DipACVA (Hon), FRCA, FRCVS (deceased)
Reader in Comparative Anaesthesia,
University of Cambridge, UK

Sonia M. Hernandez DVM, PhD, DipACZM
Assistant Professor of Wildlife Disease
Daniel B. Warnell School of Forestry and Natural Resources and Southeastern Cooperative Wildlife Disease Study
College of Veterinary Medicine
University of Georgia
Athens, Georgia, USA

Cynthia M. Trim BVSc, DVA, DipACVAA, DipECVAA, MRCVS
Professor Emeritus of Anesthesiology
Josiah Meigs Distinguished Teaching Professor
College of Veterinary Medicine
University of Georgia
Athens, Georgia, USA

Preface

In this eleventh edition of *Veterinary Anaesthesia* we have attempted to continue Dr Leslie Hall's tradition of providing 'how to' advice on anaesthetizing animals. In addition, our goal has been to expand the evidence-based theme and provide published justification for most of our conclusions, particularly in relation to clinical advice, while also including information based on our own experiences. There are now hundreds of relevant published papers, and we have to acknowledge that in the space available we cannot cite all.

The aim of the book has always been to provide a text for veterinary students, a reference work for veterinarians in practice or working with laboratory animals, and a stimulating introduction to the subject for those wishing to specialize in veterinary anaesthesia. While following the format of previous editions, we have made several major changes in this edition. We have invited other authors to contribute chapters, and are grateful for their excellent reviews which provide added dimensions to the book. A chapter specifically devoted to analgesia recognizes the importance of pain relief and the major advances in the physiology and practice in this area. A new chapter is devoted to wild animal anaesthesia and another discusses anaesthetic management of small mammals, exotic pets and small wildlife. A chapter has been added to provide current information on cardiopulmonary cerebral resuscitation. We would also like to acknowledge valuable contributions to Chapter 1 by Craig Johnson (electroencephalography) and Daniel Pang (mechanisms of action of general anaesthetic agents) to ensure accuracy in these specialized and fast advancing areas.

We would wish to express our appreciation to David Gunn (AIIP) and to Charlotte Hall for many of the figures re-used from previous editions, and to those who have provided new figures for this edition and are acknowledged in the text. We also thank Kim Stevens and Flint Buchanan for their expert assistance with some of the figures. Our warmest thanks are due to the publishers for their patience, and in particular to Nicola Lally and Alison McMurdo for their constant encouragement. Finally, we must thank our families, who tolerated our constant 'absence', and carried out our day-to-day duties for us enabling us to concentrate on writing. Without them, the book would never have been completed.

K. W. Clarke
C. M. Trim

In memoriam

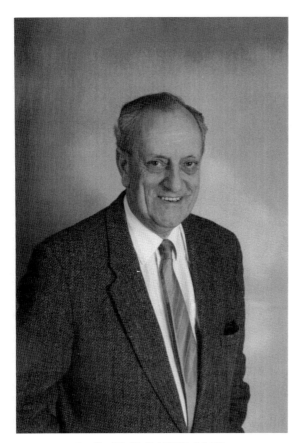

Leslie W. Hall (1927–2010)
MA, BSc, PhD, DVA, Dr (Hons Causa) Utrecht, DipECVAA, DipACVA (Hon),
FRCA, FRCVS

Dr Leslie Hall's foresight and drive led to the development of veterinary anaesthesia as a speciality. His contributions to the veterinary profession as a scientist, clinician, teacher and author have been matched by very few.

Dr Hall qualified as a veterinary surgeon at the Royal Veterinary College, London in 1950, remaining there to obtain his PhD. At that time, anaesthesia was produced in most animals by administering large doses of the few drugs available, with no specific perianaesthetic care. He recognized that animals needed better care under anaesthesia and set out to address their most pressing needs.

Dr Hall developed suitable dosage regimens, promoted the use of endotracheal intubation, oxygen administration, and artificial ventilation. He also instituted the practice of monitoring the animals during and after anaesthesia and, importantly, began administering analgesics postoperatively, an approach that was not considered necessary for animals at that time.

Dr Hall then moved to Cambridge where he excelled as a scientist, a clinician and as a teacher and worked tirelessly to promote veterinary anaesthesia as a speciality. He developed liaisons with the human medical (physician) anaesthetists, and became an active member of their national and local associations. In 1977, he was honoured with the Faculty Medal of the Faculty of Anaesthesia of the Royal College of Surgeons and, in 2001, was awarded an Honorary Fellowship of the Royal College of Anaesthetists.

Of the many highlights in Dr Hall's career, we believe the following deserve specific mention. In 1964, with six of his colleagues, Dr Hall founded the Association of Veterinary Anaesthetists (AVA). This association now has members world-wide, and is the 'base society' for the European College of Veterinary Anaesthesia and Analgesia (ECVAA). On his retirement, Dr Hall was made an Honorary Fellow of AVA. Working with his colleague, Dr Barbara Weaver, Dr Hall helped develop the Diploma of Veterinary Anaesthesia (DVA) of the Royal College of Veterinary Surgeons, the first 'specialist' veterinary qualification in anaesthesia. For the first examination in 1968, they organized a syllabus, created a robust examination, and included a medical (physician) anaesthetist on the examination panel. The DVA provided the foundation for the current Diploma of the ECVAA and served as a model for the Diploma of the American College of Veterinary Anesthesia and Analgesia (ACVAA). Dr Hall was awarded an Honorary Diploma from the ACVAA in 1985.

While teaching at Cambridge, Dr Hall provided postgraduate training in veterinary anaesthesia through research scholarships and through a clinical position of University Assistant Anaesthetist, a post equivalent to what is now termed a 'Residency'. He also used his influence to establish a career structure for those who entered the speciality. For example, he convinced surgeons that their clinical practice and the outcomes of their patients would be improved by including a trained anaesthetist. He also promoted the concept to veterinary school administrators that future veterinary surgeons needed a high standard of anaesthesia training before venturing into practice. As a result, university positions of Lecturer (and later, Professorships) in Veterinary and Comparative Anaesthesia started to appear.

In 1982, under Dr Hall's guidance, the first International (now World) Congress of Veterinary Anaesthesia was held at Cambridge. Due to the overwhelming success of that meeting, Congresses have been held, in several continents, every three years since that time. In the mid-1990s, Dr Hall served as one of the founding members of the ECVAA, the authority that grants certification for the speciality of veterinary anaesthesia and analgesia in Europe.

Leslie Hall was not just a clinician – but a brilliant scientist – indeed, he believed strongly in what is now called 'evidence-based medicine'. He authored more than 80 papers now cited in PubMed, and many more in other veterinary journals. Much of his work focused on the physiological responses to anaesthesia, particularly in horses and many of his publications are now considered 'classics'. Examples of the latter include an investigation of muscle relaxants in dogs (1953), recognition of malignant hyperthermia in pigs (1966), and the first demonstration of ventilation/perfusion mismatch in the anaesthetized horse (1968). Many anaesthetic agents were introduced into veterinary practice as a direct result of his experimental work and clinical trials. Classical examples include the introduction of halothane (1957), xylazine (1969), alphaxalone (as Saffan) (1972, 1975), and propofol (1985, 1987). Dr Hall's vision was far-reaching and involved research students from all over the world.

In addition to his scientific publications, Leslie was author/joint author of many review articles and several books. For more than 50 years he served as the primary author of this book. However, he also published a small book 'Fluid balance in canine surgery' in 1967, which includes information from some otherwise unpublished research studies, and 'Anaesthesia of the cat' in 1994 in collaboration with Dr Polly Taylor.

Leslie Hall was a knowledgeable and enthusiastic teacher of anaesthesia to veterinary and postgraduate clinical and research students. His enthusiasm for his subject was infectious, and postgraduate students were impressed by his unique ability to link clinical care with evidence-based research, and with his integrity within his research, always looking for the reason for an unexpected result. He was a superb clinician, a self-confessed workaholic, a hard taskmaster but a loyal mentor.

He imparted knowledge regardless of the venue, whether it was the surgery theatre or the local pub. Furthermore, he did all this with loving support of his family.

Although Leslie Hall had many opportunities to move elsewhere and upwards in rank, he preferred to remain Reader in Comparative Anaesthesia at Cambridge. Despite this reticence, he received many honours in the UK and elsewhere, including honorary degrees from Utrecht and the RCVS, the Francis Hogg Prize for advancing small animal practice, the Livesey Medal for alleviating pain and fear in animals, the Blaine award from the British Small Animal Veterinary Association, and Fellowship from the RCVS by election.

A fitting summation of his influence and impact comes from a note from one of his previous postgraduate students, now a Professor:

'Leslie was responsible for setting clinical standards that were rigorous and science-based and those of us lucky enough to be taught by him were the fortunate beneficiaries. Of course, Leslie's home-made beer was also legendary!'

K. W. Clarke
Cynthia Trim

Parts of this Eulogy, and the picture, were published as an 'Obituary to Dr L.W. Hall', in Veterinary Anaesthesia and Analgesia 2010 (37): 387–389, published by Wiley-Blackwell.

Section | 1 |

Principles and procedures

Chapter | **1** |

An introduction to anaesthesia and general considerations

INTRODUCTION

Anaesthesia is one of the greatest 'discoveries' there has ever been – there are few scientific advances which have reduced pain and suffering in so many people and animals. It is difficult to remember that the first anaesthetic was administered only in the 1840s (there is argument as to who was first to administer it clinically), although analgesics (for example opiates) have been available for many centuries. The term *anaesthesia* was coined by Oliver Wendell Holmes in 1846 to describe using ether to produce insensibility in a single word and it comes from the Greek 'without feeling'. The term 'analgesia' is Greek for 'without pain'.

While anaesthesia has precisely the same meaning as when it was first coined, i.e. the state in which an animal is insensible to pain resulting from the trauma of surgery, it is now used much more widely. Starting with the premise that 'pain is the conscious perception of a noxious stimulus', two conditions may be envisaged: *general anaesthesia* where the animal is unconscious and apparently unaware of its surroundings, and *analgesia* or *local anaesthesia* where the animal, although seemingly aware of its surroundings, shows diminished or no perception of pain. Perioperative analgesia, a subject once much neglected by veterinarians, is now recognized as an essential component of the process, and the physiology of pain and mechanisms of how it can be controlled and treated are discussed in Chapter 5, Analgesia.

VETERINARY ANAESTHESIA

The clinical discipline of veterinary anaesthesia is essentially a practical subject based on science. In addition to the scientific base for human anaesthesia, the veterinarian has to contend with species differences, particularly in anatomy and in metabolism that effects the actions and elimination of drugs.

In clinical veterinary anaesthesia, the major requirements of the anaesthetist are:

- Humane treatment of the animal
  - This includes prevention of awareness of pain, relief of anxiety and sympathetic animal handling
- Provision of adequate conditions for the procedure
  - This includes adequate immobility and relaxation
  - Ensuring neither the animal, nor the personnel are injured in any way.

All patients require an adequate standard of monitoring (Chapter 2), and of general care throughout the anaesthetic process. However, other than this, there is a myriad of acceptable methods from which the anaesthetist can choose to satisfy the above aims. Certain drugs and/or systems may be put forward as 'best practice' but, in veterinary anaesthesia, there is rarely the 'evidence base' to prove that they are so. Choice of methods used may be limited by a number of factors. Legal requirements, which will depend on the country concerned, need to be observed. Examples include laws involving the control of dangerous drugs, or the choice of drugs in animals destined for human consumption. In the European Union, currently, the 'cascade' is a major barrier to anaesthetists' choice. This law implies that if there is a drug licensed for a species, it is criminal to use another unlicensed agent for the same purpose, unless the veterinary surgeon can prove that their alternative choice was justified for welfare of the specific individual animal concerned. Facilities may be limited, and while expense should not be the governing factor, it does need to be considered; animals throughout the world require anaesthesia and if the owners cannot afford the cost, the animal will be denied treatment. The objective of this book is to give the reader the information enabling them to make an informed choice of the best method of anaesthesia and care for their patient in their circumstances.

GENERAL ANAESTHESIA

General anaesthesia is and has been given many different definitions (reviewed by Urban & Bleckwenn, 2002), but a simple practical one that has been used in the previous editions of this book is 'the reversible controlled drug induced intoxication of the central nervous system (CNS) in which the patient neither perceives nor recalls noxious or painful stimuli'. Professors Rees and Grey (1950) introduced the concept that the requirements from general anaesthesia were analgesia, muscle relaxation and 'narcosis', these being known as the 'Liverpool Triad'. This idea has been expanded to add suppression of reflexes (motor and autonomic) and unconsciousness or at least amnesia and, most importantly, that these requirements should be achieved without causing harm to the patient. For over 100 years anaesthesia was achieved mainly with a single drug, most commonly ether. Now, as well as a number of anaesthetic drugs which are administered by inhalation as is ether (see Chapter 7), single-agent drugs that are given by injection (see Chapter 6) are also employed. However, in clinical practice, it is now usual to use many different agents, which act at multiple receptors, in the CNS and peripherally, in order to achieve the goals required to provide good anaesthesia.

Currently, when considering single-agent anaesthetics, many authorities now believe that the state of general anaesthesia requires only two features: immobility in response to noxious stimulation and amnesia (the latter often taken as unconsciousness) (Eger et al., 1997; Urban & Bleckwenn, 2002). The argument is that the immobility is required for surgery; if the patient is unconscious they cannot perceive pain (although the autonomic system may still react to noxious stimuli), and if they don't remember the pain, it is similar to lack of perception. This theory ignores evidence and theories relating to pain and hypersensitization as described in Chapter 5. However, it considers that analgesia is desirable but is not an essential feature of the state of 'general anaesthesia'. Thus the 'definition' of a single-agent anaesthetic drug, such as the injectable agent, propofol or the volatile anaesthetic agents is that they have these two actions of preventing movement and causing amnesia (Franks, 2006). Some compounds which from structure and lipophility might be expected to be anaesthetics can cause amnesia without immobility; these are sometimes termed 'non-anaesthetics' (Johansson & Zou, 2001), their major interest being related to studies of mechanism of anaesthetic action.

Mechanisms of action of general anaesthetic agents

The central nervous system control of the functions altered by anaesthesia and related drugs is incredibly complex. Sherrington in 1906 pointed out the importance of the synapse in the CNS in providing connections between multiple neuronal systems (Fig. 1.1). At synapses, transmission involves release of transmitter that will 'trigger' the action of the next neuron. Receptors sensitive to the transmitter may be postsynaptic, or presynaptic feeding back on the original nerve terminal and modulating further action. Transmitters act through two main types of receptor: ionotropic and metabotropic. With inotropic or

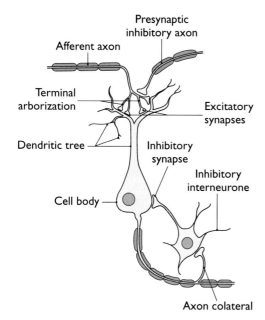

Figure 1.1 Schematic diagram of the organization of a synaptic relay within the CNS.

'ligand-gated' receptors, the transmitter binds directly with the ion-channel proteins, allowing the channel to open and the ions to pass. Binding of a transmitter to metabotropic receptors involves G-proteins as secondary messengers. Recent roles for voltage-gated channels, where changes in cellular membrane potential triggers a response, such as two-pore potassium channels have also been identified.

In the CNS, three major transmitters are considered most directly relevant to general anaesthesia. Gamma-amino-butyric acid (GABA) is inhibitory and decreases the excitability of neurons. Glycine is inhibitory in most circumstances and is the most important inhibitory transmitter at the spinal cord. The main excitatory transmitter in the CNS is glutamate. Anaesthetic drugs that are thought to act at the N-methyl d-aspartate (NMDA) receptor, one of at least three types of ligand-gated glutamate receptor, inhibit the effect of glutamate, thus again inhibiting the CNS. However, there are many other relevant transmitters, for example acetylcholine, dopamine, norepinephrine, endogenous opioids and others (Sonner et al., 2003) and their resultant actions may influence (modulate) the actions, directly or indirectly, of the GABA, glycine and glutamate pathways.

In the 1900s, for the inhalation agents (no injectable had been discovered), Meyer and Overton independently noted the correlation between anaesthetic potency and solubility in oil, which led to the 'lipid theory' that general anaesthetics acted through a non-specific mechanism by changing the lipid bilayer of nerve cells. There are exceptions which disprove the hypothesis but, nevertheless, for most the correlation is amazing, and this theory, with modifications, held sway until Franks and Lieb (1984) showed that inhalational general anaesthetics inhibited protein activity in the absence of lipids. This finding led to the explosion of studies on (a) where in the CNS anaesthetics act, (b) differences between motor and amnesic actions and, finally, (c) the molecular targets for action. (Franks (2006) quotes a review that cites 30 possible such targets.) All these three points are inextricably interlinked. A full discussion is beyond the remit of this book, but the following very simplified summary is based on reviews by Urban & Bleckwenn (2002), Sonner et al. (2003), Rudolph & Antikowiak (2004), Franks (2006) and Perouansky et al. (2012).

All anaesthetic agents do not act in the same way or in the same place. Classified by their mode and place of actions, there appear to be four main types of anaesthetic agent: (1) injectable agents such as propofol, etomidate and alfaxalone; (2) volatile anaesthetic agents such as halothane, isoflurane and sevoflurane; (3) the injectable dissociative agents such as ketamine; and (4) the gaseous agents, nitrous oxide and xenon.

It is now considered that the inhibition of motor actions occurs at the spinal cord, at least for the volatile anaesthetic agents, while amnesia and unconsciousness are the remit of the higher centres in the brain (Eger et al., 1997) – these two aspects of anaesthesia being separate. Most anaesthetics can cause amnesia at subhypnotic doses, although the relative dose for amnesia in relationship to that required for unconsciousness varies between drugs. The area of brain critical for amnesia appears to be the hippocampus and basal nucleus of the amygdala. Other centres are involved in the production of sedation and unconsciousness. For example, functional neuroimaging demonstrated that when propofol was administered at sedative doses and a noxious stimulus applied, evoked responses were attenuated only in the somatosensory cortex, but once doses reached hypnotic levels, thalamic and cortical responses ceased. Ketamine, a dissociative anaesthetic, however, did not depress sensory inflow through the thalamus. Perouansky et al. (2012) summarize by pointing out that anaesthesia is a very complex state, and that current evidence shows that general anaesthetics produce separate 'agent specific' substates, probably at different areas of the CNS.

Three very differing molecular targets have been suggested as the major sites of anaesthetic actions: GABA$_A$ receptors, NMDA receptors and glycine receptors. Anaesthetic drugs that act at the GABA$_A$ receptors are the classical IV anaesthetics; these potentiate the action of GABA, hence increase overall CNS inhibition. The volatile anaesthetic agents have similar actions at GABA$_A$ receptors in addition to actions at other targets, and their mode of action is more complex. Dissociative anaesthetics such as ketamine and the gaseous anaesthetic agents are thought to be antagonistic at the NMDA receptor, thus blocking the action of the excitatory glutamate, but again, this does not explain all their actions.

A great deal is known about the $GABA_A$ receptor (there are also $GABA_B$ and $GABA_C$). It is a polymeric receptor with five subunits; there have been at least 30 types of subunit cloned so the potential for heterogenicity is enormous. Different arrangements of subunits are sensitive to different anaesthetic agents. For example, genetically engineered 'knock-out mice' in which one particular subunit was missing were insensitive to the anaesthetic effects of the steroid anaesthetic, alfaxalone, but not to propofol suggesting that these two apparently similar IV anaesthetics were working through different configurations of $GABA_A$ receptor. The mode of action of the volatile anaesthetic agents, in particular in the brain, is less proven (and more complex) than for the IV agents; the volatile anaesthetic agents do have some actions at the $GABA_A$ receptor but at a much lower potency. Subunits of $GABA_A$ essential for efficacy differ between the volatile and IV agents. It is thought that glycine receptors are involved in the actions of the volatile agents, in particular those in the spinal cord which inhibit movement. The reason for giving these examples (there are very many more) of differing modes of actions between apparently similar types of anaesthetics is to point out that to say 'an anaesthetic acts at the $GABA_A$ receptor' is certainly not the whole story.

Knowledge of the mode of action of the anaesthetics that work at the NMDA receptor is less well developed. The anaesthetics (ketamine and the gaseous agents) are thought to cause their effects on memory and consciousness at least partly through these receptors. Sonner et al. (2003) consider that NMDA receptors in the spinal cord might be a target for all inhalation anaesthetic agents (not just those those termed 'gaseous') in the production of immobility. However, once again, action at the NMDA receptor does not explain all the actions seen.

The methods of investigation used to study anaesthetic actions are multiple, and readers are referred to the reviews cited above. All reviews point out the number of other potential molecular, ion or voltage-gated possible sites which might be the target for anaesthetic action. Other routes of investigation have examined the modulating influence of alternative CNS pathways. Following the findings of Franks and Lieb (1984), it was anticipated that a (relatively) simple pharmacological pathway for anaesthetic action might be found to explain anaesthetic actions, as has been for many other systems (e.g. opioids, see Chapter 5, α_2-adrenoceptor agonists, see Chapter 4). This has not happened, although our knowledge is greatly expanded. However, we have yet really to know how general anaesthetics work, and indeed Sonner et al. (2003) raise a question that, at least for volatile agents, some variant of the Overton–Meyer lipid theory may yet play a partial role.

DEPTH OF ANAESTHESIA

Many authorities consider that 'depth of anaesthesia' is impossible to define, but anaesthesiologists need some guidelines to ensure that the patient comes to no harm. Only two years after the first demonstration of general anaesthesia, John Snow (1847) stated, quite emphatically, that the point requiring most skill in the administration of anaesthetics is to determine when it has been carried far enough. Snow described five stages of anaesthesia produced by diethyl ether, the last stage in his experiments with animals being characterized by feeble and irregular respiratory movements heralding death – clearly a stage too far. A major problem faced by all anaesthetists since that time is to avoid both 'too light' anaesthesia with the risk of sudden violent movement, and the dangerous 'too deep' stage. Snow suggested guidelines whereby anaesthetists could reduce the risk of either too light or too deep ether anaesthesia. Guedel, in 1918, devised a scheme involving observation of changes in respiratory rate, limb movement and eye signs which formed the basis of his celebrated 'Signs and Stages of Ether Anaesthesia' which has been included until very recently in all text books of anaesthesia, and is the basis for that described in Chapter 2.

The introduction of neuromuscular blocking drugs, which remove all the somatic responses on which Guedel's scheme is based, completely changed the picture and the emphasis swung from the danger of too deep anaesthesia to that of too light anaesthesia with the risk of conscious awareness and perception of pain. Cullen et al. (1972), in an attempt to produce new guidelines indicating depth of anaesthesia, were forced to conclude that it was difficult to categorize the clinical signs of anaesthesia for any one inhalation anaesthetic let alone for inhalation agents in general. The signs also differed markedly when the dissociative anaesthetic agents such as ketamine were used. Today a very much broader range of different drugs are employed during anaesthesia. These include agents to give analgesia, amnesia, unconsciousness and relaxation of skeletal muscles as well as suppression of somatic, cardiovascular, respiratory and hormonal responses to surgical stimulation. All may influence the classical signs of 'depth' of anaesthesia.

Electroencephalography (EEG)

It is only possible to describe the EEG changes related to anaesthesia in the most general terms. The responsive alpha rhythm associated with awareness changes on induction of anaesthesia in terms of frequency and amplitude. The most common pattern seen with light general anaesthesia has low amplitude and is dominated by high frequency activity; it is often referred to as desynchronized. Increasing concentrations of anaesthetics tend to produce increasing amplitude and decreasing frequency, a phenomenon known as synchronization. In addition, some anaesthetics produce periods of burst suppression where the EEG is isoelectric, repetitive high amplitude spikes and complexes or even the epileptoid activity characteristic of the anaesthetic ethers.

The majority of attempts to monitor the depth of anaesthesia objectively have focused on the EEG, but the raw data are of limited practical value to the clinical anaesthetist. To simplify the extraction of useful information from complex waveforms, a number of methods of compressing, processing and displaying EEG signals have been developed and these techniques have, in many cases, been applied to a limited number of channels of EEG rather than the 16 channels normally studied.

Power spectrum analysis

In this technique, the EEG signal, after being digitalized, is subjected to Fast Fourier Transformation (FFT) in which it is separated into a series of sine waves. The sum of these sine waves represents the original integrated signal. Breaking up the original waveform in this way makes it possible to compare one non-standard wave form with another and, in particular, to extract the distribution of components of different frequency within the EEG signal. The power in each frequency band is derived from the sum of the squares of the amplitude of the sine waves into which the FFT has separated the original signal. Power spectrum analysis has been used in a number of experimental situations related to veterinary anaesthesia (e.g. Otto & Short, 1991; Murrell et al., 2003; Johnson et al., 2005, 2009).

Cerebral function monitors

A number of monitors, including the Bispectral Index (BIS), the Cerebral Function Monitor (CFM) and the Patient State Index (PSI) feed the EEG signals from a limited number of leads into a 'black box' which, on the basis of an algorithm derived from analysis of EEGs from a large number of human patients, produces a number which is related to depth of anaesthesia. All these monitors have a number of limitations in clinical use. They may be influenced by other electrical 'noise' such as the electromyogram (EMG). The algorithms are based mainly on anaesthetic drugs that have their hypnotic effect through actions at the GABA$_A$ receptors. The monitors are ineffective for the anaesthetic agents that act at the NMDA receptors such as nitrous oxide, xenon or ketamine. Of great concern is the fact that when neuromuscular blocking drugs were given to conscious human volunteers, BIS reduced to values suggestive of very deep anaesthesia (Messner et al., 2003). The use of these monitors may reduce the incidence of awareness under anaesthesia but has not eliminated it. The most common of these monitors is the BIS; its use and limitations in veterinary anaesthesia are described in Chapter 2.

Evoked responses

Evoked responses are changes in the EEG produced by external stimuli, surgical or otherwise. Anaesthetic depth is a balance between cerebral depression and surgical (or other) stimulation. Thus, cerebral function during anaesthesia is most easily assessed by putting in a stimulus – auditory or somatic or visual – and observing the EEG response. That response can then be compared for amplitude and latency with the response to the same stimulus in the presence of differing brain concentrations of any anaesthetic. Evoked responses can be used as monitors of anaesthetic depth when agents acting at the NMDA receptor are being employed.

The 'classic' signs of anaesthesia

Use of the term 'depth of anaesthesia' is now so ingrained in common usage that it must be accepted since it probably cannot be eradicated. It is important, however, to realize that it commonly refers to depression of brain function beyond that necessary for the production of 'general anaesthesia'.

The so-called 'classic signs' of anaesthesia, such as described in Chapter 2 for convenience of newcomers to the subject, were provided by the presence or absence of response of the anaesthetized subject to stimuli provided by the anaesthetist or surgeon. Particular signs of anaesthesia were, therefore, equated with particular anatomical levels or 'planes' of depression of the central nervous system. These signs were often likened to a series of landmarks used to assess the progress made on a journey. Such empirical, traditional methods of assessing the progress of anaesthesia and the anatomical implications that went with these methods incorporated a fallacy, because they took no account of the fact that the changing function of any biological system can only be made in terms of magnitude and time. A depth of unconsciousness is really a particular moment in a continuous temporal stream of biological or neurological phenomena to be interpreted by the magnitude and quality of these phenomena obtaining to that moment.

In general, the volatile anaesthetic agents halothane, enflurane, isoflurane, sevoflurane and desflurane produce a dose-dependent decrease in arterial blood pressure and many veterinary anaesthetists use this depression to assess the depth of anaesthesia. The effect is not so marked during anaesthetic techniques involving the administration of opioid analgesics and nitrous oxide. If the depth of unconsciousness is adequate, surgical stimulation does not cause any change in arterial blood pressure. There are, however, many other factors which influence the arterial blood pressure during surgery such as the circulating blood volume, cardiac output and the influence of drug therapy given before anaesthesia. If ketamine or high doses of opioids are given, arterial blood pressure may change very little if the depth of unconsciousness is increased by the administration of higher concentrations of inhalation anaesthetics.

Changes in heart rate alone are a poor guide to changes in the depth of unconsciousness. The heart rate may increase under isoflurane and desflurane anaesthesia due to the agents' effects. Arrhythmias are common during light levels of unconsciousness induced by halothane, when they are usually due to increased sympathetic activity. In general, however, tachycardia in the absence of any other cause may be taken to represent inadequate anaesthesia for the procedure being undertaken.

Anaesthetic agents affect respiration in a dose-dependent manner and this was responsible for the original classification of the 'depth of anaesthesia'. In deeply anaesthetized animals, tidal and minute volumes are decreased but, depending on the species of animal and on the anaesthetic agents used, respiratory rate may increase before breathing eventually ceases once the animal is close to death. As inadequate anaesthesia also is often indicated by an increase in the rate and/or depth of breathing the unwary may be tempted to administer more anaesthetic agent to the deeply anaesthetized animal in the mistaken impression that awareness is imminent. Laryngospasm, coughing or breath-holding can indicate excessive airway stimulation or inadequate depth of unconsciousness.

All anaesthetic agents, other than the dissociative drugs such as ketamine, cause a dose-related reduction in muscle tone and overdosage produces complete respiratory muscle paralysis. In the absence of complete neuromuscular block produced by neuromuscular blocking drugs, the degree of muscle relaxation may, therefore, usually be used as a measure of the depth of anaesthetic-induced unconsciousness. However, even in the presence of muscular paralysis due to clinically effective doses of neuromuscular blockers, it is not uncommon to observe movements of facial muscles, swallowing or chewing movements in response to surgical stimulation if the depth of unconsciousness becomes inadequate.

When animals are breathing spontaneously, there are several signs which are generally recognized as indicating that the depth of unconsciousness is adequate for the performance of painful procedures, i.e. the animal is unaware of the environment and of the infliction of pain – it is anaesthetized.

Unfortunately, there are many differences between the various species of animal in the signs which are usually used to estimate the depth of unconsciousness. One fairly reliable sign is that of eyeball movement, especially in horses and cattle, although even this may be modified in the presence of certain other drugs, such as the α_2-adrenoceptor agents (see Chapter 11). Unless neuromuscular blocking drugs are in use, very slow nystagmus in both horses and cattle and downward inclination of the eyeballs in pigs and dogs usually indicates a satisfactory level of unconsciousness and, at this level, breathing should be smooth although its rate and depth may alter depending on the prevailing severity of the surgical stimulation. Rapid nystagmus is usually a sign that anaesthesia is light but it is a common feature of ketamine anaesthesia and it also seen sometimes seen in horses just before death. Absence of the lash or palpebral reflex (closure of the eyelids in response to light stroking of the eyelashes) is another reasonably reliable guide to satisfactory anaesthesia. In dogs and cats, it is safe to assume that if the mouth can be opened without provoking yawning or curling of the tongue, central depression is adequate. In all animals, salivation and excessive lacrimation usually indicate a returning awareness.

Disappearance of head shaking or whisker twitching in response to gentle scratching of the inside of the ear pinna is a good sign of unawareness in pigs, cats, rabbits and guinea pigs. Pupil size is a most unreliable guide to anaesthetic depth as various ancillary agents (e.g. opioids, atropine) may influence it. The pupils do, however, dilate when an overdose of an anaesthetic has been given or when awareness is imminent.

The experienced anaesthetist relies most of the time on an animal's response to stimuli produced by the surgeon or procedure to indicate adequate depth of unconsciousness. The most effective depth is taken to be that which obliterates the animal's response to pain and/or discomfort without depressing respiratory and circulatory function.

Computer control in anaesthesia

With the current sophistication of computers, there have been many attempts to obtain a method of anaesthesia totally controlled by the computer; various parameters being monitored, results fed back into the system, and the system then altering the dose of anaesthetic administered accordingly – i.e. a closed-loop system.

The use of computers (including microprocessors) has improved many aspects of anaesthesia. Monitoring can be more sophisticated, and give more accurate results. Ventilators can be programmed to provide very specific requirements of, for example, tidal volume, or respiratory pressures. Constant infusion pumps provide a very accurate flow rate which is useful for fluid administration, but also can be utilized to provide targeted plasma levels of intravenous anaesthetic agents (this is known as Target Controlled Infusion or TCI). The most validated versions of this are the Propofusor® and the Remifusor®, which will deliver infusions to achieve set plasma levels of propofol and remifentanil respectively. Their programming is based on a very accurate knowledge of the pharmacokinetics in humans of these drugs so their algorithms are not necessarily correct for other animals, although the Propofusor has been modified successfully for use in dogs (Beths et al., 2001; Musk et al., 2006). There is computer-software available to use with other agents (RugloopII); it can be used for research projects (Ribeiro et al., 2009) but, as it classifies as a 'medical device', there may be legal limitations (country specific) to its clinical use in humans. It is also possible to have target controlled inhalation anaesthesia; the volatile anaesthetic is injected into the circuit so as to maintain a targeted end-tidal anaesthetic concentration. The anaesthetic machine named 'Zeus' from Draeger has this facility as well as programmable infusion syringes and the advertisement talks of *target controlled anaesthesia*. However, neither of these systems involves a feedback loop within the computer; the feedback loop is the anaesthetist who asks it for a different target, 'up or down' according to the patient requirements.

In order to have a feedback loop, there have to be patient data measured and returned to the computer. To date, the most common parameter used for this purpose is the 'anaesthetic depth monitor', BIS (see Electroencephalography). As has been discussed, this is a monitor based on the 'hypnosis' resulting from the anaesthetic agents that act primarily on the $GABA_A$ receptor, and therefore is most accurate with propofol anaesthesia. Not surprisingly, computer-controlled anaesthesia has been most effective with systems involving propofol infusions (Hemmerling et al., 2010). Recently, Liu et al. (2011) used computer-controlled infusion of propofol together with remifentanil, and found it more effective in maintaining a steady BIS target than was manual control. However, as discussed previously, in any one individual, steady BIS does not always represent the ideal 'depth' of anaesthesia so the anaesthetist is still needed to assess the patient's overall response, in particular cardiopulmonary changes and autonomic responses to stimulation. Absalom et al. (2011) have reviewed the current status of computer-controlled anaesthesia and consider that the limitations are such that it is a goal not yet achieved.

Minimum Alveolar Concentration (MAC) and Minimum Infusion Rate (MIR)

Minimum alveolar concentration

In 1963, Merkel & Eger proposed the concept of MAC, and Eger et al. (1965) expanded the idea further, suggesting that it would be useful as a measurement of volatile anaesthetic potency. MAC is defined as the alveolar concentration of an anaesthetic that prevents muscular movement in response to a painful stimulus in 50% of the test subjects. It is therefore what is known in pharmacology as the ED_{50} (effective dose). If adequate time is allowed for the anaesthetic in the brain to equilibrate with the anaesthetic agent in the blood, the alveolar partial pressure of the anaesthetic (which can be measured) is a reasonably accurate expression of the anaesthetic state. The stimulus, standardized as far as possible to be 'supramaximal', usually consists of tail clamping or an electrical stimulus

in animals and is usually measured in triplicate, concentration of anaesthetic being lowered until there is a response, then raised again until the response is lost. In humans, the most common stimulus is a single surgical incision; if the patient responds the next patient gets a higher dose and so on, until the ED_{50} is found. A single stimulus of this type is certainly not supramaximal, and the difference in measurement techniques may explain why MAC in humans usually is less than in experimental animals. End-tidal anaesthetic gas concentration is taken as an approximation of alveolar gas. With a forced expiration (as is requested when similar technology is used for the alcohol 'breathalyser'), this is reasonable, but under anaesthesia a forced breath cannot be obtained. For really accurate experimental results, sampling should be via a catheter passed down the trachea but, in the clinical situation, sampling at the ET tube suffices.

A number of factors affect MAC. It is not affected by the duration of anaesthesia, hyperkalaemia, hypokalaemia, hypercarbia or metabolic acid–base changes, but is reduced by hyponatraemia. MAC is reduced by 8% for every °C reduction in body temperature, and similarly, raised by hyperthermia. Young animals have high MAC values, but MAC decreases with age (Mapleson, 1996; Eger, 2001). MAC is measured as vol%, and so is dependent on atmospheric pressure, thus explaining the increased doses of volatile agents required to maintain anaesthesia at high altitudes (Quasha et al., 1980). MAC is reduced by many other anaesthetic related agents which add to neuronal depression. The MACs of two volatile and/or inhalation agents are themselves additive (Eger et al., 2003), hence the use of nitrous oxide as part of the carrier gas for volatile agents.

It is now considered that MAC is a measurement that relates to the spinal cord, and not to the brain (Eger et al., 1997). Its end-point is movement and, as discussed above (mode of action), it is movement that is considered to be prevented by the actions at the spinal cord. Interestingly, in relation to analgesia, volatile anaesthetic agents do prevent 'wind-up' of nociceptive neurons in the cord, and it is suggested that this may play a part in preventing movement.

Despite its limitations, however, the concept of MAC has now been used for more than five decades to enable the relative potencies of anaesthetics to be compared (Antognini & Carstens, 2005). This reproducible method may be contrasted with the difficulty in using physiological parameters as an indication of anaesthetic depth, or the EEG, which varies according to the agent used. Although the MAC value represents the anaesthetizing dose for only 50% of subjects, the anaesthetist can be reasonably certain that increasing the alveolar concentration to between 1.1 or 1.2 times MAC will ensure satisfactory anaesthesia in the vast majority of individuals because the dose–response curve is relatively steep. In veterinary practice, it is also important to note that, according to Eger, the variability of MAC is remarkably low between mammalian species and, as long as conditions remain the same, is quite constant in any one animal. Finally, it is important to remember that MAC is determined in healthy animals under laboratory conditions in the absence of other drugs and circumstances encountered during clinical anaesthesia which may alter the requirement for anaesthesia.

Minimum infusion rate

The accurate control of depth of unconsciousness is more difficult to achieve with intravenous anaesthetic agents. To obtain unconsciousness, they must be administered at a rate which produces a concentration of drug in the bloodstream sufficient to result in the required depth of depression of the central nervous system. The concept of minimum infusion rate (MIR) was introduced by Sears in 1970 to define the median ED_{50} of an intravenous anaesthetic agent which would prevent movement in response to surgical incision (or in experimental animals, a supramaximal stimulus). Unlike MAC, in which alveolar concentrations can be considered to equate to arterial, blood cannot be analysed rapidly for injectable anaesthetic concentrations. MIR is therefore measured similarly to MAC using movement as an end-point. However, MIR may change with time if the drug is cumulative; a lower infusion rate being required as the tissues become saturated. The term 'context sensitive MIR' is used to describe these changes with duration of infusion. As changes with context depend on pharmacokinetic parameters, MIR may differ markedly between species depending on rate of drug metabolism and elimination. In veterinary anaesthesia, to date, the greatest knowledge of MIRs in anaesthesia has been with propofol infusions (Beths et al., 2001; Bettschart-Wolfensberger et al., 2001; Oku et al., 2005; Boscan et al., 2010; Rezende et al., 2010), but the same concept (using different end-points) has been employed for choosing suitable infusion rates of sedative drugs (see Chapter 4).

ANAESTHETIC RISK

General anaesthesia and local analgesia do not occur naturally and their induction with drugs that even today are never completely devoid of toxicity must constitute a threat to the life of the patient. This can be a major or trivial threat depending on the circumstances, but no owner must ever be assured that anaesthesia does not constitute a risk. When an animal owner raises the question of risk involved in any anaesthetic procedure the veterinarian needs, before replying, to consider:

1. The state of health of the animal. Animals presented for anaesthesia may be fit and healthy or suffering from disease; they may be presented for elective ('cold') surgery or as emergency cases needing

Table 1.1 American Society of Anesthesiologists' physical status classification system

Category 1	Normal healthy patient
Category 2	A patient with mild systemic disease
Category 3	A patient with severe systemic disease
Category 4	A patient with severe systemic disease that is a constant threat to life
Category 5	A moribund patient who is not expected to survive without the operation

American Society of Anesthesiologists (2010).

immediate attention for obstetrical crises, intractable haemorrhage or thoracic injuries. In the USA, the American Society of Anesthesiologists (ASA) has adopted a classification of physical status into categories, 'E' being added after the number when the case is presented as an emergency (Table 1.1). This is a useful classification but, most importantly, it refers only to the physical status of the patient and is not necessarily a classification of risk because additional factors such as its species, breed and temperament contribute to the risk involved for any particular animal. Moreover, the assessment of a patient's 'correct' ASA classification varies between different anaesthetists (Haynes & Lawler, 1995; Wolters et al., 1996; McMillan & Brearley, 2013).

2. The influence of the surgeon. Inexperienced surgeons may take much longer to perform an operation and by rough technique produce intense and extensive trauma to tissues, thereby causing a greater metabolic disturbance (and increased postoperative pain). Increased danger can also arise when the surgeon is working in the mouth or pharynx in such a way as to make the maintenance of a clear airway difficult, or is working on structures such as the eye or larynx and provoking autonomic reflexes.

3. The influence of available facilities. Crises arising during anaesthesia are usually more easily overcome in a well-equipped veterinary hospital than under the primitive conditions which may be encountered on farms.

4. The influence of the anaesthetist. The competence, experience and judgement of the anaesthetist have a profound bearing on the degree of risk to which the patient is exposed. Familiarity with anaesthetic techniques leads to greater efficiency and the art of anaesthetic administration is only developed by experience.

General considerations in the selection of the anaesthetic method

The first consideration will be the nature of the operation to be performed, its magnitude, site and duration. In general, the use of local infiltration analgesia may suffice for simple operations such as the incision of superficial abscesses, the excision of small neoplasms, biopsies and the castration of immature animals. Nevertheless, what seems to be a simple interference may have special anaesthetic requirements. Subdermal fibrosis may make local infiltration impossible to effect. Again, the site of the operation in relation to the complexity of the structures in its vicinity may render operation under local analgesia dangerous because of possible movement by the conscious animal, e.g. operations in the vicinity of the eyes.

When adopting general anaesthesia, the likely duration of the procedure to be performed will influence the selection of the anaesthetic. Minor, very short operations may be performed after IV administration of a small dose of an agent such as propofol or thiopental sodium. For longer operations, anaesthesia may be induced with an ultra-short acting agent and maintained with an inhalation agent with or without endotracheal intubation. However, the ability to perform endotracheal intubation, to administer oxygen and to apply some form of ventilation must always be available and to hand for use should an emergency arise. Similarly, the fact that anaesthesia is brief does not remove the need for minimal monitoring. For most operations under general anaesthesia, preanaesthetic medication ('premedication') will need to be considered, particularly when they are of long duration and the animal must remain quiet and pain-free for several hours after the operation. Undesirable effects of certain agents (e.g. ketamine) may need to be countered by the administration of 'correcting' agents (e.g. α_2 adrenoceptor agonists, atropine). Although sedative premedication may significantly reduce the amount of general anaesthetic required, it may also increase the duration of recovery from anaesthesia.

The species of animal involved is a pre-eminent consideration in the selection of the anaesthetic method (see later chapters). The anaesthetist will be influenced not only by size and temperament but also by any anatomical or physiological features peculiar to a particular species or breed. Experience indicates that the larger the animal, the greater are the difficulties and dangers associated with the induction and maintenance of general anaesthesia. Methods which are safe and satisfactory for the dog and cat may be quite unsuitable for horses and cattle. In vigorous and heavy creatures the mere upset of locomotor coordination may entail risks, as also may prolonged recumbency.

Individual animals

The variable reaction of the different species of animals, and of individuals, to the various agents administered by anaesthetists will also influence the choice of anaesthetic technique. In addition, factors causing increased susceptibility to the toxic actions of anaesthetic agents must be borne in mind. These include:

1. Prolonged fasting. This, by depleting the glycogen reserves of the liver, greatly reduces its detoxicating power and when using parenterally administered agents in computed doses, allowance must be made for increased susceptibility to them.
2. Diseased conditions. Toxaemia causes degenerative changes in parenchymatous organs, particularly the liver and the heart, and great care must be taken in giving computed doses of agents to toxaemic subjects. Quite often it is found that a toxaemic animal requires very much less than the 'normal' dose. Toxaemia may also be associated with a slowing of the circulation and unless this is recognized it may lead to gross overdosing of IV anaesthetics.

EVALUATION OF THE PATIENT BEFORE ANAESTHESIA

It is probable that most veterinary operations are performed on normal, healthy animals. The subjects are generally young and represent good 'anaesthetic risks'. Nevertheless, enquiry should be made to ensure that they are normal and healthy – bright, vigorous and of hearty appetite. Should there be any doubt, operations are best delayed until there is assurance on this point. Many a reputation has been damaged by performing simple operations on young animals which are in the early stages of some acute infectious disease or which possess some congenital abnormality.

When an operation is to be performed for the relief of disease, considerable care must be exercised in assessing the factors which may influence the choice or course of the anaesthetic. Once these are recognized, the appropriate type of anaesthesia can be chosen and preoperative measures adopted to diminish or, where possible, prevent complications. The commonest conditions affecting the course of anaesthesia are those involving the cardiovascular and respiratory systems, but the state of the liver and kidneys cannot be ignored.

The owner or attendant should always be asked whether the animal has a cough. A soft, moist cough is associated with airway secretions that may give rise to respiratory obstruction and lung collapse when the cough reflex is suppressed by general anaesthesia. Severe cardiovascular disease may be almost unnoticed by the owner and enquiry should be made to determine whether the animal appears to suffer from respiratory distress after exertion, or indeed appears unwilling to take exercise, since these signs may precede other signs of cardiac and respiratory failure by many months or even years. Dyspnoea is generally the first sign of left ventricular failure and a history of excessive thirst may indicate the existence of advanced renal disease, diabetes mellitus or diabetes insipidus.

The actual examination may be restricted to one which is informative yet will not consume too much time nor unduly disturb the animal. While a more complete examination may sometimes be necessary, attention should always be paid to the pulse, the position of the apex beat of the heart, the presence of cardiac thrills, the heart sounds and the jugular venous pressure. Examination of the urine for the presence of albumin and reducing substances may also be useful.

Tachycardia is to be expected in all febrile and in many wasting diseases and, under these circumstances, is indicative of some myocardial weakness. It can, however, also be due to nervousness and where this is so it is often associated with rather cold ears and/or feet. Bradycardia may be physiological or it may indicate complete atrioventricular block. In horses, atrioventricular block that disappears with exercise is probably of no clinical significance. In all animals, the electrocardiogram may be the only way of determining whether bradycardia is physiological or is due to conduction block in the heart.

The jugular venous pressure is also important. When the animal is standing and the head is held so that the neck is at an angle of about 45° to the horizontal, distension of the jugular veins should, in normal animals, be just visible at the base of the neck. When the distension rises above this level, even in the absence of other signs, it indicates an obstruction to the cranial vena cava or a rise in right atrial or ventricular pressures. The commonest cause of a rise in pressure in these chambers is probably right ventricular hypertrophy associated with chronic lung disease, although congenital conditions such as atrial septal defects may also be indicated by this sign and it should be remembered that cattle suffering from constrictive pericarditis, or bacterial endocarditis, may have a marked increase in venous pressure.

The presence of a thrill over the heart is always a sign of cardiovascular disease and suggests an increased risk of complications arising during anaesthesia. More detailed cardiological examination is warranted when a cardiac thrill is detected during the preoperative examination.

Auscultation of the heart should never be omitted, particularly when the animal's owner is present because owners expect this to be carried out. Accurate location of the apex beat is an important observation in assessing the state of the cardiovascular and respiratory systems. It is displaced in many abnormal conditions of the lungs (e.g. pleural effusion, pneumothorax, lung collapse) and in the presence of enlargement of the left ventricle. In the absence of any pulmonary disorder, a displaced apex beat indicates cardiac hypertrophy or dilatation.

Pulmonary disorders provide particular hazards for an animal undergoing operation and any examination, no matter how brief, must be designed to disclose their presence or absence. On auscultation, attention should be directed towards the length of the expiratory sounds and the discovery of any rhonchi or crepitations. If rhonchi or crepitations are heard, excessive sputum is present, and the animal is either suffering from, or has recently suffered, a pulmonary infection. Prolongation of the expiratory sounds, especially when accompanied by high-pitched rhonchi, indicate narrowing of the airways or bronchospasm. Respiratory sounds may be absent in animals with pneumothorax, extensive lung consolidation, or severe emphysema; they are usually faint in moribund animals.

Uneven movement between the two sides of the chest is a reliable sign of pulmonary disease and one which is easily and quickly observed. The animal should be positioned squarely while the examiner stands directly in front of it and then directly behind it. In small animals, uneven movement of the two sides of the chest is often better appreciated by palpation rather than by inspection.

The mouth should be examined for the presence of loose teeth which might become dislodged during general anaesthesia and enter the tracheobronchial tree. Other mucous membranes should be inspected for evidence of anaemia, denoted by paleness.

Biochemical tests prior to anaesthesia

The question as to whether preanaesthetic urine and blood analysis should be performed routinely before every elective anaesthetic is, and has always been, controversial. While targeted tests are essential to confirm or exclude disease conditions suspected as a result of clinical history and examination, the cost/benefit of their use in animals which appear perfectly healthy can be argued on the basis that the results rarely would alter the anaesthetic protocol to be employed. Urine testing is simple, inexpensive and is particularly important in dogs for, in these animals, renal disease and previously undiagnosed diabetes mellitus are common. Urine samples may be less readily obtainable from other species of animal. The Association of Veterinary Anaesthetists (AVA) debated (Spring Meeting, 1998) the question as to the need for routine preanaesthetic checks on haematological and biochemical profiles, and voted that they were unnecessary if the clinical examination was adequate. In a more recent AVA debate led by medical anaesthetists, they pointed out that a major disadvantage of non-targeted screening was 'over-diagnosis' when an apparent abnormality of no significance was found. An advantage of prescreening, however, is that abnormalities occurring early in the course of a disease without current clinical symptoms may be identified. These values then become the baseline for comparison if abnormalities occur following anaesthesia and surgery. There may well be a place for routine screening older animals. Although in a very occasional case (e.g. the detection of a partial hepato-portal shunt in a young dog) biochemical tests may detect an unsuspected disease state, in the vast majority of young apparently fit healthy animals, they constitute an unnecessary expense and, indeed, the extra cost involved may prevent an owner from agreeing to continuation of treatment necessary for the well-being of the patient.

Provided a brief examination such as that described is carried out thoroughly, and that the examiner has sufficient skill and experience to recognize the significance or lack of significance of the findings, most of the conditions that have a bearing on the well-being of an animal in the perioperative period will be brought to light so that appropriate measures can be taken to protect it from harm.

SIGNIFICANCE OF CONDITIONS FOUND BY PREANAESTHETIC EXAMINATION

Cardiovascular and respiratory disease

The cardiovascular and respiratory systems are those which govern the rate at which oxygen can be made available to the tissues of the body. Oxygen supply is equal to the product of the cardiac output and the oxygen content of the arterial blood. Since the arterial oxygen content approximates to the product of the oxygen saturation and the quantity of oxygen which can be carried by the haemoglobin (about 1.34 mL/g of haemoglobin when fully saturated), the oxygen made available to the body can be expressed by a simple equation:

Available oxygen (mL/min) = cardiac output (mL/min)
× arterial saturation (%) × haemoglobin (g/mL) × 1.34

This equation makes no allowance for the small quantity of oxygen which is carried in physical solution in the plasma, but it serves to illustrate the way in which three variables combine to produce an effect which is often greater than is commonly supposed. If any one of the three determining variables on the right-hand side of the equation is changed, the rate at which oxygen is made available to the tissues of the body is altered proportionately. Thus, if the cardiac output is halved, the available oxygen is also halved. If two determinants are lowered simultaneously while the third remains constant, the effect on the available oxygen is the product of the individual changes. For example, if the cardiac output and the haemoglobin concentration are both halved while the arterial oxygen saturation remains at about the normal 95%, only one-quarter of the normal amount of oxygen is made available to the body tissues. If all three variables are reduced the effect is, of course, even more dramatic.

Drug metabolism and disease states

Drugs are usually metabolized through several pathways so that they are changed from fat-soluble, active, unexcretable drugs into water-soluble, inactive drugs that can be excreted by the kidneys and in the bile. Since the mammalian body metabolizes many thousands of compounds every day and has far fewer enzymes, each enzyme metabolizes many substrates. Only very rarely, if ever, will one enzyme metabolize only one substrate. Many things change enzyme function. Mechanisms for enzyme induction are poorly understood, unlike inhibition, which has been much more extensively studied. Enzyme induction is a slow process involving an increased amount of enzyme in the cell over about 24 to 48 hours, whereas inhibition is quick and sometimes occurs after only one dose of an inhibitor. Since enzymes are proteins their concentrations inside cells may be changed by a variety of factors (Fig. 1.2).

There is now an increasing amount of information about how enzymes change in response to one stressful stimulus but it is important to recognize that usually several stimuli exist at the same time in each critically ill animal. Most chemical reactions are sensitive to temperature, speeding up as the temperature increases and slowing

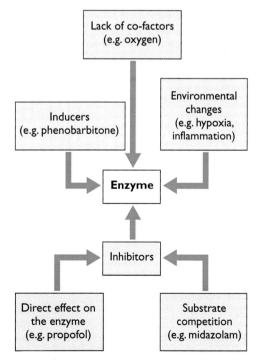

Figure 1.2 Factors which may change enzyme function.

with a decrease in temperature but, in spite of this, all fevers do not increase the rate of metabolism of drugs: the cause of the fever is important. Infections and pyrogens cause the release of inflammatory mediators which reduce the expression and activity of many enzymes. Non-traumatic stress has been shown to reduce enzyme function, possibly by decreased hepatic blood flow resulting in hypoxaemic-induced reduction in metabolizing enzymes. Endogenous corticosteroid secretion as part of the stress response or exogenous steroid given to treat disease will change the expression of drug metabolizing enymes, and metabolic activity also varies with age. The anaesthetist must be aware of these factors so that any increase or decrease in the duration of drug action may be anticipated.

Factors affecting transport of drugs in the body

Most drugs are carried in the bloodstream partly bound, usually by electrostatic bonds, to the proteins of the plasma, albumin being far the most important for the majority of agents. Light or moderate protein binding has relatively little effect on drug pharmacokinetics or pharmacodynamics. Heavy protein binding with drugs such as thiopental results in a low free plasma concentration of the drug, which may become progressively augmented as the available binding sites become saturated. The bound drug is, of course, in dynamic equilibrium with free (active) drug in the plasma water. The bonds are generally reversible and conform to the law of mass action:

The association and dissociation processes take place very quickly, and can generally be taken to be instantaneous. The equilibrium association constant K_A is defined as the ratio of rate constants, and of bound to the product of unbound concentrations.

This simple relationship is often obscured by the fact that one protein molecule may possess several binding sites for any particular drug, which may or may not have the same association constant. It can generally be assumed, however, that so long as the plasma proteins remain unchanged, the ratio of 'free' to 'bound' drug will remain constant. This ratio depends on the nature of the drug molecule. Small, neutral, water-soluble drugs will not bind to protein at all but larger lipophilic molecules may exhibit very high binding ratios.

Anaemia is often associated with hypoproteinaemia and this can have marked effects in anaesthesia. In conditions where there is anaemia and hypoalbuminaemia, a greater fraction of a given dose of a drug will be unbound and this will be even greater if other bound drugs have already occupied many of the binding sites. This can result in an increased peak activity of the drug. Liver disease giving rise to hypoalbuminaemia can result in reduced binding of drugs such as morphine so that smaller than normal doses of this analgesic will be effective when pain relief is

needed. A rapid intravenous injection of an albumin-bound drug may also lead to increased pharmacological activity because the binding capacity of the albumin in the limited volume of blood with which the drug initially mixes is exceeded and more free (active) drug is presented to the receptor sites. Plasma protein binding enhances alimentary absorption of drugs by lowering the free plasma concentration, thereby increasing the concentration gradient for diffusion from the gut lumen.

Not surprisingly, for a protein with a molecular weight of about 65 000, there are several genetically acquired variants of albumin. Furthermore, the configuration of the albumin molecule also changes during illness and, for example, in renal failure. These changes can be demonstrated by electrophoresis but their significance for the binding of drugs *in vivo* is not known.

Renal disease

Chronic renal disease is common in dogs and cats, and affected animals cannot produce concentrated urine. Dehydration from any cause deprives the kidneys of sufficient water for excretory purposes. To ensure that these animals receive an adequate fluid intake over the anaesthetic period, it is usually necessary to administer fluid by intravenous infusion. A uraemic circle can also be set up in animals suffering from chronic renal disease if the arterial blood pressure is allowed to decrease because of anaesthetic overdose or haemorrhage and renal ischaemia ensues. The maintenance of the circulating fluid volume is most important in all animals with chronic renal disease and it is important that adequate venous access is assured before anaesthesia and operation.

Acute renal failure can be defined as an abrupt decline in renal function with a decrease in glomerular filtration rate (GFR) resulting in the retention of nitrogenous waste products. Acute renal failure is classified into:

1. Pre-renal failure, denoting a disorder in the systemic circulation that causes renal hypoperfusion. Implicit here is that correction of the underlying circulatory disturbance (e.g. by improvement in cardiac function or repletion of volume) restores the GFR. However, pre-renal failure is often followed by transition to:
2. Intrinsic renal failure, where correction of the underlying circulatory impairment does not restore the GFR to normal levels. Intrinsic renal failure generally includes tubular necrosis or the blocking of tubules by cell debris or precipitated proteins and there is no question of unaffected nephrons compensating for failing nephrons as there is in chronic renal failure. Instead, all are involved in a massive disturbance of renal function with diversion of blood flow away from the renal cortex towards the medulla and an overall reduction in renal perfusion. There is, however, a potential for complete recovery, whereas chronic renal failure invariably progresses

over a variable period of time with no hope of recovery of renal function.

3. Post-renal failure (obstructive) is a third possibility and urethral obstruction is not uncommon in some species, becoming a cause for emergency anaesthesia and surgery.

Excessive reliance on blood pressure maintenance to between the 'autoregulatory range' by infusion or the use of vasoactive drugs overlooks the fact that renal blood flow is labile since the kidneys contribute to the regulation of blood pressure. The incidence of acute renal failure is high after the use of intravenous contrast radiological media, or of nephrotoxic drugs (e.g. non-steroidal anti-inflammatory drugs, gentamycin, amphotericin).

PREPARATION OF THE PATIENT

Certain operations are performed as emergencies when it is imperative that there shall be no delay and little preparation of the patient is possible. Among these operations are repair of thoracic injuries, the control of severe, persistent haemorrhage, and certain obstetrical interferences where the delivery of a live, healthy neonate is of paramount importance. For all other operations, time and care spent in preoperative preparation are well worthwhile since proper preparation not only improves the patient's chances of survival, but also prevents the complications which might otherwise occur during and after operation. When operations are to be performed on normal, healthy animals, only the minimum of preparation is required before the administration of a general anaesthetic, but operations on dehydrated, anaemic, hypovolaemic or toxic patients should only be undertaken after careful preoperative assessment and preparation.

Food and water

The time for which food should be withheld from the animal on the day it is to undergo an elective operation under general anaesthesia is species dependent. A distended stomach may interfere with the free movement of the diaphragm and hinder breathing. In dogs, cats and pigs, a full stomach predisposes to vomiting under anaesthesia but, in dogs, it has now been shown that prolonged starvation increases the incidence of gastro-oesophageal reflux (Savvas et al., 2009) so it might be time to reconsider the teaching of many years to starve for at least 12 hours. In horses, a full stomach may rupture when the horse falls to the ground as unconsciousness is induced; except in cases of colic this is unlikely with current methods of anaesthetic induction, but a full stomach will exert pressure on the diaphragm, in particular in dorsal recumbency, resulting in hypoventilation and bloat in some cases. In ruminants, a few hours of starvation will

not result in an appreciable reduction in the volume of the fluid content of the rumen but it seems to reduce the rate of fermentation within this organ, thus delaying the development of tympany when eructation is prevented by recumbency.

Excessive fasting exposes the patient to risks almost as great as those associated with lack of preparation and should not be adopted. Any fasting of birds and small mammals is actually life threatening. Many clinicians are of the opinion that prolonged fasting in horses predisposes to postanaesthetic colic by encouraging gut stasis. In horses, it is now usual practice to allow free access to water until right up to the time premedication is given.

Fluid and electrolytes

The water and electrolyte balance of an animal is a most important factor in determining uncomplicated recovery or otherwise after operation. The repair of existing deficits of body fluid, or of one of its components, is complex because of the interrelations between the different electrolytes and the difficulties imposed by the effects of severe sodium depletion on the circulation and renal function.

An anaesthetic should not be administered to an animal which has a depleted circulating blood volume for the vasodilatation caused by anaesthetic agents may lead to acute circulatory failure, and every effort should be made to repair this deficit by the infusion of crystalloid or colloid solutions, blood, or plasma, as appropriate, before anaesthesia is induced. In many instances, anaesthesia and surgery may be safely postponed until the total fluid deficit is made good and an adequate renal output is achieved but, in cases of intestinal obstruction, operation should be carried out as soon as the blood volume has been restored. Attempts to restore the complete extracellular deficit before the intestinal obstruction is relieved result in further loss of fluid into the lumen of the obstructed bowel and, especially in horses, make subsequent operation more difficult. When in doubt about the nature and volume of fluid to be administered, it is as well to remember that, with the exception of toxic conditions and where severe hypotension due to hypovolaemia is present, an animal's condition should not deteriorate further if sufficient fluid is given to cover current losses. These current losses include the inevitable loss of water through the skin and respiratory tract (approximately 20–60mL/kg/day depending on the age and species of the animal), the urinary and faecal loss, and any abnormal loss such as vomit.

Haemoglobin level

As already mentioned earlier (cardiovascular and respiratory disease), anaemia reduces oxygen content and also makes injectable anaesthetic drugs more potent by reducing overall blood protein. Where surgery is not an emergency and there is a medical cause that can be treated, then this should be done. For more immediate surgical needs, in human anaesthesia, it used to be routine to transfuse red blood cells, but the potential disadvantages (Shander et al., 2012; Theusinger et al., 2012) now mean that where blood volume is adequate, low levels of haemoglobin are tolerated unless extreme. There is no equivalent evidence relating to blood transfusions in animals but it is probable that this is also a reasonable approach to veterinary anaesthesia.

INFLUENCE OF PRE-EXISTING DRUG THERAPY

Modern therapeutic agents are often of considerable pharmacological potency and animals presented for anaesthesia may have been exposed to one or more of these. Some may have been given as part of the preoperative management of the animal but, whatever the reason for their administration, they may modify the animal's response to anaesthetic agents, to surgery and to drugs given before, during and after operation. In some cases, drug interactions are predictable and these may form the basis of many of the combinations used in modern anaesthesia, but effects which are unexpected may be dangerous.

In an ideal situation, a drug action would occur only at a desired site to produce the sought-after effect. In practice, drugs are much less selective and are prone to produce 'side effects' which have to be anticipated and taken into account whenever the drug is administered. (A 'side effect' may be defined as a response not required clinically, but which occurs when a drug is used within its therapeutic range.) Apart from these unavoidable side effects which are inherent, adverse reactions to drugs may occur in many different ways which are of importance to the anaesthetist. These include:

1. *Overdosage.* For some drugs, exact dosing may be difficult. Overdosage may be absolute as when an amount greater than the intended dose is given in error, or a drug is given by an inappropriate route, e.g. a normal intramuscular dose may constitute a serious overdose if given intravenously. Relative overdose may be due to an intrinsic difference in the animal, for example, newborn animals are sensitive to non-depolarizing neuromuscular blocking drugs. The use in dogs and cats of flea collars containing organophosphorus compounds may reduce the plasma cholinesterase. Overdose manifestations may also be due to side effects (e.g. morphine producing respiratory depression).

2. *Intolerance.* This is exhibiting a qualitatively normal response but to an abnormally low or high dose. It is usually simply explained by the Gaussian distribution of variation in the animal population.

3. *Allergy.* Allergic responses are, in general, not dose related and the allergy may be due to the drug itself or to the vehicle in which it is presented. The reaction may take a number of forms: shock, asthma or bronchospasm, hepatic congestion from hepatic vein constriction, blood disorders, rashes or pyrexia. Terms such as 'allergic', 'anaphylactic', 'anaphylactoid' or 'hypersensitive' have specific meanings to immunologists but, unfortunately, they are often used interchangeably. Strictly speaking, it is inaccurate to use any of these terms until evidence of the immunological basis of a reaction has been established. Many of these reactions are histamine related but other mediators such as prostaglandins, leucotrienes or kinins may be involved. Some immunologists consider that where either the mediator or the mechanism involved is uncertain, reactions are best described as 'histaminoid' or 'anaphylactoid' (Armitage-Chan, 2010).

4. *Drug interactions.* Despite the importance of drug interactions, there is little information in the veterinary literature on this subject. Drug interaction can occur outside the body, as when two drugs are mixed in a syringe before they are administered, or inside the body after administration by the same or different routes. It is generally unwise to mix products or vehicles in the same syringe (although frequently done). If drugs are to be administered into an IV infusion, it must be certain that some combination is compatible and, for example, does not result in precipitation of one or both drugs (Kanji et al., 2010). The result of the interaction between two drugs inside the body may be an increased or decreased action of one or both or even an effect completely different from the normal action of either drug. The result of interaction may be simply the sum of the actions of the two drugs (1 + 1 = 2), or greater (1 + 1 > 2), when it is known as synergism. When one agent has no appreciable effect but enhances the response to the other (0 + 1 > 1), the term 'potentiation' is used to describe the effect of the first on the action of the second. An agent may also antagonize the effects of another and the antagonism may be 'chemical' if they form an inactive complex, 'physiological' if they have directly opposing actions although at different sites, or 'competitive' if they compete for the same receptors. Non-competitive antagonism may result from modification by one drug of the transport, biotransformation or excretion of the other. In the liver, the non-specific metabolic degradation of many drugs occurs and many different agents have the ability to cause an 'enzyme induction' while a few decrease the activity – 'enzyme inhibition'. Analgesics such as phenylbutazone cause enzyme induction and can produce a great increase in the rate of

metabolism of substrates. Barbiturate treatment of epilepsy may almost halve the half-life of dexamethasone with a consequent marked deterioration in the therapeutic effect of this steroidal substance. Competition for binding sites and the displacement of one drug from the bound (inactive) form may lead to increased toxicity.

PHARMACOGENETICS

Throughout this chapter there has been reference made to the existence of species differences, both anatomical and physiological. However, within a species, and even within a breed, there are also differences. Many of these result in different metabolism of drugs; for example the cat's inability to conjugate many agents; rabbits' rapid metabolism of atropine, differences between species in

pseudocholine-esterase. Aside from these more generalized species/breed differences, some individual animals may respond to a drug in an unexpected manner that is qualitatively different to that of normal individuals. Many such reactions are genetically determined. Examples related to veterinary anaesthesia include malignant hyperthermia in pigs and horses, hyperkalaemia in quarter horses and the response to surgery and anaesthesia of dogs suffering from von Willebrands's disease.

Since the knowledge of the human genome, the genetics of many such problems in humans has been clarified, enabling tests to be carried out prior to anaesthesia. Although knowledge of animal genomes is not as complete, there are now genetic tests for the most common of these disorders in animals. For non-emergency surgery, in the future preanaesthetic testing in potentially susceptible animals (from breed or family history) may allow the anaesthetist to be prepared for the previously termed 'idiosyncratic reaction'.

REFERENCES

Absalom, A.R., De Keyser, R., Struys, M.M., 2011. Closed loop anesthesia: are we getting close to finding the holy grail? Anesth Analg 112, 516–518.

American Society of Anesthesiologists, 2010. http://www.asahq.org/Home/For-Members/Clinical-Information/ASA-Physical-Status-Classification-System. Accessed 18/10/2012.

Antognini, J.F., Carstens, E., 2005. Measuring minimum alveolar concentration: more than meets the tail. Anesthesiology 103, 679–680.

Armitage-Chan, E., 2010. Anaphylaxis and anaesthesia. Vet Anaesth Analg 37, 306–310.

Beths, T., Glen, J.B., Reid, J., et al., 2001. Evaluation and optimisation of a target-controlled infusion system for administering propofol to dogs as part of a total intravenous anaesthetic technique during dental surgery. Vet Rec 148, 198–203.

Bettschart-Wolfensberger, R., Freeman, S.L., Jaggin-Schmucker, N., et al., 2001. Infusion of a combination of propofol and medetomidine for long-term anesthesia in ponies. Am J Vet Res 62, 500–507.

Boscan, P., Rezende, M.L., Grimsrud, K., et al., 2010. Pharmacokinetic profile in relation to anaesthesia characteristics after a 5% micellar microemulsion of propofol in the horse. Br J Anaesth 104, 330–337.

Cullen, D.J., Eger 2nd, E.I., Stevens, W.C., et al., 1972. Clinical signs of anesthesia. Anesthesiology 36, 21–36.

Eger 2nd, E.I., 2001. Age, minimum alveolar anesthetic concentration, and minimum alveolar anesthetic concentration-awake. Anesth Analg 93, 947–953.

Eger 2nd, E.I., Koblin, D.D., Harris, R.A., et al., 1997. Hypothesis: inhaled anesthetics produce immobility and amnesia by different mechanisms at different sites. Anesth Analg 84, 915–918.

Eger 2nd, E.I., Saidman, L.J., Brandstater, B., 1965. Minimum alveolar anesthetic concentration: a standard of anesthetic potency. Anesthesiology 26, 756–763.

Eger 2nd, E.I., Xing, Y., Laster, M., et al., 2003. Halothane and isoflurane have additive minimum alveolar concentration (MAC) effects in rats. Anesth Analg 96, 1350–1353.

Franks, N.P., 2006. Molecular targets underlying general anaesthesia. Brit J Pharmacol 147 (Suppl 1), S72–S81.

Franks, N.P., Lieb, W.R., 1984. Do general anaesthetics act by competitive binding to specific receptors? Nature 310, 599–601.

Haynes, S.R., Lawler, P.G., 1995. An assessment of the consistency of ASA physical status classification allocation. Anaesthesia 50, 195–199.

Hemmerling, T.M., Charabati, S., Zaouter, C., et al., 2010. A randomized controlled trial demonstrates that a novel closed-loop propofol system performs better hypnosis control than manual administration. Can J Anaesth 57, 725–735.

Johansson, J.S., Zou, H., 2001. Nonanesthetics (nonimmobilizers) and anesthetics display different microenvironment preferences. Anesthesiology 95, 558–561.

Johnson, C.B., Sylvester, S.P., Stafford, K.J., et al., 2009. Effects of age on the electroencephalographic response to castration in lambs anaesthetized with halothane in oxygen from birth to 6 weeks old. Vet Anaesth Analg 36, 273–279.

Johnson, C.B., Wilson, P.R., Woodbury, M.R., et al., 2005. Comparison of analgesic techniques for antler removal in halothane-anaesthetized red deer (Cervus elaphus): electroencephalographic responses. Vet Anaesth Analg 32, 61–71.

Kanji, S., Lam, J., Johanson, C., et al., 2010. Systematic review of physical and chemical compatibility of commonly used medications administered by continuous infusion in intensive care units. Crit Care Med 38, 1890–1898.

Liu, N., Chazot, T., Hamada, S., et al., 2011. Closed-loop coadministration of propofol and remifentanil guided by bispectral index: a randomized multicenter study. Anesth Analg 112, 546–557.

Mapleson, W.W., 1996. Effect of age on MAC in humans: a meta-analysis. Br J Anaesth 76, 179–185.

McMillan, M., Brearley, J., 2013. Assessment of the variation in American Society of Anaesthesiologist's Physical Status Classification assignment in small animal anaesthesia. Vet Anaesth Analges, 40, 229–236.

Merkel, G., Eger 2nd, E.I., 1963. A comparative study of halothane and halopropane anesthesia including method for determining equipotency. Anesthesiology 24, 346–357.

Messner, M., Beese, U., Romstock, J., et al., 2003. The bispectral index declines during neuromuscular block in fully awake persons. Anesth Analg 97, 488–491.

Murrell, J.C., Johnson, C.B., White, K.L., et al., 2003. Changes in the EEG during castration in horses and ponies anaesthetized with halothane. Vet Anaesth Analg 30, 138–146.

Musk, G.C., Pang, D.S., Beths, T., et al., 2006. Target-controlled infusion of propofol in dogs – evaluation of four targets for induction of anaesthesia. Vet Rec 157, 766–770.

Oku, K., Ohta, M., Yamanaka, T., et al., 2005. The minimum infusion rate (MIR) of propofol for total intravenous anesthesia after

premedication with xylazine in horses. J Vet Med Sci 67, 569–575.

Otto, K., Short, C.E., 1991. Electroencephalographic power spectrum analysis as a monitor of anesthetic depth in horses. Vet Surg 20, 362–371.

Quasha, A.L., Eger 2nd, E.I., Tinker, J.H., 1980. Determination and applications of MAC. Anesthesiology 53, 315–334.

Perouansky, M., Pearce, R.A., Hemmings, H.C., 2012. Inhaled Anesthetics: Mechanisms of action. In: Millar, R.D., Erikson, L.I., Fleisher, L.A., et al. (Eds.), Miller's Anaesthesia, seventh ed. Churchill Livngstone-Elsevier, ch 20.

Rees, G.J., Gray, T.C., 1950. Methyl-n-propyl ether. Br J Anaesth 22, 83–91.

Rezende, M.L., Boscan, P., Stanley, S.D., et al., 2010. Evaluation of cardiovascular, respiratory and biochemical effects, and anesthetic induction and recovery behavior in horses anesthetized with a 5% micellar microemulsion propofol formulation. Vet Anaesth Analg 37, 440–450.

Ribeiro, L.M., Ferreira, D.A., Bras, S., et al., 2009. Correlation between clinical signs of depth of anaesthesia and cerebral state index responses in dogs during induction of anaesthesia with propofol. Res Vet Sci 87, 287–291.

Rudolph, U., Antikowiak, B., 2004. Molecular and neuronal substrates for general anaesthetics. Nat Rev Neurosci 5, 709–720.

Savvas, I., Rallis, T., Raptopoulos, D., 2009. The effect of pre-anaesthetic fasting time and type of food on gastric content volume and acidity in dogs. Vet Anaesth Analg 36, 539–546.

Sears, D.A., 1970. Disposal of plasma heme in normal man and patients with intravascular hemolysis. J Clin Invest 49, 5–14.

Shander, A., Van Aken, H., Colomina, M.J., et al., 2012. Patient blood management in Europe. Br J Anaesth 109, 55–68.

Sherrington, C.S., 1906. The Integrative Action of the Nervous System. Yale University Press, New Haven, ch 1, pp. 1–200.

Snow, J., 1847. On the inhalation of the vapour of ether in surgical operations. John Churchill, London.

Sonner, J.M., Antognini, J.F., Dutton, R.C., et al., 2003. Inhaled anesthetics and immobility: mechanisms, mysteries, and minimum alveolar anesthetic concentration. Anesth Analg 97, 718–740.

Theusinger, O.M., Felix, C., Spahn, D.R., 2012. Strategies to reduce the use of blood products: a European perspective. Curr Opin Anesthesiol 25, 59–65.

Urban, B.W., Bleckwenn, M., 2002. Concepts and correlations relevant to general anaesthesia. Br J Anaesth 89, 3–16.

Wolters, U., Wolf, T., Stutzer, H., et al., 1996. ASA classification and perioperative variables as predictors of postoperative outcome. Br J Anaesth 77, 217–222.

Chapter 2

Patient monitoring and clinical measurement

INTRODUCTION

From the earliest days of anaesthesia, the anaesthetist has monitored the patient's pulse rate, pattern of breathing and general condition. Advances in electronic technology have made reasonably reliable, easily attached, non-invasive monitoring devices available for clinical practice. Observations and measurements of certain parameters before, during, and after anaesthesia provide important data to support the clinical assessment of the animal's condition and improve the chances of survival of the very ill by indicating what treatment is needed, as well as the response to treatment already given.

It is necessary to know what to measure as well as how to measure it and not all anaesthetists may agree on the priority ranking of the monitoring devices available. However, for major surgery, for anaesthesia and surgery of poor-risk patients, and for equine anaesthesia, it would be difficult to defend the failure to use monitoring equipment, especially if it were available. Recommendations for monitoring of anaesthetized patients are available on the web sites for the Association of Veterinary Anaesthetists, American College of Veterinary Anesthesia and Analgesia, and the American Animal Hospital Association.

GENERAL CONSIDERATIONS RELATING TO MONITORING

Complications, including death, may occur in healthy patients at all stages of anaesthesia and monitors provide early warning of life-threatening developments. Anaesthetic mishaps may be caused by mechanical malfunction, disconnection of equipment, or human error. Judgemental error frequently occurs when the anaesthetist is in a hurry and circumvents basic practices and procedures, or when a decision must be made in an emergency. The prevalence of complications may also be associated with inadequate training or experience of the anaesthetist. Knowledge and experience are a function of the nature of the training received and the years of practice, but proper vigilance at all times can only be generated by self-motivation.

Routines should be developed to ensure that each aspect of apparatus function is checked before use. Failure to follow a simple checklist in every case features high on the list of causes of anaesthetic disasters. All anaesthetic equipment, including monitoring devices, should be maintained in good functioning order. It should be a matter of course to maintain monitors with a battery back up fully charged in case of need in an area without a convenient electricity outlet nearby, failure of electricity supply, or the need to disconnect from the main supply to minimize electrical interference with other monitoring equipment.

Proficiency with methods of electronic surveillance must be acquired during minor procedures so that they can be applied properly in circumstances where their use is mandatory (e.g. during major surgery or a cardiovascular crisis). Routine use ensures that probes, sensors, electrodes, etc. can be applied quickly to the animal and increases the likelihood that the information obtained is reliable.

Although current practice is to establish monitoring only after the animal has been anaesthetized, it must be recognized that many complications occur during induction of anaesthesia. Ideally, especially for poor-risk patients, monitoring should begin when the drugs for premedication are administered. Dogs and cats may vomit after administration of an opioid and the quantity and content of the vomit may warn that the animal was fed recently and so may be at risk for regurgitation and pulmonary aspiration of gastric material. Brachycephalic breeds and animals with respiratory problems should always be observed after administration of preanaesthetic drugs because sedation may cause partial or complete airway obstruction or serious respiratory depression and

hypoxaemia. In any animal, evaluation of the degree of sedation produced by premedicant drugs may indicate that the anaesthetic plan should be reassessed and either drug doses reduced or additional agents included.

Careful observation of the patient during induction of anaesthesia may allow precise titration of drugs to achieve the desired depth of anaesthesia and ensure early recognition of a complication that requires immediate specific treatment, such as cyanosis, anaphylaxis, or cardiac arrest. Where possible, patients at risk for complications may be attached to specific monitoring equipment before induction of anaesthesia. Appropriate equipment for this would be the electrocardiograph (ECG), a device for measurement of blood pressure, or a pulse oximeter.

Recording drugs, dosages and responses for each patient is essential and provides valuable information for any subsequent time that anaesthesia may be needed. Noting all measurements on an anaesthetic record provides a pictorial description of changes that can be used to predict complications and plan treatment (Fig. 2.1). Retrospective evaluation of difficult cases and of series of records, perhaps of patients with similar surgical procedures, or to compare different anaesthetic protocols, can be used to monitor the anaesthetist's performance and identify difficult situations that require further thought and improved management. For research purposes, data can be acquired into a computer for accurate data summaries.

Monitoring animals during anaesthesia must include observation of behaviour and reflexes and measurement of various physiological parameters at regular intervals to accomplish two objectives. The first objective is to ensure that the animal survives anaesthesia and surgery. The second objective is to obtain information that can be used to adjust anaesthetic administration and management to minimize physiological abnormalities, which is especially important for animals that have already compromised organ systems. The goal is to prevent development of preventable adverse consequences 1 hour, 12 hours, or even 3 days after anaesthesia.

Monitoring should continue into the recovery period to determine the need for additional analgesic drugs, adequacy of ventilation, and to record serious deviations in body temperature. Mucous membrane colour should be checked for at least 20 minutes after the animal has been disconnected from oxygen as it may take that long for hypoxaemia to develop in animals that are moderately hypoventilating and breathing air.

A variety of methods using inexpensive or expensive equipment can be used to monitor parameters determined by the species of animal to be anaesthetized and by the abnormalities already present in the patient. Not all monitoring techniques need to be applied to every patient. A recommendation for three levels of monitoring is presented in Table 2.1; level 1 monitoring information should be obtained from all anaesthetized animals, level 2 monitors are affordable and recommended for routine use in

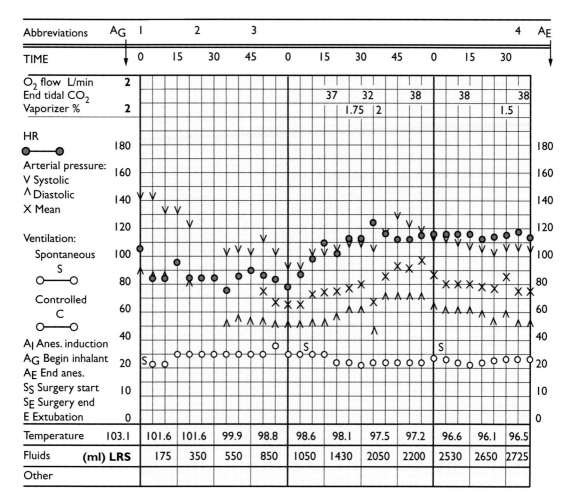

Figure 2.1 Anaesthetic record of a 61 kg, 6-year-old female Great Dane anaesthetized for exploratory laparotomy because of torsion of the spleen. Anaesthesia was induced by intravenous administration of ketamine, 200 mg, and diazepam, 10 mg, and maintained with isoflurane. Heart rate, blood pressure and respiratory rate were recorded at regular intervals to facilitate early recognition of adverse trends.

DETAILED COMMENTS:

1. Oxymorphone 4.5mg slowly IV
2. Move to O.R. 1200mg Cefotetan IV
3. Change from indirect to direct arterial BP monitoring
4. Morphine 30mg IM

some groups of patients, and level 3 monitors individually offer improved monitoring for patients with specific problems.

This chapter will describe the techniques of monitoring using a systems approach, and offer guidelines for interpretation of the information obtained. Further recommendations are given in the chapters devoted to species anaesthesia and the chapter on management of complications.

CLINICAL ASSESSMENT OF THE PATIENT

Monitoring the central nervous system

Monitoring the depth of anaesthesia is not easy (see Chapter 1). An early attempt at definition through

Table 2.1 Prioritization of monitoring

Monitor	Information obtained	Specific use
Level 1 (Basic monitoring)		
Palpebral and pedal reflexes, eye position	Depth of anaesthesia	All anaesthetized animals
Respiratory rate and depth of chest or bag excursion	Adequacy of ventilation	All anaesthetized animals
Oral mucous membrane colour	Oxygenation	All anaesthetized animals
Heart rate, rhythm, pulse strength, capillary refill time	Assessment of circulation	All anaesthetized animals
Temperature	Temperature	Dogs and cats anaesthesia greater than 30 min; all inhalation anaesthesia
Level 2 (Routine use recommended for some patients)		
Arterial blood pressure measurement (indirect or direct methods)	Blood pressure; pulse pressure variation	All inhalation anaesthesia; cardiovascular disease or depression
Blood glucose	Blood glucose	Paediatric patients; diabetics; septicaemia; insulinoma
Electrocardiography	Cardiac rate and rhythm; diagnosis of arrhythmia or cardiac arrest	All inhalation anaesthesia; thoracic trauma or cardiac disease
Pulse oximetry	Haemoglobin oxygen saturation; pulse rate	Animals breathing air during anaesthesia; recovery from anaesthesia; thoracic trauma or pulmonary disease; septicaemia/endotoxaemia
Capnography	End-tidal carbon dioxide concentration; estimate of adequacy of ventilation; warning of circuit disconnect/malfunction or cardiac arrest	All inhalation anaesthesia; patients at risk for complications
Urine output, either by expression of urinary bladder or by urethral catheterization	Urine volume produced during anaesthesia	Dogs and cats; renal disease; some urinary tract surgery; multiorgan failure
Level 3 (Use for specific patients or problems)		
Anaesthetic gas analyser	Inspired and end-tidal anaesthetic agent concentration; evaluation of depth of inhalation anaesthesia	Any patient on inhalation anaesthesia
Blood gases and pH	$PaCO_2$, PaO_2, pH, HCO_3, base excess/deficit	Suspected hypoventilation or hypoxaemia; measurement of metabolic status
Cardiac output measurement	Cardiac output	Sick animals with decreased perfusion; complicated surgeries
Central venous pressure	Indicator of central blood volume	Dehydrated/hypovolaemic patients
Packed cell volume and total protein	Haemodilution and protein concentration	Haemorrhage; large volume infusion of crystalloid solution
Peripheral nerve stimulator	Neuromuscular transmission	Use of neuromuscular blocking agents

observation of changes in reflexes, muscle tone, and respiration with administration of increased concentration of ether resulted in classification of anaesthesia into four stages (Fig. 2.2). The animal was said to make the transition from consciousness to deep anaesthesia by passing sequentially through Stage I (in which voluntary excitement might be observed), Stage II (when the animal appeared to be unconscious but exhibited involuntary muscle movement, such as limb paddling, and vocalization), Stage III (surgical anaesthesia), and Stage IV (anaesthetic overdose immediately prior to death). Stage III was further divided into Plane 1 (light anaesthesia sufficient

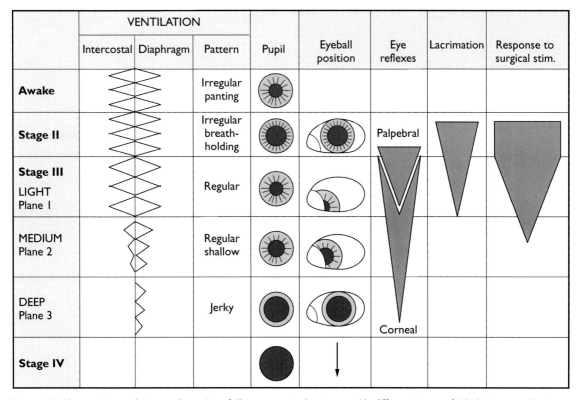

Figure 2.2 Changes in ventilation and eye signs follow recognized patterns with different stages of inhalation anaesthesia. The progression of these changes will be influenced by inclusion of injectable anaesthetic agents.
Adapted from Soma, 1971.

only for non-painful procedures), Plane 2 (medium depth anaesthesia employed for most surgical procedures), Plane 3 (deep anaesthesia), and Plane 4 (excessively deep anaesthesia). Although the progression of changes described in Fig. 2.2 are generally accurate representations of the transition from light to deep anaesthesia, the rate of changes are altered by concurrent administration of injectable drugs. Thus, in clinical practice, depth of anaesthesia is judged by a number of methods, including altered somatic and autonomic reflexes in response to nociceptive stimulation and by knowledge of the amount of anaesthetic and analgesic agents administered.

Eye position and reflexes

Eye movements are similar with thiopental, propofol, etomidate, alfaxalone, and inhalant anaesthetics in that the eyeball rotates rostroventrally during light and moderate depths of surgical anaesthesia, returning to a central position during deep anaesthesia (Fig. 2.3). Muscle tone is retained during ketamine anaesthesia and the eye remains centrally placed in the orbit in dogs and cats (Fig. 2.4),

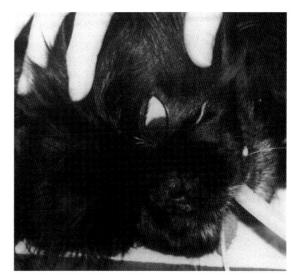

Figure 2.3 The rostroventral rotation of the eye in this dog is consistent with light and medium planes of isoflurane or sevoflurane anaesthesia.

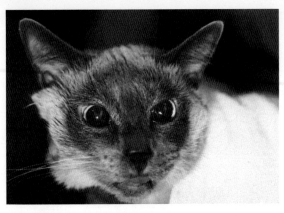

Figure 2.4 The central position of the eye, with a brisk palpebral reflex and pupillary dilation, is observed typically during ketamine anaesthesia in cats.

Table 2.2 Approximate MAC* values for isoflurane and sevoflurane in several species

Anaesthetic agent	Dogs	Cats	Horses
Isoflurane	1.4	1.6	1.3
Sevoflurane	2.4	2.6	2.3

*MAC: minimum alveolar concentration of anaesthetic agent required to prevent purposeful movement in 50% of animals in response to a standard painful stimulus; see species chapters for ranges of values.

and only slightly rotated in horses and ruminants. Fine nystagmus may be present in horses anaesthetized with ketamine (see Chapter 11). The palpebral reflex, which is partial or complete closure of the eyelids (a blink) elicited by a gentle tap at the lateral canthus of the eye or gentle stroking of the eyelashes, is frequently a useful guide to depth of anaesthesia. At a plane of anaesthesia satisfactory for surgery, the palpebral reflex is present but weak and nystagmus is absent. A brisk palpebral reflex develops when anaesthesia lightens. Ketamine anaesthesia is associated with a brisk palpebral reflex.

A corneal reflex is a similar lid response elicited by gentle pressure on the cornea. The presence of a corneal reflex is no indicator of depth of anaesthesia and may still be present for a short time after cardiac arrest has occurred.

The pedal reflex is frequently tested in dogs, cats and small laboratory animals to determine if depth of anaesthesia is adequate for the start of surgery. Pinching the web between the toes or firm pressure applied to a nail bed will be followed by withdrawal of the limb if analgesia is inadequate. Other species-specific reflexes that have been found useful include the whisker reflex in cats, where pinching of the pinna elicits a twitch of the whiskers, and tickling the inside of a pig's ear, where a shake of the head indicates inadequate anaesthesia for surgery. It must be remembered that administration of neuromuscular blocking agents blocks somatic reflexes and respiratory responses, and that the eye position will be central.

Increasing the depth of anaesthesia by increasing administration of an anaesthetic agent in most cases produces increased respiratory and cardiovascular depression. However, more than one anaesthetic or preanaesthetic agent is generally administered and the cardiopulmonary effects are determined by the combination of agents used and their dose rates. Thus measurements of respiratory rates, heart rates, and blood pressure are not reliable guides to depth of anaesthesia. It is not uncommon for an unstimulated dog or horse anaesthetized with an inhalation agent to have a low arterial blood pressure and yet in the next minute start moving its legs in response to a skin incision, all accompanied by a dramatic increase in blood pressure. Nevertheless, significant increases in heart rate and/or arterial blood pressure in response to surgical stimulation are an indication of inadequate analgesia. In certain circumstances, surgical pain can induce a vasovagal response resulting in bradycardia, decreased peripheral perfusion and pale mucous membranes. An example is traction on the ovarian ligament during ovariohysterectomy in a bitch. Preanaesthetic administration of an anticholinergic may prevent bradycardia but may also obscure heart rate responses to painful stimuli.

Anaesthetic gas analysers

The anaesthetic gas analyser measures the concentration of inhalation anaesthetic agent in inspired and expired gases (Fig. 2.5). The gases are sampled at the junction of the endotracheal tube and breathing circuit by continuous aspiration of gases at a rate of 150 mL/min to a monitor placed at some distance from the patient. To assess the depth of anaesthesia, the end-tidal concentration of inhalation agent is measured (alveolar concentration is measured at the end of exhalation) and compared with the Minimum Alveolar Concentration (MAC) value for that inhalant anaesthetic and species (Table 2.2). Using MAC for monitoring depth of anaesthesia is not precise as MAC is only an approximation of the predicted response in 50% of a population and MAC is decreased in very young and in old patients. Higher than MAC values will be required to prevent movement in all patients, and to block autonomic responses and increases in cortical electrical activity in response to a painful stimulus (March & Muir, 2003a), usually 1.2–1.5 times MAC, when anaesthesia is maintained almost entirely by inhalation agent. Less than MAC value may be sufficient when the patient is receiving continuous or intermittent administration of an adjunct agent(s) such as an opioid, lidocaine, ketamine, propofol,

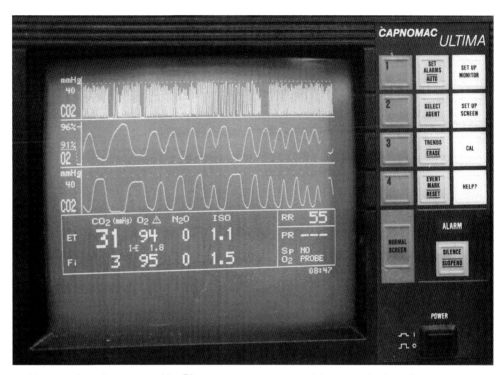

Figure 2.5 This gas analyser (Capnomac Ultima™, Datex-Engstrom Inc., Tewksbury, Maryland, USA) is monitoring a 27 kg female English Bulldog that was premedicated with glycopyrrolate and butorphanol and anaesthesia induced with propofol. She has been breathing oxygen and isoflurane at a vaporizer setting of 2.5% for 5 minutes. The monitor indicates that the inspired (Fi) isoflurane concentration is less than the vaporizer setting and that the end-tidal (ET) isoflurane concentration is less than MAC value.

or medetomidine/dexmedetomidine. For these animals, the anaesthetic administration must be adjusted according to observation of reflexes and lack of significant cardiovascular response to surgical stimulus.

It should be noted that the gas analyser also accurately measures inspired anaesthetic concentration, which may be substantially lower than the vaporizer setting in rebreathing systems during anaesthesia in large dogs, horses and ruminants (see Fig. 2.5). A situation may arise where administration of an anaesthetic agent may be inadequate despite an apparently adequate vaporizer setting. In a retrospective study of equine anaesthesia, it was found that horses were four times more likely to move during anaesthesia when an anaesthetic agent analyser was not used (Parviainen & Trim, 2000).

Some monitors using the principles of infrared absorption spectrometry cannot be used for horses or ruminants as they will measure exhaled methane and record the concentration as halothane, for example the Datex Capnomac/ Normac (Taylor, 1990). There may be minimal effect with isoflurane but negligible with sevoflurane and desflurane. Analysers that use higher wavelengths of infrared light should be unaffected by methane (Moens et al., 1991).

EEG and Bispectral index

The subject of encephalogram (EEG) guidance to depth of anaesthesia has been discussed in Chapter 1 and Murrell and Johnson (2006) have published a review of the techniques using bispectral index and somatosensory evoked potentials for assessment of pain in animals.

Intraoperative awareness occurs when a patient becomes conscious during general anaesthesia. Significant psychological effects have been identified in humans after episodes of awareness that later are associated with changed behaviour (Apfelbaum et al., 2006). The American Society of Anesthesiologists (ASA) task force identified certain procedures and anaesthetic techniques during anaesthesia of human patients that may be associated with intraoperative awareness and these included caesarian section, cardiac surgery, trauma surgery, rapid-sequence induction, total intravenous anaesthesia, and use of reduced anaesthetic drug dosages with or without neuromuscular paralysis. Awareness has been reported in the absence of tachycardia or hypertension. Nonetheless, clinical techniques such as observation for lack of movement, the palpebral reflex, and other monitors are useful to assess anaesthetic unconsciousness.

Monitoring of brain electrical activity has clinical application and a number of monitors have been developed. Various signal processing algorithms can be applied to the frequency, amplitude, and latency of the EEG to generate a number. This number, or 'index', is scaled 0 to 100 with a value of 100 associated with wakefulness and 0 referring to an isoelectric EEG. One monitor, the Bispectral Index (BIS) has become the one most used. BIS is a proprietary algorithm based on a large number of EEG recordings taken during human anaesthesia that converts a single channel frontal EEG to an index 0 to 100, of which a range of 40 to 60 is reported to be associated with anaesthesia without awareness or decreased incidence of awareness when compared with anaesthesia monitored by other means. It has also been proposed that targeting a specific BIS index range may avoid excessive depth of anaesthesia such that the patients enter recovery at a lighter plane of anaesthesia with less respiratory depression and experience shorter recovery times. Concerns are that the numeric value may be influenced by other factors such as bolus administration of anaesthetic drugs, electrocautery, or cerebral hypoxia, and may not accurately reflect the depth of anaesthesia and initiate an inappropriate change in anaesthetic administration. Further, that use of a brain function monitor may result in excessively deep anaesthesia to the detriment of organ blood flow and function. Several prospective multicentre controlled trials involving human patients have evaluated the role of BIS monitoring in determining depth of anaesthesia and reliability for prevention of awareness during intravenous or inhalant general anaesthesia (Bruhn et al., 2005; Avidan et al., 2008; Ellerkmann et al., 2010; Kertai et al., 2011). The results thus far have not supported a unified view, however, it appears that BIS monitoring may have an impact on incidence of awareness but not influence the amount of anaesthetic agents administered or influence postoperative mortality.

The use of BIS monitoring is being investigated in animals. Electrodes manufactured for human patients may require modification and reconfiguration to adjust to the differences in shape and nature of animals' heads. Decreasing BIS values have been recorded with increasing concentrations of isoflurane and sevoflurane in dogs and cats (March & Muir, 2003b; Lamont et al., 2004; Campagnol et al., 2007). Burst suppression of the EEG, characterized by periods of low amplitude waves interspersed with bursts of high amplitude waves, occurs during deep anaesthesia (2.0 MAC) resulting in paradoxical increases in BIS values (Lamont et al., 2004; Henao-Guerrero et al., 2009). Concern has been expressed that the BIS range for animals may not be the same as the accepted range for anaesthesia in humans. A study in experimental cats found that pedal and palpebral reflexes were lost at BIS values 66 to 67, however, these values may not be associated with a surgical depth of anaesthesia (March & Muir, 2003b). BIS values increased significantly

in anaesthetized cats in response to a noxious stimulus (March & Muir, 2003a). The relationship between BIS and clinically evaluated anaesthetic depth in dogs was found to be unsatisfactory (Bleijenberg et al., 2011). Although BIS decreased significantly between sedation and anaesthesia, BIS values overlapped significantly between light and deep anaesthesia. Similarly, in horses anaesthetized with isoflurane, BIS monitoring was not found to be a useful predictor of depth of anaesthesia or warning of patient movement (Haga & Dolvik, 2002). In another investigation in horses anaesthetized with sevoflurane and undergoing a variety of surgical procedures, the mean BIS value was >60 and changes in BIS values were not detected in all horses that moved during anaesthesia (Belda et al., 2010). Further investigations are needed to define the recommendations for BIS monitoring in veterinary medicine.

Another monitor used in human anaesthesia is the cerebral state index (CSI) monitor. The CSI is not dependent on algorithms derived from human patients (see Chapter 1) and, consequently, was hoped to be more reliable in domestic species. However, Ribeiro et al. (2009) investigating induction of anaesthesia with propofol in dogs concluded that CSI monitoring was not consistent with the clinical observations observed in different stages of depth of anaesthesia.

Monitoring the circulation

The heart rate, pulse rate and rhythm, tissue perfusion, and blood pressure of all anaesthetized animals should be assessed at frequent regular intervals (Table 2.3).

Pulse rate and rhythm

The peripheral pulse rate and rhythm may be counted by palpation of a peripheral arterial pulse, such as the femoral artery in dogs and cats, lingual artery in dogs (Fig. 2.6), facial, median or metatarsal arteries in horses (Fig. 2.7), and femoral, median, or auricular arteries in ruminants and pigs. The pulse rate and rhythm can also be determined from the audible sound of blood flow from a Doppler ultrasound probe (see later) and as a digital number and waveform generated by a pulse oximeter. The physiological relationship between the heart sounds, ECG, and arterial pulse is depicted in Figure 2.8. Pulse deficits are identified by palpation of a peripheral pulse that has an irregular rhythm, pauses, or a pulse rate that is less than the heart rate determined by auscultation of the heart using a stethoscope. Pulse deficits may be associated with any of several cardiac dysrhythmias, such as sinoatrial heart block, atrioventricular heart block, premature ventricular depolarizations, or atrial fibrillation, and will require an ECG for diagnosis.

Table 2.3 Methods of assessing cardiovascular function in anaesthetized clinical patients

Heart rate and rhythm

Palpation of arterial pulse
Oesophageal stethoscope
Electrocardiogram
Blood pressure monitor
Pulse oximeter

Tissue perfusion

Mucous membrane colour
Capillary refill time
Blood pressure
Bleeding at operative site
Observation of intestine colour
Urine output

Arterial blood pressure

Palpation of arterial pulse
Doppler ultrasound method
Oscillometric method
Arterial catheterization

Blood volume

Pulse pressure variation
Central venous pressure
Assess blood loss

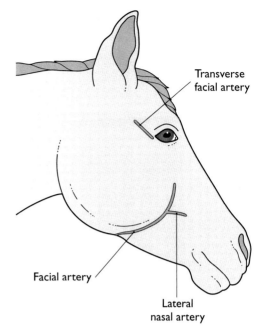

Figure 2.7 Sites for palpation of arterial pulse or catheter placement for blood pressure measurement in horses.

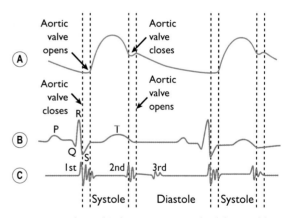

Figure 2.8 Relationship between aortic pulse (A), ECG (B), and heart sounds as auscultated with a stethoscope (C). *Modified from Guyton, 1986.*

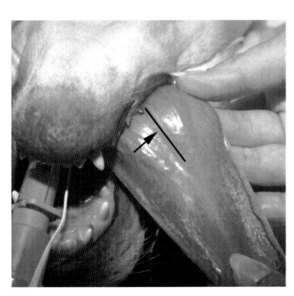

Figure 2.6 The lingual artery is easily palpated in dogs midline on the ventral surface of the tongue, adjacent to the nerve and between the lingual veins. The arrow in the photograph points to a line drawn adjacent to the lingual artery.

Heart rate monitors

Heart rates measured before anaesthesia are greatly influenced by the environment. Means (standard deviations, range) of heart rates obtained by palpation from healthy cats at home were 118 mean (SD 11, range 80–160) beats per minute compared with mean 182 (SD 20, range 142–222) when obtained by electrocardiography in the veterinary hospital (Sawyer et al., 1991).

The lowest acceptable heart rates during anaesthesia are controversial, but reasonable guidelines are 55 beats/min

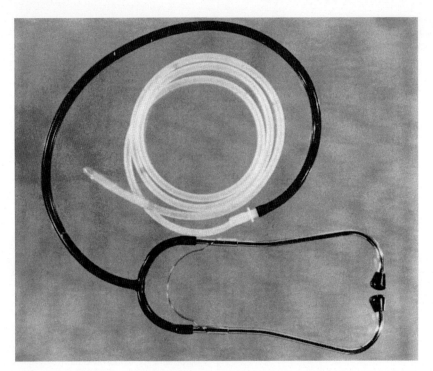

Figure 2.9 The oesophageal stethoscope. It may be used with a single earpiece or with a conventional stethoscope headpiece. This is a simple and inexpensive monitoring device for heart beat and respiratory activity.

for large dogs, 65 beats/min for adult cats, 26 beats/min for horses, and 50 beats/min for cattle. Heart rates should be higher in small breed dogs and much higher in immature animals. Heart rates may be less than these values when medetomidine/dexmedetomidine has been administered. It should be remembered that heart rate is a major determinant of cardiac output, consequently, bradycardia should be treated if blood pressure and peripheral perfusion are also decreased.

Oesophageal stethoscope

The oesophageal stethoscope (Fig. 2.9) is a simple method of monitoring heart rate in dogs and cats. This monitor consists of a tube with a balloon on the end which is passed dorsal to the endotracheal tube and into the oesophagus until the tip is level with the heart. The open end of the tube is connected to an ordinary stethoscope headpiece, to a single earpiece that can be worn by the anaesthetist or surgeon, or connected to an amplifier that makes the heart sounds audible throughout the room. This monitor provides only information about heart rate and rhythm; the intensity of sound is not reliably associated with changes in blood pressure or cardiac output. Other electronic oesophageal probes are available to provide heart rate, and some also may produce an ECG and oesophageal temperature.

Electrocardiography

Heart rate and rhythm can be obtained from an ECG using standard limb leads in small animals, clip electrodes and ECG paste or gel, and selecting ECG Lead II on the oscilloscope (Fig. 2.10A). Poor contact of the electrodes to the skin from hair bunched in the clips, or close proximity to another electrical apparatus, such as the hot water circulating pad, can result in electrical interference that obscures the ECG. The leads should not be placed over the thorax as breathing will move the electrodes and result in a wandering ECG baseline (Fig. 2.10B).

A frequently used monitor lead in equine anaesthesia is the 'base-apex' lead. The right arm electrode is clipped on the neck in the right jugular furrow and the left arm electrode is passed between the forelimbs and clipped at the apex of the heart over the left fifth intercostal space several inches from the midline. The left leg electrode is clipped on the neck or on the shoulder. Good electrical contact is achieved with alcohol or electrode paste. Lead I is selected on the electrocardiograph and the normal configuration includes a negative R wave (see Fig. 2.10C). A bifid P wave is frequently observed in the normal equine ECG. Sinus arrhythmia in dogs and cats is abolished when atropine or glycopyrrolate has been administered. Other arrhythmias, for example second degree atrioventricular heart block and ventricular premature depolarizations (VPD) or

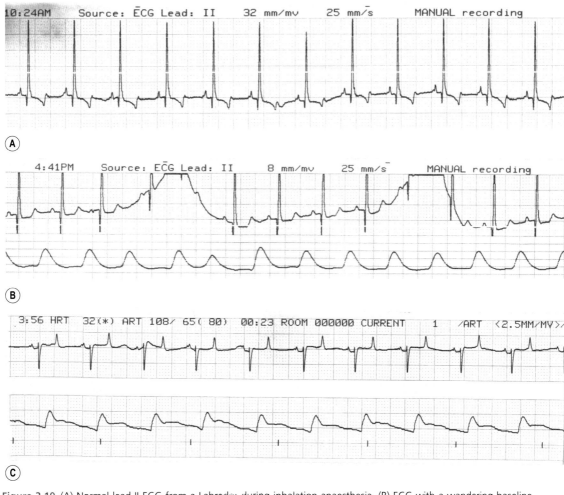

Figure 2.10 (A) Normal lead II ECG from a Labrador during inhalation anaesthesia. (B) ECG with a wandering baseline induced by movement of leads as the dog breathes. The bottom trace is arterial blood pressure. This dog has a heart rate of 114 beats per minute, systolic arterial pressure of 96 mmHg, diastolic pressure of 46 mmHg, and mean pressure of 61 mmHg. (C) Normal base apex ECG and blood pressure recorded from a horse anaesthetized with isoflurane.

premature ventricular complexes (PVC), may or may not require specific treatment (see Chapter 21).

There is a high incidence of sinus arrhythmia and first and second degree atrioventricular (AV) heart block in conscious unsedated horses (Robertson, 1990). In contrast, AV block during anaesthesia is uncommon except when the horse has been premedicated with detomidine, or supplemental intravenous injections of xylazine are given during anaesthesia. The appearance of this arrhythmia during anaesthesia on any other occasion is cause for concern as this rhythm may progress within a few minutes to advanced heart block (P waves only, no ventricular complexes) and cardiac arrest. Atrial fibrillation and PVCs occur rarely in horses but may require specific treatment if associated with hypotension.

Tissue perfusion

Evaluation of tissue perfusion can be done by considering gum or lip mucous membrane colour, the capillary refill time, and the blood pressure. High mean arterial pressure does not guarantee adequate tissue perfusion. For example, when blood pressure increases during anaesthesia in response to a surgical stimulus, cardiac output may be decreased due to increased afterload from peripheral vasoconstriction.

Tissue perfusion is usually decreased when the gums are pale, rather than pink, sometimes when very pink, and the capillary refill time (CRT) exceeds 1.5 seconds, or the mean arterial pressure (MAP) is less than 60 mmHg. When MAP is above 60 mmHg, palpation of the strength

Abbreviations	
NIBP	Non-invasive blood pressure
IBP	Invasive blood pressure
SAP	Systolic arterial pressure
DAP	Diastolic blood pressure
MAP	Mean arterial pressure
CVP	Central venous pressure
CO	Cardiac output

Myths about blood pressure in anaesthetized animals
If you can feel a strong pulse the blood pressure is adequate
Heart rate will increase during hypotension

of the peripheral pulse and observation of oral membrane colour and CRT should be used to assess adequacy of peripheral perfusion and cardiac output. During laparotomy, intestinal colour should be bright pink and intestines that are pale pink, white, or grey may be an indicator of inadequate tissue perfusion. Measurement of central venous O_2 saturation may provide further information in sick patients, as described later.

Arterial blood pressure

Systolic (SAP), mean (MAP), and diastolic (DAP) arterial pressures in awake healthy animals are approximately 125–160 mmHg, 90–110 mmHg, and 75–95 mmHg, respectively. Excepting when premedication has included detomidine or medetomidine or when anaesthesia was induced with ketamine or tiletamine, arterial blood pressure is decreased from the awake value during anaesthesia. Arterial blood pressure is lower in paediatric patients than in mature animals. For example, healthy 5- or 6-day-old foals anaesthetized with isoflurane had an average MAP of 58 mmHg. When the same foals were reanaesthetized 4–5 weeks later, the average MAP had increased to 80 mmHg, with a corresponding decrease in cardiac index (Hodgson et al., 1990).

Hypotension may be defined as MAP less than 65 mmHg in mature animals. A MAP as low as 60 mmHg may be allowed in dogs and cats provided that the mucous membrane colour is pink and CRT is 1 second. This combination of values may occur during inhalation anaesthesia at the time of minimal stimulation during preparation of the operative site and before the onset of surgery. MAP is not usually allowed to fall below 65–70 mmHg for any length of time in anaesthetized horses because of the increased risk for postanaesthetic myopathy. When hypotension is documented, appropriate treatment can be instituted, such as decreasing anaesthetic depth or commencing or increasing the intravenous administration of fluids or administration of a vasoactive drug such as dopamine, dobutamine, or ephedrine. The outcome of untreated severe or prolonged hypotension may be unexpected cardiac arrest during anaesthesia or neurological deficits, blindness or renal failure after recovery from anaesthesia.

An approximate estimate of blood pressure can be made from palpation of a peripheral artery. However, strength of a palpated pulse is determined by the pulse pressure (difference between systolic and diastolic pressures) and, in states associated with vasodilatation, a peripheral pulse can be palpated at MAP as low as 40 mmHg so that, in some cases, palpation alone does not suggest the urgency for treatment. The turgidity of the artery will provide further information because pressure is likely to be low if the artery is soft or collapsible rather than solid like a pencil. Bear in mind that it is not uncommon for heart rates to be within an accepted normal range while blood pressure is low or decreasing (Fig. 2.11).

Measurement of blood pressure can be made easily; equipment cost varies. The investment in time and money is worthwhile in animals at risk for hypotension, such as small animals and horses anaesthetized with inhalation agents, and in animals with abnormalities likely to give rise to complications during anaesthesia. The least expensive techniques are the Doppler ultrasound technique in dogs and cats, and direct blood pressure measurement using an anaeroid manometer in horses, however, purchase of a unit that monitors more than one parameter, for example, ECG, blood pressure, and temperature, is more economical than acquiring monitors individually.

Doppler ultrasound for indirect measurement of blood pressure

Hair is first clipped from the skin on the palmar surface of the paw of dogs and cats (Fig. 2.12). A probe covered with contact gel is placed over the artery and taped in place with the electrical lead pointing down towards the toes (Fig. 2.13). Ultrasound waves emitted from one of the two piezoelectric crystals embedded in the probe pass through the skin and deeper tissues. A structure that is stationary will reflect sound back to the second crystal without any frequency change (Stegall et al., 1968). Moving objects, such as erythrocytes and the artery wall, will reflect some of the sound at a different frequency (Doppler-shift). The change in frequency can be heard through a loudspeaker as an audible swooshing sound with each pulse.

A cuff is wrapped snugly around the extremity proximal to the probe, in dogs and cats with the centre of the inflatable part of the cuff, or an arrow or dot, on the medial aspect of the limb and the air tube positioned on the distal end of the cuff. The cuff is connected to an anaeroid

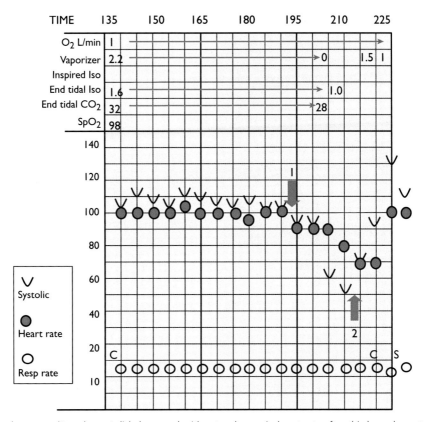

Figure 2.11 Blood pressure (Doppler systolic) decreased without a change in heart rate after this hound was turned over (Arrow 1) during anaesthesia. Blood pressure continued to decrease after isoflurane was discontinued. Infusion of dobutamine (Arrow 2) produced a rise in blood pressure.

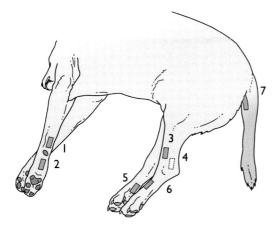

Figure 2.12 Sites for application of the Doppler probe for indirect measurement of arterial blood pressure in dogs. 1 & 2: Ulnar artery on the caudal surface of the forelimb, above and below the carpal pad; 3: cranial tibial artery on the craniolateral surface of the hindlimb; 4 & 5: saphenous artery on the medial surface of the flexor tendons and on the plantar surface of the paw proximal to the foot pad; 6: dorsal pedal artery; 7: coccygeal artery on the ventral surface of the tail.

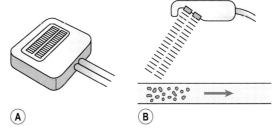

Figure 2.13 Doppler-shift pulse detector. One piezoelectric crystal emits incident ultrasound signal while the other receives the reflected signal from cells in flowing blood. The frequency shift between the incident and reflected sound is converted to audible sound.

manometer and a bulb for manual inflation of the cuff with air (Fig. 2.14). In horses, the cuff is wrapped around the base of the tail with the cuff air bladder centred over the ventral surface of the tail. The probe is taped distal to the cuff over the coccygeal artery in the ventral midline groove. The coccygeal artery can be used for this technique in adult cattle but the results are not reliable. In foals, the probe and cuff are commonly attached to the tail. In foals

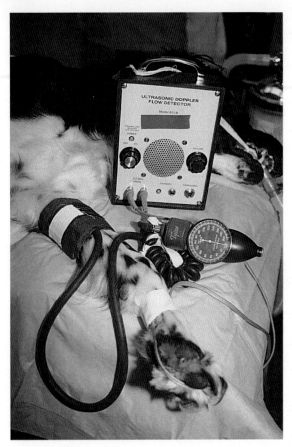

Figure 2.14 Measurement of arterial pressure in a dog by taping a Doppler probe over an artery distal to the carpal pad so that audible sounds of arterial pulses are emitted from the box. A blood pressure cuff is applied higher up the limb and the anaeroid manometer attached to the cuff is used to identify systolic and diastolic pressures.

and small ruminants in lateral recumbency, the probe can be taped over the metatarsal artery on the lateral surface of the hind limb or the common digital artery on the medial side of the forelimb distal to the carpus. The cuff is secured around the limb above the hock or carpus and positioned level with the sternum. In pigs, the probe is most reliable when taped over the common digital artery on the caudomedial aspect of the forelimb. The cuff should be placed between the carpus and the elbow but, because of the triangular shape of the forearm, it may be unable to occlude blood flow when inflation of the cuff causes it to slip down over the carpus. For all animals, the width of the air bladder within the cuff is important for accuracy; a bladder that is too narrow will overestimate blood pressure and one that is too wide will underestimate it. The cuff (air bladder) width should be 40% of the circumference of the extremity and the leg positioned so

that the cuff is level with the manubrium. Furthermore, a cuff that is attached too loosely or slips down the extremity and becomes loose, or situated over a joint such as the carpus will result in an erroneously high value.

To measure blood pressure, the cuff is inflated to above systolic pressure to occlude the artery and no sound is heard. The pressure in the cuff is gradually released until the first sounds of blood flow are detected at systolic pressure. As additional pressure is released from the cuff, diastolic pressure is heard as a change in character of sound from a one or two beat sound to a multiple beat sound, to a muffling of sound, or to a growl. This will occur 15–40 mmHg below systolic pressure. The sounds associated with diastolic pressure are well defined in some animals but not at all clear in others. In some animals, a first muffling of beat signals may occur 10–15 mmHg above the true diastolic pressure. In this event, the second change in beat signal will be more abrupt or distinct. Mean pressure can be calculated as one third of the pulse pressure (systolic–diastolic) plus diastolic pressure.

A decrease in intensity of the pulsing sound, when the attachment and setting have been unchanged, is a reliable indication of decreased blood flow. Furthermore, changes in cardiac rhythm are easily detected by listening to this monitor.

The Doppler ultrasonic method was observed to provide both overestimated and underestimated values over a wide range of systolic pressures in conscious and anaesthetized dogs, with a tendency for overestimation when MAP <80 mmHg and underestimation at high pressures (Haberman et al., 2006; Bosiack et al., 2010). An investigation in cats comparing the Doppler ultrasonic method, using a cuff placed halfway between the carpus and the elbow, with measurements obtained from a femoral artery catheter revealed that the indirect method consistently underestimated systolic pressure by an average of 14 mmHg (Grandy et al., 1992). Caulkett et al. (1998) also determined that the Doppler method both overestimated and underestimated systolic blood pressure in anaesthetized cats but that it proved to be an accurate predictor of MAP. Using this technique of measuring blood pressure in mature horses using a cuff width 48% of the circumference of the tail (bladder width 10.4 cm) systolic pressure was underestimated and diastolic pressure overestimated by approximately 9% (Parry et al., 1982). In another investigation, measurements of systolic arterial pressure in horses anaesthetized in dorsal recumbency with halothane using a cuff 41% of the tail circumference was reasonably accurate but, in 5% of the horses, this technique had an error range of ±20 mmHg (Bailey et al., 1994).

Oscillometry for indirect measurement of blood pressure

Devices that non-invasively measure peripheral blood pressure using the oscillometric method operate by

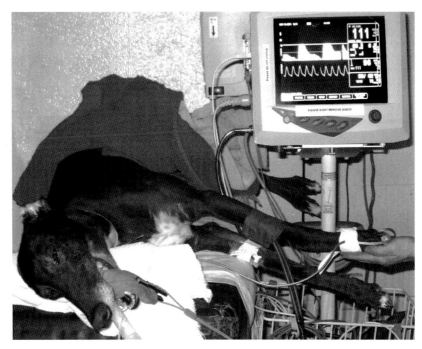

Figure 2.15 Non-invasive measurement of blood pressure by oscillometry. The cuff should be positioned level with the manubrium or sternum, and for big dogs it may be necessary to hold the limb elevated during measurement to achieve alignment. A Doppler ultrasound probe is also attached to the limb of this dog for audible recognition of blood flow.

automatically inflating a cuff placed around an extremity, either above or below the carpus, above or below the hock, or the tail (Fig 2.15). The monitor measures and records the amplitude of pressure changes in the cuff caused by pulses in underlying arteries. The cuff is inflated to above systolic pressure and deflated slowly. The pressure oscillations in the cuff start small and increase to a maximum value (corresponding with MAP) and then decrease. Each monitor uses fixed or variable parameter identification points based on the MAP value to calculate electronically systolic and diastolic pressures. The algorithm determining systolic and diastolic pressures varies between models and thus measurement results are not the same for all models. There is a also small difference in the recorded MAP and MAP calculated from the systolic and diastolic pressures using the formula MAP = diastolic pressure + 0.33 (systolic − diastolic) and this value is dependent on the measurement device (Kiers et al., 2008). Values for SAP, DAP, MAP, and heart rate are digitally displayed and the monitor can be programmed to measure automatically at a specified time interval. The cuff should be situated approximately level with the heart (manubrium or sternum if in lateral recumbency) for accurate measurement. Artefactual pressure changes induced in the cuff by movement of the extremity, for example, during preparation of the surgical site, will either induce abnormal readings or prevent the monitor from obtaining a measurement

(Haberman et al., 2006; Bosiack et al., 2010). Closest correlations between direct and indirect measurements have been measured using cuff widths of 40% of the circumference of the animal's leg or tail.

By far the highest number of published articles comparing NIBP and IBP measurements have been in dogs. Not all investigations have produced similar results, in part influenced by use of different models from several manufacturers, measurement in awake versus anaesthetized animals, increased variability attributed to haemodynamic alterations imposed by disease, differences in size and gender, sites of measurement, patient body position, pharmacological methods used to alter blood pressure, and the investigators varied definitions of hypotension or hypertension. The 'take home' message is that NIBP does not accurately predict IBP all of the time and that no treatment decision should be made based solely on one measurement. Investigations of specific models have employed the average of three to six consecutive readings taken 30–60 seconds apart to increase accuracy. Frequently during anaesthesia, the site of surgery and accessibility dictates the site for application of the cuff. Different sites have been investigated with the result that the forelimb in dogs was determined to be more accurate when compared with lingual artery pressure and the hind limb more accurate when compared with dorsal pedal artery pressure (McMurphy et al., 2006), no difference between measurements was recorded between the fore and hind limbs (Sawyer et al., 1991), or that the tibial or coccygeal arteries provided better correlation than the metacarpal artery when compared with aortic or anterior tibial artery pressure (Sawyer et al., 2004; Haberman et al., 2006). Most oscillometric monitors provide a reasonable approximation of MAP in normotensive animals.

The greatest concern during most anaesthetic episodes is the accurate identification of hypotension to avoid cardiac arrest or postoperative organ malfunction. The Surgivet V60046, with the cuff placed distal to the hock, provided accurate information for MAP in normotensive and hypotensive dogs, with 90.6% of the dogs with MAP <70 mmHg being accurately diagnosed as hypotensive (Deflandre & Hellebrekers, 2007). The monitor was less accurate at high pressures. The Cardell 9401, DINAMAP (Device for Indirect Noninvasive Automatic Mean Arterial Pressure) 8100, DINAMAP 8300 and PetMAP overestimated pressures during hypotension (Sawyer et al., 1991; Meurs et al., 1996; Bosiack et al., 2010; Shih et al., 2010), and did not reliably predict the severity of hypotension in animals with acute haemorrhage or in critically-ill patients in the ICU. Wernick et al. (2010) compared measurements in anaesthetized dogs between pressures recorded from the dorsal pedal artery and from a cuff around the antebrachium using the DINAMAP 8300. The DINAMAP slightly underestimated SAP and DAP and overestimated MAP; comparisons that fell just short of the validation requirement proposed by the American College of Veterinary Internal Medicine (Brown et al., 2007). In contrast, the DINAMAP 8300 underestimated all BP parameters in awake experimental Beagles, and to a greater extent at high pressures generated by administration of phenylephrine (Haberman et al., 2006). Comparisons with the Cardiocap II in clinical canine patients using premedication to alter blood pressure (acepromazine or medetomidine) generated a smaller bias than previously reported (Sawyer et al., 2004; McMurphy et al., 2006) but greater limits of agreement (variability) that was attributed to variation in clinical population (MacFarlane et al., 2010).

In clinical practice, it may be necessary to identify hypertension before anaesthesia and to measure accurately high pressures during anaesthesia in patients at risk, such as phaeochromocytoma, renal or endocrine disease. Oscillometric methods tend to underestimate systolic blood pressures during hypertension (Haberman et al., 2006; McMurphy et al., 2006; Deflandre & Hellebrekers, 2007; Bosiack et al., 2010), consistently underestimate MAP or DAP (Haberman et al., 2006), overestimated MAP or DAP (Bosiack et al., 2010), or underestimated SAP and DAP with close agreement with MAP (McMurphy et al., 2006).

The Cardell 9301V with 2.5 cm-wide neonatal pressure cuff placed around the forelimb above the carpus, with the monitor set at 'small cuff' mode has been evaluated in cats (Pedersen et al., 2002). Low pressure MAP <60 mmHg was achieved by increasing depth of anaesthesia with isoflurane and high pressures MAP >140 mmHg were created by administration of medetomidine. Mean differences between NIBP and IBP were <5 mmHg for MAP and DAP in all pressure ranges; SAP differences increased as pressure increased from hypotension to hypertension resulting in underestimation of SAP. The DINAMAP had good correlation with IBP systolic pressure in anaesthetized cats (Caulkett et al., 1998), however, the Datascope Passport did not accurately estimate direct blood pressure in cats (Branson et al., 1997).

In horses, the oscillometric method of blood pressure measurement is used when direct measurement of arterial pressure is not possible, for total intravenous anaesthesia, and for awake animals. The cuff is wrapped around the tail of mature horses and foals or around the hind limb near the metatarsal artery in foals. The cuff should not be wrapped tightly. Some investigators have recommended that the tail cuff be placed close to the base of the tail but, in this author's opinion, more accurate readings are obtained with the cuff applied approximately 10 cm from the base of the tail, where the tail diameter is constant for the length of the cuff. In standing horses, cuff placement may be higher than the atrium, resulting in a measurement that is lower than the actual pressure. Early investigations of the DINAMAP confirmed accurate and clinically useful values for arterial pressure using a cuff width 24% of the tail circumference in ponies (Geddes et al., 1977) and 25–35% in horses (Latshaw et al., 1979; Muir et al., 1983). However, measurements were inaccurate at heart rates of less than 25 beats/minute. Our experience using a Model 8300 DINAMAP and a cuff width 35–40% of the tail circumference ratio (child or small adult cuff for a mature horse depending on tail thickness and the amount of hair) has been that MAP value obtained from this monitor is usually the same as that obtained by direct blood pressure measurement. Occasionally, the DINAMAP recorded pressures 10–20 mmHg higher than the true MAP. An evaluation of the Cardell Model 9402 and the DINAMAP Pro 100 in anaesthetized foals of less than 7 days of age using cuff sizes recommended by the manufacturers revealed that both monitors had similar performance (Giguère et al., 2005b). Analysis of MAP values confirmed acceptable accuracy with the cuffs on the tail or metatarsus for conditions of normotension and hypotension, although the Cardell was most accurate over the coccygeal artery and the DINAMAP over the metatarsal artery. Cuffs placed over the median artery produced less accurate values and wider variability. This study also confirmed that blood pressure did not correlate well with cardiac output, i.e. a good MAP does not guarantee that cardiac output is also acceptable. In summary, indirect method of measurement of blood pressure provides useful information in most horses, but may produce erroneous values in a small number. Consequently, blood pressure should be measured by direct means whenever possible in horses at risk of developing low blood pressure, for example, during inhalation anaesthesia.

Standards have been set for automated sphygmoma-nometers in human medicine by several organizations, including the British Hypertension Society, the Association for the Advancement of Medical Instrumentation (AAMI) and the American National Standards Institute, Inc. (ANSI). Devices validated for use in humans must have a correlation of ≥0.9 across a range of measurements with specific % of readings to be within 5, 10, or 15 mmHg of the standard measurement. Requirements for validation were tightened in 2011. These standards have been met for MAP at low and normal pressures in dogs with the Surgivet V60046 (Deflandre & Hellebrekers, 2007), for MAP and DAP in cats with the Cardell 9301V (Pedersen et al., 2002), and for MAP in foals using the Cardell 9402 and DINAMAP Pro 100 (Giguère et al., 2005b). For the most part, oscil-lometric blood pressure monitors provide useful information for management of the clinical patient. Trends in pressures can be used to direct management of anaesthesia and, although hypotension may not be accurately diagnosed, a decrease in measurements to low values should be a warning that action should be taken. A single abnormal measurement should be confirmed by taking two more readings. Failure of the monitor to achieve a reading ('timed out') when it had just previously been recording may indicate a change in peripheral blood flow. It must be remembered that although on average there is reasonable correlation between direct and indirect pressure measurements, in individual patients the difference in readings can be up to 20 mmHg and a patient may not be identified as having a MAP outside an accepted range. Therefore, NIBP readings must be assessed together with other observations of cardiovascular performance and depth of anaesthesia.

High-definition oscillometry

In contrast to previously described oscillometric techniques, high-definition oscillometric (HDO) technology discriminates between pressure waveform changes that are characteristic for systolic, mean, and diastolic pressures. The technology allows much more rapid assessments that minimize the impact of outside factors, and is able to accommodate fast heart rates and weak pulse signals. The expectation is for increased accuracy at high and low blood pressures and increased reliability for use in ill patients. In anaesthetized dogs, comparison between IBP measured at the dorsal pedal artery and a high-definition oscillometric device, Memodiagnostic MD_15/90 Pro, revealed that values for SAP, MAP, and DAP were all overestimated by HDO and the overestimation increased for SAP and DAP with increasing pressures (Wernick et al., 2010). The precision exceeded the 15 mmHg limit required for validation and only 50–60% of readings were within 10 mmHg. In a group of conscious experimental Beagles with implanted aortic devices for telemetry of blood pressures, measurement of pressures from a cuff around the base of the tail using HDO revealed that MAP most closely

paralleled the telemetered pressures (Meyer et al., 2010). The standards set by AAMI were not met in this study. The authors noted that the mean standard deviations were substantially decreased by use of six averaged measurements at any time point compared with a single measurement.

Direct measurement of blood pressure

Measurement of arterial blood pressure directly is accomplished by insertion of a 20 gauge, 22 gauge or, in very small animals, a 24 gauge catheter aseptically into a peripheral artery; the dorsal pedal, anterior tibial, femoral, coccygeal, metacarpal, auricular or lingual artery in dogs (Fig. 2.16), the dorsal pedal, femoral or coccygeal artery in cats, the lateral nasal, facial, transverse facial, or metatarsal artery in horses (see Fig. 2.7), or an auricular artery in ruminants, pigs and rabbits (Fig. 2.17). Placement of a catheter in an artery in most animals is not difficult with experience. Complications are rare provided there is strict attention to asepsis during insertion, wrapping to maintain cleanliness, use of sterile solutions for flushing, and appropriate pressure on the artery when the catheter is removed to avoid a haematoma. The cap or extension must be secured firmly to the arterial catheter to prevent accidental disconnection and blood loss. The catheter is connected by saline-filled tubing to either an anaeroid manometer (Fig. 2.18) or an electrical pressure transducer (Fig. 2.19) for measurement of arterial pressure. Either an air gap or a connector containing a latex diaphragm

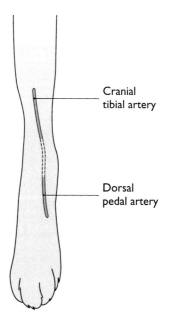

Figure 2.16 Sites for insertion of arterial catheters on the cranial aspect of the right hind limb of a dog.

Cranial tibial artery

Dorsal pedal artery

should be maintained next to the anaeroid manometer to prevent saline entering the manometer and to maintain sterility. An optional addition to the electrical transducer is a continuous flushing device (Fig. 2.20) that can be inserted between the transducer and the artery. This device is connected to a bag of saline that has been pressurized to 200 mmHg and will deliver 2–4 mL saline/hour to help prevent clotting of blood in the catheter. Extension tubing

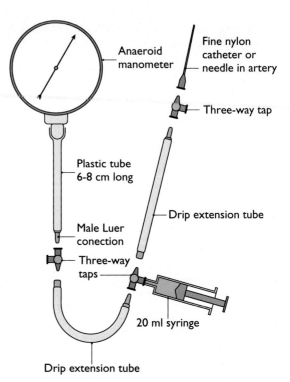

Figure 2.18 Inexpensive apparatus for the direct measurement of mean arterial blood pressure.

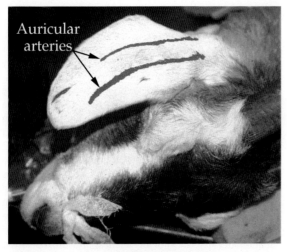

Figure 2.17 Ink lines have been drawn over the auricular arteries in this goat.

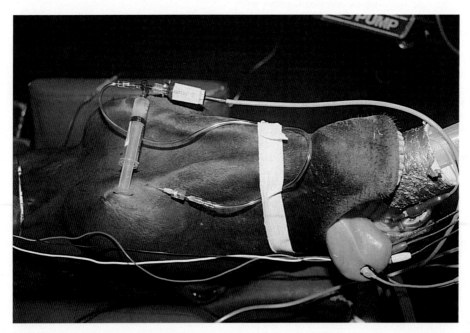

Figure 2.19 Direct measurement of blood pressure in a horse using a catheter in the facial artery connected by saline-filled tubing to an electrical transducer.

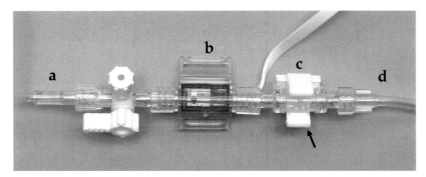

Figure 2.20 Continuous infusion valve (c) for attachment to a pressure transducer (b). A pressurized bag of intravenous fluid (d) is connected to the device to give a continuous infusion of 3 mL per hour. With this particular version, rapid flushing of the saline-filled tubing (a) to the arterial catheter is achieved by squeezing the tabs (arrow) around the valve.

sold specifically for arterial pressure measurement is non-distensible to preserve an accurate waveform.

For accurate measurement, the electrical transducer, or the air–saline junction in the tubing connected to the manometer, are zero reference points and should be placed level with the right atrium that approximately corresponds to the manubrium; the point of the shoulder or thoracic inlet when the animal is in dorsal recumbency or level with the sternum or spine when in lateral recumbency.

The anaeroid manometer costs very little but provides only MAP. The needle of the anaeroid manometer deflects slightly with each beat and the value at the upper deflection of the needle is slightly less than the MAP value obtained by direct measurement (Riebold & Evans, 1985). The electrical transducer provides values for SAP, MAP and DAP, heart rate, and a waveform that can be observed on the oscilloscope or paper printout (Fig. 2.21). Values may be slightly different when recorded from different sites, for example comparison of lingual artery and dorsal pedal artery pressures in dogs revealed that systolic pressure was higher and the diastolic pressure was lower in the pedal artery (McMurphy et al., 2006). Mean pressures should be similar in most arteries but systolic pressure increases by up to 30% and diastolic pressure decreases by 10–15% with increasing distance of measurement site from the heart due to enhancement of the peripheral pulse pressure (Guyton, 1986).

Important advantages of direct measurement of blood pressure are the reliability of measurement compared with NIBP, independence from observer error, and the ability continuously to observe the pressure and immediately detect an abnormality (Fig. 2.22). Systolic pressure variation (pulse pressure variation, 'cycling') caused by controlled ventilation is an indication of decreased cardiovascular function (Fig. 2.23). Artificial ventilation is key to inducing cycling in that the increase in thoracic pressure during inspiration causes a significant decrease in stroke volume in situations of decreased venous return to the heart. A

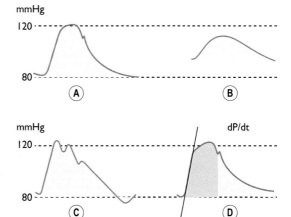

Figure 2.21 Waveforms from direct measurement of the arterial pressure. (A) Good trace. (B) Recording of the same pressure but with excessive damping, systolic pressure low, diastolic pressure high, mean arterial pressure unchanged. (C) Recording of same pressures but with resonance, systolic pressure apparently increased while diastolic pressure reduced, mean pressure unchanged. (D) Illustration of how left ventricular contractility may be estimated from the rate of rise of pressure during early systole (dP/dt) while the shaded area gives an index of stroke volume.

significant relationship has been documented between pulse pressure variation and volume loss and measurement of pulse pressure variation has been used to predict responsiveness of a patient by increased cardiac output to volume loading with IV crystalloid and/or colloid fluid (Durga et al., 2008; Pizov et al., 2010; Cannesson et al., 2011). One multicentre study of human patients noted that approximately 25% of patients with small pulse pressure variation still experienced a clinically significant increase in cardiac output in response to fluid loading (Cannesson et al., 2011). Pulse pressure variation has been determined to be better than measurement of central

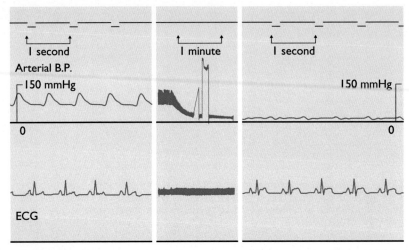

Figure 2.22 Top: pressure trace from a dog's femoral artery. Bottom: Lead II electrocardiogram. Circulatory failure from an overdose of pentobarbital. Note that while the pressure trace shows the circulation to be ineffective, the ECG trace is little different from normal – heart rate monitors relying on the QRS complex for detection of the heart beat would, under these circumstances, show an unchanged heart rate and, in the absence of a blood pressure record, encourage the erroneous belief that all was well with the circulatory system.

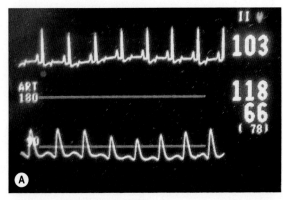 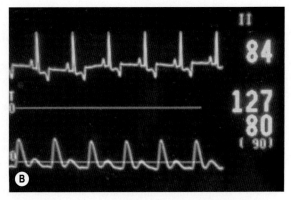

Figure 2.23 (A) Variations in the height of systolic arterial pressure and pulse pressures corresponding to positive pressure ventilation as seen in this arterial waveform of a dog anaesthetized with isoflurane are predictive of decreased preload or hypovolaemia. Note that hypovolaemia was present even when the arterial pressures were within accepted ranges. (B) Expansion of blood volume using an IV fluid bolus resulted in improvement in cardiovascular function as demonstrated by disappearance of systolic pressure and pulse pressure variations increased blood pressure, and decreased heart rate.

venous pressure for optimizing fluid therapy. Not all animals with hypovolaemia may show systolic pressure or pulse pressure variations. Each patient with obvious pulse pressure variation should be evaluated for the potential adverse effect of volume loading before administration of IV fluids. It must be remembered that cycling will not be observed in animals that are spontaneously breathing or are ventilated with small (6 mL/kg) tidal volumes.

Central venous pressure

The apparatus for measurement of central venous pressure (CVP) can include a commercially available plastic venous manometer set or be constructed from venous extension tubes and a centimetre ruler (Fig. 2.24). A catheter of sufficient length is introduced into the jugular vein and advanced until its tip lies in the cranial vena cava. The distance the catheter tip has to be introduced is, initially, estimated by measurement of length from the jugular vein to the third rib and, once the catheter is connected to the manometer, its position may be adjusted until the level of fluid in the manometer tube moves in time with the animal's respiratory movements. In dogs and cats, the introduction of a catheter into the jugular vein is often greatly facilitated by laying the animal on its side and extending its head and neck over a rolled up towel or sandbag. Care

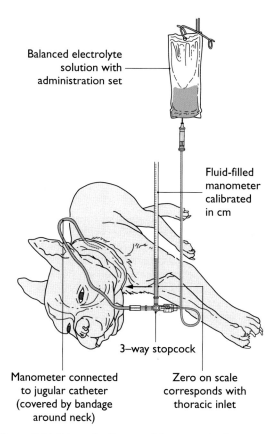

Balanced electrolyte solution with administration set

Fluid-filled manometer calibrated in cm

3–way stopcock

Manometer connected to jugular catheter (covered by bandage around neck)

Zero on scale corresponds with thoracic inlet

Figure 2.24 Schematic diagram of the apparatus for measurement of central venous pressure.

must be taken to avoid entrainment of air during insertion of the catheter. Air embolism will occur through an open-ended catheter that is inserted with the animal in sternal or standing position or during inspiration in a recumbent animal. If the catheter is to be left in position for a long time, it is kept patent with a drip infusion or the catheter is kept filled with heparin–saline solution (10 units/mL) between measurements. Readings may be taken at any time. If an intravenous drip is used, it is turned full on and the stopcock manipulated first to fill the manometer tube from the bag or bottle and then to connect the manometer tube to the catheter. The fall of fluid in the manometer is observed and should be 'step-like' in response to respiratory pressure changes. The CVP is read off when fluid fall ceases.

Central venous pressure may also be measured by attaching an electrical transducer to the jugular catheter. Venous pressures being low, the margin of error introduced by inaccuracies in obtaining a suitable reference point to represent zero pressure may be clinically significant. Whatever apparatus is used, the zero of the scale should be carefully located, either by placing the patient

and manometer in close proximity or by using a spirit level to ensure accuracy. The ideal reference point is the mean pressure in the right atrium but, for practical purposes, the most appropriate is the sternal manubrium which is easily located and is related to the position of the right atrium in all animals, irrespective of body position. Measurements of CVP are not significantly affected by positioning the animal in right or left recumbency or by catheter size, although oscillations are more easily observed with a 16 gauge catheter (Oakley et al., 1997).

CVP is used in the evaluation of adequacy of blood volume, with the normal range being 0–5 cmH_2O or 0–4 mmHg in small animals. Hypovolaemia is indicated when the CVP is less than 0 cmH_2O. An increase in pressure above 12 cmH_2O or 9 mmHg may be caused by fluid overload or cardiac failure. A recent study measured mean CVP of 9.4 ± 3.6 cmH_2O in standing horses with their heads in a neutral position (Norton et al., 2011). Head height exerted a significant effect on CVP in that the CVP decreased by 2.0 ± 6.5 cmH_2O when the horses' heads were elevated and increased by 3.7 ± 5.5 cmH_2O when the heads were lowered to the ground. The authors suggested to increase accuracy of comparison of measurements to be made over several hours that the zero reference point be identified by a small line of clipped hair.

Left atrial pressure (pulmonary arterial occlusion pressure)

Left heart failure may precede that of the right side and precipitate pulmonary oedema without a rise in central venous pressure. The pulmonary arterial occlusion pressure (PAOP) is used as a measure of the left atrial filling pressure. A balloon-tip catheter is introduced into the jugular vein and its tip advanced into the heart. Inflation of the balloon with 0.5 mL air facilitates floating the catheter in the bloodstream into the pulmonary artery and then the catheter can be advanced until the tip is wedged in a small pulmonary vessel. The measurement is made using the same apparatus as is used for the measurement of central venous pressure or using an electrical pressure transducer. Care must be taken to ensure that vessel occlusion is not maintained between measurements or pulmonary infarction may occur. If a balloon catheter is used, the balloon should only be inflated while measurements are made and, if a simple catheter is used, it should be slightly withdrawn from the wedged position between measurements.

Cardiac output

The measurement of cardiac output is not one that has been routinely carried out in clinical veterinary anaesthesia. Invasive methods are commonly employed in research and there are minimally invasive and non-invasive methods available for use in research and clinical patients.

The cost of the equipment, as always, is a limiting factor. Various sources of inaccuracy are likely to influence results of cardiac output measurements and personnel using these techniques should first read relevant literature.

Fick method

The Fick method was one of the earliest methods to be used to calculate cardiac output (CO) and utilized oxygen as the indicator. The method used the formula $CO = O_2$ consumption per minute/(arterial O_2 content − mixed venous O_2 content) × 100 because the size of a fluid stream can be calculated when the amount of a substance entering the stream and the concentration difference between entry and removal are known (Lake, 1990). This method has a number of technical difficulties and, more recently, a non-invasive technique using CO_2 has been used in clinical patients. The non-invasive cardiac output (NICO) method employs a differential Fick partial rebreathing technique that eliminates the need to measure mixed venous CO_2 by assuming that the value remains constant (Jaffe, 1999). A combined mainstream capnometer and fixed orifice differential pressure pneumotachometer (to measure flow) adapter is inserted next to the endotracheal tube adapter (Fig. 2.25). An adjustable (rebreathing) loop of tubing with an automatic valve is then attached before connecting the patient to the circle anaesthesia system. The animal must be on controlled ventilation and the rebreathing loop is expanded or contracted so that the volume of the loop matches 35–70% of the ventilator's tidal volume setting. The NICO has a 3-minute cycle within which the rebreathing valve is activated for 35 seconds so that the animal's breathing is rerouted from the anaesthesia circle into the rebreathing loop. Typically, the patient's $PaCO_2$ increases up to 5 mmHg during rebreathing. Concurrent input from the pulse oximeter allows the NICO to calculate stroke volume and manual entry of the patient's weight produces CO in mL/kg. Accuracy of the NICO is unsatisfactory in patients <18 kg bodyweight (Yamashita et al., 2007). This technique is contraindicated in any animal for which a small increase in $PaCO_2$ would be deleterious, such as conditions at risk for increased intracranial pressure. Cardiac output measurements obtained by NICO are useful to assess trends but should not be considered as absolute values (Giguère et al., 2005a).

Indicator dilution method

The principle involves injection of an indicator substance into a central or peripheral vein and blood is withdrawn from an artery continuously with a pump and directed through an electrical cuvette densitometer where the concentration of the indicator is measured. This blood is then delivered back to the patient. The electrical input from the densitometer is proportional to the indicator concentration and the monitor generates an indicator–dilution curve that is plotted against time. The area under the curve, with some modifications, is proportional to the cardiac output. The original technique used indocyanine green, a non-toxic dye, but this technique is complicated by a gradual increase in baseline due to recycling. Thermodilution cardiac output measurement (TDCO) is an indicator dilution method that has replaced dye dilution and is the technique that is used for comparing all new methods of cardiac output measurement. A multilumen catheter with a thermistor approximately 4 cm from the tip (Swan–Ganz catheter) is inserted into the jugular vein and

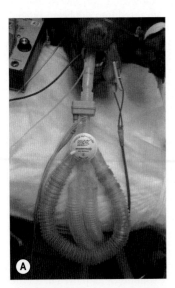
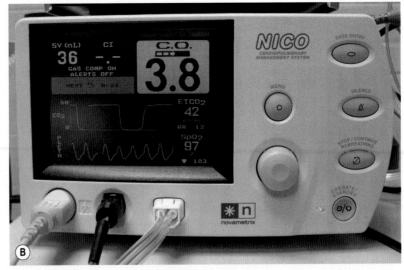

Figure 2.25 (A) Rebreathing circuit of the NICO™ (Novametrix Medical Systems, Inc. Wallingford, CT, USA). (B) NICO™ monitor measuring cardiac output in an anaesthetized dog.

advanced through the heart until the tip lies in the pulmonary artery. Correct placement of the catheter is confirmed by connecting a pressure transducer to the lumen that exits at the tip of the catheter and observation of the distinctive pressures and waveforms as the catheter passes through the atrium, ventricle and pulmonary artery. The catheter is designed such that one lumen of the catheter exits in the right atrium and that port is used for injection of cooled saline or 5% dextrose. The time of injection and temperature of injectate is recorded by the monitor, the temperature changes in the pulmonary artery are detected, and the time lapse from injection to measured temperature change allow calculation of cardiac output. Different lengths of catheter and varying volumes of injectate are chosen to accommodate various sizes of animals, from cats to horses. Either the ventilator is temporarily shut off or each injection is made at the same time in the respiratory cycle and two to three measurements are performed in quick succession and averaged to improve accuracy. Problems associated with insertion of a Swan–Ganz catheter include prolongation of anaesthesia time, initiation of premature ventricular depolarizations, and potential complications of laceration of a blood vessel, knotting of the catheter, and infection.

Lithium dilution cardiac output (LiDCO™) technique mimics the dye dilution technique by injection of lithium chloride into a central or peripheral vein and a pump withdraws blood from an artery pulling it through a lithium sensor to measure blood concentration. Advantages of this system include no major invasive catheterization and a small volume of injectate that is easily injected by hand and which causes minimal haemodynamic effect. The patient's haemoglobin and sodium concentrations must be entered into the monitor because lithium is distributed only in plasma. Some blood loss may occur even though the sampled blood is returned to the patient. A close correlation between the LiDCO and thermodilution techniques has been verified in several animal species (Linton et al., 2000; Mason et al., 2001; Beaulieu et al., 2005). One experimental study in anaesthetized neonatal foals discovered that the LiDCO technique overestimated TDCO measurements when CO <10 L/min and that the correlations changed over time, however, the authors concluded that LiDCO was an acceptable alternative to TDCO (Corley et al., 2002).

In anaesthetized healthy experimental dogs weighing 22–25.4 kg ventilated with tidal volumes of 10–15 mL/kg, cardiac outputs ranged from 50 to 303 mL/kg/min and the average difference between the LiDCO and NICO was 9.3 mL/kg/min, indicating that NICO would be acceptable for clinical use (Gunkel et al., 2004). Comparison of the NICO and LiDCO techniques in foals 1–6 days old and weighing 32–61 kg identified a good correlation for CO measurements between the two techniques over a wide range of values (Valverde et al., 2007). The NICO technique tended to overestimate the LiDCO values at low

cardiac outputs but have a closer agreement at higher values.

Pulse contour method

Monitors have been developed for assessing changes in cardiac output by analysis of the arterial pulse waveform. The LiDCO™*plus* monitor includes the PulseCO™ system that analyses the arterial waveform following initial calibration by measuring cardiac output by lithium dilution and calculates stroke volume and CO. The PiCCO™ system's initial calibration uses transpulmonary thermal dilution and requires cardiac catheterization. The FloTrac™/Vigileo™ is 'self-calibrated' based on an algorithm derived from measurements in humans. These systems have been increasingly used for tracking the haemodynamic status of human patients in the ICU or postoperative recovery areas. Studies in human patients have determined that the monitors lose accuracy with time and require recalibration, particularly when major changes in cardiovascular status have occurred, and that values obtained by one monitor differ from values obtained from a monitor from a different manufacturer. Although good agreement was obtained between LiDCO™ and PulseCO™, cardiac output measurements in dogs anaesthetized with fentanyl and pentobarbital, the PulseCO™ was unable to measure accurately the decrease in CO after severe haemorrhage and the authors concluded that recalibration was necessary after any major alteration in haemodynamic status (Cooper & Muir, 2007). Investigations of the PulseCO™ in dogs with systemic inflammatory response syndrome (SIRS) (Duffy et al., 2009) and in horses using inotropes to change cardiovascular dynamics (Schauvliege et al., 2009) revealed failure of accuracy when compared with LiDCO™ and the need for frequent recalibration. In anaesthetized neonatal foals, values for CO recorded using PulseCO™ agreed significantly better with values from LiDCO™ than measurements using the PiCCO™ method (Shih et al., 2009). Comparison of the FloTrac™/Vigileo™ with TDCO in experimental dogs documented overestimations, sometimes excessive, influenced by MAP which led to the conclusion that FloTrac™/Vigileo™ was not suitable for CO measurement in dogs (Bektas et al., 2012).

Flow method

Transoesophageal Doppler echocardiography cardiac output (TEECO) is increasingly used as a cardiovascular monitor in anaesthetized human patients. The technique involves insertion of a probe into the oesophagus to the level of the left ventricular outflow tract. The pulsed-wave Doppler crystal emits an ultrasound wave and moving objects (red blood cells) change the frequency resulting in a curved waveform. Cardiac output is calculated from the velocity-time integral (VTI, area under the curve) of the ascending aorta × aortic cross-sectional area × heart rate. Comparison with TDCO measurements has identified no significant differences between measurements from both techniques in horses and dogs (Young et al., 1996; Yamashita et al., 2007). Probe size has been a problem, and the technique requires operator training.

Impedance cardiography

Transthoracic bioimpedance (BICO) involves placement of electrodes, continuous output of high-frequency, low magnitude current, measurement of electrical resistance, and a monitor that calculates CO using an algorithm. BICO did not produce acceptable values in Beagle dogs (Yamashita et al., 2007).

Blood loss

Monitoring blood loss should include measuring the volume of blood aspirated into a suction bottle, estimating free blood on drapes around the surgical site, and counting blood-soaked gauze squares. Placing a bucket under the surgical site to catch free-flowing blood, for example during rhinotomy in large animals, will assist assessment of blood loss. Gauze squares of different sizes absorb varying amounts of blood from 5–8 mL to 12–14 mL. The volume of blood lost on the gauze squares may be estimated or the gauzes weighed and, after the weight of the same number of dry gauzes has been subtracted, applying the formula that 1 g weight equals 1 mL blood. Measurement of packed cell volume is not useful during acute blood loss as this value will not change initially. Once an increased volume of balanced electrolyte solution with or without colloid has been infused, the packed cell volume and total protein concentrations will decrease to a value of use during assessment. When evaluating packed cell volume changes, it is important to consider that anaesthesia *per se* will result in sequestration of red blood cells in the spleen and decrease the packed cell volume by up to 20%.

In the conscious animal, loss of blood volume is initially compensated for by increased heart rate and cardiac contractility, together with peripheral vasoconstriction. These physiological responses are blunted or abolished during anaesthesia. Consequently, the significance of the blood loss may not be appreciated owing to maintenance of a normal heart rate. Furthermore, it should be remembered that when MAP is decreasing in response to haemorrhage, cardiac output decreases to a greater extent (Fig. 2.26) (Weiskopf et al., 1981).

Measurement of arterial pressure is an important step in the management of blood loss as oxygen delivery to tissues is impaired when mean arterial pressure decreases below 60 mmHg. The potential impact of blood loss on the patient may be evaluated better by assessing the volume of blood loss against the total blood volume. The blood volume varies between species and is usually assessed in mature animals as 86 mL/kg body weight in dogs, 56 mL/kg in cats, 72 mL/kg in draught horses and ponies, 100 mL/kg in Thoroughbreds and Arabians, 60 mL/kg in sheep.

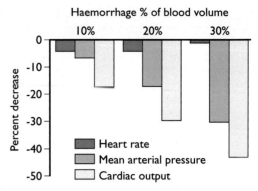

Figure 2.26 Cardiovascular responses to graded haemorrhage in five splenectomized isoflurane-anaesthetized dogs. Results are presented as percent change from values measured before blood loss
Adapted from Weiskopf et al., 1981.

Blood volume of paediatric patients may be 50% greater than the blood volume of the mature animal. The percentage of this volume that the animal can lose before circulatory shock ensues depends to a large extent on the physical status of the patient, the preanaesthetic PCV, the depth of anaesthesia, and the support treatment provided. Significant cardiovascular changes occur after loss of 15% of the blood volume. The maximum blood loss allowed before giving a blood transfusion is usually 20% of the estimated blood volume, however, in some animals up to 30% of the total blood volume may be lost without onset of hypotension or hypoxia if the patient has no major preanaesthetic illness, is ventilated with oxygen, the depth of anaesthesia is lightened, balanced electrolyte and colloid solutions are infused intravenously, and vasoactive drugs are administered as needed.

Monitoring the respiratory system

Visual observation of respiratory rate and depth of breathing is a basic estimate of adequacy of breathing. The respiratory rate may be counted by observation of chest movement or movement of the reservoir bag on the anaesthesia machine. The excursion of the chest, abdomen, or bag should be observed to gain an impression of the depth of breathing. In general, except possibly in horses, a spontaneous rate of 6 breaths/min or less is likely indicative of hypoventilation. Respiratory rates of 10 breaths/min or greater may provide adequate ventilation or be associated with hypoventilation when the breaths are shallow. Chest wall movement with no corresponding movement of the reservoir bag is indicative of airway obstruction or tension pneumothorax.

Rate monitors and apnoea alarms

Rate monitors and apnoea alarms may use a thermistor either connected to the endotracheal tube or placed in front of a dog's nose. The thermistor detects temperature differences between inspired and exhaled gases to produce a signal that drives a digital rate meter to make a noise which varies in intensity or pitch in time with the animal's breathing. An alarm sounds if a constant gas temperature is detected. Like the oesophageal stethoscope that counts only heart rate, the respiratory rate monitor registers rate only and not adequacy of ventilation.

Tidal and minute volume monitors

The volume of each breath (tidal volume) and the volume of gas inhaled or exhaled per minute (minute volume) can be measured in small animals by attaching a gas meter such as a Wright's respirometer within the circle circuit or to the endotracheal tube. The respirometer has a low resistance to breathing and is reasonably accurate over volumes ranging from 4 L/min to 15 L/min but under reads below 4 L/min.

Blood gas analysis

Measurement of the partial pressure of carbon dioxide in a sample of arterial blood ($PaCO_2$) using blood gas analysis is the best monitor of ventilation. Arterial blood may be collected from any peripheral artery used for invasive blood pressure measurement. Commonly for clinical patients, a small amount of 1 : 1000 heparin is drawn into a 3 mL plastic syringe using a 25 gauge needle and the plunger withdrawn to wash the inside of the syringe with heparin. Excess heparin is then squirted from the syringe leaving only syringe dead space filled with heparin and no bubbles. A larger volume of heparin will increase the acidity of the sample. A 2 mL sample of blood is collected from most dogs and 2–3 mL from horses (collecting the same volume for sequential samples). Individually packaged 1 mL syringes containing a dry lithium heparin pellet (to decrease dilution) can also be used (for example, Portex® Line Draw Arterial Blood Sampling Kit, Smiths Medical ASD, Inc., Keene, NH, USA). After removing the cap from the nozzle of the syringe, the plunger should be pushed fully forward before allowing the syringe to fill with blood. Larger plastic syringes containing lyophilized heparin are also commercially available.

Blood may be collected by percutaneous puncture or from a catheter. The contents of the catheter should be aspirated using a separate syringe before a sample of blood is collected for analysis. This mixture of saline and blood may be discarded or, if collected into a syringe containing some heparinized saline, can be returned into the animal through a venous catheter. The blood sample should be collected anaerobically slowly over several respiratory cycles and without aspirating any air bubbles. Excessive negative pressure should be avoided as oxygen can be extracted from the blood sample. After expressing a drop of blood and any bubbles from the needle, the syringe should be sealed either with a special cap or by inserting the tip of the needle into a rubber stopper. Leaving an air bubble in the syringe for any length of time allows diffusion of gases between the blood and bubble such that PCO_2 will decrease and PO_2 will decrease if the animal is breathing O_2 and increase if the animal is breathing air. The syringe should be inverted several times over 20 seconds to mix the blood with the heparin. The temperature of the animal should be measured at the time of sampling. Firm pressure should be applied to the artery for 3 minutes after percutaneous needle puncture to avoid haematoma formation.

Ideally, blood gas analysis should be performed immediately after blood collection into plastic syringes because there is a significant change in PO_2, an increase if PO_2 is 12 kPa (90 mmHg) and a decrease when the PO_2 is >33.3 kPa (>250 mmHg), due to diffusion of O_2 into or out of the syringe and metabolism in white blood cells and platelets that consumes O_2 and produces CO_2 (Beaulieu et al., 1999). Not all plastic syringes are the same, even those marketed specifically for blood gas analysis, and the magnitude of PO_2 change depends on the manufacturer and characteristics of the syringe (Wu et al., 1997). Investigations have discovered that the change in PO_2 over time is greater with a 3 mL syringe than a 5 mL syringe (Wu et al., 1997) and inaccuracy is greater when <1.8 mL is collected into a 3 mL syringe compared with >2 mL (Hedberg et al., 2009). Furthermore, accuracy of PO_2 measurement is related to the method of storage of the syringe before analysis, in iced water at 0°C or at ambient temperature of 20–25°C, and the time lapse between collection and analysis (Pretto & Rochford, 1994; Deane et al., 2004, Picandet et al., 2007). Iced water decreases the rate of metabolism in blood and the lower temperature promotes increased PO_2 by facilitating diffusion of O_2 from water into the plastic syringe through increased gas solubility and increased haemoglobin O_2 affinity (Wu et al., 1997). A significant change in PO_2 has been measured by 10 minutes after blood collection (Pretto & Rochford, 1994; Picandet et al., 2007). PCO_2 undergoes a clinically insignificant but statistically significant change. Picandet et al. (2007) suggested that although the PCO_2 appeared to be stable, the value may have been a balance between leakage of CO_2 out of the blood and increased CO_2 from metabolism. Values other than PO_2 may be relied upon from plastic syringes stored at room temperature up to 60 minutes. It has been suggested that blood from different species may require different handling but published data reveal differences in results even within the same species. Despite differences in findings between investigations, it appears that with an expected PO_2 of about 13.3 kPa (100 mmHg), the increase may be less if the plastic syringe is kept at room temperature until analysis (Deane et al., 2004; Picandet et al., 2007) whereas the decrease may be less in blood with a high PO_2 when the syringe is stored in a slurry of ice and water (Pretto & Rochford, 1994). Plastic syringes for blood gas analysis

43

have largely replaced use of glass syringes due to decreased cost and increased convenience. Glass syringes are non-disposable items that must be sterilized before use and not infrequently the plunger becomes immoveable or the glass breaks. However, when blood is collected into glass syringes and stored in an ice and water slurry at $0°C$, PO_2 and PCO_2 values are minimally changed for 90 minutes (Pretto & Rochford, 1994; Beaulieu et al., 1999; Deane et al., 2004; Picandet et al., 2007; Noël et al., 2010).

Plastic vacutainer tubes containing lyophilized heparin have been used to collect blood from conscious horses for blood gas and acid–base analysis. A detailed investigation of this practice revealed that PO_2 increases significantly, more than 6.65 kPa (50 mmHg) within 15 minutes, due to diffusion of O_2 through the wall of the tube with a greater change occurring when tubes are stored at $0°C$ than $22°C$ before analysis (Noël et al., 2010). The change in PCO_2 was less dramatic but statistically significant and was greater when the vacutainer is stored at $22°C$ than $0°C$. The calculated values of bicarbonate (HCO_3), total CO_2 (TCO_2), standard base excess (SBE) were minimally affected. The authors also noted that the design of the vacutainer tube does not allow collection of an anaerobic blood sample and concluded that plastic vacutainer tubes do not produce accurate results for PO_2 and PCO_2 but can be used when HCO_3, TCO_2 and SBE are the main interest, in which case the tubes should be stored at $0°C$ when analysis is delayed.

The blood sample is introduced into equipment incorporating electrodes measuring pH, PCO_2 and PO_2. The machine uses the measured values to compute HCO_3, TCO_2, SBE and oxygen saturation (SaO_2). The patient's temperature is entered into the blood gas analyser for appropriate adjustment of pH and PO_2. The patient's haemoglobin concentration must be known for an accurate measure of base excess. Fully automated pH and blood gas analysers are highly accurate but expensive. Portable and less expensive equipment is available, for example, STATPAL® (Sendx Medical Inc., Carlsbad, California, USA) and i-STAT® (Abbott Laboratories, Abbott Park, Illinois, USA), although the cost of individual analyses may be higher.

Hypercarbia, hypocarbia

Normal values for $PaCO_2$ in conscious unsedated animals are given in Table 2.4. Increased $PaCO_2$ (hypercarbia, hypercapnia) is a direct consequence of hypoventilation and commonly occurs during anaesthesia. An increase of 10 mmHg above normal is mild hypoventilation, an increase of 10–20 mmHg is moderate hypoventilation, and an increase >20 mmHg is severe hypoventilation. Thus, $PaCO_2$ values exceeding 8 kPa (60 mmHg) are indicative of severe respiratory depression. A decrease in $PaCO_2$ (hypocarbia) will occur with increased ventilation. A $PaCO_2$ less than 2.6 kPa (20 mmHg) causes cerebral vasoconstriction and cerebral hypoxia.

Table 2.4 Mean normal values for pH, $PaCO_2$, and PaO_2 in mature conscious unsedated animals

Species	pHa	$PaCO_2$	PaO_2	References
Dogs	7.40	4.67 (35)	13.6 (102)	Horwitz et al., 1969
	7.38	5.3 (40)	13.3 (100)	Haskins et al., 2005
Cats	7.34	4.5 (34)	13.3 (100)	Middleton et al., 1981
Horses	7.38	5.05-6.1 (38-46)	13.3 (100)	Steffey et al., 1987; Wagner et al., 1991; Wan et al., 1992
	7.41	4.8 (36)	12.2 (91)	Clarke et al., 1991; Tate et al., 1993
Cattle	7.40	5.28 (39)	11.8 (89)	Gallivan et al., 1989
Sheep	7.48	4.4 (33)	12.2 (92)	Wanner & Reinhart, 1978
Goats	7.45	5.45 (41)	12.6 (95)	Forster et al., 1981
Pigs	7.50	5.4 (41)	10.5 (79)	Hannon, 1983

Values for $PaCO_2$ and PaO_2 given as kPa (mmHg)

Hypercarbia in some anaesthetized dogs and cats during anaesthesia may be associated with tachycardia with or without increased blood pressure. In these animals, intermittent positive pressure ventilation (IPPV) will result in decreased heart rate within a few minutes. In other patients, hypercarbia may be associated with hypotension. Hypercarbia in horses during anaesthesia may also cause stimulation of the sympathetic nervous system, increased blood pressure and cardiac output (Wagner et al., 1990, Khanna et al., 1995). Adverse effects of hypercarbia are observed in some horses as tachycardia of 60–70 beats/min, or hypotension caused by decreased myocardial contractility. These abnormalities are corrected within 5–10 minutes of initiating IPPV. More frequently, the effects of hypoventilation during inhalation anaesthesia are manifested as an inadequate depth of anaesthesia despite a vaporizer setting that should provide a sufficient depth of anaesthesia. In these animals, controlled ventilation expands the lungs, thereby improving uptake of anaesthetic agent and resulting in increased depth of anaesthesia (Fig. 2.27).

Oxygenation

PaO_2 values are influenced by the inspired oxygen tension (PIO_2), adequacy of ventilation, cardiac output, and blood

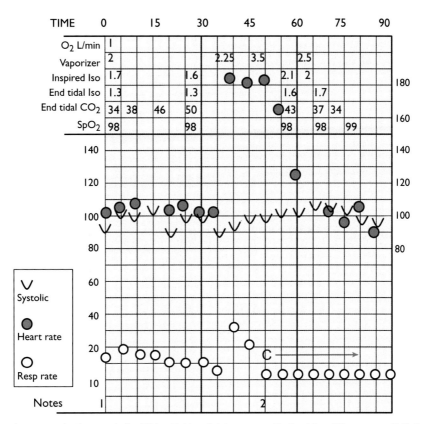

TIME	0		15		30		45		60		75		90
O$_2$ L/min	1												
Vaporizer	2						2.25	3.5		2.5			
Inspired Iso	1.7				1.6				2.1	2			
End tidal Iso	1.3				1.3					1.6	1.7		
End tidal CO$_2$	34	38	46		50				43		37	34	
SpO$_2$	98				98					98		98	99

Figure 2.27 Part of an anaesthetic record of a 32 kg Golden Retriever anaesthetized for stifle surgery. At Note 1 the dog was moved into the operating room. The increase in ETCO$_2$ from 34 to 50 mmHg (4.5 to 6.65 kPa) over the next 30 minutes indicated increasing hypoventilation. An abrupt increase in heart rate from 102 to 180 beats/min was presumed a response to increased surgical stimulation. Increasing the vaporizer setting to 3.5% was slow to change the circuit isoflurane concentration. Institution of controlled ventilation quickly increased the depth of anaesthesia (ET isoflurane concentration increased to 1.6%), decreasing heart rate. Subsequently the vaporizer setting could be decreased.

pressure. A PaO$_2$ of 12–14.6 kPa (90–110 mmHg) is normal in unsedated animals at sea level and PaO$_2$ values less than 8 kPa (60 mmHg) constitute hypoxaemia.

The maximum possible PaO$_2$ is governed by the inspired O$_2$ % and animals breathing oxygen may have PaO$_2$ values up to five times greater than when breathing air. The partial pressure of oxygen at the alveolar level (P$_A$O$_2$) can be calculated from the following formula:

$$PaO_2 = [(\text{barometric pressure} - P_{\text{water vapour}}) \times FIO_2] - (PaCO_2/0.8)$$

where the value for water vapour is 6.25 kPa (47 mmHg), FIO$_2$ is the fractional concentration of O$_2$ in inspired gas, and 0.8 is the respiratory exchange ratio. Values for PaO$_2$ greater than 53.2 kPa (400 mmHg) are expected in healthy dogs and cats breathing oxygen. Horses and ruminants are subject to lung collapse during recumbency and anaesthesia and, consequently, ventilation and perfusion are mismatched within the lung, resulting in a lower PaO$_2$ in some individuals.

Hypoxaemia may develop in dogs and cats during anaesthesia or recovery as a result of hypoventilation when breathing air. This situation is most likely to occur in old animals, animals with hypotension, pneumothorax, pulmonary disease, CNS depression from metabolic disease, or after administration of opioids. Hypoxaemia may also develop during general anaesthesia as a result of severe lung collapse. Patients at greatest risk are small animals during thoracotomy or repair of a ruptured diaphragm, foals with pneumonia and horses with abdominal distension from pregnancy or colic. Hypoxaemia may be suspected but is not always obvious as the mucous membranes may be less pink than desired but not cyanotic.

Oxygen content

Oxygen delivery to tissues is dependent on tissue blood flow and arterial blood oxygen content (CaO$_2$). Oxygen content comprises O_2 carried by haemoglobin (Hb) and a small amount of dissolved O_2. The formula for calculating CaO_2 shows that the Hb concentration of the blood, the Hb oxygen affinity and the PO_2 are important determinants of O_2 content:

$$CaO_2 \text{ mL/dL} = [\text{total Hb} - (\text{COHb} + \text{metHb})] \times SaO_2 \\ \times 1.39 + PaO_2 \times 0.003$$

where SaO_2 (oxygen saturation) is a decimal fraction of 1, Hb concentration in g/dL, and 1.39 mL/g is the volume of O_2 in mL that can be bound to 1 g of human Hb. The number 1.31 or 1.34 is often substituted for 1.39 as being a practical rather than theoretical value. Correct calculation of SaO_2 should refer to the ratio of oxyhaemoglobin (O_2Hb) to active Hb (O_2Hb + deoxyhaemoglobin, HHb). Inactive Hb has lost the ability to bind O_2 and this most commonly refers to carboxyhaemoglobin (COHb) and methaemoglobin (metHb) (Toffaletti & Zijlstra, 2007). Most gas analysers calculate saturation from PO_2 by computer and do not actually measure saturation. When the total Hb value is used in the formula (as with blood gas analyser results) measured values for SaO_2 may be accurate in most anaesthetized patients because their quantities of COHb and metHb are small. For accuracy, the different forms of Hb must be measured by an automated multiwavelength spectrophotometer commonly referred to as a cooximeter. Critical care management may include animals exposed to carbon monoxide poisoning or animals with methaemoglobinaemia from acetominophen or benzocaine toxicity, for example. Carbon monoxide displaces O_2 from Hb with an affinity approximately 300× that of Hb affinity for O_2. Animals with carbon monoxide poisoning do not have decreased PO_2 so that, unless the different forms of Hb are measured, the decrease in blood O_2 content may not be realized. A value for O_2 saturation obtained from a pulse oximeter (SpO_2) will not be decreased in these patients because the wavelengths used by the monitors are not sensitive to COHb as a consequence of COHb absorbing as much light at 660 nm as does O_2Hb. A patient with increased concentration of metHb would be reported as having an abnormally low SpO_2. MetHb absorbance is high at both wavelengths used by pulse oximeters and the resultant effect is to decrease SpO_2 down to 85% regardless of the PaO_2 and SaO_2 values (Tremper & Barker, 1990).

Oxygen affinity

The O_2 affinity of blood is usually described by the oxygen dissociation curve (ODC) at standard values of pH = 7.40, pCO_2 = 5.33 kPa (40 mmHg), and temperature of 37°C (Fig. 2. 28). The relationship between PaO_2 and SaO_2 is not linear because Hb changes its affinity for O_2 at increasing levels of saturation. Several factors cause the normal ODC to shift to the right or left along the x-axis, for example, an increase in PCO_2, decrease in pH, increase

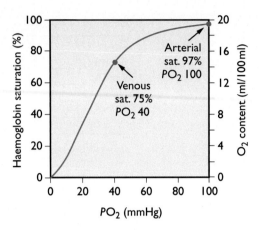

Figure 2.28 Graph depicting the relationship between PaO_2, haemoglobin oxygen saturation SaO_2, and oxygen content in humans.

in temperature, and increased concentration of 2,3-diphosphoglycerate (DPG) in the red cells will produce a shift to the right, and vice versa. Comparison of O_2 dissociation curves is possible by using the P_{50} value that is the PO_2 required for 50% Hb saturation.

The haemoglobin O_2 affinity varies between species. Human Hb P_{50} is 3.5 kPa (26.3 mmHg) (Lumb, 2000; Toffaletti & Zijlstra, 2007). The canine ODC is similar to human with a range of P_{50} reported as 3.5–4.2 kPa (26–31.5 mmHg), however, the small difference may result in small errors in measurement of canine PO_2 produced by a blood gas analyser using human P_{50} (Scott et al., 2005). Bovine, equine, and camelid ODC have lower P_{50} values indicating higher O_2 affinity. Thus, the llama ODC, P_{50} 3.3 kPa (24.6 mmHg), is to the left of sheep such that the O_2 content of llama blood at a PO_2 of 6.7 kPa (50 mmHg) is similar to that of a PO_2 of 8 kPa (60 mmHg) in sheep (Moraga et al., 1996). Fetal ODC is shifted to the left of the maternal curve so that the Hb is adapted to operate at lower PO_2 levels present in the fetus. Fetal Hb concentrations are significantly higher than maternal in both llama and sheep, increasing O_2 content, and the camelid placenta is very thin compared with others, facilitating O_2 diffusion (Moraga et al., 1996). In animals genetically adapted to high altitude, the left shift of the ODC improves oxygenation of arterial blood that outweighs the decrease in offloading of O_2 at the tissues.

The high O_2 affinity and increased Hb concentration in llamas are not different whether the animals are at high or low altitude, a similarity shared with guinea pigs that are also considered to be genetically adapted to high altitude (Pairet & Jaenicke, 2010). The high blood-O_2 affinity in camelids (llama, vicuna, alpaca, guanaco) is partly due to amino acid substitutions in the Hb molecule that reduce the DPG effect and resists shift of the ODC to the right (Weber, 2007). Thus, although the intrinsic O_2 affinity of llama Hb is lower than camel (lowland species), the effect on DPG binding results in greater O_2 affinity. Vicunas have a different amino acid substitution on Hb that affects Cl binding and increases Hb O_2 affinity in vicuna over llama.

Reduced P_{50} is critical for maintenance of arterial oxygenation in animals at high altitude. Thus, factors that oppose that state and cause the ODC to shift to the right, such as hypoventilation and decreased pH, oppose this effect and are deleterious to tissue oxygen delivery (Winslow, 2007). Where O_2 extraction is high, as in exercise, hyperventilation, increased cardiac output, and vasodilation are important for maintaining tissue oxygenation.

High altitude human residents do not have Hb genetically adapted to high altitude but a variety of other physiological adaptations that include increased Hb concentration, hyperventilation, blunted response of the chemoreceptors to hypoxia, and higher catecholamine levels (Hainsworth & Drinkhill, 2007). Hyperventilation to a $PaCO_2$ 3.3 kPa (25 mmHg) is normal at high altitude and the alkalinization further improves O_2 loading in the lungs. The reduction in O_2 release to tissues is partly offset by a more efficient O_2 extraction in the tissues by mechanisms including an increase in tissue capillarization.

Mixed venous, central venous, and venous PO₂

Mixed venous PO_2 ($PmvO_2$) is obtained from a blood sample collected from the pulmonary artery after placement of a cardiac catheter. The information obtained is interpreted based on the fact that $PmvO_2$ is representative of total body O_2 extraction. Factors that influence $PmvO_2$ are: (1) arterial O_2 content (CaO_2); (2) cardiac output; (3) distribution of peripheral blood flow; and (4) tissue O_2 extraction. Decreases in the first three factors or an increase in the fourth will cause decreased $PmvO_2$. O_2 saturation of pulmonary artery blood is generally around 70–75%. A decrease in $SmvO_2$ to less than 65% is significant and indicates an abnormality in the patient, whereas a decrease to 50% is significantly low. Small variations in $PmvO_2$ exert little influence on PaO_2. As the $PmvO_2$ decreases further, extraction of oxygen from alveolar gas is increased decreasing PaO_2, especially in patients with compromised ventilation such as hypoventilation or ventilation–perfusion mismatches. Conditions lowering $PmvO_2$ are low cardiac output and hypotension or increased oxygen extraction created by sepsis and postoperative shivering, although the opposite effect may occur when sepsis results in impaired tissue oxygen extraction. An abrupt decrease in $PmvO_2$ may occur following a sudden decrease in cardiac output, decreased venous return, for example, following repositioning, and increased O_2 consumption during muscle movement. $PmvO_2$ may be higher than normal in animals in which endotoxaemia has induced a hyperdynamic circulation with increased cardiac output.

Central venous O_2 saturation measurement ($ScvO_2$) may be used as a surrogate for $SmvO_2$. For greatest accuracy, $ScvO_2$ should be measured from blood collected from the tip of a central venous catheter placed close to, or within, the right atrium (Walley, 2010). The site of sampling is important because sampling from the tip of a catheter some distance away from the right atrium produces inaccurate results when compared to $SmvO_2$.

Peripheral venous blood collected from the cephalic, femoral, or jugular veins is not comprised of blood from major organs and cannot be used to evaluate tissue oxygen extraction but may be used as a screening method for arterial pH and PCO_2.

Measurement of pH and blood gases in lingual venous blood from healthy normotensive, anaesthetized dogs slightly overestimated arterial pH and overestimated PCO_2 and base excess when compared to values measured in arterial blood (Pang et al., 2009). The differences were not large and unlikely to significantly alter therapeutic management. Most of the lingual PO_2 values were excessively lower than PaO_2 values particularly during administration of medetomidine. Significant differences were obtained when comparing mean values for jugular venous and arterial pH and PCO_2. The ranges of values for both parameters from all three sampling sites were almost identical.

Pulse oximetry

Pulse oximetry is a non-invasive method of continuously measuring haemoglobin oxygen saturation (SpO_2). The abbreviation SpO_2 is used to identify the method of measurement of SaO_2. The pulse oximeter sensor consists of light-emitting diodes (LEDs) that emit light in the red (660 nm) and infrared (940 nm) wavelengths and a photodetector that measures the amount of light that has been transmitted through tissues (Tremper & Barker, 1990). The principles of measurement are based on the different light absorption spectra of oxyhaemoglobin and reduced haemoglobin, and the detection of a pulsatile signal. Pulse oximeters are available as single parameter monitors or in combination, for example, pulse oximetry and NIBP or pulse oximetry and capnography.

Pulse oximeters display a digital record of saturation and pulse rate, with an audible beep, and some monitors display the oxygen saturation waveform (Fig. 2.29). A limit for acceptable saturation can be entered into the monitor, allowing an alarm to sound when lower values are sensed. The pulse rate displayed on the oximeter must correspond to the rate obtained by palpation or ECG, and the sensor should be in position for at least 30 seconds before the measurement can be assumed to be accurate. The shape of the sensor, thickness of tissue placed within the sensor, the presence of pigment and hair, and movement of the patient, can be responsible for the oximeter failing to measure oxygen saturation. Ambient light may interfere with probe function and covering it with gauze may produce a reading. It may be impossible to obtain a

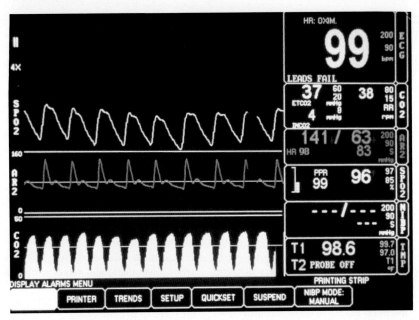

Figure 2.29 Multiparameter monitor displays haemoglobin oxygen saturation (SpO2) waveform and value (96%), arterial blood pressure (systolic 141 mmHg, diastolic 63 mmHg, mean 83 mmHg), and CO2 waveform and values (inspired 4 mmHg (0.5 kPa), end-tidal 37 mmHg (4.9 kPa), respiratory rate 38 breaths/minute), and temperature of 98.6°F in an anaesthetized dog (Advisor®, Surgivet™, Smiths Medical PM, Inc., Norwell, MA, USA). Heart rate of 99 beats/minute is obtained from pulse oximeter and blood pressure. ECG and NIBP are not connected.

reading from a pulse oximeter when peripheral vasoconstriction is severe, for example, after administration of medetomidine in dogs or patients in circulatory shock. The pulse oximeter will not accurately reflect blood O_2 content in patients with carbon monoxide or methaemoglobin poisoning (see earlier). Oxygen delivery to tissues may be compromised by low blood O_2 content, cardiac output, or blood flow. Thus a patient with low Hb concentration may display normal values for SpO_2 and yet suffer tissue hypoxia. Anaesthetic management of anaemic patients should, therefore, include administration of supplemental inspired O_2 and cardiovascular support.

Pulse oximetry saves lives by detecting desaturation before clinically apparent. SpO_2 >90% does not guarantee adequate oxygenation of tissues

A pulse oximeter detects inadequate blood oxygenation, which should be taken as an indication to supplement the animal's inspired oxygen concentration and to search for the cause. Hypoxaemia is defined as PaO_2 of 8 kPa (60 mmHg) or SaO_2 ≤90% (Table 2.5). A pulse oximeter is a valuable monitor for use on all anaesthetized animals and specifically for animals anaesthetized with injectable anaesthetic agents and breathing air, or during inhalation anaesthesia in patients with pulmonary disease or

Table 2.5 Relationship between PaO_2 and haemoglobin saturation in humans

PaO_2		SaO_2	Interpretation
kPa	mmHg	%	
≥13.3	≥100	100	Oxygenated
10.6	80	94	
9.3	70	92	
8.0	60	90	Hypoxaemia
6.7	50	80	
5.3	40	70	Venous

traumatic pulmonary contusions or pneumothorax, and during thoracotomy or major surgery in the cranial abdomen. It is also important to keep track of oxygenation in animals during recovery from anaesthesia, in patients with partial airway obstruction, or when ventilation is depressed or impaired by systemic opioid administration or residual pneumothorax after thoracotomy or ruptured diaphragm repair.

The pulse oximeter is particularly valuable because it provides an immediate monitor of decreased oxygen saturation, so that corrective treatment can be initiated before respiratory or cardiovascular failure develops. Use of pulse oximetry is associated with reduction in odds of anaesthetic-related death (Brodbelt, 2009). Evaluation of the patient should take into account the fact that the pulse oximeter does not measure CO_2 concentration or blood pressure and may continue to read satisfactorily in the presence of hypotension. However, it can provide a warning of a severe decrease in tissue blood flow caused by hypotension or decreased cardiac output by abruptly failing to obtain a signal. Loss of signal may also occur spontaneously with no change in the patient's condition due to local blood vessel compression and measurement is restored by changing the position of the probe. Compression of the base of the tongue between the endotracheal tube and the jaw may decrease blood flow and signal acquisition from a probe clipped to the tongue.

Although pulse oximetry saves lives by identifying low SpO_2 before desaturation is clinically apparent, it must be realized that the number observed on the pulse oximeter is not always accurate and that different results may be obtained from different probe types, different sites on the body, different models, and different species of animals. Most models are reasonably accurate for saturations >90% but for some models that consistently overestimate SaO_2 (Dolphin Voyager in dogs), a higher threshold of 93% has been suggested (Burns et al., 2006).

Different body sites in dogs have been evaluated for accuracy of measurement of SaO_2. In one investigation, a multisite clip probe placed on the lip, tongue, toe web, and the tip of the tail gave accurate and reliable estimations of SaO_2 values during conditions of full haemoglobin saturation and moderate haemoglobin desaturation (92%) (Huss et al., 1995). In this study, the human finger probe was accurate only when placed on the dog's lip and when haemoglobin saturation was complete. The lip was found to be the best site in conscious animals. Another study of conscious dogs in an intensive care unit found that a circumferential pulse oximeter probe around a digit or the metatarsus produced excellent correlations between pulse oximeter and SaO_2 values (Fairman, 1993). An evaluation of the Ohmeda Biox 3700 with a human ear probe applied to the tongue provided an accurate evaluation of SaO_2 (Jacobsen et al., 1992). The pulse oximeter underestimated SaO_2 at higher saturations and overestimated SaO_2 at saturations <70%. However, as the authors pointed out, detection of hypoxaemia is more important than measurement of the exact degree of hypoxaemia. One evaluation of four Nellcor models and the Surgivet V3304 with the probe applied at five sites in anaesthetized dogs and cats achieved arterial saturations of 98%, 85%, and 72% by varying inspired O_2 % (Matthews et al., 2003). SpO_2 measurements were reasonably accurate at SaO_2 >90%. The study revealed in dogs that measurements

obtained from the lip and ear were less accurate and, although all sites in the cats had low correlation, the hind paw was the most accurate. Failure to achieve readings was most frequent with the Surgivet V3304.

Different monitors, types of sensors, and alternative sites for measurement have been evaluated in horses (Whitehair et al., 1990; Chaffin et al., 1996; Matthews et al., 2003). The Ohmeda Biox 3700 pulse oximeter and the Physio-Control Lifestat 1600 pulse oximeter were evaluated in mature horses using the human ear lobe probe (Whitehair et al., 1990). Measurements were obtained from the tongue and the ear, with the most accurate measurements obtained from the tongue; the oximeters failed to detect a pulse at the nostril, lip, or vulva. The results revealed that both oximeters tended to underestimate saturation by 3.7%, with 95% of the oxygen saturation values within 1% above or 8% below SaO_2 (Whitehair et al., 1990). The Nellcor N-200 pulse oximeter was evaluated in anaesthetized foals using a fingertip probe (Durasensor DS-100A) (Chaffin et al., 1996). Attachment of the probe to the tongue or ear of the foals slightly underestimated SaO_2 within the range of 80–100% saturation. Evaluation of four Nellcor models and the Surgivet V3304 in anaesthetized horses with the probe on the tongue lip, ear, nostril and prepuce or vulva found that correlations between SpO_2 and SaO_2 were fairly high at all sites except the ear (Matthews et al., 2003). All monitors except the Nellcor NPB-290 failed to produce readings at some times, with the V3304 failing 60% of the times.

Reflectance pulse oximeters detect changes in absorption of light reflected from tissues, rather than transmitted through tissues as just described (Watney et al., 1993; Chaffin et al., 1996). Attachment of a reflectance probe designed for the human forehead to the ventral surface of the base of the tail in foals had 100% sensitivity for detecting SaO_2 <90% but consistently underestimated the actual value (Chaffin et al., 1996). Therefore, this probe site combination will incorrectly identify some foals as being hypoxaemic.

Capnography

Capnography indirectly estimates $PaCO_2$ by measuring the concentration of CO_2 in expired gas. Capnography is also useful for diagnosis of mechanical problems in anaesthetic circuits, airway obstruction, and cardiogenic shock. There are two types of gas sampling. Sidestream sampling is when gas is aspirated from an adapter inserted between the endotracheal tube and anaesthetic circuit (Matthews et al., 1990) and delivered to the capnometer (see Figs. 2.5, 2.29, 2.30). Gases leaving the analyser should be directed back into the anaesthetic circuit or into the scavenging system. Mainstream gas sampling occurs when the measuring device is placed between the endotracheal tube and delivery circuit (Fig. 2.31). Measurement of CO_2 directly exhaled from the patient provides more accurate

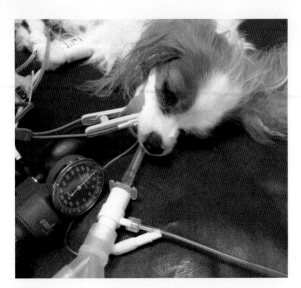

Figure 2.30 Gases are aspirated from a T-adapter inserted between the endotracheal tube and the delivery circuit, and the capnogram and end-tidal CO_2 are displayed on a monitor distant from the patient. Also attached to this dog is a pulse oximeter probe on the tongue and blood pressure cuff and Doppler probe on a forelimb.

measurement in patients with small tidal volumes or for non-rebreathing circuits where alveolar gas is diluted by the fresh gas flow. The CO_2 concentration is measured by infrared absorption and the capnometer provides breath-by-breath numerical values for CO_2 concentration and usually a CO_2 waveform (capnograph). The upward slope of the waveform represents expiration and the highest value is the end-tidal CO_2 ($ETCO_2$). The downward slope occurs during inspiration and the inspiratory baseline should be zero (Fig. 2.32). An increase in baseline to 0.5 kPa (4 mmHg) will occur with rebreathing due to an increase in apparatus dead space, such as the endotracheal tube extending beyond the incisors and inclusion of the sampling adaptor and a humidity and moisture exchanger (see Fig. 2.29). This degree of rebreathing is not significant to the patient. A greater increase in baseline to 1.3-1.9 kPa (10-14 mmHg) indicates equipment malfunction, such as a unidirectional valve on a circle circuit stuck in the open or closed position, exhaustion of CO_2 absorbent, incorrect assembly of a non-rebreathing circuit, or disconnection of a coaxial circuit (Fig. 2.33A). Respiratory rate may increase, sometimes panting in dogs, despite eye signs indicating adequate depth of anaesthesia. Signs of sympathetic stimulation from hypercarbia such as tachycardia and increased blood pressure may be present.

Falsely low measurements of $ETCO_2$ using side-stream sampling may occur with the use of non-rebreathing circuits, because the high gas flow results in dilution of expired gases, and in animals with very small tidal

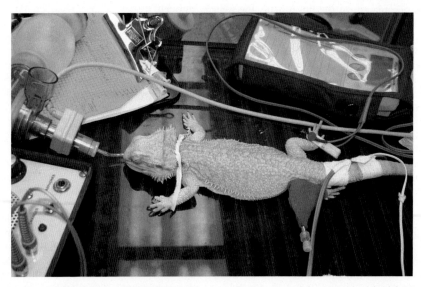

Figure 2.31 A CO_2 sensor inserted next to the endotracheal tube will more accurately measure end-tidal CO_2 in animals with small tidal volumes (Tidal Wave™, Novametrix, Wallingford, CT, USA). Other monitors on this Bearded Dragon are a pulse oximeter probe on a foot, Doppler probe on the ventral surface of the tail over the coccygeal artery and a cloacal temperature probe. After induction of anaesthesia an intraosseous needle was inserted in a femur for fluid therapy and drug administration. The patient is lying on a heated pad.

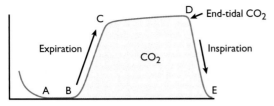

Figure 2.32 Schematic diagram of a capnogram. AB = Initial expiration (dead space), BC = expiration, CD = alveolar gas plateau, D = end-tidal CO_2 value, DE = inspiration.

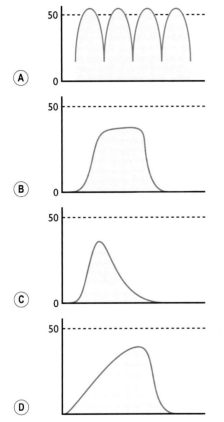

Figure 2.33 Interpretation of capnograms. (A). Dog is panting and inspiratory CO_2 is 14 mmHg indicating significant rebreathing. (B) Normal appearance of an $ETCO_2$ waveform during controlled ventilation. (C) Inspiratory waveform is sloping indicating a leak during inspiration, dilution with fresh gas during a long pause between breaths, or prolonged inspiration. (D) Waveform has a sloping expiration indicating partial airway obstruction or impaired lung deflation y-axis = 0-50 mmHg (0-6.65 kPa).

Table 2.6 Troubleshooting the capnogram

Unexpectedly low ETCO₂

Cardiac arrest
Significant decrease in cardiac output
Abrupt onset hypotension
Air embolism
Pulmonary embolism
Sampling line disconnected or broken
Endotracheal tube cuff deflated
Tidal volume too small

Absent ETCO₂

Apnoea
Endotracheal tube disconnect
Airway obstruction
Oesophageal intubation

Failure to read zero on inspiration (rebreathing)

Large apparatus dead space
Expiratory valve in circle stuck open or closed
Exhausted CO_2 absorbent
In and out tubes of NRB attached backwards
NRB circuit assembled incorrectly
Breathing rapid and shallow

Prolonged inspiratory or expiratory slope

Gas sampling rate too low
Partial airway obstruction
Leak around endotracheal tube cuff
Bronchoconstriction
Obstruction or crack in the sampling line

NRB = non-rebreathing circuit

volumes, breathing slowly, or that are panting. Falsely low CO_2 measurements will be obtained in animals that are ventilating with small tidal volumes, or in small animals that have significant lung collapse such as diaphragmatic hernia or thoroscopy, and during spontaneous ventilation in large animals. Bumps and dips in the expiratory plateau may be caused by spontaneous respiratory efforts, heartbeats, and movements of the animal by the surgeon (Fig. 2.34).

Measurement of high $ETCO_2$ confirms respiratory acidosis. $PaCO_2$ can be high when $ETCO_2$ is normal or low. CO_2 waveform is essential aid for alerting and troubleshooting abnormalities.

Changes in $ETCO_2$ or waveform are useful indicators of significant alteration in physiological status or equipment malfunction (Table 2.6, see Fig. 2.33). A sudden decrease in $ETCO_2$ to 1.6-2.7 kPa (12-20 mmHg) is cause for concern and the patient should be checked for hypotension or cardiac arrest. Absence of CO_2 may indicate equipment leaks and disconnection, pulmonary embolism or air embolism. Detection of CO_2 >5 mmHg immediately after endotracheal intubation may rule out accidental oesophageal intubation. Exhaled water vapour condenses

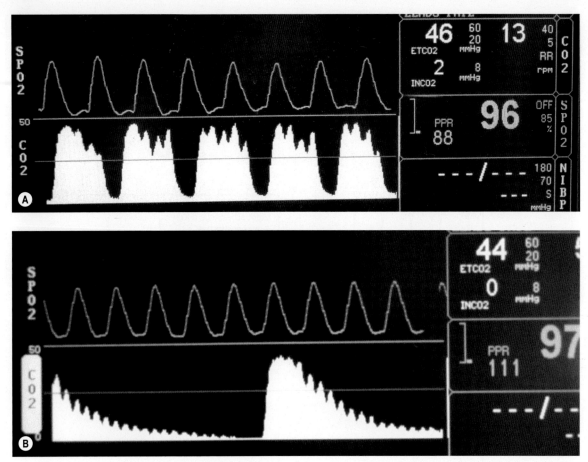

Figure 2.34 Cardiac oscillations are seen as regular small dips in the CO_2 waveform generated by heartbeats causing small air movements within the airways. (A) Dog is breathing 13/minute with an end-tidal CO_2 concentration of 46 mmHg (6.1 kPa) indicating mild hypoventilation. (B) Dog is breathing only 5/minute with the same degree of hypoventilation. In both patients, inspired CO_2 of 0–2 mmHg is normal.

in the sampling tubing and water trap but unpredictable and bizarre values are obtained when water enters the monitor.

Abrupt decrease ETCO$_2$ to 1.6-2.7 kPa (12-20 mmHg) occurs with decreased cardiac output or cardiac arrest.

Significant correlation between $ETCO_2$ and $PaCO_2$ has been recorded in dogs and horses, with the $PaCO_2$ exceeding the $ETCO_2$ by 1.00–4.65 kPa (1–35 mmHg) depending on the degree of pulmonary shunting and lung collapse. The difference between $PaCO_2$ and $ETCO_2$ is usually less in dogs than in horses. In a group of mechanically ventilated dogs in intensive care, the $ETCO_2$ was on average 0.67 kPa (5 mmHg) less than $PaCO_2$ (Hendricks & King, 1994). In anaesthetized healthy mature horses, an average difference of 1.6 kPa (12 mmHg), range 0–4.3 kPa (0–32 mmHg) was recorded during halothane and 1.9 kPa

(14 mmHg) during isoflurane anaesthesia (Meyer & Short, 1985; Cribb, 1988; Moens, 1989). In one study of 110 horses, the $PaCO_2$–$ETCO_2$ difference was greater in heavier horses and was increased when horses were in dorsal recumbency compared with lateral recumbency (Moens, 1989). Institution of controlled ventilation from the start of anaesthesia in horses may preserve the $PaCO_2$–$ETCO_2$ difference to less than 10 mmHg. A mean $PaCO_2$–$ETCO_2$ difference of 1.8 ± 0.9 kPa (13.4 ± 6.9 mmHg; range 0–37.5 mmHg) was measured in 125 horses anaesthetized with isoflurane in dorsal recumbency for colic surgery (Trim, 1998). Spontaneously breathing foals anaesthetized with isoflurane had a mean $PaCO_2$–$ETCO_2$ difference in the first hour of anaesthesia of 0.9 kPa (7 mmHg) which increased over 90 minutes of anaesthesia to 1.7 kPa (13 mmHg), coincident with an increase in $PaCO_2$ (Geiser & Rohrbach, 1992). This study emphasized

the limitations of capnometry in spontaneously breathing anaesthetized foals.

In conditions in which hypoventilation is expected and the $ETCO_2$ value is normal or low, for example in dogs with pulmonary disease or during thoracotomy, and anaesthetized horses at risk for severe lung collapse, such as colic patients or foals, one direct measurement of $PaCO_2$ by blood gas analysis is advisable, if available. $ETCO_2$ values exceeding 6.7 kPa (50 mmHg) represent increased $PaCO_2$ and significant hypoventilation. The $ETCO_2$ value at which controlled ventilation is recommended varies between clinicians and is also dependent on the patient's disease or procedure.

Transcutaneous CO_2 analysis

Carbon dioxide diffuses through tissues and can be detected by a sensor on the skin. Transcutaneous capnometry is proposed as a non-invasive method of detecting respiratory depression in patients after anaesthesia and surgery and in the ICU. The transcutaneous CO_2 ($TcPCO_2$) sensor is warmed electrically and creates a local hyperaemia resulting in a measurement that is usually slightly higher than $PaCO_2$ (Eberhard, 2007). Published investigations in human patients have cited conflicting results, with some studies confirming good correlation between $TcPCO_2$ and $PaCO_2$ and others significant bias and limits of agreement with a low degree of correlation. Studies are needed to determine the value of this monitor in veterinary medicine.

Acid–base analysis

Maintaining blood pH within a normal range is important for adequate cellular function. The most dominant buffer system is the bicarbonate $[HCO_3^-]$/carbonic acid, a relationship that is described by the Henderson–Hasselbalch equation where the ratio of $[HCO_3^-]$ to dissolved CO_2 is 20:1

$$pH = 6.1 + \log[HCO_3^-]/(PaCO_2 \times 0.03)$$

HCO_3^- is an important buffer because it is volatile, being eliminated or retained as CO_2 in the lungs, and is effective at a range of pH values. As a primary acid–base abnormality develops there is a physiological compensation in the opposite direction. Thus, when acid is added to the system, it combines with HCO_3 generating CO_2 that can be eliminated through the lungs. In contrast, added base combines with carbonic acid (H_2CO_3) generating HCO_3^- that can be eliminated via the kidneys. Respiratory compensation may occur within hours but renal compensation takes days. Other important buffers include proteins and haemoglobin. When interpreting acid–base status in an anaesthetized animal, it should be remembered that anaesthetic agents depress respiration such that

the compensatory respiratory response is eliminated. Thus a patient may have normal acid–base status, respiratory acidosis or alkalosis, metabolic acidosis or alkalosis, or a mixture of two or three respiratory and metabolic components.

Acid–base analysis is underpinned by complex mathematical formulae (Wooten, 2010). The following information is a simplified and abbreviated version for clinical evaluation.

Blood gas and acid-base values

pH: The normal arterial pH of humans is 7.40. A pH <7.35 is referred to as an acidaemia and a pH >7.45 as an alkalaemia. Blood pH of some other species differs slightly from pH 7.40 and clinical assessment must take into account the normal range of values for that species (see Table 2.4).

$PaCO_2$: This value is representative of the rate and depth of breathing and metabolic CO_2 production. The normal average value for $PaCO_2$ is 5.3 kPa (40 mmHg) in most species, except cats where pCO_2 is lower. Venous blood PCO_2 will be approximately 0.8 kPa (6 mmHg) higher than $PaCO_2$. An increase in $PaCO_2$ (hypercarbia, hypercapnia) results in a decrease in pH and is most frequently due to hypoventilation. A decrease in $PaCO_2$ results in increased pH and is due to increased ventilation.

HCO_3^-: This value as reported by an automated blood gas analyser is calculated from pH and PCO_2, thus it is representative of both respiratory and metabolic status. For example, a high $[HCO_3^-]$ may be due to metabolic alkalosis or to a severe respiratory acidosis.

TCO_2: Total CO_2 (TCO_2) is also representative of both respiratory and metabolic status as it includes $[HCO_3^-]$ and dissolved CO_2, although the contribution by dissolved CO_2 is small (PCO_2 mmHg × 0.003 mEq/L). Sometimes chemical determination of TCO_2 in serum or plasma is used as an estimate of blood bicarbonate concentration, however, results obtained from biochemical autoanalysers may be significantly different from that obtained by calculation from pH and PCO_2. Errors arise from differences in handling the samples, such as exposure to air, underfilling of blood collection tubes, delay in analysis, and renewing reagents. A combination of these factors may decrease the TCO_2 by as much as 5.3 mEq/L in canine blood and 4.6 mEq/L in feline blood.

Base excess (BE): The BE value describes the buffering capacity (bicarbonate and haemoglobin) of the blood and provides a calculated assessment of the metabolic status of the patient that is almost independent of respiratory changes. There are a variety of formulae used to calculate BE and automated blood gas analysers compute BE. The value of BE describes the amount of acid or base (mEq/L) that must be added *in vitro* to return the blood to pH 7.40 under standard conditions of PCO_2 5.3 kPa (40 mmHg), and temperature 37°C. Consequently, BE of zero is neither acidotic nor alkalotic, positive BE describes a metabolic alkalosis and negative BE (base deficit) describes a metabolic acidosis. Standard BE (SBE, also called BE_{ecf}) is the BE value when haemoglobin is at 5 g/dL to represent more clearly the BE of the entire extracellular fluid *in vivo*.

SBE can indicate the presence of a metabolic acidosis or alkalosis but may be misleading in cases of mixed acid–base abnormalities. It also does not provide information about the cause(s) of the metabolic abnormalities. A corrected formula for SBE (SBEc) can be applied that includes values for albumin and phosphate (PO_4) (Kellum, 2005).

$$SBEc = (HCO_3^- - 24.4) + ([8.3 \times \text{Albumin g/dL}] \times 0.15] + [0.29 \times \text{Phosphate mg/dL} \times 0.32]) \times (pH - 7.4).$$

In humans,

Normal SBE of 0 (range, ± 2.5 mEq/L) is used for human patients, however, normal values differ between species (Table 2.7). Since metabolic status is influenced by diet, in general, species that are carnivores usually have a mild metabolic acidosis, whereas metabolic alkalosis is normal in species that are herbivores, as determined by blood gas analysers using reference values for human blood. The SBE of venous blood can be used to evaluate

acid–base status because the difference between arterial and venous PCO_2 is small.

Acid–base charts (Siggaard–Andersen) and a PO_2 – PCO_2 diagram are available for easy interpretation of blood gas analyses at sea-level and at high altitude (Paulev & Zubieta-Calleja, 2005).

Anion gap (AG): The AG is calculated from measured serum cations and anions as follows:

$$AG = (Na^+ + K^+) - (Cl^- + HCO_3^-)$$

The gap is mainly due to weak acids, primarily albumin and some PO_4, and a minor part due to strong ions, such as lactate and sulphate (SO_4). Plasma proteins other than albumin can be positive or negative but the final composition is generally neutral. AG may or may not be helpful because it can be normal in the face of opposing metabolic abnormalities. A change in [Na^+] without concurrent change in [Cl^-], and vice versa, will alter the AG. Dehydration can widen the gap by increasing the concentrations of the measured ions and hypoalbuminaemia decreases the anion gap. Changes in albumin and PO_4 commonly occur in critically ill patients and must be considered when interpreting AG (Kellum, 2007; Fidkowski & Helstrom, 2009). A corrected formula for AG (AGc) is used for human patients with metabolic acidosis (Kellum, 2005, 2007):

$$AGc = ([Na^+ + K^+] - [Cl^- + HCO_3^-]) - (2[\text{albumin in g/dL}] + 0.5[\text{phosphate in mg/dL}]) - \text{lactate}$$

or

$$AGc = ([Na^+ + K^+] - [Cl^- + HCO_3^-]) - (2[\text{albumin in g/dL}] + 1.5[\text{phosphate in mmol/L}]) - \text{lactate}$$

Using these formulae, AGc should be approximately zero.

Strong ion difference (SID): SID is defined as the difference between the sum of the strong cations (Na^+, K^+, Ca^{2+}, and Mg^{2+}) and the sum of the strong anions (Cl^- and lactate). Ionized concentrations of Mg and Ca are used in the formula but are sometimes omitted for simplicity. The apparent SID is defined as:

$$SIDa = (Na^+ + K^+ + Ca^{2+} + Mg^{2+}) - (Cl^- + \text{lactate})$$

An increase in SID is the result of metabolic alkalosis and a decrease in SID the result of a metabolic acidosis. Changes in SID not attributable to sodium or chloride fall into a category called unidentified ions (UA) that includes substances such as ketoacids. Strong ion difference effective (SIDe) is calculated from a formula that includes

Table 2.7 Reference ranges for acid–base and biochemical parameters

Parameter	Dogs	Cats	Horses
HCO_3^- (mEq/L)	22.2 (18.8–25.6)	18 (14.4–21.6)	24–30
SBE (mEq/L)	−1.8 (−0.2–+3.4) −2.1 ± 2.3	−6 ± 4.8	−6 ± 6 5 ± 2
Lactate (mmol/L)	<2	<1.46	<2
Anion gap (mEq/L)	12–25 17 ± 2.0	15–28	11.6 ± 5.06
Strong ion difference* (mEq/L)	34–44		40 ± 8.4
Strong ion gap (mEq/L)	−8 ± 2		−2 ± 6 0.36 ± 1.84
$A_{TOT}^†$ (mEq/L)			12–15 13.5 ± 0.55

* SID = (Na^+ + K^+) − (Cl^- + lactate)
† A_{TOT} = 2.25 × albumin (g/dL) + 1.4 × globulin (g/dL) + 0.59 × P_i (mg/dL)
Navarro et al., 2005; Hopper and Haskins, 2008; Valverde et al., 2008; Viu et al., 2010

albumin and PO_4 and requires use of a computer program (Moviat et al., 2008).

$$SIDe = 2.46 \times 10^{pH-8} \times PCO_2 \text{ mmHg} + (\text{albumin g/dL})$$
$$\times (0.123 \times pH - 0.631) + (\text{phosphate mEq/L})$$
$$\times (0.309 \times pH - 0.469)$$

Strong ion gap (SIG): SIG is the sum of unmeasured ions and is equal to SIDe – SIDa. SIG is normally zero, although a range of values has been reported for healthy human patients, and does not change with changes in pH or albumin concentration. Administration of colloids that include gelatin are known to elevate the SIG. A high SIG >2 mEq/L indicates accumulation of unmeasured anions as a cause of acidosis. SIG ≥5 mEq/L has been associated with increased mortality in human patients (Moviat et al., 2008). AGc has a strong correlation with SIG, even when the formula is simplified by omitting PO_4 (Gunnerson, 2005).

A simplified calculation of SIG has also been used (Constable, 2000):

$$SIG \text{ mEq/L} = (2.2 [\text{Total protein g/dL}] / 1 + 10^{6.7-pH}) - AG$$

Total weak acid concentration (A_{TOT}): The 'weak' acids are mostly proteins, especially albumin, and inorganic phosphate, and are not completely dissociated at physiological pH. They can act as non-volatile buffers, switching between forms that are associated or dissociated with a proton, i.e. A^- vs HA, in response to pH. These non-volatile buffers are not in as large a quantity as the volatile buffer, HCO_3^-, but still have significant effects on pH. Hypoproteinaemia results in a non-respiratory alkalosis, whereas hyperproteinaemia causes non-respiratory acidosis.

Free water effect: The free water concentration is identified by sodium concentration, such that a deficit of free water causes hypernatraemia and alkalosis (concentration alkalosis) and excess of free water causes hyponatraemia and acidosis (dilutional acidosis). The free water effect is calculated by subtracting normal sodium concentration from measured sodium and multiplying the change in concentration by 0.25 in dogs and 0.22 in cats (Hopper & Haskins, 2008).

Interpretation of acid base abnormalities

Step 1: Identification of the critical nature of the patient's acid–base status. pH values less than 7.25 and greater than 7.55 can be associated with significant effects on physiological function. Extreme values warrant immediate management.

> **pH is determined by changes in PCO2, AGc or SID, and ATOT.**

Step 2: Determine whether a respiratory abnormality exists. An increase in $PaCO_2$ above normal is called a respiratory acidosis because increased CO_2 causes the carbonic acid equilibrium equation to move to the right:

$$CO_2 + H_2O \rightleftharpoons H_2CO_3 \rightleftharpoons H^+ + HCO_3^-$$

If the $PaCO_2$ and pH are deviated from normal in opposite directions then a respiratory component is present. If the $PaCO_2$ and pH are changed in the same direction, then respiratory and metabolic components are present. Increased $PaCO_2$ most frequently occurs due to decreased ventilation caused by CNS depression from anaesthetic agents or trauma, or to decreased ventilation from partial airway obstruction, pulmonary disease, lung collapse, or failure of intercostal or diaphragmatic muscle function. A decrease in $PaCO_2$ from normal is a respiratory alkalosis and commonly occurs as a result of hyperventilation when the patient is anxious or distressed, as a physiological response to metabolic acidosis or hypoxia in conscious patients, or due to mechanical overventilation. In human patients, the change in pH expected from a change in $PaCO_2$ can be calculated:

- pH decreases by 0.05 unit and $[HCO_3^-]$ increases 1 mEq/L for every acute 1.33 kPa (10 mmHg) increase in PCO_2
- pH increases 0.10 unit and $[HCO_3^-]$ decreases 2 mEq/L for every acute 1.33 kPa (10 mmHg) decrease in PCO_2

Hopper & Haskins (2008) reported expected compensation in dogs as:

- $[HCO_3^-]$ increases 1.5 mEq/L for every acute 1.33 kPa (10 mmHg) increase in PCO_2
- $[HCO_3^-]$ decreases 2.5 mEq/L for every acute 1.33 kPa (10 mmHg) decrease in PCO_2

Chronic hypercarbia or hypocarbia generate greater changes in $[HCO_3^-]$ so that pH gradually returns to normal.

Step 3: Determine the metabolic component using blood gas and laboratory results. Complete assessment of acid–base balance will require knowledge of electrolyte and lactate values, patient history and immediate details (i.e. anaesthesia, ventilatory and circulatory status). It has been proposed that non-respiratory acid–base abnormalities fall into four categories: (1) free water deficit or excess; (2) increased or decreased $[Cl^-]$; (3) changes in protein; and (4) presence of unmeasured organic anions (Fidkowski & Helstrom, 2009).

SBE will determine the direction and magnitude of metabolic abnormality in most patients. It is less accurate when abnormal levels of lactate, phosphate, or proteins are present. Calculation of the AG may or may not reveal the presence of unmeasured anions as the AG is influenced by electrolyte abnormalities and hypoproteinaemia.

Diagnosis of hyperchloraemic metabolic acidosis is determined by measurement of Na and Cl, the absolute value for Cl, and the ratio of Na to Cl. The ratio of sodium to chloride is important because the Cl may be within the accepted normal range but calculation of SBE or SIDa will reveal a significant change in metabolic status. Calculation of AGc or SIG more specifically detects changes in unmeasured strong ions, e.g. lactate. Elevated blood lactate may have several origins but should always be investigated for unsuspected pathology. Many unmeasured anions have been identified, including citrate, isocitrate, ketoglutarate, succinate, and malate.

Simple cases may be managed using pH and blood gas analysis and routine laboratory tests to provide information on pH, PCO_2, SBE, and AG or AGc. Accurate determination of metabolic abnormalities in complex cases can be made using AGc or SIG when the essential laboratory test results and computerized formulae are available.

Monitoring body temperature

In the normal animal, body heat is unevenly distributed with the core temperature being 2–4°C higher than the peripheral. General anaesthesia inhibits vasoconstriction, allowing generalized redistribution of body heat. An additional decrease in body temperature occurs as heat is lost to the environment by exposure to cold operating room conditions, skin preparation with cold solutions, and abdominal surgical exposure. Furthermore, anaesthetics inhibit thermoregulation, vasoconstriction, and shivering, thereby decreasing the thresholds for cold responses. Administration of unwarmed IV fluid contributes substantially to the decrease in body temperature.

One method used in research animals to monitor temperature non-invasively involves subcutaneous injection of temperature-sensitive microchips. One study in experimental goats compared different sites with core (abdominal) and rectal temperatures (Torrao et al., 2011). The results determined that temperature measured from probes in the shoulder, flank or muscle varied from core temperature by up to 3.5°C and the differences varied inconsistently. Microchips implanted in the retroperitoneum most closely approximated core and rectal body temperatures with little variability.

Hypothermia

There does not seem to be a generally accepted definition of hypothermia and the definition should be appropriate to the species concerned. One study group has defined mild hypothermia in human patients to be between 34°C (93.2°F) and 36°C (96.8°F) (Reynolds et al., 2008). A decrease in temperature of 1–3°C below normal has been demonstrated to provide substantial protection against cerebral ischaemia and hypoxaemia in anaesthetized dogs (Wass et al., 1995). However, perioperative hypothermia is associated with several significant adverse effects (Table

Table 2.8 Adverse effects of perianaesthetic hypothermia

Impaired cardiovascular function
Hypoventilation
Decreased metabolism and detoxification of anaesthetic drugs
Weakness during recovery from anaesthesia
Decreased resistance to infection
Increased incidence of surgical wound infection
Increased postoperative protein catabolism

2.8) (Carli et al., 1991; Sheffield et al., 1994; Kurz et al., 1996; Reynolds et al., 2008). Mild hypothermia has been associated with triple the incidences of adverse myocardial events in elderly human patients and postoperative surgical infection; effects that apply to other species. Body temperature <35.6°C (96°F) appears to be associated with increased ataxia in horses during recovery from inhalation anaesthesia. Life-threatening cardiovascular depression may develop when the temperature decreases below 32.8°C (91°F).

Rectal or oesophageal temperature should be monitored at regular intervals during inhalation anaesthesia, during protracted total intravenous anaesthesia, and during recovery from anaesthesia. Small animals can be insulated from a cool environment by a variety of methods, including plastic covered foam pads and hot water circulating pads to lie on, and wrapping of extremities with towels or plastic bubble-wrap or cling-film. Heat loss from the respiratory tract may be minimized by ensuring that the inspired air remains warm and humidified. This can be accomplished by employing rebreathing circuits and low flow administration, or by attachment of a humidifier to the endotracheal connection of the anaesthetic circuit.

Active skin warming of the limbs may be the most effective method of preventing heat loss (Cabell et al., 1997). This can be accomplished by application of hot water or hot air circulating devices (e.g. Bair Hugger), or warmed towels, warmed fluid bags identified for this purpose by injection of food colour, and gel-filled packs. Special care should be taken to avoid skin sloughing from burns caused by application of devices that are too hot. Electrical heating pads and packs heated in a microwave oven are frequently to blame for tissue damage. It should also be remembered that warming devices placed over the site of an intramuscular injection, or an opioid-filled patch applied to the skin, may alter local blood flow and speed absorption of the drug. Fluids to be administered IV should be warm, either in the bag or bottle by storage in an incubator or at the time of administration by attaching a warming block or device to the administration line.

Table 2.9 Causes of hyperthermia

Causes	Examples
Fever	
Increased hypothalamic set point	Infection, inflammation, septicaemia, endotoxaemia
Hyperthermia	
Increased heat generation: increased basal metabolic rate, increased muscle activity, increased thyroid hormone, increased sympathetic activity	Adverse drug reaction including amphetamines, neuroleptic syndrome, serotonin syndrome Seizures Thyrotoxicosis Phaeochromocytoma Malignant hyperthermia syndrome
Decreased heat dissipation	Increased ambient temperature Old age Decreased cardiac output
McAllen & Schwartz, 2010	

Prevention of heat loss should be started at the beginning of anaesthesia. Preparation of the surgical site is often the time of greatest heat loss if active warming is not present and alcohol and cold solutions are used in skin preparation. An overhead hospital infant radiant heat warmer has proven effective at preventing hypothermia in cats and small dogs.

Hyperthermia

Increased body temperature is occasionally measured in anaesthetized animals. Hyperthermia developing in dogs and cats is most often caused by either excessive application of heat in an attempt to prevent hypothermia or by a pyrogenic reaction to a bacterial infection or inflammation, a contaminant in IV fluids, or drugs. Other causes of intraoperative hyperthermia are loss of central nervous system temperature regulation, thyrotoxicosis, or phaeochromocytoma (Table 2.9). Symptomatic treatment includes wetting the coat or hair with cold water, IV administration of cold fluids, and sedation if applicable. Determination of the cause of hyperthermia may indicate other specific treatment. Hyperthermia (40.5°C; 105°F) quite frequently develops in cats during recovery from anaesthesia that included administration of tiletamine–zolazepam. In these animals, the increase in temperature is associated with increased muscle activity such as paddling, uncoordinated movements, or purposeful movements directed at restraints or bandages. Treatment that is usually effective includes directing a flow of air over the cat from a fan placed outside the

cage and providing sedation, for example, butorphanol, 0.2 mg/kg IM, with or without acepromazine, 0.05–0.1 mg/kg IM. Circulating iced water through a rigid plastic pad placed in the cage with the cat is an effective method of reducing body temperature. Administration of ketamine or hydromorphone and other opioids to cats has also been associated with hyperthermia developing during recovery from anaesthesia (Posner et al., 2010). Rarely, hyperthermia is a manifestation of the malignant hyperthermia syndrome (MH) which is a life-threatening hypermetabolic condition triggered by stress and certain anaesthetic agents.

Malignant hyperthermia

Malignant hyperthermia (MH) occurs most frequently during anaesthesia of human beings and pigs (McGrath, 1986; Roewer et al., 1995), but has been reported to occur in dogs (O'Brien et al., 1990; Nelson, 1991; Roberts et al., 2001), cats (Bellah et al., 1989), and horses (Manley et al., 1983; Klein et al., 1989; Aleman et al., 2009). Clinical signs of MH in pigs (see Chapter 14) usually include an increase in temperature, increased respiratory rate and depth, increased $ETCO_2$ and $PaCO_2$, metabolic acidosis, tachycardia, hypertension, and arrhythmias. Purple blotches may be observed in the skin of the abdomen and snout. The soda lime canister on the anaesthesia machine may become excessively hot to touch and the absorbent changes colour rapidly, reflecting massive carbon dioxide production. Rigidity of the jaw and limb muscles may be observed as the condition progresses. The animal dies unless the condition is treated early.

The clinical appearance of dogs developing MH during anaesthesia may differ from pigs. Tachycardia may not be a feature, skeletal muscle rigidity may not occur, and rectal temperature may not increase until the syndrome is well established (Nelson, 1991). The earliest signs may be related to increased CO_2 production. These signs include an increased respiratory rate and depth, rapid changing of CO_2 absorbent colour, a hot CO_2 absorbent canister, and increased $ETCO_2$ in the absence of hypoventilation or malfunctioning one-way valves. Increased respiratory rate would be the only one of these signs present in a dog that was merely overheated.

The clinical picture of MH in horses is not clear cut. Abnormal measurements may not be observed for some time after induction of anaesthesia. Observed signs may be suggestive that the horse is in a light plane of anaesthesia, however, the earliest changes are usually increased $PaCO_2$ and $ETCO_2$. Heart rates may be mildly elevated and arterial blood pressure is often within the normal range for inhalation anaesthesia (Manley et al., 1983; Klein et al., 1989). Changes in anaesthetic management may permit the horse to survive anaesthesia but severe rhabdomyolysis developing during recovery from anaesthesia may necessitate euthanasia.

Monitoring urine volume

The urinary output depends on the renal blood flow that, in turn, depends on cardiac output and circulating blood volume, and thus it is a relatively sensitive indicator of the circulatory state during anaesthesia. Measurement of urine production is advisable in animals with severe chronic renal disease, renal failure, or circulatory failure from non-renal causes. The urinary bladder may be catheterized using aseptic technique before anaesthesia or after induction of anaesthesia, and the catheter connected to a plastic bag for continuous collection of urine. In event of inadequate urine flow, the catheter should be checked for blockage by mucus or blood and that urine is not pooling in the bladder and cannot drain because of the relationship between the catheter tip and positioning of the animal. Alternatively, urine may be collected and measured at the end of anaesthesia. Urine output of less than 1 mL/kg/hour is considered to be inadequate. However, urine flow during anaesthesia is very variable, for example, one group of healthy dogs anaesthetized for orthopaedic procedures with oxymorphone, propofol, and isoflurane produced 0–2.2 mL/kg/h (mean 0.46 mL/kg/h) (Boscan et al., 2010).

Failure of patients to produce an adequate urine volume over the course of anaesthesia may be unrelated to intraoperative cardiovascular function. Indeed, fluid retention is now a recognized complication of surgery in human patients and has been documented to occur in anaesthetized dogs (Boscan et al., 2010; Cagini et al., 2011). Fluid retention has been measured by a variety of methods including weighing patients before and after anaesthesia, calculation of the discrepancy between the volume of fluid administered and the volume of urine produced, and bioimpedance analysis. The latter method involves passing a small undetectable alternating current through the body, from hand to foot electrodes in humans, and bioimpedance analysis measures the resistance to flow of the current. This technique has detected increases in total body water and extracellular fluid volume after anaesthesia in dogs (Boscan et al., 2010). The tendency to retain fluid has been documented in human patients to be greater on the second postoperative day and apparently unrelated to age or sex of the patient, early mobilization after surgery and early oral intake (Cagini et al., 2011). Fluid retention occurs even with intraoperative fluid restriction, although the amount is increased with high volume fluid therapy. The cause of fluid retention is thought to be multifactorial. Decreased arterial pressure or hypovolaemia during anaesthesia causes release of vasopressin (antidiuretic hormone) and that increases free water absorption in distal tubules of the kidney (Hauptman et al., 2000). Some anaesthetic agents may influence urine output, for example, decreased urine production was measured in dogs receiving morphine for premedication when compared with dogs without

morphine (Robertson et al., 2001). A study of healthy and traumatized dogs in the ICU receiving LRS 60 mL/kg/day with a continuous infusion of either morphine, 0.12 mg/kg/h, or fentanyl, 3 µg/kg/h, confirmed that both opioids decreased urine flow significantly (Anderson & Day, 2008). Healthy control dogs receiving only LRS produced urine at a rate of 1.23 ± 0.13 mL/kg/h. Morphine or fentanyl infusion decreased urine production to approximately 0.7 mL/kg/h and urine specific gravity increased.

Monitoring blood glucose

Clinical signs of hypoglycaemia may not be obvious during anaesthesia and the condition may go unrecognized. Consequences of hypoglycaemia are coma, hypotension, or prolonged recovery from anaesthesia with depression, weakness, or even seizures.

Animals at risk for developing hypoglycaemia during anaesthesia include paediatric patients, diabetics, and animals with hepatic disease, portosystemic shunt, insulinoma, and septicaemia or endotoxaemia. Occasionally, healthy adult sheep, goats, and even horses develop hypoglycaemia which manifests as a prolonged or weak recovery from anaesthesia. Routine monitoring of patients at risk for hypoglycaemia should include measurement of blood glucose at the start and the end of anaesthesia. Blood glucose can be determined rapidly using reagent strips and a glucometer. Animals with low blood glucose concentrations initially or those undergoing major or prolonged surgery, should have their blood glucose monitored at approximately 1 hour intervals during anaesthesia.

Patients at risk for hypoglycemia should be given 5% dextrose in water (D5W) as part of the intraoperative IV fluid therapy. D5W should be infused at a rate of 3 (2–5) mL/kg/hour to maintain blood glucose between 5.5 and 11.0 mmol/L (100 and 200 mg/dL). Balanced electrolyte solution should also be infused at the usual rate of 5–10 mL/kg/hour.

Monitoring neuromuscular blockade

The mechanical response to nerve stimulation (i.e. muscular contraction) may be observed following the application of supramaximal single, tetanic or 'train-of-four' electrical stimuli to a suitable peripheral motor nerve, usually a foot twitch in response to stimulation of the peroneal, tibial, or ulnar nerves. During general anaesthesia the response obtained may be influenced by the anaesthetic agents and any neuromuscular blocking drugs which have been used. Details about neuromuscular blocking drugs and the monitoring technique are given in Chapter 8.

REFERENCES

Aleman, M., Nieto, J.E., Magdesian, K.G., 2009. Malignant hyperthermia associated with ryanodine receptor 1 (C7360G) mutation in Quarter Horses. J Vet Intern Med 23, 329–334.

Anderson, M.K., Day, T.K., 2008. Effects of morphine and fentanyl constant rate infusion on urine output in healthy and traumatized dogs. Vet Anaesth Analg 35, 528–536.

Apfelbaum, J.L., Arens, J.F., Cole, D.J., et al., 2006. Practice advisory for intraoperative awareness and brain function monitoring A report by the American Society of Anesthesiologists task force on intraoperative awareness. Anesthesiology 104, 847–864.

Avidan, M.S., Zhang, L., Burnside, B.A., et al., 2008. Anesthesia awareness and the bispectral index. N Engl J Med 358, 1097–1108.

Bailey, J.E., Dunlop, C.I., Chapman, P.L., et al., 1994. Indirect Doppler ultrasonic measurement of arterial blood pressure results in a large measurement error in dorsally recumbent anaesthetised horses. Equine Vet J 26, 70–73.

Beaulieu, K.E., Kerr, C.L., McDonell, W.N., 2005. Evaluation of a lithium dilution cardiac output technique as a method for measurement of cardiac output in anesthetized cats. Am J Vet Res 66, 1639–1645.

Beaulieu, M., Lapointe, Y., Vinet, B., 1999. Stability of PO_2, PCO_2, and pH in fresh blood samples stored in a plastic syringe with low heparin in relation to various blood-gas and hematological parameters. Clin Biochem 32, 101–107.

Bektas, R.N., Kutter, A.P.N., Jud, R.S., et al., 2012. Evaluation of a minimally invasive non-calibrated pulse contour cardiac output monitor (FloTrac/Vigileo) in anaesthetized dogs. Vet Anaesth Analg 39, 464–471.

Belda, E., Blissitt, K.J., Duncan, J.C., et al., 2010. The bispectral index during recovery from halothane and sevoflurane anaesthesia in horses. Vet Anaesth Analg 37, 25–34.

Bellah, J.R., Robertson, S.A., Buergelt, C.D., et al., 1989. Suspected malignant hyperthermia after halothane anesthesia in a cat. Vet Surg 18, 483–488.

Bleijenberg, E.H., van Oostrom, H., Akkerdaas, L.C., et al., 2011. A study into the relationship between the bispectral index and the clinically evaluated anaesthetic depth in dogs. Vet Anaesth Analg 38, 536–543.

Boscan, P., Pypendop, B.H., Siao, K.T., et al., 2010. Fluid balance, glomerular filtration rate, and urine output in dogs anesthetized for an orthopedic surgical procedure. Am J Vet Res 71, 501–507.

Bosiack, A.P., Mann, F.A., Dodam, J.R., et al., 2010. Comparison of ultrasonic Doppler flow monitor, oscillometric, and direct arterial blood pressure measurements in ill dogs. J Vet Emerg Crit Care 20, 207–215.

Branson, K.R., Wagner-Mann, C.C., Mann, F.A., 1997. Evaluation of an oscillometric blood pressure monitor on anesthetized cats and the effect of cuff placement and fur on accuracy. Vet Surg 26, 347–353.

Brodbelt, D., 2009. Perioperative mortality in small animal anaesthesia. Vet J 182, 152–161.

Brown, S.A., Atkins, C., Bagley, R., et al., 2007. Guidelines for the identification, evaluation and management of systemic hypertension in dogs and cats. J Vet Intern Med 21, 542–558.

Bruhn, J., Kreuer, S., Bischoff, P., et al., 2005. Bispectral index and A-line AAI index as guidance for desflurane-remifentanil anaesthesia compared with a standard practice group: a multicentre study. Br J Anaesth 94, 63–69.

Burns, P.M., Driessen, B., Boston, R., et al., 2006. Accuracy of a third (Dolphin Voyager) versus first generation pulse oximeter (Nellcor N-180) in predicting arterial oxygen saturation and pulse rate in the anesthetized dog. Vet Anaesth Analg 33, 281–295.

Cabell, L.W., Perkowski, S.Z., Gregor, T., et al., 1997. The effects of active peripheral skin warming on perioperative hypothermia in dogs. Vet Surg 26, 79–85.

Cagini, L., Capozzi, R., Tassi, V., et al., 2011. Fluid and electrolyte balance after major thoracic surgery by bioimpedance and endocrine evaluation. Eur J Cardiothorac Surg 40, e71–76.

Campagnol, D., Teixeira Neto, F.J., Monteiro, E.R., et al., 2007. Use of bispectral index to monitor depth of anesthesia in isoflurane-anesthetized dogs. Am J Vet Res 68, 1300–1307.

Cannesson, M., Le Manach, Y., Hofer, C.K., et al., 2011. Assessing the diagnostic accuracy of pulse pressure variations for the prediction of fluid responsiveness: A 'Gray Zone' approach. Anesthesiology 115, 231–241

Carli, F., Webster, J., Pearson, M., et al., 1991. Postoperative protein metabolism: effect of nursing elderly patients for 24 h after abdominal surgery in a thermoneutral environment. Anaesthesia 66, 292–299.

Caulkett, N.A., Cantwell, S.L., Houston, D.M., 1998. A comparison of indirect blood pressure monitoring techniques in the anesthetized cat. Vet Surg 27, 370–377.

Chaffin, M.K., Matthews, N.S., Cohen, N.D., et al., 1996. Evaluation of pulse oximetry in anaesthetised foals using multiple combinations of transducer type and transducer attachment site. Equine Vet J 28, 437–445.

Clarke, K.W., England, G.C.W., Goosens, L., 1991. Sedative and cardiovascular effects of romifidine, alone and in combination with butorphanol, in the horse. J Vet Anaesth 18, 25–29.

Constable, P.D., 2000. Clinical assessment of acid-base status: Comparison of the Henderson-Hasselbalch and strong ion approaches. Vet Clin Pathol 29, 115–128.

Cooper, E.S., Muir, W.W., 2007. Continuous cardiac output monitoring via arterial pressure waveform analysis following severe hemorrhagic shock in dogs. Crit Care Med 35, 1724–1729.

Corley, K.T.T., Donaldson, L.L., Furr, M.O., 2002. Comparison of lithium dilution and thermodilution cardiac output measurements in anaesthetised neonatal foals. Equine Vet J 34, 598–601.

Cribb, P.H., 1988. Capnographic monitoring during anesthesia with controlled ventilation in the horse. Vet Surg 17, 48–52.

Deane, J.C., Dagleish, M.P., Benamou, A.E., et al., 2004. Effects of syringe material and temperature and duration of storage on the stability of equine arterial blood gas variables. Vet Anaesth Analg 31, 250–257.

Deflandre, C.J.A., Hellebrekers, L.J., 2007. Clinical evaluation of the Surgivet V60046, a non invasive blood pressure monitor in anaesthetized dogs. Vet Anaesth Analg.35, 13–21.

Duffy, A.L., Butler, A.L., Radecki, S.V., et al., 2009. Comparison of continuous arterial pressure waveform analysis with the lithium dilution technique to monitor cardiac output in conscious dogs with systemic inflammatory response syndrome. Am J Vet Res 70, 1365–1373.

Durga, P., Jonnavittula, N., Muthuchellappan, R., et al., 2008. Measurement of systolic pressure variation during graded volume loss using simple tools on Datex Ohmeda S/5 monitor. J Neurosurg Anesthesiol 21, 161–164.

Eberhard, P., 2007. The design, use, and results of transcutaneous carbon dioxide analysis: Current and future directions. Anesth Analg 105, S48–S52.

Ellerkmann, R.K., Soehle, M., Riese, G., et al., 2010. The Entropy Module and Bispectral Index as guidance for propofol-remifentanil anaesthesia in combination with regional anaesthesia compared with a standard clinical practice group. Anaesth Intensive Care 38, 159–166.

Fairman, N., 1993. Evaluation of pulse oximetry as a continuous monitoring technique in critically ill dogs in the small animal intensive care unit. Vet Emerg Crit Care 2, 50–56.

Fidkowski, C., Helstrom, J., 2009. Diagnosing metabolic acidosis in the critically ill: bridging the anion gap, Stewart, and base excess methods. Can J Anaesth 56, 247–256.

Forster, H.V., Bisgard, G.E., Klein, J.P., 1981. Effect of peripheral chemoreceptor denervation on acclimatization of goats during hypoxia. J Appl Physiol 50, 392–398.

Gallivan, J.G., McDonell, W.N., Forrest, J.B., 1989. Comparative ventilation and gas exchange in the horse and cow. Res Vet Sci 46, 331–336.

Geddes, L.A., Chaffee, V., Whistler, S.J., et al., 1977. Indirect mean blood pressure in the anesthetized pony. Am J Vet Res 38, 2055–2057.

Geiser, D.R., Rohrbach, B.W., 1992. Use of end-tidal CO_2 tension to predict arterial CO_2 values in isoflurane-anesthetized equine neonates. Am J Vet Res 53, 1617–1621.

Giguère, S., Bucki, E., Adin, D.B., et al., 2005a. Cardiac output measurement by carbon dioxide rebreathing, 2-dimentional echocardiography, and lithium dilution method in anesthetized neonatal foals. J Vet Intern Med 19, 737–743.

Giguère, S., Knowles, H.A., Valverde, A., et al., 2005b. Accuracy of indirect measurement of blood pressure in neonatal foals. J Vet Intern Med 19, 571–576.

Grandy, J.L., Dunlop, C.I., Hodgson, D.S., et al., 1992. Evaluation of the doppler ultrasonic method of measuring systolic arterial blood pressure in cats. Am J Vet Res 53, 1166–1169.

Gunkel, C.I., Valverde, A., Morey, T.E., et al., 2004. Comparison of non-invasive cardiac output measurement by partial carbon dioxide rebreathing with the lithium dilution method in anesthetized dogs. J Vet Emerg Crit Care 14, 187–195.

Gunnerson, K.J., 2005. Clinical review: The meaning of acid-base abnormalities in the intensive care unit – epidemiology. Crit Care 9, 508–516.

Guyton, A.C., 1986. Textbook of Medical Physiology. W.B. Saunders, Philadelphia, pp. 218–229.

Haberman, C.E., Kang, C.W., Morgan, J.D., et al., 2006. Evaluation of oscillometric and Doppler ultrasonic methods of indirect blood pressure estimation in conscious dogs. Can J Vet Res 70, 211–217.

Haga, H.A., Dolvik, N.I., 2002. Evaluation of the bispectral index as an indicator of degree of central nervous system depression in isoflurane-anesthetized horses. Am J Vet Res 63, 438–442.

Hainsworth, R., Drinkhill, M.J., 2007. Cardiovascular adjustments for life at high altitude. Resp Physiol Neurobiol 158, 204–211.

Hannon, J.P., 1983. Blood acid-base curve nomogram for immature domestic pigs. Am J Vet Res 44, 2385–2390.

Haskins, S., Pascoe, P.J., Ilkiw, J.E., et al., 2005. Reference cardiopulmonary values in normal dogs. Comp Med 55, 156–161.

Hauptman, J.G., Richter, M.A., Wood, S.L., et al., 2000. Effects of anesthesia, surgery, and intravenous administration of fluids on plasma antidiuretic hormone concentrations in healthy dogs. Am J Vet Res 61, 1273–1276.

Hedberg, P., Majava, A., Kiviluoma, K., et al., 2009. Potential preanalytical errors in whole-blood analysis: effect of syringe sample volume on blood gas, electrolyte and lactate values. Scand J Clin Lab Invest 69, 585–591.

Henao-Guerrero, P.N., McMurphy, R.M., KuKanich, B., et al., 2009. Effect of morphine on the bispectral index during isoflurane anesthesia in dogs. Vet Anaesth Analg 36, 133–143.

Hendricks, J.C., King, L.G., 1994. Practicality, usefulness, and limits of end-tidal carbon dioxide monitoring in critical small animal patients. J Vet Emerg Crit Care 4, 29–39.

Hodgson, D.R., Dunlop, C.I., Chapman, P.L., et al., 1990. Cardiopulmonary effects of isoflurane in foals (abstract). Vet Surg 19, 316.

Hopper, K., Haskins, S.C., 2008. A case-based review of a simplified quantitative approach to acid-base analysis. J Vet Emerg Crit Care 18, 467–476.

Horwitz, L.D., Bishop, V.S., Stone, H.L., et al., 1969. Cardiovascular effects of low-oxygen atmospheres in conscious and anaesthetized dogs. J Appl Physiol 27, 370–373.

Huss, B.T., Anderson, M.A., Branson, K.R., et al., 1995. Evaluation of pulse oximeter probes and probe placement in healthy dogs. J Am Anim Hosp Assoc 31, 9–14.

Jacobsen, J.D., Miller, M.W., Matthews, N.S., et al., 1992. Evaluation of accuracy of pulse oximetry in dogs. Am J Vet Res 53, 537–540.

Jaffe, M.B., 1999. Partial CO_2 rebreathing cardiac output – operating principles of the NICO™ system. J Clin Monit 15, 387–401.

Kellum, J.A., 2005. Clinical review: Reunification of acid-base physiology. Crit Care 9, 500–507.

Kellum, J.A., 2007. Disorders of acid-base balance. Crit Care Med 35, 2630–2636.

Kertai, M.D., Palanca, B.J.A., Pal, N., et al., 2011. Bispectral index monitoring, duration of bispectral index below 45, patient risk factors, and intermediate-term mortality after noncardiac surgery in the B-Unaware trial. Anesthesiology 114, 545–556.

Khanna, A.K., McDonell, W.N., Dyson, D.H., et al., 1995. Cardiopulmonary effects of hypercapnia during controlled intermittent positive pressure ventilation in the horse. Can J Vet Res 59, 213–221.

Kiers, H.D., Hofstra, J.M., Wetsels, J.F.M., 2008. Oscillometric blood pressure measurements: differences between measured and calculated mean arterial pressure. Neth J Med 66, 474–479.

Klein, L., Ailes, N., Fackelman, G., et al., 1989. Postanesthetic equine myopathy suggestive of malignant hyperthermia. A case report. Vet Surg 18, 479–482.

Kurz, A., Sessler, D.I., Lenhardt, R., 1996. Perioperative normothermia to reduce the incidence of surgical-wound infection and shorten hospitalization. New Engl J Med 334, 1209–1215.

Lake, C.L. (Ed.), 1990. Monitoring of ventricular function. In: Clinical Monitoring. W.B. Saunders Company, Philadelphia, pp. 237–279.

Lamont, L.A., Greene, S.A., Grimm, K.A., et al., 2004. Relationship of bispectral index to minimum alveolar concentration multiples of sevoflurane in cats. Am J Vet Res 65, 93–98.

Latshaw, H., Fessler, J.F., Whistler, S.J., et al., 1979. Indirect measurement of mean blood pressure in the normotensive and hypotensive horse. Equine Vet J 11, 191–194.

Linton, R.A., Young, L.E., Martin, D.G., et al., 2000. Cardiac output measured by lithium dilution, thermodilution, and transesophageal Doppler echocardiography in anesthetized horses. Am J Vet Res 61, 731–737.

Lumb, A.B., 2000. Nunn's Applied Respiratory Physiology. Elsevier Limited, Philadelphia.

MacFarlane, P.D., Grint, N., Dugdale, A., 2010. Comparison of invasive and non-invasive blood pressure monitoring during clinical anaesthesia in dogs. Vet Res Commun 34, 217–227.

Manley, S.V., Kelly, A.B., Hodgson, D., 1983. Malignant hyperthermia-like reactions in three anesthetized horses. J Am Vet Med Assoc 183, 85–89.

March, P.A., Muir III, W.W., 2003a. Minimum alveolar concentration measures of central nervous system activation in cats anesthetized with isoflurane. Am J Vet Res 64, 1528–1533.

March, P.A., Muir III, W.W., 2003b. Use of the bispectral index as a monitor of anesthetic depth in cats anesthetized with isoflurane. Am J Vet Res 64, 1534–1541.

Mason, D.J., O'Grady, M., Woods, J.P., et al., 2001. Assessment of lithium dilution cardiac output as a technique for measurement of cardiac output in dogs. Am J Vet Res 62, 1255–1261.

Matthews, N.S., Hartke, S., Allen, J.C.J., 2003. An evaluation of pulse oximeters in dogs, cats, and horses. Vet Anaesth Analg 30, 3–14.

Matthews, N.S., Hartsfield, S.M., Cornick, J.L., et al., 1990. A comparison of end-tidal halothane concentration measurement at different locations in the horse (Abstract). Vet Surg 19, 317.

McAllen, K.J., Schwartz, D.R., 2010. Adverse drug reactions resulting in hyperthermia in the intensive care unit. Crit Care Med 38, S244–S251.

McGrath, C., 1986. Malignant hyperthermia. Semin Vet Med Surg (Small animal) 1, 238–244.

McMurphy, R.M., Stoll, M.R., McCubrey, R., 2006. Accuracy of an oscillometric blood pressure monitor during phenylephrine-induced hypertension in dogs. Am J Vet Res 67, 1541–1545.

Meurs, K.M., Miller, M.W., Slater, M.R., 1996. Comparison of indirect oscillometric and direct arterial methods for blood pressure measurements in anesthetized dogs. J Am Anim Hosp Assoc 32, 471–475.

Meyer, O., Jenni, R., Greiter-Wilke, A., et al., 2010. Comparison of telemetry and high-definition oscillometry for blood pressure measurements in conscious dogs: Effects of torcetrapib. J Am Assoc Lab Anim Sci 49, 464–471.

Meyer, R.E., Short, C.E., 1985. Arterial to end-tidal CO_2 tension and alveolar dead space in halothane- or isoflurane-anesthetized horses. Am J Vet Res 46, 597–599.

Middleton, D.J., Ilkiw, J.E., Watson, A.D.J., 1981. Arterial and venous blood gas tensions in clinically healthy cats. Am J Vet Res 42, 1609–1611.

Moens, Y., 1989. Arterial-alveolar carbon dioxide tension difference and alveolar dead space in halothane anaesthetised horses. Equine Vet J 21, 282–284.

Moens, Y., Gootjes, P., Lagerweij, E., 1991. The influence of methane on the infrared measurement of halothane in the horse. J Vet Anaesth 18, 4–7.

Moraga, F., Monge, C., Riquelme, R., et al., 1996. Fetal and maternal blood oxygen affinity: A comparative study in llamas and sheep. Comp Biochem Physiol 115A, 111–115.

Moviat, M., Terpstra, A.M., Ruitenbeek, W., et al., 2008. Contributions of various metabolites to the 'unmeasured' anions in critically ill patients with metabolic acidosis. Crit Care Med 36, 752–758.

Muir, W.W., Wade, A., Grospitch, B.J., 1983. Automatic noninvasive sphygmomanometry in horses. J Am Vet Med Assoc 182, 1230–1233.

Murrell, J.C., Johnson, C.B., 2006. Neurophysiological techniques to assess pain in animals. J Vet Pharmacol Ther 29, 325–335.

Navarro, M., Monreal, L., Segura, D., et al., 2005. A comparison of traditional and quantitative analysis of acid-base and electrolyte imbalances in horses with gastrointestinal disorders. J Vet Intern Med 19, 871–877.

Nelson, T.E., 1991. Malignant hyperthermia in dogs. J Am Vet Med Assoc 198, 989–994.

Noël, P.G., Couëtil, L., Constable, P.D., 2010. Effects of collecting blood into plastic heparinised vacutainer tubes and storage conditions on blood gas analysis values in horses. Equine Vet J 42 (Suppl 38), 91–97.

Norton, J.L., Nolen-Walston, R.D., Underwood, C., et al., 2011. Repeatability, reproducibility, and effect of head position on central venous pressure measurement in standing adult horses. J Vet Intern Med, 575–578.

O'Brien, D., Pook, H.A., Klip, A., et al., 1990. Canine stress syndrome/malignant hyperthermia susceptibility: calcium hemostasis defect in muscle and lymphocytes. Res Vet Sci 48, 124–128.

Oakley, R.E., Olivier, B., Eyster, G.E., et al., 1997. Experimental evaluation of central venous pressure monitoring in the dog. J Am Anim Hosp Assoc 33, 77–82.

Pairet, B., Jaenicke, E., 2010. Structure of the altitude adapted hemoglobin of guinea pig in the R2-state. PLoS ONE 5, e12389.

Pang, D.S.J., Allaire, J., Rondenay, Y., et al., 2009. The use of lingual venous blood to determine the acid-base and blood-gas status of dogs under anaesthesia. Vet Anaesth Analg 36, 124–132.

Parry, B.W., McCarthy, M.A., Anderson, G.A., et al., 1982. Correct occlusive bladder width for indirect blood pressure measurement in horses. Am J Vet Res 43, 50–54.

Parviainen, A.K., Trim, C.M., 2000. Complications associated with anaesthesia for ocular surgery: a retrospective study 1989–1996. Equine Vet J 32, 555–559.

Paulev, P.E., Zubieta-Calleja, G.R., 2005. Essentials in the diagnosis of acid-base disorders and their high altitude application. J Physiol Pharm 56 (Supp 4), 155–170.

Pedersen, K.M., Butler, M.A., Ersbøll, A.K., et al., 2002. Evaluation of an oscillometric blood pressure monitor for use in anesthetized cats. J Am Vet Med Assoc 221, 646–650.

Picandet, V., Jeanneret, S., Lavoie, J.P., 2007. Effect of syringe type and storage temperature on results of blood gas analysis in arterial blood of horses. J Vet Intern Med 21, 476–481.

Pizov, R., Eden, A., Bystritski, D., et al., 2010. Arterial and plethysmographic waveform analysis in anesthetized patients with hypovolemia. Anesthesiology 113, 83–91.

Posner, L.P., Pavuk, A.A., Rokshar, J.L., et al., 2010. Effects of opioids and anesthetic drugs on body temperature in cats. Vet Anaesth Analg 37, 35–43.

Pretto, J.J., Rochford, P.D., 1994. Effects of sample storage time, temperature and syringe type on blood gas tensions in samples with high oxygen partial pressures. Thorax 49, 610–612.

Reynolds, L., Beckmann, J., Kurz, A., 2008. Perioperative complications of hypothermia. Best Prac Res Clin Anesth 22, 645–657.

Ribeiro, L.M., Ferreira, D.A., Brás, S., et al., 2009. Correlation between clinical signs of depth of anaesthesia and cerebral state index responses in dogs during induction of anaesthesia with propofol. Res Vet Sci 87, 287–291.

Riebold, T.W., Evans, A.T., 1985. Blood pressure measurements in the anesthetized horse: comparison of four methods. Vet Surg 14, 332–337.

Roberts, M.C., Mickelson, J.R., Patterson, E.E., et al., 2001. Autosomal dominant canine malignant hyperthermia is caused by a mutation in the gene encoding the skeletal muscle calcium release channel (RYR1). Anesthesiology 95, 716–725.

Robertson, S.A., 1990. Practical use of ECG in the horse. In Practice 12, 59–67.

Robertson, S.A., Hauptman, J.G., Nachreiner, R.F., et al., 2001. Effects of acetylpromazine or morphine on urine production in halothane-anesthetized dogs. Am J Vet Res 62, 1922–1927.

Roewer, N., Dziadzka, A., Greim, C.A., et al., 1995. Cardiovascular and metabolic responses to anesthetic-induced malignant hyperthermia in swine. Anesthesiology 83, 141–159.

Sawyer, D.C., Brown, M., Striler, E.L., et al., 1991. Comparison of direct and indirect blood pressure measurement in anesthetized dogs. Lab Anim Sci 41, 134–138.

Sawyer, D.C., Guikema, A.H., Siegel, E.M., 2004. Evaluation of a new oscillometric blood pressure monitor in isoflurane-anesthetized dogs. Vet Anaesth Analg 31, 27–39.

Schauvliege, S., Van den Eede, A., Duchateau, L., et al., 2009. Comparison between lithium dilution and pulse contour analysis techniques for cardiac output measurement in isoflurane anaesthetized ponies: influence of different inotropic drugs. Vet Anaesth Analg 36, 197–208.

Scott, N.E., Haskins, S.C., Aldrich, J., et al., 2005. Comparison of measured oxyhemoglobin saturation and oxygen content with analyzer-calculated values and hand-calculated values obtained in unsedated healthy dogs. Am J Vet Res 66, 1273–1277.

Sheffield, C.W., Sessler, D.I., Hunt, T.K., 1994. Mild hypothermia during isoflurane anesthesia decreases resistance to E. coli dermal infection in guinea pigs. Acta Anaesth Scand 38, 201–205.

Shih, A., Robertson, S., Vigani, A., et al., 2010. Evaluation of an indirect oscillometric blood pressure monitor in normotensive and hypotensive anesthetized dogs. J Vet Emerg Crit Care 20, 313–318.

Shih, A.C., Giguère, S., Sanchez, L.C., et al., 2009. Determination of cardiac output in anesthetized neonatal foals by use of two pulse wave analysis methods. Am J Vet Res 70, 334–339.

Soma, L.R. (Ed.), 1971. Depth of general anesthesia. In: Textbook of Veterinary Anaesthesia. Williams & Wilkins Company, Baltimore, pp. 178–187.

Steffey, E.P., Dunlop, C.I., Farver, T.B., et al., 1987. Cardiovascular and respiratory measurements in awake and isoflurane-anesthetized horses. Am J Vet Res 48, 7–12.

Stegall, H.E., Kardon, M.B., Kemmerer, W.T., 1968. Indirect measurement of arterial blood pressure byDoppler ultrasonic sphygmomanometry. J Appl Physiol 25, 793–798.

Tate, L.P., Corbett, W.T., Foreman, J.H., et al., 1993. Instrumentation of exercising Thoroughbreds to determine blood gas tensions and acid-base status. Vet Surg 22, 171–176.

Taylor, P.M., 1990. Interference with the Datex Normac anaesthetic agent monitor for halothane in horses and sheep. J Assoc Vet Anaesth 17, 32–34.

Toffaletti, J., Zijlstra, W.G., 2007. Misconceptions in reporting oxygen saturation. Anesth Analg 105, S5–S9.

Torrao, N.A., Hetem, R.S., Meyer, L.C.R., et al., 2011. Assessment of the use of temperature-sensitive microchips to determine core body temperature in goats. Vet Rec 168, 328.

Tremper, K.K., Barker, S.J., 1990. Monitoring of oxygen. In: Lake, C.L. (Ed.), Clinical Monitoring. W. B. Saunders Company, Philadelphia, pp. 283–313.

Trim, C.M., 1998. Monitoring during anaesthesia: techniques and interpretation. Equine Vet Educ 10, 207–218.

Valverde, A., Giguère, S., Morey, T.E., et al., 2007. Comparison of noninvasive cardiac output measured by use of partial carbon dioxide rebreathing or the lithium dilution method in anesthetized foals. Am J Vet Res 68, 141–147.

Valverde, A., Hatcher, M.E., Stämpfli, H.R., 2008. Effects of fluid therapy on total protein and its influence on calculated unmeasured ions in the anesthetized dog. J Vet Emerg Crit Care 18, 480–487.

Viu, J., Jose-Cunilleras, E., Armengou, L., et al., 2010. Acid-base imbalances during a 120 km endurance race compared by traditional and simplified strong ion difference methods. Equine Vet J 42 (suppl 38), 76–82.

Wagner, A.E., Bednarski, R.M., Muir, W.W., 1990. Hemodynamic effects of carbon dioxide during intermittent positive-pressure ventilation in horses. Am J Vet Res 51, 1922–1929.

Wagner, A.E., Muir, W.W., Hinchcliff, K.W., 1991. Cardiovascular effects of xylazine and detomidine in horses. Am J Vet Res 52, 651–657.

Walley, K.R., 2010. Use of central venous oxygen saturation to guide therapy. Am J Respir Crit Care Med, 184, 514–520.

Wan, P.Y., Trim, C.M., Mueller, P.O., 1992. Xylazine-ketamine and detomidine-tiletamine-zolazepam anesthesia in horses. Vet Surg 21, 312–318.

Wanner, A., Reinhart, M.E., 1978. Respiratory mechanics in conscious sheep: response to methacholine. J Appl Physiol 44, 479–482.

Wass, C.T., Lanier, W.L., Hofer, R.E., et al., 1995. Temperature changes of >1 or =1°C alter functional neurologic outcome and histopathology in a canine model of complete cerebral ischemia. Anesthesiology 83, 325–335.

Watney, G.C.G., Norman, W.M., Schumacher, J.P., et al., 1993. Accuracy of a reflectance pulse oximeter in anesthetized horses. Am J Vet Res 54, 497–501.

Weber, R.E., 2007. High-altitude adaptations in vertebrate hemoglobins. Resp Physiol Neurobiol 158, 132–142.

Weiskopf, R.B., Townsley, M.I., Riordan, K.K., et al., 1981. Comparison of cardiopulmonary responses to graded hemorrhage during enflurane, halothane, isoflurane, and ketamine anesthesia. Anesth Analg 60, 481–491.

Wernick, M., Doherr, M.G., Howard, J., et al., 2010. Evaluation of high-definition and conventional oscillometric blood pressure measurement in anaesthetised dogs using ACVIM guidelines. J Small Anim Pract 51, 318–324.

Whitehair, K.J., Watney, G.C.G., Leith, D.E., et al., 1990. Pulse oximetry in horses. Vet Surg 19, 243–248.

Winslow, R.M., 2007. The role of hemoglobin oxygen affinity in oxygen transport at high altitude. Resp Physiol Neurobiol 158, 121–127.

Wooten, E.W., 2010. The standard strong ion difference, standard total titratable base, and their relationship to the Boston compensation rules and the Van Slyke equation for extracellular fluid. J Clin Monit Comput 24, 177–188.

Wu, E.Y., Barazanji, K.W., Johnson Jr., R.L., 1997. Sources of error in A-aDO$_2$ calculated from blood stored in plastic and glass syringes. J Appl Physiol 82, 196–202.

Yamashita, K., Ueyama, Y., Miyoshi, K., et al., 2007. Minimally invasive determination of cardiac output by transthoracic bioimpedance, partial carbon dioxide rebreathing, and transesophageal Doppler echocardiography in Beagle dogs. J Vet Med Sci 69, 43–47.

Young, L.E., Blissett, K.J., Bartram, D.H., et al., 1996. Measurement of cardiac output by transoesophageal Doppler echocardiography in anaesthetized horses: Comparison with thermodilution. Br J Anaesth 77, 773–780.

Chapter | 3 |

An introduction to pharmacokinetics

INTRODUCTION

The term pharmacodynamics refers to the relationship between drug concentration and its clinical or pharmacological effect, while pharmacokinetics refers to the mathematical description of the various processes relating to drug movement from the site of its administration, followed by distribution to the tissues and, finally, elimination from the body. To paraphrase, pharmacokinetics is 'what the body does to the drug' whereas pharmacodynamics is 'what the drug does to the body'. However, they cannot be regarded as separate processes for drugs produce effects *in vivo* which alter their own kinetic and dynamic profiles, for example acute haemodynamic effects will influence distribution (Fig. 3.1).

Physical principles

In the account of the pharmacokinetics of inhaled drugs that follows, frequent reference is made to tensions, solubilities and concentrations of gases in solution. These terms may perhaps be best explained by considering specific examples.

Tension (partial pressure), units and atmospheric pressure

The tension of a gas in a liquid is the pressure of the agent in the gas with which the liquid should be in equilibrium. A liquid and a gas, or two liquids, are in equilibrium if, when separated by a permeable membrane, there is no exchange between them. The statement that 'the tension of nitrous oxide in the blood is 50.5 kPa (380 mmHg)'

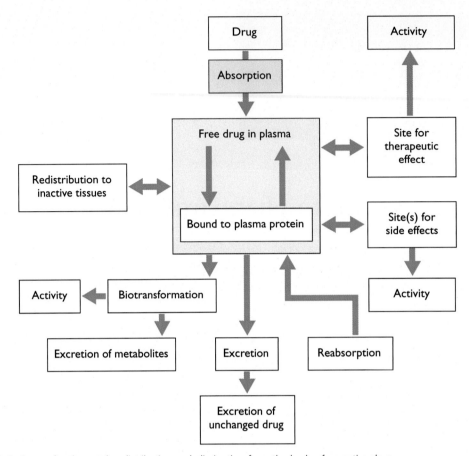

Figure 3.1 Pathways for the uptake, distribution and elimination from the body of an active drug.

means that if a sample of blood were placed in an ambient atmosphere containing nitrous oxide at a concentration of 50% v/v (and, therefore according to Dalton's law, exerting a partial pressure of 50.5 kPa (380 mmHg), there would be no movement of nitrous oxide into or out of the blood. 'Tension' is a term used by physiologists and anaesthetists, while physicists speak of 'partial pressure'.

In the example above, tensions (partial pressures) are given in two units, mmHg, but also in kilopascals (kPa) which is the SI unit and which, as veterinary scientists, we should be using. Reluctance to change is partly due to the fact that atmospheric pressure in weather forecasts is presented in a variety of different units depending on the country. For many years, atmospheric pressure was given to us in mmHg (before that in inches Hg). In Europe, SI units are used, and atmospheric pressure is presented as millibars. A millibar is, in fact, a hectopascal, so 10 millibars = 1 kPa. 'Standard' atmospheric pressure at sea level is approximately 760 mmHg or 1013 millibars (101.3 kPa).

With an inhalation anaesthetic, anaesthesia depends on the tension (partial pressure) of the agent. Minimum alveolar concentration (MAC, see Chapter 1) is expressed as volume %. For example, if at sea level MAC was 1%, a tension of 1% of standard atmospheric, i.e. 7.6 mmHg or 1.01 kPa is what is required to prevent movement in response to stimulation in 50% of animals. However, if anaesthesia is carried out at an elevation of 2000 metres, atmospheric pressure is approximately 80 kPa, so the % of anaesthetic gas required to give a tension of 1.01 kPa is now 1.25 %. Thus, MAC expressed as vol% has to be corrected for the atmospheric pressure (Mapleson, 1996). Fortunately, in clinical practice, most calibrated vaporizers are compensated such that, at any dial setting, they put out a specific partial pressure of the agent, even although the dial says % (see Chapter 10) and so the anaesthetist may not realize that they are administering a higher % (but the same mass) of anaesthetic.

Solubility coefficients of gases

At any given temperature, the mass of a gas dissolved in a solution, i.e. its concentration in the solution, varies directly with its tension (Henry's law) and is governed by the solubility of the gas in the particular solvent. The solubility of anaesthetics varies widely and, therefore, at any one tension, the quantities of the different anaesthetics in the solvent are not equal. The solubility of anaesthetics in the blood and tissues are best expressed in terms of their partition, or distribution, coefficients. For example, the blood–gas partition coefficient of nitrous oxide is 0.47. This means that when blood and alveolar air containing nitrous oxide at a given tension are in equilibrium, there will be 47 parts of nitrous oxide per unit volume (say per litre) of blood for every 100 parts of nitrous oxide per unit volume (litre) of alveolar air. In general, the partition coefficient of a gas at a stated temperature is the ratio, at equilibrium, of the gas's concentration on the two sides of a diffusing membrane or interface.

Tissue solubility does not necessarily correlate with blood–gas solubility. The newer volatile agents (e.g. isoflurane, desflurane, sevoflurane) may have a low blood–gas partition coefficient but their brain–blood partition coefficient is not necessarily lowered to the same extent. The brain–blood partition coefficient can be estimated by dividing the brain–gas with the blood–gas partition coefficient. The brain–blood partition coefficients for halothane, enflurane, isoflurane and desflurane calculate to be 1.86, 1.73, 1.67 and 1.27, respectively. Hence desflurane has a more rapid uptake in the brain tissue. For simplicity, in many theoretical calculations, it is often assumed that in the brain and all other tissues (except fat) gases have very nearly the same solubility as they have in blood because their tissue–blood partition coefficients are sufficiently close to unity.

Concentration of a gas in solution

The concentration of a gas in solution may be expressed in a variety of ways including:

1. The volume of gas which can be extracted from a unit of volume of solution under standard conditions (v/v)
2. The weight of dissolved gas per unit volume of solvent (w/v)
3. The molar concentration, i.e. the number of gram–molecules of gas per litre of solvent. The molar concentration is the most useful – equimolar solutions of gases of different molecular weights contain equal concentrations of molecules. This would not be so if their concentrations in terms of w/v were equal.

PHARMACOKINETICS OF INHALED ANAESTHETICS

Inhaled anaesthetics have a pharmacokinetic profile which results in ease in controlling the depth of anaesthesia as a result of rapid uptake and elimination: a knowledge of this profile can facilitate their use in clinical practice. They cannot be introduced into the brain without at the same time being distributed through the entire body, and this distribution exerts a controlling influence over the rate of the uptake or elimination of the anaesthetic by brain tissue. Even if the inhalation agent is metabolized to a considerable extent (e.g. halothane), such metabolism does not play a clinically significant part in removal of the anaesthetic. Thus, all inhalation anaesthetics may be regarded as essentially inert gases as far as uptake and elimination are concerned.

Uptake of inhaled anaesthetics

If some factors are reduced to their simplest possible terms, and certain assumptions are made, it is possible to give approximate predictions relating to inert gas exchange in the body (Bourne, 1964). These predictions are sufficiently realistic for practical purposes and serve to illustrate the main principles involved. Once these are understood more elaborate expositions found elsewhere (Eger, 1974; 2010; Mapleson, 1989) should become reasonably easy to follow.

For simplicity, the physiological variables such as cardiac output and tidal volume must be assumed to be unaffected by the presence of the gas, and to remain uniform throughout the administration. Allowance cannot be made for alterations in the tidal volume as administration proceeds. The blood supply to the grey matter of the brain must be assumed to be uniform and the gas to be evenly distributed throughout the grey matter. Finally, although in practice anaesthetics are seldom administered in this way, the anaesthetic must be assumed to be given at a fixed inspired concentration, and, what is more, it must be assumed that no rebreathing of gases occurs.

The tensions of the gas in the alveolar blood and tissues all tend to move towards inspired tension (Kety, 1951), but a number of processes, each of which proceeds at its own rate, intervene to delay the eventual saturation of the tissues. The tension of the gas in the brain follows, with a slight delay, its tension in the alveolar air. Since both the rate of induction and recovery from inhalation anaesthesia are governed by the rate of change of the tension of the anaesthetic in the brain, and this in turn is governed by the rate of change of tension in the alveoli, the factors that determine the anaesthetic tension in the alveoli are obviously of very great importance.

The rate at which the tension of an anaesthetic in the alveolar air approaches its tension in the inspired air depends on the pulmonary ventilation, the uptake of the anaesthetic by the blood and tissues, and the inspired concentration. First, by means of pulmonary ventilation the gas is inhaled, diluted with functional residual air, and enters the alveoli. This is where diffusion occurs and normally the alveolar gas equilibrates almost immediately with the pulmonary blood, which is then distributed throughout the body. A second diffusion process occurs across the capillary membranes of the tissues into the interstitial fluid and from there through the cell membranes into the cells themselves. Venous blood leaving the tissues is in equilibrium with the tissue tension. The blood from the tissues returns to the lungs, still carrying some of its original content of anaesthetic, and is again equilibrated with alveolar gas which now contains a slightly higher tension of the anaesthetic. It is in this manner that the alveolar (or arterial) and venous (or tissue) tensions of the anaesthetic in question gradually, and in that order, rise towards eventual equilibrium with the inspired tension.

As this complex process proceeds, the tension of the anaesthetic in the alveolar air increases continuously, but not at a uniform rate. Plotted against time, alveolar tension rises in a curve that is, in general, the same for every inert gas (Fig. 3.2). This curve tails off and slopes gradually upwards until, after several hours or even days, depending on the anaesthetic in question, complete equilibrium is reached. The steep initial rise represents movement of anaesthetic into the lungs, i.e. the pulmonary wash-in phase. The slowly rising tail represents more gradual tissue saturation. The change from steep part of the curve to the tail marks the point at which lung wash-in gives place to tissue saturation as the most important influence. The tail can be very long if the anaesthetic in question has a very high fat/blood partition coefficient.

Blood solubility and alveolar tension

The shape of curve obtained with any given anaesthetic depends on a number of factors. These include such things as minute volume of respiration, the functional residual capacity of the lungs, the cardiac output and the blood flow to the main anaesthetic absorbing bulk of the body – muscles and fat. However, one physical property of the anaesthetic itself is considerably more important than all of these factors – the solubility of the anaesthetic in the blood. This is the factor that determines the height of the 'knee' in the alveolar uptake curve. With anaesthetics of low blood solubility the knee is high; with high solubility the knee is low. This may be illustrated by consideration of the hypothetical extremes of solubility.

A totally insoluble gas would not diffuse into the pulmonary blood and would not be carried in it away from the lungs. If such a gas were inhaled at a constant inspired tension in a non-rebreathing system, its alveolar tension would increase exponentially as lung washout proceeded until, after a very short time, alveolar tension equalled inspired tension (Fig. 3.3). The curve obtained would be all initial rise and there would be no tail. Such a gas could not ever be an anaesthetic, since none would ever reach the brain.

A gas of extremely low blood solubility (see Fig. 3.3, curve B) would give an almost identical curve. The loss into the pulmonary bloodstream of only a minute amount of the gas contained in the lungs at any moment would bring the tension of the gas in the blood into equilibrium with that in the alveolar air. The capacity of the blood for such a gas would be extremely small. Likewise, the capacity of the entire body tissue (with the possible exception of fat) would be small, since as already pointed out, the tissue–blood partition coefficients of most anaesthetics are

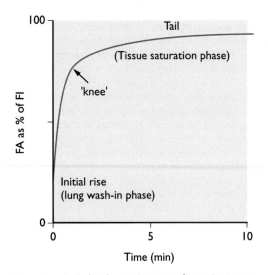

Figure 3.2 Typical alveolar tension curve for an inert gas inhaled at a fixed concentration from a non-rebreathing system.

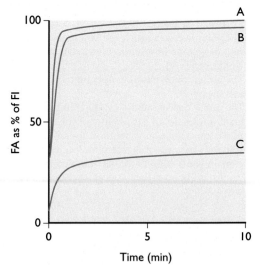

Figure 3.3 Alveolar tension curves for a totally insoluble gas (A), of low solubility (B), (nitrous oxide) and a gas of extremely high solubility (C), all breathed at a constant inspired concentration from a non-rebreathing system.

Table 3.1 Partition coefficients of some inhalation anaesthetics at 37°C

Partition coefficient	Desflurane	Isoflurane	Sevoflurane	Enflurane	Halothane
Blood–gas	0.42	1.40	0.60	2.00	1.94
Tissue–blood					
Brain	1.29	1.57	1.70	2.70	1.94
Heart	1.29	1.61	1.78	1.15	1.84
Liver	1.31	1.75	1.85	3.70	2.07
Muscle	1.02	1.92	3.13	2.20	3.38
Fat	27.20	44.90	47.59	83.00	51.10

close to unity. If such an agent, even when given at the highest permissible concentration of 80% with 20% of oxygen, only produced a faint depression of the central nervous system, it could nevertheless be looked upon as a very active agent because it would be deriving its effect through the presence in the brain of only a minute trace.

At the other hypothetical extreme would be a gas of very nearly infinite solubility in blood. All but a very small fraction of the gas in the lungs at any one moment would dissolve in the pulmonary blood as soon as the blood arrived at the alveoli. The capacity of the blood and body tissues for such a gas would be vast. The alveoli tension curve (see Fig. 3.3, C) would be very flat, with virtually no rapid initial rise and a very slowly rising tail. Given enough time for full equilibrium, it might be possible to achieve very deep anaesthesia by using a minute inspired tension but, of course, in one sense, the gas would be a very weak anaesthetic, since its concentration in the brain would be enormous.

Ranging between these hypothetical extremes of solubility are the gaseous and volatile anaesthetics. Their solubilities in blood and tissues for humans and some animals (figures taken from various sources but mainly from data sheets) are shown in Table 3.1. The effect of the different solubilities on the alveolar tension when the agents are administered at a constant inspired tension are shown in Figure 3.4.

The tension of anaesthetic agents in brain tissue

In addition to the alveolar tensions, the anaesthetist is also concerned with the tension of anaesthetic agents in the grey matter of the brain. In the lungs (unless pathological changes are present), diffusion from the alveolar air to the blood is almost instantaneous, so that for theoretical purposes the tension in the arterial blood leaving the lungs can be regarded as equal to the tension in the alveolar air. Only when the body has become absolutely saturated does the arterial tension equal the tissue tension. During the saturation process, and after the administration is stopped, the tissue tension is accurately represented by the

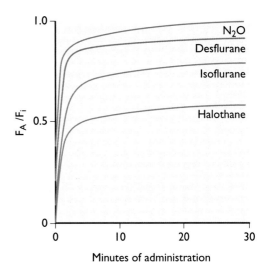

Figure 3.4 Increase in alveolar tension (FA) towards inspired tension (FI) during administration at a fixed concentration in a non-rebreathing system. Effect of blood solubility. The curves are not drawn accurately and only represent approximate, relative curves.

tension of the agent in the venous blood leaving that tissue. This lags behind the arterial tension by an amount that depends mainly upon the blood supply to the tissue. Fatty tissues are exceptions to this rule for, in them, the relative solubilities play an important part. In organs with a rich blood supply such as the brain and heart, the venous tension rises quite quickly to the arterial tension. After about 20 minutes (in humans) with anaesthetics whose solubility in grey matter is about equal to that in blood, or perhaps 40 minutes in the case of agents like halothane which are a little more soluble in grey matter, arterial and grey matter tensions, during uptake and during elimination, are almost equal (see Fig. 3.3).

It follows from these considerations that if a gas has a low blood solubility, any change in its tension in the alveolar air is quickly reflected in the grey matter in the brain, whereas if the blood solubility is high there will be a considerable delay because the whole body will act as a very large buffer. Thus, with an inhalation anaesthetic, the speed with which induction of anaesthesia can be carried out (when the inspired tension is kept constant) is governed by the solubility of the anaesthetic in the blood. Low solubility (e.g. desflurane) favours rapid induction, whereas high blood solubility (e.g. methoxyflurane) leads to slow induction. The important point to note here is, of course, that so far all arguments have been based on the assumption that the inspired concentration is maintained constant. In fact, alteration of the inspired tension can do much to overcome the slow induction with agents of high blood solubility. For example, if in animals, methoxyflurane were given at concentrations that would give satisfactory anaesthesia after full equilibration, induction might take many hours. It would be a very long time before the animal even lost consciousness. In practice, this difficulty is overcome by starting the administration with a much higher concentration, which would, if administered indefinitely, kill the animal. As the desired level of anaesthesia is reached, the inspired concentration is reduced. However, the maximum concentration that can be administered is limited by the volatility of the anaesthetic, and its pungency.

Recovery from anaesthesia

When the administration of the anaesthetic is terminated, its concentration in the inspired air cannot be reduced (wash-out phase) to below zero. Although the full buffering effect of the body tissues will not be seen after accelerated inductions and brief administration (those tissues with a poor blood supply or high tissue–blood partition coefficient will then be only very incompletely saturated), elimination of the more soluble anaesthetics will take time and recovery will be slow. Low blood solubility leads to rapid elimination of anaesthetics like desflurane and rapid recovery from anaesthesia.

At the end of anaesthesia, the volume of nitrous oxide eliminated causes the minute volume of expiration to exceed the inspired volume and this outpouring of nitrous oxide dilutes the alveolar content of oxygen. If the animal is breathing room air, the alveolar oxygen tension can fall to low levels, resulting in a severe reduction in PaO_2. This phenomenon, called 'diffusion hypoxia' can also happen if nitrous oxide is cut off during anaesthesia. Theoretically, it can happen with any agent, but it is unlikely to have any ill effects with very soluble agents, because of the small volumes involved and the slow excretion of the agent. The danger is greatest if two insoluble agents (e.g. nitrous oxide and desflurane) are administered together.

Speed of uptake and elimination related to safety of inhalation agents

Blood solubility is not only important as a factor influencing the speed of induction and recovery. It has wider implications; it determines (in an inverse manner) the extent to which tissue tensions keep pace with alterations in inspired tension and thus it controls the rate at which anaesthesia can be deepened or lightened. With a very soluble agent, such as diethyl ether or methoxyflurane, no sudden change in tissue tension is possible; if gross overdosage is given, the anaesthetist has plenty of time in which to observe the signs of deepening unconsciousness and to reduce the concentration of the inhaled mixture. With an anaesthetic of low blood solubility, such as sevoflurane, however, increase in tissue tension follows very quickly after an increase in the inspired tension; anaesthesia may deepen rapidly and a gross overdose may result. It is, therefore, very important with the less soluble anaesthetics to consider carefully the factors that favour the giving of an overdose, the chief of which must be volatility and potency.

Volatility

Volatility governs the potential strength of the inspired mixture for, obviously, the more volatile the anaesthetic, the greater the risk of its being administered at a high concentration. Gaseous anaesthetics and liquid anaesthetics which have low boiling points are, therefore, potentially dangerous.

Potency

With most drugs, potency determines the magnitude of a possible overdose. With inhalation anaesthetics, however, usually MAC is taken as a measure of potency (Eger et al., 1965; White, 2003). However, MAC is not a measurement of the potential to overdose, as the physical characteristics of some anaesthetics mean that it is impossible to obtain many multiples of MAC. With a weak anaesthetic such as nitrous oxide, overdose is impossible; if it were not for lack of oxygen, nitrous oxide could be given at 100% concentration without danger. However, depending on species, isoflurane has a MAC of 1.3 % (i.e. a tension of 1.3 kPa or approximately 10 mmHg); its saturated vapour pressure at 20°C is 31.5 kPa (236 mmHg) so, theoretically, it is possible to give approximately 25× MAC. Fortunately, modern calibrated vaporizers prevent this from happening.

Uptake and elimination of inhalation anaesthetics in clinical practice

The various assumptions made for the purpose of theoretical or mathematical predictions of inhalational anaesthetic uptake and elimination cannot be made in everyday practice. Many of the factors which have to be regarded as constant if any mathematical prediction is to be made, do, in fact, vary considerably during the course of anaesthesia. These factors include the tidal volume, the physiological dead space, the functional residual capacity (FRC – that volume of gas in the lungs which dilutes each single breath of anaesthetic), the thickness and permeability of the alveolar–capillary membrane, the cardiac output and pulmonary blood flow (which may be different, especially in pathological conditions of the lungs), regional variations in ventilation/perfusion relationships in the lungs, the blood flow through the tissues of the body, the partition coefficients of the anaesthetic between the gaseous or vapour state and lung tissue or blood, and between blood and the body tissues, and the blood flow diffusion coefficient and diffusion distance for each of the tissues of the body.

In addition, the anaesthetics themselves may modify many of the variables as administration proceeds. For example, most anaesthetics depress breathing and reduce the cardiac output. Considerations such as these indicate only too clearly why it is not yet possible to give a complete account of the uptake and elimination of inhalation anaesthetics as encountered in clinical practice.

Other factors affecting inhalation anaesthetic administration

The vaporizer

Modern vaporizers are capable of delivering very accurate concentrations; limitations are described in Chapter 10 (see also Fig. 3.5). The vaporizers are designed so that, at maximal output, they give the number of MAC multiples that are considered safe for induction of anaesthesia in humans. This is, however, an inspired concentration that can kill if maintained for too long. Older vaporizers which may be inaccurate or non-compensated vaporizers are still in use in veterinary anaesthesia and these will not provide the same safety factor.

The breathing system

The fresh gas that flows into the breathing system (circuit) is diluted by the expired alveolar gas, causing a difference between the concentration of the inflowing gas and the

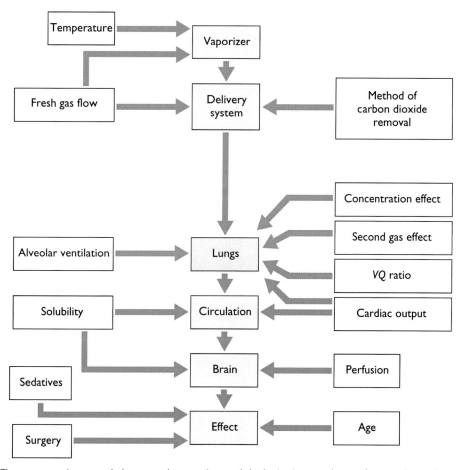

Figure 3.5 The concentration cascade between the vaporizer and the brain tissue and some factors which influence it.

concentration which is actually inspired. The lower the fresh gas flow rates, the greater this difference becomes. Absorption by tubing and any absorbent used to remove carbon dioxide, as well as high anaesthetic uptake by the animal, may also increase this difference. At the beginning of anaesthesia, anaesthetic agent may be 'taken up' by the soda lime. Wet soda lime absorbs much less of volatile anaesthetics than when it is relatively dry. A variable amount of the anaesthetic may be absorbed in the tubing of the breathing system. There is a large difference between materials.

In a circle system, the fresh gas utilization will vary widely depending on the arrangement of the system components. An arrangement with the spill-off valve between the fresh gas inlet and the lungs will result in lower fresh gas utilization. Better characteristics with greater utilization are found where the spill-off valve closes during inspiration and is as close to the lungs as possible.

The lungs

Depending on how much fresh gas reaches the lungs and how much anaesthetic is carried away in the arterialized blood, there will be a variable concentration difference between the inspired and arterial concentrations of the anaesthetic. The inspired concentration of the agent is the easiest parameter to be changed by the anaesthetist in order to influence the uptake and elimination of the anaesthetic.

With higher alveolar ventilation, there is a more rapid increase in the alveolar uptake curve. Depending on the properties of the anaesthetic agent (see Chapter 7), during spontaneous ventilation the animal has some limited protection against overdosage because volatile anaesthetics depress ventilation, but although this reduces the speed of further uptake, it also reduces the elimination of any overdose that has already occurred. Respiratory depression should not be relied upon to prevent overdosage (as has been suggested when draw-over non-compensated vaporizers are employed 'in circle'), as such respiratory depression is likely also to be accompanied by cardiovascular depression.

Nitrous oxide, because it can be given in high concentration, increases alveolar ventilation and thus its own uptake via the concentration effect, in particular when the animal is hypoventilated and highly soluble agents are used (Eger, 1963). For example, if halothane or sevoflurane is used in low concentrations, its uptake is increased as well (second gas effect) due to the additional inspiratory inflow by the concentration effect of the nitrous oxide (Epstein et al., 1964; Peyton et al., 2008).

Cardiac output

Cardiac output is another major determinant of inhaled anaesthetic uptake. The higher the cardiac output the more anaesthetic agent is removed from the alveolar gas and the slower is the rise in alveolar concentration. The volatile anaesthetic agents all depress cardiac output and, while with spontaneous ventilation a protective negative feed back exists with respect to high concentrations, the reverse is true for the circulation because, due to the depressed circulation, less of the agent is removed from the alveoli so that alveolar concentration rises more rapidly.

PHARMACOKINETICS OF INTRAVENOUS ANAESTHETICS

The pharmacokinetics of the intravenous agents, i.e. the processes by which drug concentrations at effector sites are achieved, maintained and diminished after intravenous (IV) injection, is of increasing importance today because of the use of computer models to study drug uptake and elimination, and the use of microprocessors to control anaesthetic administration. For a more detailed account of their pharmacokinetics than follows here reference should be made to standard textbooks of pharmacology (e.g. Shafer et al., 2010; Buxton & Benet, 2011).

Pharmacokinetic variables commonly reported for IV or otherwise parenterally administered drugs are total apparent volume of distribution, total elimination clearance, and elimination half-life.

Total apparent volume of distribution

The total apparent volume of distribution (V_d) relates the amount of drug in the body to the plasma or blood concentration:

$$V_d = \text{amount of drug/drug concentration}$$

A frequently reported total volume of distribution is the volume of distribution at steady state, V_{dss}, the total apparent volume a drug would have if it were in equilibrium with all body tissues. Another commonly reported, and usually larger, total volume of distribution is $V_{d\beta}$ which, together with elimination clearance (Cl_E), determines the elimination half-life.

In theory, a volume of distribution is measured by injecting a known quantity of the drug and, after allowing an adequate period of time for it to distribute, determining its concentration (both free and combined) in the plasma. In practice, the equilibrium necessary is seldom attained because, before it is complete, the opposing processes of metabolism or excretion come into operation.

A knowledge of the apparent volume of distribution makes it possible to calculate the doses to be administered initially and subsequently to achieve desired concentrations in the blood and tissues.

Total elimination clearance (Cl$_E$) and elimination half-life (t$_{1/2\beta}$)

Cl$_E$ is an independent variable relating the rate of irreversible drug removal from the body to the plasma or blood concentration:

$$Cl_E = \text{rate of elimination/drug concentration}$$

Thus, Cl$_E$ is the sum of the elimination clearances of all the organs and tissues of the body, principally the liver and the kidneys. The elimination half-life, t$_{1/2\beta}$, is a dependent variable and is the time required for the amount of drug in the body to decrease by one-half:

$$t_{1/2\beta} = \ln 2 \times V_{d\beta}/Cl_E$$

$$\text{or, } t_{1/2\beta} = 0.693 \times V_{d\beta}/Cl_E.$$

These pharmacokinetic variables can be useful for drugs with a rapid onset of action, such as IV administered propofol, but they do not provide a complete description of their pharmacokinetics. The total volume of distribution is not realized until after extensive drug distribution and redistribution has occurred. Thus, predicted early drug concentrations based on the dose and V$_{dss}$ will be very low. Although elimination clearance begins from the time the drug arrives at the clearing organs, the relatively slow decline in drug concentrations due to elimination clearance becomes a significant factor in the relationship of plasma (or blood) concentration with time only after the initial rapid decline due to the distribution and redistribution phase is over (Fig. 3.6).

It is now appreciated that the offset of clinical effect is not simply a function of half-life. It may be affected by the rate of equilibration between plasma and effector site and duration of infusion. Hughes et al. (1992) proposed the use of context-sensitive half-time (t$_{1/2}$ context) and defined this as the time for the plasma concentration to decrease by 50% after termination of an IV infusion designed to maintain a constant plasma concentration. Context refers to the duration of infusion. They demonstrated that context-sensitive half-lives of commonly used IV anaesthetic agents and opioids could differ markedly from elimination half-lives and were dependent on duration of infusion.

Compartmental models

Drugs injected into a vein are distributed directly in the bloodstream to the brain and the other tissues of the body. Those given by the alimentary route (by mouth or high into the rectum) must first be absorbed into the blood and they then pass through the liver before reaching the central nervous system. Passage through the liver (the 'first pass') is avoided if the drugs are given via the mucous membranes of the nose, the terminal rectum, or sublingually, so that administration of suitable drugs by these routes renders the effective dose similar to that needed by the intravenous route. Elimination of these drugs from the body is not a reversal of the process of absorption; they are broken down, mostly in the liver, and are then excreted mainly by the kidneys.

When a drug is administered by IV injection, the onset and duration of its effect depend on the distribution to the tissues, tissue binding and access to those tissues where the pharmacological effect takes place, interaction with receptor sites, and elimination by various routes (see Fig. 3.1). Since the body is composed of innumerable tissue zones, each with a unique blend of perfusion, binding affinity, etc. for the drug, quantification of the whole process is nearly impossible unless some gross simplifications can be made. For any particular drug, the body can be thought of as comprising one or more compartments, each of which can be considered as a space throughout which the substance is uniformly distributed and has uniform kinetics of distribution or transport.

Secondary dispersion of highly lipid-soluble drugs such as the IV anaesthetic agents occurs as they cross cell membranes and the limiting factor to this process is the rate at which they are delivered to the cells – the blood flow to the tissues. Thus, organs with a rapid blood flow (e.g. brain, heart, liver, kidney) initially receive a high concentration of the drug but, with time, this is depleted as the agent redistributes into moderately and slowly perfused tissues (the muscles and fat, respectively). The greater the lipid solubility of the drug the more rapid its redistribution, but even charged drugs can be redistributed. Redistribution also means that repeated doses of the drug can exert prolonged effects due to the gradual passage over an extended period from saturated sites where it is inactive, back into the plasma. Plasma and the organs where blood

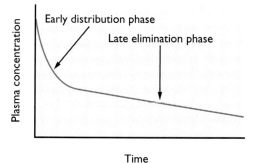

Figure 3.6 Plasma concentration versus time relationship following rapid intravenous administration of a drug such as propofol, illustrating the rapid decline in plasma drug concentration during the early distributional (α) phase and the much slower decline in the terminal (β) elimination phase.

flow is rapid can be taken to represent one 'compartment', while moderately and poorly perfused tissues represent second and third compartments.

The one compartment model

When drugs behave as if they were distributed into a single uniform compartment, excretion takes place according to 'first order' kinetics, i.e. in any time period a constant proportion of the remaining drug will be eliminated; the elimination rate is proportional to the concentration. When a drug concentration decreases in this constant proportion manner, the concentration curve can be defined by a simple exponential equation:

$$C/C^0 = e^{-kt}$$

where C = drug concentration at time t; C^0 = drug concentration at time 0 (i.e. immediately after IV administration); k = a constant; t = time elapsed; and e = the base of the natural logarithm (2.718).

Taking the natural logarithm of both sides of the equation, a linear equation results:

$$\ln(C/C^0) = -kt \text{ or } \ln(C/C^0)/t = -k$$

Thus, the natural logarithm of the proportion by which C has decreased to time is a constant (k) which has the dimension of rate and will be stated in reciprocal units (t^{-1}). From this it follows that a graph of $\ln(C/C^0)$ against time will yield a straight line, of gradient −k. In practice, very few drugs behave according to one compartment kinetics, since some initial redistribution from the circulation to other tissues is almost inevitable. The majority of drugs can be regarded as obeying what are known as zero order or first order kinetics.

A zero order process is one that occurs at a constant rate and is, therefore, independent of the quantity of drug present at the particular sites of absorption or removal. A zero order process requires a large excess of drug available on the entry side (e.g. intravenous infusion) or, on the removal side, a system of limited capacity.

A first order process is considered to be the most common for both drug absorption and elimination. In a first order process, the rate of the reaction is exponentially related to the amount of drug available. In other words, a constant fraction of the drug is absorbed or eliminated in constant time. The rate constants (k_{ab} and k_{el}) are measurements of these fractions since they represent the fraction of the drug present which is absorbed or eliminated in unit time (usually in 1 minute or 1 hour).

A very simplified example of a first order elimination is shown in Figure 3.7 where the natural logarithm (ln) of the plasma concentration of a drug given by a single IV injection is plotted against time. Under these conditions, a plot of ln plasma concentration versus time is linear. The

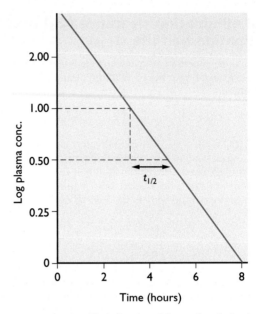

Figure 3.7 Simplified diagram of first order elimination from the plasma of an intravenous drug. The plot of log plasma concentration versus time is linear.

time taken for the plasma concentration to halve ($t_{1/2}$) is known as the plasma half-life. V_d can be calculated for the initial concentration (i.e. that at zero time) and from this, by assuming V_d to be constant over the whole time period (which, in practice, it seldom is), the clearance from the plasma can be calculated. A more accurate method assumes (usually incorrectly) that the clearance from the plasma is a constant fraction of the instantaneous level, thus:

Plasma clearance (C_1)

$$= \frac{\text{Original dose}}{\text{Area under curve to complete elimination.}}$$

The area under the curve (AUC) is obtained from a graph of the actual (not log concentration) against time. A drug with a high C_1 will have a lower AUC than one with a lower C_1 given at the same dose. A drug given to an animal with a reduced C_1 resulting from disease will have a higher AUC than the same drug administered to an animal with a normal C_1. It follows from this that the diseased animal will be exposed to a higher drug concentration for a longer period of time and greater and more persistent drug effects can be produced unless the dose of the drug is reduced.

What is known as 'the plateau principle' applies when a drug undergoes zero order absorption and first order elimination. Under these conditions, it can be shown that when the concentration of the drug being administered is changed, the time taken to reach a steady state (plateau)

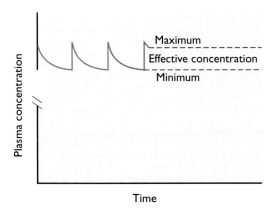

Figure 3.8 Intermittent intravenous dosage to maintain an effective anaesthetic concentration. Single compartment model.

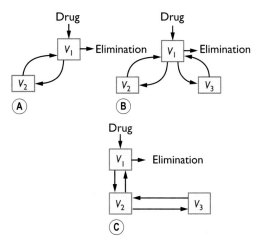

Figure 3.9 (A) Two compartment model. (B) Mamillary three compartment model. (C) Catenary three compartment model. In the mamillary three compartment model, both V_2 and V_3 exchange with V_1, whereas in the catenary model, V_3 is 'deep' to V_2 and is not connected in any way to V_1. This catenary model has been proposed for some drug metabolites and has characteristics of its own.

level is determined solely by the reciprocal of k_{el}. The height of the plateau reached depends on the concentration of the drug administered and when this height is attained, the amount of drug given is reduced to maintain it. Similar principles apply when a loading dose is followed by subsequent doses to maintain this level (Fig. 3.8). About 97% of a drug will be eliminated from the plasma in about $5 \times t_{1/2}$ (i.e. 50% + 25% + 12.5% + 6.25% + 3.125%).

The two compartment model

Frequently, the serial plasma concentrations after the intravenous administration of a drug show an initial rapid decay (the α phase), followed by a linear decline (the β phase) when plotted on the same semi-logarithmic axes. The curve of best fit is a bi-exponential decay, which is characteristic of drug concentration in the central compartment (V_1) of a two compartment system where the drug is assumed to enter V_1, from which it is also eliminated. A second peripheral compartment (V_2) receives drug by redistribution from V_1 but elimination of the drug does not take place except by transfer back to V_1 (Fig. 3.9).

In the two compartment model, the half-life is expressed as $t_{1/2\beta}$ which makes it clear that it is limited to the β (elimination) phase of the decay, but it depends on both elimination and distribution rates so that it cannot be regarded as a direct indicator of elimination rate.

The multicompartment model

A three compartment model has been used to explain a curve of declining drug concentration which does not fit in a conveniently bi-exponential fashion and better fits a three-exponential equation. However, great care must

be exercised when expanding the number of terms, since the 'degrees of freedom' in the regression equations are progressively reduced, thus widening the confidence interval for the line. In other words, although a more complex curve may fit measured concentration points better, the probability of it being correct diminishes. There are two types of three compartment models. In one, the 'mamillary' model, both peripheral compartments (V_2 and V_3) connect to the central compartment (V_1). For some drug metabolites, a different, 'catenary', model has been proposed where V_3 is 'deep' to V_2, but is not connected to V_1 and has quite different characteristics.

Rarely can a plasma decay curve be defined so precisely as to permit justification of more than three exponential terms. Moreover, the compartments cannot be equated with true anatomical volumes. The use of 'perfusion models' overcomes many difficulties to some extent, but these require much more information. The perfusion model takes a number of anatomically defined compartments and, by consideration of their volumes, blood flow rates through them and tissue/blood partition coefficients computes the movement of drug between them. Unfortunately, with the possible exception of propofol in the dog, for most agents, there is inadequate information available for accurate prediction. Moreover, the tissue/blood partition coefficients vary widely because of the wide range of solubilities in the various tissues, and in different species. Thus, the perfusion model is limited by the number of identifiable tissues or organs for which reliable data are available.

Practical methods of drug delivery during intravenous anaesthesia

It is possible to improve the titration of intravenous drugs by administering continuous variable rate infusions rather than by injecting intermittent bolus doses. Continuous infusion is the logical extension of the more traditional incremental bolus dose method which inevitably leads to fluctuations in blood (and hence brain) concentrations that follow each bolus dose (see Fig. 3.8). To achieve an effective blood concentration rapidly, a 'loading dose' is administered; the loading dose is then continued by infusions at suitable rates to maintain anaesthesia at the depth required.

In practice, intravenous infusions are generally titrated on an empirical basis depending on the response of the animal to the infusion rate. However, the aim for the future is to predict the dosage requirements from pharmacokinetic data. The smaller the loading dose, the greater the initial maintenance infusion rate needed because the amount of drug infused must be equal to that which is removed from the brain by both distribution and elimination processes. With time, distribution assumes less importance, and the infusion rate required to maintain any given blood concentration becomes solely dependent on the elimination rate. Thus, the infusion rate needed to maintain a given concentration in the body decreases as a function of the infusion period. In other words, the minimal infusion rate becomes 'context sensitive'.

Ideally, the anaesthetist would like to know the concentration of the anaesthetic agent attained and maintained at its site of effect (i.e. the brain) but, as may be guessed from the above considerations, this is rarely possible. All that can be said is that the plasma or blood drug concentration is often related to, and is a valid measure of, the required quantity so that $t_{1/2}$ is, usually, the paramount determinant of dose frequency when intermittent administration is practised. The main difficulties in devising suitable computer controlled infusion regimens for the induction and maintenance of IV anaesthesia arise from the variable response of individual subjects (Fig. 3.10). The future of computer-controlled infusions for administering intravenous anaesthetics will depend on their safety, reliability, cost-effectiveness and 'user friendliness'.

Target controlled infusions (TCI)

Considerations of the points discussed above have led to the establishment of two or three stages in computer

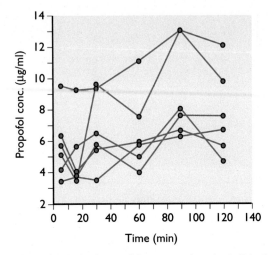

Figure 3.10 Blood propofol concentrations (μg/mL) in 6 dogs (Beagles) after an induction dose of 7 mg/kg followed by an infusion of 0.4 mg/kg/min, illustrating the tendency of blood concentrations to rise when the infusion rate is kept constant throughout 120 minutes of anaesthesia.

controlled infusion regimens following a loading dose or initial high infusion rate. In human anaesthesia, a syringe-driven system was specifically designed for propofol, the Diprifusor (Glen, 1998), and later a similar version for remifentanil, the Remifusor (Hoymork et al., 2003). These drug-specific syringe-drivers have increased in sophistication over the last few years and are accepted 'medical technology'. Their computer base uses pharmacokinetic data coupled with patient data of weight/agent etc. to calculate the infusion rates necessary to reach and maintain a set plasma propofol level. TCI with propofol and remifentanil using this apparatus have been investigated in dogs (Beths et al., 2001; Musk et al., 2005; Musk & Flaherty, 2007).

The dedicated TCI infusers are expensive. Another method of TCI is to use a special Windows-based computer program (Rugloop©) to drive the syringe. The company claims that the program contains a complete TCI model database for most common IV anaesthetic drugs. Its claim is only to be for marketed for experimental use only, but it includes veterinary software, and has been used experimentally with propofol in dogs (Bras et al., 2009).

REFERENCES

Beths, T., Glen, J.B., Reid, J., et al., 2001. Evaluation and optimisation of a target-controlled infusion system for administering propofol to dogs as

part of a total intravenous anaesthetic technique during dental surgery. Vet Rec 148, 198–203.

Bourne, J.G., 1964. Uptake, elimination and potency of the inhalational anaesthetics. Anaesthesia 19, 12–32.

Bras, S., Bressan, N., Ribeiro, L., et al., 2009. A step towards effect-site target-controlled infusion with propofol in dogs: a k(e0) for propofol. J Vet Pharmacol Ther 32, 182–188.

Buxton, I.L.O., Benet, L.Z., 2011. Pharmacokinetics. In: Brunton, L.L. (Ed.), Goodman & Gilmans's The Pharmacological Basis of Therapeutics, twelfth ed. McGraw Hill Medical, New York.

Eger II, E.I., 1963. Effect of inspired anesthetic concentration on the rate of rise of alveolar concentration. Anesthesiology 24, 153–157.

Eger 2nd, E.I., Saidman, L.J., Brandstater, B., 1965. Minimum alveolar anesthetic concentration: a standard of anesthetic potency. Anesthesiology 26, 756–763.

Eger II, E.I., 1974. Anesthetic Uptake and Action. Williams and Wilkins, Baltimore.

Eger II, E.I., 2010. Inhaled anaesthetics: Uptake and distribution. In: Millar, R.D. (Ed.), Miller's Anesthesia, seventh ed. Churchill Livingstone, New York, pp. 539–560.

Epstein, R.M., Rackow, H., Salanitre, E., Wolf, G.L., 1964. Influence of the concentration effect on the uptake of anesthetic mixtures: the second gas effect. Anesthesiology 25, 364–371.

Glen, J.B., 1998. The development of 'Diprifusor': a TCI system for propofol. Anaesthesia 53 (Suppl 1), 13–21.

Hoymork, S.C., Raeder, J., Grimsmo, B., et al., 2003. Bispectral index, serum drug concentrations and emergence associated with individually adjusted target-controlled infusions of remifentanil and propofol for laparoscopic surgery. Br J Anaesth 91, 773–780.

Hughes, M.A., Glass, P.S.A., Jacobs, J.R., 1992. Context-sensitive half-time in multicompartment pharmacokinetic models for intravenous anaesthetic drugs. Anesthesiology 76 (3), 334–341.

Kety, S.S., 1951. The theory and applications of the exchange of inert gas at the lungs and tissues. Pharmacol Rev (Baltimore) 3, 1–41.

Mapleson, W.W., 1989. Pharmacokinetics of inhalational anaesthetics. In: General Anaesthesia, fifth ed. Nunn, Utting & Brown, London, pp. 44–59.

Mapleson, W.W., 1996. Effect of age on MAC in humans: a meta-analysis. Br J Anaesth 76, 179–185.

Musk, G.C., Flaherty, D.A., 2007. Target-controlled infusion of propofol combined with variable rate infusion of remifentanil for anaesthesia of a dog with patent ductus arteriosus. Vet Anaesth Analg 34, 359–364.

Musk, G.C., Pang, D.S., Beths, T., et al., 2005. Target-controlled infusion of propofol in dogs – evaluation of four targets for induction of anaesthesia. Vet Rec 157, 766–770.

Peyton, P.J., Horriat, M., Robinson, G.J., et al., 2008. Magnitude of the second gas effect on arterial sevoflurane partial pressure. Anesthesiology 108, 381–387.

Shafer, S.L., Flood, P., Schwinn, D.A., 2010. Basic principles of pharmacology. In: Millar, R.D. (Ed.), Miller's Anesthesia, seventh ed. Churchill Livingstone, New York, pp. 479–495.

White, D., 2003. Uses of MAC. Br J Anaesth 91, 167–169.

Chapter | 4 |

Principles of sedation, anticholinergic agents, and principles of premedication

TERMINOLOGY

The terminology used in pharmacology and medical anaesthesia textbooks to describe drugs which act on the central nervous system undergoes regular change as understanding of the modes of action evolves. The term *hypnotic* is used regularly for a depressant of the central nervous system, which enables the animal to go to sleep more easily, or a drug used to intensify the depth of sleep. The animal may be aroused by stimulus. However, the term 'hypnosis' is also used for the 'sleep' component of anaesthesia (see Chapter 1). The term *sedative* appears to be rarely used in medical literature, but can be considered to be a drug which relieves anxiety and, as a result, tends to make it easier for the patient to rest or sleep – they are usually associated with drowsiness. Many drugs fall into both the sedative and the hypnotic categories, the differentiation usually being related to dose. They are best considered as one group, exemplified by α_2-adrenoceptor agonists (α_2-agonists) such as dexmedetomidine where low doses cause drowsiness and higher doses cause sleep. The term *tranquillizer* (or *ataractic*) appears now used only in the veterinary texts but previously was considered to be a drug with a predominant action in relieving anxiety without producing undue sedation and that will affect mood and behaviour.

There is considerable overlap between the action of CNS depressant drugs. Benzodiazepines are considered to be both anxiolytics and sedative/hypnotics. Drugs such as phenothiazines, now classified as antipsychotic in the medical literature, are those previously termed *neuroleptics*. They reduce psychomotor agitation, exerting their effects by blocking dopamine-mediated responses in the central nervous system. Overdose causes marked extrapyramidal symptoms and parkinsonian-type tremor. However, the dopamine-blocking effects of such drugs mean that they are now also considered to contribute to anaesthesia (see Chapter 1). The term 'tranquillizer' is still loosely used in clinical anaesthesia to cover both the anxiolytics and antipsychotics and will continue to be used in places in this and later chapters.

The multiplicity of definitions is confusing, but understanding of the major actions of the drugs is important in order to appreciate their limitations. For example, if drugs such as the benzodiazepines are used for premedication, they will not quieten a fit animal, but may make it more difficult to handle by removing its inhibitions, so that vicious animals become more likely to bite or kick. By reducing nervousness, phenothiazine derivatives may make an animal more liable to sleep, but will not make the vicious animal easier to handle, no matter what dose is given. Effective sedation depends on selection of the drug appropriate for the procedure, the species of animal, its temperament and condition, and must allow for possible side effects. Drug combinations are often more effective in controlling animals than high doses of an individual drug. Where 'sedative' and 'tranquillizing' drugs are used for premedication, low doses are usually utilized and their effects on the subsequent depth and duration of anaesthesia must be taken into account. In all cases, it is important that the animal is left undisturbed for an adequate period of time after administration of the sedative because stimulation during the onset of the drug's action may prevent the full effect from developing. To sedate an animal that is in pain, a suitable analgesic must be used, possibly in combination with a sedative drug, because most sedative drugs themselves have little or no analgesic activity and may cause exaggerated reactions to painful stimulation.

During the past three decades, major pharmacological advances have been made in the recognition of specific drug receptor sites and of the actions resulting from their stimulation or blockade. These advances have been followed by synthesis of potent drugs, which act as agonists or as antagonists at such sites. These advances have resulted in a better understanding of the actions of existing drugs, in newer and more potent agonist drugs, and of antagonists enabling the reversal of some sedative agent effects.

PHENOTHIAZINE DERIVATIVES

This group of drugs still has a major role both in human psychiatric medicine and in veterinary anaesthesia. They are classified as antipsychotic drugs (or in older terminology 'neuroleptics'). They are dopamine antagonists, but also block α_1-adrenoceptors. The degree of activity in different pharmacological actions varies from one compound to another. All have a wide range of central and peripheral effects which have been well reviewed (Tobin & Ballard, 1979; Lees, 1979).

Being dopamine antagonists, they have calming and mood-altering (antipsychotic) effects, and also a powerful antiemetic action, particularly against opioid induced vomiting. The degree of sedation produced varies between drugs. They are metabolized by the liver, and long-term dosage can lead to liver damage. In medical practice, sedation is an unwanted side effect but, in veterinary medicine, the phenothiazine derivatives are used primarily for this purpose. In general, they are not considered to have analgesic activity, although methotrimeprazine is claimed to be a powerful analgesic in humans. Their major cardiovascular side effects are related to their ability to block α_1-adrenoceptors, and thus having an antiepinephrine (antiadrenaline) effect. This results in a fall in arterial blood pressure primarily due to peripheral vasodilatation, and a decrease in packed cell volume caused by splenic dilation. Phenothazines exert an antiarrhythmic effect on the heart (Muir et al., 1975; Muir, 1981) that was originally thought to be due to a quinidine action on the cardiac membrane (Lees, 1979) but may be caused by a blocking action on the cardiac α-arrhythmic receptors (Maze et al., 1985; Dresel, 1985). The phenothiazines have a spasmolytic action on the gut although, at least in horses, gut motility is not reduced (Davies & Gerring, 1983). However, as they cause relaxation of the cardiac sphincter, in ruminants they increase the chance of regurgitation should an animal become recumbent. Phenothiazines have varying degrees of antihistamine activity and also produce a partial cholinergic block. All cause a fall in body temperature partly due to increased heat loss through dilated cutaneous vessels and partly through resetting of thermoregulatory mechanisms. In spite of all their side effects, the phenothiazines are well tolerated by the majority of normovolaemic animals.

Although promethazine is used as an antihistamine, the most commonly used phenothiazine today in the UK, North America and Australasia is acepromazine. Other derivatives such as chlorpromazine, propionylpromazine and promazine are or have been used elsewhere.

Acepromazine

Acepromazine, also known as ACP (its original trade name) or as ace, is the 2-acetyl derivative of promazine and has the chemical name 2–acetyl-10-(3-dimethylaminopropyl) phenothiazine. It is prepared as the maleate, a yellow crystalline solid. It is metabolized in the liver and both conjugated and non-conjugated metabolites are excreted in the urine. Some of these metabolites are detectable for a considerable period (McGree et al., 2013). Although available for over 50 years, it remains widely used in veterinary medicine for sedation, premedication, and a range of non-anaesthetic related indications. It continues to be the subject of a huge number of scientific publications.

Like all phenothiazine drugs, with low doses there are effects on behaviour and, as the dose is increased, sedation occurs but the dose–response curve rapidly reaches a plateau after which higher doses do not increase, but only lengthen sedation and increase side effects (Tobin & Ballard, 1979). Further increase in doses may cause excitement and extrapyramidal signs. In many animals, sedation may be achieved with intramuscular (IM) doses as low as 0.03 mg/kg, although the drug has been used safely at ten times this dose when prolonged effects were required. A calming effect on the behaviour of excitable animals can be seen at doses even below 0.03 mg/kg, making acepromazine a drug liable to abuse especially in the greyhound and the equine sporting field. The length of action is dose dependent but can be prolonged. Clinically obvious sedation lasts 4–6 hours after doses of 0.02 mg/kg. In horses, Parry et al. (1982) considered that there were detectable residual effects for 12 hours after doses of 0.1 mg/kg, and for 16–24 hours after 0.15 mg/kg IM. In general, the apparent sedation is not as great as that which can been achieved with α_2-agonists, although owners of giant breeds of dog often complain that their animals are sedated for several days following acepromazine administration. Despite this, there are many situations where acepromazine is the sedative drug of choice.

In practice, the dose is chosen in relation to the length of sedation required and the purpose for which it is needed. However, the drug cannot be relied upon to give sedation in all animals; some individuals fail to become sedated and, in these, other drugs or drug combinations must be employed. Excitement reactions are rare but have been reported following intravenous (IV) or IM injection of the drug (MacKenzie & Snow, 1977; Tobin & Ballard, 1979). Other central effects of acepromazine include

hypothermia and a moderate antiemetic effect, especially against opioid-induced vomiting (Valverde et al., 2004).

Clinical doses of acepromazine have little effect on respiration; sedated animals may breathe more slowly but the minute volume of respiration is unchanged. In all species, acepromazine, as all phenothiazines, causes a dose-related fall in arterial blood pressure mediated through vasodilation. The lowering of blood pressure is well tolerated in fit patients but may not be so in shocked or hypovolaemic animals. The effects of clinical dose rates of acepromazine on heart rate are generally minimal, most investigators having found a slight rise (Kerr et al., 1972; MacKenzie & Snow, 1977; Parry et al., 1982) or no change (Muir et al., 1979). However, Popovic et al. (1972) reported that, in dogs, doses of 0.1 mg/kg IM acepromazine caused bradycardia and even sinoatrial arrest. Changes in cardiac output appear to be minimal (Maze et al., 1985) even when in association with anaesthetic agents (Sinclair & Dyson, 2012).

Fainting and cardiovascular collapse have been reported to occur occasionally in all species of animal following the use of even low doses of acepromazine. In some cases, it may have been due to administration to a hypovolaemic animal but, in others, it has not been explained. Some strains of Boxer dogs (particularly those in the UK) are renowned for collapsing after a very small dose of acepromazine given by any route, and it has been suggested that this may be due to vasovagal syncope.

Acepromazine has little antihistamine activity. It has a powerful spasmolytic effect on smooth muscle including that of the gut, which may explain why it can give some visceral analgesia (Sanchez et al., 2008) and is effective in treatment of equine spasmodic colic. Acepromazine is not thought to have specific analgesic properties. Although it reduces amount of inhalation anaesthetic agents required (Heard et al., 1986; Doherty et al., 1997), it is not effective against experimentally applied nociceptive stimuli (Sanchez et al., 2008; Bergadano et al., 2009).

Acepromazine has some very specific properties, which increase its usefulness as a premedicant agent:

- It reduces the dose required of anaesthetic agents for induction and maintenance
- It has antiarrhythmic effects and protects against epinephrine-induced fibrillation (Muir, 1981)
- When used as a premedicant in horses, it significantly reduces the incidence of death associated with anaesthesia and surgery (Johnston et al., 1995; 2002). In dogs, its use also significantly reduces anaesthetic-related deaths when compared with no premedication (Brodbelt et al., 2008a,b)
- It has been shown to be a free radical scavenger (Serteyn et al, 1999)
- Its use in anaesthetized horses reduces the 'shunt fraction' and increases arterial oxygenation (Marntell et al., 2005).

Relative contraindications to use of acepromazine include:

- Hypovolaemia
- Liver damage. Low doses can be used but have increased duration
- Renal hypertension
- Boxer dogs (see above)
- Stallions, because of the danger of priapism (see below). However, the advantage of a 50% reduction in anaesthetic death rate is generally considered to outweigh the very small risk (Driessen et al., 2011).

Acepromazine causes paralysis of the retractor penis muscle and protrusion of the flaccid penis from the prepuce in bulls and stallions; it is often given to facilitate examination of the penis. In horses, however, physical damage to the dangling penis may result in swelling and failure of the organ to return within the prepuce when the drug action ceases. This event, which may eventually necessitate amputation of the penis, has been reported following the use of several phenothiazine derivatives. There were several reported incidences of priapism, where there is an erection of the penis (rather than a flaccid paralysis) in stallions following administration of the neuroleptanalgesic mixture 'Large Animal Immobilon' which contains acepromazine (Pearson & Weaver, 1978). There are also very occasional reports of priapism occurring following the administration of acepromazine alone (van der Harst et al., 2002; Taylor & Bolt, 2011). Priapism in adult geldings has been effectively treated by the administration of 8 mg of benztropinemesylate (Wilson et al., 1991), a drug used in the treatment of Parkinson's disease. However, this drug is not readily available. As both priapism and flaccid paralysis with subsequent physical injury are equally calamitous in valuable breeding stallions, the manufacturers specifically contraindicate use of acepromazine in these animals. The risk is very low (Driessen et al., 2011). Should priapism occur, the condition must be treated quickly and efficiently; an Esmarch's bandage will reduce the erection and allow the penis to be returned to the sheath where it can be retained, but should this fail, or in case of a flaccid paralysis, the penis must be supported to prevent further damage.

At one time, it was thought that acepromazine might reduce the threshold at which epileptiform seizures occurred and therefore should not be used in dogs with epilepsy, or prior to myelography. With doses in the clinical range, there was no good evidence to support this theory (Tobias et al., 2006; da Costa et al., 2011; Drynan et al., 2012) and, in Europe, this contraindication has been removed from the product information.

Solutions of acepromazine for injection are available at different concentrations (country dependent). Tablets for oral use in dogs and cats and a paste for oral use in horses are also available. The injectable forms are non-irritant, painless and are effective by IV, IM or subcutaneous (SC)

routes. Following IV injection, sedation is usually obvious within 5 minutes but full effects may not be apparent for 20 minutes and, when the drug is used for premedication, at least this period should be allowed to elapse before anaesthetic agents are given. Maximal effects are seen 30–45 minutes after IM and SC injection.

Very small doses of acepromazine have been used to treat behavioural problems in dogs and horses but the dose required in any individual case can only be found by trial and error. Parenteral doses of acepromazine for sedative and premedicant purposes in most domestic animals are in the range of 0.025–0.1 mg/kg. In horses, oral availability is good (Hashem & Keller, 1993) and the recommended dose is 0.15 mg/kg; this contrasts with dogs where there is marketing authorization for oral dosage up to 3 mg/kg, although whether this dose is required or is desirable is doubtful. Recommended doses for specific purposes will be discussed in the chapters relating to the individual species of animal.

Propionylpromazine

Propionylpromazine, 10-(3-dimethyl aminopropyl)-2-propionylphenothiazine, has been used widely in some countries for sedation and premedication of both small and large animal patients. Its actions, the sedation it produces and its side effects are very similar to those of acepromazine. In horses, it is used in doses of 0.15–0.25 mg/kg and, in dogs, the dose ranges from 0.2 to 0.3 mg/kg. It has also been widely used in combination with methadone.

Fluphenazine

Fluphenazine is a very long acting (several weeks) agent that has a licence for use in humans to treat certain psychiatric diseases. It has a great affinity to dopamine D_2 receptors, thus acting as a dopamine antagonist. It has been used to produce long-term sedation for horses stabled through injury, but also 'abused' as a 'calmer' for horses in competition, although this is strictly against competition rules. There are no published trials relating to its pharmacokinetics or clinical use in animal species, but several detailing side effects in the horse. These can be dramatic, and include sweating, ataxia, and extrapyramidal signs, the latter being reported to continue for some days after dosing. The toxicity is well reviewed by Brashier (2006). Although this drug has no direct use in anaesthesia, if the animal has been pretreated there may be additive effects with drugs used for anaesthesia.

Other phenothiazine agents

Chlorpromazine was used extensively in veterinary practice but has largely been replaced. Its actions and side effects are similar to those of acepromazine, but it is less potent (doses of up to 1 mg/kg were used in all species of animal), has a longer duration of action and produces less sedation. *Promazine* has actions similar to those of chlorpromazine but is claimed to give better sedation with fewer side effects. For premedication, it was administered at doses of up to 1 mg/kg. *Methotrimeprazine* is a typical phenothiazine but it is also a potent analgesic, having a potency about 0.7 times that of morphine. In veterinary practice in the UK, it was combined with etorphine as the neuroleptanalgesic mixture 'Small Animal Immobilon'. *Promethazine* is used in veterinary medicine primarily for its potent antihistamine activity, although recently there has been renewed interest in relation to its actions in decreasing reactive oxygen species (Péters et al., 2009). Solutions of this drug are irritant to the tissues.

BUTYROPHENONES

As with phenothiazines, the primary action of butyrophenones is as dopamine antagonists and, in humans, they were classed as major tranquillizers (neuroleptics), and currently as antipsychotics. Used alone, they can cause very unpleasant side effects, including hallucinations, mental agitation, and feelings of aggression. These side effects often are not obvious to an observer and only become known when a human patient recovers from the drug and complains. The incidence is dose related and increases with increased dose rate. Overdose results in dystonic reactions. We do not know whether the subjective effects produced in animals are similar to those that occur in humans, but the unpredictable aggressive behaviour occasionally observed in animals given a butyrophenone suggests they may be.

Cardiovascular and respiratory effects of the butyrophenones are minimal, although arterial hypotension may result from α_1-adrenergic blockade. They are potent antiemetics, acting on the chemoemetic trigger zone to prevent drug-induced vomiting, such as may be caused by opioid analgesics, thus making them the drug of choice for the neuroleptic component of neuroleptanalgesia (Brown et al., 2011). Some texts even categorize butyrophenones as injectable anaesthetic agents (Reves et al., 2010), although they can only contribute to the anaesthetic state when in combination with other agents.

In veterinary medicine, drugs in this group are used as sedatives, in neuroleptanalgesic combinations, and may be a useful part of other anaesthetic combinations.

Azaperone

Azaperone, 4'-fluoro-4 [4-(2 pyridyl)-1-piperazinyl] butyrophenone, is a drug licensed in Europe in pigs where its

IM administration produces a good, dose-related sedative effect up to the maximum recommended dose for clinical use (4 mg/kg). Pigs may show excitement during the first 20 minutes following injection, particularly if disturbed during this period. Intravenous use of this drug frequently results in a vigorous excitement phase.

Azaperone in clinical doses has minimal effects on respiration; such effect as there is being that of slight stimulation. Clarke (1969) reported a consistent small fall in arterial blood pressure in pigs following the IM injection of 0.3–3.5 mg/kg of the drug. Reductions in cardiac output and heart rate are clinically insignificant (MacKenzie & Snow, 1977).

Azaperone is used both as a sedative and as a preanaesthetic medicant in pigs. It is also used on the farm to sedate pigs before transportation, and to prevent fighting following the mixing of calves or pigs in one pen. When azaperone is used to assist in vaginal delivery of piglets or for caesarean section, the piglets may appear sleepy for some hours after delivery. However, provided they are kept warm they breathe well.

Use in horses, although documented, is not advisable. Doses of 0.4–0.8 mg/kg IM sometimes give good sedation, but some horses develop muscle tremors and sweat profusely (Lees & Serrano, 1976). Intravenous use frequently results in extreme excitement which can cause injury to the horse and/or its handlers (Dodman & Waterman, 1979). The fact that pigs show a similar reaction, coupled with the known central nervous effect in humans, suggests that the excitement is due to a direct effect of the drug.

Droperidol

Droperidol is a potent neuroleptic agent, which is an extremely effective antiemetic and is said to antagonize the respiratory depressant effects of morphine-like compounds by increasing the sensitivity of the respiratory centre to carbon dioxide. Although it was claimed that extrapyramidal side effects were rare, they are produced by overdosing but are sometimes delayed for up to 24 hours after administration of the drug. In humans, droperidol has recently had a resurgence in popularity for premedication (Sneyd, 2009) because of its effect in reducing postoperative vomiting and for counteracting pruritus induced by epidural injection of morphine (Horta et al., 2006). In veterinary medicine, droperidol has been most frequently used in combination, although it has also been used as a sedative in pigs.

Fluanisone

This is 4'-fluoro-4-[4-(o-methoxy)phenyl]-1-piperazinyl] butyrophenone. It is used in the neuroleptanalgesic combination 'Hypnorm' (p. 93).

BENZODIAZEPINES

Chlordiazepoxide was first introduced in 1955 and since that time drugs of the benzodiazepine group have been widely used in human and veterinary medicine. Many different compounds now exist differing primarily in bioavailability, permissible route of administration and duration of action. Drugs of this group are utilized to provide:

- an antianxiety action
- sedation and hypnosis
- anticonvulsant effects
- muscle relaxation
- anterograde amnesia.

Benzodiazepine compounds exert their main sedative effects through depression of the limbic system, and their muscle relaxing properties through inhibition of the inter-nuncial neurons at spinal levels. They act selectively at $GABA_A$ receptors within the central nervous system. They do not activate the receptor directly, but enhance the response to GABA by increasing the frequency of Cl^- channel opening and, therefore, enhance the potentiation of the neural inhibition that is mediated by this transmitter (Olkkola & Ahonen, 2008). The effect of benzodiazepines can be antagonized by inverse agonists or competitive antagonists such as flumazenil. The point of action within the $GABA_A$ receptor is not identical to that at which general anaesthetic agents such as thiopental are thought to exert part of their effect (see Chapter 1). Knowledge of the molecular structure of the $GABA_A$ receptor and its subunits is advancing rapidly and is beyond the scope of this book, but order of arrangement of 'subunits' appears to be responsible for different facets of the overall action (at least in transgenic rats) leading to the future possibility of 'designer' drugs with more specific actions (Sneyd & Rigby-Jones, 2010).

It is impossible to induce anaesthesia with benzodiazepine drugs alone in fit healthy animals (Lees, 1979). The benzodiazepines are generally employed in combination with other central nervous depressant drugs to produce anaesthesia and to counteract the convulsant and hallucinatory properties of ketamine and tiletamine. Used for premedication, they improve the quality of induction of anaesthesia and reduce the dose required of subsequent anaesthetic agents. Benzodiazepines cause minimal cardiovascular and respiratory depression, although they may add to the depressant effects of the other anaesthetics.

Many benzodiazepines can be given by the IM, IV, transmucous membrane, oral and rectal routes. Maximal effects may not be apparent for several minutes following IV administration and there are marked differences between individuals in sensitivity. Metabolism is in the liver and, in many instances, metabolites are as active or more active than the parent compound; actions therefore tend to be prolonged.

In a variety of animals, benzodiazepines have the property of stimulating appetite (Van Miert et al., 1989). Diazepam has been particularly widely used for this in cats showing anorexia following illness.

Of the available benzodiazepine drugs, diazepam, midazolam, climazolam and zolazepam have been most utilized in veterinary anaesthesia.

Diazepam

Diazepam is insoluble in water and solutions for injections contain solvents such as propylene glycol, ethanol, and sodium benzoate in benzoic acid. Intravenous injection of many preparations causes thrombophlebitis due to these solvents. An emulsion preparation is non-irritant to veins and is less painful to inject. Diazepam is highly protein bound, and is metabolized by the liver, many of the metabolites being active. In humans, half-life of elimination has been reported as 43 hours. In contrast, in the dog it is shorter at 3.2 hours (Loscher & Frey, 1981) but an active metabolite is longer lasting. In horses, Muir et al. (1982) reported half-lives between 2.52 and 21.6 hours. At clinical dosage rates, diazepam has no significant effect on the circulation or respiratory activity but does produce some muscular relaxation. It has very low toxicity and large doses given to dogs for prolonged periods do not produce changes in metabolic function.

Diazepam has a major role in veterinary practice in the control of convulsions of any origin. However, as with most benzodiazepines, the sedative and hypnotic effects of diazepam alone appear to be minimal and in fit, healthy dogs attempts to use it alone for hypnosis have been unsuccessful. In horses, Muir et al. (1982) did find that at doses exceeding 0.2 mg/kg IV there was some sedation lasting for around 2 hours, but this was accompanied by muscle weakness. This dose of 0.2 mg/kg is used to sedate foals, which will tend to lie down.

The major anaesthetic use of diazepam is a part of an anaesthetic combination protocol, either as premedication, or in combination with other agents. In sick animals (which are more likely to sedate), it reduces the dose of anaesthetic agents subsequently required and its combination with opioids for induction of anaesthesia provides good cardiovascular stability (Psatha et al., 2011). It is particularly useful prior to or in combination with ketamine as it appears to reduce the hallucinations, which seem to be associated with this dissociative anaesthetic agent, and it has been used in this combination in very many species.

Midazolam

Midazolam, (8-chloro-6 (2-flurophenol)-1–methyl-4H imidazo (1,5-a) (1,4)) benzodiazepine is a water-soluble compound yielding a solution with a pH of 3.5. Above pH values of 4.0, the chemical configuration of the molecule changes so that it becomes lipid soluble. The aqueous solution is not painful on IV injection and does not cause thrombophlebitis. Midazolam is metabolized in the liver. In humans, its half-life of elimination is considerably shorter than that of diazepam thus it is less cumulative and recovery is more rapid. In dogs, half-life of elimination has been measured at 77–98 minutes (Hall et al., 1988; Court & Greenblatt, 1992), also shorter than that of diazepam. Midazolam has good biovailability by non-IV routes including oral and transmucous membrane. In humans, it is used to treat seizures, for premedication, as an infusion for sedation in intensive care, and as an IV injection to induce deep sedation and often, amnesia. The dose required in humans is approximately half to one third that of diazepam (Court & Greenblatt, 1992) and the onset of action is slower than a circulation time. In contrast to humans, in adult fit healthy animals, it is difficult to induce sedation with IV midazolam alone, and aberrant excitement reactions can occur (Covey-Crump & Murison, 2008). However, in sick animals, or when combined with agents such as opioids or ketamine, good hypnosis can be achieved, and midazolam, in combination with other agents, now has a major role in the anaesthesia of all species.

The lack of guaranteed sedation with midazolam alone means that there are few animal studies on its use as a sole agent but there are very many publications detailing its use in combination with other analgesic/anaesthetic agents for sedation, as a premedicant and for anaesthesia. This wide literature provides a basis for the recommendations that will be given in the chapters on the individual species.

Climazolam

Climazolam is a potent benzodiazepine which, following IV administration, has a very rapid onset of effect. It has a marketing authorization in Switzerland for use in dogs, but has been used in a wide variety of animals including cattle, sheep, horses and dogs (Rehm & Schatzmann, 1984). It is used as part of anaesthetic combinations. It is particularly effective for use with ketamine and, in horses, this combination has been used by constant rate infusion (CRI) to produce total intravenous anaesthesia (TIVA), the climazolam being reversed with sarmazenil (see below) at the end of surgery to produce a rapid recovery (Bettschart-Wolfensberger et al., 1996). Climazolam (1.0–1.5 mg/kg) has also been used in combination with fentanyl (0.005–0.015 mg/kg) for anaesthesia in the dog (Erhardt et al., 1986).

Zolazepam

This drug is used in animals combined, in a fixed ratio, with the dissociative agent, tiletamine (see Chapter 6).

BENZODIAZEPINE ANTAGONISTS

Flumazenil

Flumazenil is a potent and specific competitive benzodiazepine antagonist and, in human medical practice, is now being widely employed to reverse midazolam sedation in 'day case' patients.

Flumazenil has been reported to reverse diazepam or climazolam sedation in sheep and cattle (Rhem & Schatzmann, 1984) and has also been used in combination with naloxone to reverse climazolam/fentanyl combination anaesthesia (Erhardt et al., 1986). Although to date the veterinary use of flumazenil has been limited by cost, it may be employed in any situation where it may become necessary to reverse the effects of a benzodiazepine drug (Heniff et al., 1997; Wismer, 2002).

Sarmazenil

This antagonist has marketing authorization in Switzerland for use in dogs and cats. It has been used to reverse the effects of climazolam in a number of species (Rehm & Schatzmann, 1984; Bettschart-Wolfensberger et al., 1996). Midazolam-induced ataxia in a horse was effectively reversed with sarmazenil (author KC).

α_2-ADRENOCEPTOR AGONISTS

Xylazine has been used as a sedative in animals since 1968 but, at that time, the mechanisms of its complex actions and side effects were not understood. When it was described as 'both excitatory and inhibitory of adrenergic and cholinergic neurons' (Kronberg et al., 1966), this statement appeared more than a little confusing. A similar drug, clonidine, was originally used in humans for its powers of local peripheral vasoconstriction but now is used as an antihypertensive and also, off label, as a sedative and analgesic.

These actions and the correctness of the above description only became explicable when Langer (1974) suggested the existence of receptor sites situated presynaptically on the noradrenergic neurons which, when stimulated by noradrenaline, inhibited the further release of this transmitter, thus forming a negative feedback mechanism. Langer suggested further that these presynaptic inhibitory receptors differed from the previously recognized α-adrenoceptors and should therefore be termed α_2-adrenoceptors. There are postsynaptic and presynaptic α_2-adrenoceptors in both central and peripheral sites. The distinction between α_1- and α_2-adrenoceptors is made on sensitivity to specific agonist and antagonists. Epinephrine (adrenaline) and norepinephrine (noradrenaline)

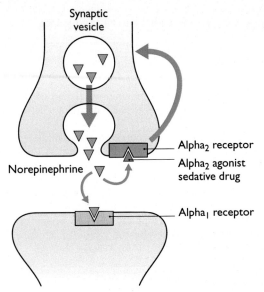

Figure 4.1 This represents a noradrenergic neuron in the central nervous system (CNS). Norepinephrine is the natural ligand and acts at the effector sites (α_1- and, peripherally, also α_2-receptors). However, in the central nervous system, there are α_2-receptors on the noradrenergic neuron; stimulation of these acts as a negative feedback system and prevents further release of norepinephrine. The α_2-agonist sedative drugs act at this point, and therefore block release of norepinephrine.

Box 4.1 Actions of α_2-adrenoceptor agonists with clinical significance

Central

- Sedation
- Cardiovascular
  - Depression of cardiovascular centre
  - 'Late' vasodilation (after peripheral vasoconstriction has waned)
- Analgesia
  - Central and spinal
- Pituitary – hormonal
  - Reduced ADH, increased urination
  - Reduced ACTH, decreased cortisol

Central and peripheral

- Bradycardia

Peripheral

- Cardiovascular
  - Vasoconstriction
- Intestinal relaxation, decreased motility
- Uterine stimulation.
- Reduced renin and insulin secretions
  - Hyperglycaemia
- Platelets
  - Aggregation

---

stimulate both types. For α_1-adrenoceptors, phenylephrine and methoxamine are considered to be fairly specific agonists and prazosin to be a specific antagonist. Classically, for pharmacological tests, clonidine was considered a specific α_2-agonist and yohimbine an antagonist. Current research utilizes newer and more selective agents.

Norepinephrine is the natural ligand for both α_1- and α_2-adrenoceptors. When norepinephrine is released from a 'sympathetic 'neuron, it acts on both these receptors at the effector site, resulting in 'sympathetic' stimulation. However, there are α_2-adrenoceptors on the sympathetic neuron which, when stimulated by the released norepinephrine, exert a negative feedback and prevent further release of norepinephrine (Fig. 4.1). Simplistically, the α_2-adrenoceptor agonists (α_2-agonists) exert their central effects by stimulating these presynaptic α_2-receptors, thus preventing the release of norepinephrine and damping or preventing sympathetic drive from the central nervous system.

As the presynaptic α_2-adrenoceptors inhibit norepinephrine release, it might be expected that the action of agonists would be the opposite of the classic effects of sympathetic stimulation. However, postsynaptic α_2-adrenoceptors often exert a stimulating action similar to

that exerted by α_1-adrenoceptors at the same site. Peripheral postsynaptic α_2-receptors are spread widely in many tissues explaining many of the actions of α_2-agonists (Box 4.1). Receptor distribution, concentration and subtypes (Bylund, 1988; Bylund et al., 1988) vary with species, which may explain some of the species differences that occur. The most dramatic of the peripheral effects is that of both arterial and venous vasoconstriction, over-riding the centrally induced reduction in sympathetic drive.

Few drugs are absolutely specific in their actions but just show selectivity, thus at higher doses, the alternative α-receptors may also be stimulated or blocked, a factor possibly explaining some of the side effects and aberrant reactions occasionally seen with their clinical use. All the α_2-agonists other than xylazine have an imidazole ring, and it is thought that stimulation of imidazole receptors may have a major role in their actions (Kahn et al., 1999), but it is possible that there is also some activity at muscarinic, opioid and dopamine receptors. Knowledge of the molecular biology and genetic basis of the receptors is increasing at a rate to make it beyond the scope of this book, and readers are advised to consult recent pharmacological reviews.

Clinically relevant actions of α_2-adrenoceptor agonist drugs

In recent years, new potent and highly selective α_2-agonists have been developed for both medical and veterinary use. Advantages of use in humans are just beginning to be appreciated (Sanders & Maze, 2007). There are now several thousand publications describing the clinical actions of these drugs. The major actions of clinical importance are summarized in Box 4.1. This section will cover the general principles of the actions and use of α_2-agonists – specifics of drug doses will be discussed in the relevant chapters for the species.

In veterinary practice, the drugs with marketing authorizations in either Europe or North America are xylazine, detomidine, medetomidine, dexmedetomidine and romifidine. The major actions and side effects of all these drugs are similar, although there may be differences in length of action and in the extent and significance of some of the side effects seen. There are variations between the drugs in their specificity for α_2- and α_1-receptors and this explains some of the differences in observed clinical effects. There is also marked variation in species sensitivity to their actions. For example, cattle are approximately 10 times more sensitive to xylazine than horses or dogs, but are equally sensitive to medetomidine as are dogs, and equally or less sensitive to detomidine than horses. Pigs appear very resistant to xylazine, but only a little less so to medetomidine. Generalized comparisons of their potency are meaningless except in the context of a stated species of animal.

Pharmacokinetics: routes of administration

Most α_2-agonists are metabolized by the liver to the extent that oral administration is not very effective, although clonidine is administered orally to people and there are reports of xylazine toxicity in people who have eaten meat from animals recently darted with this drug. Bioavailability is high for most other routes of administration – including across mucous membranes. Consequently, the more potent agents must be handled with care to avoid accidental self-administration.

Sedation: hypnosis

All α_2-agonists produce a dose-related degree of sedation up to a maximum, after which any increase in dose only increases duration. Whether or not it is possible to induce recumbency depends on the species and the drug. For example, ruminants assume recumbency when only moderately sedated while horses try to stay standing. In horses, detomidine at doses of 10 or more times the dose used for clinical sedation does not induce recumbency (Di Concetto et al., 2007), while even low doses of medetomidine may make the horse so ataxic that it falls (Bryant et al., 1991).

Animals deeply sedated with any of the α_2-agonists may still demonstrate marked, even enhanced reflex responses. This is most obvious in the horse when the apparently deeply sedated horse can respond to a simple touch with a well-directed kick. This reflex response can occur in all species, for example, dogs apparently heavily sedated with medetomidine may abruptly rise and bite a person in the hand when touched. The message is never to trust sedation! The addition of opioids reduces or removes these responses.

When α_2-agonists are used for premedication, they greatly reduce the dose requirements of inhalation anaesthetics or intravenous agents. They also combine with opioids to produce deep sedation or even anaesthesia.

Analgesia

α_2-Agonists are potent analgesics through both spinal and central actions and even in subsedative doses (Vainio et al., 1986; Nolan et al., 1986; Scheinin & Macdonald, 1989; Kahn et al., 1999; Murrell & Hellebrekers, 2005). α_2-Agonists provide excellent analgesia when given by the epidural or intrathecal routes through a direct action on the receptors in the dorsal horn of the spinal cord.

Cardiovascular effects

The major side effects of α_2-adrenoceptor agonists are on the cardiovascular system. With all the agents and in all species there is marked bradycardia, due to suppression of the central cardiovascular centre and mediated through the vagus nerve. There may be a reflex component in response to the early hypertensive phase, but this is not the major cause – the bradycardia lasts long after the hypertensive phase has waned, and also occurs when peripheral antagonism has prevented the early phase rise in blood pressure (Bryant et al., 1998; Enouri et al., 2008; Honkavaara et al., 2008).

The administration of an anticholinergic drug to prevent the bradycardia induced by α_2-agonists has been suggested. However, when anticholinergic agents are used in animals sedated with α_2-agonists, although the fall in heart rate is prevented, there is tachycardia, and the hypertensive phase of the α_2-agonist's action is enhanced (Alibhai et al., 1996). In cats sedated with xylazine, administration of glycopyrrolate further decreased cardiac output (Dunkle et al., 1986). Heart rates of normal sleeping dogs (Hall et al., 1991) and horses (Hall, unpublished data) drop to values similar to those seen in animals sedated by α_2-adrenoceptor agonists. The bradycardia in the sedated animal can be over-ridden by toxaemia or by the administration of some anaesthetics. Thus, although anticholinergics may be used in emergency, it is generally accepted that their routine use is not advisable.

The effects of α_2-agonists on arterial blood pressure depend on the relative effects of the central and peripheral stimulation. There is often an initial hypertensive phase, the extent and duration of which depend on the particular drug, its dose, route of administration, and the species of animal concerned. The hypertensive phase is followed by a more prolonged period of lower blood pressure, again dependent on the drug, route of administration and the species of animal. Cardiac output falls as a result of the bradycardia. The circulation appears to be slowed; the veins take time to fill and IV anaesthetic agents take longer than expected to exert their effects. The exact state of the peripheral circulation is more complicated and dose dependent. During the early phase of arterial hypertension with bradycardia, peripheral resistance is increased, presumably through vasoconstriction. How long this poor peripheral perfusion lasts is difficult to ascertain, as blood pressure may fall below pre-dosing values as a result of the bradycardia. In the later hypotensive phase, peripheral resistance is reduced.

Vasconstriction may result in changes in organ blood flow which may in turn have other effects. Cerebral vasoconstriction induced by α_2-agonists may lead to a decrease in intracranial pressure (McCormick et al., 1993). Administration of α_2-agonists decreases intraocular pressure (Trim et al., 1985; Virkkila et al., 1994).

The question of the possible direct effects of α_2-agonists on the myocardium is an open one. There have been anecdotal reports of animals which were in a very excited state at the time of xylazine or detomidine administration suffering sudden cardiac arrest and the suggestion has been made that this drug might sensitize the heart to epinephrine-induced arrhythmias. Muir & Piper (1977) showed this to be the case in halothane anaesthetized dogs, but other studies have failed to show the same effect in horses, or with the other α_2-agonist agents (Pettifer et al., 1996). α_2-Adrenoceptors are present in the coronary vessels but, despite the potential for reduced myocardial blood flow, in humans, the use of α_2-agonist agents during cardiac surgery reduces the overall morbidity and mortality from the procedures (Wijeysundera et al., 2009).

Respiratory and pulmonary actions

Respiratory effects of α_2-agonists are dose and depth of sedation related and differ between species of animal. In dogs, cats and horses respiratory rates are reduced, but unless there is very deep sedation, any fall in PaO_2 is not usually clinically relevant (Hsu et al., 1985; Short et al., 1986; Clarke & Taylor, 1987). Dogs deeply sedated with medetomidine or dexmedetomidine may breathe intermittently – gaps of up to 45 seconds being followed by 20 rapid respiratory movements, and individual animals may become hypoxic. In ruminants, however, tachypnoea may occur, breathing appears to require a considerable effort and the PaO_2 falls to levels causing desaturation of the haemoglobin (Celly et al., 1997). This hypoxaemia does not seem to be due to changes in blood pressure or in

ventilation and, indeed, has been shown to occur following clonidine injection in anaesthetized artificially ventilated sheep (Eisenach & Grice, 1988). The problem seems greatest in sheep (Kästner, 2006) but can occur with all ruminants. Celly et al. (1999) demonstrated that within 10 minutes of xylazine injection there was extensive pulmonary damage, with intra-alveolar haemorrhage and interstitial and alveolar oedema.

Very occasionally, a horse will show tachypnoea for a short period of time. This phase seems to pass rapidly (15 minutes) without treatment. The cause is unknown. Kendall et al. (2010) documented that this is a common occurrence in febrile horses. However, it can occur in healthy horses and Bettschart-Wolfensberger et al. (1999) documented an experimental pony that always responded in this manner despite all cardiopulmonary parameters, including arterial blood gas values, being normal.

Other actions

All α_2-agonist drugs cause an increase in urination, thought to be through inhibition of antidiuretic hormone (ADH) release. In some species, high dose rates induce hyperglycaemia which might contribute to diuresis. Intestinal motility ceases almost completely. These side effects must be taken into account when these drugs are used to facilitate radiological investigations and glucose tolerance tests. Some of the α_2-agonists cause significant uterine stimulation and their administration is contraindicated in very early or late pregnancy for they may induce abortion.

In doses that produce clinical sedation, most of these drugs cause hypothermia but the mechanism by which this is produced appears to differ between drugs and species of animal. Xylazine-induced hypothermia has been shown to be antagonized by idazoxan while clonidine-induced hypothermia is intensified (Livingstone et al., 1984). In rats, low doses of detomidine cause hypothermia that can be reversed by yohimbine (Virtanen, 1989), but higher doses cause hyperthermia probably due to an α_1-adrenoceptor-stimulating action.

Xylazine

Xylazine, 2-(2,6-dimethylphenylamino)-4H-5,5 dihydro-1,3-thiazine, was enthusiastically received as a sedative and, over the past 40 years, it has maintained its popularity as a generally reliable sedative and premedicant in a wide range of animal species (Clarke & Hall, 1969). The drug is a typical α_2-adrenoceptor agonist and exerts its effects accordingly as described above. It has some major differences from the newer agents:

• Its structure does not have an imidazole ring and, to our knowledge, there are no studies documenting xylazine activity at imidazole receptors

- There are marked variations in susceptibility to xylazine between the various species of domestic animals. Horses, dogs and cats require 10 times the dose needed in cattle. Pigs are even more resistant. Lesser variations in sensitivity may occur in breeds within a single species and that this might contribute to the occasional failure of the drug to produce sedation
- The ecbolic effect (increased uterine contractions) at equisedative doses appears greater than for the newer agents
- When given to dogs, vomiting is more frequent and more prolonged than that seen following medetomidine administration.

Xylazine is non-irritant and can be given by IV, IM or SC injection, although the SC route is less reliable. Although not proved by laboratory testing, anecdotally there are suggestions that the potency of available commercial solutions may decrease with time after first use of the bottle, and this deterioration may be enhanced by increased environmental temperature (Van Dieten, 1988, personal communication). In horses, the drug is usually used in doses that enable the animal to remain standing (although with marked ataxia). In ruminants and in small animals, sedation is dose dependent and higher doses are used which may cause recumbency, unconsciousness and a state close to general anaesthesia. Although the drug can be a potent analgesic, where surgery is to be performed, local analgesia must be used to supplement its effects. The cardiopulmonary and other effects of xylazine are typical of this group of drugs, as described above. Doses and reactions specific to various species will be discussed in the relevant chapters.

Xylazine has proved to be a very safe sedative in a wide variety of animals but some serious reactions have been reported. There have been reports of violent excitement or collapse in horses associated with its IV injection, although some may have been due to inadvertent intra-arterial injection. Deaths have also been reported in cattle possibly as a result of the drug-induced hypoxaemia. The availability of antagonists such as atipamezole increases the safety of xylazine. In small animals, deaths have mainly occurred in relation to other anaesthetic agents when xylazine has been used in anaesthetic combinations (Clarke & Hall, 1990; Dyson et al., 1998).

Xylazine is a useful drug for premedication prior to induction of anaesthesia with one of a wide variety of agents. Its use greatly reduces the dose of anaesthetic required. In heavily sedated animals, circulation is slowed, the effects of subsequent anaesthetic agents is delayed and overdose of the anaesthetic may result. Xylazine is particularly useful in combination with ketamine for its muscle relaxing properties help to reduce the rigidity caused by the dissociative agent and, for many years, xylazine/ketamine combinations have proved useful in a wide range of animal species.

Detomidine

Detomidine, 4-(2,3-dimethylphenyl)methyl-1H-imidazole hydrochloride, is an imidazole derivative which has been developed as a sedative/analgesic for animals. It is supplied in multidose bottles, currently at a concentration of 10 mg/mL and may be given by the IV and IM routes. It is effective if given sublingually and there is now a gel form marketed for this route in horses. Unlike xylazine, its relative potency in most domestic animals is fairly similar.

The properties of detomidine are well documented in *Acta Veterinaria Scandinavica*, Supplement 82/1986 (20 papers). Its analgesic effects have been shown in a number of pain models and it is particularly effective as an analgesic in equine colic (Jochle et al., 1989). Cardiopulmonary and other changes are typical of an α_2-agonist as described above.

One difference between xylazine and detomidine appears to be in their effects on the uterus. Whereas xylazine appears to have marked ecbolic effects, detomidine, at IV doses of 20 µg/kg, slows electrical activity in the pregnant bovine uterus, although higher doses (40–60 µg/kg) will increase this activity (Jedruch & Gajewski, 1986).

Detomidine is now used widely as a sedative and premedicant for horses but is also marketed for use in cattle in Europe. Detomidine has a high therapeutic index. The early investigations in horses used dose rates between 10 (the dose currently used for short duration sedation) and 300 µg/kg, and horses remained standing after the highest doses, although with unacceptable prolongation of sedation and side effects (bradycardia, arterial hypertension, ataxia, sweating, piloerection, muscle tremor and diuresis). Action of detomidine is prolonged in patients with abnormal liver function (Chambers et al., 1996). A more detailed description of the effects and uses of detomidine in horses is given in Chapter 11.

The doses of detomidine required in cattle appear to be similar to those in horses. Again, early experimental work suggested that high doses were needed for adequate sedation but subsequent trials have shown that doses of up to 30 mg/kg are satisfactory. In the authors' experience, doses of 10 µg/kg IV produce sedation in cattle very similar to that seen in horses, i.e. cattle remain standing but show marked ataxia. Detomidine has two advantages over xylazine in cattle: less stimulation of uterine contraction and decreased likelihood of recumbency.

Medetomidine

This compound, 4-(1-(2,3-dimethylphenyl) ethyl)-1H-imidazole, is a very potent, efficacious and selective agonist for α_2-adrenoreceptors in the central and peripheral nervous system (Virtanen, 1989). It is a mixture of two sterioisomers and the preparation marketed currently for small animal use contains 1 mg/mL of the racemic mixture.

The dextrorotatory isomer (dexmedetomidine) is the active component and is now marketed as a separate product. Medetomidine solution is non-irritant and can be administered by IV, IM, SC or transmucous membrane. It is metabolized rapidly in the liver, and has a half-life of elimination of approximately 0.5–1.5 hours in dogs, cats and horses (Salonen, 1989; Bettschart-Wolfensberger et al., 1999; Grimsrud et al., 2012).

Medetomidine induces sedation, hypnosis and analgesia, and significant cardiovascular effects of bradycardia, arterial hypertension followed by hypotension and reduced cardiac output. Its actions in dogs and cats have been well reviewed (Murrell & Hellebrekers, 2005; Cullen, 1996). In most animals, medetomidine slows respiration (Clarke & England, 1989). Nevertheless, at normal sedative doses in healthy non-ruminant animals the $PaCO_2$ does not rise to an excessive level (Vainio et al., 1989; Cullen, 1996). Cyanosis has been reported in up to one third of dogs sedated with medetomidine (Clarke & England, 1989; Vaha-Vahe, 1989) and, in most cases, this has been attributed to decreased tissue blood flow with increased oxygen extraction leading to cyanosis from venous desaturation. In bitches, the electrical activity of the uterine muscle is depressed at doses of 20 µg/kg while, at higher doses (40–60 µg/kg), there is an initial increase in this activity for some 5–7 minutes followed by depression; it is reported that pregnant bitches do not abort (Jedruch et al., 1989). When medetomidine is used for premedication, it severely reduces the dose of IV agents needed for anaesthetic induction or maintenance, and also the MAC of volatile agents (Lerche & Muir, 2006).

The marketing authorization for medetomidine is for use in cats and dogs, and details of dose and effect in these species are given in the relevant chapters. However, the drug has been used in a very large variety of other species. In rodents and other laboratory animals, there are marked variations in susceptibility to its effects, the guinea pig being most resistant. Combinations with opioids or ketamine are more effective than the sedative alone. Medetomidine has been used also in sheep and cattle; IV doses of 10–20 µg/kg causing sedation similar to that seen after 0.1–0.2 mg/kg of xylazine (Kästner, 2006). In wild animals, higher doses are required and the drug is usually used in combination with ketamine when administered by dart gun for immobilization. Indeed, medetomidine/ketamine combinations have been found to provide excellent immobilization and relaxation in a wide range of species of animals, while the ability to reverse the sedation with $α_2$-adrenoceptor antagonists has proved to be particularly useful (Jalenka, 1989). In horses, despite the risk of recumbency, use of medetomidine has become popular as a continuous rate infusion given following a small (5–7 µg/kg) loading dose either for standing sedation (Bettschart-Wolfensberg et al., 1999) or, more frequently, during anaesthesia (Ringer et al., 2007; Valverde et al., 2010).

Dexmedetomidine

Dexmedetomidine ((+)-4-(S)-[1-(2,3-dimethylphenyl)ethyl]-1H-imidazole monohydrochloride) is the S-enantiomer of medetomidine, and the active component of the racemic agent. It is the most potent and specific $α_2$-agonist available and was originally developed for use in humans.

Dexmedetomidine now has veterinary marketing authorization for use in dogs and cats in many countries. Dose rates, which are essentially half of those used with medetomidine, are given in terms of body surface area rather than as weight (as were originally those for medetomidine). It is claimed that its specificity results in less side effects (Murrell & Hellebrekers, 2005). However, many veterinary studies have found no clinically significant differences other than dose between use of dexmedetomidine and that of the racemic mixture for cats and dogs (Granholm et al., 2006, 2007), or when used off-label in other species (Kästner et al., 2001). There are now many publications detailing the effects of dexmedetomidine in a wide range of species.

Romifidine

Romifidine (N-(2-bromo-6-fluorophenyl)-4,5-dihydro-1H-imidazol-2-amine) was developed from clonidine and has all the usual properties of an $α_2$-agonist. It is used primarily for sedation and premedication for horses (reviewed by England & Clarke, 1996), although it has or has had a marketing licence for cats and dogs in some countries. After injection in the horse, plasma levels fall so rapidly that a half-life of elimination cannot be calculated, but experiments using radioactive romifidine have documented detectable radioactivity for 37 hours, suggesting residual metabolites. In contrast, in dogs, the plasma half-life of the parent drug is 2 hours (European Medicines Agency, Safety report; Summary 2010). Romifidine's actions differ in some ways from the other $α_2$-agonists in veterinary use. Romifidine appears to be less hypnotic, certainly than medetomidine. In horses, when compared to IV xylazine (1 mg/kg) or detomidine (20 µg/kg), romifidine at 40 µg/kg and 80 µg/kg produced less ataxia and the horses' heads were held higher. The response to imposed stimuli was reduced to the same degree by all three drugs. The duration of effect was longest with romifidine. There is controversy as to the degree of analgesia produced by romifidine (England & Clarke, 1996). For example, in cats, analgesia appeared to be less than that of xylazine (Selmi et al., 2004) and, in clinical horses, when given as a constant rate infusion during isoflurane anaesthesia, it did not appear to reduce the concentration of inhalant required (Devisscher et al., 2010). In contrast, with electrical nociceptive testing, romifidine had good analgesic properties (Spadavecchia et al., 2005) and it has the expected analgesic activity when given by the epidural or spinal route (Amarpal et al., 2002).

The lack of ataxia with romifidine has made it very popular for use to sedate horses for standing procedures, and it is also widely used for a premedication or with ketamine for anaesthetic induction in this species. In contrast, it clinical use in small animal practice is not widespread as a greater degree of hypnosis is preferred in these species. As with all α_2-agonists, it has been used in many other species with anticipated results.

Clonidine

Clonidine (N-(2,6-dichlorophenyl)-4,5-dihydro-1H-imidazol-2-amine) is an α_2-agonist agent which, in humans, has been used primarily as an antihypertensive agent, sedation being an unwanted side effect. Publications detail its use in other areas such as control of opioid withdrawal symptoms. It has been used in animals, but the many agents in this class holding veterinary marketing licences are better researched for suitable dosage and effects.

α_2-ADRENOCEPTOR ANTAGONISTS

The central and peripheral effects of α_2-agonists can be reversed by equally specific antagonists. These include atipamezole, yohimbine, tolazoline and idazoxan. Other actions, for which they might have clinical use, include:

- Antidepressant
- Aphrodisiac
- Antiobesity
- Antidiabetic (type 2).

In veterinary practice, the α_2-antagonists are used to terminate sedation induced by an α_2-agonist in situations such as at the end of a non-painful procedure in small animals and horses, in ruminants, where prolonged recumbency may be detrimental, after capture of wild animals (Kock et al., 1989), or following accidental overdose of the sedative agonists (Di Concetto et al., 2007).

There are some general considerations when using α_2-antagonists in clinical practice (Box 4.2). It is important to realize that reversal of sedation includes reversal of analgesia. Depending on the agents chosen, re-sedation may occur and this could have serious consequences in wild animals that are no longer under observation and vulnerable to predators. The dose rates of antagonist drugs for reversing sedation will vary with the dose of sedative used and the elapsed time after its administration. Higher doses are required to reverse cardiopulmonary effects than to reverse sedation (Vainio et al., 1989). Selection of optimum dose of antagonist is not easy and adverse side effects of the antagonist may be revealed. Convulsions have been reported after yohimbine, idazoxan and atipamezole but, in most reports, ketamine, which is not

> **Box 4.2 Considerations when using atipamezole (or other α_2-adrenergic antagonists)**
>
> - Analgesia is reversed as well as sedation
> - Only the α_2-agonists reversed
>   - Ketamine convulsive action may be revealed
> - Dose required will depend on the residual degree of sedation
> - Duration of action of agonist and antagonist must match
>   - Re-sedation can occur. Dangerous for wild animals

influenced by the α_2-antagonists, was part of the sedative combination used and may have been the cause of this side effect.

Atipamezole

Atipamezole, 4-(2-ethyl-2,3-dihydro-1H-inden-2-yl)-1H-imidazole hydrochloride, is a specific α_2-antagonist that was developed to reverse the actions of medetomidine (and, more recently, dexmedetomidine) (Virtanen, 1989), and has marketing authorization for dogs and cats. In dogs, to reverse recently given medetomidine sedation, doses of five times that of the medetomidine dose are required (Vainio & Vahe-Vahe, 1989); the marketed solutions of atipamezole are five times the strength of the marketed medetomidine (and 10 times that of dexmedetomidine) so that equal volumes of agonist and antagonist can be employed. Cats sedated with medetomidine are usually given a lower dose (50% in volume) of antagonist. Medetomidine and antagonism with atipamezole is now very widely used in small animal practice (Sinclair, 2003; Murrell & Hellebrekers, 2005). Serious relapse into sedation has not been noted. Atipamezole also reverses the cardiopulmonary effects of the α_2-agonists although, in dogs, there is a transient fall in blood pressure (Vainio, 1990) and in sheep, although respiration is improved, PaO_2 may still be lower than prior to sedation (unpublished observations, KC). Overdose of atipamezole does not appear to cause major problems in most species of animal. Cats may appear hyper-alert, and injection into the unsedated dog (Clarke & England, 1989) causes mild muscular tremors but little else. Convulsions have never been noted in the absence of ketamine. Atipamezole will also antagonize all α_2-agonists (see species chapters).

Yohimbine

Yohimbine, an extract from a plant, historically has been used as an aphrodisiac. Although it has actions at many receptor sites (thus many side effects), numerous studies have demonstrated its effectiveness in antagonizing α_2-agonist-induced sedation and analgesia in laboratory animals and dogs. Doses of 0.1 mg/kg generally have been employed to reverse xylazine sedation in small animals; high doses have caused excitement in dogs.

Tolazoline

This is used at doses of 4 mg/kg to antagonize the effects of xylazine in horses. The rate of IV administration needs to be controlled to approximately 100 mg/min to avoid hypotension. It is a mixed α_1- and α_2-antagonist and also has a direct peripheral vasodilator action. Temporary side effects, which usually last not more than 1–2 hours, include changes in blood pressure, tachycardia, peripheral vasodilatation and sweating.

Idazoxan

Idazoxan ((±)-2-(2,3-dihydro-1,4-benzodioxin-2-yl)-4,5-dihydro-1H-imidazole) is a very specific α_2- adrenoceptor antagonist that has been used widely as a tool in research. Clinically, the main veterinary experience has been in free-ranging animals, where it has been effective in reversing xylazine-induced sedation.

Peripheral α_2-antagonist MK-467

This agent, also known as L-659,066, is an exciting prospect as it does not cross the blood–brain barrier, and therefore can be used to reverse the unwanted peripheral effects (such as the vasoconstriction) of the α_2-agonist, while leaving the sedation and analgesia intact. Bryant et al. (1998) first reported its effective use in sheep; effects in ponies were disappointing as doses were too low. Recently, interest has been revived and a number of recent publications have detailed the effects of MK-467 in reducing the peripheral cardiovascular and other effects of medetomidine and dexmedetomidine, while leaving sedation unchanged (Enouri et al., 2008; Honkavaara et al., 2012; Restitutti et al., 2012). The drug has also proved useful in pharmacological research to elucidate which actions of the agonists are mediated peripherally.

OTHER AGENTS USED FOR SEDATION

Some older and less specific agents are still used to produce sedation, albeit without marketing authorizations. *Chloral hydrate* produces excellent sedation in horses and cattle with minimal cardiopulmonary side effects. The limitations of its use were poor analgesia (but that can be provided by other means) and the fact that large volumes of an irritant solution were required. The use of IV catheters reduces the importance of this latter problem. *Barbiturates*

used at subanaesthetic doses have also been used to sedate. *Reserpine*, an agent that works by depleting the sympathetic neurons of noradrenaline, is still used to calm horses. It has a long action (up to three weeks) and is useful for horses that need to be kept quiet following injury. *Magnesium*, once used in an anaesthetic combination for large animals, together with chloral and barbiturate is making a 'comeback'. Magnesium is given orally to horses as a 'calmer' and this (currently – 2012) does not infringe competition rules. However, in human anaesthesia, it is being used as an intra-anaesthetic infusion where it appears to contribute to analgesia and hypnosis, reducing the other agents required (James, 2009). However, a magnesium infusion failed to reduce anaesthetic requirements in anaesthetized dogs undergoing surgery (Rioja et al., 2012).

SEDATIVE–OPIOID COMBINATIONS

The combination of two drugs with actions at different receptors often results in synergism where the overall effect is greater than the sum of their individual actions. In contrast, combinations of agents that work at the same receptor can only be additive. This is the basis for the combination of sedative and opioid agents. The sedative has an additional use of counteracting undesired opioid side effects, in particular, excitement reactions and opioid-induced vomiting. There is nothing new about the use of such combinations, veterinarians having used them for many years to render animals more manageable.

The range of sedative/opioid mixtures in use for sedation and control of animals is extensive, including α_2-agonists, phenothiazines, butyrophenones (neuroleptic agents) and benzodiazepines all having been combined with a wide variety of agonist and partial agonist opioids. Where high doses of potent opioids such as fentanyl or alfentanil (see chapter 5) are used, a state similar to anaesthesia is achieved. Unfortunately, severe respiratory depression may accompany the use of these high dose opioid techniques.

Thus, in veterinary anaesthesia, sedative/opioid combinations are used in three ways:

- To obtain more reliable sedation
- To induce anaesthesia, or a state close to this.
- Commercially available fixed-dose combinations.

Reliable sedation is achieved usually with acepromazine or α_2-agonists combined with an opioid such as butorphanol, buprenorphine, hydromorphone, oxymorphone, methadone or moderate doses of morphine. The improved sedation (e.g. reduction of 'kick' response to touch in horses) can be achieved at opioid doses well below those required for analgesia but, if more potent opioids are used, they will contribute to pain relief. Fentanyl is the most popular opioid for anaesthetic indications; combinations with benzodiazepines, or with α_2-agonists inducing unconsciousness. The ultra-potent opioids such as etorphine or carfentanil have been used in regimens for darting wild animals (see Chapter 18).

Suitable regimens for these indications for each species of animal are given in later chapters of this book.

The original concept of neuroleptanalgesia and neuroleptanaesthesia was used specifically to describe the combination of opioids with phenothiazines or butyrophenones (neuroleptics). The neuroleptic agents have the specific property of reducing opioid-induced vomiting in dogs (and humans). As many of the sedatives used (e.g. the α_2-agonists) are not 'neuroleptic' agents, the term 'sedative–opioid' combination is preferred.

The fixed ratio combinations date back to the concept of neuroleptanaesthesia. *Hypnorm*, *Thalamonal* and *Innovar – VET* are (or were) commercially available mixtures of fentanyl and butyrophenone tranquillizer (flu-anisone or droperidol). They have been used in dogs, pigs, primates, rabbits and rodents, particularly in the experimental laboratory situation. The advantages of the mixtures include ease of administration, reasonable safety margin, quiet postoperative state, and reversibility with narcotic antagonists (such as naloxone). Disadvantages include variable response in certain breeds, the spontaneous movements that occur, the need to employ further analgesia and anaesthesia when major surgery is to be performed, and respiratory depression.

Immobilon®

Immobilon® is now marketed only for horses and deer. It consists of a very potent and long acting μ agonist etorphine (2.45 mg/mL) together with acepromazine (10 mg/mL). When the procedure is completed, the effects of the etorphine (but not acepromazine) can be reversed by the use of the specific antagonist diprenorphine (3.0 mg/mL, LA Revivon®).

After IV injection of Immobilon®, horses become recumbent within one minute and, although excitement may occur, it is much less severe than following IM administration. Once recumbent, intense muscular activity makes the animal very stiff and violent continuous tremors occur for up to 20 minutes. Hypertension and tachycardia are present but respiration is severely depressed. Horses regain the standing position within a few minutes of IV injection of Revivon®. Occasionally, horses become excited shortly after standing and a further excitement phase may occur several hours later due to enterohepatic recycling of the etorphine.

Immobilon® and other etorphine-containing combinations have been used extensively for the capture of wild game. Modern use is as 'knockdown', as in horses, but the historical reports (Harthoorn, 1972) used much lower dose rates whereby the animals (elephants and giraffes) became sedated but remain standing. Immobilon® is not recommended for wild felidae.

In humans, etorphine is extremely potent and its use constitutes a danger to the anaesthetist and assistants. Should an accident occur, naloxone is recommended as the drug of choice for treatment of humans, but many doses may be needed to maintain respiration until medical help can be obtained (see Chapter 18). It is important that the naloxone is not expired. Although not licensed for use in humans, there are anecdotal reports of diprenorphine being used effectively in emergency situations, but this drug does cause hallucinations in humans.

ANTICHOLINERGIC AGENTS

Anticholinergic agents are used widely in anaesthesia to antagonize the muscarinic effects of acetylcholine and thus to block transmission at parasympathetic postganglionic nerve endings. The main purposes are:

- To reduce salivation and bronchial secretions
- To block the effects of impulses in the vagus nerves
- To block certain of the effects produced by drugs that stimulate the parasympathetic system.

The reduction of salivation and bronchial secretion is necessary if irritant volatile anaesthetics such as ether are used. Ruminants produce large quantities of saliva but anticholinergic drugs merely make their saliva more viscid and thick and more likely to create respiratory obstruction.

Some drugs, in particular the α_2-agonists and, in high doses, the opioids, can cause marked vagally-mediated bradycardia. Under light anaesthesia, surgery of the head and neck is prone to trigger vagal reflexes, and the horse, dog and cat seem to be most at risk from these disturbances. In cats, dogs, and cattle, the oculocardiac reflex is well known to result in bradycardia and even cardiac arrest; stimulation of the nose or other similarly sensitive structures can have the same effect or cause laryngospasm. In horses, stimulation about the head and neck can produce sudden cardiac arrest without a prior warning of bradycardia.

Anticholinesterase drugs such as neostigmine are used to antagonize the block produced by competitive neuromuscular blocking drugs and their use must be preceded or combined with one of the anticholinergic drugs to block the muscarinic effects of the released acetylcholine. Also, the depolarizing agent suxamethonium has effects similar to those of acetylcholine and, at least in dogs and cats, an anticholinergic 'cover' should be employed when this relaxant is used (see Chapter 8).

In recent years, the advisability of routine premedication with anticholinergic drugs has been questioned. These drugs certainly have side effects; for example the tachycardia they induce may be undesirable and disturbance of vision may cause a cat to panic. Reduced gut motility may cause colic in horses.

Current practice seems to be not to use anticholinergic drugs for routine premedication unless there is a specific reason (e.g. intention to use high dose opioids), but to reserve them for corrective measures should bradycardia occur during the course of the anaesthetic. This, of course, assumes that monitoring is adequate to detect the bradycardia. However, IV injection of small doses of atropine may cause further bradycardia before increasing heart rate. At one time it was said that this was a central effect, but this is no longer thought to be the case and the reason is unknown (Glick, 2010). Glycopyrrolate, said not to cross the blood–brain barrier, can also cause this further bradycardia (Richards et al., 1989). Thus, the decision to include an anticholinergic agent in premedication may be based on the species of animal concerned, its size, the drugs to be used for and during anaesthesia, the likelihood of complications from bradycardia or vagal reflexes, the level of monitoring in use and any specific contraindications. The main contraindications are in conditions associated with tachycardia and in certain forms of glaucoma that are aggravated by dilatation of the pupil.

Atropine

Atropine, the most important of the alkaloids obtained from *Atropa belladonna* (deadly nightshade), is used in anaesthesia as its water-soluble sulphate. Its metabolism is not the same in all species of animal. When administered to dogs, atropine disappears very rapidly from the bloodstream (half-life of elimination 30–40 minutes). Part of the dose is excreted unchanged in the urine, part appears in the urine as tropine and the remainder is apparently broken down in the body to as yet unidentified substances. In cats, atropine is hydrolysed by either of two esterases which are found in large quantities in the liver and kidneys. These esterases are also found in rats and at high levels in some strains of rabbits, thus making atropine very short acting in this species.

Atropine inhibits transmission of postganglionic cholinergic nerve impulses to effector cells but inhibition is not equally effective all over the body and atropine has less effect upon the urinary bladder and intestines than upon the heart and salivary glands.

The drug has unpredictable effects on the central nervous system. Certain cerebral and medullary functions are initially stimulated then later depressed, so that the final outcome depends on the dose used and the route of administration. Clinical doses may produce an initial slowing of the heart due to stimulation of vagal centres in the brain before its peripheral anticholinergic effects occur. Atropine overdose causes a 'central cholinergic effect' with fluctuations between hyperexcitability and depression. Although atropine is, in general, a very safe drug with a wide therapeutic margin, occasional cases have been reported where an individual person or animal has appeared unduly sensitive to the central effects.

The main action of the drug is on the heart rate, which usually increases due to peripheral inhibition of the cardiac vagus; the initial slowing due to central action is only seen before the onset of peripheral inhibition. The minute volume of respiration is slightly increased due to central stimulation. Bronchial musculature is relaxed and bronchial secretions are reduced.

Atropine has marked ocular effects. Mydriasis results from the local or systemic administration of atropine.

Although atropine reduces muscle tone in the gastrointestinal tract, at the doses usually used for premedication this effect is minimal. The passage of barium meals along the gut of the dog is not appreciably slowed by atropine premedication. It is possible that the incidence of postanaesthetic colic in horses is increased by the use of this drug, although historically very large doses (more than 10 times the 0.01 mg/kg now recommended) were used, and such high doses did cause impacted colic. Because of the different ways in which they metabolize the drug, the effectiveness of a given dose varies according to the species of animal and will be discussed in the relevant species chapters.

Hyoscine

Hyoscine is an alkaloid resembling atropine, found in the same group of plants but usually obtained from the shrub henbane (*Hyoscyamus niger*). The peripheral actions of hyoscine resemble those of atropine. Hyoscine has a marketing licence for use in the horse as an antispasmolytic in cases of equine colic and is used to relax the intestine before rectal examinations. It has been used during anaesthesia in horses at doses of 0.1 mg/kg IV when it has increased heart rate for around 15 minutes (Borer & Clarke, 2006). In dogs, it has been used in doses of 5-20 µg/kg IM.

Glycopyrrolate

Glycopyrrolate is a quaternary ammonium anticholinergic agent with powerful and prolonged antisialagogue activity. As an antisialagogue, it is about five times as potent as atropine. It is particularly useful for combination with anticholinesterases for antagonizing the effects of non-depolarizing neuromuscular blocking agents. It has a slower onset of action than atropine and, as neostigmine also has a slow onset of action, a preparation of neostigmine with glycopyrrolate is available for when combined use is required. Work on anaesthetized human patients showed no difference in the cardiovascular effects of atropine and glycopyrrolate other than in the time of onset of action.

Glycopyrrolate has now been used widely in veterinary practice in doses of 0.01–0.02 mg/kg and a big advantage is that there is not the species-related pharmacokinetic disadvantages of atropine and it is effective in rabbits. However other potential advantages have not materialized. A comparison (Richards et al., 1989) of atropine given IV at doses of 0.02–0.04 mg/kg with IV glycopyrrolate (0.01 and 0.02 mg/kg) in dogs with drug-induced bradycardia showed that both agents caused a high incidence of cardiac arrhythmia, including atrioventricular block, during the first three minutes after injection, and the tachycardia that followed was equal with both agents. It has been suggested that as the drug does not readily cross the blood–brain barrier, it might have less effect on vision than other anticholinergic agents, but it still causes pupillary dilation in the cat.

Fenpipramide

A combination of levomethadone with fenpipramide is marketed in Europe under the trade name 'Polamivet'. Fenpipramide is an anticholinergic agent, and is included to prevent methadone-induced bradycardia. It appears to do this satisfactorily (Tunsmeyer et al., 2012), but there appears to be no information available concerning veterinary use of fenpipramide alone.

PREMEDICATION

Preanaesthetic medication or 'premedication' helps both the anaesthetist and the animal, for it makes induction and maintenance of anaesthesia easier for the anaesthetist while, at the same time, rendering the experience safer and more comfortable for the patient. It implies the administration, usually before, but sometimes at or immediately after, the induction of anaesthesia, of sedatives, anxiolytics and analgesics, with or without anticholinergics. The classical aims of using premedication are listed in Box 4.3.

The use of anticholinergic agents for premedication has been discussed in the previous section. Analgesic agents are essential if the patient is in pain in the preoperative period but, even when pain is absent, analgesics may increase preoperative sedation, reduce the dose of anaesthetic drugs needed, contribute to analgesia during surgery and even, if sufficiently long acting, contribute to analgesia postoperatively. The use of long-acting analgesics such as buprenorphine is particularly popular for the contribution they make to all stages of the anaesthetic process. Very potent but short-acting opioids, such as fentanyl and alfentanil, will reduce the dose of anaesthetic required, but their short action means that further analgesia must be provided during recovery.

Box 4.3 **Classical aims of premedication**

- To relieve anxiety, apprehension, fear and resistance to anaesthesia
- To counteract unwanted side effects of agents used in anaesthesia
  - Side effects depend on species and on drugs used
  - Examples – vomiting (mainly in dogs and cats), poor quality of recovery, bradycardia, salivation and excessive muscle tone
- To reduce the dose of anaesthetic
  - In many (but not all) cases, drug combinations may have a lower incidence of side effects than a high dose of the anaesthetic would have on its own
- To contribute to perioperative analgesia
  - Long-acting analgesics at premedication may contribute to pain relief before, during and after surgery

---

The sedative and anxiolytic drugs play the major role in premedication, improving the quality of anaesthesia and recovery, contributing to anaesthesia and, in some cases, counteracting unwanted side effects such as the muscle rigidity produced by ketamine. By calming the animal in the preoperative period, the necessary clipping and cleaning is made more pleasant for both the animal and nursing staff. Moreover, by controlling emotional disturbance, the release of catecholamines is reduced, thus decreasing the chance of epinephrine-induced cardiac arrhythmias, smoothing the course of anaesthesia and (usually) ensuring a quiet recovery.

The degree of activity of the CNS at the time when anaesthesia is induced determines the amount of anaesthetic that has to be administered to produce surgical anaesthesia. Sedatives and analgesics enhance the effects of the anaesthetic agents. In general, the depressant effects of the drugs used in premedication summate (or are even synergistic) with those of the anaesthetic and, unless this is clearly understood, overdosage may occur. Most sedative drugs depress respiration and, if given in large doses before anaesthetics that also produce respiratory depression (e.g. propofol), respiratory failure may occur before surgical anaesthesia is attained. Premedication must, therefore, be regarded as an integral part of the whole anaesthetic technique.

The type of sedative drug chosen for premedication will depend on a variety of factors. Acepromazine is a good anxiolytic and reduces the incidence of vomiting in dogs and cats, so is particularly useful if morphine, hydromorphone, or oxymorphone is also to be given. However, acepromazine increases the chance of regurgitation at induction of general anaesthesia in ruminants. The α_2-agonists provide profound sedation and are useful in the

95

animal which is particularly difficult to handle. It is important to remember that the potent opioids have a major effect in reducing the dose of subsequent anaesthetic drugs otherwise overdosage will occur. Some sedatives may provide muscle relaxation and these are especially effective in counteracting the muscle tension associated with the use of ketamine. Benzodiazepines provide little obvious preoperative sedation in healthy animals, but may provide good premedication for the sick, and their muscle relaxing properties are useful when ketamine is to be used for induction. Often, more than one sedative drug is used in premedication. For example, α_2-adrenoceptor agonists and benzodiazepines may be combined prior to the use of ketamine. However, such polypharmacy must be used with care, as many such combinations have synergistic activity and it is easy to administer an overdose of anaesthetic agents given subsequently. Premedicant drugs can be given by any one or more of the usual routes of drug administration. The choice is governed both by the nature of the drug and the time available before anaesthesia is to be induced.

In the past, it was fairly simple to define the limits of premedication and when anaesthesia began. Today, with the wide range of different types of drugs available, such distinctions are no longer clear. α_2-Agonists or benzodiazepines may be given 30 minutes prior to anaesthesia as premedicants or IV as part of the anaesthetic induction process (co-induction). Dissociative agents, such as ketamine, may be regarded as being drugs for premedication or for the induction or maintenance of general anaesthesia. In clinical practice, exact definitions of terminology are unimportant as long as the anaesthetist clearly understands the role played by each drug used, be it 'premedicant', 'dissociative agent' or 'anaesthetic', in the total process in bringing the animal to a state suitable for the performance of surgery, examination, or whatever else is required. Anxiolytics, sedatives, hypnotics and analgesics all have their place in this process. In any particular case, the choice of drugs, their dose and route of administration depends on the circumstances and gives the anaesthetist the opportunity to demonstrate their clinical assessment skills based on their scientific knowledge.

REFERENCES

Alibhai, H.I., Clarke, K.W., Lee, Y.H., et al., 1996. Cardiopulmonary effects of combinations of medetomidine hydrochloride and atropine sulphate in dogs. Vet Rec 138, 11–13.

Amarpal, Kinjavdekar, P., Aithal, H.P., et al., 2002. Analgesic, sedative and haemodynamic effects of spinally administered romifidine in female goats. J Vet Med A, Physiol Pathol Clin Med 49, 3–8.

Bergadano, A., Andersen, O.K., Arendt-Nielsen, L., et al., 2009. Modulation of nociceptive withdrawal reflexes evoked by single and repeated nociceptive stimuli in conscious dogs by low-dose acepromazine. Vet Anaesth Analg 36, 261–272.

Bettschart-Wolfensberger, R., Clarke, K.W., Vainio, O., et al., 1999. Pharmacokinetics of medetomidine in ponies and elaboration of a medetomidine infusion regime which provides a constant level of sedation. Res Vet Sci 67, 41–46.

Bettschart-Wolfensberger, R., Taylor, P.M., Sear, J.W., et al., 1996. Physiologic effects of anesthesia induced and maintained by intravenous administration of a climazolam-ketamine combination in ponies premedicated with

acepromazine and xylazine. Am J Vet Res 57, 1472–1477.

Borer, K.E., Clarke, K.W., 2006. The effect of hyoscine on dobutamine requirement in spontaneously breathing horses anaesthetized with halothane. Vet Anaesth Analg 33, 149–157.

Brashier, M., 2006. Fluphenazine-induced extrapyramidal side effects in a horse. Vet Clin N Am Equine Pract 22, e37–45.

Brodbelt, D.C., Blissitt, K.J., Hammond, R.A., et al., 2008a. The risk of death: the confidential enquiry into perioperative small animal fatalities. Vet Anaesth Analg 35, 365–373.

Brodbelt, D.C., Pfeiffer, D.U., Young, L.E., et al., 2008b. Results of the confidential enquiry into perioperative small animal fatalities regarding risk factors for anesthetic-related death in dogs. J Am Vet Med Assoc 233, 1096–1104.

Brown, E.N., Purdon, P.L., Van Dort, C.J., 2011. General anaesthesia and altered states of arousal: A systems neuroscience analysis. Ann Rev Neurosci 34, 601–628.

Bryant, C.E., England, G.C., Clarke, K.W., 1991. Comparison of the sedative effects of medetomidine and

xylazine in horses. Vet Rec 129, 421–423.

Bryant, C.E., Thompson, J., Clarke, K.W., 1998. Characterisation of the cardiovascular pharmacology of medetomidine in the horse and sheep. Res Vet Sci 65, 149–154.

Bylund, D.B., 1988. Subtypes of alpha 2-adrenoceptors: pharmacological and molecular biological evidence converge. Trends Pharmacol Sci 9, 356–361.

Bylund, D.B., Ray-Prenger, C., Murphy, T.J., 1988. Alpha-2A and alpha-2B adrenergic receptor subtypes: antagonist binding in tissues and cell lines containing only one subtype. J Pharmacol Exp Ther 245, 600–607.

Celly, C.S., Atwal, O.S., McDonell, W.N., et al., 1999. Histopathologic alterations induced in the lungs of sheep by use of alpha2-adrenergic receptor agonists. Am J Vet Res 60, 154–161.

Celly, C.S., McDonell, W.N., Young, S.S., et al., 1997. The comparative hypoxaemic effect of four alpha 2 adrenoceptor agonists (xylazine, romifidine, detomidine and medetomidine) in sheep. J Vet Pharmacol Ther 20, 464–471.

Chambers, J.P., Waterman, A.E., Livingston, et al., 1996. Prolonged action of detomidine in TB horses with abnormal liver function. J Assoc Vet Anaesth 23, 27–28.

Clarke, K.W., 1969. Effect of azaperone on the blood pressure and pulmonary ventilation in pigs. Vet Rec 85, 649–651.

Clarke, K.W., England, G.C.W., 1989. Medetomidine, a new sedative-analgesic for use in the dog and its reversal with atipamezole. J Small Anim Pract 30, 343–348.

Clarke, K.W., Hall, L.W., 1969. 'Xylazine' – a new sedative for horses and cattle. Vet Rec 85, 512–517.

Clarke, K.W., Hall, L.W., 1990. A survey of anaesthetic practice in small animals. J Assoc Vet Anaesth 17, 4–10.

Clarke, K.W., Taylor, P.M., 1987. Detomidine; a new sedative for horses. Equine Vet J 18, 366–370.

Court, M.H., Greenblatt, D.J., 1992. Pharmacokinetics and preliminary observations of behavioral changes following administration of midazolam to dogs. J Vet Pharmacol Ther 15, 343–350.

Covey-Crump, G.L., Murison, P.J., 2008. Fentanyl or midazolam for co-induction of anaesthesia with propofol in dogs. Vet Anaesth Analg 35, 463–472.

Cullen, L.K., 1996. Medetomidine sedation in dogs and cats: a review of its pharmacology, antagonism and dose. Br Vet J 152, 519–535.

da Costa, R.C., Parent, J.M., Dobson, H., 2011. Incidence of and risk factors for seizures after myelography performed with iohexol in dogs: 503 cases (2002–2004). J Am Vet Med Assoc 238, 1296–1300.

Davies, J.V., Gerring, E.L., 1983. Effect of spasmolytic analgesic drugs on the motility patterns of the equine small intestine. Res Vet Sci 34, 334–339.

Devisscher, L., Schauvliege, S., Dewulf, J., et al., 2010. Romifidine as a constant rate infusion in isoflurane anaesthetized horses: a clinical study. Vet Anaesth Analg 37, 425–433.

Di Concetto, S., Michael Archer, R., Sigurdsson, S.F., et al., 2007. Atipamezole in the management of detomidine overdose in a pony. Vet Anaesth Analg 34, 67–69.

Dodman, N.H., Waterman, A.E., 1979. Paradoxical excitement following the intravenous administration of

azaperone in the horse. Equine Vet J 11, 33–35.

Doherty, T.J., Geiser, D.R., Rohrbach, B.W., 1997. Effect of acepromazine and butorphanol on halothane minimum alveolar concentration in ponies. Equine Vet J 29, 374–376.

Dresel, P.E., 1985. Cardiac alpha receptors and arrhythmias. Anesthesiology 63, 582–583.

Driessen, B., Zarucco, L., Kalir, B., et al., 2011. Contemporary use of acepromazine in the anaesthetic management of male horses and ponies: a retrospective study and opinion poll. Equine Vet J 43, 88–98.

Drynan, E.A., Gray, P., Raisis, A.L., 2012. Incidence of seizures associated with the use of acepromazine in dogs undergoing myelography. J Vet Emerg Crit Care (San Antonio) 22, 262–266.

Dunkle, N., Moise, N.S., Scarlett-Kranz, J., et al., 1986. Cardiac performance in cats after administration of xylazine or xylazine and glycopyrrolate: echocardiographic evaluations. Am J Vet Res 47, 2212–2216.

Dyson, D.H., Maxie, M.G., Schnurr, D., 1998. Morbidity and mortality associated with anesthetic management in small animal veterinary practice in Ontario. J Am Anim Hosp Assoc 34, 325–335.

Eisenach, J.C., Grice, S.C., 1988. Epidural clonidine does not decrease blood pressure or spinal cord blood flow in awake sheep. Anesthesiology 68, 335–340.

England, G.C., Clarke, K.W., 1996. Alpha 2 adrenoceptor agonists in the horse – a review. Br Vet J 152, 641–657.

Enouri, S.S., Kerr, C.L., McDonell, W.N., et al., 2008. Effects of a peripheral alpha2 adrenergic-receptor antagonist on the hemodynamic changes induced by medetomidine administration in conscious dogs. Am J Vet Res 69, 728–736.

Erhardt, W., Stephen, M., Schatzmann, U., et al., 1986. Reversal of anaesthesia by simultaneously administered benzodiazpine and opioid antagonists in the dog. J Assoc Vet Anaesth 14, 90–99.

European Medicines Agency 2010. Romifidine, Safety report; Summary www.ema.europa.eu/ema accessed 4/3/2013.

Glick, D.B., 2010. The autonomic system. In: Millar, R.D., Erikson, L.I., Fleisher, L.A., et al. (Eds.), Miller's Anesthesia, seventh ed. Churchill Livingston-Elsevier.

Granholm, M., McKusick, B.C., Westerholm, F.C., et al., 2006. Evaluation of the clinical efficacy and safety of dexmedetomidine or medetomidine in cats and their reversal with atipamezole. Vet Anaesth Analg 33, 214–223.

Granholm, M., McKusick, B.C., Westerholm, F.C., et al., 2007. Evaluation of the clinical efficacy and safety of intramuscular and intravenous doses of dexmedetomidine and medetomidine in dogs and their reversal with atipamezole. Vet Rec 160, 891–897.

Grimsrud, K.N., Mama, K.R., Steffey, E.P., et al., 2012. Pharmacokinetics and pharmacodynamics of intravenous medetomidine in the horse. Vet Anaesth Analg 39, 38–48.

Hall, L.W., Dunn, J.K., Delaney, M., et al., 1991. Ambulatory electrocardiography in dogs. Vet Rec 129, 213–216.

Hall, R.I., Szlam, F., Hug, C.C., Jr, 1988. Pharmacokinetics and pharmacodynamics of midazolam in the enflurane-anesthetized dog. J Pharmacokinet Biopharm 16, 251–262.

Harthoorn, A.M., 1972. Restraint and neuroleptanalgesia in ungulates. Vet Rec 91, 63–67.

Hashem, A., Keller, H., 1993. Disposition, bioavailability and clinical efficacy of orally administered acepromazine in the horse. J Vet Pharmacol Ther 16, 359–368.

Heard, D.J., Webb, A.I., Daniels, R.T., 1986. Effect of acepromazine on the anesthetic requirement of halothane in the dog. Am J Vet Res 47, 2113–2115.

Heniff, M.S., Moore, G.P., Trout, A., et al., 1997. Comparison of routes of flumazenil administration to reverse midazolam-induced respiratory depression in a canine model. Acad Emerg Med 4, 1115–1118.

Honkavaara, J., Restitutti, F., Raekallio, M., et al., 2012. Influence of MK-467, a peripherally acting alpha2-adrenoceptor antagonist on the disposition of intravenous dexmedetomidine in dogs. Drug Metab Disposit Biol Fate Chem 40, 445–449.

Honkavaara, J.M., Raekallio, M.R., Kuusela, E.K., et al., 2008. The effects of L-659,066, a peripheral alpha2-adrenoceptor antagonist, on dexmedetomidine-induced sedation and bradycardia in dogs. Vet Anaesth Analg 35, 409–413.

Horta, M.L., Morejon, L.C., da Cruz, A.W., et al., 2006. Study of the prophylactic effect of droperidol, alizapride, propofol and promethazine on spinal morphine-induced pruritus. Br J Anaesth 96, 796–800.

Hsu, W.H., Lu, Z.X., Hembrough, F.B., 1985. Effect of xylazine on heart rate and arterial blood pressure in conscious dogs, as influenced by atropine, 4-aminopyridine, doxapram, and yohimbine. J Am Vet Med Assoc 186, 153–156.

Jalenka, H.H., 1989. The use of medetomidine and medetomidine-keatmine combinations and atipamezole at Helsinki Zoo – a review of 240 cases. Acta Vet Scand Suppl 85, 193–198.

James, M.F., 2009. Magnesium: an emerging drug in anaesthesia. Br J Anaesth 103, 465–467.

Jedruch, J., Gajewski, Z., 1986. The effect of detomidine hydrochloride (Domosedan) on the electrical activity of the uterus in cows. Acta Vet Scand Suppl 82, 189–192.

Jedruch, J., Gajewski, Z., Ratajska-Michalczak, K., 1989. Uterine motor responses to an alpha 2-adrenergic agonist medetomidine hydrochloride in the bitches during the end of gestation and the post-partum period. Acta Vet Scand Suppl 85, 129–134.

Jochle, W., Moore, J.N., Brown, J., et al., 1989. Comparison of detomidine, butorphanol, flunixin meglumine and xylazine in clinical cases of equine colic. Equine Vet J Suppl, 111–116.

Johnston, G.M., Eastment, J.K., Wood, J.L.N., et al., 2002. The confidential enquiry into perioperative equine fatalities (CEPEF): mortality results of Phases 1 and 2. Vet Anaesth Analg 29, 159–170.

Johnston, G.M., Taylor, P.M., Holmes, M.A., et al., 1995. Confidential enquiry of perioperative equine faalities (CEPEF-1): preliminary results. Equine Vet J 27, 193–200.

Kästner, S.B., 2006. A2-agonists in sheep: a review. Vet Anaesth Analg 33, 79–96.

Kästner, S.B., Von Rechenberg, B., Keller, K., et al., 2001. Comparison of medetomidine and dexmedetomidine as premedication in isoflurane anaesthesia for orthopaedic surgery in domestic sheep. J Vet Med A, Physiol Pathol Clin Med 48, 231–241.

Kendall, A., Mosley, C., Brojer, J., 2010. Tachypnea and antipyresis in febrile horses after sedation with alpha-agonists. J Vet Intern Med/Am Coll Vet Intern Med 24, 1008–1011.

Kerr, D.D., Jones, E.W., Holbert, D., et al., 1972. Comparison of the effects of xylazine and acetylpromazine maleate in the horse. Am J Vet Res 33, 777–784.

Khan, Z.P., Ferguson, C.N., Jones, R.M., 1999. Alpha-2 and imidazoline receptor agonists. Their pharmacology and therapeutic role. Anaesthesia 54, 146–165.

Kock, R.A., Iago, M., Gulland, F.M.D., et al., 1989. The use of two novel alpha 2 adrenceptor antagonists, idazoxan and its analogue, RX821002A in zoo and wildlife animals. J Assoc Vet Anaesth 16, 4–10.

Kronberg, G., Oberdorf, A., Hoffmeister, F., et al., 1966. Adrenergich-cholinergische neuronenhemmstoffe. Naturwissenschafaten 53, 502.

Langer, S.Z., 1974. Presynaptic regulation of catecholamine release. Biochem Pharmacol 23, 1793–1800.

Lees, P., 1979. Chemical Restraint of Large Animals In Pharmacological Basis of Small Animal Medicine. In: Bogan, J.A., Lees, P., Yoxall, A.T. (Eds.).Blackwell Scientific Publications, London.

Lees, P., Serrano, L., 1976. Effects of azaperone on cardiovascular and respiratory functions in the horse. Br J Pharmacol 56, 263–269.

Lerche, P., Muir, W.W., 2006. Effect of medetomidine on respiration and minimum alveolar concentration in halothane- and isoflurane-anesthetized dogs. Am J Vet Res 67, 782–789.

Livingston, A., Low, J., Morris, B., 1984. Effects of clonidine and xylazine on body temperature in the rat. Br J Pharmacol 81, 189–193.

Livingstone, A., Nolan, A., Waterman, A., 1986/87. The pharmacology of the alpha 2 adrenergic agonist drugs. J Assoc Vet Anaesth 14, 3–10.

Loscher, W., Frey, H.H., 1981. Pharmacokinetics of diazepam in the dog. Arch Int Pharmacodynam Ther 254, 180–195.

Mackenzie, G., Snow, D.H., 1977. An evaluation of chemical restraining agents. Vet Rec 101, 30–33.

Marntell, S., Nyman, G., Funkquist, P., et al., 2005. Effects of acepromazine on pulmonary gas exchange and circulation during sedation and dissociative anaesthesia in horses. Vet Anaesth Analg 32, 83–93.

Maze, M., Hayward, E., Jr, Gaba, D.M., 1985. Alpha 1-adrenergic blockade raises epinephrine-arrhythmia threshold in halothane-anesthetized dogs in a dose-dependent fashion. Anesthesiology 63, 611–615.

McCormick, J.M., McCormick, P.W., Zabramski, J.M., et al., 1993. Intracranial pressure reduction by a central alpha-2 adrenoreceptor agonist after subarachnoid hemorrhage. Neurosurgery 32, 974–979; discussion 979.

McGree, J.M., Noble, G., Schneiders, F., et al., 2013. A Bayesian approach for estimating detection times in horses: exploring the pharmacokinetics of a urinary acepromazine metabolite. J Vet Pharmacol Ther. 36, 31–42.

Muir, W.W., 1981. Drugs used to produce standing chemical restraint in horses. Vet Clin N Am Large Anim Pract 3, 17–44.

Muir, W.W., Piper, F.S., 1977. Effect of xylazine on indices of myocardial contractility in the dog. Am J Vet Res 38, 931–934.

Muir, W.W., Sams, R.A., Huffman, R.H., et al., 1982. Pharmacodynamic and pharmacokinetic properties of diazepam in horses. Am J Vet Res 43, 1756–1762.

Muir, W.W., Skarda, R.T., Sheehan, W., 1979. Hemodynamic and respiratory effects of a xylazine-acetylpromazine drug combination in horses. Am J Vet Res 40, 1518–1522.

Muir, W.W., Werner, L.L., Hamlin, R.L., 1975. Effects of xylazine and acetylpromazine upon induced ventricular fibrillation in dogs anesthetized with thiamylal and halothane. Am J Vet Res 36, 1299–1303.

Murrell, J.C., Hellebrekers, L.J., 2005. Medetomidine and dexmedetomidine: a review of cardiovascular effects and antinociceptive properties in the dog. Vet Anaesth Analg 32, 117–127.

Nolan, A.M., Waterman, A.E., Livingston, A., 1986. The analgesic activity of alpha-2 adrenoceptor agonists in sheep: A comparison with opioids. J Assoc Vet Anaesth 14, 14–15.

Olkkola, K.T., Ahonen, J., 2008. Midazolam and other benzodiazepines. Handbook Exp Pharmacol 335–360.

Parry, B.W., Anderson, G.A., Gay, C.C., 1982. Hypotension in the horse induced by acepromazine maleate. Aust Vet J 59, 148–152.

Pearson, H., Weaver, B.M., 1978. Priapism after sedation, neuroleptanalgesia and anaesthesia in the horse. Equine Vet J 10, 85–90.

Péters, F., Franck, T., Pequito, M., et al., 2009. In vivo administration of acepromazine or promethazine to horse decreases the reactive oxygen species production response of subsequently isolated neutrophils to stimulation with phorbol myristate acetate. J Vet Pharmacol Ther 32, 541–547.

Pettifer, G.R., Dyson, D.H., McDonell, W.N., 1996. An evaluation of the influence of medetomidine hydrochloride and atipamezole hydrochloride on the arrhythmogenic dose of epinephrine in dogs during halothane anesthesia. Can J Vet Res 60, 1–6.

Popovic, N.A., Mullane, J.F., Yhap, E.O., 1972. Effects of acetylpromazine maleate on certain cardiorespiratory responses in dogs. Am J Vet Res 33, 1819–1824.

Psatha, E., Alibhai, H.I., Jimenez-Lozano, A., et al., 2011. Clinical efficacy and cardiorespiratory effects of alfaxalone, or diazepam/fentanyl for induction of anaesthesia in dogs that are a poor anaesthetic risk. Vet Anaesth Analg 38, 24–36.

Rehm, W.F., Schatzmann, U., 1984. Benzodiazepines as sedatives for large animals. J Assoc Vet Anaesth 12, 93–106.

Restitutti, F., Raekallio, M., Vainionpaa, M., et al., 2012. Plasma glucose, insulin, free fatty acids, lactate and cortisol concentrations in dexmedetomidine-sedated dogs with or without MK-467: A peripheral alpha-2 adrenoceptor antagonist. Vet J 193, 481–485.

Reves, J.G., Glass, P.S.A., Lubarski, D.A., McEvoy, M.D., Martinez-Ruiz, R., 2010. Intravenous anaesthetics. In: Millar, R.D., Erikson, L.I., Fleisher, L.A., et al. (Eds.), Miller's Anesthesia, seventh ed. Churchill Livingston-Elsivier.

Richards, D.L.S., Clutton, R.E., Boyd, C., 1989. Electrocardiographic findings following intravenous glycopyrrolate to sedated dogs: a comparison with atropine. J Assoc Vet Anaesth 16, 46–50.

Ringer, S.K., Kalchofner, K., Boller, J., et al., 2007. A clinical comparison of two anaesthetic protocols using lidocaine or medetomidine in horses. Vet Anaesth Analg 34, 257–268.

Rioja, E., Dzikiti, B.T., Fosgate, G., et al., 2012. Effects of a constant rate infusion of magnesium sulphate in healthy dogs anaesthetized with isoflurane and undergoing ovariohysterectomy. Vet Anaesth Analg 39, 599–610.

Salonen, J.S., 1989. Pharmacokinetics of medetomidine. Acta Vet Scand Suppl 85, 49–54.

Sanchez, L.C., Elfenbein, J.R., Robertson, S.A., 2008. Effect of acepromazine, butorphanol, or N-butylscopolammonium bromide on visceral and somatic nociception and duodenal motility in conscious horses. Am J Vet Res 69, 579–585.

Sanders, R.D., Maze, M., 2007. Alpha2-adrenoceptor agonists. Curr Opin Investig Drugs 8, 25–33.

Scheinin, M., MacDonald, E., 1989. An introduction to the pharmacology of alpha 2-adrenoceptors in the central nervous system. Acta Vet Scand Suppl 85, 11–19.

Selmi, A.L., Barbudo-Selmi, G.R., Mendes, G.M., et al., 2004. Sedative, analgesic and cardiorespiratory effects of romifidine in cats. Vet Anaesth Analg 31, 195–206.

Serteyn, D., Benbarek, H., Deby-dupont, G., et al., 1999. Effects of acepromazine on equine polymorphonuclear neutrophil activation: a chemiluminescence study. Vet J 157, 332–335.

Short, C.E., Matthews, N., Harvey, R., et al., 1986. Cardiovascular and pulmonary function studies of a new sedative/analgetic (detomidine/ Domosedan) for use alone in horses or as a preanesthetic. Acta Vet Scand Suppl 82, 139–155.

Sinclair, M.D., 2003. A review of the physiological effects of alpha2-agonists related to the clinical use of medetomidine in small animal practice. Can Vet J 44, 885–897.

Sinclair, M.D., Dyson, D.H., 2012. The impact of acepromazine on the efficacy of crystalloid, dextran or ephedrine treatment in hypotensive dogs under isoflurane anesthesia. Vet Anaesth Analg 39, 563–573.

Sneyd, J.R., 2009. Droperidol: past, present and future. Anaesthesia 64, 1161–1164.

Sneyd, J.R., Rigby-Jones, A.E., 2010. New drugs and technologies, intravenous anaesthesia is on the move (again). Br J Anaesth 105, 246–254.

Spadavecchia, C., Arendt-Nielsen, L., Andersen, O.K., et al., 2005. Effect of romifidine on the nociceptive withdrawal reflex and temporal summation in conscious horses. Am J Vet Res 66, 1992–1998.

Taylor, A.H., Bolt, D.M., 2011. Persistent penile erection (priapism) after acepromazine premedication in a gelding. Vet Anaesth Analg 38, 523–525.

Tobias, K.M., Marioni-Henry, K., Wagner, R., 2006. A retrospective study on the use of acepromazine maleate in dogs with seizures. J Am Anim Hos Assoc 42, 283–289.

Tobin, T., Ballard, S., 1979. Pharmacological review – the phenothiazine tranquilizers. J Equine Med Surg 3, 460–466.

Trim, C.M., Colbern, G.T., Martin, C.L., 1985. Effect of xylazine and ketamine on intraocular pressure in horses. Vet Rec 117, 442–443.

Tunsmeyer, J., Vaske, B., Bosing, B., et al., 2012. Cardiovascular effects of a proprietary l-methadone/ fenpipramide combination (Polamivet) alone and in addition to acepromazine in healthy Beagle dogs. Vet Anaesth Analg 39, 451–463.

Vaha-Vahe, T., 1989. Clinical evaluation of medetomidine, a novel sedative and analgesic drug for dogs and cats. Acta Vet Scand 30, 267–273.

Vainio, O., Palmu, L., Virtanen, R., et al., 1986. Medetomidine: A new sedative and analgesic drug for dogs and cats. J Assoc Vet Anaesth 14, 53–55.

Vainio, O., Vahe-Vahe, T., 1989. Reversal of medetomidine sedation by atipamezole in dogs. J Vet Pharmacol Ther 13, 15–22.

Vainio, O., 1990. Reversal of medetomidine-induced cardiovascular and respiratory changes with atipamezole in dogs. Vet Rec 127, 447–450.

Vainio, O., Vaha-Vahe, T., Palmu, L., 1989. Sedative and analgesic effects of medetomidine in dogs. J Vet Pharmacol Ther 12, 225–231.

Valverde, A., Cantwell, S., Hernandez, J., et al., 2004. Effects of acepromazine on the incidence of vomiting associated with opioid administration in dogs. Vet Anaesth Analg 31, 40–45.

Valverde, A., Rickey, E., Sinclair, M., et al., 2010. Comparison of cardiovascular function and quality of recovery in isoflurane-anaesthetised horses administered a constant rate infusion of lidocaine or lidocaine and medetomidine during elective surgery. Equine Vet J 42, 192–199.

van der Harst, M.R., van der Velden, M.A., Ensink, J.M., 2002. [Priapism in the stallion]. Tijdschr diergeneeskunde 127, 746–751.

Van Miert, A.S., Koot, M., Van Duin, C.T., 1989. Appetite-modulating drugs in dwarf goats, with special emphasis on benzodiazepine-induced hyperphagia and its antagonism by flumazenil and RO 15-3505. J Vet Pharmacol Ther 12, 147–156.

Virkkila, M., Ali-Melkkila, T., Kanto, J., et al., 1994. Dexmedetomidine as intramuscular premedication for day-case cataract surgery. A comparative study of dexmedetomidine, midazolam and placebo. Anaesthesia 49, 853–858.

Virtanen, R., 1989. Pharmacological profiles of medetomidine and its antagonist, atipamezole. Acta Vet Scand Suppl 85, 29–37.

Wijeysundera, D.N., Bender, J.S., Beattie, W.S., 2009. Alpha-2 adrenergic agonists for the prevention of cardiac complications among patients undergoing surgery. Cochrane Database Syst Rev, CD004126.

Wilson, D.V., Nickels, F.A., Williams, M.A., 1991. Pharmacologic treatment of priapism in two horses. J Am Vet Med Assoc 199, 1183–1184.

Wismer, T.A., 2002. Accidental ingestion of alprazolam in 415 dogs. Vet Hum Toxicol 44, 22–23.

Chapter | 5 |

Analgesia

Kate Borer-Weir

Analgesia is one component of the triad of anaesthesia (with narcosis and muscle relaxation) and some anaesthetic drugs have analgesic properties. Analgesia must be provided before surgery in animals with pre-existing injuries as well as in the intra- and postoperative periods.

It is difficult to define pain satisfactorily. Everyone has their own idea of 'what pain is' but it can be hard to put this experience into words. The International Association for the Study of Pain (IASP) has the following definition: 'Pain is an unpleasant sensory and emotional experience associated with actual or potential tissue damage or described in terms of such damage.' This definition relates to human experience and may not be accurate when applied to animals, as they cannot describe emotions brought about by pain. However, the IASP also recommends that 'the inability to communicate verbally does not negate the possibility that an individual is experiencing pain and is in need of appropriate pain-relieving treatment'. It is now generally accepted that animals feel pain in the same way as humans, as the physiological mechanisms are similar. Controversy exists about whether neonatal animals and fetuses in utero feel pain and which procedures are acceptable to perform on neonates of what age without analgesia.

PHYSIOLOGY OF PAIN

Nociception describes the sensory processes by which noxious stimuli are transmitted to the brain. Stimulation of peripheral nerve endings (nociceptors) generates action potentials in sensory nerves. Different nociceptors respond to different stimuli: mechanoreceptors respond to pressure and stretch; thermoreceptors to heat and cold; and chemoreceptors to inflammatory mediators such as H^+, K^+ and prostaglandins. Nociceptive impulses are transmitted in Aδ and C fibres. Aδ fibres are small myelinated fibres which transmit the sensation of fast, sharp pain. C fibres are the smallest unmyelinated fibres which detect slow, dull pain. Sensory neurons enter the spinal cord via the dorsal horn (ending preferentially on cells in laminae 1, 2 and 5) where they may stimulate a simple withdrawal reflex, passing the information directly to motor nerves to cause movement of a limb away from a painful surface for example.

Concurrently, information passes up the spinal cord in pathways including the spinothalamic and spinoreticular tracts (in the ventrolateral white matter), through many interneurons to reach the brain, particularly the thalamus. From here, information passes to higher centres in the cerebral cortex.

In the spinal cord, many receptors and mediators modulate the information passing to the brain. Excitatory transmitters, including glutamate, substance P and prostaglandins, propagate the pain impulse. Inhibitory transmitters, such as endorphins, norepinephrine, serotonin (5-hydroxytryptamine; 5-HT) and γ-aminobutyric acid (GABA), reduce the painful stimuli reaching the brain. This forms the basis of the 'gate theory', an adaptive method of controlling the painful stimuli which reach the brain. It evolved to allow escape from life-threatening situations and means that the brain does not perceive the true amount of pain until the concentrations of inhibitory neurotransmitters, such as epinephrine and norepinephrine, drop sufficiently to allow nociceptive transmission to resume. Descending pathways from the brain (particularly the periaqueductal grey; PAG) also contribute to this inhibitory control. Stimulation of non-nociceptive neurons (e.g. by touch or pressure) can inhibit transmission in nociceptive neurons.

The nervous system demonstrates 'functional plasticity' and numerous changes occur after continued nociceptive stimulation. The products of tissue breakdown and damage have direct and indirect effects on sensory neurons. Neurotransmitters are released in the periphery from nociceptive nerve terminals, including substance P, bradykinin, neurokinin A and calcitonin gene-related peptide (CGRP). These substances cause vasodilation, extravasation of plasma proteins, stimulation of inflammatory cells to release more mediators and excitation of other sensory and sympathetic neurons. This produces an 'inflammatory soup', sensitizing nociceptors and sensory nerves causing peripheral sensitisation (primary hyperalgesia: increased sensitivity to painful stimulation at the site of injury). Prostaglandins in particular increase the sensitivity to pain by lowering the threshold at which nociceptive neurons fire. Other changes in the peripheral nervous system include spontaneous, ectopic activity in primary afferent nerves and sprouting of sympathetic nerves around the dorsal root ganglion.

Glutamate, one of the primary excitatory neurotransmitters in the CNS usually acts via AMPA (α-amino-3-hydroxy-5-methyl-4-isoxazole propionic acid) and neurokinin receptors. However, continued nociceptive stimulation within the spinal cord releases glutamate and substance P and removes the Mg^{2+} plug which usually blocks the N-methyl-d-aspartate (NMDA) receptor for glutamate, allowing priming of this receptor. Once the NMDA receptor is active, glutamate binding allows Ca^{2+} entry and stimulates second messenger release. Continued nociceptive stimulation alters the distribution of AMPA receptors within the dorsal horn and there may be loss of inhibitory neurons containing GABA. These changes within the CNS are known as central sensitization (secondary hyperalgesia), representing the spread of pain sensitivity (a lowered threshold to pain) outside the area of the original injury. The development of central sensitization may be regulated by the c-fos gene, which is expressed rapidly in spinal and supraspinal neurons following nociceptive stimulation.

Allodynia describes altered pain perception, whereby non-painful stimuli, such as touch, are perceived as painful by the patient. It commonly occurs during neuropathic or chronic pain and can be very hard to control with analgesic drugs. The mechanism behind allodynia may include sprouting of non-nociceptive A fibres into areas of the dorsal horn where C fibres normally terminate.

Optimal pain management should include preventing the development of chronic or neuropathic pain and the associated changes in the nervous system associated with hyperalgesia. Pre-emptive analgesia describes the provision of analgesia before any painful stimuli have occurred. This prevents the development of hypersensitization during surgery and should result in less postoperative pain that is easier to manage with lower doses of analgesic drugs. In animals with pre-existing injuries, such as those with orthopaedic problems or after road traffic accidents, provision of analgesia as soon as possible may reduce the development of sensitization but not completely eliminate it. There are conflicting reports on the benefits of pre-emptive analgesia and differences between experimental and clinical studies. Meta-analyses in human medicine have demonstrated both a positive effect (Ong et al., 2005) and no benefit (Moiniche et al., 2002).

The goal of multimodal analgesia is to block the pain pathways at multiple sites, using agents with different modes of action, thus providing more effective pain control with decreased dose rates and reduced prevalence or severity of toxic side effects. Drugs can be used to inhibit transduction and peripheral sensitization, inhibit transmission of sensory impulses, modulate the spinal pathways involved in central sensitization and to inhibit perception of a noxious stimulus in the brain.

In humans, analgesia is considered to be effective when the clinical signs of pain disappear. Similarly, a drug may be considered to be analgesic in an animal if signs associated with pain are ameliorated following administration. It is important to be sure that the drug effect is truly analgesia and not merely preventing the animal displaying the behavioural signs of pain. An extreme example would be administration of a neuromuscular blocking drug that causes paralysis without affecting the perception of a painful stimulus.

PAIN ASSESSMENT

Pain assessment is a crucial component of effective analgesia. Clinical signs of pain (Box 5.1) are unreliable, nonspecific, and differ between species. Heart rate, respiratory rate and pupil dilation were not useful indicators of pain in dogs recovering from surgery (Holton et al., 1998a). Furthermore, these parameters were poorly correlated with subjective pain scores in dogs after orthopaedic surgery (Conzemius et al., 1997). In horses following orthopaedic surgery, measurement of blood pressure, but not heart

---

Box 5.1 Clinical signs and behaviours commonly associated with pain

Clinical signs

Tachycardia
Tachypnoea
Hypertension
Pale mucous membranes
Cardiac arrhythmias
Dilated pupils
Salivation
Teeth grinding
Sweating
Poor body or coat condition

Observed behaviours

Abnormal postures: hunched up, guarding abdomen, praying position
Abnormal movement (increased or decreased): restlessness, circling, rolling)
Abnormal gait: stiffness, lameness
Reluctance to move or lie down
Aggression
Paying attention to an injured area: licking, chewing
Vocalization: whining, crying, howling
Head hanging down, low tail carriage
Depression, inappetance, dullness
Not grooming, poor hair coat
Increased urination and defaecation
Trembling
Poor interaction with people or animals, hiding
Unaware of surroundings

Note: Not all these are specific to pain, and may not be displayed by all species in all circumstances.

---

rate, was correlated with behavioural assessment of pain (Bussieres et al., 2008).

Pain assessment often relies on behavioural indicators of pain (see Box 5.1), but these vary between species, breeds, and individuals. Behaviour is also modified when the animal is in a hospital environment. Behavioural signs of pain depend on the origin of the pain, for example, visceral or somatic pain, and the type of procedure performed. Much of the early research on pain assessment was performed on dogs in the acute postoperative period. Now research includes behaviours associated with chronic pain (including cancer), medical pain and pain in domestic, agricultural, and exotic species. Behavioural assessment of pain in horses and donkeys (Ashley et al., 2005) and laboratory animals (Roughan & Flecknell, 2004; Roughan et al., 2009) have been reviewed.

Measurement of 'stress hormones' including epinephrine, cortisol, endorphins, glucose and insulin have not proved useful in diagnosing pain in individual animals in the clinical setting, although they can be supportive in research studies to distinguish between treatment and control groups. They are increased by conditions causing stress such as hospitalization and general anaesthesia.

When assessing behaviour, the animal should first be observed undisturbed and then during a series of interactions. Some behaviours arising from poor general health, medical problems, anxiety or fear may be mistakenly assessed as pain behaviour, and other behaviours such as aggression may be normal for the individual. Pain may also be evident through the suppression of normal behaviour, rather than additional pain-related behaviour. Prey animals in particular are unlikely to display overt pain behaviours as an evolutionary survival mechanism, and pain assessment in these animals can be difficult. Pain behaviours are useful to detect the presence of pain but they may not indicate the severity of pain.

Pain scales

Pain scales were created to increase objectivity in pain assessment and to decrease variability between scorers and animals. Pain scales are not infallible but use of a pain score helps to monitor changes in the same animal over time, providing information for adjustments in the analgesic regimen. During preanaesthetic evaluation, the patient should be assessed for pre-existing pain and a judgement made regarding the degree of pain likely to be experienced during the procedure. For example, minor procedures such as laceration repair would be expected to cause less pain than major orthopaedic surgery or thoracotomy.

A simple descriptive score (SDS) uses a scale from 0 to 3 to score no pain (0), mild pain (1), moderate pain (2) and severe pain (3). This is simple and quick to perform during a busy working day but is subjective and relatively imprecise. Inter-observer variability using an SDS was fair for dogs post-surgery assessed by three or four vets (Holton et al., 1998b).

The visual analogue scale (VAS) is a line 100 mm long anchored at either end with 0 = no pain and 100 = worst pain possible (Fig. 5.1). The observer places a mark on the line at their assessment of the patient's pain and the distance from 0 to the mark is measured. There is considerable inter-individual variability in the score assigned by different observers using a VAS (Holton et al., 1998b), but a single observer can become consistent with practice.

A simple numerical rating scale (NRS) can be used to assign a score from 0 to 10 for the assessed degree of pain. This score is commonly used to assess equine lameness. The numbers do not have specific descriptors, and there is often considerable inter-observer variability in scoring. A more involved NRS uses multiple categories containing specific descriptors of different types of behaviour, each of which has a numerical score. One descriptor from each category is selected and the total score from each category added to give an overall pain score. This gives a more thorough pain evaluation, but is also more time consuming. It can be limiting if the behaviour displayed by the individual animal does not match exactly any of the descriptors in the scale. An example is the University of Melbourne Pain Scale (UMPS), which includes both behavioural responses and physiological data (Firth & Haldane, 1999). A similar composite pain scale based on the NRS has been developed to assess orthopaedic pain in horses (Bussieres et al., 2008).

The previous pain scores are all unidimensional, assessing only pain intensity. However, it is well known from human experience that pain has additional significant sensory and affective qualities. These are addressed in multidimensional pain scores. The McGill pain questionnaire uses a series of descriptive words, categorized according to their sensory, affective or evaluative capacity, each of which is anchored to a numerical score to assess pain in humans (Melzack, 2005). The Glasgow Composite Pain Tool was developed in a similar way to assess acute surgical pain in dogs (Holton et al., 2001). A series of expressions and descriptions of behaviour were reduced to specific words and phrases to describe different aspects of the pain experience. The aim was to reduce inter-observer variability and bias. The Short Form of the Glasgow Pain Scale is an extension of this, incorporating a numerical score to aid clinical use (Reid et al., 2007). Many of the problems associated with pain assessment in animals and limitations of some of the scores currently available, including validation of the score and linearity of the scale used, have been reviewed (Flecknell & Roughan, 2004).

Analgesiometry systems (nociceptive threshold testing) are commonly used in the initial testing of analgesic drugs to assess relative potency, onset and duration of action. These involve the use of a controlled and repeatable stimulus, often a pressure or thermal stimulus, applied before and after administration of an analgesic (Dixon et al., 2002). The animal is observed for a specific aversion response, such as turning of the head, at which point the stimulus is stopped and the maximum value noted. This provides a very useful starting point for the comparison of different analgesics in animals, but it must be appreciated that clinical pain is much more complex and the performance of a drug in an analgesiometry system may not be representative of its efficacy as an analgesic in different clinical pain scenarios (Melzack, 2005).

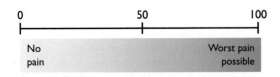

Figure 5.1 Visual analogue scale (VAS).

Specific pain scores for different species are discussed further in the relevant species chapters.

NON-STEROIDAL ANTI-INFLAMMATORY DRUGS (NSAIDS)

NSAIDS have anti-inflammatory, analgesic and antipyretic actions. They are among the most commonly used drugs in veterinary medicine to relieve pain and inflammation in all species. Many can be given initially by injection and then prescribed orally for longer-term use. They are not subject to controlled drugs legislation and there are many different agents licensed for use in different species and in different countries. Salicylate is a naturally occurring NSAID found in willow which has been used for thousands of years. However, the first synthetic NSAID was synthesized in the 1870s (Lees et al., 2004b). Acetylsalicylate (acetylsalicylic acid; aspirin) still has an annual consumption of approximately 80 billion tablets per year.

Pharmacology

NSAIDS inhibit production of prostaglandins (PGs) and thromboxane (TX) via inhibition of cyclo-oxygenase (COX; Fig. 5.2). PGs, TX and leukotrienes (LTs) are generated from arachidonic acid which is a 20-carbon fatty acid, released from cell membrane phospholipids after cell damage. The conversion of cell membrane phospholipid to arachidonic acid is catalysed by phospholipase A_2, which is inhibited by glucocorticoids (Fig. 5.2).

PGs have many homeostatic functions in the body, including maintenance of the gastric mucosal barrier and protection against gastric ulceration. PGs also help to maintain adequate renal blood flow, especially in situations where this is reduced. As well as their physiological functions, PGs are key inflammatory mediators, acting synergistically with other mediators, such as histamine and bradykinin, to increase pain, capillary permeability and oedema.

In general, NSAIDs are well absorbed after oral administration, are highly protein bound in plasma and have a large volume of distribution (Lees et al., 2004b; Curry et al., 2005). There are significant species differences in pharmacokinetics, including clearance, half-life and COX selectivity, meaning that extrapolation between different species is not recommended (Lees et al., 2004b). Genetic polymorphisms in response to NSAIDS exist, for example clearance and elimination half-life of celecoxib in Beagles differed by more than twofold in animals with hepatic microsomal enzyme differences (Paulson et al., 1999). Disease states may also reduce clearance and thus increase the effective half-life of NSAIDS (Lohuis et al. 1991). The pharmacokinetics can also differ depending on whether NSAIDs are administered before or after general anaesthesia (Lascelles et al., 1998).

COX-1 and COX-2

Two iso-enzymes of COX with slightly different chemical structures were discovered in 1991. Initially, these two iso-forms were thought to have quite separate and different roles. COX-1 was regarded as the *constitutive* enzyme, responsible for the production of PGs with physiological or 'housekeeping' functions including gastric and renal protection. COX-2 was thought to be the *inducible* enzyme, found at sites of injury producing PGs with inflammatory functions.

Classical NSAIDs inhibit both COX-1 and COX-2 with COX-1 inhibition resulting primarily in the side effects of these drugs including gastric ulceration and renal failure. Drug manufacturers sought to develop NSAIDs with COX-2 selective inhibitory activity. They hoped this would remove the risk of side effects, but retain the beneficial anti-inflammatory effects.

NSAIDs are thus classified into:

- Non-selective drugs which inhibit both COX-1 and COX-2 equally (classical NSAIDs)
- COX-2 selective which selectively or preferentially inhibit COX-2
- COX-1 selective which selectively or preferentially inhibit COX-1
- COX-2 specific which inhibit COX-2 exclusively and have almost no effect on COX-1 at therapeutic doses. These are also known as 'coxib' drugs.

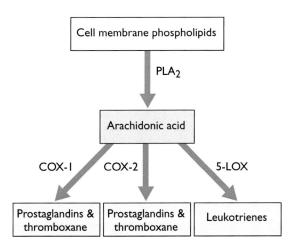

PLA$_2$ = Phospholipase A$_2$
COX = Cyclo-oxygenase
LOX = Lipoxygenase

Figure 5.2 Metabolism of phospholipids to form arachidonic acid, prostaglandins, thromboxane and leukotrienes.

Coxib drugs are large molecules which fit into the binding pocket of the COX-2 receptor, but are too large to fit into the smaller COX-1 receptor, resulting in their selectivity (Bergh & Budsberg, 2005).

The COX-1:COX-2 ratio describes the selectivity of the NSAID and refers to the dose of drug which must be given to inhibit each of the two isoforms. Non-selective agents have a COX-1:COX-2 ratio close to 1. COX-2 selective inhibitors have a ratio greater than 1 (i.e. a higher dose of drug must be given to inhibit COX-1 compared to the dose required to inhibit COX-2). The specific COX-2 inhibitors typically have a COX-1:COX-2 ratio of 100 or more. This means you would need to give 100× more drug to inhibit COX-1 than you would to inhibit COX-2.

The COX-1:COX-2 ratio varies depending on the type of assay used. The whole blood assay is considered the most applicable to the *in vivo* situation. Ratios also vary between different tissues and species. For example, in the dog, carprofen is thought to be COX-2 selective; in the horse, it is non-selective, whereas in humans, it is COX-1 selective (Brideau et al., 2001; Lees et al., 2002, 2004b). Many COX-1:COX-2 ratios are based on the IC_{50} for each isoform (the concentration of drug giving 50% inhibition of COX). However, it is more relevant to look at the ratio that reflects the clinically desirable degree of inhibition for each enzyme. This is believed to be 20% or less for COX-1 inhibition and 80% or more for COX-2 inhibition, resulting in an IC_{20} COX-1:IC_{80} COX-2 ratio. This ratio is often quite different from the IC_{50} ratio for a given drug.

Initially, the roles of COX-1 and COX-2 were thought to be quite separate with little overlap in the functions of the PGs produced by each isoform. However, we now know that there is a considerable overlap between the two (Wallace, 1999; Curry et al., 2005). In particular, COX-1 is upregulated at sites of injury and catalyses the production of inflammatory PGs. COX-1 is involved in spinal cord pain processing and hypersensitization, and COX-1 inhibition in the spinal cord reduces postoperative pain in rats (Zhu et al., 2005). COX-2 has physiological roles in the body, including gastric ulcer healing and it is constitutively expressed in many tissues, including the kidney, brain, reproductive tract and ciliary body of the eye. The role of COX-2 in different tissues and the effects of COX-2 inhibition have been reviewed (Bergh & Budsberg, 2005). Therefore, selective COX-2 inhibition does not completely eliminate the side effects associated with classical NSAIDS.

There is continuing debate over the presence of a third isoform of COX, COX-3, within the CNS (Kis et al., 2005). Some consider this to be a separate isoform, others feel that it is merely a splice variant of COX-1 and should not be considered separately from COX-1, while others question its existence at all (Kis et al., 2005). COX-3 was first described in dogs where it was primarily found in the cerebral cortex and was produced by the COX-1 gene (Chandrasekharan et al., 2002). Others have reported that it has a low expression level, limiting its clinical importance (Kis et al., 2005). Some NSAIDs may have a central component to their analgesic actions mediated by COX-3. Most NSAIDs cross the blood–brain barrier poorly, with the exception of paracetamol, which appears to exert its main antipyretic and analgesic effects in the CNS. Paracetamol has minimal inhibitory effects on peripheral COX activity *in vitro*, but produces analgesia in different animal models of pain and nociception (Warner & Mitchell, 2002). It also lacks ulcerogenic potential in the gastrointestinal tract. It may be a potent inhibitor of COX-3 (Chandrasekharan et al., 2002) with weak activity against COX-1 and COX-2. However, in humans, the existence of COX-3 has not been proven and, as a result, interest and research in the area has waned. The target site of action of paracetamol is still unclear. On a similar note, some studies have reported that carprofen is only a weak inhibitor of COX in the periphery (Lees et al., 2002), yet it is a powerful analgesic agent. It has been hypothesized that central inhibition of COX-3 may contribute to carprofen's analgesic actions.

Other studies have hypothesized that the central analgesic effect of NSAIDs is mediated by activation of descending inhibitory pathways (both opioidergic and adrenergic) within the spinal cord (Lizarraga & Chambers, 2006).

NSAIDs may also exert anti-inflammatory actions through a variety of COX-independent mechanisms, including key signaling pathways involving phosphatidylinositol 3-kinase (PI3K), peroxisome proliferator-activated receptors (PPAR), nuclear factor kappa B (NFκB) and mitogen-activated protein kinases (MAPK) among others. These mechanisms have been recently reviewed (Little et al., 2007b; KuKanich et al., 2012).

Side effects

The side effects of NSAIDs are mainly related to undesirable inhibition of COX-1 and are generally common to the group although the likelihood of each varies slightly depending on the COX-1:COX-2 selectivity ratio of the specific drug and the particular species concerned. Gastrointestinal ulceration is one of the commonest side effects in both humans and animals. PGs increase blood flow to the gastric mucosa and also increase secretion of protective mucous and bicarbonate. COX-2 is upregulated around existing gastric ulcers and this isoenzyme may play a key role in ulcer healing. In humans and small animals, gastric lesions and gastric ulcerations are commonest. In horses, while gastric ulceration occurs in response to NSAIDs, lesions involving the colon resulting in right dorsal colitis may also occur, particularly after an NSAID overdose. Combination therapy with two different NSAIDs or administration above the recommended dose also increases the risk of serious GI side effects (Reed et al., 2006).

Both carprofen and meloxicam had minimal effects on gastrointestinal permeability in healthy dogs, however, individual variation was apparent, with permeability increasing in some (Craven et al., 2007), while gastric lesions on endoscopy and occult blood on faecal examination have been reported in experimental dogs (Luna et al., 2007). In horses, non-selective COX inhibitors such as flunixin slow the recovery of ischaemic-damaged intestinal mucosa (Campbell & Blikslager, 2000; Tomlinson & Blikslager, 2004), mainly by affecting the integrity of tight junctions between intestinal cells and thus increasing paracellular permeability. This effect was not seen with meloxicam, a COX-2 selective inhibitor in the horse (Little et al., 2007a).

COX-inhibiting nitric oxide donors (CINODs) are nitrosoesters of classical NSAIDs, which may have a better GI safety profile than NSAIDS. In the body, CINODs are broken down to release the parent NSAID and nitric oxide (NO). NO is a vasodilator which may help to prevent local ischaemia in the GI tract associated with COX inhibition or, alternatively, NO may prevent neutrophil attachment to gastric mucosal blood vessels. The pharmacology of the first CINOD to be developed, naproxcinod, has been reviewed (Wallace et al., 2009), although there have been no reports of the use of CINODs in veterinary medicine.

In the kidney, PGs are released from the macula densa in response to vasoconstriction of the afferent arteriole. The resultant vasodilation helps to maintain adequate renal blood flow and glomerular filtration rate (GFR). Adverse renal effects of NSAIDS are most likely to occur during periods when renal blood flow is already compromised, such as hypotension due to haemorrhage, shock or general anaesthesia. These effects appear to be similar with both non-selective NSAIDs and selective COX-2 inhibitors as both COX-1 and COX-2 are constitutively expressed in the kidney. Perioperative carprofen had no effect on GFR or renal blood flow in experimental, healthy anaesthetized Beagles (Frendin et al., 2006) and meloxicam had no significant effect on renal function in otherwise healthy dogs rendered hypotensive under anaesthesia (Bostrom et al., 2006). NSAID-induced nephrotoxicity in humans is more likely in patients also receiving diuretics and/or ACE inhibitors (Weir, 2002).

The different COX isoforms are responsible for producing PGs and TX with different vascular effects. Prostacyclin (PGI_2) is produced under the action of COX-2 in the vascular endothelium. PGI_2 inhibits platelet aggregation, causes vasodilation and inhibits the proliferation of vascular smooth muscle. Thromboxane A_2 (TXA_2) is produced by COX-1 in platelets and causes platelet aggregation, vasoconstriction and proliferation of vascular smooth muscle. Usually, the body is able to maintain equilibrium in the production of PGI_2 and TXA_2. Aspirin primarily inhibits COX-1, reducing production of TXA_2. This can result in bleeding, but is also the reason for the use of low-dose aspirin to prevent thrombosis in susceptible human patients after heart attacks and strokes. Conversely, specific COX-2 inhibitors reduce production of PGI_2 and leave the body in a 'pro-aggregatory' state, with an increased susceptibility to thrombotic events in humans. The risk of these vascular thrombotic events led to the withdrawal of many coxib drugs from the human market. The thrombotic risk to animals treated with coxib drugs is unclear at the moment, as long-term treatment was necessary in humans before the risk became evident. Animals have a different vascular wall structure to humans and tend to have a lower risk of thrombotic vascular events overall, so there may be minimal risk associated with the use of coxib drugs in veterinary species.

Drugs available

The use of NSAIDs in the cat (Lascelles et al., 2007) and dog (KuKanich et al., 2012) have been comprehensively reviewed. Most clinical studies comparing the analgesic efficacy of different NSAIDs in veterinary species have concluded that there are minor, if any, differences in efficacy between the commonly used drugs (Slingsby & Waterman-Pearson, 2000a, 2002; Deneuche et al., 2004; Laredo et al., 2004; Erkert et al., 2005; Leece et al., 2005). This may reflect true equivalency between different drugs or may be due to limitations in pain assessment scores to detect subtle differences in analgesia in animals. The evidence for long-term use of NSAIDs to treat canine osteoarthritis has recently been reviewed (Innes et al., 2010) with the authors concluding that longer-term treatment had beneficial effects compared to acute treatment, with a low incidence of adverse effects. Drug doses of commonly used NSAIDs licensed in veterinary species in the UK are listed in Table 5.1.

Carprofen

At clinically effective doses, carprofen is a weak inhibitor of COX iso-enzymes in the periphery (Brideau et al., 2001; Lees et al., 2002, 2004a). Its anti-inflammatory actions may be due to a number of different mechanisms, including inhibition of reactive oxygen species and lysosomal enzymes, stimulation of proteoglycan synthesis and modification of the release of cytokines such as IL-1 and IL-6 (Armstrong & Lees, 2002; Lees et al., 2002). Central inhibition of COX-3 has also been proposed to explain carprofen's analgesic effect. Other studies have shown that carprofen is mildly COX-2 preferential in dogs (Kay-Mugford et al., 2000; Wilson et al., 2004). In cats, the recommended dose of carprofen causes 95% inhibition of COX-2 for 42 hours (Giraudel et al., 2005). The COX-1:COX-2 ratio in the horse is around 1.6–2, making carprofen non-selective or very mildly COX-2 selective (Brideau et al., 2001; Beretta et al., 2005).

Table 5.1 Drug doses of some commonly used NSAIDs licensed in veterinary species in the UK

	Dog	Cat	Horse	Cow	Pig
Carprofen	2–4 mg/kg q 24 h IV, SC, PO	4 mg/kg ONCE IV, SC	0.7 mg/kg q 24 h IV, PO	1.4 mg/kg IV, SC	N/A
Meloxicam	0.2 mg/kg on day 1; 0.1 mg/kg q 24 h thereafter IV, SC, PO	0.3 mg/kg once SC OR 0.1 mg/kg on day 1; 0.05 mg/kg q 24 h thereafter SC, PO	0.6 mg/kg q 24 h IV, PO	0.5 mg/kg once IV, SC	0.4 mg/kg once IM
Ketoprofen	2 mg/kg q 24 h or followed by 0.25–1 mg/kg q 24 h IV, IM, SC, PO	2 mg/kg q 24 h or followed by oral admin 1 mg/kg q 24 h for 5 days SC, PO	2.2 mg/kg q 24 h IV	3 mg/kg q 24 h IV, IM	3 mg/kg once IM
Phenylbutazone	N/A	N/A	4.4 mg/kg q 12 h for 4 days followed by 2.2 mg/kg q 24–48 h IV, PO	N/A	N/A
Flunixin	N/A	N/A	1.1 mg/kg q 24 h IV, PO	2.2 mg/kg q 24 h IV	2.2 mg/kg once IM
Suxibuzone	N/A	N/A	6.25 mg/kg q 12 h for 2 days, then ½ dose. Ponies: use ½ horse dose PO	N/A	N/A
Tepoxalin	10 mg/kg q 24 h PO	N/A	N/A	N/A	N/A
Firocoxib	5 mg/kg q 24 h PO	N/A	0.09 mg/kg IV then 0.1 mg/kg PO q 24 h for up to 14 days	N/A	N/A
Mavacoxib	2 mg/kg q 1 month PO	N/A	N/A	N/A	N/A
Robenacoxib	2 mg/kg SC 1 mg/kg PO q 24 h	2 mg/kg SC 1 mg/kg PO q 24 h	N/A	N/A	N/A
Tolfenamic acid	4 mg/kg q 24 h for 3 days IM, SC, PO	4 mg/kg q 24 h for 3 days SC, PO	N/A	2–4 mg/kg IV, SC	2 mg/kg once IM
Vedaprofen	N/A	N/A	2 mg/kg followed by 1 mg/kg q 12 h PO	N/A	N/A

N/A: Not applicable; q: Every; IV: intravenous; SC: subcutaneous; IM: intramuscular; PO: per os. Recommended licensed dosing regimens change frequently and readers are urged to consult up-to-date data sheets before use

Meloxicam

Meloxicam is COX-2 selective (Kay-Mugford et al., 2000). It reduced production of inflammatory mediators in synovial fluid (PGE_2, substance P and bradykinin) and reduced activity of matrix metalloprotease (MMP) enzymes and markers of cartilage catabolism such as glycosaminoglycans (de Grauw et al., 2009). Meloxicam administered to dogs for 10 days had no effect on platelet function or blood clotting (Brainard et al., 2007). A possible adverse drug reaction to meloxicam has been reported in a dog which developed cutaneous and ocular lesions 24–48 hours after administration (Niza et al., 2007).

Ketoprofen

Ketoprofen is a non-selective or COX-1 selective NSAID, licensed for use in a variety of species. It is not generally considered a very potent analgesic or anti-inflammatory drug, but has a good antipyretic action.

Phenylbutazone

Phenylbutazone is most commonly used in horses where it is frequently used orally for long-term treatment of chronic musculoskeletal conditions. It is slightly COX-1 selective in the horse, with a COX-1:COX-2 ratio around 0.5 (Beretta et al., 2005).

Suxibuzone

Suxibuzone is a prodrug for phenylbutazone in horses and is rapidly converted to phenylbutazone and oxyphenbutazone after absorption. Suxibuzone and phenylbutazone had comparable efficacy (Sabate et al., 2009), but suxibuzone had lower gastric ulcerogenic potential than phenylbutazone (Monreal et al., 2004). The difference in ulcerogenic potential between the two drugs was hypothesized to be due to a local toxic effect of phenylbutazone in the gastric mucosal cells and unrelated to COX inhibition; however, both drugs were administered at more than twice their respective recommended doses (Monreal et al., 2004).

Flunixin

Flunixin is COX-1 selective in the horse, with a COX-1:COX-2 ratio of 0.4 (Beretta et al., 2005). It is commonly used in the treatment of orthopaedic and soft tissue conditions and is a particularly good analgesic for equine colic. There is concern that flunixin may mask increasing levels of pain indicative of the need for surgical intervention in colic, and it should thus be used with caution until a diagnosis has been reached.

Firocoxib

Firocoxib has an IC_{50} COX-1:COX-2 selectivity ratio (in a canine whole blood assay) of 384, making it highly COX-2 specific (Brideau et al., 2001; McCann et al., 2004). Although not currently licensed in cats, experimentally it has a COX-1:COX-2 ratio of 58 in this species (McCann et al., 2005). According to the manufacturer's data, after oral administration, firocoxib is detected in plasma within 15 minutes and peak plasma concentrations are reached within 90 minutes. Plasma concentrations are maintained for 24 hours, making once daily dosing possible. The safety of firocoxib has been evaluated in experimental dogs (Steagall et al., 2007). In dogs with arthritis, firocoxib was as efficacious (Pollmeier et al., 2006) or more efficacious (Hazewinkel et al., 2008) than carprofen.

The pharmacokinetics of firocoxib have been described in the horse (Kvaternick et al., 2007). In horses with arthritis, firocoxib had similar efficacy to phenylbutazone (Doucet et al., 2008). Both firocoxib and flunixin produced effective analgesia in horses after gastrointestinal surgery but, unlike flunixin, firocoxib did not impair gastrointestinal mucosal healing after ischaemia (Cook et al., 2009a).

Robenacoxib

Robenacoxib is a novel specific COX-2 inhibitor licensed for use in dogs and cats (King et al., 2009), producing good anti-inflammatory, analgesic and antipyretic effects in experimentally-induced inflammation in cats (Giraudel et al., 2009). The drug has a short residence time in blood but accumulates in inflammatory exudate (King et al., 2009). Using *in vitro* whole blood assays, the IC_{50} COX-1:COX-2 ratio in cats was 502 and in dogs was 129; whereas the more clinically relevant IC_{20} COX-1:IC_{80} COX-2 ratio in cats was 17 and in dogs was 20 (Giraudel et al., 2009b; King et al., 2010). The use of 2 mg/kg in cats resulted in 5% inhibition of COX-1 and 90% inhibition of COX-2 over 12 hours (Giraudel et al., 2009b). Bioavailability was 84–88% after SC or PO administration in fasted dogs, but dropped to 62% in fed dogs (Jung et al., 2009).

Mavacoxib

Mavacoxib has been recently marketed in dogs as a long-term oral drug administered once monthly. It has a low rate of elimination in the bile, resulting in a prolonged plasma half-life. The elimination half-life was longer in client-owned dogs (39 days) than experimental Beagles (19 days). Five percent of client-owned dogs had an elimination half-life greater than 80 days, making this subgroup at increased risk of toxic side effects after repeated monthly dosing. Its COX-1:COX-2 ratio is 40, making mavacoxib COX-2 selective, rather than specific. In manufacturer's data involving a comparison of mavacoxib with carprofen in 600 dogs, the incidence of GI side effects was similar with both drugs.

Dual Inhibitors: tepoxalin

Tepoxalin inhibits both COX iso-enzymes as well as 5-lipoxygenase (5-LOX) resulting in reduced formation of PGs, TX and leukotrienes (LTs). The leukotrienes are important inflammatory mediators in their own right, involved in many different inflammatory, allergic and neoplastic conditions (Goodman et al., 2008) so inhibition of 5-LOX should contribute to the anti-inflammatory and analgesic properties of these drugs (Curry et al., 2005). Leukotrienes cause neutrophil recruitment and activation in the endothelium and the gastric lining, contributing to gastric irritation and ulceration (Moreau et al., 2005). One of the theories about the side effects of NSAIDs is that when COX is inhibited, arachidonic acid is shunted into the 5-LOX pathway, increasing production of leukotrienes and thus increasing the risk of gastric ulceration (Kirchner et al., 1997). The dual inhibitors should avoid this biological imbalance by inhibiting both enzyme pathways.

At present, there is little evidence about the clinical use of tepoxalin in dogs. Most published evidence has been conducted in a laboratory setting using rats

(Wallace et al., 1993). Tepoxalin was compared to meloxicam in experimental dogs, although clinical efficacy or side effects were not evaluated (Agnello et al., 2005). Tepoxalin was more effective than carprofen or meloxicam at inhibiting the inflammation (increased PGE_2 concentrations) due to experimentally-induced uveitis in dogs (Gilmour & Lehenbauer, 2009). After its initial launch, there were anecdotal reports from vets of gastrointestinal complications (vomiting and diarrhoea) associated with tepoxalin treatment in dogs, in contrast to the experimental GI safety demonstrated with rats. There is still a need for large scale published clinical trials in dogs. In dogs, tepoxalin has a high first pass effect after oral administration resulting in rapid conversion to an acid metabolite (Homer et al., 2005). This acid metabolite is a potent inhibitor of COX. As a result, tepoxalin in dogs only inhibits 5-LOX for a short period of time, whereas the inhibition of COX is much longer lasting, so the drug is actually acting as a non-selective classical NSAID, or even a COX-1 selective drug. This may be the reason for the side effects reported in dogs.

Licofelone is another dual inhibitor which reduces lameness in experimental dogs, although it is not currently commercially available in the UK (Moreau et al., 2005, 2007).

OPIOIDS

Opioids have been used as painkillers in humans for at least 2000 years. Opium is the prototype opioid, derived from the poppy (*Papaver somniferum*), its major active constituent being morphine. There is now a wide range of both naturally occurring and synthetic opioids available, so that the clinician has an enormous range of choice. They are principally used to provide analgesia but some are cough suppressants. Unfortunately, these drugs have a wide range of side effects and, in humans, they cause euphoria and addiction, rendering them liable to abuse and resulting in controls on their supply and use. Abuse is not a feature of their use in veterinary patients. At least in humans, it seems that the euphoric effects of opioids contribute to their analgesia as patients are unconcerned by any residual pain. Whether this is also true in animals can only remain a speculation.

Pharmacology

Endogenous opioid ligands, such as the endorphins, dynorphins and enkephalins, are found in the CNS. Opioids, both natural and synthetic, bind to opioid receptors (Martin et al., 1976). The main opioid receptors are known as μ (mu, OP3, MOP), κ (kappa, OP2, KOP) and δ (delta, OP1, DOP). Opioid receptor terminology is still the subject of considerable debate, and a unanimous

decision has not yet been reached on the naming of the receptors. Initially, Martin et al. (1976) hypothesized that there was also a σ (sigma) receptor, although this is now thought not to be a true opioid receptor. Recently, another receptor has been included in the family: the nociceptin orphanin FQ receptor (N/OFQ, OP4, NOP). Opioid receptors are G-protein coupled receptors causing cellular hyperpolarization due to potassium efflux, closing of calcium channels and reduced cyclic adenosine monophosphate (cAMP) production via inhibition of adenylate cyclase. These cellular effects reduce cell excitability and inhibit release of neurotransmitters.

The μ receptor is found throughout the CNS, particularly in the dorsal horn of the spinal cord and in areas of the brain (such as the periaqueductal grey; PAG) responsible for descending inhibitory control of nociceptive transmission. Binding to the μ receptor is responsible for the majority of opioid-related side effects, including euphoria and addiction in humans. The μ receptor is the main receptor responsible for the analgesic actions of opioids, although there is evidence, at least in humans and rodent models, for some analgesia mediated by the κ receptor, possibly acting in the dorsal horn of the spinal cord. However, analgesia induced by κ agonists is relatively weak and has a ceiling effect. The κ receptor may be responsible for dysphoria. There is some evidence that κ agonists can antagonize some of the side effects induced by μ agonists. The δ receptor may modify the actions of opioids at other receptors. The N/OFQ receptor has a pronociceptive (i.e. antianalgesic) action supraspinally and endogenous N/OFQ may be responsible for setting a pain threshold. The role of N/OFQ in modulation of analgesia is incompletely understood, although N/OFQ receptor antagonists show potential as long-lasting analgesics (Zaveri, 2003).

Drugs may be agonists or antagonists at all opioid receptors, or may exert their actions through one specific type of receptor. Furthermore, some drugs are agonists at one type of receptor and antagonists at another (agonist–antagonists). Partial opioid agonists also exist which exert agonist actions at the specific receptor, although not usually as profound as a pure agonist. Partial agonists often provide sufficient analgesia for clinical use and may also be able to antagonize some of the side effects of pure agonists. Partial agonists are less liable to abuse and so are subject to less stringent controls over their use. They are discussed further under buprenorphine below.

In humans, oral opioids often have reasonably good bioavailability and long elimination half-lives, whereas in dogs, opioids such as methadone and morphine have short elimination half-lives and are rapidly cleared from the circulation. Oral opioids in animals generally have very poor bioavailability due to high first pass metabolism in the liver (KuKanich et al., 2005) making oral administration unfeasible in most veterinary species. Care is necessary when administering systemic opioids to animals with significant hepatic disease as the metabolism of opioids is reduced and thus their half-life extended (Waterman & Kalthum, 1990). There is currently increasing interest in encapsulation of different opioids into liposome formulations to provide sustained release preparations for use in humans, enabling prolongation of dosing intervals.

Opioids have synergistic actions with most sedatives and anaesthetic agents. In general, opioids have an anaesthetic sparing effect (minimum alveolar concentration [MAC] sparing effect; see Chapters 1 and 7) in small animals, allowing lower doses of injectable and inhalational agents to be used, thus reducing the side effects of these agents. In horses, studies have generally failed to find a MAC sparing effect of opioids (Bennett et al., 2004) and this may be related to the central excitatory effects of opioids in horses. However, clinical studies have noted that horses administered opioids as part of an anaesthetic regimen were easier to maintain at a stable plane of anaesthesia and required fewer supplementary doses of injectable anaesthetic agents (Clark et al., 2005).

Side effects

The side effects of opioids vary with species and drug. Side effects are much more common when high doses are given experimentally to pain-free animals, and many side effects are less serious when used clinically in painful animals.

Respiratory depression is commonly cited as the most important side effect of opioids, but this is generally much less of a problem in animals than in humans. High doses of the potent full μ agonists, especially administered IV or in an anaesthetized animal are most likely to cause problematic respiratory depression, necessitating the use of intermittent positive pressure ventilation (IPPV). During the recovery period, or postoperatively, when IPPV cannot be used, highly respiratory depressant opioids are best avoided. Respiratory depression may be more problematic in patients which cannot tolerate even mild increases in $PaCO_2$, such as animals with head trauma or raised intracranial pressure. In animals with thoracic pain, opioids may actually improve respiratory function as a result of their analgesic effect. The cough reflex is depressed and this may increase the risk of aspiration.

In dogs, opioids usually produce sedation. However, historically, there has been a great deal of concern that in cats and horses, especially pain-free animals, opioids cause excitement (Muir et al., 1978), including box-walking in horses. This stems from pharmacological studies which used much higher doses of opioids than would be used clinically. Sensible clinical doses of opioids can be used quite safely in these species, as excitement is particularly unlikely to occur when pain is present. Dysphoria may occur after higher doses of opioids in all species. Use of sedatives such as acepromazine (ACP) or the α_2-agonists may help to minimize the excitatory or dysphoric effects of opioids.

Vomiting is most likely to occur after the use of morphine in dogs and cats (KuKanich et al., 2005) and is less likely after administration of other opioids. Vomiting is thought to be due to stimulation of the chemoreceptor trigger zone. Administration of morphine as a premedicant also significantly increases the risk of gastro-oesophageal reflux during general anaesthesia in dogs (Wilson et al., 2005). Administration of ACP 15 minutes before the opioid significantly reduced the incidence of vomiting in dogs (Valverde et al., 2004a). Opioids reduce gastrointestinal motility in most species causing constipation and reduced faecal output (Boscan et al., 2006a). These GI alterations may predispose horses to colic due to pelvic flexure and caecal impactions. Some studies have indicated that perianaesthetic morphine does not increase the incidence of colic in horses (Mircica et al., 2003; Andersen et al., 2006), whereas others have reported an increased risk (Senior et al., 2004, 2006). However, other drugs, such as the α_2-agonists and general anaesthetic agents, as well as pain itself, will also cause significant reductions in GI motility.

In general, opioids do not have profound cardiovascular effects. Bradycardia may occur, particularly after high doses of the full μ agonists, thought to be due to activation of the parasympathetic nervous system and can thus usually be treated successfully with anticholinergics. There may be a direct negative chronotropic effect of some potent full μ agonists such as remifentanil in humans which is resistant to anticholinergic administration (Tirel et al., 2005), but otherwise there are minimal direct cardiac effects attributed to opioid administration. In horses, hypertension often occurs after opioids (Muir et al., 1978).

Hyperthermia (up to 40°C) after use of opioids has been reported in cats (Posner et al., 2007, 2010). Mydriasis occurs in cats, whereas opioids cause miosis in dogs.

Pruritus has been reported after epidural opioids (especially morphine) and is a major problem in humans. There are occasional reports of epidural morphine-induced pruritus in veterinary species (Burford & Corley, 2006). Urinary retention may also occur after epidural opioids. It is usually self-limiting, but requires careful nursing care and bladder expression until normal function resumes. Delayed hair regrowth over the site of epidural opioid administration is also commonly reported.

Histamine release occurs after IV injection of pethidine (meperidine) and occasionally after rapid IV injection of morphine, resulting in hypotension (Guedes et al., 2006). The other opioids are much less likely to induce histamine release after IV injection.

All opioids cross the placental barrier and may result in respiratory depression and sedation in the neonate if used at parturition. An opioid antagonist such as naloxone may be used to antagonize these effects in the neonate.

Many of the side effects are thought to be mediated by peripheral opioid receptors, raising the possibility of the use of peripheral opioid antagonists which are unable to cross the blood–brain barrier, such as methylnaltrexone, to reduce side effects without affecting the degree of analgesia produced (van Hoogmoed & Boscan, 2005; Boscan et al., 2006b).

Opioid-induced hyperalgesia (OIH) is a recognized phenomenon in humans and rodents associated with both acute and chronic opioid use, resulting in a paradoxical increased sensitivity to pain after opioid administration (Angst & Clark, 2006; Lee et al., 2011). The underlying pathophysiological mechanisms are complex and involve many different pathways and receptors, including interactions between the NMDA receptor, 5-HT receptors, substance P and nitric oxide among others. In humans and rodents, it is thought to have a genetic basis, associated with alterations in genes encoding for peripheral β_2-adrenoceptors and drug transporters. It has not been investigated to any great extent in veterinary species.

Drugs available

Doses of commonly used opioids are listed in Table 5.2.

Morphine

Morphine is still considered the 'gold standard' opioid to which all other drugs are compared. It produces profound analgesia mediated via μ (and possibly κ) agonist activity. It produces euphoria and is addictive in humans and thus falls into Schedule 2 of the UK controlled drugs legislation.

Onset time is around 10–15 minutes after IV administration and up to 30 minutes after IM administration. Morphine is most commonly administered every 4 hours in dogs and horses and every 4–6 hours in cats. Individual variations in duration of action reinforce the need for frequent pain assessment to titrate an analgesic regimen to effect.

The major metabolite in humans is morphine-6-glucuronide which may contribute to morphine's analgesic efficacy. Morphine-6-glucuronide has not been detected in dogs following morphine administration (KuKanich et al., 2005).

Methadone

Methadone is a synthetic full μ agonist, with an onset and duration of action similar to morphine. The pharmacokinetics in dogs have been reported (KuKanich & Borum, 2008; Ingvast-Larsson et al., 2010). It is much less likely to induce vomiting than morphine and histamine release is unlikely, making methadone safer for IV injection. There are conflicting opinions on the relative sedative potency of morphine and methadone. Methadone has been recently licensed for use in cats and dogs in the UK.

Methadone exists as a racemic mixture and the R(−) enantiomer (levo-methadone) appears to be responsible for most of the μ agonist actions (McCance-Katz, 2011). In humans, levo-methadone also has a lower cardiac toxicity (QT interval prolongation, increasing the risk of torsades de pointes) (Grilo et al., 2010).

Table 5.2 Drug doses of some commonly used opioids in veterinary species

	Dog	Cat	Horse	Cow	Pig
Morphine IV, IM	0.2–0.5 mg/kg q 4 h CRI: 0.1–0.3 mg/kg/h	0.1–0.3 mg/kg q 4-6 h CRI: 0.05–0.2 mg/kg/h	0.1–0.15 mg/kg q 4 h CRI: 0.1 mg/kg/h	0.1 mg/kg q 4 h	0.1–0.2 mg/kg q 4 h
Methadone IV, IM	0.2–0.5 mg/kg q 4 h	0.1–0.3 mg/kg q 4 h	0.1–0.15 mg/kg q 4 h	?	?
Pethidine (meperidine) IM, *never* IV	3–5 mg/kg q 2 h	3–5 mg/kg q 2 h	2 mg/kg q 1-2 h	?3–5 mg/kg q 2 h	?1–2 mg/kg q 1–2 h
Buprenorphine IV, IM, ?SC	0.01–0.02 mg/kg q 4–6 h	0.01—0.02 mg/kg q 6–8 h	0.005–0.01 mg/kg q 6–8 h	0.005–0.01 mg/kg q 6–8 h	?0.01 mg/kg q 6–8 h
Butorphanol IV, IM	0.1–0.5 mg/kg q 2–4 h	0.1–0.5 mg/kg q 2–4 h	0.1 mg/kg q 2–4 h	?0.05–0.1 mg/kg q 2–4 h	0.2 mg/kg q 2–4 h
Fentanyl IV	Bolus 1–10 µg/kg CRI: 0.1–0.7 µg/kg/min	Bolus 1–10 µg/kg CRI: 0.1–0.4 µg/kg/min	4 µg/kg	?	?
Remifentanil IV	0.1–0.6 µg/kg/min	?	?	?	?

N/A: Not applicable; q: Every; CRI:= Continuous rate (intravenous) infusion; IV: intravenous; SC: subcutaneous; IM: intramuscular. Note: Not all of these agents are licensed for use in animals. Many doses are empirical and evidence based recommendations are still required, particularly in large animal species. ? indicates uncertainty over optimal dosage

Some have reported that the S(+) enantiomer of methadone (dextro-methadone) is an NMDA antagonist, whereas others have reported NMDA antagonism by both enantiomers, although higher doses are required to block NMDA receptors than to achieve μ opioid effects (Matsui & Williams, 2010).

There is little published veterinary literature on levo-methadone, although it is commercially available in Europe formulated with fenpipramide (an anticholinergic) as 'Polamivet', which has been investigated in dogs (Tunsmeyer et al., 2012). Levo-methadone provided good analgesia in cats after ovariectomy (Rohrer Bley et al., 2004).

Pethidine (meperidine)

Pethidine has a rapid onset of action (approximately 10 minutes) and a short duration of action of up to 2 hours in small animals but less in large animals. Pethidine administered IV causes histamine release and signs of anaphylaxis. For this reason, it should only be administered IM. Pethidine is less likely to produce bradycardia than the other opioids, as its chemical structure is similar to atropine.

Papaveretum

Papaveretum is a mixture of opioids, containing morphine, papaverine and codeine (253 parts morphine, 23 papaverine, 20 codeine). Papaveretum is most useful for providing analgesia along with profound sedation and control of vicious dogs when used in conjunction with a sedative. Vomiting is a common side effect. Doses used are similar to those for morphine, as are speed of onset and duration of action.

Buprenorphine

Buprenorphine falls onto Schedule 3 of the UK Misuse of Drugs Act 1971 and is licensed for administration in dogs, cats and horses in the UK. It produces minimal sedation and respiratory depression when used at clinical doses.

Buprenorphine is classically described as a partial μ agonist. The drug has a 'bell-shaped' dose–response curve, where initially increasing the dose increases the analgesic effect until a threshold is reached, after which further dose increases result in a decreasing analgesic effect, i.e. the drug is antagonizing its own analgesic effect. There was concern that administration of high doses of buprenorphine could potentially result in 'anti-analgesia'. These concerns appear unfounded, as the doses required to produce this effect are well above those which are used clinically. Clinically, increasing the dose may improve the quality of analgesia, although no increased analgesic effect was demonstrated by increasing the dose from 0.02 to 0.04 mg/kg in dogs undergoing ovariohysterectomy (Slingsby et al., 2011).

Recently, the drug has been described as a high affinity/high avidity μ agonist. Buprenorphine binds very tightly to the μ receptor and demonstrates slow receptor kinetics, resulting in a long onset of action of around 45 minutes and a long duration of up to 6–8 hours. However, thermal antinociceptive thresholds were increased in cats from 4 to 12 hours after injection (Robertson et al., 2003a). Conversely, following ovariohysterectomy, dogs required further analgesia 4–5 hours after administration of 0.02-0.04 mg/kg (Slingsby et al., 2011).

The high affinity and slow dissociation from the μ receptor has led to concerns that if the analgesia produced by buprenorphine is insufficient, it may be difficult to top-up with a full μ agonist. However, a large dose of morphine can displace buprenorphine from the μ receptor if more profound analgesia is required.

The high affinity of buprenorphine for the μ receptor can be used to advantage if unacceptable opioid-related side effects occur in a painful patient. Administration of a pure μ antagonist would antagonize the side effects seen but would leave the animal without any opioid-related analgesia. Buprenorphine can displace the original opioid from the receptor, thus reducing the side effects seen, but still produce opioid-related analgesia. This process is known as *sequential analgesia* and is used to antagonize some of the effects of very potent full μ agonists such as sedation and respiratory depression. Buprenorphine is commonly used for this purpose in laboratory animal anaesthesia to antagonize the adverse effects of fentanyl, while maintaining postoperative analgesia (Flecknell et al., 1989). Nalbuphine (see below) has been recommended in humans to produce sequential analgesia.

Administration of buprenorphine onto the oral mucous membranes of cats resulted in equivalent plasma concentrations and degree of thermal antinociception to that achieved after injection (Robertson et al., 2003b, 2005a), and this route is suitable for more prolonged analgesia in animals that are difficult to inject. However, clinically, the transmucosal route may be inferior to IV or IM administration in cats undergoing ovariohysterectomy, with increased pain scores in cats administered buprenorphine transmucosally compared to the other routes (Giordano et al., 2010). The alkaline pH of cat saliva improves absorption, and transmucosal administration may be less effective in species with neutral salivary pH. A case report of transmucosal buprenorphine administration in a horse reported good analgesia (Walker, 2007), although a pharmacokinetic study failed to detect plasma concentrations of buprenorphine after sublingual administration (Messenger et al., 2011).

Buprenorphine is also available in a transdermal patch formulation, utilizing a matrix formulation. A 35 μg/h patch has been evaluated in cats and did not result in changes in thermal thresholds, although signs of euphoria, sedation and mydriasis were observed (Murrell et al., 2007).

Butorphanol

Butorphanol is a mixed agonist–antagonist drug, being an agonist at κ receptors and an antagonist at μ receptors. As a result, it does not produce profound analgesia and is best reserved for use in non-painful conditions. In the UK, it is currently not subject to controls under the Misuse of Drugs Act 1971. It is used in cats, dogs and horses in sedative combinations with α_2-agonists and to produce mild analgesia. Butorphanol is also used in dogs for its antitussive effect. Onset time is around 5–15 minutes and duration of action is controversial, although thought by many to be around 2 hours (Robertson et al., 2003a; Lascelles & Robertson, 2004). Data provided by the manufacturer indicates that butorphanol provides analgesia for 4–6 hours. Butorphanol has been administered as a continuous rate infusion (CRI) to conscious horses (Sellon et al., 2001, 2004).

Fentanyl

Fentanyl is a pure μ agonist with a potency around 50 times greater than morphine, enabling the use of small doses to produce profound analgesia. After IV injection, it has a rapid onset of action (around 1–2 minutes), although a single dose will only last around 20 minutes. It can be used as part of an induction protocol in cardiovascularly unstable small animal patients in association with a benzodiazepine, such as diazepam or midazolam. It is often used as a CRI, although cumulation will occur after prolonged infusions. It is a relatively potent respiratory depressant, especially when used in high doses as a CRI under anaesthesia and IPPV may be required. Bradycardia may also occur with the use of high doses, but is rapidly reversible by reduction of the infusion rate or treatment with anticholinergics.

Fentanyl is well absorbed across intact skin and is available in a transdermal patch formulation, designed to release fentanyl gradually. The patch contains a reservoir of fentanyl which is released across a rate controlling membrane. Damage to the patch can result in more rapid release of fentanyl and the potential for overdose and toxicity. A case of profound sedation in a dog has been reported due to suspected ingestion or transmucosal absorption of fentanyl (Schmiedt & Bjorling, 2007). In dogs and cats, there is a significant lag time (up to 24 hours) after application of the patch before plasma concentrations begin to rise, however, in horses, plasma fentanyl increases around 2 hours after patch application (Maxwell et al., 2003; Orsini et al., 2006). A skin depot of the drug is produced and fentanyl continues to be absorbed into the circulation for some time after removal of the patch. The duration of action in dogs and horses is up to 72 hours after patch application and up to 104 hours in cats. However, frequent pain assessment is still necessary as breakthrough pain may occur, necessitating further opioid or non-opioid analgesic administration.

Remifentanil

Remifentanil is an ultra-short acting full μ agonist. It is a fentanyl derivative with an ester linkage which undergoes rapid metabolism by hydrolysis by non-specific blood and tissue esterases without involvement of the liver. Its rapid onset and offset of action make remifentanil most suitable for use as a CRI. Its context sensitive half-life is unaffected by duration of infusion, giving it a short, predictable duration of action without cumulative effects. Recovery from remifentanil is more rapid than from any other opioid and, as such, provision for postoperative analgesia must be made well in advance of termination of remifentanil infusion.

In dogs undergoing orthopaedic surgery, remifentanil reduced isoflurane requirements by 40–50% (Allweiler et al., 2007). Pre-emptive administration of an anticholinergic is recommended as remifentanil can cause profound bradycardia. Remifentanil is also more respiratory depressant than the other opioids and IPPV is usually required.

Alfentanil

This fentanyl derivative is only one-quarter as potent an analgesic as fentanyl itself. It has a rapid onset of action, although it may accumulate following repeated doses. Analgesia is accompanied by respiratory depression and severe bradycardia.

Etorphine

Etorphine is a very potent derivative of morphine. It has similar properties to morphine but is more respiratory depressant. Its very great potency means that a small volume can be used in dart gun projectiles for immobilizing large, wild game animals. However, this makes it a dangerous drug to handle and constitutes a safety hazard to the anaesthetist.

Etorphine is extremely long acting and recovery is also delayed by enterohepatic recycling. Its action is usually terminated by the use of diprenorphine, a specific antagonist, but relapse into deep sedation may occur. The drug produces CNS stimulation before depression, resulting in excitement before the onset of anaesthesia. In an attempt to overcome this, etorphine is marketed in fixed ratio combinations with phenothiazine tranquillizers ('Large Animal Immobilon' with acepromazine and 'Small Animal Immobilon' with methotrimeprazine). Should accidental self-administration occur, death can result if the human antidote (naloxone) is not readily available.

Sufentanil and carfentanil

Sufentanil is approximately 10 times as potent as fentanyl. It is not used extensively in veterinary medicine. Carfentanil is one of the most potent opioids known. It is said to be three to eight times as potent as etorphine and is useful for anaesthesia of elephants, although it is a dangerous drug to handle since it is rapidly absorbed across mucous membranes. An antagonist drug suitable for use in humans should be readily available whenever carfentanil is used.

Opioid antagonists

Naloxone is a pure antagonist at all opioid receptors and will antagonize the effect of all opioid agonists but it is less effective against partial agonists. In humans, reversal of opioid actions with naloxone is sometimes accompanied by tachycardia, but there are no reports of this in the veterinary literature. The drug is fairly short acting and its effects may wear off before those of the previously administered agonist so that repeated doses of antagonist may be required. This is particularly important in veterinary medicine where large and frequent doses of naloxone are necessary to counter the accidental self-administration of etorphine.

Naltrexone is a long-acting derivative of naloxone and, although not often used in veterinary practice, it is useful should a long-acting pure antagonist be required.

Some partial agonists, which either produce poor analgesia or cause dysphoria sufficient to preclude their use as analgesics, are used for their antagonistic properties. *Nalorphine* was the first partial agonist to be used as an antagonist but it has now been superseded by naloxone because of the psychomimetic effects of nalorphine. *Nalbuphine* is a κ agonist and μ antagonist similar to butorphanol. It is used in humans to reverse opioid-induced respiratory depression with the aim of maintaining some κ-mediated analgesia. *Diprenorphine* is marketed as a specific antagonist for etorphine and, in animals, it appears to be very efficient in this role. However, as it causes hallucinations in humans; it is only licensed for use in animals and in humans naloxone remains the drug of choice for countering the effects of etorphine.

LOCAL ANAESTHETICS

The terms 'local anaesthetic' and 'local analgesic' are often used interchangeably and there is considerable debate over which is the more appropriate term to use. In this chapter, drugs which act by blocking Na^+ channels are described as local anaesthetics. Local anaesthetic techniques are considered as those which can be used to provide the sole means of anaesthesia and analgesia for a surgical procedure. For example, standing surgical procedures can be performed in large animals after performing a paravertebral block with a local anaesthetic drug for flank surgery. Conversely, local analgesic techniques are used to provide analgesia but do not produce complete anaesthesia. They are often used as an adjunct to general anaesthesia to produce a MAC sparing effect and contribute to multimodal analgesia. Local analgesia can be produced using drugs such as opioids as well as the local anaesthetic drugs.

Many surgical procedures can be satisfactorily performed under local anaesthesia. It enables protracted operations to be performed on standing animals and, in large animals, this avoids the dangers associated with prolonged recumbency. Whether or not sedation is employed as an adjunct will depend on the species, temperament and health of the animal, as well as the magnitude of the procedure. In adult cattle and horses, sedation may induce the animal to lie down and it is thus often better avoided. In other animals, sedation should be adopted since efficient surgery is greatly facilitated by the reduction of fear and liability to sudden movement. Local anaesthetics may exert a sedative action when they are absorbed from sites of injection and for surgery on the standing animal the dose of any sedative drug should be reduced to allow for this.

Anatomy and physiology

The unit of nervous tissue consists of the nerve cell (neuron) and its processes, the dendrites, and axon. The neuronal surface is almost entirely covered by supporting cells. The larger neurons are surrounded by a coat of fatty material known as the myelin sheath. The thickness of this sheath increases with the diameter of the axon it encloses, and it is composed of a number of lipoprotein lamellae. These are laid down from Schwann cells that enclose the axons. The myelin sheath is not continuous along the entire length of the fibre, but is interrupted at more or less regular intervals (the nodes of Ranvier) to leave short segments of the axon covered only by the Schwann cells. At these nodal areas in myelinated fibres and throughout the entire length of the unmyelinated fibres, the axon is separated from the surrounding tissue fluid only by the thickness of the Schwann cell. In the internodal segments of myelinated fibres, the axon is separated from surrounding fluid by the myelin sheath as well.

Peripheral nerves are composed of fibres of many different diameters, the smallest of which have no surface myelin coating, while the larger fibres are surrounded by increasing numbers of myelin lamellae. There is some correlation between fibre size and function, with the largest diameter fibres (15–25 μm) transmitting somatic motor efferent information. Smaller fibres (5–15 μm) carry proprioceptive and cutaneous afferent messages and the smallest fibres (<5 μm) transmit afferent and efferent nociceptive information.

Not all nerve fibres are equally sensitive to local anaesthetics. When a peripheral nerve is exposed to a local anaesthetic, conduction in its constituent fibres is blocked at a rate that is inversely proportional to their diameters. Function fails first in the smallest, unmyelinated fibres

115

followed by the smaller myelinated fibres and finally larger myelinated fibres. This is because the Schwann cells containing myelin are relatively impervious to local anaesthetic solutions compared to those which contain little or no myelin. Once a drug has penetrated through the connective tissues of the nerve, it can act upon the entire length of any unmyelinated fibre but only on the short segments at the nodes of Ranvier in myelinated fibres. The number of nodes of Ranvier per unit length of an axon is greater in small fibres than in thick ones. The most sensitive nerve fibres are B fibres, conveying sympathetic information. Next most sensitive are sensory Aδ fibres, conveying painful information. The least sensitive are the largest, Aα motor fibres. The sensitivity of the unmyelinated C fibres, also conveying painful sensory information, overlaps with these. This raises the possibility of producing a differential block where only sensory fibres are blocked, leaving motor function unaffected. Sensations are lost in the following order: pain, followed by cold and warmth, then touch and deep pressure.

Pharmacology

Local anaesthetics reversibly block the transmission of action potentials along a nerve axon by blocking Na^+ channels and stabilizing excitable cell membranes. They prevent movement of Na^+ ions down their concentration gradient from the extracellular surface through specific channels into cells and thus prevent cells depolarizing and reaching threshold potential for propagation of the action potential. The drug binds to the internal surface of a Na^+ channel on the cell membrane.

Most local anaesthetics consist of an aromatic lipophilic end and a hydrophilic (amine) end, joined by an intermediate chain. Some compounds lack the hydrophilic tail (e.g. benzocaine) and are nearly insoluble in water so that they are unsuitable for injection but they can be applied to mucosal surfaces. The intermediate chain may be either ester or amide linked which affects drug metabolism. Ester-linked drugs (procaine and amethocaine) are metabolized by esterases (plasma pseudo-cholinesterases). They have shorter durations of action and their metabolism is not affected by liver dysfunction. Amide-linked drugs are metabolized in the liver. The metabolites of local anaesthetics are of clinical importance since they may exert both pharmacological and toxicological effects similar to those of their parent compounds. The excretion of both ester- and amide-linked compounds occurs through the kidneys. Less than 5% of the drug is excreted unchanged. The renal clearance of the amide-type drugs appears to be inversely related to their protein-binding abilities. Renal clearance is also inversely proportional to urinary pH, suggesting that urinary excretion occurs by non-ionic diffusion.

Modification of the chemical structure alters activity and the physical properties of the molecule. Lengthening of the intermediate chain or addition of carbon atoms to the aromatic or amine groups increases potency up to a ceiling, beyond which any further increase in molecular weight is followed by a decrease in activity.

Lipid solubility of a local anaesthetic determines its potency as axonal membranes are predominantly lipid. However, this relationship is clearer *in vitro* than *in vivo* and other factors also affect local anaesthetic potency *in vivo*. Protein binding determines duration of action as the binding site (Na^+ channel) is protein. Finally, pKa (the pH at which the solution contains equal proportions of charged and uncharged molecules) determines speed of onset. Local anaesthetics are weak bases (proton acceptors) with pKas ranging from 7.7 to 8.9. At body pH (7.4), weak bases such as local anaesthetics become ionized by accepting protons: $B + H^+ \rightarrow BH^+$. However, local anaesthetics must diffuse across the axon sheath to bind to the internal side of the Na^+ channel in their uncharged free base form. Local anaesthetics with a pKa closest to body pH (such as mepivacaine: pKa 7.6) have the fastest onset of action as proportionally more drug is present in its uncharged form. Local anaesthetics with a higher pKa, such as bupivacaine (pKa 8.1), have a longer onset of action as proportionally more of the drug is in its ionized form. In infected tissue, the pH generally drops, resulting in a greater proportion of local anaesthetic becoming ionized and thus unable to penetrate the cell membrane. As a result, local anaesthetics are often ineffective in infected tissues. Once inside the cell, the local anaesthetic must be ionized in order to bind to the internal surface of the Na^+ channel.

Warming local anaesthetics to 40°C reduces the pKa (e.g. for lidocaine from 7.92 at 25°C to 7.57 at 40°C), thus hastening the speed of onset and potentially improving quality of analgesia (Arai et al., 2006).

Local anaesthetics are unusual in that they are applied directly at their site of action and systemic absorption therefore controls offset and duration of action. Some local anaesthetics, such as lidocaine, cause vasodilation and are thus commercially available with epinephrine added as a vasoconstrictor to reduce local blood flow and prolong duration of action. Conversely, cocaine is a potent vasoconstrictor as it inhibits neuronal uptake of catecholamines and also inhibits monoamine oxidase. The systemic absorption of a local anaesthetic is affected by:

1. The site of injection
2. The dosage
3. The addition of a vasoconstrictor
4. The pharmacological profile of the drug itself.

Side effects

Local anaesthetics affect not only neurons but all types of excitable tissue including skeletal, smooth and cardiac muscle. Cardiovascular and central nervous disturbances are the commonest side effects but allergic reactions

Table 5.3 Commonly used and toxic doses of some local anaesthetics

	Normal dose (mg/kg)	Toxic dose (mg/kg)
Lidocaine	5	10–20
Bupivacaine	2	3.5–4.5
Ropivacaine	3	5

Note: Not all of these agents are licensed for use in animals

occasionally occur with ester-type agents. Toxicity most commonly occurs following inadvertent intravascular injection resulting in high systemic plasma concentrations of the drug. Before injection, it is essential to draw back on the plunger of the syringe to check it has not accidentally penetrated a blood vessel. Simple overdose is also common in small animals as many of the commercially available presentations are very concentrated. It is essential to weigh accurately the animal and calculate the safe dose before using a local anaesthetic. Many local anaesthetics have a narrow margin of safety before toxic doses are reached (Table 5.3). Toxicity is more common after performing some blocks, such as intercostal and interpleural blocks, which have a high degree of systemic absorption.

The CNS is the first body system to be affected by toxicity. Signs include depression or sedation, muscle tremors and seizures depending on the dose of local anaesthetic reaching the brain. These effects may be missed during perioperative use in a sedated or anaesthetized animal. These paradoxical and conflicting effects are explained by the fact that local anaesthetics preferentially block inhibitory interneurons, resulting in excitatory effects. As the concentration of local anaesthetic increases, both inhibitory and excitatory neurons are blocked, resulting in overall depressant effects. Lidocaine has anticonvulsant activity as well as the ability to produce seizures. In general, the dose giving rise to anticonvulsant activity is less than that associated with convulsions.

The cardiovascular system is next to be affected by toxicity and arguably the most important. Local anaesthetics have direct actions on the heart and peripheral vasculature through blocking Na^+ channels and indirect actions via blockade of sympathetic nerve fibres resulting in vasodilation. Sympathetic blockade is particularly marked after epidural injection of local anaesthetics, resulting in pooling of blood in the pelvic and splanchnic circulations. This can result in reduced venous return to the heart and systemic hypotension.

Toxic concentrations of local anaesthetics are associated with a reduction in the rate of rise of phase 0 of the cardiac action potential (the phase of rapid cellular depolarization due to Na^+ conductance across the cell membrane). This causes a decrease in the rate of depolarization in Purkinje fibres and ventricular muscle, a reduction in amplitude of the action potential, and a marked decrease in conduction velocity. On the ECG, there is an increase in the P–R interval and in QRS complex duration. This causes a suppression of automaticity, decreased electrical excitability of the myocardium and reduced myocardial contractility. Severe arrhythmias and cardiac arrest are possible. In experimentally-induced toxicity in anaesthetized dogs, a reduction in systolic function occurred before the onset of arrhythmias (Coyle et al., 1994).

The cardiovascular toxicity of the local anaesthetics differs and is most potent with bupivacaine, which is slower to dissociate from Na^+ channels than ropivacaine or lidocaine, thus allowing the development of re-entry arrhythmias. Conversely, lidocaine at low doses is used to treat ventricular tachyarrhythmias (it is a class Ib antiarrhythmic drug) because of its effects on the cardiac action potential. It shortens the duration of the action potential and refractory period by reducing the repolarization phase and can thus prevent re-entry arrhythmias.

There is currently a lot of interest in human medicine in the use of lipid infusions to treat local anaesthetic cardiovascular toxicity. Initial studies were performed in experimental dogs administered an overdose of bupivacaine, causing circulatory arrest. Cardiopulmonary resuscitation was initiated with internal cardiac massage followed by a bolus and CRI of 20% lipid infusion (Weinberg et al., 2003). All the dogs treated with lipid infusion survived, whereas none of the saline control animals did. Subsequent case reports from human medicine have recommended bolus doses of 1 mL/kg every 3–5 minutes during resuscitation, up to a maximum of 3 mL/kg followed by 0.25 mL/kg/min. The mechanism of this effect is currently unknown. It has been hypothesized that the lipid infusion creates a 'lipid plasma phase' which attracts the lipid soluble bupivacaine molecules and makes them unavailable to tissues (Weinberg et al., 2003). The lipids may also interact with bupivacaine directly at the tissue level or may alter metabolic energy utilization in the heart. Further investigation of the optimal dose, rate and duration of infusion is still required and the safety of rapid infusion of high doses of lipid still requires investigation. Currently, recommendations are that lipid infusion should only be used alongside other conventional treatments such as cardiac massage and epinephrine in case of cardiac arrest or anticonvulsant drugs to treat local anaesthetic-induced seizures.

Methaemoglobinaemia is also possible after use of local anaesthetics. It occurs when Fe^{2+} in haemoglobin is oxidized to Fe^{3+} which is unable to bind and carry oxygen, resulting in cyanosis. Methaemoglobin production occurs particularly after use of prilocaine but also with lidocaine, procaine and benzocaine (Lagutchik et al., 1992).

Local analgesics can enhance the duration of action of both depolarizing and non-depolarizing neuromuscular blocking agents. Drugs such as the phenothiazine derivatives and pethidine (meperidine) may lower the threshold at which the convulsant actions of local anaesthetics are encountered.

Drugs available

Cocaine is an alkaloid obtained from the leaves of *Erythroxylum coca*, a South American plant, and is an ester-linked local anaesthetic first introduced by Koeller in 1884. Its toxicity and addictive properties in humans led to a search for synthetic substitutes and reference to it now has become largely historical. Its one remaining use is for nasal surgery, where its intense vasoconstriction shrinks the mucous membrane, allowing more room for the surgeon and aiding haemostasis.

Cinchocaine is a potent, toxic local anaesthetic. It is now mainly used as part of a commercially available euthanasia mixture for large animals (Somulose; with the potent barbiturate, quinalbarbitone). Cinchocaine is added to the mixture in large enough quantities to produce cardiac arrest and the barbiturate is used to produce CNS depression.

Procaine

Procaine was introduced in 1905. It has a high pKa (8.9), therefore onset of action is slow. Lipid solubility is low resulting in low potency and due to its ester linkage it has a short duration of action. It is licensed for use in food-producing animals in the UK.

Amethocaine

Amethocaine is an ester-linked local anaesthetic which is particularly useful for desensitizing mucous membranes. It can be instilled into the conjunctival sac instead of proxymetacaine (proparacaine) and it can also be applied to the pharyngeal, laryngeal and nasal mucous membranes. An ointment is available for desensitization of intact skin.

Lidocaine

Lidocaine (lignocaine) was introduced in 1944. Lidocaine is an amide-linked local anaesthetic, with a pKa of 7.9 and a rapid onset of action. It is only around 70% protein bound so it has a limited duration of action of around 2 hours. Duration of action is also reduced by absorption away from the site of application due its profound vasodilatory properties, unless formulated with epinephrine. Its lipid solubility and potency are lower than some of the other newer local anaesthetic agents such as bupivacaine. It spreads well throughout tissues and penetrates mucosal surfaces well, making it a suitable agent for topical application.

Prilocaine

Prilocaine has a pKa similar to lidocaine (7.7) resulting in a rapid onset of action. Potency is similar to lidocaine although the degree of protein binding is lower (55%). It is the most rapidly metabolized amide and its metabolism releases o-toluidine, which causes methaemoglobinaemia. It is most commonly utilized in EMLA cream (Eutectic Mixture of Local Anaesthetics), which is a mixture of 2.5% lidocaine and 2.5% prilocaine, used for topical anaesthesia of intact skin. A eutectic mixture describes two compounds which, when mixed under specific conditions, produce a substance that now behaves with a single set of physical characteristics.

Mepivacaine

Mepivacaine is an amide-linked local anaesthetic with a pKa of 7.6 and a rapid onset of action (around 10 minutes). It is around 75% protein bound with a duration of action of around 2 hours. It is commonly utilized for diagnostic and therapeutic local analgesia in equine lameness investigation, as specific nerve blocks of the distal limbs performed with mepivacaine produce less tissue swelling and oedema than those performed with lidocaine.

Bupivacaine

Bupivacaine is an amide-linked local anaesthetic with a high pKa of 8.1 resulting in a slow onset of action of around 40 minutes. However, it is around 95% protein bound and has a very long duration of action of 6–8 hours. It is also very lipid soluble and has a high potency. Bupivacaine is not licensed for use in veterinary species although it is commonly used to provide long-acting intra- and postoperative analgesia. It is also the most toxic local anaesthetic with a narrow margin of safety (see Table 5.3).

Levo-bupivacaine

Levo-bupivacaine is the S(−) enantiomer of bupivacaine and was developed for use in human medicine as a less toxic alternative to bupivacaine. The concentrations needed to produce CNS toxicity and myocardial depression are higher for levo-bupivacaine compared to racemic bupivacaine.

Ropivacaine

Ropivacaine was also developed as a less toxic alternative to bupivacaine. It has a propyl group attached to the amine end of the molecule, compared to a butyl group in bupivacaine. It is formulated as a pure S(−) enantiomer, which is less toxic and more potent than the R-enantiomer. The pKa of ropivacaine is the same as bupivacaine, as is the protein binding, meaning that the two compounds have similar onsets and durations of action. Ropivacaine has a slightly lower lipid solubility than bupivacaine which may reduce penetration of the drug into large motor fibres. The motor blockade produced by ropivacaine is less profound and of shorter duration than that produced by bupivacaine, meaning that ropivacaine may be more able to produce a differential nerve block. The margin of safety in dosing of ropivacaine is slightly greater than for bupivacaine, but accurate dosing is still essential to avoid overdosage.

Routes of administration

The techniques of local anaesthetic administration are generally not difficult to learn and do not involve the use of expensive or complicated equipment.

Topical local analgesia

Proparacaine (proxymetacaine) and amethocaine are used to produce corneal anaesthesia (Herring et al., 2005). Caution is required as repeated use of these drugs may slow corneal healing. Topical local anaesthetics also reduce tear production, due to a reduction in corneal sensation. Topical anaesthesia of the larynx in cats is usually performed before intubation using lidocaine spray , but there is concern that the propellents in some formulations may be irritant. Topical anaesthesia of intact skin is achieved using EMLA (lidocaine and prilocaine) or amethocaine cream. They are useful adjuncts to venous catheterization in fractious animals including cats and rabbits. Caution over the amount applied is necessary due to the potential to induce methaemoglobinaemia with prilocaine.

Lidocaine is formulated in a patch for long-term use to treat conditions such as osteoarthritis in humans, with the aim of achieving high local lidocaine concentrations and minimal systemic absorption. In humans, it is recommended that the patches are applied for 12 hours per day over the site of injury. The patches have been used anecdotally in veterinary species, although the bioavailability is poor (around 3%) and the lidocaine is rapidly metabolized after absorption. In horses, lidocaine was not detected in the plasma after patch application (Bidwell et al., 2007).

Splash blocks are currently receiving increased interest. It was always assumed that local anaesthetics should not be used close to wound edges as they would cause tissue swelling, oedema and inhibit wound healing. However, modern local anaesthetics are much less likely to cause these problems. Application of bupivacaine into the peritoneal cavity and along the incisional surfaces of the abdominal muscles reduced pain scores in dogs after ovariohysterectomy without any side effects (Carpenter et al., 2004).

'Wound soaker' or diffusion catheters (Fig. 5.3) are increasingly used to provide postoperative analgesia to areas which are not suitable for a specific peripheral nerve block (Wolfe et al., 2006; Abelson et al., 2009). The catheters have small holes, known as micropores, and are buried within the wound during surgical closure. They are particularly suitable for use after amputations, mammary strips and ear surgery for example.

Regional local analgesia

Simple regional blocks include the 'inverted-L' block used to anaesthetize the flank to allow standing surgery in large animals, where two linear infiltrations are made of the whole thickness of the abdominal wall, one cranial to and one dorsal to, the line of incision. Ring block of an extremity involves infiltration of a transverse plane around the whole extremity, paying particular attention to the sites of large nerve trunks. In limbs, the technique is more effective when the injection is made distal to a tourniquet. When used for operations on a cow's teats, it is important

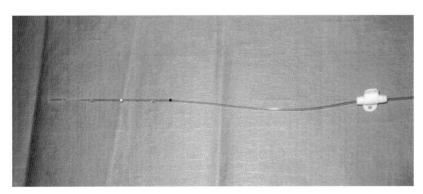

Figure 5.3 The catheter usually is placed by the surgeons before wound closure but can be placed later via an introducer catheter. The area with the 'infusion' holes (to the left of the black dot as you look at the picture) is situated so it is totally contained within the wound, and in the area requiring analgesia. The 'non-infusion' end of the catheter is firmly anchored to the skin. In veterinary medicine, a long acting local anaesthetic is usually injected via this catheter at 4-6 hour intervals. For analgesia in humans, a continuous infusion may be used.
Photograph courtesy of Elizabeth Armitage-Chan.

that vasoconstrictors are not added to the local anaesthetic solutions, as prolonged vasoconstriction may result in ischaemic necrosis of the teat end.

More commonly, regional analgesia is performed by blocking conduction in the sensory nerve or nerves innervating the operation site. The operative field itself is not touched while its sensations are abolished and good analgesia results from the use of small quantities of solution. The solution must, however, be brought into the closest possible contact with the nerve which is to be blocked. Specific nerve blocks can produce analgesia of a region or area of the body. These include blockade of a single nerve, or groups of nerves such as the brachial plexus (radial, median, ulnar, musculocutaneous and axillary nerves) to provide anaesthesia of the distal forelimb.

The accuracy of local anaesthetic placement when performing specific nerve blocks can be improved by use of a nerve stimulator and a dedicated, insulated needle (Mahler & Reece, 2007; Mahler & Adogwa, 2008). After inserting the needle, a small current is passed through it. The technique relies on the fact that the nerve to be blocked contains motor fibres as the stimulating current produces a muscle twitch. The needle is redirected until a twitch can still be observed with the lowest possible current as this implies that the tip of the needle is in close proximity to the nerve sheath. Recently, ultrasound guided techniques for local anaesthetic blocks (brachial plexus, femoral and sciatic nerves) have been described (Campoy et al., 2010) which should aid accuracy in placement. Continuous peripheral nerve blockade can be achieved with catheters placed subcutaneously around peripheral nerves to enable postoperative blockade in a conscious patient without the need for repeated injections (Mahler & Reece, 2007; Driessen et al., 2008).

Intrapleural local anaesthesia describes the placement of local anaesthetics in the pleural space, usually via an indwelling chest drain placed following thoracic procedures. Intermittent instillation of long-acting local anaesthetics, such as bupivacaine or ropivacaine, into the chest drain provided effective analgesia after thoracotomy in humans (Tetik et al., 2004). In dogs post-thoracotomy, intrapleural bupivacaine was as effective as systemic morphine or intercostal nerve blocks with bupivacaine (Thompson & Johnson, 1991). The drug diffuses across the pleura and blocks the intercostal nerves. After instillation of local anaesthetic, the patient should be placed incision-side down to allow gravity dependent pooling of the drug near the intercostal nerves on the affected side and aid development of analgesia there. The presence of an open pericardium, and thus direct contact between the local anaesthetic and the heart, did not increase the cardiac toxicity or induce arrhythmias (Bernard et al., 2006).

Intratesticular anaesthesia is commonly used during castration of large animals, involving injection of a short-acting local anaesthetic into the testicle and subcutaneously in the scrotum. Injection may also be performed higher in the spermatic cord.

Intravenous regional analgesia (IVRA)

In 1908, Bier first reported a technique of 'venous anaesthesia'. A small venous catheter is inserted at the distal extremity of a limb and secured. The limb is exsanguinated, usually with an Esmarch bandage, a tourniquet is inflated or tied to occlude the arterial supply at the top of the limb and the local anaesthetic solution is injected via the catheter. Analgesia of the limb up to the lower limit of the tourniquet occurs rapidly, and when the tourniquet is released it wears off with almost equal rapidity.

The mode of action of this technique is unclear but it seems to be both safe and simple for operations on the digits, especially in ruminants where the procedure can be carried out on the standing animal and in dogs, usually as an analgesic adjunct to general anaesthesia. The good analgesia and bloodless field are appreciated by the surgeon. Analgesia develops distally and progresses proximally so it is important that the injection is made as distally as possible. If the tourniquet is left in place for more than about 1.5 hours ischaemic damage may follow and pain is severe. It is also important that the tourniquet is not released immediately after local anaesthetic injection as this may result in high plasma concentrations of the drug and systemic toxicity. Bupivacaine should not be used for this technique at all because, due to its toxicity, cardiovascular collapse and death may occur when the tourniquet is released. Major advantages of this technique are that it requires no precise knowledge of anatomy and only one injection is required.

Intra-articular analgesia

Intra-articular analgesia (or intrasynovial in tendon sheaths) is used to provide profound local analgesia with minimal systemic side effects. It is important to use preservative free drugs as the preservatives may have toxic effects on articular cartilage and a sterile injection technique is essential to avoid introducing infection into the joint. Many drugs have a prolonged duration of action when injected into synovial cavities, and a single injection may produce 24 hours of analgesia due to slow systemic absorption. Morphine has a low lipid solubility and is thus retained within the synovial cavity for a prolonged period of time (Lindegaard et al., 2010a). Low doses are also required to produce comparable analgesia compared to systemic recommendations, and this may be further limited by the size of the joint space restricting the volume that can be comfortably injected.

Upregulation of opioid receptors occurs in inflamed joints (Keates et al., 1999; Sheehy et al., 2001) and both opioids and local anaesthetics produce analgesia when injected intra-articularly (Day et al., 1995; Lindegaard et al., 2010b). In general, local anaesthetics produce more profound intra-articular analgesia than opioids, although superior analgesia can be produced by using a combination of the two (Sammarco et al., 1996; Santos et al., 2009). However, the effects of intra-articular morphine are controversial and a meta-analysis of human studies concluded that intra-articular morphine produced a definite but mild analgesic effect, although systemic absorption of morphine could not be excluded (Gupta et al., 2001).

Recent evidence indicates that local anaesthetics may be toxic to chondrocytes. After 30 minutes exposure to bupivacaine *in vitro*, less than 30% of cultured equine chondrocytes were viable (Park et al., 2011). Cell viability after exposure to lidocaine was 66% and mepivacaine 86%.

Ketamine has been used intra-articularly in humans producing analgesia for up to 24 hours without psychomimetic side effects, although the analgesia produced was not as effective as that due to intra-articular bupivacaine (Dal et al., 2004). NMDA receptors are found on peripheral sensory axons which may be responsible for the analgesic effect of peripheral ketamine. Other agents used intra-articularly in humans, and occasionally animal studies, include corticosteroids, NSAIDS, α_2-agonists and neostigmine.

Epidural and intrathecal analgesia

Epidural analgesia describes the administration of drugs into the extradural space (outside the dura mater but underneath the ligamentum flavum). Intrathecal (spinal, subdural or subarachnoid) analgesia is more commonly utilized in human medicine, and describes injection of drugs into the cerebrospinal fluid (CSF), where diffusion of the drugs is aided by movement of CSF.

Advantages of epidural analgesia include fewer side effects of the drugs compared to systemic administration, long-lasting analgesia from a single injection and its contribution to a multimodal analgesic plan. Most epidural injections have a MAC sparing effect, reducing inhalational agent requirements by 30–40% (Golder et al., 1998). Epidurals are also useful to produce profound muscle relaxation of the affected area. Epidural analgesia in small animals has been reviewed (Jones, 2001; Campoy, 2004).

In small animals, epidural injections are most commonly performed at the lumbosacral (L-S) space. In large animals, the sacrococcygeal (S-Co) or first intercoccygeal (Co1-Co2) spaces are more commonly employed, described as 'caudal block' producing analgesia over the tail and croup as far as the mid-sacral region, the anus, vulva, perineum and the caudal aspect of the thigh, without affecting motor function of the hind limb and allowing the animal to remain standing. In animals at parturition, 'straining' or 'bearing down' ceases while uterine contractions are unaffected. With L-S injections, motor function of the hind limbs is usually affected, but the area of analgesia produced is greater, extending from the tail and perineal area caudally, including the hind limbs and abdominal area. Epidural morphine injected at the L-S space may also produce analgesia of the thorax.

Anatomy of the epidural space

The epidural space is not a cavity in the undisturbed state *in vivo*; it contains blood vessels, lymphatics, nerves and fat in dorsal and lateral compartments, i.e. it is only a *potential* space.

The spinal cord lies within the spinal canal and is covered by three membranes: the outer layer is the dense dura mater, with the arachnoid mater underneath and the delicate pia mater immediately surrounding the spinal cord. The wall of the spinal canal is formed by the vertebral arches and bodies, the intervertebral discs and the intervertebral ligaments. The spinal cord and dura mater end at the lumbar enlargement and the canal itself tapers off caudal to this, to end at the fourth or fifth coccygeal vertebra. Spinal nerves caudal to the end of the dural sac are known as the cauda equina. The dural sac ends between L6 and L7 in most dogs and between L7 and S3 in cats. In each vertebral segment, the canal has lateral openings between the vertebral arches, the intervertebral foraminae, through which pass blood vessels and the spinal nerves.

The venous plexuses of the spinal canal lie in the epidural space to form a network and can be subdivided into:

1. A pair of ventral venous plexuses lying on either side of the dorsal longitudinal ligament of the vertebra, into which the basivertebral veins drain.
2. A single dorsal venous plexus which connects with the dorsal external veins. All interconnect with one another and form a series of venous rings at the level of each vertebra. The accidental injection of drugs into these veins may occur during epidural injection and result in toxicity.

In addition to the venous plexuses, branches from vertebral, ascending cervical, deep cervical, intercostal, lumbar and iliolumbar arteries enter the intervertebral foramina and anastomose with one another, chiefly in the lateral parts of the epidural space. The spaces between the nerves, arteries and veins in the epidural space are filled with fatty tissue, the amount of which corresponds with the adiposity of the subject.

For drugs to be effective after epidural injection, they must diffuse into neuronal tissue. There have been many different suggestions as to the fate of epidurally injected drugs including: uptake into epidural fat, leakage out through the intervertebral foramina, diffusion into nerve roots outside the meninges or removal by epidural blood flow. The most likely explanations are probably diffusion into the dorsal roots of spinal nerves within the dura mater or direct diffusion through the meninges to reach the CSF and superficial layers of the spinal cord.

Drugs used for epidural injection

Epidural analgesia can be produced using local anaesthetics, opioids, ketamine (Rédua et al., 2002; Hamilton et al., 2005), α_2-agonists, NSAIDS and other agents. A commonly used clinical combination is a local anaesthetic plus an opioid. This combination usually produces better quality analgesia with a shorter onset time and a longer duration than the use of a single agent (Ganidagli et al., 2004). Local anaesthetics cause temporary loss of sensation in those parts of the body supplied by affected sensory nerves and, when more concentrated solutions are used, paralysis of those parts supplied by the motor fibres.

Morphine is the most commonly used epidural opioid as its low lipid solubility ensures that it is retained within the spinal canal for a prolonged period of time, providing analgesia for up to 24 hours after a single injection. The low lipid solubility may also result in a high potency when administered spinally (Dickenson et al., 1990), but does mean that epidural morphine has a prolonged onset of action of 1 hour or more. Spinally administered opioids may act at presynaptic sites in the dorsal horn to prevent the release of substance P and at postsynaptic receptors to hyperpolarize nerve cells. Thus, they diminish nociception without having any noticeable effect on motor function.

Epidural xylazine produces profound analgesia in some animals without interfering with motor activity (Caulkett et al., 1993) although sedation, decreased intestinal activity and mild ataxia are reported in horses and cattle (Lee et al., 2004). Lidocaine and xylazine combinations have been used to good effect in horses and cattle (Grubb et al., 1992, 2002). Medetomidine has been used epidurally in small animals at the L–S space, however, injection is usually accompanied by cardiopulmonary changes (hypertension followed by hypotension, bradycardia and respiratory depression) suggesting that much of the epidural drug is absorbed systemically.

The spread of solutions injected epidurally is most likely a function of the volume of drug used (Freire et al., 2010) and the site of injection. During late pregnancy and parturition, epidural blockade tends to spread further. This may be due to the space occupying and massaging effects of distended venous plexuses in the epidural space causing rhythmic pressure waves which tend to disperse solutions lying around them. Increased vascularity of the meninges and changes in the CSF may also contribute to the increased spread during pregnancy. Spread can be increased in obese patients as the increased epidural fat reduces the volume of the epidural space. Local anaesthetic concentration affects the efficacy and selectivity of the block (sensory versus motor blockade).

Hyperbaric solutions of local anaesthetics have been used epidurally by the addition of glucose (50 mg/mL). In humans, hyperbaric (compared to plain) ropivacaine increased the speed of onset of block, spread and reliability of analgesia, duration of analgesic effects and also hastened recovery from the motor effects of the block (Fettes et al., 2005).

All drugs injected epidurally should be preservative free to avoid neurotoxic effects of preservatives. Use of a sterile surgical technique is also essential to avoid the risk of introducing infection. Different techniques have been used to determine correct location of the spinal needle before drug injection. These include the 'hanging drop', lack of resistance to a test injection of air or sterile saline and the presence of epidural pressure waves (Iff et al., 2007). These are discussed in more detail in specific species chapters.

Continuous epidural block

Epidural catheters can be used to provide long-term analgesia and, with the correct choice of drugs and concentrations, animals can be kept both ambulatory and pain free (Hansen, 2001). The technique can also be used to prevent straining in cases of rectal and vaginal prolapse. Use of epidural catheters in 43 horses has been reported (Martin et al., 2003). The introduction of commercially available sterile packs of catheters and suitable needles has made the use of continuous blocks attractive in many species.

Risks associated with continuous epidural block include technical difficulties in catheter placement and management, the potential for damaging the spinal cord, meninges and nerves and introducing infection. However, practice should render the technique safer and its accomplishment less formidable in all species.

Contraindications to epidural injections

Contraindications include anatomical abnormalities (including pelvic fractures which may increase the risk of inadvertent intrathecal injection), uncontrolled hypovolaemia, coagulopathies, infection or skin disease at site of needle insertion, bacteraemia or septicaemia and raised intracranial pressure (inadvertent intrathecal injection may result in brain herniation).

Side effects

Motor blockade is a common complication of epidural injection. Urinary retention can occur, particularly with the use of epidural opioids and may require manual expression of the bladder until normal function returns. Pruritus has been reported occasionally after epidural opioids in animals (Haitjema & Gibson, 2001; Burford & Corley, 2006), although this complication is much commoner in humans. Unlike in humans, respiratory depression attributable to epidural opioids is uncommon in animals. Neurological damage due to spinal nerve trauma has been reported and infection can occur. Delayed hair regrowth commonly occurs over the injection site and can be very distressing for owners.

Inadvertent intrathecal injection is possible at the L–S space. In cats, the subarachnoid space extends into the sacral area, meaning that CSF can be obtained after placement of a needle in the L–S space. It is also possible to obtain CSF from the L–S space in dogs, even though theoretically the subarachnoid space ends at L6–L7. Puncture of the dura is not a problem as long as it is recognized. Before injection, the spinal needle should be carefully observed for any sign of CSF in the hub. If the needle has been placed in the subarachnoid space, it is common to halve the proposed doses of drugs to be injected, as the presence of CSF will aid cranial spread of the drugs and could result in cardiopulmonary toxicity if the normal epidural doses were used. Intrathecal morphine has been reported to cause myoclonus in two dogs (Kona-Boun et al., 2003; da Cunha et al., 2007).

Before epidural injections, the spinal needle should also be carefully observed for any signs of blood in the needle hub. A 'bloody tap' indicates perforation of a spinal blood vessel, and systemic toxicity could result if injection was completed. The spinal needle should be withdrawn in this case.

Hypotension is possible, as a result of either sympathetic blockade or cardiovascular depression from high systemic plasma concentrations of local anaesthetics. Local anaesthetics should not be injected epidurally in cardiovascularly unstable animals and some authors recommend pre-emptively fluid loading every patient before any epidural injection to avoid the risk of hypotension. Bradycardia and hypotension has also been reported as a consequence of large increases in epidural pressure during injection (Iff & Moens, 2008).

Systemic administration of lidocaine

Low dose lidocaine CRI is commonly used intra- and postoperatively in dogs and horses, but not cats due to unacceptable cardiopulmonary depression (Pypendop & Ilkiw, 2005). Suggested doses are in Table 5.4. Lidocaine has a profound dose-dependent MAC sparing effect (Doherty & Frazier, 1998; Dzikiti et al., 2003; Valverde et al., 2004b) and can obtund the EEG changes associated with the noxious stimulation of castration (Murrell et al., 2005). The analgesic mechanism is not completely

understood but may involve both spinal and supra-spinal effects through lidocaine's actions at voltage-gated Na^+ channels which are upregulated by both inflammatory and neuropathic pain. Experimentally, lidocaine CRI increases thermal thresholds in horses (Robertson et al., 2005b).

Lidocaine is an effective pro-kinetic agent in humans and horses (Rimback et al., 1990; Groudine et al., 1998; Brianceau et al., 2002; Malone et al., 2006). This may be partly attributed to its analgesic effect as pain and nociception inhibit gastrointestinal motility due to stimulation of sympathetic innervation of the GI tract. Alternatively, lidocaine may affect release of neurotransmitters and inflammatory mediators and reduce peritoneal irritation affecting GI motility (Rimback et al., 1990). In normal horses, lidocaine CRI had no effect on duodenal or rectal distension thresholds suggesting minimal effects on visceral antinociception (Robertson et al., 2005b). However, lidocaine effects on visceral pain in animals with abnormal gastrointestinal function and inflammatory changes may be quite different from normal pain-free horses. Lidocaine CRI improved the barrier function of ischaemic jejunal mucosa in experimental horses, preventing the deleterious effects on GI barrier function caused by NSAIDS such as flunixin (Cook et al., 2008).

Systemic lidocaine has anti-inflammatory effects, inhibiting neutrophil functions, such as release of lysosomal enzymes and reactive oxygen species (ROS) (Rimback et al., 1990), attenuating leucocyte adhesion to endothelial cells, reducing microvascular permeability and extravasation of fluid induced by endotoxin in rats (Schmidt et al., 1997; Hollmann & Durieux, 2000) and reduced haemodynamic and cytokine responses to endotoxin in rabbits (Taniguchi et al., 2000). Lidocaine inhibits accumulation, adhesion, activation and migration of human neutrophils (Hollmann & Durieux, 2000) but, in horses,

Table 5.4 Doses of other analgesic agents commonly used in animals

	Dog	Cat	Horse
Lidocaine	Bolus 1–2 mg/kg IV over 15 mins CRI: 50–100 µg/kg/min	Not suitable	Bolus 1.3–1.5 mg/kg IV over 15 mins CRI: 50 µg/kg/min
Ketamine	Bolus 0.5 mg/kg IV; CRI intraop: 10–20 µg/kg/min; postop: 2 µg/kg/min	As dogs	Bolus 0.6 mg/kg IV; CRI: 10–25 µg/kg/min
Tramadol	2–3 mg/kg IV CRI: 1.3–2.6 mg/kg/h PO: 2–10 mg/kg q 6–12 h	2 mg/kg IV, SC 2–10 mg/kg PO	2 mg/kg IM q 4 h
Gabapentin	10 mg/kg PO q 12 h	10 mg/kg PO q 8 h*	2.5–5 mg/kg PO q 8–24 h

q: Every; CRI = Continuous rate (intravenous) infusion; IV: intravenous; SC: subcutaneous; IM: intramuscular; PO = per os. Note: Not all of these agents are licensed for use in animals. Many doses are empirical and evidence based recommendations are still required
*After Vettorato & Corletto (2011)

effects have only been noted at concentrations greater than those likely to be reached after lidocaine CRI (Cook et al., 2009b). The anti-inflammatory effects of local anaesthetics have been comprehensively reviewed (Hollmann & Durieux, 2000) and there is a great deal of research interest in this area in both human and veterinary medicine. The anti-inflammatory actions are thought to be mediated by G-protein (particularly G_q) coupled receptors rather than Na^+ channels (Hollmann et al., 2001). Theoretically, the anti-inflammatory effects and inhibition of neutrophil response to bacteria may increase the risk of systemic infection, although experimentally, no adverse effects on host defence mechanisms have been observed (Hollmann & Durieux, 2000).

Although intravenous local anaesthetics can cause CNS and cardiovascular toxicity, low doses of lidocaine at a slow infusion rate minimize the likelihood of toxicity developing. The first signs of toxicity are usually sedation or muscle fasciculations (Meyer et al., 2001), which disappear rapidly upon discontinuation of the infusion.

KETAMINE

Ketamine, as well as being an injectable anaesthetic agent, has analgesic properties at subanaesthetic doses. Ketamine is a non-competitive NMDA antagonist. The NMDA receptor is a crucial part of the mechanism of CNS hypersensitization and wind-up. Ketamine exists as a racemic mixture and the S(+) isomer has a greater inhibitory effect at the NMDA receptor than R(−) ketamine, resulting in increased analgesic potency with fewer side effects than the racemic mixture (Kohrs & Durieux, 1998). In humans, there are conflicting studies on the benefits of ketamine as an analgesic, with some reporting a reduction in postoperative opioid requirement and improved analgesia (Michelet et al., 2007) while others have reported beneficial effects only after the development of unacceptable side effects (Max et al., 1995). Direct comparison between studies is often difficult due to differences in anaesthetic and analgesic techniques utilized and the surgical procedures undertaken (Elia & Tramer, 2005). Ketamine may reduce the occurrence of phantom limb pain in humans (Dertwinkel et al., 2002). Ketamine may also have anti-inflammatory effects through reducing neutrophil activation and release of cytokines, such as tumour necrosis factor (TNF-α) and interleukin-6 (IL-6) (Lankveld et al. 2005).

In dogs undergoing forelimb amputation, ketamine intra- and postoperatively reduced pain scores and increased activity levels with no adverse cardiorespiratory effects (Wagner et al., 2002). However, others have reported dysphoria and excitation in experimental dogs receiving ketamine CRI (Boscan et al., 2005; Solano et al., 2006; Bergadano et al., 2009) and have questioned the analgesic effects of low doses in dogs (Bergadano et al.,

2009). A single dose of 2.5 mg/kg ketamine IM at the time of anaesthetic induction significantly improved postoperative analgesia in dogs undergoing ovariohysterectomy (Slingsby & Waterman-Pearson, 2000b). Suggested doses are in Table 5.4. The optimal dose of ketamine to produce clinical analgesia requires further investigation.

Ketamine CRI has been used at varying doses in experimental horses with conflicting anti-nociceptive and adverse effects (Fielding et al., 2006; Lankveld et al., 2006; Peterbauer et al., 2008), reflecting the difficulties of using experimental, pain-free subjects to investigate a drug thought to act on chronic pain.

A combined CRI of morphine, lidocaine and ketamine (MLK) or lidocaine and ketamine is frequently used to provide profound, multimodal analgesia in dogs and horses (Muir et al., 2003; Enderle et al., 2008).

Other NMDA antagonists, such as amantadine, dextromethorphan and magnesium, may prove useful for neuropathic pain management, although further research into their efficacy is required. Amantadine is an antiviral drug also used for treatment of Parkinson's disease in humans. It has been used as an adjunctive treatment (with meloxicam) in dogs with osteoarthritis at a dose of 3–5 mg/kg every 24 hours PO and improved activity scores (Lascelles et al., 2008).

Perzinfotel, a selective NMDA antagonist reported to be 10 times as potent as ketamine, has been investigated in dogs and had a potent MAC-sparing effect without adverse cardiopulmonary side effects (Kushiro et al., 2007; Ueyama et al., 2009).

TRAMADOL

Tramadol is a synthetic analogue of codeine, used for more than 20 years to treat pain in humans. Tramadol is not a controlled drug in the UK, and has a low potential for abuse, which has made it popular in human medicine. It is not licensed for use in veterinary species. It is a weak opioid receptor agonist and inhibits reuptake of noradrenaline and serotonin, giving it an α_2-adrenergic effect. Tramadol exists as a racemic mixture with (+)-Tramadol acting via μ, κ and δ opioid receptors as well as α_2- and serotonin receptors. The other enantiomer, (−)-Tramadol acts via α_2- receptors. In humans, tramadol is primarily metabolized to O-desmethyltramadol, an active metabolite known as M1, which is a more potent μ receptor agonist, thought to be responsible for the main analgesic effects. This demethylation reaction is controlled by cytochrome P-450 2D6 which displays genetic polymorphism in humans, resulting in individual variation in efficacy between extensive and poor metabolizers. In veterinary species, metabolism varies and therapeutic concentrations of M1 may not be produced (Giorgi et al., 2009a) resulting in debate over the mechanisms of analgesia produced by tramadol. Higher concentrations of N-O-didesmethyl-tramadol (M5) are measured in veterinary species (Giorgi et al., 2009a,b). This metabolite also has a higher affinity for the μ opioid receptor than the parent compound, but may not produce clinically significant analgesia as it does not easily penetrate the blood–brain barrier. N-desmethyltramadol (M2) is also produced in large quantities in animals but is thought to be an inactive metabolite (Giorgi et al., 2009a).

The pharmacokinetics have been investigated most completely in the dog, with conflicting results between different studies, perhaps depending on the individual animals used and their P2D6 capacity. For example, three-fold differences in volume of distribution and area under plasma concentration curve were reported after IV administration of similar doses to Beagle dogs (KuKanich & Papich, 2004; Giorgi et al., 2009b). The elimination half-life in dogs after PO or IV administration is much shorter than in humans, suggesting frequent administration would be necessary to maintain therapeutic plasma concentrations (KuKanich & Papich, 2004; McMillan et al., 2008; Giorgi et al., 2009b). Tenfold differences in the plasma M1 concentrations have been reported in different studies and M1 is not reliably detected in all individuals (McMillan et al., 2008; Giorgi et al., 2009c). Tramadol is available as a sustained release oral formulation but, in dogs, the pharmacokinetics are highly variable, with plasma concentrations only reliably detected in 50% of individuals (Giorgi et al., 2009c). These pharmacokinetic studies appear to be at odds with the few clinical studies which have reported good analgesia after tramadol administration in the dog (Mastrocinque & Fantoni, 2003; Kongara et al., 2009; Seddighi et al., 2009; Vettorato et al., 2009). Doses are given in Table 5.4.

Pharmacokinetics have been reported in the cat (Pypen-dop & Ilkiw, 2008). Clearance was slower in cats than dogs, reflecting species differences in liver biotransformation, particularly as elimination of M1 requires glucuronidation. The effects of tramadol on nociceptive (thermal and pressure) thresholds in cats have been investigated (Steagall et al., 2008; Pypendop et al., 2009) and tramadol has been used epidurally (Castro et al., 2009). Tramadol in cats preanaesthesia reduced the MAC of sevoflurane by 40% (Ko et al., 2008) and produced good analgesia in cats undergoing ovariohysterectomy (Brondani et al., 2009). Chronic administration of oral tramadol in cats has not been investigated, although anecdotally good results can be obtained in animals where NSAIDs are ineffective or contraindicated. The tablets are unpalatable to cats, however.

The main side effect in dogs is mild sedation, although nausea, salivation and retching are occasionally seen (McMillan et al., 2008; Monteiro et al., 2009). Direct administration of M1 in dogs produces more consistent signs of nausea and sedation (KuKanich & Papich, 2004). Clinically, there are minimal cardiorespiratory side effects,

although increased apnoeic threshold and reduced total CO_2 sensitivity are reported in cats, mediated by effects at opioid receptors (Teppema et al., 2003; Monteiro et al., 2009).

In horses, very low plasma concentrations of M1 or M2 are reported after administration (Giorgi et al., 2006; Shilo et al., 2008). However, these metabolites and M5 can be detected by sensitive liquid chromatography/mass spectrometry techniques (De Leo et al., 2009). The elimination half-life in the horse was very short, suggesting that frequent administration (probably 2 mg/kg IM every 4 hours) would be necessary to maintain effective plasma concentrations in horses (Shilo et al., 2008). The bioavailability in horses was very low (3%) thus precluding oral administration. The clinical efficacy in the horse has not been investigated, although experimentally there was no effect on thermal threshold after IV administration (Dhanjal et al., 2009) although epidural administration increased electrical thresholds (Natalini & Robinson, 2000). The pharmacokinetics have also been investigated in goats (de Sousa et al., 2008).

GABAPENTIN

There is increasing evidence that many conditions in animals are associated with neuropathic pain, including syringomyelia in dogs (Rusbridge & Jeffery, 2008) and laminitis in horses (Jones et al., 2007). Management of neuropathic pain is of major importance in human medicine and is receiving increasing attention in veterinary medicine, although good experimental evidence for many of the drugs used to treat neuropathic pain in animals is lacking.

Gabapentin is an antiepileptic drug which is a structural analogue of GABA, although gabapentin does not exert its effects via GABA receptors. It is currently thought to bind to the $\alpha_2\delta$ subunit protein associated with voltage-dependent calcium channels, reducing calcium influx into presynaptic nerve terminals and inhibiting release of excitatory amino acids in the CNS. It has also been hypothesized to act via NMDA receptors, Na^+ channels, opioid receptors or monoaminergic pathways (Rose & Kam, 2002). Most of the reports of its use in veterinary species are anecdotal, case reports or small case series (Cashmore et al., 2009) and it is not licensed in animals. Suggested doses are given in Table 5.4.

The pharmacokinetics have been studied in horses (Dirikolu et al., 2008; Terry et al., 2010). Gabapentin was used in a single case report to treat suspected neuropathic pain following femoral nerve paresis in a horse. (Davis et al., 2007).

Preliminary studies in cats have indicated that oral gabapentin had no effect on thermal thresholds

(Pypendop et al., 2010), despite the drug having good oral bioavailability in this species (Siao et al., 2010). Gabapentin also did not cause a reduction in isoflurane MAC in experimental cats (Reid et al., 2010). However, it should be noted that these animals were not suffering from neuropathic pain. In dogs undergoing intervertebral disc surgery, gabapentin reduced pain scores, although the effect was not significant until 3 days after surgery, suggesting that gabapentin may have a delayed analgesic effect (Aghighi et al., 2009).

Pregabalin is a derivative of gabapentin, thought to have the same mechanism of action. Pharmacokinetics have been studied in dogs (Salazar et al., 2009). Other anticonvulsants, such as carbamazepine, may have a role to play in specific types of neuropathic pain such as treatment of headshaking in horses, thought to have a similar pathogenesis to post-herpetic (trigeminal) neuralgia in humans. The use, efficacy and side effects of drugs used to treat neuropathic pain require a great deal more research in veterinary species.

OTHER ANALGESIC AGENTS

Nitrous oxide (N_2O), xenon and the α_2-agonists have analgesic properties and are discussed further in the relevant chapters on the pharmacology of these agents.

REFERENCES

Abelson, A.L., McCobb, E.C., Shaw, S., et al., 2009. Use of wound soaker catheters for the administration of local anesthetic for post-operative analgesia: 56 cases. Vet Anaesth Analg 36, 597–602.

Aghighi, S.A., Tipold, A., Kastner, S.B.R., 2009. Effects of gabapentin as add-on medication on pain after intervertebral disc surgery in dogs- preliminary results. Proceedings of the 10th World Congress of Veterinary Anaesthesia, Glasgow, UK, 133.

Agnello, K.A., Reynolds, L.R., Budsberg, S.C., 2005. In vivo effects of tepoxalin, an inhibitor of cyclooxygenase and lipoxygenase, on prostanoid and leukotriene production in dogs with chronic osteoarthritis. Am J Vet Res 66, 966–972.

Allweiler, S., Brodbelt, D.C., Borer, K., et al., 2007. The isoflurane-sparing and clinical effects of a constant rate infusion of remifentanil in dogs. Vet Anaesth Analg 34, 388–393.

Andersen, M.S., Clark, L., Dyson, S.J., et al., 2006. Risk factors for colic in horses after general anaesthesia for MRI or nonabdominal surgery: absence of evidence of effect from perianaesthetic morphine. Equine Vet J 38, 368–374.

Angst, M.S., Clark, J.D., 2006. Opioid-induced hyperalgesia: a qualitative systematic review. Anesthesiology 104, 570–587.

Arai, Y.C., Ikeuchi, M., Fukunaga, K., et al., 2006. Intra-articular injection of warmed lidocaine improves intraoperative anaesthetic and postoperative analgesic conditions. Br J Anaesth 96, 259–261.

Armstrong, S., Lees, P., 2002. Effects of carprofen (R and S enantiomers and racemate) on the production of IL-1, IL-6 and TNF-alpha by equine chondrocytes and synoviocytes. J Vet Pharmacol Ther 25, 145–153.

Ashley, F.H., Waterman-Pearson, A.E., Whay, H.R., 2005. Behavioural assessment of pain in horses and donkeys: application to clinical practice and future studies. Equine Vet J 37, 565–575.

Bennett, R.C., Steffey, E.P., Kollias-Baker, C., et al., 2004. Influence of morphine sulfate on the halothane sparing effect of xylazine hydrochloride in horses. Am J Vet Res 65, 519–526.

Beretta, C., Garavaglia, G., Cavalli, M., 2005. COX-1 and COX-2 inhibition in horse blood by phenylbutazone, flunixin, carprofen and meloxicam: an in vitro analysis. Pharmacol Res 52, 302–306.

Bergadano, A., Andersen, O.K., Arendt-Nielsen, L., et al., 2009. Plasma levels of a low-dose constant-rate-infusion of ketamine and its effect on single and repeated nociceptive stimuli in conscious dogs. Vet J 182, 252–260.

Bergh, M.S., Budsberg, S.C., 2005. The coxib NSAIDs: potential clinical and pharmacologic importance in veterinary medicine. J Vet Intern Med 19, 633–643.

Bernard, F., Kudnig, S.T., Monnet, E., 2006. Hemodynamic effects of interpleural lidocaine and bupivacaine combination in anesthetized dogs with and without an open pericardium. Vet Surg 35, 252–258.

Bidwell, L.A., Wilson, D.V., Caron, J.P., 2007. Lack of systemic absorption of lidocaine from 5% patches placed on horses. Vet Anaesth Analg 34, 443–446.

Boscan, P., Pypendop, B.H., Solano, A.M., et al., 2005. Cardiovascular and respiratory effects of ketamine infusions in isoflurane-anesthetized dogs before and during noxious stimulation. Am J Vet Res 66, 2122–2129.

Boscan, P., Van Hoogmoed, L.M., Farver, T.B., et al., 2006a. Evaluation of the effects of the opioid agonist morphine on gastrointestinal tract function in horses. Am J Vet Res 67, 992–997.

Boscan, P., Van Hoogmoed, L.M., Pypendop, B.H., et al., 2006b. Pharmacokinetics of the opioid antagonist N-methylnaltrexone and evaluation of its effects on gastrointestinal tract function in horses treated or not treated with morphine. Am J Vet Res 67, 998–1004.

Bostrom, I.M., Nyman, G., Hoppe, A., et al., 2006. Effects of meloxicam on renal function in dogs with hypotension during anaesthesia. Vet Anaesth Analg 33, 62–69.

Brainard, B.M., Meredith, C.P., Callan, M.B., et al., 2007. Changes in platelet function, hemostasis, and prostaglandin expression after treatment with nonsteroidal anti-inflammatory drugs with various cyclooxygenase selectivities in dogs. Am J Vet Res 68, 251–257.

Brianceau, P., Chevalier, H., Karas, A., et al., 2002. Intravenous lidocaine and small-intestinal size, abdominal fluid, and outcome after colic surgery in horses. J Vet Intern Med 16, 736–741.

Brideau, C., Van Staden, C., Chan, C.C., 2001. In vitro effects of cyclooxygenase inhibitors in whole blood of horses, dogs, and cats. Am J Vet Res 62, 1755–1760.

Brondani, J.T., Loureiro Luna, S.P., Beier, S.L., et al., 2009. Analgesic efficacy of perioperative use of vedaprofen, tramadol or their combination in cats undergoing ovariohysterectomy. J Feline Med Surg 11, 420–429.

Burford, J.H., Corley, K.T., 2006. Morphine-associated pruritus after single extradural administration in a horse. Vet Anaesth Analg 33, 193–198.

Bussières, G., Jacques, C., Lainay, O., et al., 2008. Development of a composite orthopaedic pain scale in horses. Res Vet Sci 85, 294–306.

Campbell, N.B., Blikslager, A.T., 2000. The role of cyclooxygenase inhibitors in repair of ischaemic-injured jejunal mucosa in the horse. Equine Vet J Suppl, 59–64.

Campoy, L., 2004. Epidural and spinal anaesthesia in the dog. In Practice 26, 262–269.

Campoy, L., Bezuidenhout, A.J., Gleed, R.D., et al., 2010. Ultrasound-guided approach for axillary brachial plexus, femoral nerve, and sciatic nerve blocks in dogs. Vet Anaesth Analg 37, 144–153.

Carpenter, R.E., Wilson, D.V., Evans, A.T., 2004. Evaluation of intraperitoneal and incisional lidocaine or bupivacaine for analgesia following ovariohysterectomy in the dog. Vet Anaesth Analg 31, 46–52.

Cashmore, R.G., Harcourt-Brown, T.R., Freeman, P.M., et al., 2009. Clinical diagnosis and treatment of suspected neuropathic pain in three dogs. Aust Vet J 87, 45–50.

Castro, D.S., Silva, M.F., Shih, A.C., et al., 2009. Comparison between the analgesic effects of morphine and tramadol delivered epidurally in cats receiving a standardized noxious stimulation. J Feline Med Surg 11, 948–953.

Caulkett, N., Cribb, P.H., Duke, T., 1993. Xylazine epidural analgesia for cesarian section in cattle. Can Vet J 34, 674–676.

Chandrasekharan, N.V., Dai, H., Roos, K.L., et al., 2002. COX-3, a cyclooxygenase-1 variant inhibited by acetaminophen and other analgesic/antipyretic drugs: cloning, structure, and expression. Proc Natl Acad Sci USA 99, 13926–13931.

Clark, L., Clutton, R.E., Blissitt, K.J., et al., 2005. Effects of peri-operative morphine administration during halothane anaesthesia in horses. Vet Anaesth Analg 32, 10–15.

Conzemius, M.G., Hill, C.M., Sammarco, J.L., et al., 1997. Correlation between subjective and objective measures used to determine severity of postoperative pain in dogs. J Am Vet Med Assoc 210, 1619–1622.

Cook, V.L., Jones Shults, J., McDowell, M., et al., 2008. Attenuation of ischaemic injury in the equine jejunum by administration of systemic lidocaine. Equine Vet J 40, 353–357.

Cook, V.L., Meyer, C.T., Campbell, N.B., et al., 2009a. Effect of firocoxib or flunixin meglumine on recovery of ischemic-injured equine jejunum. Am J Vet Res 70, 992–1000.

Cook, V.L., Neuder, L.E., Blikslager, A.T., et al., 2009b. The effect of lidocaine on in vitro adhesion and migration of equine neutrophils. Vet Immunol Immunopathol 129, 137–142.

Coyle, D.E., Porembka, D.T., Sehlhorst, C.S., et al., 1994. Echocardiographic evaluation of bupivacaine cardiotoxicity. Anesth Analg 79, 335–339.

Craven, M., Chandler, M.L., Steiner, J.M., et al., 2007. Acute effects of carprofen and meloxicam on canine gastrointestinal permeability and mucosal absorptive capacity. J Vet Intern Med 21, 917–923.

Curry, S.L., Cogar, S.M., Cook, J.L., 2005. Nonsteroidal Antiinflammatory Drugs: A Review. J Am Anim Hosp Assoc 41, 298–309.

da Cunha, A.F., Carter, J.E., Grafinger, M., et al., 2007. Intrathecal morphine overdose in a dog. J Am Vet Med Assoc 230, 1665–1668.

Dal, D., Tetik, O., Altunkaya, H., et al., 2004. The efficacy of intra-articular ketamine for postoperative analgesia in outpatient arthroscopic surgery. Arthroscopy 20, 300–305.

Davis, J.L., Posner, L.P., Elce, Y., 2007. Gabapentin for the treatment of neuropathic pain in a pregnant horse. J Am Vet Med Assoc 231, 755–758.

Day, T.K., Pepper, W.T., Tobias, T.A., et al., 1995. Comparison of intra-articular and epidural morphine for analgesia following stifle arthrotomy in dogs. Vet Surg 24, 522–530.

de Grauw, J.C., van de Lest, C.H., Brama, P.A., et al., 2009. In vivo effects of meloxicam on inflammatory mediators, MMP activity and cartilage biomarkers in equine joints with acute synovitis. Equine Vet J 41, 693–699.

De Leo, M., Giorgi, M., Saccomanni, G., et al., 2009. Evaluation of tramadol and its main metabolites in horse plasma by high-performance liquid chromatography/fluorescence and liquid chromatography/electrospray ionization tandem mass spectrometry techniques. Rapid Commun Mass Spectrom 23, 228–236.

de Sousa, A.B., Santos, A.C., Schramm, S.G., et al., 2008. Pharmacokinetics of tramadol and o-desmethyltramadol in goats after intravenous and oral administration. J Vet Pharmacol Ther 31, 45–51.

Deneuche, A.J., Dufayet, C., Goby, L., et al., 2004. Analgesic comparison of meloxicam or ketoprofen for orthopedic surgery in dogs. Vet Surg 33, 650–660.

Dertwinkel, R., Heinrichs, C., Senne, I., et al., 2002. Prevention of severe phantom limb pain by perioperative administration of ketamine – an observational study. Acute Pain 4, 9–13.

Dhanjal, J.K., Wilson, D.V., Robinson, E., et al., 2009. Intravenous tramadol: effects, nociceptive properties, and pharmacokinetics in horses. Vet Anaesth Analg 36, 581–590.

Dickenson, A.H., Sullivan, A.F., McQuay, H.J., 1990. Intrathecal etorphine, fentanyl and buprenorphine on spinal nociceptive neurones in the rat. Pain 42, 227–234.

Dirikolu, L., Dafalla, A., Ely, K.J., et al., 2008. Pharmacokinetics of gabapentin in horses. J Vet Pharmacol Ther 31, 175–177.

Dixon, M.J., Robertson, S.A., Taylor, P.M., 2002. A thermal threshold testing device for evaluation of analgesics in cats. Res Vet Sci 72, 205–210.

Doherty, T.J., Frazier, D.L., 1998. Effect of intravenous lidocaine on halothane minimum alveolar concentration in ponies. Equine Vet J 30, 300–303.

Doucet, M.Y., Bertone, A.L., Hendrickson, D., et al., 2008. Comparison of efficacy and safety of paste formulations of firocoxib and phenylbutazone in horses with naturally occurring osteoarthritis. J Am Vet Med Assoc 232, 91–97.

Driessen, B., Scandella, M., Zarucco, L., 2008. Development of a technique for continuous perineural blockade of the palmar nerves in the distal equine thoracic limb. Vet Anaesth Analg 35, 432–448.

Dzikiti, T.B., Hellebrekers, L.J., van Dijk, P., 2003. Effects of intravenous lidocaine on isoflurane concentration, physiological parameters, metabolic parameters and stress-related hormones in horses undergoing surgery. J Vet Med A Physiol Pathol Clin Med 50, 190–195.

Elia, N., Tramer, M.R., 2005. Ketamine and postoperative pain – a quantitative systematic review of randomised trials. Pain 113, 61–70.

Enderle, A.K., Levionnois, O.L., Kuhn, M., et al., 2008. Clinical evaluation of ketamine and lidocaine intravenous infusions to reduce isoflurane requirements in horses under general anaesthesia. Vet Anaesth Analg 35, 297–305.

Erkert, R.S., MacAllister, C.G., Payton, M.E., et al., 2005. Use of force plate analysis to compare the analgesic effects of intravenous administration of phenylbutazone and flunixin meglumine in horses with navicular syndrome. Am J Vet Res 66, 284–288.

Fettes, P.D., Hocking, G., Peterson, M.K., et al., 2005. Comparison of plain and hyperbaric solutions of ropivacaine for spinal anaesthesia. Br J Anaesth 94, 107–111.

Fielding, C.L., Brumbaugh, G.W., Matthews, N.S., et al., 2006. Pharmacokinetics and clinical effects of a subanesthetic continuous rate infusion of ketamine in awake horses. Am J Vet Res 67, 1484–1490.

Firth, A.M., Haldane, S.L., 1999. Development of a scale to evaluate postoperative pain in dogs. J Am Vet Med Assoc 214, 651–659.

Flecknell, P.A., Roughan, J.V., 2004. Assessing pain in animals putting research into practice. Anim Welfare 13, S71–S75.

Flecknell, P.A., Liles, J.H., Wootton, R., 1989. Reversal of fentanyl/fluanisone neuroleptanalgesia in the rabbit using mixed agonist/antagonist opioids. Lab Anim 23, 147–155.

Freire, C.D., Torres, M.L., Fantoni, D.T., et al., 2010. Bupivacaine 0.25% and methylene blue spread with epidural anesthesia in dog. Vet Anaesthes Analges 37, 63–69.

Frendin, J.H., Bostrom, I.M., Kampa, N., et al., 2006. Effects of carprofen on renal function during medetomidine-propofol-isoflurane anesthesia in dogs. Am J Vet Res 67, 1967–1973.

Ganidagli, S., Cetin, H., Biricik, H.S., et al., 2004. Comparison of ropivacaine with a combination of ropivacaine and fentanyl for the caudal epidural anaesthesia of mares. Vet Rec 154, 329–332.

Gilmour, M.A., Lehenbauer, T.W., 2009. Comparison of tepoxalin, carprofen, and meloxicam for reducing intraocular inflammation in dogs. Am J Vet Res 70, 902–907.

Giordano, T., Steagall, P.V., Ferreira, T.H., et al., 2010. Postoperative analgesic effects of intravenous, intramuscular, subcutaneous or oral transmucosal buprenorphine administered to cats undergoing ovariohysterectomy. Vet Anaesth Analg 37, 357–366.

Giorgi, M., Saccomanni, G., Daniello, M.R., et al., 2006. In vitro metabolism of tramadol in horses: preliminary data. J Vet Pharmacol Ther 29, 124.

Giorgi, M., Del Carlo, S., Saccomanni, G., et al., 2009a. Pharmacokinetic and urine profile of tramadol and its major metabolites following oral immediate release capsules administration in dogs. Vet Res Commun 33, 875–885.

Giorgi, M., Del Carlo, S., Saccomanni, G., et al., 2009b. Pharmacokinetics of tramadol and its major metabolites following rectal and intravenous administration in dogs. NZ Vet J 57, 146–152.

Giorgi, M., Saccomanni, G., Lebkowska-Wieruszewska, B., et al., 2009c. Pharmacokinetic evaluation of tramadol and its major metabolites after single oral sustained tablet administration in the dog: a pilot study. Vet J 180, 253–255.

Giraudel, J.M., King, J.N., Jeunesse, E.C., et al., 2009a. Use of a pharmacokinetic/pharmacodynamic approach in the cat to determine a dosage regimen for the COX-2 selective drug robenacoxib. J Vet Pharmacol Ther 32, 18–30.

Giraudel, J.M., Toutain, P.L., King, J.N., et al., 2009b. Differential inhibition of cyclooxygenase isoenzymes in the cat by the NSAID robenacoxib. J Vet Pharmacol Ther 32, 31–40.

Giraudel, J.M., Toutain, P.L., Lees, P., 2005. Development of in vitro assays for the evaluation of cyclooxygenase inhibitors and predicting selectivity of nonsteroidal anti-inflammatory drugs in cats. Am J Vet Res 66, 700–709.

Golder, F.J., Pascoe, P.J., Bailey, C.S., et al., 1998. The effect of epidural morphine on the minimum alveolar concentration of isoflurane in cats. Vet Anaesth Analg 25, 52–56.

Goodman, L., Coles, T.B., Budsberg, S., 2008. Leukotriene inhibition in small animal medicine. J Vet Pharmacol Ther 31, 387–398.

Grilo, L.S., Carrupt, P.A., Abriel, H., 2010. Stereoselective Inhibition of the hERG1 Potassium Channel. Front Pharmacol 1, Article 137, 1–11.

Groudine, S.B., Fisher, H.A., Kaufman, R.P., Jr., et al., 1998. Intravenous lidocaine speeds the return of bowel function, decreases postoperative pain, and shortens hospital stay in patients undergoing radical retropubic prostatectomy. Anesth Analg 86, 235–239.

Grubb, T.L., Riebold, T.W., Crisman, R.O., et al., 2002. Comparison of lidocaine, xylazine, and lidocaine & xylazine for caudal epidural analgesia in cattle. Vet Anaesth Analg 29, 64–68.

Grubb, T.L., Riebold, T.W., Huber, M.J., 1992. Comparison of lidocaine, xylazine, and xylazine/lidocaine for caudal epidural analgesia in horses. J Am Vet Med Assoc 201, 1187–1190.

Guedes, A.G., Rude, E.P., Rider, M.A., 2006. Evaluation of histamine release during constant rate infusion of morphine in dogs. Vet Anaesth Analg 33, 28–35.

Gupta, A., Bodin, L., Holmstrom, B., et al., 2001. A systematic review of the peripheral analgesic effects of intraarticular morphine. Anesth Analg 93, 761–770.

Haitjema, H., Gibson, K.T., 2001. Severe pruritus associated with epidural morphine and detomidine in a horse. Aust Vet J 79, 248–250.

Hamilton, S.M., Johnston, S.A., Broadstone, R.V., 2005. Evaluation of analgesia provided by the administration of epidural ketamine in dogs with a chemically induced synovitis. Vet Anaesth Analg 32, 30–39.

Hansen, B.D., 2001. Epidural catheter analgesia in dogs and cats: technique and review of 182 cases. J Vet Emerg Crit Care 11, 95–103.

Hazewinkel, H.A., van den Brom, W.E., Theyse, L.F., et al., 2008. Comparison of the effects of firocoxib, carprofen and vedaprofen in a sodium urate crystal induced synovitis model of arthritis in dogs. Res Vet Sci 84, 74–79.

Herring, I.P., Bobofchak, M.A., Landry, M.P., et al., 2005. Duration of effect and effect of multiple doses of topical ophthalmic 0.5% proparacaine hydrochloride in clinically normal dogs. Am J Vet Res 66, 77–80.

Hollmann, M.W., Durieux, M.E., 2000. Local anesthetics and the inflammatory response: a new therapeutic indication? Anesthesiology 93, 858–875.

Hollmann, M.W., Gross, A., Jelacin, N., et al., 2001. Local anesthetic effects on priming and activation of human neutrophils. Anesthesiology 95, 113–122.

Holton, L., Reid, J., Scott, E.M., et al., 2001. Development of a behaviour-based scale to measure acute pain in dogs. Vet Rec 148, 525–531.

Holton, L.L., Scott, E.M., Nolan, A.M., et al., 1998a. Relationship between physiological factors and clinical pain in dogs scored using a numerical rating scale. J Small Anim Pract 39, 469–474.

Holton, L.L., Scott, E.M., Nolan, A.M., et al., 1998b. Comparison of three methods used for assessment of pain in dogs. J Am Vet Med Assoc 212, 61–66.

Homer, L.M., Clarke, C.R., Weingarten, A.J., 2005. Effect of dietary fat on oral bioavailability of tepoxalin in dogs. J Vet Pharmacol Ther 28, 287–291.

Iff, I., Moens, Y., 2008. Two cases of bradyarrhythmia and hypotension after extradural injections in dogs. Vet Anaesth Analg 35, 265–269.

Iff, I., Moens, Y., Schatzmann, U., 2007. Use of pressure waves to confirm the correct placement of epidural needles in dogs. Vet Rec 161, 22–25.

Ingvast-Larsson, C., Holgersson, A., Bondesson, U., et al., 2010. Clinical pharmacology of methadone in dogs. Vet Anaesth Analg 37, 48–56.

Innes, J.F., Clayton, J., Lascelles, B.D., 2010. Review of the safety and efficacy of long-term NSAID use in the treatment of canine osteoarthritis. Vet Rec 166, 226–230.

Jones, E., Vinuela-Fernandez, I., Eager, R.A., et al., 2007. Neuropathic changes in equine laminitis pain. Pain 132, 321–331.

Jones, R.S., 2001. Epidural analgesia in the dog and cat. Vet J 161, 123–131.

Jung, M., Lees, P., Seewald, W., et al., 2009. Analytical determination and pharmacokinetics of robenacoxib in the dog. J Vet Pharmacol Ther 32, 41–48.

Kay-Mugford, P., Benn, S.J., LaMarre, J., et al., 2000. In vitro effects of nonsteroidal anti-inflammatory drugs on cyclooxygenase activity in dogs. Am J Vet Res 61, 802–810.

Keates, H.L., Cramond, T., Smith, M.T., 1999. Intraarticular and periarticular opioid binding in inflamed tissue in experimental canine arthritis. Anesth Analg 89, 409–415.

King, J.N., Dawson, J., Esser, R.E., et al., 2009. Preclinical pharmacology of robenacoxib: a novel selective inhibitor of cyclooxygenase-2. J Vet Pharmacol Ther 32, 1–17.

King, J.N., Rudaz, C., Borer, L., et al., 2010. In vitro and ex vivo inhibition of canine cyclooxygenase isoforms by robenacoxib: A comparative study. Res Vet Sci 88, 497–506.

Kirchner, T., Aparicio, B., Argentieri, D.C., et al., 1997. Effects of tepoxalin, a dual inhibitor of cyclooxygenase/5-lipoxygenase, on events associated with NSAID-induced gastrointestinal inflammation. Prostaglandins Leukot Essent Fatty Acids 56, 417–423.

Kis, B., Snipes, J.A., Busija, D.W., 2005. Acetaminophen and the cyclooxygenase-3 puzzle: sorting out facts, fictions, and uncertainties. J Pharmacol Exp Ther 315, 1–7.

Ko, J.C., Abbo, L.A., Weil, A.B., et al., 2008. Effect of orally administered tramadol alone or with an intravenously administered opioid on minimum alveolar concentration of sevoflurane in cats. J Am Vet Med Assoc 232, 1834–1840.

Kohrs, R., Durieux, M.E., 1998. Ketamine: teaching an old drug new tricks. Anesth Analg 87, 1186–1193.

Kona-Boun, J.J., Pibarot, P., Quesnel, A., 2003. Myoclonus and urinary retention following subarachnoid morphine injection in a dog. Vet Anaesth Analg 30, 257–264.

Kongara, K., Chambers, P., Johnson, C.B., 2009. Glomerular filtration rate after tramadol, parecoxib and pindolol following anaesthesia and analgesia in comparison with morphine in dogs. Vet Anaesth Analg 36, 86–94.

KuKanich, B., Borum, S.L., 2008. The disposition and behavioral effects of methadone in Greyhounds. Vet Anaesth Analg 35, 242–248.

KuKanich, B., Papich, M.G., 2004. Pharmacokinetics of tramadol and the metabolite O-desmethyltramadol in dogs. J Vet Pharmacol Ther 27, 239–246.

KuKanich, B., Bidgood, T., Knesl, O., 2012. Clinical pharmacology of nonsteroidal anti-inflammatory drugs in dogs. Vet Anaesth Analg 39, 69–90.

KuKanich, B., Lascelles, B.D., Papich, M.G., 2005. Pharmacokinetics of morphine and plasma concentrations of morphine-6-glucuronide following morphine administration to dogs. J Vet Pharmacol Ther 28, 371–376.

Kushiro, T., Wiese, A.J., Eppler, M.C., et al., 2007. Effects of perzinfotel on the minimum alveolar concentration of isoflurane in dogs. Am J Vet Res 68, 1294–1299.

Kvaternick, V., Pollmeier, M., Fischer, J., et al., 2007. Pharmacokinetics and metabolism of orally administered firocoxib, a novel second generation coxib, in horses. J Vet Pharmacol Ther 30, 208–217.

Lagutchik, M.S., Mundie, T.G., Martin, D.G., 1992. Methemoglobinemia induced by a benzocaine-based topically administered anesthetic in eight sheep. J Am Vet Med Assoc 201, 1407–1410.

Lankveld, D.P., Bull, S., Van Dijk, P., et al., 2005. Ketamine inhibits LPS-induced tumour necrosis factor-alpha and interleukin-6 in an equine macrophage cell line. Vet Res 36, 257–262.

Lankveld, D.P., Driessen, B., Soma, L.R., et al., 2006. Pharmacodynamic effects and pharmacokinetic profile of a long-term continuous rate infusion of racemic ketamine in healthy conscious horses. J Vet Pharmacol Ther 29, 477–488.

Laredo, F.G., Belda, E., Murciano, J., et al., 2004. Comparison of the analgesic effects of meloxicam and carprofen administered preoperatively to dogs undergoing orthopaedic surgery. Vet Rec 155, 667–671.

Lascelles, B.D., Robertson, S.A., 2004. Use of thermal threshold response to evaluate the antinociceptive effects of butorphanol in cats. Am J Vet Res 65, 1085–1089.

Lascelles, B.D., Court, M.H., Hardie, E.M., et al., 2007. Nonsteroidal anti-inflammatory drugs in cats: a review. Vet Anaesth Analg 34, 228–250.

Lascelles, B.D., Cripps, P.J., Jones, A., et al., 1998. Efficacy and kinetics of carprofen, administered preoperatively or postoperatively, for the prevention of pain in dogs undergoing ovariohysterectomy. Vet Surg 27, 568–582.

Lascelles, B.D., Gaynor, J.S., Smith, E.S., et al., 2008. Amantadine in a multimodal analgesic regimen for alleviation of refractory osteoarthritis pain in dogs. J Vet Intern Med 22, 53–59.

Lee, I., Yamagishi, N., Oboshi, K., et al., 2004. Comparison of xylazine, lidocaine and the two drugs combined for modified dorsolumbar epidural anaesthesia in cattle. Vet Rec 155, 797–799.

Lee, M., Silverman, S.M., Hansen, H., et al., 2011. A comprehensive review of opioid-induced hyperalgesia. Pain Physician 14, 145–161.

Leece, E.A., Brearley, J.C., Harding, E.F., 2005. Comparison of carprofen and meloxicam for 72 hours following ovariohysterectomy in dogs. Vet Anaesth Analg 32, 184–192.

Lees, P., Aliabadi, F.S., Landoni, M.F., 2002. Pharmacodynamics and enantioselective pharmacokinetics of racemic carprofen in the horse. J Vet Pharmacol Ther 25, 433–448.

Lees, P., Giraudel, J., Landoni, M.F., et al., 2004a. PK-PD integration and PK-PD modelling of nonsteroidal anti-inflammatory drugs: principles and applications in veterinary pharmacology. J Vet Pharmacol Ther 27, 491–502.

Lees, P., Landoni, M.F., Giraudel, J., et al., 2004b. Pharmacodynamics and pharmacokinetics of nonsteroidal anti-inflammatory drugs in species of veterinary interest. J Vet Pharmacol Ther 27, 479–490.

Lindegaard, C., Frost, A.B., Thomsen, M.H., et al., 2010a. Pharmacokinetics of intra-articular morphine in horses with lipopolysaccharide-induced synovitis. Vet Anaesth Analg 37, 186–195.

Lindegaard, C., Gleerup, K.B., Thomsen, M.H., et al., 2010b. Anti-inflammatory effects of intra-articular administration of morphine in horses with experimentally induced synovitis. Am J Vet Res 71, 69–75.

Little, D., Brown, S.A., Campbell, N.B., et al., 2007a. Effects of the cyclooxygenase inhibitor meloxicam on recovery of ischemia-injured equine jejunum. Am J Vet Res 68, 614–624.

Little, D., Jones, S.L., Blikslager, A.T., 2007b. Cyclooxygenase (COX) inhibitors and the intestine. J Vet Intern Med 21, 367–377.

Lizarraga, I., Chambers, J.P., 2006. Involvement of opioidergic and alpha2-adrenergic mechanisms in the central analgesic effects of non-steroidal anti-inflammatory drugs in sheep. Res Vet Sci 80, 194–200.

Lohuis, J.A., van Werven, T., Brand, A., et al., 1991. Pharmacodynamics and pharmacokinetics of carprofen, a non-steroidal anti-inflammatory drug, in healthy cows and cows with Escherichia coli endotoxin-induced mastitis. J Vet Pharmacol Ther 14, 219–229.

Luna, S.P., Basilio, A.C., Steagall, P.V., et al., 2007. Evaluation of adverse effects of long-term oral administration of carprofen, etodolac, flunixin meglumine, ketoprofen, and meloxicam in dogs. Am J Vet Res 68, 258–264.

Mahler, S.P., Adogwa, A.O., 2008. Anatomical and experimental studies of brachial plexus, sciatic, and femoral nerve-location using peripheral nerve stimulation in the dog. Vet Anaesth Analg 35, 80–89.

Mahler, S.P., Reece, J.L., 2007. Electrical nerve stimulation to facilitate placement of an indwelling catheter for repeated brachial plexus block in a traumatized dog. Vet Anaesth Analg 34, 365–370.

Malone, E., Ensink, J., Turner, T., et al., 2006. Intravenous continuous infusion of lidocaine for treatment of equine ileus. Vet Surg 35, 60–66.

Martin, C.A., Kerr, C.L., Pearce, S.G., et al., 2003. Outcome of epidural catheterization for delivery of analgesics in horses: 43 cases (1998–2001). J Am Vet Med Assoc 222, 1394–1398.

Martin, W.R., Eades, C.G., Thompson, J.A., et al., 1976. The effects of morphine and nalorphine- like drugs in the nondependent and morphine-dependent chronic spinal dog. J Pharmacol Exp Ther 197, 517–532.

Mastrocinque, S., Fantoni, D.T., 2003. A comparison of preoperative tramadol and morphine for the control of early postoperative pain in canine ovariohysterectomy. Vet Anaesth Analg 30, 220–228.

Matsui, A., Williams, J.T., 2010. Activation of mu-opioid receptors and block of Kir3 potassium channels and NMDA receptor conductance by L- and D-methadone in rat locus coeruleus. Br J Pharmacol 161, 1403–1413.

Max, M.B., Byas-Smith, M.G., Gracely, R.H., et al., 1995. Intravenous infusion of the NMDA antagonist, ketamine, in chronic posttraumatic pain with allodynia: a double-blind comparison to alfentanil and placebo. Clin Neuropharmacol 18, 360–368.

Maxwell, L.K., Thomasy, S.M., Slovis, N., et al., 2003. Pharmacokinetics of fentanyl following intravenous and transdermal administration in horses. Equine Vet J 35, 484–490.

McCance-Katz, E.F., 2011. (R)-methadone versus racemic methadone: what is best for patient care? Addiction 106, 687–688.

McCann, M.E., Andersen, D.R., Zhang, D., et al., 2004. In vitro effects and in vivo efficacy of a novel cyclooxygenase-2 inhibitor in dogs with experimentally induced synovitis. Am J Vet Res 65, 503–512.

McCann, M.E., Rickes, E.L., Hora, D.F., et al., 2005. In vitro effects and in vivo efficacy of a novel cyclooxygenase-2 inhibitor in cats with lipopolysaccharide-induced pyrexia. Am J Vet Res 66, 1278–1284.

McMillan, C.J., Livingston, A., Clark, C.R., et al., 2008. Pharmacokinetics of intravenous tramadol in dogs. Can J Vet Res 72, 325–331.

Melzack, R., 2005. The McGill pain questionnaire: from description to measurement. Anesthesiology 103, 199–202.

Messenger, K.M., Davis, J.L., LaFevers, D.H., et al., 2011. Intravenous and sublingual buprenorphine in horses: pharmacokinetics and influence of sampling site. Vet Anaesth Analg 38, 374–384.

Meyer, G.A., Lin, H.C., Hanson, R.R., et al., 2001. Effects of intravenous lidocaine overdose on cardiac electrical activity and blood pressure in the horse. Equine Vet J 33, 434–437.

Michelet, P., Guervilly, C., Helaine, A., et al., 2007. Adding ketamine to morphine for patient-controlled analgesia after thoracic surgery: influence on morphine consumption, respiratory function, and nocturnal desaturation. Br J Anaesth 99, 396–403.

Mircica, E., Clutton, R.E., Kyles, K.W., et al., 2003. Problems associated with perioperative morphine in horses: a retrospective case analysis. Vet Anaesth Analg 30, 147–155.

Moiniche, S., Kehlet, H., Dahl, J.B., 2002. A qualitative and quantitative systematic review of preemptive analgesia for postoperative pain relief: the role of timing of analgesia. Anesthesiology 96, 725–741.

Monreal, L., Sabate, D., Segura, D., et al., 2004. Lower gastric ulcerogenic effect of suxibuzone compared to phenylbutazone when administered orally to horses. Res Vet Sci 76, 145–149.

Monteiro, E.R., Junior, A.R., Assis, H.M., et al., 2009. Comparative study on the sedative effects of morphine, methadone, butorphanol or tramadol, in combination with acepromazine, in dogs. Vet Anaesth Analg 36, 25–33.

Moreau, M., Daminet, S., Martel-Pelletier, J., et al., 2005. Superiority of the gastroduodenal safety profile of licofelone over rofecoxib, a COX-2 selective inhibitor, in dogs. J Vet Pharmacol Ther 28, 81–86.

Moreau, M., Lussier, B., Doucet, M., et al., 2007. Efficacy of licofelone in dogs with clinical osteoarthritis. Vet Rec 160, 584–588.

Muir, W.W., 3rd, Wiese, A.J., March, P.A., 2003. Effects of morphine, lidocaine, ketamine, and morphine-lidocaine-ketamine drug combination on minimum alveolar concentration in dogs anesthetized with isoflurane. Am J Vet Res 64, 1155–1160.

Muir, W.W., Skarda, R.T., Sheehan, W.C., 1978. Cardiopulmonary effects of narcotic agonists and a partial

agonist in horses. Am J Vet Res 39, 1632–1635.

Murrell, J.C., Robertson, S.A., Taylor, P.M., et al., 2007. Use of a transdermal matrix patch of buprenorphine in cats: preliminary pharmacokinetic and pharmacodynamic data. Vet Rec 160, 578–583.

Murrell, J.C., White, K.L., Johnson, C.B., et al., 2005. Investigation of the EEG effects of intravenous lidocaine during halothane anaesthesia in ponies. Vet Anaesth Analg 32, 212–221.

Natalini, C.C., Robinson, E.P., 2000. Evaluation of the analgesic effects of epidurally administered morphine, alfentanil, butorphanol, tramadol, and U50488H in horses. Am J Vet Res 61, 1579–1586.

Niza, M.M., Felix, N., Vilela, C.L., et al., 2007. Cutaneous and ocular adverse reactions in a dog following meloxicam administration. Vet Dermatol 18, 45–49.

Ong, C.K., Lirk, P., Seymour, R.A., et al., 2005. The efficacy of preemptive analgesia for acute postoperative pain management: a meta-analysis. Anesth Analg 100, 757–773.

Orsini, J.A., Moate, P.J., Kuersten, K., et al., 2006. Pharmacokinetics of fentanyl delivered transdermally in healthy adult horses – variability among horses and its clinical implications. J Vet Pharmacol Ther 29, 539–546.

Park, J., Sutradhar, B.C., Hong, G., et al., 2011. Comparison of the cytotoxic effects of bupivacaine, lidocaine, and mepivacaine in equine articular chondrocytes. Vet Anaesth Analg 38, 127–133.

Paulson, S.K., Engel, L., Reitz, B., et al., 1999. Evidence for polymorphism in the canine metabolism of the cyclooxygenase 2 inhibitor, celecoxib. Drug Metab Dispos 27, 1133–1142.

Peterbauer, C., Larenza, P.M., Knobloch, M., et al., 2008. Effects of a low dose infusion of racemic and S-ketamine on the nociceptive withdrawal reflex in standing ponies. Vet Anaesth Analg 35, 414–423.

Pollmeier, M., Toulemonde, C., Fleishman, C., et al., 2006. Clinical evaluation of firocoxib and carprofen for the treatment of dogs with osteoarthritis. Vet Rec 159, 547–551.

Posner, L.P., Gleed, R.D., Erb, H.N., et al., 2007. Post-anesthetic

hyperthermia in cats. Vet Anaesth Analg 34, 40–47.

Posner, L.P., Pavuk, A.A., Rokshar, J.L., et al., 2010. Effects of opioids and anesthetic drugs on body temperature in cats. Vet Anaesth Analg 37, 35–43.

Pypendop, B.H., Ilkiw, J.E., 2005. Assessment of the hemodynamic effects of lidocaine administered IV in isoflurane-anesthetized cats. Am J Vet Res 66, 661–668.

Pypendop, B.H., Ilkiw, J.E., 2008. Pharmacokinetics of tramadol, and its metabolite O-desmethyl-tramadol, in cats. J Vet Pharmacol Ther 31, 52–59.

Pypendop, B.H., Siao, K.T., Ilkiw, J.E., 2009. Effects of tramadol hydrochloride on the thermal threshold in cats. Am J Vet Res 70, 1465–1470.

Pypendop, B.H., Siao, K.T., Ilkiw, J.E., 2010. Thermal antinociceptive effect of orally administered gabapentin in healthy cats. Am J Vet Res 71, 1027–1032.

Rédua, M.A., Valadão, C.A., Duque, J.C., et al., 2002. The pre-emptive effect of epidural ketamine on wound sensitivity in horses tested by using von Frey filaments. Vet Anaesth Analg 29, 200–206.

Reed, S.K., Messer, N.T., Tessman, R.K., et al., 2006. Effects of phenylbutazone alone or in combination with flunixin meglumine on blood protein concentrations in horses. Am J Vet Res 67, 398–402.

Reid, J., Nolan, A.M., Hughes, J.M.L., et al., 2007. Development of the short-form Glasgow Composite Measure Pain Scale (CMPS-SF) and derivation of an analgesic intervention score. Anim Welfare 16, 97–104.

Reid, P., Pypendop, B.H., Siao, K.T., et al., 2010. The effects of intravenous gabapentin administration on the minimum alveolar concentration of isoflurane in cats. Anesth Analg 111, 633–637.

Rimback, G., Cassuto, J., Tollesson, P.O., 1990. Treatment of postoperative paralytic ileus by intravenous lidocaine infusion. Anesth Analg 70, 414–419.

Robertson, S.A., Lascelles, B.D., Taylor, P.M., et al., 2005a. PK-PD modeling of buprenorphine in cats: intravenous and oral transmucosal administration. J Vet Pharmacol Ther 28, 453–460.

Robertson, S.A., Sanchez, L.C., Merritt, A.M., et al., 2005b. Effect of systemic lidocaine on visceral and somatic nociception in conscious horses. Equine Vet J 37, 122–127.

Robertson, S.A., Taylor, P.M., Lascelles, B.D., et al., 2003a. Changes in thermal threshold response in eight cats after administration of buprenorphine, butorphanol and morphine. Vet Rec 153, 462–465.

Robertson, S.A., Taylor, P.M., Sear, J.W., 2003b. Systemic uptake of buprenorphine by cats after oral mucosal administration. Vet Rec 152, 675–678.

Rohrer Bley, C., Neiger-Aeschbacher, G., Busato, A., et al., 2004. Comparison of perioperative racemic methadone, levo-methadone and dextromoramide in cats using indicators of post-operative pain. Vet Anaesth Analg 31, 175–182.

Rose, M.A., Kam, P.C., 2002. Gabapentin: pharmacology and its use in pain management. Anaesthesia 57, 451–462.

Roughan, J.V., Flecknell, P.A., 2004. Behaviour-based assessment of the duration of laparotomy-induced abdominal pain and the analgesic effects of carprofen and buprenorphine in rats. Behav Pharmacol 15, 461–472.

Roughan, J.V., Wright-Williams, S.L., Flecknell, P.A., 2009. Automated analysis of postoperative behaviour: assessment of HomeCageScan as a novel method to rapidly identify pain and analgesic effects in mice. Lab Anim 43, 17–26.

Rusbridge, C., Jeffery, N.D., 2008. Pathophysiology and treatment of neuropathic pain associated with syringomyelia. Vet J 175, 164–172.

Sabate, D., Homedes, J., Salichs, M., et al., 2009. Multicentre, controlled, randomised and blinded field study comparing efficacy of suxibuzone and phenylbutazone in lame horses. Equine Vet J 41, 700–705.

Salazar, V., Dewey, C.W., Schwark, W., et al., 2009. Pharmacokinetics of single-dose oral pregabalin administration in normal dogs. Vet Anaesth Analg 36, 574–580.

Sammarco, J.L., Conzemius, M.G., Perkowski, S.Z., et al., 1996. Postoperative analgesia for stifle surgery: a comparison of intra-articular bupivacaine, morphine, or saline. Vet Surg 25, 59–69.

Santos, L.C., de Moraes, A.N., Saito, M.E., 2009. Effects of intraarticular ropivacaine and morphine on lipopolysaccharide-induced synovitis in horses. Vet Anaesth Analg 36, 280–286.

Schmidt, W., Schmidt, H., Bauer, H., et al., 1997. Influence of lidocaine on endotoxin-induced leukocyte-endothelial cell adhesion and macromolecular leakage in vivo. Anesthesiology 87, 617–624.

Schmiedt, C.W., Bjorling, D.E., 2007. Accidental prehension and suspected transmucosal or oral absorption of fentanyl from a transdermal patch in a dog. Vet Anaesth Analg 34, 70–73.

Seddighi, M.R., Egger, C.M., Rohrbach, B.W., et al., 2009. Effects of tramadol on the minimum alveolar concentration of sevoflurane in dogs. Vet Anaesth Analg 36, 334–340.

Sellon, D.C., Monroe, V.L., Roberts, M.C., et al., 2001. Pharmacokinetics and adverse effects of butorphanol administered by single intravenous injection or continuous intravenous infusion in horses. Am J Vet Res 62, 183–189.

Sellon, D.C., Roberts, M.C., Blikslager, A.T., et al., 2004. Effects of continuous rate intravenous infusion of butorphanol on physiologic and outcome variables in horses after celiotomy. J Vet Intern Med 18, 555–563.

Senior, J.M., Pinchbeck, G.L., Allister, R., et al., 2006. Post anaesthetic colic in horses: a preventable complication? Equine Vet J 38, 479–484.

Senior, J.M., Pinchbeck, G.L., Dugdale, A.H., et al., 2004. Retrospective study of the risk factors and prevalence of colic in horses after orthopaedic surgery. Vet Rec 155, 321–325.

Sheehy, J.G., Hellyer, P.W., Sammonds, G.E., et al., 2001. Evaluation of opioid receptors in synovial membranes of horses. Am J Vet Res 62, 1408–1412.

Shilo, Y., Britzi, M., Eytan, B., et al., 2008. Pharmacokinetics of tramadol in horses after intravenous, intramuscular and oral administration. J Vet Pharmacol Ther 31, 60–65.

Siao, K.T., Pypendop, B.H., Ilkiw, J.E., 2010. Pharmacokinetics of gabapentin in cats. Am J Vet Res 71, 817–821.

Slingsby, L.S., Taylor, P.M., Murrell, J.C., 2011. A study to evaluate buprenorphine at 40 mug kg(-1) compared to 20 mug kg(-1) as a post-operative analgesic in the dog. Vet Anaesth Analg 38, 584–593.

Slingsby, L.S., Waterman-Pearson, A.E., 2000a. Postoperative analgesia in the cat after ovariohysterectomy by use of carprofen, ketoprofen, meloxicam or tolfenamic acid. J Small Anim Pract 41, 447–450.

Slingsby, L.S., Waterman-Pearson, A.E., 2000b. The post-operative analgesic effects of ketamine after canine ovariohysterectomy – a comparison between pre- or post-operative administration. Res Vet Sci 69, 147–152.

Slingsby, L.S., Waterman-Pearson, A.E., 2002. Comparison between meloxicam and carprofen for postoperative analgesia after feline ovariohysterectomy. J Small Anim Pract 43, 286–289.

Solano, A.M., Pypendop, B.H., Boscan, P.L., et al., 2006. Effect of intravenous administration of ketamine on the minimum alveolar concentration of isoflurane in anesthetized dogs. Am J Vet Res 67, 21–25.

Steagall, P.V., Mantovani, F.B., Ferreira, T.H., et al., 2007. Evaluation of the adverse effects of oral firocoxib in healthy dogs. J Vet Pharmacol Ther 30, 218–223.

Steagall, P.V., Taylor, P.M., Brondani, J.T., et al., 2008. Antinociceptive effects of tramadol and acepromazine in cats. J Feline Med Surg 10, 24–31.

Taniguchi, T., Shibata, K., Yamamoto, K., et al., 2000. Effects of lidocaine administration on hemodynamics and cytokine responses to endotoxemia in rabbits. Crit Care Med 28, 755–759.

Teppema, L.J., Nieuwenhuijs, D., Olievier, C.N., et al., 2003. Respiratory depression by tramadol in the cat: involvement of opioid receptors. Anesthesiology 98, 420–427.

Terry, R.L., McDonnell, S.M., Van Eps, A.W., et al., 2010. Pharmacokinetic profile and behavioral effects of gabapentin in the horse. J Vet Pharmacol Ther 33, 485–494.

Tetik, O., Islamoglu, F., Ayan, E., et al., 2004. Intermittent infusion of 0.25% bupivacaine through an intrapleural catheter for post-thoracotomy pain relief. Ann Thorac Surg 77, 284–288.

Thompson, S.E., Johnson, J.M., 1991. Analgesia in dogs after intercostal thoracotomy. A comparison of morphine, selective intercostal nerve block, and interpleural regional analgesia with bupivacaine. Vet Surg 20, 73–77.

Tirel, O., Chanavaz, C., Bansard, J.Y., et al., 2005. Effect of remifentanil with and without atropine on heart rate variability and RR interval in children. Anaesthesia 60, 982–989.

Tomlinson, J.E., Blikslager, A.T., 2004. Effects of ischemia and the cyclooxygenase inhibitor flunixin on in vitro passage of lipopolysaccharide across equine jejunum. Am J Vet Res 65, 1377–1383.

Tunsmeyer, J., Vaske, B., Bosing, B., et al., 2012. Cardiovascular effects of a proprietary L-methadone/fenpipramide combination (Polamivet) alone and in addition to acepromazine in healthy beagle dogs. Vet Anaesth Analg 39, 451–463.

Ueyama, Y., Lerche, P., Eppler, C.M., et al., 2009. Effects of intravenous administration of perzinfotel, fentanyl, and a combination of both drugs on the minimum alveolar concentration of isoflurane in dogs. Am J Vet Res 70, 1459–1464.

Valverde, A., Cantwell, S., Hernandez, J., et al., 2004a. Effects of acepromazine on the incidence of vomiting associated with opioid administration in dogs. Vet Anaesth Analg 31, 40–45.

Valverde, A., Doherty, T.J., Hernandez, J., et al., 2004b. Effect of lidocaine on the minimum alveolar concentration of isoflurane in dogs. Vet Anaesth Analg 31, 264–271.

van Hoogmoed, L.M., Boscan, P.L., 2005. In vitro evaluation of the effect of the opioid antagonist N-methylnaltrexone on motility of the equine jejunum and pelvic flexure. Equine Vet J 37, 325–328.

Vettorato, E., Corletto, F., 2011. Gabapentin as part of multi-modal analgesia in two cats suffering multiple injuries. Vet Anaesth Analg 38, 518–520.

Vettorato, E., Zonca, A., Isola, M., et al., 2010. Pharmacokinetics and efficacy of intravenous and extradural tramadol in dogs. Vet J 183, 310–315.

Wagner, A.E., Walton, J.A., Hellyer, P.W., et al., 2002. Use of low doses of ketamine administered by constant rate infusion as an adjunct for postoperative analgesia in dogs. J Am Vet Med Assoc 221, 72–75.

Walker, A.F., 2007. Sublingual administration of buprenorphine for long-term analgesia in the horse. Vet Rec 160, 808–809.

Wallace, J.L., 1999. Selective COX-2 inhibitors: is the water becoming muddy? Trends Pharmacol Sci 20, 4–6.

Wallace, J.L., McCafferty, D.M., Carter, L., et al., 1993. Tissue-selective inhibition of prostaglandin synthesis in rat by tepoxalin: anti-inflammatory without gastropathy? Gastroenterology 105, 1630–1636.

Wallace, J.L., Viappiani, S., Bolla, M., 2009. Cyclooxygenase-inhibiting nitric oxide donors for osteoarthritis. Trends Pharmacol Sci 30, 112–117.

Warner, T.D., Mitchell, J.A., 2002. Cyclooxygenase-3 (COX-3): filling in the gaps toward a COX continuum? Proc Natl Acad Sci USA 99, 13371–13373.

Waterman, A.E., Kalthum, W., 1990. The effect of clinical hepatic disease on the distribution and elimination of pethidine administered post-operatively to dogs. J Vet Pharmacol Ther 13, 137–147.

Weinberg, G., Ripper, R., Feinstein, D.L., et al., 2003. Lipid emulsion infusion rescues dogs from bupivacaine-induced cardiac toxicity. Reg Anesth Pain Med 28, 198–202.

Weir, M.R., 2002. Renal effects of nonselective NSAIDs and coxibs. Cleve Clin J Med 69 (Suppl 1), SI53–58.

Wilson, D.V., Evans, A.T., Miller, R., 2005. Effects of preanesthetic administration of morphine on gastroesophageal reflux and regurgitation during anesthesia in dogs. Am J Vet Res 66, 386–390.

Wilson, J.E., Chandrasekharan, N.V., Westover, K.D., et al., 2004. Determination of expression of cyclooxygenase-1 and -2 isozymes in canine tissues and their differential sensitivity to nonsteroidal anti-inflammatory drugs. Am J Vet Res 65, 810–818.

Wolfe, T.M., Bateman, S.W., Cole, L.K., et al., 2006. Evaluation of a local anesthetic delivery system for the postoperative analgesic management of canine total ear canal ablation – a randomized, controlled, double-blinded study. Vet Anaesth Analg 33, 328–339.

Zaveri, N., 2003. Peptide and nonpeptide ligands for the nociceptin/orphanin FQ receptor ORL1: research tools and potential therapeutic agents. Life Sci 73, 663–678.

Zhu, X., Conklin, D.R., Eisenach, J.C., 2005. Preoperative inhibition of cyclooxygenase-1 in the spinal cord reduces postoperative pain. Anesth Analg 100, 1390–1393.

Chapter | 6 |

General pharmacology of the injectable agents used in anaesthesia

INTRODUCTION

Injectable anaesthetic agents may be used either just to induce anaesthesia prior to maintenance with an inhalant, or as the only anaesthetic agent for as long as required. In human anaesthesia, such use is almost always by intravenous (IV) injection, duration being extended by infusion. This is termed 'total intravenous anaesthesia' or TIVA. Many injectable agents are poor analgesics so additional analgesia is usually necessary. While in veterinary anaesthesia achievement of TIVA by infusion is ideal (see Chapter 3), practicality may mean that prolongation is by bolus injections. Some agents can be given by the intramuscular (IM) route and, in veterinary practice, may be used (often with sedatives or analgesics) at a dose which gives anaesthesia of sufficient duration for some surgery. This is only practicable with agents with minimal cardiac depressant effects, such as ketamine. Other routes which have been employed with suitable agents include subcutaneous (SC), intraperitoneal (not recommended for routine use), transmucous membrane and even oral or rectal. The IV route gives the anaesthetist some control over anaesthetic depth; the other routes do not.

Injectable anaesthesia is often claimed to be 'easy' and to require less equipment than do inhalant anaesthetics, but this is not so. Some factors that the anaesthetist has to consider concerning the drugs they are using are listed in Box 6.1. Not all agents given IV produce loss of consciousness in one injection site–brain circulation time and, if not, it becomes more difficult to titrate the dose to the animal's requirements. Once the agent has been injected, it cannot be removed other than by the metabolic process so there is no margin for error. Duration of action depends both on redistribution and on metabolism (see

---

Box 6.1 Some considerations when using injectable anaesthetic agents

Legal Requirements

Country dependent

- Laws concerning storage, handling and recording
- In European Union, the 'Cascade'

Pharmacokinetics (see Chapter 3)

Speed of onset of action

- Does the drug work in a circulation time or is there a delay in action, even with IV use?
- If a delay, is it due to slow crossing of the blood–brain barrier, reaching the receptors, or is it a prodrug?
- Allowance for delay is necessary to avoid overdosage

Initial volume of distribution

- Redistribution is often the reason for initial termination of anaesthesia from a single IV dose
- Differences between thin and fat animals
- Is the drug highly protein bound? Does ionization influence the activity?

Clearance

- Context-sensitive half-life and route of elimination
- Is the drug cumulative?
- Is it suitable for TIVA?
- Is metabolism in the cat (or any other species) different?
- Effect of disease?

Routes of administration

- Only IV or other routes?
- If only IV, why? Duration of action too short? Irritant (see formulation)?

Formulation

Maximal available concentration

- Limits use in large animals
- Limits non-IV use

Irritancy

- Limits route of injection
- Tissue damage if not IV?
- Thrombotic potential; erythrocyte damage

Pain on injection

- This may be the formulation or the drug itself

Shelf-life once open

- Does it contain a preservative?
- Is the vial 'single use only'?

Side effects of carrier?

- Histamine release by cremophor EL
- Hyperlipidosis following lipid infusions

Combination with other drugs

- Some formulations may be incompatible with infusion fluids and/or other ancillary drugs

Pharmacodynamics

Quality of anaesthesia

- Smooth passage to unconsciousness
- Lack of response to stimuli (analgesia)
- Muscle relaxation

Cardiovascular: myocardial depression, heart rate and rhythm, peripheral vascular resistance

- The major factor in overall safety
- Limits level of overdose before death occurs (LD 50)
- CV effects are not always easily reversible until drug metabolized

Respiratory effects

- Ability to give oxygen and ventilate should *always* be available

Other side effects

Examples:

- Myoclonic movement; vomiting; hallucinatory effects

Quality of recovery

- Is it quiet; examples
  - Do dogs vocalize?
  - Are horses able to get up quietly and without ataxia?

Chapter 3) and agents which are short acting with a single injection given for induction of anaesthesia may become long acting when used for TIVA as context-sensitive half-life increases. Table 6.1 gives relevant comparative pharmacokinetic data for humans for the drugs discussed in this chapter. However, there are many species differences, not all of which are well documented. In particular, cats, because of their inability to conjugate many agents (see

Chapter 16) may metabolize the drug and/or the solvent differently. Knowledge of pharmacodynamics of the agents is also essential for safe use. Almost all of the injectable agents cause respiratory depression, so endotracheal intubation, oxygen and the ability to ventilate should still be available. It is more difficult to compensate for cardiovascular effects resulting from overdose. Specific side effects, for example myoclonus, may be more problematic in

Table 6.1 Pharmacokinetic parameters of IV anaesthetic agents in humans as there is good comparative data available

Agent	Elimination half-life (hours)	Clearance (mL/kg/min)	Apparent volume of distribution at steady state (L/kg)	Protein binding (%)
Thiopental	7–17	3–4	1.5–3	85
Methohexital	2–6	10–15	1.5–3	85
Propofol	1.8–7	20–30	2–10	98
Etomidate	2.9–5.3	18–25	2.5–4.5	76
Ketamine	2.5–3	12–17	3.1	60

These values differ in other species (see text). Note the wide variation in some reported values.
After Hijazi & Boulier (2002), Evers et al. (2006); Reves et al. (2012).

different species. For example, a quiet calm non-ataxic recovery is essential for horses so only agents (or combinations) that will ensure this should be used. Most IV anaesthetics are used in perioperative combination with sedatives and analgesics to overcome the shortcomings of the anaesthetic agent, but the combinations may further alter the pharmacodynamics.

Formulation of injectable anaesthetic agents

There is not yet an ideal injectable anaesthetic and the search continues for new drugs, or new, improved formulations of existing drugs. The technology involved in formulation (or pharmaceutics) is advancing rapidly and a full resume is beyond the scope of this chapter. Useful reviews include Baker & Naguib (2005) and Loftsson & Brewster (2010). MacPherson (2001) also explains the various preservatives that may be added, their potential side effects and neurotoxicity. Formulations must allow the drug to be available once injected; even small changes can change bioavailability. They should not be irritant if injected extravascularly, not cause pain on injection, have no cardiopulmonary effects themselves, not be toxic, and should not release histamine or cause anaphylactic reactions. A further consideration is to ensure that the final product remains sterile in use; this is of particular importance in small animal practice where economics prefer the use of multidose bottles. Generic versions of drugs may differ in formulation from the original branded product. The following are the most common methods of formulating IV anaesthetic drugs.

Water based

The agent may be presented as a 'salt' to improve solubility. Examples include thiopental (as the sodium salt) and

ketamine (the hydrochloride). Such solutions may or may not have additive preservatives and antibacterial agents.

Lipid emulsion

Many drugs used in anaesthesia use lipid emulsion carriers, the most notable being propofol. The emulsions used may vary in their source and percentage of lipid, each component having a technical reason for its presence, and in their droplet size. Macroemulsions (droplet size 0.1–100 μm) such as used for Diprivan® (the original propofol) appear white while microemulsions (droplet size >0.1 μm) are translucent or opalescent. Lipid emulsions are an excellent growth medium for bacteria, and this has caused clinical problems (Bennett et al., 1995). Some formulations of propofol now contain EDTA or sodium metabisulphite to retard (but not prevent) bacterial growth. Lipid infusions may cause hyperlipaemia. This might contribute to the propofol infusion syndrome (see below). Cats do not metabolize lipids as rapidly as other species (see Chapter 16).

Cyclodextrins

These are complex polysaccharides, derived from starch, that have a hydrophobic centre and 'wrap round' lipophilic drugs – described as 'guest–host complexes' (Sneyd, 2004). There are a number of different forms which are suitable for solubilizing a wide range of drugs. In veterinary anaesthesia, they are the carrier for alfaxalone (see below) but are/have been trialled for several other IV anaesthetic agents including propofol. Although nontoxic, the concern in human use is that they may possible trigger anaphylactic reactions; time will tell.

Propylene glycol

This is used as a solvent for a number of agents in anaesthesia, these being etomidate and diazepam. It is miscible with water at all concentrations and also has some preservative action. It does cause pain on injection and a high incidence of thrombophlebitis.

Micelle formulations

Nanotechnology to produce polymeric micelle formulations of a number of drugs, including propofol, has been investigated. The micelles are so small that solutions appear clear.

Solvents no longer used

Cremophor EL, which is polyethylated castor oil, was tried as a solvent for a number of anaesthetic drugs, but can cause anaphylaxis and, since the withdrawal of the steroid combination Saffan® or Althesin® (see steroid anaesthesia below), is now no longer used.

Polysorbate 80, derived from sorbitol, was considered a possibility, but propofol in polysorbate 80 caused major cardiopulmonary depression when tested in goats (Bettschart-Wolfensberger et al., 2000).

Sites of action of injectable anaesthetic agents

The state of consciousness we term 'general anaesthesia', and the receptor theories of how drugs cause this are discussed in Chapter 1. To summarize an extremely simplified view, the injectable (and some inhalation) anaesthetics that cause dose-dependent hypnosis are agonists at the GABA$_A$ receptors, but do not necessarily effect the same site on that receptor. They may also act at other central and peripheral ion channels and/or receptors; hence the difference in properties between the agents. The dissociative agents, such as ketamine, act primarily as antagonists at NMDA receptors. It is also possible to obtain a state resembling anaesthesia by the combination of opioid agonists, α_2-agonists and dopamine antagonists (Brown et al., 2011); these agents are discussed in Chapters 4 and 5.

IV AGENTS ACTING PRIMARILY AT THE GABA$_A$ RECEPTORS

The barbiturates

Currently, four barbiturate drugs are used in veterinary medicine. Phenobarbital is very long acting and is used as an anticonvulsant. Within anaesthesia, agents used are pentobarbital, thiopental and methohexital. All three exert their hypnotic properties primarily by actions at the GABA$_A$ receptor (see Chapter 1). Properties in common are that all are very respiratory depressant and are poor analgesics. All are metabolized by the liver, with species differences in rate.

Thiopental

Thiopental (thiopentone) was introduced into veterinary practice in the 1930s and over the next 60 years became the most widely used agent for induction of anaesthesia. Thiopental was originally licensed at a dose of up to 30 mg/kg, now considered a massive overdose, but which gave prolonged hypnosis. Previous editions of this book review the veterinary studies. Thiopental's primary use in human and in veterinary anaesthesia is for the induction of anaesthesia. However, all barbiturates are neuroprotective, are excellent antiepileptics and infusions of thiopental still have place for prolonged sedation, for example in poisoning cases causing fits and, in humans, in cases of head injury (Majdan et al., 2013).

Thiopental sodium is presented as a yellow solid, to be dissolved in water before use, the concentration to be made being as low as practicable in relation to volume required. Thus, 1.25% or less is recommended for cats and small dogs, 2.5% for larger dogs and up to 10 % for horses and cattle. The preparation contains anhydrous sodium carbonate to prevent precipitation of the insoluble free acid by atmospheric CO_2. Aqueous solutions are strongly alkaline and are incompatible to mix with many analgesics and sedative drugs, but do seem compatible with propofol (Chilvers et al., 1999; Ko et al., 1999). Depending on concentration, the solution is highly irritant. It can only be used IV and even 1.25% causes skin sloughs if accidentally injected extravascularly; 10% solutions can result in major damage to surrounding tissues. Solutions of thiopental may be kept for several days; bacterial growth does not easily occur (Strachan et al., 2008).

The pharmacokinetics of thiopental are typical of a cumulative agent. Following a single IV injection, blood and brain levels rise then fall rapidly as the drug is redistributed into other tissues, in particular fat. From a single 'induction' dose of thiopental, recovery of consciousness is as rapid as for propofol as both are very lipophilic and have a large volume of distribution. However, for thiopental, metabolism by the liver is slow, so if larger or multiple doses are given, it accumulates in the tissues; recovery now depends on metabolism and can be very prolonged. With only an induction dose of thiopental, there is residual sedation following recovery. In animals with little fat, or in which liver enzymes may not be fully functional (e.g. greyhounds; neonates), recovery is even slower (Sams et al., 1985; Robinson et al., 1986). In mixed-breed dogs, the half-lives of elimination have been reported as from approximately 2.5 to 7 hours and plasma clearances as from 1.5 to 97 mL/kg/minute (Brandon & Baggot, 1981; Ilkiw et al., 1991). It has always been claimed (and is the author's experience) that barbiturates are shorter acting in herbivores than in cats and dogs but, with the range of reported values from different laboratories, it is not possible to find evidence to prove this (Ilkiw et al., 1991; Abass et al., 1994). Thiopental is highly protein bound (more than 75%); it is the non-bound fraction that is active, so animals with hypoproteinaemia (including anaemia) are very sensitive to its effects. The drug also is partially ionized and acts as a weak organic acid; the dissociation constant is such that a small change in pH will markedly affect the degree of ionization, and this in turn can alter distribution.

When thiopental is injected IV, it results in a smooth induction of anaesthesia within a circulation time: in the unpremedicated animal, this is very rapid (with fast injection, it can be as little as 20 seconds in a horse). If premedication reduces cardiac output (as do the α_2-agonists), then speed of induction will be slowed. The induction dose of thiopental required for endotracheal intubation in an unpremeditated animal (most domestic species) can be over 15 mg/kg; after acepromazine premedication with rapid injection in dogs, the dose is 7–10 mg/kg and, after α_2-agonists, the dose reduces further depending on the sedation achieved (Young et al., 1990; England & Hammond, 1997). Doses used to induce anaesthesia in horses premedicated with acepromazine are 11 mg/kg, while after moderate α_2-premedication, 7 mg/kg suffices (Clarke & Gerring, 1990). Previously, the recommendation (for humans and dogs) was to give thiopental very rapidly, but current advice for small animals is that the drug should be injected more slowly, over around one minute, in order to reduce the initial cardiorespiratory depression. A major reason for fast administration was to avoid an excitement phase at induction; effective sedative premedication negates this problem.

Thiopental is very respiratory depressant. Rapid IV injection of the drug causes apnoea and a fall in blood pressure, even in normovolaemic animals, through a decrease in systemic vascular resistance. In hypovolaemic animals, rapid injection of thiopental can be fatal. After the initial fall, in normovolaemic animals, the blood pressure returns to about the normal level but there is a persistent tachycardia. The drug has a dose-dependent direct depressant effect on the myocardium but, at normal induction doses, cardiac output is maintained by the increase in heart rate. Thiopental is a poor analgesic; very deep levels of anaesthesia are necessary to prevent response to noxious stimulation so, if used other than as an induction agent, additional analgesia, such as fentanyl, is required. Muscle relaxation is poor, possibly partly the effect of increased $PaCO_2$ through respiratory depression. Shivering is common in all species of animal in the recovery period and may be due to persistent cutaneous vasodilation in a cold environment.

The only absolute contraindication to the use of thiopental as an induction agent is porphyria, a disease characterized by progressive acute demyelination of nerves, that is well documented in humans. Porphyria is very rare but has been diagnosed in cattle, pigs and cats (Tobias, 1964). Partial contraindications for thiopental include neonates, caesarean section with a live fetus, very thin animals, uraemia, untreated hypovolaemia and hypoproteinaemia. In small animals, there are several agents available which are preferable to thiopental for longer periods of anaesthesia, although the drug can be useful for this purpose in small ruminants.

Thiopental's current limited availability relates to its replacement in human anaesthesia by propofol (see below) but, where available, it remains a useful agent in veterinary anaesthesia.

Methohexital

Methohexital sodium is a racemic mixture of the α-d and a-l isomers of sodium 5-allyl-1-methyl-5-(1-methyl-2-pentynyl) barbiturate, and differs from thiopental in having no sulphur in the molecule. It is supplied as a colourless solid and, when dissolved in water, forms a colourless solution which is stable for at least six weeks kept at room temperature.

Methohexital is approximately twice as potent as thiopental, and it is less irritant if accidentally given outside the vein. As for thiopental, when given by rapid IV injection, it rapidly crosses the blood–brain barrier and causes anaesthesia in a circulation time. As for thiopental, initial lowering of plasma levels and awakening is due to redistribution, but it differs from thiopental in that metabolism is much faster, is relatively non-cumulative and complete recovery is rapid, seldom exceeding 30 minutes even after prolonged infusion. Hepatic metabolism breaks methohexital down to non-active metabolites which are rapidly excreted. Cardiorespiratory actions and lack of analgesia are similar to those of thiopental. Sedative premedication avoids muscle tremors during the induction of and recovery from anaesthesia. Suitable doses will be discussed in the relevant species chapters.

Methohexital has been superseded by propofol for most indications but, where it is still available, it can prove a useful agent both for anaesthetic induction and for the maintenance of hypnosis.

Pentobarbital sodium

Pentobarbital sodium in the form of a racemic mixture of sodium 5-ethyl-5-(1-methylbutyl) barbiturate is marketed as a sterile 6.5% solution containing propylene glycol. Pentobarbital has been, and in some areas still is, used to provide total injectable anaesthesia. It is relatively non-irritant and, although the best results are obtained with IV administration, it has been used by intraperitoneal injection in laboratory animals. In humans, it can be used for sedation by the oral or rectal routes. When given IV, it is slow to cross the blood–brain barrier, so anaesthetic induction is slow. The usual mode of administration is to give two-thirds the calculated dose rapidly, so that there is not an excitement phase on induction (one of its isomers has an excitatory effect). Following induction, the anaesthetist must wait some time (a minute or more) to ensure full effect before giving the next increment, or overdose may occur. Doses in unpremedicated dogs and cats to give anaesthesia long enough for 30 minutes of surgery (with additional analgesia) are up to 30 mg/kg IV. Full recovery is accompanied by excitement and, in dogs, vocalization, and takes up to 24 hours. Premedication reduces the dose needed, reduces the chance of excitement at induction or recovery, and speeds recovery. Use of the intraperitoneal route, which is not recommended, often results in a major excitement reaction during the induction period.

The side effects of pentobarbital anaesthesia are as of thiopental; dose dependent respiratory depression, hypotension, and myocardial depression although, at minimally effective dose rates, an increased pulse rate may sustain cardiac output. Analgesia is very poor. Contraindications and partial contraindications are as for thiopental.

As for thiopental, pentobarbital appears to be metabolized more rapidly in horses, sheep and goats than in pigs, dogs and cats, although the authors have been unable to locate evidence to confirm this. Pentobarbital is used to control seizures (e.g. caused by poisons of unknown origins). It is used also in very concentrated forms for euthanasia. The euthanasia solutions contain preservatives and must not be used for anaesthesia, even in large animals. Many of the euthanasia solutions (e.g. Somulose®) are combined with an agent to stop the heart. They should be given very slowly to ensure that the pentobarbital has time to cross the blood–brain barrier and induce anaesthesia before cardiac arrest occurs. In pregnant animals, anaesthesia prior to administration of such euthanasia solutions is preferable to ensure that the fetus is anaesthetized prior to the cardiac arrest in the dam, as it is probable that transport of pentobarbital across the placenta is slow.

Other barbiturates

Thiamylal sodium

Thiamylal closely resembles thiopental in chemical structure except that while the latter is the ethyl derivative of the series, the former is the allyl compound. It is also similar to thiopental in its actions as an anaesthetic. It is no longer available.

Phenols

Propofol

The active ingredient of propofol, 2,6 di-isopropylphenol (Fig 6.1), exists as an oil at room temperatures. Propofol is presented for anaesthetic use as a free flowing oil-in-water milk-coloured macro-emulsion, the original format (Diprivan®) containing 1% w/v soya bean oil, 1.2% w/v purified egg phosphatide and 2.25% w/v glycerol (see 'Formulation' above). Contamination of syringes of propofol was implicated in a high incidence of postoperative infection (Bennett et al., 1995) and so some preparations now contain preservatives. The first clinical trials of propofol were reported for humans in 1977, for dogs in 1984 (Hall, 1984) and 1987 (Watkins et al., 1987) and for cats in 1988 (Brearley et al., 1988). Since this time, propofol has become the IV induction agent most widely used in human anaesthesia, as well as being used for TIVA and for sedation in intensive care.

Propofol is licensed for IV use as an anaesthetic agent in humans, cats and dogs. There is occasionally pain on injection. Although propofol is non-irritant, it can only be used IV as its elimination is too rapid for use by other routes. A number of generic versions of propofol are available. Currently (2012) in the USA and in Europe, there are two formats with veterinary licences. Propoflo® is similar to the original, and vials are for single use only. Propofol™ Plus (PropoFlo™28) contains benzyl alcohol as preservative, and its multidose bottles may be used for up to 28 days after the vial is first broached. PropoClear™ was a formulation as a micelle but, unfortunately, in clinical use, it proved painful on injection (Michou et al., 2012) and possibly caused local tissue damage and has been withdrawn.

Following IV injection of propofol, hypnosis is induced in a circulation time with anaesthetic depth reaching maximal after around 90 seconds (Reves et al., 2012). Recovery is extremely rapid and complete. The initial recovery from a bolus injection is through redistribution, as is thiopental. Also, as for thiopental, propofol is highly protein bound. The difference between the two agents is that the clearance of propofol as it is released from these tissues is very rapid (see Table 6.1), so residual sedation is not seen. Propofol is highly lipophilic and rapidly metabolized primarily to inactive glucuronide conjugates, involving cytochrome P450 systems, the metabolites being excreted in the urine. However, clearance can be greater than liver blood flow, and extrahepatic mechanisms (e.g. lung and kidney) are thought to contribute.

Pharmacokinetic studies in animals have shown species, breed and individual variations, and also variations depending on other anaesthetic and sedative agents given, in speed of elimination of propofol. In dogs, half-life of elimination, depending on other drugs administered, has been reported as between 75 and 486 minutes, volume of distribution as from 3.7 to 6.5 L/kg and clearance as between 34 and 58 mL/kg/minute (Nolan et al., 1993; Reid & Nolan, 1993, 1996; Zoran et al., 1993; Hall et al., 1994; Hughes & Nolan, 1999); the values of clearance and volume of distribution being considerably higher than the human values (see Table 6.1). Zoran et al. (1993) compared the pharmacokinetics of propofol in greyhounds with mixed breed dogs; half-life of elimination

Table 6.2 Mean utilization rate of propofol	
Species	**Mean utilization rate (mg/kg/min)**
Mouse	2.22
Rabbit	1.55
Rat	0.61
Pig	0.28
Cat	0.19
Data supplied to L Hall by JB Glen	

was longer (175 minutes cf 122 minutes) and clearance less (54 cf 115 mL/kg/minute) in greyhounds. *In vitro* studies have shown breed and gender differences in metabolic utilization of propofol (Hay Kraus et al., 2000) and also suggest that the canine kidney (in contrast to humans) does not metabolize the drug (Soars et al., 2001). In the goat, half-life of elimination is very rapid (15 minutes) and clearance very high (275 mL/kg/minute) (Rigby-Jones et al., 2002).

The cat, however, because of its inability to conjugate phenols, metabolizes both propofol and the lipid solvent more slowly than other carnivores. Table 6.2 gives data from the original developmental work (JB Glen, personal communication to LWH), and demonstrates that the utilization of propofol is very slow in cats. Very recent, as yet unpublished (2012) work has investigated the pharmacokinetics of a single dose of 8 mg/kg propofol in the cat. Early analysis of the results (a one compartmental model) suggests that the volume of distribution is 14 ± 6 L/kg; the half-life of elimination 5.9 ± 3.6 hours, and the clearance 115 ± 45 mL/kg/minute (Khursheed Mama, also on behalf of colleagues, personal communication to KC, October 2012).

In cats, considerable first pass extraction of propofol occurs in the lung (Matot et al., 1993), but it is uncertain whether all of the drug is released back into the circulation or is metabolized in the pulmonary tissue.

Propofol causes dose-dependent respiratory and cardiovascular depression, equivalent to that resulting from thiopental injection. As such, it is not safer than thiopental (as has been claimed) but has the advantage of the rapid recovery of consciousness. Heart rate changes with propofol vary. Propofol is a very poor analgesic and, if used for surgery, additional analgesia is required. Details of early pharmacological studies performed in rabbits, cats, pigs and monkeys (Glen, 1980; Glen & Hunter, 1984) showed that propofol is compatible with a wide range of drugs used for premedication, inhalation anaesthesia and neuromuscular block. It lacks any central anticholinergic effect, is not potentiated by other non-anaesthetic drugs,

does not affect bronchomotor tone or gastrointestinal motility, and decreases the risk for catecholamine-induced cardiac arrhythmias. None of the hundreds of clinical and scientific studies carried out since has negated these original findings. Propofol does not trigger malignant hyperthermia in susceptible pigs (Raff & Harrison, 1989).

The pharmacokinetics of propofol make it the ideal agent for use as TIVA and, in human anaesthesia, it is used widely in this manner in combination with infusions of potent opioids, such as fentanyl or remifentanil, to provide the necessary analgesia (see Chapter 3). The respiratory depressant effects of these combinations mean that IPPV is essential. Similar opioid combinations are used in dogs (Andreoni & Hughes, 2009); in horses, ketamine or α_2-agonists are used to provide analgesia with propofol infusions (Nolan et al., 1996; Bettschart-Wolfensberger et al., 2001). In humans, low dose propofol infusion is used for prolonged sedation for intensive (critical) care. Some unexpected deaths in children on this regimen led to the contraindication of prolonged propofol for paediatric use, but it is now realized that the *propofol infusion syndrome* (PRIS) is not limited to this age group. PRIS is defined as the occurrence of bradycardia resistant to treatment, together with lipaemic plasma, metabolic acidosis and often rhabdomyolysis (Fudickar & Bein, 2009). PRIS is usually fatal. Its aetiology is not fully understood.

Propofol is now accepted as a most useful agent in all domestic animals (Short & Bufalari, 1999), although volume and cost limit use in large animals. The dose for induction of anaesthesia in unpremedicated dogs is around 6 mg/kg; recovery from this is complete (awake, walking, no ataxia) in around 20 minutes. Premedication reduces this dose depending on degree of sedation; for example 0.02–0.04 mg/kg of acepromazine reduces the necessary propofol dose by about 30%. Premedication with 10 or 20 µg/kg of medetomidine decreases the anaesthetic induction dose in dogs to about 5 mg/kg and 3 mg/kg respectively (Hall et al., 1994, 1997). There is a suggestion that some families of Boxer dogs may be more susceptible to propofol since recovery was prolonged in some related animals of this breed (Hall & Chambers, 1987). In dogs, excitatory phenomena, mainly muscle twitching, extensor rigidity and opisthotonus, occur occasionally associated with the use of propofol (Davies & Hall, 1991).

In unpremedicated cats, the IV dose for induction is around 8 mg/kg, recovery after this single dose is less rapid – presumably because of relative inability to conjugate phenols. In cats, the incidence of postanaesthetic side effects such as vomiting/retching and sneezing or pawing at the mouth is about 15%, but this can be reduced by acepromazine premedication (Brearley et al., 1988). Propofol, however, is cumulative in cats. Pascoe et al. (2006) showed that while complete recovery (walking without ataxia) was similar to that in dogs (means of 74–80 minutes) after just induction or a 30-minute infusion of propofol, if infusion continued for 150 minutes, recovery was significantly delayed to 148 minutes. Of more concern is the report from Andress et al. (1995) where cats received daily administration of a 30-minute propofol infusion. Recovery time increased significantly after the second day. On the basis of pre-set criteria, no cat completed the intended 10-day trial. Haematology showed an increase in Heinz bodies but, more importantly, the cats had stopped eating, had diarrhoea, general malaise and two had facial oedema. Whether these toxic signs relate to the propofol or the lipid, and whether there is any relation to PRIS is not known. Bley et al. (2007) used propofol infusions of 5–20 minutes twice daily for 5 days for radiotherapy in cats and did not note clinically serious adverse effects. Nevertheless, there are other agents suitable for anaesthesia in cats (see Chapter 16), and these authors would not recommend use of daily infusions of propofol in cats unless no other regimen is available.

Propofol has been used for anaesthesia in many species of animal, both as an induction agent and for TIVA. Suitable dosage regimens will be discussed in the relevant species chapters.

Fospropofol

Fospropofol (phosphono-O-methyl-2,6-diisopropyl-phenol,disodium salt) is a water-soluble prodrug of propofol (see Fig 6.1). It is broken down by endothelial alkaline phosphatases to propofol, formaldehyde and phosphate (Fechner et al., 2008). It has been developed, and is licensed in some countries, for sedation for surgical procedures and in intensive care, the rationale being that, by avoiding a lipid 'carrier', propofol infusion syndrome might be avoided.

There is now quite considerable experience with the use of fospropofol in humans for sedation. As a prodrug, induction of sedation from a single bolus dose (6.5 mg/kg) takes 4–8 minutes (Bengalorkar et al., 2011). Reported side effects at induction are paraesthesia and pruritus but not pain on injection. Monitoring as for anaesthesia is considered as mandatory. Duration from a single dose is a little longer than that of propofol. Side effects reported at recovery are similar to those seen after propofol infusion (Candiotti et al., 2011).

A study in rabbits (Li et al., 2012) compared the pharmacokinetics of prolonged infusion (2, 4, 6 or 8 hours) of propofol (emulsion formulation) and fospropofol. Minimal infusion rate (MIR) ranged from 0.75 to 1.08 mg/kg/minute for propofol and 1.8–2.4 mg/kg /minute for fospropofol. Induction was smooth in both cases; time to loss of righting reflex was 6–8 minutes for propofol and 17–19 minutes for fospropofol. Recovery times increased with increasing length of infusion; after 2, 4, 6 and 8 hours being 10,19, 36 and 48 minutes for propofol, and 15, 26, 52 and 84 minutes for fospropofol. These times demonstrate the context sensitive recovery time of both propofol and fospropofol. Of concern, one rabbit in the 8-hour fospropofol group died during the recovery phase. Rabbits received oxygen supplementation, breathed spontaneously and, although respiratory rate was reduced, SpO_2 never fell below 90%.

The place of fospropofol in veterinary medicine has yet to be elucidated. In humans, there is concern that formate accumulation following fospropofol could be toxic, although there are no such reports to date. There are no publications concerning fospropofol or its metabolites in cats. However, there is a need for long-term sedation for intensive care in animals, and fospropofol may prove useful for this purpose.

Steroid anaesthesia

A number of neurosteroid compounds have been investigated as hypnotics in humans, although currently none remain in clinical use. Hydroxydione (Anderson, 1956) was slow to take effect and very irritant to the veins; others which at least reached clinical trial include minaxolone, eltanalone, and pregnanolone (Kumar et al., 1993; Sear, 1996, 1998). Alfaxalone (alphaxalone) has always been

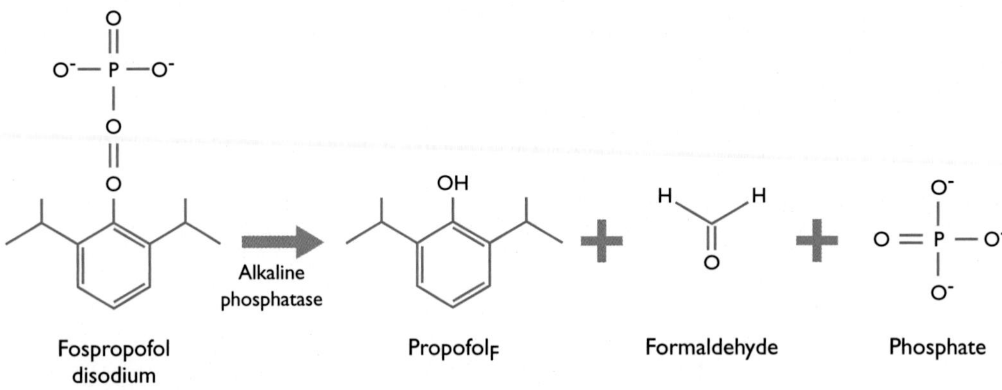

Fospropofol
disodium

Alkaline
phosphatase

Propofol$_F$

Formaldehyde

Phosphate

Figure 6.1 Chemical structure of fospropofol disodium and the scheme of its enzymolysis to propofol$_F$.

one the most promising steroids, but is virtually insoluble in water. However, in combination with another weakly hypnotic steroid, alphadolone, it was dissolved in cremophor EL, and the combination marketed as 'Althesin®' in human anaesthesia and as 'Saffan®' for use in cats. Althesin was withdrawn from medical clinical use in 1984, because of concerns of reaction to the cremophor, but Saffan remained available in veterinary practice until the advent of the alfaxalone in cyclodextrins, discussed in detail below.

Saffan contained 9 mg of alfaxalone and 3 mg of alphadolone per mL, and therefore most studies, referenced in previous editions of this book, expressed the dose in terms of total steroid. Saffan was non-irritant, and was licensed for use in cats by either IV or IM injection. It was non-cumulative and was used to extend anaesthesia without unduly lengthening recovery times. Its specific advantage was that, in cats, it was not very respiratory depressant and could be given at a single dose that was sufficient to enable the surgery of ovariohysterectomy. Analgesia, judged lack of movement or cardiovascular responses to surgery, appeared adequate. Interestingly, a study suggested that alfaxalone was responsible for the hypnotic effect but alphadolone for the antinociception (Nadeson & Goodchild, 2000); if this is so, the current formulation of alfaxalone may not provide such good surgical conditions. Following Saffan injection, blood pressure fell through vasodilation. Cardiac index was well maintained (Dyson et al., 1987). Saffan's disadvantages were a 'twitchy' recovery (it was essential to keep the cats in a quiet environment) with face-rubbing, paddling, and even opisthotonus. Reactions to the cremophor manifest by swollen paws, ears, larynx and occasionally pulmonary oedema. Despite these side effects, which did lead directly to the death of some cats, the overall death rate in practice in cats anaesthetized with Saffan was considerably less than with other methods of anaesthesia employed (Clarke & Hall, 1990), presumably due to the limited degree of cardiac depression when compared to other agents.

Saffan was licensed only for cats. Dogs were specifically contraindicated because of their sensitivity to histamine release in response to the cremophor, although there were reports of its use in this species in combination with antihistamine agents. However, Saffan was used satisfactorily in a very wide range of domestic and exotic species, the main limitation being size in relation to volume of the drug combination.

Alfaxalone

Alfaxalone, solubilized in 2-hydroxypropyl β-cyclodextrin (Alfaxan®; henceforth termed alfaxalone) has been developed, initially in Australia by Jurox Pty Ltd, and (2012) is licensed as an anaesthetic drug for use in cats and dogs in Australia, New Zealand, South Africa and Europe. It is presented as an aqueous solution of 10 mg/mL, in bottles.

There is no preservative, and it is recommended that an opened bottle vial be used within a day.

Alfaxalone is relatively short acting, non-irritant and is non-cumulative, making it suitable both for IV induction of anaesthesia and TIVA by bolus injection or by infusion. The dose recommended by Jurox for induction of anaesthesia in non-premedicated dogs is 2 mg/kg IV given slowly over 60 seconds, although the current European data sheet suggests that up to 3 mg/kg might be needed on occasions. In premedicated dogs, reduced doses are used depending on the degree of sedation. For maintenance of anaesthesia, recommended doses are, in non-premedicated dogs, 0.13–0.16 mg/kg/minute or boluses of 1.3–1.5 mg/kg and, in premedicated dogs, 0.1–0.12 mg/kg/minute or boluses of 1–1.2 mg/kg. Cats appear to need higher doses, 5 mg/kg, again given slowly IV, being recommended for induction of anaesthesia. Suggested doses for maintenance in cats are, for non-premedicated 0.16–0.18 mg/kg/minute or boluses of 1.6– 1.8 mg/kg and for premedicated cats, 1.1–1.3 mg/kg/minute or boluses of 1.1–1.3 mg/kg. There appear no contraindications to use of alfaxalone with any of the usually used premedicant sedative, analgesic or anticholinergic agents, but administration together with other injectable anaesthetic agents is specifically contraindicated. Some of the experimental work supporting these claims has yet (2012) to be published in peer-reviewed journals but abstracts of presentations are available (www.Alfaxan.co.uk).

Alfaxalone is rapidly metabolized in the liver. The pharmacokinetics in dogs have been investigated (Ferre et al., 2006) at both the usual IV induction dose (2 mg/kg) and at a supramaximal dose (10 mg/kg). At 2 mg/kg and 10 mg/kg respectively, the mean duration of anaesthesia until the dog responded to the presence of an endotracheal tube was 6.4 and 26.2 minutes; plasma clearance 59.4 and 52.9 mL/kg/minute, plasma terminal half-life ($t_{1/2}$) 24.0 and 37.4 minutes, and for both, volume of distribution between 2 and 3 L/kg. The authors concluded there was no clinically significant difference in pharmacokinetic parameters between the doses. In greyhounds (Pasloske et al., 2009), following 2 mg/kg alfaxalone IV, $t_{1/2}$ was 34.3 minutes and plasma clearance 48.4 mL/kg/minute, suggesting alfaxalone is slightly longer acting in this breed, but the difference is unlikely to be of major clinical significance. A similar study in cats (Whittem et al., 2008) examined the pharmacokinetics of 5 mg/kg and 25 mg/kg IV; results for these two doses were, respectively; plasma clearance 25.1 and 14.8 mL/kg/minute and $t_{1/2}$ 45.2 and 76.6 minutes. The cat study also investigated continuing anaesthesia by four incremental doses; the duration of subsequent anaesthesia resulting from each increment did not change, suggesting that at least over this dosage schedule there were no clinically evident cumulative effects.

Safety studies, giving the intended dose, and three and ten times its multiple in both dogs and cats have been published (Muir et al., 2008, 2009). In dogs, this dosing schedule was 0 (placebo), 2, 6 and 20 mg/kg; in cats 0, 5, 15 and 50 mg/kg of alfaxalone. Rescue IPPV was allowed if necessary.

In dogs, induction of anaesthesia was smooth and rapid; for 2, 6 and 20 mg/kg respectively, the duration of lack of response to noxious stimuli was 9.3, 32 and 69.7 minutes and duration of anaesthesia (to extubation) 9.8, 31.4 and 75.1 minutes. Quality of anaesthesia appeared excellent and, from the results, antinociception appeared to last throughout the whole period. Recovery was not described, but scores did not differ between doses. Alfaxalone caused an increase in heart rate, and a fall in arterial blood pressure, cardiac output and systemic vascular resistance, but the changes were minimal except at 20 mg/kg and, even at this dose, were clinically acceptable. Respiratory depression occurred at all doses; apnoea was common particularly at the higher doses.

In cats, induction of anaesthesia was smooth and rapid; for 5, 15 and 50 mg/kg respectively, the duration of lack of response to noxious stimuli was 15.3, 48.4 and 143.7 minutes and duration of anaesthesia 26, 75.4 and 172 minutes. Thus, in contrast to dogs, antinociception did not appear to last for the whole period of anaesthesia. Recovery quality was scored as excellent after doses of 5 and 15 mg/kg, but 5 hours after receiving 50 mg/kg, five (of eight) cats had not fully recovered and were euthanized. Alfaxalone caused a dose dependent fall in heart rate, arterial blood pressure, cardiac output and systemic vascular resistance, but the changes at 5 and 15 mg/kg were rarely statistically and unlikely to be clinically significant. At 50 mg/kg (i.e. a 10× overdose), cardiovascular depression was very marked. Apnoea was common at all doses. Even at 5 mg/kg, PaO_2 fell and 5/8 cats required IPPV at some period; by 15 mg/kg all cats received IPPV. In summary, in cats, doses of up to 15 mg/kg produced minimal or clinically acceptable cardiovascular changes, but respiratory depression was a potential problem even at 5 mg/kg. The dose of 50 mg/kg was obviously an unacceptably high overdose but, even then, no cat died at the time of drug administration.

The peer-reviewed publication of the pharmacokinetic and safety studies described above demonstrate that IV alfaxalone produces good quality anaesthesia in dogs and cats, is non-cumulative, at clinically applicable doses cardiovascular effects are minimal but (in contrast to Saffan in cats), dose-dependent apnoea and respiratory depression may occur. In clinical practice, however, it is usual to use ancillary sedative and analgesic agents. There are now a number of publications, both clinical and experimental, investigating such combinations for induction of anaesthesia, and often comparing alfaxalone with other anaesthetic regimens. In dogs, alfaxalone did not cause pain on injection (Michou et al., 2012). To compare the incidence of apnoea induced by alfaxalone or propofol in dogs

(Keates & Whittem, 2012), a dose-escalation study found the median dose of alfaxalone which induced apnoea was 10 mg/kg (i.e. 5× recommended doses) and for propofol was 13 mg/kg (i.e. twice the normal induction dose). Amengual et al. (2013), however, found that, in premedicated dogs, the incidence of post-induction apnoea was high (around 50%) with either alfaxalone (1.5 mg/kg) or propofol (3 g/kg) given by fast IV injection, reinforcing the data sheet advice for Alfaxan® that it should be given slowly. An experimental study in non-premedicated dogs (Rodriguez et al., 2012), compared the cardiorespiratory effects of a mean of 4.15 mg/kg alfaxalone (i.e. above the recommended dose) with a mean of 2.91 mg/kg etomidate; at these doses alfaxalone increased (statistically but not clinically significantly) heart rate and cardiac index, with a non-significant fall in arterial blood pressure and systemic vascular resistance. Quality of induction and recovery were better than those of etomidate. Maddern et al. (2010) showed that, in dogs, the mean dose of alfaxalone needed for anaesthetic induction was 1.2 mg/kg after premedication with medetomidine 4 µg/kg or butorphanol 0.1 mg/kg but, in dogs receiving both premedicants, the alfaxalone dose was significantly reduced to 0.8 mg/kg. Psatha et al. (2011) compared the use of alfaxalone to a diazepam/ketamine/propofol combination for methadone-premedicated dogs in ASA grade 3 or worse; they found that 1–2 mg/kg alfaxalone gave satisfactory induction of anaesthesia, systolic arterial blood pressure did not fall from pre-induction values and that cardiovascular parameters throughout the subsequent gaseous maintenance of anaesthesia did not differ between treatments. Alfaxalone can be used satisfactorily for induction of anaesthesia in premedicated (acepromazine, morphine and atropine) puppies aged 6–12 weeks (O'Hagan et al., 2012a); dose rates were similar to those seen in adult dogs.

In cats premedicated with acepromazine and meloxicam, mean doses of alfaxalone required for induction of anaesthesia and endotracheal intubation were 4.7 mg/kg (Taboada & Murison, 2010). In young cats (>12 months), the mean dose needed to induce anaesthesia in non-premedicated cats was 4.2 mg/kg but, in cats premedicated with acepromazine and butorphanol, was 2.7 mg/kg (Zaki et al., 2009). Recovery quality was better in premedicated cats. O'Hagan et al. (2012b) found that the mean dose of alfaxalone required for induction for endotracheal intubation in heavily premedicated kittens (acepromazine, morphine and atropine) under 12 weeks of age was 4.7 mg/kg.

The studies described above all support the information supplied by the manufacturers that IV alfaxalone administered over a minute leads to a smooth induction of anaesthesia, cardiovascular changes are minimal (increased heart rate and sometimes a small fall in arterial blood pressure) even in dogs with a compromised circulation;

there may be transient apnoea but this is no more, and probably less, likely to occur than after propofol. However, in many of the above mentioned studies, although recovery was usually classified as excellent or acceptable, there is mention of occasional incidences of twitching and paddling in recovery, even following relatively prolonged anaesthesia with inhalant agents (Jimenez et al., 2012; Mathis et al., 2012).

Alfaxalone for TIVA is of particular interest as this was one of the major uses of Saffan in cats. In an experimental study in dogs sedated with acepromazine and hydromorphone, Ambros et al. (2008) compared alfaxalone and propofol for TIVA. Cardiovascular parameters (including cardiac output) did not differ between treatments. Respiratory depression was greater with propofol. Recovery times and quality did not differ between treatments. Two studies have examined alfaxalone TIVA for ovariohysterectomy in dogs, in each case the dogs received oxygen supplementation. Suarez et al. (2012) premedicated the bitches with acepromazine (0.01 mg/kg) and morphine (0.4 mg/kg) then used alfaxalone or propofol for induction and for maintenance of anaesthesia. Doses required for maintenance were 0.1–0.02 mg/kg/minute for alfaxalone and 0.3–0.5 mg/kg/minute for propofol. Both agents provided adequate anaesthesia for the purpose. There were no significant differences in cardiopulmonary parameters or recovery parameters between treatments, but both caused marked respiratory depression. Herbert et al. (2013) compared premedication with buprenorphine (0.02 mg/kg) and either acepromazine (0.05 mg/kg) or dexmedetomidine (approximately 0.01 mg/kg) prior to induction and TIVA with alfaxalone. Alfaxalone infusion rate was significantly lower after dexmedetomidine (median 0.08 range 0.06–0.19 mg/kg/minute) than after acepromazine (median 0.11 range 0.07–0.33). Beths et al. (2012) premedicated cats with medetomidine (0.02 mg/kg) and morphine (0.3–0.5 mg/kg); mean induction and infusion rates were 1.8 mg/kg and 0.18 mg/kg/minute and apnoea and hypoventilation were common. Quality of anaesthesia was better, but quality of recovery worse in the medetomidine group. In cats, alfaxalone as a total intravenous anaesthetic was used in eight very young (<12 weeks) premedicated kittens (O'Hagan et al., 2012b) to enable ovariohysterectomy; following induction dose the first increment was required at 5.5 minutes; bolus administrations to maintain anaesthesia amounted to 0.18 mg/kg/minute. Mean recovery time (in some cases after atipamezole) was 40 minutes. Apnoea did not occur. Noise induced twitching was noted in three of 37 cats. In all these studies, premedication used moderately high doses of opioid, and/or α_2-agonists; these were considered necessary to contribute to perioperative analgesia but may well have influenced both respiratory depression and time and quality of recovery. There is still need to elucidate the best combination with alfaxalone to enable surgery.

Alfaxalone has been used in rabbits, doses of 2–3 mg/kg IV providing satisfactory conditions for endotracheal intubation prior to administration of inhalation agents (Grint et al., 2008). Alfaxalone can be used by IM injection. Saffan was used by this route routinely in cats. For alfaxalone, it is probable that combinations with sedatives will be needed to ensure a practicable volume. Alfaxalone has already been used by a variety of routes in exotic animals. IM administration of 20 mg/kg to red-eared sliders (turtles) resulted in a smooth induction of sedation/anaesthesia of short duration (Kischinovsky et al., 2013). Alfaxalone by immersion followed by branchial/transcutaneous irrigation proved adequate for surgery on an axolotl (McMillan & Leece, 2011). In the green iguana, 10 mg/kg alfaxalone IM provides light sedation, 20 mg/kg short duration anaesthesia and 30 mg/kg anaesthesia for 40 minutes (Bertelsen & Sauer, 2011). Approximately 10 mg/kg IM in marmosets provides adequate sedation to allow mask induction or IV injection (Thomas et al., 2012). Combinations with medetomidine have been used IM to immobilize wallabies (Bouts et al., 2011). These early studies suggest that alfaxalone will have a major role to play in the immobilization of exotic animals.

In larger animals, IV alfaxalone, in combination with heavy sedation, has been used successfully to anaesthetize horses, both as an induction agent and as 'top ups' to enable castration (Leece et al., 2009; Kloppel & Leece, 2011; Keates et al., 2012). The pharmacokinetics have been investigated in adult horses and in foals (Goodwin et al., 2011, 2012). Alfaxalone has also been used in pigs (Keates, 2003) and sheep (Andaluz et al., 2012; Torres et al., 2012; Walsh et al., 2012), in all cases providing satisfactory short duration anaesthesia.

Alfaxalone in cyclodextrin has been available in veterinary practice in Australia for some years and, by August 2010 it was licensed in Australia, New Zealand, Thailand and in six European countries. Its use in small animals as an induction agent has become very popular; studies in use as TIVA are less well developed. Its potential for causing respiratory depression is accepted but, to date, there have been no published reports of any unexpected side effects. It is anticipated that this agent will prove very useful in small animal and other areas of veterinary anaesthetic practice.

Imidazole derivatives

Etomidate

Etomidate (R-1-(1-ethylphenyl)imidazole-5-ethyl ester) is an imidazole derivative that exists in a chiral form. The formulations for clinical use are the R (+) enantiomer (Forman, 2011). Currently, there are two commercial preparations available, one in propylene glycol, the other as a lipid, but formulations in cyclodextrins have also been developed. When injected into the bloodstream, etomidate becomes approximately 75% protein bound. It has a large volume of distribution both centrally and peripherally and so, as for thiopental, it quickly enters the brain and leaves rapidly as it becomes redistributed in the body. It is quickly hydrolysed by esterases in the liver and plasma to pharmacologically inert metabolites. The clearance is 15–20 mL/kg/minute and the context sensitive half-life in humans is shorter than that of propofol. The pharmacokinetics of etomidate in cats have been investigated (Wertz et al., 1990) and are best described by a three-compartment open model similar to those determined in people.

In effective doses, etomidate causes loss of consciousness in one injection site–brain circulation time. There may be some pain on injection. In dogs, doses of 1.5–3 mg/kg produce hypnosis, in a dose dependent manner, lasting from 10 to 20 minutes. Intravenous injection is associated with a high incidence of involuntary muscle movement, tremor and hypertonus, although these can be reduced by sedative premedication. The EEG changes produced by etomidate at induction are similar to those seen with barbiturates and no specific epileptogenic or convulsive activity is observed, so the muscle movements cannot be attributed to central nervous activity. Lack of cardiovascular depression is the outstanding feature of etomidate; there is minimal effect on cardiac function. The drug does release significant amounts of histamine and there is a very low incidence of thrombosis after injection.

In 1983, Ledingham & Watt reported an increase in mortality among human intensive care patients receiving prolonged etomidate infusion. This led to the realization that the drug inhibits increases in plasma cortisol and aldosterone concentrations during surgical stress, even when adrenocorticotropic hormone levels are normal or increased. As a result, in human anaesthesia and sedation, etomidate is no longer used for infusions. The safety or otherwise of etomidate as an IV induction agent in patients in shock has been debated frequently (Flynn & Shehabi, 2012), but its lack of cardiovascular effects ensures that it remains in use as an anaesthetic induction agent.

Etomidate is used quite widely for induction of anaesthesia in cats and dogs (see Chapters 15 and 16), in particular in animals with cardiovascular compromise. In normal dogs, induction doses of 3 mg/kg caused no significant changes in blood pressure, cardiac output or heart rate (Rodriguez et al., 2012). Following premedication with midazolam, 4 mg/kg etomidate had less effect on blood pressure than did 8 mg/kg propofol (Sams et al., 2008). In studies in models of hypovolaemia (induced by haemorrhage), etomidate had minimal cardiovascular effects in dogs (Pascoe et al., 1992) and in swine (Johnson et al., 2003). In canine surgical patients, adrenocortical function is suppressed for 2–6 hours after 2 mg/kg IV etomidate (Kruse-Elliott et al., 1987; Dodam et al., 1990), but that suppression is not total.

Etomidate has been used in other species, being most useful in pigs (Clutton et al., 1997), although volumes required are large. Volume and the tendency for myoclonic episodes limit potential for use in large animals.

Metomidate

Metomidate, an imidazole derivative similar to etomidate, was marketed for use, in combination with the butyrophenone, azaperone, as a hypnotic in pigs. Anaesthetic properties are very similar to those of etomidate, minimal cardiac depression, and very poor (or non-existent) analgesia. At the doses used, duration of action is longer than that of etomidate. Metomidate has also been given by intraperitoneal injection at the same time as an intramuscular injection of azaperone but the results were unpredictable. Although introduced as a hypnotic for pigs, it has also been used for restraint for a variety of species of birds (Cooper, 1974). Metomidate is no longer available commercially.

New etomidate derivatives

The desire to find an IV hypnotic agent with the cardiovascular sparing and pharmacokinetic advantages of etomidate, but which does not result in adrenocortical suppression has led to the synthesis of a number of etomidate derivatives; an example of how knowledge of structure in relation to function has led to 'designer' drugs (Sneyd & Rigby-Jones, 2010). Those that appear furthest in development include methyoxycarbonyl-etomidate (MOC-etomidate), carboetomidate and methoxycarbonyl-carboetomidate (Sneyd & Rigby-Jones, 2010; Forman, 2011; Pejo et al., 2012a,b,c; Sneyd, 2012). MOC-etomidate is an exceptionally short-acting hypnotic that is metabolized by non-specific plasma esterases; it still depresses adrenocortical function, but for a much shorter time than does etomidate. Carboetomidate has been designed (by removal of a binding nitrogen atom from etomidate) not to inhibit adrenocortical function, but is metabolized a little slower. Pejo et al. (2012a) explain how they hypothesized that by incorporating MOC-etomidate's labile ester into etomidate, they might obtain the best qualities of both the etomidate derivatives – rapid elimination with no inhibition of adrenocortical function; methoxycarbonyl-carboetomidate is the result.

Eugenols

The eugenols are related to oil of cloves. A eugenol, propanidid (Epontol), became available in the UK in 1967. Epontol was found to produce profound hypotension, probably because propanidid was dissolved in cremophor EL. Recently, a new eugenol agent, AZD3043, has undergone trials in humans (Sneyd, 2012). Clove oil is used widely as an anaesthetic in fish, although it has proved lethal in cane toads (Hernandez et al., 2012).

DRUGS ACTING PRIMARILY AT THE NMDA RECEPTOR

Dissociative agents

Three cyclohexylamine derivatives, phencyclidine (no longer in regular use), ketamine and tiletamine, have been used to produce 'anaesthesia'. The type of anaesthesia they produce differs markedly from that produced by the agents discussed above and they have been described as having cataleptic, analgesic and anaesthetic action, but no hypnotic properties. Catalepsy is defined as a characteristic akinetic state with loss of orthostatic reflexes but without impairment of consciousness in which the extremities appear to be paralysed by motor and sensory failure. Another definition of the state produced by these agents is 'dissociative anaesthesia' which is characterized by complete analgesia combined with only superficial sleep. In humans, hallucinations and emergence delirium phenomena are known to occur, and, although it cannot be established whether similar phenomena are experienced by animals, behaviour suggests that it might be so. Spontaneous involuntary muscle movement and hypertonus are not uncommon during induction and purposeless tonic–clonic movements of the extremities may be mistaken to indicate an inadequate level of anaesthesia and, unless this possibility is recognized, overdoses may be given. Animals may remain with their eyes open and have a good tone in the jaw muscles with active laryngeal and pharyngeal reflexes, while analgesia is excellent. In practice, these agents are usually used in combination with sedatives, which reduce or prevent the hallucinatory side effects and improve muscle relaxation.

It is now known that these three agents are antagonists at the NMDA receptor, and therefore have good analgesic properties, but they have no actions at the GABA receptor, hence their lack of the more usual form of hypnosis.

Ketamine

Ketamine is a dissociative anaesthetic agent that is used widely throughout veterinary anaesthesia, in combination with a variety of sedative agents. When used alone, anaesthesia is as described above. Its use in human anaesthesia has been limited by the hallucinatory effects, but it is being 'rediscovered' for anaesthesia on the battlefield (Mercer, 2009), as an analgesic and for a variety of other uses including as an antidepressant.

Veterinary preparations currently available in the UK contain racemic ketamine hydrochloride, 100 mg/mL, as a colourless aqueous solution with benzethonium chloride 0.01% as a preservative and, in some preparations, EDTA as an antioxidant. Medical preparations include less concentrated solutions, preservative free solutions, and the S (+)-ketamine isomer. Ketamine is non-irritant, and can be given by almost any route including IV, IM, SC, transmucous membrane, and transdermal. Veterinary preparations do cause pain on IM or SC injection.

Protein binding of ketamine has been reported in humans as 60-64% (Hijazi & Boulieu, 2002) and in dogs and horses, as approximately 50% (Kaka et al., 1979; Kaka & Hayton, 1980). This is considerably less than that of thiopental or propofol, making ketamine a drug of choice for hypoproteinaemic patients such as those with burns or with acute blood loss. Following IV injection of ketamine, anaesthesia does not occur in a circulation time; there is a short delay (of seconds not minutes). Ketamine is then distributed rapidly, and initial recovery is through redistribution. Elimination half-life is also relatively fast, 58–70 minutes being reported in dogs, cats and horses (Baggot & Blake, 1976; Waterman et al., 1987; Pypendop & Ilkiw, 2005). Ketamine metabolism is by hydroxylation and conjugation, but one of the metabolites, norketamine, is also active, and is probably partly responsible for prolonged behavioural effects. Certainly, infusions of ketamine in horses can have a clinical cumulative effect in relation to duration of side effects (Bettschart-Wolfensberger et al., 1996), although pharmacokinetics of infusions do not suggest that this should be so (Lankveld et al., 2006). Bioavailability of IM injection is from 50 to 90% bioavailable and plasma levels rise very quickly (Baggot & Blake, 1976; Hanna et al., 1988). In recent years, there have been many studies looking at the potential advantages of S (+)-ketamine, these being higher potency and faster elimination. However, a number of veterinary studies have failed to find any clinically significant difference between use of the S (+)-enantiomer or the racemate (Jud et al., 2010; Gerritsmann et al., 2012).

During ketamine anaesthesia, circulation is well maintained, mainly supported by sympathetic support as ketamine blocks the reuptake of norepinephrine by adrenergic nerve terminals. The direct effect of ketamine on isolated myocardium is complicated, having positive or negative inotropic actions depending on the experimental conditions (Hanouz et al., 2004; Jiang et al., 2011). Cardiac arrhythmias are uncommon under ketamine anaesthesia and the minimal arterial blood pressure is always similar to and rarely less than the preoperative level. At normal clinical doses, respiration is well maintained, but is depressed with overdosage. In cats overdosed with xylazine and ketamine, depression is sometimes manifest by rapid shallow breathing which can be misinterpreted, and apnoea follows. In veterinary anaesthesia, ketamine is combined with benzodiazepines and/or α_2-agonists in order to counteract the unwanted 'dissociative' side effects; cardiopulmonary depression may be considerably greater with these combinations than with ketamine alone. Similarly, control of the airway (usually retained with ketamine alone) is lost with the combinations.

The difficulty in assessing the depth of unconsciousness coupled with the poor muscle relaxation produced by ketamine make it doubtful that it should ever be used alone for anaesthesia for surgery. However, in combination, most effectively with α_2-agonists, the fact it can be administered by so many routes means that it has a wide range of veterinary uses. Ketamine combinations may be given IM at single doses adequate for surgical procedures and, as such, they are widely used in cats, laboratory animals, and by dart in wild animals. Ketamine can, however, be used in a more controllable manner, following premedication with the sedative, for IV anaesthetic induction and, if required, subsequent infusion to extend duration. There are very many possible anaesthetic combinations, and some suitable dose regimens will be given in the species chapters.

In veterinary anaesthesia, low dose ketamine infusions are being used for perioperative analgesia in dogs and horses (Wagner et al., 2002; Elfenbein et al., 2011), although experimental nociceptive testing does not always support the clinical belief that there is good postoperative analgesia (Bergadano et al., 2009). Ketamine (preservative free) has also been used by the epidural route as an analgesic (Robinson & Natalini, 2002; Hamilton et al., 2005; DeRossi et al., 2011). All authors consider that ketamine can only provide part of the multimodal postoperative anaesthetic regimen, and there is need for more objective assessment of its use in the postoperative period. However, although ketamine has been widely used for anaesthesia in animals over the years, it may be that, as in human medicine, new uses for this drug are now being developed in veterinary anaesthesia.

Tiletamine and Tiletamine–Zolazepam combination

Tiletamine hydrochloride is a dissociative agent similar to ketamine but at least twice as potent, and much longer lasting. Tiletamine is currently marketed in combination with the benzodiazepine agent, zolazepam ('Telazol®', 'Zoletil®') in many countries. This preparation is a 1:1 dry powder with a long shelf-life.

Lin et al. (1993) give an extensive review of the clinical pharmacology of tiletamine, of zolazepam and of the clinical use of the combination. Pharmacodynamics are very similar to those of ketamine, other than the longer duration of action. Tiletamine, as ketamine, may be administered by a wide number of different routes. Its plasma half-life in cats is 2–4 hours; that of zolazepam up to 5 hours. However, zolazepam has proved insufficient to remove the unwanted side effects of the dissociative drug; muscle rigidity is common and some seizure-like manifestations may be seen, so it is usual to administer Telzol®

together with an α_2-agonist or opioid. In domestic cats, the drug combination at clinical doses causes tachycardia with slight rises in blood pressure and cardiac output. Its use in non-domesticated cats has been well described by Lewis (1994). In dogs and horses, recovery is often violent, even with α_2-agonists, and ketamine is usually preferred. Telazol is particularly popular for use in wild animals as it can be made into highly concentrated solutions convenient for dart guns. Lin et al. (1993) give extensive documentation of doses which have been used, successfully or otherwise, in domestic, experimental and wild animals.

Miscellaneous agents

Some miscellaneous agents which still have animal use are mentioned briefly below.

Chloral hydrate

Chloral hydrate is a white, translucent, crystalline substance which volatilizes on exposure to air, producing a penetrating smell. It is not deliquescent, but it is readily soluble in water and aqueous solutions are generally stable. Solutions may be sterilized by boiling for a few minutes. Chloral hydrate is a prodrug; it is reduced to 2,2,2-trichloroethanol and its narcotic effect is generally attributed to this substance. When given by IV injection its effects are slow in appearing and this means that it is difficult to assess the degree of depression produced by a given dose as injection proceeds. Even following slow intravenous infusion of a dilute solution, narcosis continues to deepen for several minutes and additional doses should not be administered until it is clear that the maximum depth of depression from the initial dose has been reached. Perivascular injection causes severe tissue reaction, often followed by sloughing of the overlying tissues, but use of an intravenous catheter reduces the risk of this happening.

Chloral hydrate is not an anaesthetic. It has only very weak analgesic action. Hypnotic doses cause respiratory depression. At sedative, and even hypnotic doses cardiac function is well maintained, but large doses result in arterial hypotension. Death from chloral hydrate results as a result of respiratory depression. The drug was never used as an anaesthetic in dogs and cats but, formerly, it was used extensively in large animals, sometimes in combination with a barbiturate. Used as a sedative in horses, and anaesthesia induced with thiopental, the resultant period of anaesthesia was suitable for castrations and recovery occurred within the hour. Its action in cattle is similar to that in horses and recovery is quiet. It was often given, well diluted with water, by stomach tube into the rumen. It is still used occasionally as a sedative in cattle, but more recently introduced agents are more convenient to administer.

Chloralose

Chloralose is prepared by heating equal quantities of glucose and chloral hydrate under controlled conditions so that two isomers are produced. Only α-chloralose has narcotic properties; β-chloralose can produce muscular pain. α-Chloralose is available commercially as a white, crystalline powder and it is used as a 1% solution in water or saline. The solution is prepared fresh immediately before use by heating to 60°C. Heating above this temperature results in decomposition and precipitation occurs on standing. Chloralose is still extensively used in physiological and pharmacological non-survival experiments. Because large volumes of solution have to be given before consciousness is lost, anaesthesia is often induced with some other agent such as methohexital or, today, propofol.

An intravenous dose of 80–100 mg/kg of chloralose causes loss of consciousness but spontaneous muscular activity is common. The peak narcotic action of chloralose is seen some 15–20 minutes after injection. The arterial blood pressure is elevated and the activity of the autonomic nervous system is believed to be unaffected. The heart rate is often greatly increased and respiratory depression does not occur until very large doses are given. In the body, chloralose is broken down to chloral and glucose and the safety margin is relatively wide. Disadvantages are its relative insolubility, the long comparatively shallow depth of anaesthesia and the slow recovery accompanied by struggling. It has no place in veterinary practice but many experimentalists regard it as a valuable drug for maintenance of unconsciousness for long, non-survival experiments.

REFERENCES

Abass, B.T., Weaver, B.M., Staddon, G.E., et al., 1994. Pharmacokinetics of thiopentone in the horse. J Vet Pharmacol Ther 17, 331–338.

Alfaxan Research http://www.alfaxan.co.uk/Alfaxan_LearnMore/learn_AlfaxanResearch.html accessed 12/10/12.

Ambros, B., Duke-Novakovski, T., Pasloske, K.S., 2008. Comparison of the anesthetic efficacy and cardiopulmonary effects of continuous rate infusions of alfaxalone-2-hydroxypropyl-beta-cyclodextrin and propofol in dogs. Am J Vet Res 69, 1391–1398.

Amengual, M., Flaherty, D., Auckburally, A., et al., 2013. An evaluation of anaesthetic induction in healthy dogs using rapid intravenous injection of propofol or alfaxalone. Vet Anaesth Analg 40, 115–123.

Andaluz, A., Felez-Ocana, N., Santos, L., et al., 2012. The effects on cardio-respiratory and acid-base variables of the anaesthetic alfaxalone in a 2-hydroxypropyl-beta-cyclodextrin (HPCD) formulation in sheep. Vet J 191, 389–392.

Anderson, C.D., 1956. Hydroxydione sodium (viadril) for anesthesia; a report of clinical experience. Calif Med 85, 187–188.

Andreoni, V., Hughes, J.M., 2009. Propofol and fentanyl infusions in dogs of various breeds undergoing surgery. Vet Anaesth Analg 36, 523–531.

Andress, J.L., Day, T.K., Day, D., 1995. The effects of consecutive day propofol anesthesia on feline red blood cells. Vet Surg 24, 277–282.

Baggot, J.D., Blake, J.W., 1976. Disposition kinetics of ketamine in the domestic cat. Arch int Pharmacodynam Ther 220, 115–124.

Baker, M.T., Naguib, M., 2005. Propofol: the challenges of formulation. Anesthesiology 103, 860–876.

Bengalorkar, G.M., Bhuvana, K., Sarala, N., et al., 2011. Fospropofol: clinical pharmacology. J Anaesthesiol Clin Pharmacol 27, 79–83.

Bennett, S.N., McNeil, M.M., Bland, L.A., et al., 1995. Postoperative infections traced to contamination of an intravenous anesthetic, propofol. New Engl J Med 333, 147–154.

Bergadano, A., Andersen, O.K., Arendt-Nielsen, L., et al., 2009. Plasma levels of a low-dose constant-rate-infusion of ketamine and its effect on single and repeated nociceptive stimuli in conscious dogs. Vet J 182, 252–260.

Bertelsen, M.F., Sauer, C.D., 2011. Alfaxalone anaesthesia in the green iguana (Iguana iguana). Vet Anaesth Analg 38, 461–466.

Beths, T., Touzot-Jourde, T., Musk, G., et al., 2012. Total intravenous anaesthesia (TIVA) in cats. http://www.alfaxan.co.uk/Alfaxan_LearnMore/learn_AlfaxanResearch.html accessed 12/10/12.

Bettschart-Wolfensberger, R., Freeman, S.L., Jaggin-Schmucker, N., et al., 2001. Infusion of a combination of propofol and medetomidine for long-term anaesthesia in ponies. Am J Vet Res 62, 500–507.

Bettschart-Wolfensberger, R., Semder, A., Alibhai, H., et al., 2000. Cardiopulmonary side-effects and pharmacokinetics of an emulsion of propofol (Disoprivan) in comparison to propofol solved in polysorbate 80 in goats. J Vet Med A, Physiol Pathol Clin Med 47, 341–350.

Bettschart-Wolfensberger, R., Taylor, P.M., Sear, J.W., et al., 1996. Physiologic effects of anesthesia induced and maintained by intravenous administration of a climazolam-ketamine combination in ponies premedicated with acepromazine and xylazine. Am J Vet Res 57, 1472–1477.

Bley, C.R., Roos, M., Price, J., et al., 2007. Clinical assessment of repeated propofol-associated anesthesia in cats. J Am Vet Med Assoc 231, 1347–1353.

Bouts, T., Karunaratna, D., Berry, K., et al., 2011. Evaluation of medetomidine-alfaxalone and medetomidine-ketamine in semi-free ranging Bennett's wallabies (Macropus rufogriseus). J Zoo Wildlife Med 42, 617–622.

Brandon, R.A., Baggot, J.D., 1981. The pharmacokinetics of thiopentone. J Vet Pharmacol Ther 4, 79–85.

149

Brearley, J.C., Kellagher, R.E.B., Hall, L.W., 1988. Propofol anaesthesia in cats. J Small Anim Pract 29, 315–322.

Brown, E.N., Purdon, P.L., Van Dort, C.J., 2011. General anesthesia and altered states of arousal: a systems neuroscience analysis. Annu Rev Neurosci 34, 601–628.

Candiotti, K.A., Gan, T.J., Young, C., et al., 2011. A randomized, open-label study of the safety and tolerability of fospropofol for patients requiring intubation and mechanical ventilation in the intensive care unit. Anesth Analg 113, 550–556.

Chilvers, M., Jones, D., Rushmer, J., et al., 1999. Propofol-thiopentone admixture: recovery characteristics. Anaesth Intensive Care 27, 601–609.

Clarke, K.W., Gerring, E.L., 1990. Detomidine as a sedative and premedicant in the horse (1985-1990). Proceedings of the 36th Annual Convention of the American Association of Equine Practitioners, Lexington, Kentucky, December 2-5 1990, pp. 629-635.

Clarke, K.W., Hall, L.W., 1990. A survey of anaesthetic practice in small animals. J Assoc Vet Anaesth 17, 4–10.

Clutton, R.E., Blissitt, K.J., Bradley, A.A., et al., 1997. Comparison of three injectable anaesthetic techniques in pigs. Vet Rec 141, 140–146.

Cooper, J.E., 1974. Metomidate anaesthesia of some birds of prey for laparotomy and sexing. Vet Rec 94, 437–440.

Davies, C., Hall, L.W., 1991. Propofol and excitatory sequelae in dogs. Anaesthesia 46, 797–798.

DeRossi, R., Frazilio, F.O., Jardim, P.H., et al., 2011. Evaluation of thoracic epidural analgesia induced by lidocaine, ketamine, or both administered via a lumbosacral approach in dogs. Am J Vet Res 72, 1580–1585.

Dodam, J.R., Kruse-Elliott, K.T., Aucoin, D.P., et al., 1990. Duration of etomidate-induced adrenocortical suppression during surgery in dogs. Am J Vet Res 51, 786–788.

Dyson, D.H., Allen, D.G., Ingwersen, W., et al., 1987. Effects of saffan on cardiopulmonary function in healthy cats. Can J Vet Res 51, 236–239.

Elfenbein, J.R., Robertson, S.A., Corser, A.A., et al., 2011. Systemic effects of a prolonged continuous infusion of ketamine in healthy horses. J Vet Intern Med Am Coll Vet Intern Med 25, 1134–1137.

England, G.C., Hammond, R., 1997. Dose-sparing effects of romifidine premedication for thiopentone and halothane anaesthesia in the dog. J Small Anim Pract 38, 141–146.

Evers, A.S., Crowder, C.M., Balser, J.R., 2006. General anaesthesthetics. In: Brunton, L.L., Lazo, J.S., Parker, K.L., (Eds.), Goodman and Gilman's 'The Pharmacological Basis of Therapeutics'. McGraw-Hill, New York, pp. 348.

Fechner, J., Schwilden, H., Schuttler, J., 2008. Pharmacokinetics and pharmacodynamics of GPI 15715 or fospropofol (Aquavan injection) – a water-soluble propofol prodrug. Handbook Exp Pharmacol 253–266.

Ferre, P.J., Pasloske, K., Whittem, T., et al., 2006. Plasma pharmacokinetics of alfaxalone in dogs after an intravenous bolus of Alfaxan-CD RTU. Vet Anaesth Analg 33, 229–236.

Flynn, G., Shehabi, Y., 2012. Pro/con debate: Is etomidate safe in hemodynamically unstable critically ill patients? Crit Care 16, 227.

Forman, S.A., 2011. Clinical and molecular pharmacology of etomidate. Anesthesiology 114, 695–707.

Fudickar, A., Bein, B., 2009. Propofol infusion syndrome: update of clinical manifestation and pathophysiology. Minerva Anestesiol 75, 339–344.

Gerritsmann, H., Stalder, G.L., Seilern-Moy, K., et al., 2012. Comparison of S(+)-ketamine and ketamine, with medetomidine, for field anaesthesia in the European brown hare (Lepus europaeus). Vet Anaesth Analg 39, 511–519.

Glen, J.B., 1980. Animal studies of the anaesthetic activity of ICI 35 868. Br J Anaesth 52, 731–742.

Glen, J.B., Hunter, S.C., 1984. Pharmacology of an emulsion formulation of ICI 35 868. Br J Anaesth 56, 617–626.

Goodwin, W., Keates, H., Pasloske, K., et al., 2012. Plasma pharmacokinetics and pharmacodynamics of alfaxalone in neonatal foals after an intravenous bolus of alfaxalone following premedication with butorphanol tartrate. Vet Anaesth Analg 39, 503–510.

Goodwin, W.A., Keates, H.L., Pasloske, K., et al., 2011. The pharmacokinetics and pharmacodynamics of the injectable anaesthetic alfaxalone in the horse. Vet Anaesth Analg 38, 431–438.

Grint, N.J., Smith, H.E., Senior, J.M., 2008. Clinical evaluation of alfaxalone in cyclodextrin for the induction of anaesthesia in rabbits. Vet Rec 163, 395–396.

Hall, L.W., 1984. A clinical study of a new intravenous agent in dogs and cats. J Assoc Vet Anaesth 12, 115–121.

Hall, L.W., Chambers, J.P., 1987. A clinical trial of propofol infusion anaesthesia in dogs. J Small Anim Pract 28, 623–637.

Hall, L.W., Lagerweij, E., Nolan, A.M., et al., 1994. Effect of medetomidine on the pharmacokinetics of propofol in dogs. Am J Vet Res 55, 116–120.

Hall, L.W., Lagerweij, E., Nolan, et al., 1997. Disposition of propofol after medetomidine premedication in beagle dogs. J Vet Anaesth 24, 23–29.

Hamilton, S.M., Johnston, S.A., Broadstone, R.V., 2005. Evaluation of analgesia provided by the administration of epidural ketamine in dogs with a chemically induced synovitis. Vet Anaesth Analg 32, 30–39.

Hanna, R.M., Borchard, R.E., Schmidt, S.L., 1988. Pharmacokinetics of ketamine HCl and metabolite I in the cat: a comparison of i.v., i.m., and rectal administration. J Vet Pharmacol Ther 11, 84–93.

Hanouz, J.L., Persehaye, E., Zhu, L., et al., 2004. The inotropic and lusitropic effects of ketamine in isolated human atrial myocardium: the effect of adrenoceptor blockade. Anesth Analg 99, 1689–1695, table of contents.

Hay Kraus, B.L., Greenblatt, D.J., Venkatakrishnan, K., et al., 2000. Evidence for propofol hydroxylation by cytochrome P4502B11 in canine liver microsomes: breed and gender differences. Xenobiotica 30, 575–588.

Herbert, G.L., Bowlt, K.L., Ford-Fennah, V., et al., 2013. Alfaxalone for total intravenous anaesthesia in dogs undergoing ovariohysterectomy: a comparison of premedication with acepromazine or dexmedetomidine. Vet Anaesth Analg 40, 124–133.

Hernandez, S.E., Sernia, C., Bradley, A.J., 2012. The effect of three anaesthetic protocols on the stress response in cane toads (Rhinella marina). Vet Anaesth Analg 39, 584–590.

Hijazi, Y., Boulieu, R., 2002. Protein binding of ketamine and its active metabolites to human serum. Eur J Clin Pharmacol 58, 37–40.

Hughes, J.M., Nolan, A.M., 1999. Total intravenous anesthesia in greyhounds: pharmacokinetics of propofol and fentanyl – a preliminary study. Vet Surg 28, 513–524.

Ilkiw, J.E., Benthuysen, J.A., Ebling, W.F., et al., 1991. A comparative study of the pharmacokinetics of thiopental in the rabbit, sheep and dog. J Vet Pharmacol Ther 14, 134–140.

Jiang, X., Gao, L., Zhang, Y., et al., 2011. A comparison of the effects of ketamine, chloral hydrate and pentobarbital sodium anesthesia on isolated rat hearts and cardiomyocytes. J Cardiovasc Med (Hagerstown) 12, 732–735.

Jimenez, C.P., Mathis, A., Mora, S.S., et al., 2012. Evaluation of the quality of the recovery after administration of propofol or alfaxalone for induction of anaesthesia in dogs anaesthetized for magnetic resonance imaging. Vet Anaesth Analg 39, 151–159.

Johnson, K.B., Egan, T.D., Layman, J., et al., 2003. The influence of hemorrhagic shock on etomidate: a pharmacokinetic and pharmacodynamic analysis. Anesth Analg 96, 1360–1368.

Jud, R., Picek, S., Makara, M.A., et al., 2010. Comparison of racemic ketamine and S-ketamine as agents for the induction of anaesthesia in goats. Vet Anaesth Analg 37, 511–518.

Kaka, J.S., Hayton, W.L., 1980. Pharmacokinetics of ketamine and two metabolites in the dog. J Pharmacokinet Biopharm 8, 193–202.

Kaka, J.S., Klavano, P.A., Hayton, W.L., 1979. Pharmacokinetics of ketamine in the horse. Am J Vet Res 40, 978–981.

Keates, H., 2003. Induction of anaesthesia in pigs using a new alphaxalone formulation. Vet Rec 153, 627–628.

Keates, H., Whittem, T., 2012. Effect of intravenous dose escalation with alfaxalone and propofol on occurrence of apnoea in the dog. Res Vet Sci 93, 904–906.

Keates, H.L., van Eps, A.W., Pearson, M.R., 2012. Alfaxalone compared

with ketamine for induction of anaesthesia in horses following xylazine and guaifenesin. Vet Anaesth Analg 39, 591–598.

Kischinovsky, M., Duse, A., Wang, T., et al., 2013. Intramuscular administration of alfaxalone in red-eared sliders (Trachemys scripta elegans) – effects of dose and body temperature. Vet Anaesth Analg 40, 13–20.

Kloppel, H., Leece, E.A., 2011. Comparison of ketamine and alfaxalone for induction and maintenance of anaesthesia in ponies undergoing castration. Vet Anaesth Analg 38, 37–43.

Ko, J.C., Golder, F.J., Mandsager, R.E., et al., 1999. Anesthetic and cardiorespiratory effects of a 1:1 mixture of propofol and thiopental sodium in dogs. J Am Vet Med Assoc 215, 1292–1296.

Kruse-Elliott, K.T., Swanson, C.R., Aucoin, D.P., 1987. Effects of etomidate on adrenocortical function in canine surgical patients. Am J Vet Res 48, 1098–1100.

Kumar, V.L., Malhotra, J., Kumar, V., 1993. Anaesthetic steroids – a review. Indian J Med Sci 47, 87–95.

Lankveld, D.P., Driessen, B., Soma, L.R., et al., 2006. Pharmacodynamic effects and pharmacokinetic profile of a long-term continuous rate infusion of racemic ketamine in healthy conscious horses. J Vet Pharmacol Ther 29, 477–488.

Ledingham, I.M., Watt, I., 1983. Influence of sedation on mortality in critically ill multiple trauma patients. Lancet 1, 1270.

Leece, E.A., Girard, N.M., Maddern, K., 2009. Alfaxalone in cyclodextrin for induction and maintenance of anaesthesia in ponies undergoing field castration. Vet Anaesth Analg 36, 480–484.

Lewis, J.C.M., 1994. Anaesthesia of non-domestic cats. In: Hall, L.W., Taylor, P.M. (Ed.), Anaesthesia of the cat. Balliere Tindall, London, pp. 329–330.

Li, R., Zhang, W.S., Liu, J., et al., 2012. Minimum infusion rates and recovery times from different durations of continuous infusion of fospropofol, a prodrug of propofol, in rabbits: a comparison with propofol emulsion. Vet Anaesth Analg 39, 373–384.

Lin, H.C., Thurmon, J.C., Benson, G.J., et al., 1993. Telazol – a review of its

pharmacology and use in veterinary medicine. J Vet Pharmacol Ther 16, 383–418.

Loftsson, T., Brewster, M.E., 2010. Pharmaceutical applications of cyclodextrins: basic science and product development. J Pharm Pharmacol 62, 1607–1621.

MacPherson, R.D., 2001. Pharmaceutics for the anaesthetist. Anaesthesia 56, 965–979.

Maddern, K., Adams, V.J., Hill, N.A., et al., 2010. Alfaxalone induction dose following administration of medetomidine and butorphanol in the dog. Vet Anaesth Analg 37, 7–13.

Majdan, M., Mauritz, W., Brazinova, A., et al., 2013. Barbiturates use and its effects in patients with severe TBI in five European countries. J Neurotrauma 30, 23–29.

Mathis, A., Pinelas, R., Brodbelt, D.C., et al., 2012. Comparison of quality of recovery from anaesthesia in cats induced with propofol or alfaxalone. Vet Anaesth Analg 39, 282–290.

Matot, I., Neely, C.F., Katz, R.Y., et al., 1993. Pulmonary uptake of propofol in cats. Effect of fentanyl and halothane. Anesthesiology 78, 1157–1165.

McMillan, M.W., Leece, E.A., 2011. Immersion and branchial/transcutaneous irrigation anaesthesia with alfaxalone in a Mexican axolotl. Vet Anaesth Analg 38, 619–623.

Mercer, S.J., 2009. 'The Drug of War' – a historical review of the use of Ketamine in military conflicts. J Roy Naval Med Serve 95, 145–150.

Michou, J.N., Leece, E.A., Brearley, J.C., 2012. Comparison of pain on injection during induction of anaesthesia with alfaxalone and two formulations of propofol in dogs. Vet Anaesth Analg 39, 275–281.

Muir, W., Lerche, P., Wiese, A., et al., 2008. Cardiorespiratory and anesthetic effects of clinical and supraclinical doses of alfaxalone in dogs. Vet Anaesth Analg 35, 451–462.

Muir, W., Lerche, P., Wiese, A., et al., 2009. The cardiorespiratory and anesthetic effects of clinical and supraclinical doses of alfaxalone in cats. Vet Anaesth Analg 36, 42–54.

Nadeson, R., Goodchild, C.S., 2000. Antinociceptive properties of neurosteroids II. Experiments with Saffan and its components alphaxalone and alphadolone to reveal separation of anaesthetic and antinociceptive effects and the involvement of spinal cord GABA(A) receptors. Pain 88, 31–39.

Nolan, A., Reid, J., Welsh, E., et al., 1996. Simultaneous infusions of propofol and ketamine in ponies premedicated with detomidine: a pharmacokinetic study. Res Vet Sci 60, 262–266.

Nolan, A.M., Reid, J., Grant, S., 1993. The effects of halothane and nitrous oxide on the pharmacokinetics of propofol in dogs. J Vet Pharmacol Ther 16, 335–342.

O'Hagan, B., Pasloske, K., McKinnon, C., et al., 2012a. Clinical evaluation of alfaxalone as an anaesthetic induction agent in dogs less than 12 weeks of age. Aust Vet J 90, 346–350.

O'Hagan, B.J., Pasloske, K., McKinnon, B., et al., 2012b. Clinical evaluation of alfaxalone as an anaesthetic induction agent in cats less than 12 weeks of age. Aust Vet J 90, 395–401.

Pascoe, P.J., Ilkiw, J.E., Frischmeyer, K.J., 2006. The effect of the duration of propofol administration on recovery from anesthesia in cats. Vet Anaesth Analg 33, 2–7.

Pascoe, P.J., Ilkiw, J.E., Haskins, S.C., et al., 1992. Cardiopulmonary effects of etomidate in hypovolemic dogs. Am J Vet Res 53, 2178–2182.

Pasloske, K., Sauer, B., Perkins, N., et al., 2009. Plasma pharmacokinetics of alfaxalone in both premedicated and unpremedicated Greyhound dogs after single, intravenous administration of Alfaxan at a clinical dose. J Vet Pharmacol Ther 32, 510–513.

Pejo, E., Cotten, J.F., Kelly, E.W., et al., 2012a. In vivo and in vitro pharmacological studies of methoxycarbonyl-carboetomidate. Anesth Analg 115, 297–304.

Pejo, E., Feng, Y., Chao, W., et al., 2012b. Differential effects of etomidate and its pyrrole analogue carboetomidate on the adrenocortical and cytokine responses to endotoxemia. Crit Care Med 40, 187–192.

Pejo, E., Ge, R., Banacos, N., et al., 2012c. Electroencephalographic recovery, hypnotic emergence, and the effects of metabolite after continuous infusions of a rapidly metabolized etomidate analog in rats. Anesthesiology 116, 1057–1065.

Psatha, E., Alibhai, H.I., Jimenez-Lozano, A., et al., 2011. Clinical efficacy and cardiorespiratory effects of alfaxalone, or diazepam/fentanyl for induction of anaesthesia in dogs that are a poor anaesthetic risk. Vet Anaesth Analg 38, 24–36.

Pypendop, B.H., Ilkiw, J.E., 2005. Pharmacokinetics of ketamine and its metabolite, norketamine, after intravenous administration of a bolus of ketamine to isoflurane-anesthetized dogs. Am J Vet Res 66, 2034–2038.

Raff, M., Harrison, G.G., 1989. The screening of propofol in MHS swine. Anesth Analg 68, 750–751.

Reid, J., Nolan, A.M., 1993. Pharmacokinetics of propofol in dogs premedicated with acepromazine and maintained with halothane and nitrous oxide. J Vet Pharmacol Ther 16, 501–505.

Reid, J., Nolan, A.M., 1996. Pharmacokinetics of propofol as an induction agent in geriatric dogs. Res Vet Sci 61, 169–171.

Reves, J.G., Glass, P.S.A., Lubarski, D.A., McEvoy, M.D., et al., 2012. Intravenous anaesthetics. In: Millar, R.D., Erikson, L.I., Fleisher, L.A., et al. (Eds.), Miller's Anesthesia, seventh ed. Churchill Livngston-Elsivier.

Rigby-Jones, A.E., Nolan, J.A., Priston, M.J., et al., 2002. Pharmacokinetics of propofol infusions in critically ill neonates, infants, and children in an intensive care unit. Anesthesiology 97, 1393–1400.

Robinson, E.P., Natalini, C.C., 2002. Epidural anesthesia and analgesia in horses. Vet Clin N Am Equine Pract 18, 61–82, vi.

Robinson, E.P., Sams, R.A., Muir, W.W., 1986. Barbiturate anesthesia in greyhound and mixed-breed dogs: comparative cardiopulmonary effects, anesthetic effects, and recovery rates. Am J Vet Res 47, 2105–2112.

Rodriguez, J.M., Munoz-Rascon, P., Navarrete-Calvo, R., et al., 2012. Comparison of the cardiopulmonary parameters after induction of anaesthesia with alphaxalone or etomidate in dogs. Vet Anaesth Analg 39, 357–365.

Sams, L., Braun, C., Allman, D., et al., 2008. A comparison of the effects of propofol and etomidate on the induction of anesthesia and on cardiopulmonary parameters in dogs. Vet Anaesth Analg 35, 488–494.

Sams, R.A., Muir, W.W., Detra, R.L., et al., 1985. Comparative pharmacokinetics and anesthetic effects of methohexital, pentobarbital, thiamylal, and thiopental in Greyhound dogs and non-Greyhound, mixed-breed dogs. Am J Vet Res 46, 1677–1683.

Sear, J.W., 1996. Steroid anesthetics: old compounds, new drugs. J Clin Anesth 8, 91S–98S.

Sear, J.W., 1998. Eltanolone: 50 years on and still looking for steroid hypnotic agents! Eur J Anaesthesiol 15, 129–132.

Short, C.E., Bufalari, A., 1999. Propofol anesthesia. Vet Clin N Am Small Anim Pract 29, 747–778.

Sneyd, J.R., 2004. Recent advances in intravenous anaesthesia. Br J Anaesth 93, 725–736.

Sneyd, J.R., 2012. Novel etomidate derivatives. Curr Pharm Des 18, 6253–6256.

Sneyd, J.R., Rigby-Jones, A.E., 2010. New drugs and technologies, intravenous anaesthesia is on the move (again). Br J Anaesth 105, 246–254.

Soars, M.G., Riley, R.J., Findlay, K.A., et al., 2001. Evidence for significant differences in microsomal drug glucuronidation by canine and human liver and kidney. Drug Metab Dispos 29, 121–126.

Strachan, F.A., Mansel, J.C., Clutton, R.E., 2008. A comparison of microbial growth in alfaxalone, propofol and thiopental. J Small Anim Pract 49, 186–190.

Suarez, M.A., Dzikiti, B.T., Stegmann, F.G., et al., 2012. Comparison of alfaxalone and propofol administered as total intravenous anaesthesia for ovariohysterectomy in dogs. Vet Anaesth Analg 39, 236–244.

Taboada, F.M., Murison, P.J., 2010. Induction of anaesthesia with alfaxalone or propofol before isoflurane maintenance in cats. Vet Rec 167, 85–89.

Thomas, A.A., Leach, M.C., Flecknell, P.A., 2012. An alternative method of endotracheal intubation of common marmosets (Callithrix jacchus). Lab Anim 46, 71–76.

Tobias, G., 1964. Congenital porphyria in a cat. J Am Vet Med Assoc 145, 462–463.

Torres, M.D., Andaluz, A., Garcia, F., et al., 2012. Effects of an intravenous bolus of alfaxalone versus propofol on intraocular pressure in sheep. Vet Rec 170, 226.

Wagner, A.E., Walton, J.A., Hellyer, P.W., et al., 2002. Use of low doses of ketamine administered by constant rate infusion as an adjunct for postoperative analgesia in dogs. J Am VetMed Assoc 221, 72–75.

Walsh, V.P., Gieseg, M., Singh, P.M., et al., 2012. A comparison of two different ketamine and diazepam combinations with an alphaxalone and medetomidine combination for induction of anaesthesia in sheep. NZ Vet J 60, 136–141.

Waterman, A.E., Robertson, S.A., Lane, J.G., 1987. Pharmacokinetics of intravenously administered ketamine in the horse. Res Vet Sci 42, 162–166.

Watkins, S.B., Hall, L.W., Clarke, K.W., 1987. Propofol as an intravenous anaesthetic agent in dogs. Vet Rec 120, 326–329.

Wertz, E.M., Benson, G.J., Thurmon, J.C., et al., 1990. Pharmacokinetics of etomidate in cats. Am J Vet Res 51, 281–285.

Whittem, T., Pasloske, K.S., Heit, M.C., et al., 2008. The pharmacokinetics and pharmacodynamics of alfaxalone in cats after single and multiple intravenous administration of Alfaxan at clinical and supraclinical doses. J Vet Pharmacol Ther 31, 571–579.

Young, L.E., Brearley, J.C., Richards, D.L.S., et al., 1990. Medetomidine as a premedicant in dogs and its reversal by atipamezole. J Small Anim Pract 31, 554–559.

Zaki, S., Ticehurst, K., Miyaki, Y., 2009. Clinical evaluation of Alfaxan-CD(R) as an intravenous anaesthetic in young cats. Aust Vet J 87, 82–87.

Zoran, D.L., Riedesel, D.H., Dyer, D.C., 1993. Pharmacokinetics of propofol in mixed-breed dogs and greyhounds. Am J Vet Res 54, 755–760.

Chapter | 7 |

General pharmacology of the inhalation anaesthetics

INTRODUCTION

Since the first use of nitrous oxide (N_2O) by Watt in 1844, and of ether by Morton in 1846, a large number of inhalation anaesthetic agents have been investigated. Many of those once used clinically have now been discarded but, surprisingly, the first two are still in use, at least in some parts of the world. Of those covered in earlier editions of this book, chloroform (first used in 1847) was discarded as it results in dose-dependent liver toxicity and also sensitizes the heart to epinephrine-induced arrhythmias. Cyclopropane was withdrawn because it is flammable and explosive when mixed with oxygen. Trichlorethylene, an excellent analgesic, reacted with the carbon dioxide absorbent and had to be given by a non-rebreathing system. The agents discussed individually below, to the best of the authors' knowledge, all remain in clinical use (in humans and/or in animals) in some areas of the world.

The ideal inhalation anaesthetic should provide good quality anaesthesia, be practicable to give, non-flammable, stable chemically under all circumstances (in and out of the animal), allow a rapid induction and recovery from anaesthesia, have minimal effects on circulation and on the respiratory system, provide analgesia and muscle relaxation, be non-toxic and have no other unwanted side effects. No such agent exists, although xenon is coming close to meeting these targets.

The term 'volatile anaesthetic agent' can be applied to agents that are in liquid form at room temperature and 1 atmosphere of pressure and, therefore, require the use of a vaporizer. However, other agents are in gaseous form, and are presented in cylinders. The term 'inhalation agent' covers all. The mode of action of inhalation agents has been discussed in Chapter 1. Suffice it to say here that actions at any single receptor, ligand or voltage-gated channel cannot explain all the effects of inhalation anaesthetic agents.

Minimum alveolar concentration (MAC)

The concept of minimum alveolar concentration (MAC), how it is measured and factors which will effect it were discussed in Chapter 1. Variation in measurement of MAC have been reviewed by Shaughnessy & Hofmeister (2013). If a combination of inhalation anaesthetic agents is employed, their MACs are additive; this is the basis of regimens that use N_2O (since N_2O is not sufficiently potent to be used as a sole anaesthetic agent) together with a volatile agent such as isoflurane (Eger et al., 2003). It is now thought that an inhalation anaesthetic's effect in preventing movement (and that is what defines MAC) is mediated at the spinal cord (Sonner et al., 2003; Antognini et al., 2005), while higher centres influence amnesia, hypnosis, and perception of pain. However, MAC remains the standard measure of 'potency' of an anaesthetic, is the measure by which equipotent levels of inhalation anaesthetics can be compared, and gives an indication of the concentration that, depending on other agents given, will be required in the clinical situation.

Analgesia

The mode by which inhalation agents produce, or do not produce, analgesia is not clear-cut. The two gaseous agents, N_2O and xenon, produce marked analgesia, possibly through actions at the NMDA receptor. The volatile agents, ether and methoxyflurane, are not known to act at this receptor, yet have marked analgesic properties, while many other volatile agents do not.

Uptake and elimination

The pharmacokinetics of inhalation agents, the importance of the physical properties and the influence of physiological effects (e.g. cardiac output and ventilation) have been explained in Chapter 3. The important physical properties of agents in current use are given in Table 7.1. Of practical importance are:

- The lower the blood/gas solubility, the faster the induction of anaesthesia
- Speed of recovery from a short anaesthetic is fastest with agents with low blood/gas solubility, but awakening is also hastened by 'take up' of the agent by tissues other than the brain
- Recovery from a long anaesthetic will depend also on the amount of agent in the tissues, so the gas solubility in other tissues becomes an issue. A high fat solubility delays full recovery from a prolonged anaesthetic
- Induction of anaesthesia can be hastened by giving more than one MAC multiple, assuming that the saturated vapour pressure of the agent allows a sufficient concentration and that it can be given without causing hypoxia (Tables 7.1 and 7.2).

Table 7.1 Physical characteristics of some anaesthetic agents

Anaesthetic	Human blood/ gas part.coeff.	Brain/blood part.coeff.	Oil/gas part.coeff.	Fat/blood part.coeff.	Boiling point °C	Saturated vapour pressure at 20°C in mm Hg (kPa)
Xenon	1.115–1.14	0.23	1.9		−108.1	Atmospheric (gas at 20°C)
Desflurane	0.42	1.3	18.7	27	23.5	664 (88.5)
Nitrous oxide	0.47	1.1	1.4	2.3	−89.0	Atmospheric (gas at 20°C)
Sevoflurane	0.65	1.7	53.0	48	58.5	157 (20.9)
Isoflurane	1.4	1.6	97.0	45	48.5	236 (31.5)
Enflurane	1.8	1.4	98.0	36	56.5	172 (22.9)
Halothane	2.5	1.9	220.0	51	50.2	240 (32.0)
Ether	12.0	2.0	65.0		34.6	442 (58.9)
Methoxyflurane	15.0	1.4	970		104.8	23 (3.1)

NB: Atmospheric pressure may be reported in mmHg or millibar. 1 millibar = 1 hectopascal = 0.1 kPa
Order gives the lowest blood/gas solubility first. Solubilities depend on the temperature (most reported are at 37°C) and for oil/gas on oil used, hence variations in reported values. Blood/gas solubility values vary between species (Bergadano et al., 2003; Soares et al., 2012), partly, but not totally related to triglyceride value. Values compiled from Eger (1995), Jones (1990), Steffey (2002), Goto et al. (1998) and Jordan & Wright (2010).

Table 7.2 Some reported minimal alveolar concentration (MAC) values

Anaesthetic	Species	MAC (vol %)
Nitrous oxide	Humans	104
Xenon	Humans	62–71
	Dog	119
Halothane	Humans	0.75
	Dog	0.86–0.95
	Cat	0.82–1.22
	Horse	0.88
	Goat	1.3–1.4
Isoflurane	Humans	1.2
	Dog	1.28
	Cat	1.2–2.22
	Horse	1.31
	Goat	1.5–1.62
Sevoflurane	Humans	2.1
	Dog	2.09–2.36
	Cat	2.5–4.0
	Horse	2.31–2.84
	Goat	2.7
Desflurane	Humans	6
	Dog	7.2–10.32
	Cat	10.27
	Horse	8.06
	Goat	10.52

MAC values depend on measurement methods and conditions (Quasha et al., 1980) hence range reported. MACs over 80% represent a theoretical projection.

Information compiled from the following reviews: Eger (1994), Clarke (1999), Lynch et al. (2000), Alibhai, (2001), Steffey (2002), Shaughnessy & Hofmeister, 2013 and original papers: Barter et al. (2004), Goto et al. (1998), Nickalls & Mapleson (2003), Steffey et al. (2005a,h)

Flammability and chemical stability

Modern anaesthetics must be non-flammable in the range of concentrations and gas mixtures (usually of O_2 and N_2O) used in clinical practice. Non-flammability is achieved by halogenation – in particular fluorination – of the agent. In most cases, this does not greatly change the flammability limits but it does increase the energy necessary to ignite the agents and it is this which renders these agents non-flammable in normal clinical use.

Although the anaesthetic agent itself may not be easily flammable, its breakdown products may be so. N_2O increases the flammability of organic vapours because its exothermic decomposition results in production of an oxygen-rich mixture (33% O_2). Breakdown of sevoflurane with the carbon dioxide absorbent, Barolyme, leads to a massive rise in temperature (see chemical stability below), resulting in melting of the anaesthetic circuit, fires and

explosions (Fatheree & Leighton, 2004; Wu et al., 2004). Dunning et al. (2007), in *in-vitro* experiments, have demonstrated that sevoflurane breakdown with both Barolyme and soda lime can result in explosive concentrations of hydrogen, and this may have been a contributory cause of the fires that have occurred.

Anaesthetic agents need to be stable in storage and precautions required to ensure this will be discussed under the specific agents. The greatest concern is the potential for reaction of the agent with the highly alkaline compounds used for CO_2 absorption (e.g. soda lime or Barolyme) in closed breathing systems. Until relatively recently, it was thought that the fluorinated hydrocarbons, other than sevoflurane, did not react with soda lime under the conditions likely to occur clinically, but this is now known not to be true.

Sevoflurane, when used in closed systems, produces a number of breakdown products of which 'Compound A' ($CF_3=C(CF_3)-O-CH_2F$) is nephrotoxic in rats. Although toxic values (in rats) usually need to exceed 1000 ppm, under certain circumstances, levels as low as 50 ppm may cause medullary tubular necrosis (Keller et al., 1995). The concentrations of Compound A which occur are greatest at higher temperatures, with dry absorbents, with low flow or closed systems and, not surprisingly, with high concentrations of sevoflurane (Baum & Aitkenhead, 1995). Levels in humans and the dog using closed systems are usually about 20 ppm but, in certain circumstances, reach over 50 ppm in individuals (Smith et al., 1996). Nevertheless, there is no evidence that renal failure has resulted from sevoflurane anaesthesia in humans (Sahin et al., 2011) or during veterinary use in domestic animals.

The passage of some inhalation anaesthetic agents over very dry highly basic CO_2 absorbents results in accumulation of carbon monoxide (CO) and formaldehyde within a closed anaesthetic system. Of the inhalation agents in common use, desflurane produces the greatest amount of CO, and halothane probably the least (Fang et al., 1995). It was thought that breakdown of sevoflurane would not release CO until the cases mentioned above. In both those cases, the absorbent was Barolyme, which has since been withdrawn. In Fatheree & Leighton's case (2004), a low flow (not closed) system was being used. At the end of surgery, they found that the absorbent canister was very hot, and on disconnection, saw white smoke and smelt burning plastic (on later examination there was fused plastic, and burnt rubber). The patient had arterial blood carboxyhaemoglobin of 29%, oxygen saturation of only 69%, developed acute respiratory distress syndrome, but recovered with intensive care. During anaesthesia, the only point of note had been that inspired sevoflurane was low despite a vaporizer setting of 8%. An unexpectedly low delivered sevoflurane concentration appears to be a warning sign of breakdown of the agent. In the report of Wu et al. (2004), there was an explosion and fire in a machine which had been left with oxygen running and the vaporizer turned on between patients.

The problems relating to agent breakdown occur mainly with dry soda lime, and can be reduced by turning off the O_2 flow of 'fail-safe' machines when they are not in use to avoid the drying effect of continuous gas flow through the system. However, the best avoidance is to use one of the newer absorbents; those without the KOH are less likely to result in breakdown of any inhalation agents; the absorbents which do not contain any of the strong bases (see Chapter 10) reduce agent breakdown even further and are best used for sevoflurane.

Biotransformation and organ toxicity

Damage to organs as a result of inhalation anaesthetic agents may be due to direct toxic effects of the agent, to effects mediated by metabolites, or to hypoxic changes, usually from poor organ blood flow. Except in sensitivity reactions, the toxicity of the unchanged compound is often, but not always, directly related to the concentration present and decreasing the concentration and/or the duration of exposure will decrease toxicity.

Toxic effects of anaesthetic drugs are most commonly seen in the liver and kidneys. Kharasch (2008) has recently reviewed the current understanding of the mechanisms. The most commonly cited example is that of halothane. A small amount of halothane (up to 3%) is metabolized by anaerobic reduction, catalysed by CYP2A6, that results in a small increase in transaminase, which is clinically unimportant. However, large amounts (25% plus) undergo oxidation catalysed predominantly by CYP2E1. Breakdown products include trifluoroacetyl halides which can link to liver proteins. In some cases, antibodies are formed against the halothane-induced antigen, resulting in immune-mediated liver damage (so-called 'halothane hepatitis'). However, isoflurane and enflurane produce similar breakdown products to halothane to a lesser extent and, although very rare, similar autoimmune-mediated hepatitis may occur (Frink, 1995; Kenna & Jones, 1995).

The renal damage which was reported following the prolonged use of methoxyflurane was originally thought to be due to free fluoride ions formed from hepatic metabolism. This theory is now known to be incorrect. In most species, fluoride alone is nephrotoxic only at very high concentrations. Kharasch (2008) explains that methoxyflurane is O-demethylated to fluoride and to dichloracetic acid (DCAA). DCAA alone is not nephrotoxic, but appears to increase the toxicity of fluoride. Of the fluorinated inhalation agents, only methoxyflurane breaks down both to fluoride and DCAA. The incorrect interpretation of the mechanisms of methoxyflurane nephrotoxicity delayed the introduction of sevoflurane (metabolism of which results in fluoride) for many years.

Actions on vital body functions

In experiments on isolated organs, almost all anaesthetics have a dose-dependent depressant effect on the cardiovascular system but, in an intact animal, these effects may be modified or even controlled by mechanisms such as the effect of increased CO_2 or the response to surgery causing sympathetic stimulation. There are major differences between the cardiovascular actions of the agents in spontaneously breathing patients compared to those undergoing intermittent positive pressure ventilation (IPPV), when CO_2 can be controlled. Of practical clinical importance for comparison of such effects is, for the cardiovascular system, the effect of equipotent dose effects on heart rate and rhythm (including sensitivity to epinephrine), on myocardial contractility, cardiac output, and on the resistance of peripheral, pulmonary, cerebral and other organ vasculature. Of particular importance is the effect on overall blood flow (rather than just blood pressure). The effect of different anaesthetic agents on overall blood flow to specific organs, in particular brain, kidneys and heart, has been the subject of a great deal of research in human anaesthesia, in order to relate use of a specific agent to a specific type of surgery, or patient disease. For example, isoflurane causes more 'coronary steal' than enflurane (Diana et al., 1993); there are many investigations as to the relative effects of sevoflurane and desflurane on this phenomenon. With the exception of N_2O, all the inhalation anaesthetics produce a concentration-dependent depression of respiration. Although there is some difference of degree between the agents currently used, the impact on respiration is considered of less importance than cardiovascular effects as IPPV can always be employed. Some anaesthetics are irritant to the airways that may lead to breath holding when they are used for anaesthetic induction or in very lightly anaesthetized animals. Good monitoring (see Chapter 2) enables many of these depressant effects to be detected and treated.

All the halogenated volatile anaesthetic agents, (but not the gaseous agents N_2O and xenon) can trigger the condition of malignant hyperthermia. There recently have been concerns that inhalant anaesthesia may lead to prolonged cognitive dysfunction through a direct neurotoxic action (reviewed by Mandal et al., 2009).

Not all effects of inhalation agents are negative. Despite the concern over cognitive dysfunction mentioned above, most anaesthetic agents are thought to have neuroprotective properties (Matchett et al., 2009; Schifilliti et al., 2010) against hypoxic insult, as do many intravenous agents. Inhalation agents also protect the heart against hypoxic insults; most experimental evidence in animal models suggests that this protection is greater than that of intravenous agents and that this is so has been confirmed in clinical practice (De Hert et al., 2005; Landoni et al., 2007; Bein, 2011; Van Rompaey & Barvais, 2011).

Interaction with other drugs

Any drug that has CNS depressant effects, whether sedative, hypnotic or analgesic will add, or in some cases be synergistic with, the effect of inhaled anaesthetic agents. Many such drug combinations are used to reduce the dose of inhalation anaesthetic agent used, and will be described in the relevant species chapters. The basis of use is that if less inhalation agent is used, there will be less cardiovascular depression. There is little or no evidence as yet that this is always the case; blood pressure may be higher but cardiac output, and therefore blood flow, may not be improved over that which would have occurred with the inhalation agent alone. The exception is the use of some of the analgesics together with inhalation agents which themselves give poor analgesia. Local nerve blocks where practicable are particularly effective. Other techniques include infusion of opioids, lidocaine, α_2-agonists or ketamine (see Chapter 5). There are species differences between the most suitable methods.

Agents which stimulate the CNS will tend to reverse the effects of anaesthetic drugs. In veterinary patients for anaesthesia, interactions with accidental ingested of recreational drugs ('uppers or downers') may have to be considered on rare occasions.

All neuromuscular blocking drugs are potentiated by volatile anaesthetics in a dose-dependent manner (see Chapter 8), but not by the inhalation agent, xenon. Interest has been greatest in relation to anaesthesia of patients with myasthenia gravis (Blichfeldt-Lauridsen & Hansen, 2012). Sevoflurane has been reported to reduce the TOF (train of four) ratio in a dose-dependent manner in both normal and myasthenic patients (Nitahara et al., 2007).

The sensitization of the myocardium to both endogenous and exogenous epinephrine by the inhalational agents has been the subject of much investigation. Straight-chain hydrocarbons (such as halothane) tend to sensitize the heart to catecholamines; the ethers, especially if fluorinated, do not have this effect.

Occupational exposure to inhalation anaesthetic agents

Personnel exposed to trace concentrations of inhalation anaesthetics in the atmosphere inhale and retain these agents in their bodies for some hours or even days, depending on the solubility of the agents concerned. As a result of concerns raised in the 1970s that such exposure might be deleterious to health, legal requirements setting 'limits' to such exposure have been introduced in most countries. In the UK, they are governed by 'The Control of Substance Hazardous to Human Health (COSHH) regulations' and the Occupational Exposure Standards (OES) set is based on an eight hour time weighted average of 100 ppm of N_2O, 10 ppm of halothane and 50 ppm of isoflurane. The limits have not been updated to include sevoflurane and desflurane. In the USA, levels of exposure which should not be exceeded are, for example, by government recommendation 2.0 ppm for volatile agents and 25 ppm for N_2O. Other countries differ in their requirements (ISSA, 1996). The limits of exposure chosen by various authorities differ between countries have no good evidence base (ISSA, 1996). The most serious concern was that of effects on fertility and on developmental defects. ISSA (1996) summarizes a meta-analysis of the evidence available in 1996; there is evidence in experimental models that implicates nitrous oxide but there is little compelling evidence of long-lasting harm relating to the other agents. However, there is evidence of concurrent reduction in cognitive function for personnel working in an atmosphere contaminated by inhalation anaesthetics. The result of the concerns led to the introduction of waste gas scavenging, and regular monitoring of its efficacy (see Chapter 10), and the authors are in no doubt that this has improved the working environment in operating theatres.

INDIVIDUAL INHALATION ANAESTHETICS

Nitrous oxide (N_2O)

N_2O is a gaseous anaesthetic agent. Although the first original anaesthetic agent, it is still in use in medical and veterinary anaesthesia, in particular because of its outstanding analgesic effects, which are evident at subanaesthetic concentrations. Its mode of action is thought primarily to be action inhibiting the NMDA receptor (Jevtovic-Todorovic et al., 1998; Mennerick et al., 1998), which may explain its analgesic potency (see Chapter 5). As such, the use of BIS monitors are ineffective at monitoring the depth of anaesthesia with this agent, as are auditory evoked potentials (see Chapter 1) (Yagi et al., 1995).

N_2O is a colourless gas with a faint, rather pleasant smell; it is not flammable or explosive but it will support combustion, even in the absence of free O_2. Compressed into cylinders (tanks) at 40 atmospheres pressure it liquefies so is presented in cylinders (see Chapter 10). N_2O is also available in a 50% mixture with 50% oxygen, as Entanox® or Nitronox.

The MAC of N_2O is over 100% so it cannot be used alone to produce anaesthesia and must be administered with sufficient O_2 (>25%) to prevent hypoxia. However, the rapid onset and recovery from its effects, coupled with its strong analgesic properties make it a useful adjuvant to an anaesthetic protocol. The low solubility of N_2O results in rapid equilibration between inspired and expired concentrations. As a result, when used with oxygen in a low-flow rebreathing circuit, concentrations of N_2O tend to increase as, while after equilibration there is no further uptake of N_2O, oxygen is still being utilized. To prevent a hypoxic mixture, higher flows or inspired oxygen monitoring are advisable.

N_2O moves rapidly into gas-filled spaces in the body at a greater rate than nitrogen can diffuse out. This is of considerable importance in herbivores and in the presence of a closed pneumothorax. The low solubility also results in the phenomena of *'the second gas effect'* at induction of anaesthesia, and potentially in *'diffusion hypoxia'* at recovery. When N_2O is first administered to a patient, a large gradient exists between the tension in the inspired gas and the arterial blood so that initially the blood takes up large volumes of gas. Its rapid removal from the alveoli by the blood elevates the tension of any remaining (second) gas or vapour such as oxygen, or a volatile anaesthetic agent, and augments alveolar ventilation. Thus, during the first few minutes of N_2O administration, anaesthetic uptake is facilitated because the enhanced tension of the second gas ensures a steeper tension gradient for its passage into the blood. This is known as 'the second gas effect'. There is also a reverse effect speeding elimination of the accompanying volatile agent at recovery, speeding arousal (Peyton et al, 2011). The phenomenon known as 'diffusion hypoxia' occurs immediately following anaesthesia when the gas is being rapidly eliminated from the lungs; N_2O may form 10% or more of the volume of expired gas, and the outward diffusion of N_2O into the alveoli lowers the partial pressure of O_2 in the lungs, and therefore in arterial blood. Thus, 5–10 minutes of O_2 inhalation when N_2O is discontinued at the end of a lengthy procedure is advisable even in healthy animals, and essential in animals suffering from any pulmonary inadequacy.

N_2O causes minimal cardiovascular effects. It is non-irritant to inhale, and it causes increased pulmonary ventilation (Hall, 1988). Only 0.004% of N_2O is metabolized and it has no direct toxic effects on liver and kidneys. However, exposure to low levels over several days causes bone marrow depression in humans due to interference with methionine synthase giving rise to disturbances of folate metabolism (Hathout & El-Saden, 2011) and megablastosis (ISSA, 1996). It is embryotoxic in experimental animals. It is also a major 'greenhouse' gas. The use of N_2O within anaesthesia is now declining in popularity, but it still has a major role as an analgesic.

Xenon

Xenon, a gaseous agent, has been used 'experimentally' as an anaesthetic for more than 60 years. It first received a 'licence' for use in humans in Russia in 2000, and is now approved in several European countries. Its actions have been the subject of many reviews (Lynch et al., 2000; Sanders et al., 2003; Harris & Barnes, 2008; Jordan & Wright, 2010). The interest lies in the fact it is very insoluble (see Table 7.1), thus resulting in a very rapid induction and recovery, has minimal if any cardiovascular depressant

effects, is an excellent analgesic, is neuroprotective, and is non-toxic (including to the environment).

The mode of action of xenon is thought to be primarily at the NMDA receptors (as for N_2O). Xenon's analgesic effects at subanaesthetic doses are equal to or better (depending on the nociceptive stimulus used) than N_2O. Xenon has no action on GABA receptors and, as a result, many anaesthetic depth monitors such as BIS are unreliable (see Chapter 1). In contrast to N_2O, auditory evoked potentials (see Chapter 1) can be used for some assessment of depth of xenon anaesthesia (Yagi et al., 1995; Sanders & Maze, 2005).

Xenon is non-flammable, non-explosive, and is presented in cylinders as a compressed gas. Its density is 4.5 times and viscosity twice that of air. As a result, its use requires special flow meters (Baumert, 2009). It is obtained by fractional distillation of liquefied air, quantities are very small (>0.0875 ppm) and the process requires a lot of energy. Thus, although it is a by-product of production of oxygen, xenon has many uses other than anaesthesia, is very expensive and is likely to remain so. Methods of electronically controlled administration involving totally closed systems and enabling recovery of agent are being devised to make full use of what is available.

The MAC of xenon has been reported as between 63 and 71% in humans and a theoretical 119% for dogs (Lynch et al., 2000; Sanders et al., 2003). Induction and recovery are very rapid and excitement-free, from both short and long anaesthetics. The solubility characteristics of xenon are closer to those of nitrogen than are those of N_2O, so there is less (but not no) potential for xenon expanding gas-filled spaces. In humans, potential expansion of gas bubbles in the blood is of concern for surgery such as cardiopulmonary bypass. Studies investigating this (Lockwood, 2002; Casey et al., 2005; Benavides et al., 2006) suggest that although it can happen, the expansion is less than with N_2O, and clinical studies (Lockwood et al., 2006) found no problem. Nevertheless, the possibility of expansion of gut spaces needs to be considered if xenon is ever to be used in herbivores.

Xenon has minimal effects on the cardiovascular system; it does not cause depression of myocardial contractility when tested in *'in vitro'* preparations or in animal models with induced cardiac damage (Ishiguro, 2001; Sanders et al., 2003). It does not sensitize the heart to epinephrine. Preconditioning with xenon protects against subsequent cardiac ischaemia. It does have some vagotonic effects (Ishiguro, 2001). Xenon causes dose-dependent respiratory depression, resulting in apnoea at high doses (Dingley et al., 1999). The high viscosity and density of xenon are such as to increase airway resistance. Zhang et al. (1995) demonstrated that pulmonary resistance was statistically but probably not clinically significantly greater in dogs breathing with xenon than breathing N_2O.

Other advantages of xenon include that it does not trigger malignant hyperthermia. There is no evidence of toxicity, whether direct, through metabolism or through breakdown products. Its release into the environment (from where it came) causes no environmental damage.

To date, animal studies of xenon anaesthesia have been where the animal has been an experimental model. From the 'control' stages of such a dog model, and following induction of anaesthesia with propofol, Francis et al. (2008) compared three anaesthetic maintenance protocols: 1.2% isoflurane + 70% N_2O; 0.8% isoflurane + 5 µg/kg min remifentanil; and 63% xenon +5 µg/kg min remifentanil. Blood pressure fell with both isoflurane protocols, but not with the xenon protocol. However, heart rate fell with both remifentanil protocols; heart rate and cardiac output was lowest, and systemic vascular resistance, epinephrine and norepinephrine levels highest with xenon + remifentanil. Although remifentanil would have been the major cause of bradycardia, the vagotonic effect of xenon may have contributed. The veterinary clinical perspective from this study is that the high blood pressure seen with the xenon + remifentanil did not mean that cardiac output and tissue blood flow were necessarily adequate.

Diethyl ether

Diethyl ether, commonly known simply as 'ether', was one of the earliest volatile anaesthetics to be used in clinical practice. Its flammability, irritant smell, and high blood gas and blood fat solubilities, and slow induction and recovery mean it is not used in the developed world.

Ether is a transparent, colourless liquid, which is highly flammable in air and explosive in O_2-rich atmospheres. It is decomposed by air, light and heat; the liquid is, therefore, stored in amber-coloured bottles kept in a cool dark place. Its heavy vapour (twice that of air) tends to pool on the floor and, unless ventilation is good, the possibility of fires is very great. Sparks of static electricity from electrical switches and apparatus can easily ignite ether/air mixtures and ether/oxygen mixtures are explosive. Ether should not be administered in locations where electrical equipment such as radiographic apparatus or diathermy is to be used.

Ether is safe in the presence of epinephrine. Its administration is associated with sympathoadrenal stimulation which opposes its negative inotropic effect. Normally, cardiac output is well maintained even at deep levels of unconsciousness. During light levels of unconsciousness, ether does not depress respiration. The metabolites of ether are relatively non-toxic substances as ethyl alcohol, acetic acid and acetaldehyde.

The MAC of ether in humans is around 3.2%. It is very irritant to the airways and its inhalation provokes the secretion of saliva and of mucus within the respiratory tract (although this problem is counteracted by premedication with an anticholinergic agent). Postanaesthetic nausea is pronounced. However, despite its disadvantages,

the margin of safety with ether means that it is still used in humans and animals in situations where there is minimal equipment and expertise available; in such circumstances, many potential causes of fires also are not available.

Halothane

Halothane, 2-bromo-2-chloro-1,1,1-trifluoroethane, was introduced into medical and to veterinary anaesthesia in 1956 (Hall, 1957) and was so greatly superior to existing agents that it soon became used throughout the world. It was the first inhalation agent that could be used effectively in large animals; without it many advances in equine surgery would not have occurred. Although no longer 'authorized' for medical or veterinary use in North America or Europe, it is still in use in other areas of the world, and remains on the World Health Organisation's list of core medicines (WHO, 2010).

Halothane is a colourless liquid, which is broken down by ultraviolet light and so is stored in dark bottles with thymol as a preservative. Thymol collects in calibrated vaporizers, decreasing anaesthetic output and making regular service essential. Physical properties of halothane are given in Table 7.1. Its low solubility relative to ether (the agent most used prior to halothane) means that induction and recovery are calm, and relatively rapid, albeit slower than the newer agents discussed below.

Halothane does not irritate the respiratory mucosa and so, in contrast to isoflurane, it can be used to induce anaesthesia without causing breath-holding. It is for this reason that halothane has, until the advent of sevoflurane, remained available for human use. Most veterinary calibrated vaporizers will produce an inspired concentration of 5%; it is possible to induce anaesthesia in dogs and cats with it using 2–4%; anaesthesia then can be maintained with end tidal concentrations of 0.8–1.2%, as MAC is 0.8–1.4% depending on species (see Table 7.2).

Halothane causes dose-dependent respiratory depression, leading to a progressive rise in $PaCO_2$. Nevertheless, animals tend to breathe spontaneously better under halothane anaesthesia than after the more modern agents (Steffey, 2002). There is a dose-dependent depression of cardiac output and arterial blood pressure in all mammalian species due mainly to a negative inotropic effect, although it does cause some block of transmission at sympathetic ganglia. Bradycardia is common due to vagal activity. Arrhythmias are associated with CO_2 accumulation from respiratory depression, hypoxia, catecholamine release and overdosage. Halothane sensitizes the heart to epinephrine-induced tachyarrhythmias. Some adaptation of both cardiovascular and respiratory function occurs with time (Dunlop et al., 1987; Steffey et al., 1987). Blood pressure tends to increase at the start of surgery as a result of increased systemic vascular resistance (Wagner et al., 1995).

Halothane has minimal muscle relaxant effects and is a poor analgesic, so supplementation with analgesics (see Chapter 5) is often effective. It does not contribute to postoperative analgesia. Shivering is often seen in all species of domestic animals during recovery but the reason for it is not completely understood. Halothane can be a trigger for malignant hyperthermia, as can all the halogenated anaesthetic agents.

Halothane is metabolized extensively (>25%) in the liver. The pathways and potential 'immune-mediated' toxicity of the trifluoroacetyl halides have been discussed earlier (biotransformation and organ toxicity). The small increase in liver enzymes that occurs routinely on the basis of dose and time of halothane administration is clinically unimportant in most domestic species. However, there appears to be some variation between species in susceptibility to hepatic damage. The guinea pig is particularly susceptible (Lunam et al., 1985) and there being several reports of postanaesthetic fatalities in goats associated with acute liver damage (Antognini & Eisele, 1993, Alibhai, 2001). However, it is the very occasional immune-mediated fatal fulminant hepatic failure (less than 1:35 000 – as reported in the National Halothane Study, Bunker, 1968; Bunker et al, 1969) associated with repeated exposure to the drug at short intervals (Elliott & Strunin, 1993), which is the reason for the withdrawal of halothane from human anaesthsia in North America and Europe. There are no substantiated reports of this type of hepatitis resulting from halothane anaesthesia in animals.

Methoxyflurane

Methoxyflurane is a non-explosive and non-flammable anaesthetic agent that is also a potent analgesic at subanaesthetic doses and, in Australia, it is administered by paramedics as an inhalant analgesic prior to hospital admission. It was withdrawn from human anaesthetic use because of the renal toxicity discussed above (Biotransformation and organ toxicity). Its physical properties (see Table 7.1) of a high blood gas solubility results in uptake and elimination being very slow; its high boiling point and low saturated vapour pressure mean that high concentrations are not possible, and therefore it is very difficult (but not impossible) to overdose. It gives good postoperative analgesia because of its prolonged elimination. It stimulates the sympathetic system, supporting circulation; blood pressure and cardiac output are well maintained. In veterinary anaesthesia, it was popular for small animals because of these margins of safety.

Enflurane

Enflurane, is a fluorinated ether first developed by Ross Terrell in the 1960s. It provides good anaesthesia, the solubility resulting in onset and elimination times being a little shorter than those of halothane (see Table 7.1). MAC

is from 1.7% in humans to 2.4% in cats (see Table 7.2). It causes dose-related cardiovascular and respiratory depression. Comparative studies of equipotent concentrations of halothane, enflurane, isoflurane and sevoflurane dogs showed that enflurane produced the greatest falls in cardiac output and arterial blood pressure (Mutoh et al., 1997). Enflurane sensitizes the heart to catecholamines such as epinephrine, but to a lesser extent than does halothane (Stevens, 1972). The actions of the non-depolarizing relaxants are markedly enhanced. The degree of metabolic biotransformation is approximately 2–8% (Elliott & Strunin, 1993) a by-product being small quantities of inorganic fluoride, but also trifluoroacetyl chloride, so it is capable of causing immune-mediated hepatitis. Enflurane has epileptogenic properties (Stevens, 1972); muscle twitching is seen in humans and in dogs, and there can sometimes be seizure-like activity at induction and recovery (Eger, 1995).

Isoflurane

Isoflurane (Fig. 7.1) is a structural isomer of enflurane, and exists as a racemic mixture of two optical isomers (Stevens, 1972). It is a clear liquid supplied in dark coloured glass bottles and does not require the use of any preservative. Isoflurane's high volatility, coupled with its relatively low solubility in blood and tissues (see Table 7.1) mean that induction of and recovery from anaesthesia is noticeably faster than with equipotent doses of halothane, and its low solubility in fatty tissues avoids accumulation in obese subjects. During anaesthetic maintenance it is easy to maintain stability or to change depth. Clinical signs of anaesthesia resemble those of halothane. However, isoflurane has a pungent smell and is irritant to the airways,

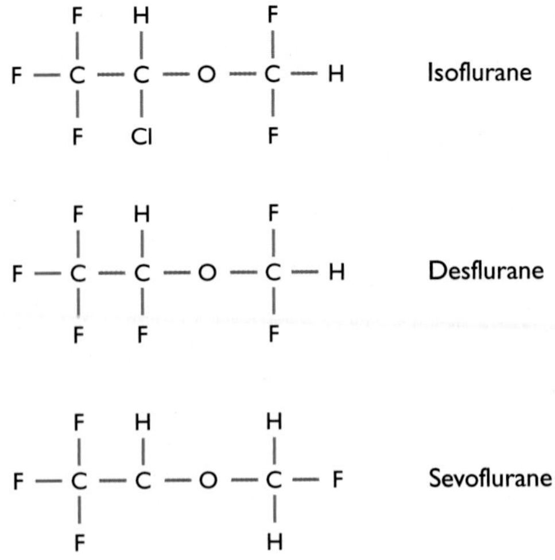

Figure 7.1 Chemical structure of isoflurane, desflurane and sevoflurane.

causing airway secretions, coughing and breath-holding. It is, therefore, not suitable for 'mask' induction in people. The problem does not appear so acute in animals; most veterinary calibrated vaporizers will provide inspired concentrations of 5% which is higher than required for mask induction, and isoflurane has been used successfully to induce and/or to maintain anaesthesia in many species.

Isoflurane is authorized as an anaesthetic agent in many animal species, and has a 'minimal residual limit' for use in food animals in Europe. It has been used widely in humans and animals for over 40 years and, as such, there is a lot of knowledge of its actions. Comprehensive reviews of its pharmacological properties are those of Wade & Stevens (1981) and Eger (1984). Respiratory depression is greater than with halothane but surgical stimulation helps to counteract this. Isoflurane causes a marked dose-dependent fall in arterial blood pressure, and systemic vascular resistance; at doses close to MAC (Fig. 7.2; see Table 7.2), there is little myocardial depression, heart rate is well maintained, or even (depending on species) increased, so that cardiac output and blood flow remain good. Compared with halothane, under isoflurane in oxygen anaesthesia, mucous membranes appear pink, a sign of good peripheral blood flow. At higher MAC values, cardiac depression does occur, although cardiac output is sometimes maintained by increased heart rate. Isoflurane does not sensitize the myocardium to epinephrine-induced arrhythmias.

For human anaesthesia, there is often concern about perfusion of specific organs in relation to disease stages or specific surgery. As isoflurane maintains cardiac output in association with vasodilation, blood flow to most vital organs is well maintained. However, with the increase in neurosurgery, of relevance to veterinary anaesthesia are the effects of anaesthetics on cerebral blood flow. In common with sevoflurane and desflurane, isoflurane, at 1 MAC or less, preserves cerebral vasculature response to CO_2 and can decrease cerebral vascular resistance and cerebral metabolic rate (Young, 1992). It is also considered that preconditioning with volatile anaesthetic agents confers some degree of neuroprotection to hypoxia (Eger, 1995), although probably less than that provided by nitrous oxide and xenon.

Isoflurane can be used satisfactorily in small animals in simple plenum vaporizers used in the 'in circle' method (Brosnan et al., 1998) (see Chapter 10) but its potency and high volatility mean that, to avoid overdose, it is usually administered from a calibrated vaporizer. As the boiling point and, therefore, the saturated vapour pressure of halothane and isoflurane are similar (see Table 7.1), recycled ex-halothane vaporizers can be recalibrated for isoflurane at service and are economical to purchase for veterinary use.

Isoflurane undergoes a small amount of biotransformation (approximately 0.2%), the main metabolites being trifluroacetic acid and inorganic fluoride, but the risk of

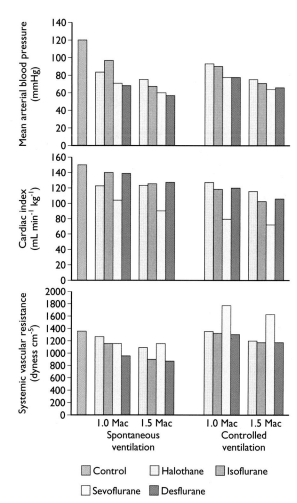

Figure 7.2 Comparison of cardiovascular parameters in goats anaesthetized with one of four volatile anaesthetic agents. Goats were anaesthetized with the inhalant at concentrations of MAC and 1.5 MAC, and breathing spontaneously or ventilated to normocapnia. Control is non-anaesthetized but in lateral recumbency. There were few statistically significant differences between agents. At MAC with spontaneous respiration, MAP with isoflurane was significantly higher than desflurane or sevoflurane and SVR was significantly lower with desflurane than either isoflurane or sevoflurane – not what was expected! This difference was not present with IPPV. Halothane is shown to demonstrate that, in this set of experiments, cardiac index was well maintained in comparison with the newer agents, even at 1.5 MAC.
Figure courtesy of HIK Alibhai, and adapted from Alibhai, 2001.

immune-mediated hepatitis in susceptible patients is much smaller than for halothane. Isoflurane can be a trigger for malignant hyperthermia. Isoflurane can interact with dry soda lime to form carbon monoxide (Kharasch, 2008), but the quantities are less than with desflurane.

Desflurane

Desflurane is a fluorinated methyl ethyl ether, differing from isoflurane only in the substitution of fluorine for chlorine at the α-ethyl carbon atom (see Fig. 7.1). It is a clear, colourless and virtually odourless fluid, with a boiling point of 23.5°C and a saturated vapour pressure of 88.53 kPa (664 mmHg) at 20°C (see Table 7.1). Desflurane has high chemical stability and does not have added preservatives. It is not degraded by artificial light but, nevertheless, is supplied in dark coloured bottles.

As desflurane boils at close to room temperature, if the bottle is inadequately sealed, all of the agent vaporizes and the bottle is found empty. The low boiling point also means that a special vaporizer, such as the Tec 6 vaporizer (see Chapter 10) is essential. In these vaporizers, desflurane is contained in a sump which is electrically heated and controlled to maintain a constant temperature of approximately 39°C, while an electronically controlled pressure regulating valve ensures a precise output from the vaporizer which is not affected by the rate of gas flow. With the Tec 6, the desflurane concentration is reduced by up to 2% by the concurrent use of N_2O in the carrier gas flow (Johnston et al., 1994), but there is no evidence as to whether other makes of vaporizer suffer from the same problem. The vaporizers are 'fail safe' in that any fault results in 'cut off' of supply of desflurane; the consequential rapid recovery of the patient can cause problems, so some other method of maintaining anaesthesia should always be available.

Desflurane has a very low solubility in blood, fat and tissues (see Table 7.1) and induces anaesthesia very rapidly, as well as permitting rapid changes in depth of anaesthesia when the inspired concentration is altered (Eger, 1992; Smiley, 1992; White, 1992; Jones & Nay, 1994). Similarly, recovery is rapid. Unfortunately, as for isoflurane, it is irritant to the airways and, therefore, in people, induction of anaesthesia is complicated by breath-holding, coughing and laryngeal spasm (Smiley, 1992; White, 1992). No similar problems have been reported when desflurane has been used to induce anaesthesia in the dog and cat and dogs recovered within 3–9 minutes following 5–9 hours of desflurane anaesthesia (Hammond et al., 1994; McMurphy & Hodgson, 1995).

The MAC of desflurane varies between species and between individuals within that species (see Table 7.2). In an individual animal, the MAC of an inhalation agent does not usually vary by more than 10% (Quasha et al., 1980) but, for desflurane, there have been reports of sudden large increases of MAC during the period of measurement (Eger et al., 1988; Clarke et al., 1996a). Such differences have not been reported for other inhalation agents.

Desflurane undergoes minimal metabolism (0.02%) and therefore the potential for toxicity is low (Kharasch et al., 2006). Desflurane can be a trigger for malignant hyperthermia. In experimental circumstances, the effects of desflurane on vital organ function are similar to those of isoflurane (Merin et al., 1991; Hartman et al., 1992) in that it causes dose-related vasodilatation, moderate impairment of myocardial function and a similar degree of respiratory depression. The heart is not sensitized to epinephrine-induced arrhythmias. However, 'sympathetic storms' have been reported in people, whereby an increase in inhaled concentration was followed by tachycardia and an increase in arterial blood pressure (Ebert & Muzi, 1993; Weiskopf et al., 1994). Variations in reported MAC may be due to a similar occurrence. Desflurane decomposes to release carbon monoxide when used with dry soda lime so, in order to use it with minimum fresh gas flows, the soda lime must be damp, or one of the less basic carbon dioxide absorbents (see Chapter 10) may be used.

The major potential advantages of desflurane in comparison with isoflurane result from its low solubilities in blood and fat. However, in most veterinary species, it is probable that the advantages are minimal once other agents have also been employed (Mohamadnia et al., 2008; Lozano et al., 2009). The exception is in the horse (see Chapter 11), where desflurane renders it exceptionally easy to maintain stable anaesthesia and, as it is possible to run in a totally closed system, it is economical in use. Clarke et al. (1996a,b) reported that, in ponies, recovery after desflurane, when coupled with low dose xylazine, proved to be extremely rapid, quiet and uneventful; without xylazine, animals tended to fall at their first attempt to stand. Subsequent clinical investigations (Bradbrook et al., 2006) have confirmed these advantages, although they become less pronounced when multiple analgesic/other anaesthetic agents are also included in the regimens. Most veterinary anaesthetists who have used desflurane to anaesthetize clinical cases are impressed by the speed and the completeness of recovery which is faster than isoflurane, although differences do not always reach statistical significance (Mohamadnia et al., 2008; Lozano et al., 2009).

Desflurane does not have any authorization for veterinary use. Its future use in animals will probably depend on availability of vaporizers and its fate in the medical anaesthetic market.

Sevoflurane

Sevoflurane is a fluorinated ether (see Fig. 7.1), which has been licensed for medical use in Japan since 1990 and is now approved for clinical use in medical practice in the USA and Europe. It has a veterinary marketing authorization (as at 2012) only for use in dogs. Nevertheless, in the last 10 years, it has become very popular for clinical anaesthesia in a wide variety of animals, anecdotally of particular note being the ease of maintaining a stable level of anaesthesia.

Sevoflurane is marketed, depending on manufacturer, in dark plastic, glass or aluminium bottles. This is because there are concerns about its stability in the presence of Lewis Acids (electron pair acceptors), which are present in various metals and in some components of glass (Baker, 2009). Some preparations have additional water content to prevent this reaction. Contaminants and damage thought to due to the Lewis-Acid reactions were found in one type of (otherwise conventional) vaporizer, which has now been redesigned to prevent any contact between the anaesthetic and metal.

Sevoflurane is non-irritant to the respiratory passages so that induction of anaesthesia is not complicated by coughing or breath-holding and, indeed, it was the ability to use it for 'mask' induction that first earned it popularity. Calibrated vaporizers will provide up to 8% sevoflurane; this high concentration in comparison with MAC (2.1–3.4%) was chosen for human use to enable very rapid mask induction. The solubility coefficients (see Table 7.1) mean that such induction is faster than with isoflurane (although not as fast as desflurane), but the differential in recovery is not so marked. It is very easy to maintain a stable level of anaesthesia, but also easy to overdose. Both induction and emergence phases usually are smooth, although there have been reports of occasional emergence excitement in children (Kuratani & Oi, 2008) and in animals (Clarke, 1999; Mohamadnia et al., 2008; Lozano et al., 2009). Sevoflurane can predispose the brain to convulsive activity (Eger, 1995; Constant et al., 2005), although not to the same extent as enflurane

The pharmacological actions of sevoflurane (Ebert et al., 1995; Clarke, 1999; Steffey, 2002) are similar to those of isoflurane and desflurane; i.e. there is dose-dependent depression of both cardiovascular and respiratory systems but, at MAC (see Table 7.2), cardiac output is usually well maintained (see Fig. 7.2). Sevoflurane does not sensitize the heart to epinephrine-induced arrhythmias. Sevoflurane can be a trigger for malignant hyperthermia.

Approximately 5% of sevoflurane is metabolized; the metabolic products include hexafluropropanol, which is rapidly conjugated, and free fluoride. The problems of sevoflurane's stability with soda lime are discussed above (flammability and chemical stability). Despite high free fluoride from biotransformation and despite compound A from breakdown with soda lime, extensive clinical experience in humans has not found cases of renal failure following its use. The (very rare) reports of the overheating and fires are more concerning; the danger can be avoided totally by use of the newer non-basic carbon dioxide absorbents (see Chapter 10).

In veterinary clinical anaesthesia, sevoflurane has now become used widely in domestic and exotic animals (see species chapters); despite the limitations of sevoflurane's chemical stability, methods to combat its breakdown have been developed, and no unexpected clinical problems have been reported. Although, as yet, epidemiological assessments are not available, it appears to be a useful and well-tolerated anaesthetic agent.

COMPARISON OF VOLATILE AGENTS FOR VETERINARY CLINICAL PRACTICE

The advent of sevoflurane and desflurane led to a very large number of studies comparing them with isoflurane, either as sole agents, or more usually in clinical studies, in combination with induction agents and with analgesics. Comprehensive reviews include (Eger, 1994; Clarke, 1999, 2008; Steffey, 2002). Alibhai (2001) compared the effects in goats of all three agents (see Fig. 7.2).

Mask induction of anaesthesia with sevoflurane in suitably sized animals is smooth and rapid; it is possible with the other two agents but may be accompanied by breath-holding or by salivation. For all three agents, although speed of induction and recovery follow the pattern as expected from solubilities (desflurane faster than sevoflurane, faster than isoflurane), in clinical studies where other agents are also being used, the difference is masked; differences are there and sometimes (Matthews et al., 1998, Bradbrook et al., 2006) but not always (Leece et al., 2008; Mohamadnia et al., 2008; Lozano et al., 2009), reach statistical significance. Nevertheless, recoveries from desflurane seem to be fastest, but whether the difference is of clinical value has yet to be evaluated. Quality of recovery is of special importance in horses and will be discussed in Chapter 11.

The cardiopulmonary changes induced by equipotent administration of any of the three agents are very similar – all three agents induce similar dose-dependent reductions in cardiac output, blood pressure, systematic vascular resistance (see Fig. 7.2) and respiratory depression. With spontaneous respiration, the circulation is supported by the induced hypercarbia. Differences between the agents may reach statistical significance in one study but not in another, and are unlikely to be of veterinary clinical relevance. All three agents can trigger malignant hyperthermia. None sensitizes the heart to epinephrine-induced arrhythmias.

The major differences between the agents lie in their biotransformation and their chemical stability. The theoretical toxicity from sevoflurane metabolism, or from its reaction with strong base carbon dioxide absorbents has not been found to occur in human or veterinary clinical practice. However, the risk of the absorbent overheating, and/or of the release of carbon monoxide, means that veterinary surgeons should consider using the new non-basic absorbents (see Chapter 10) when administering sevoflurane, and possibly desflurane, in a closed breathing system.

In summary, as long as the necessary apparatus (e.g. a desflurane vaporizer; suitable carbon dioxide absorbent) is available isoflurane, desflurane and sevoflurane are all excellent anaesthetic agents for use in veterinary clinical practice. Sevoflurane is the agent of choice for 'mask' induction but, other than this, and legal requirements allowing, the choice between them is the personal preference of the anaesthetist.

REFERENCES

Alibhai, H.I.K., 2001. Aspects of inhalation anaesthesia in the goat. Thesis for the degree of PhD. Royal Veterinary College, University of London, UK.

Antognini, J.F., Eisele, P.H., 1993. Anesthetic potency and cardiopulmonary effects of enflurane, halothane, and isoflurane in goats. Lab Anim Sci 43, 607–610.

Antognini, J.F., Barter, L., Carstens, E., 2005. Overview movement as an index of anesthetic depth in humans and experimental animals. Comp Med 55, 413–418.

Baker, M.T., 2009. Sevoflurane-Lewis acid stability. Anesth Analg 108, 1725–1726.

Barter, L.S., Ilkiw, J.E., Steffey, E.P., et al., 2004. Animal dependence of inhaled anaesthetic requirements in cats. Br J Anaesth 92, 275–277.

Baum, J.A., Aitkenhead, A.R., 1995. Low-flow anaesthesia. Anaesthesia 50 (Suppl), 37–44.

Baumert, J.-H., 2009. Xenon-based anaesthesia: theory and practice. Open Access Surg 2, 5–13.

Bein, B., 2011. Clinical application of the cardioprotective effects of volatile anaesthetics: PRO – get an extra benefit from a proven anaesthetic free of charge. Eur J Anaesthesiol 28, 620–622.

Benavides, R., Maze, M., Franks, N.P., 2006. Expansion of gas bubbles by nitrous oxide and xenon. Anesthesiology 104, 299–302.

Bergadano, A., Lauber, R., Zbinden, A., et al., 2003. Blood/gas partition coefficients of halothane, isoflurane and sevoflurane in horse blood. Br J Anaesth 91, 276–278.

Blichfeldt-Lauridsen, L., Hansen, B.D., 2012. Anesthesia and myasthenia gravis. Acta Anaesthesiol Scand 56, 17–22.

Bradbrok, C.A., Borer, K.E., Armitage-Chan, E., et al., 2006. A comparison in clinical cases of recovery from anaesthesia following maintenance with desflurane or isoflurane. Proceedings of the 9th World Congress of Veterinary Anaesthesiology, Santos, Brazil.

Brosnan, S., Royston, B., White, D., 1998. Isoflurane concentrations using uncompensated vaporisers within circle systems. Anaesthesia 53, 560–564.

Bunker, J.P., 1968. Final Report of the National Halothane Study. Anesthesiology 29, 231–232.

Bunker, J.P., Forrest, W.H., Mosteller, F., et al., (Eds.), 1969. National Halothane Study. A study of the possible association between halothane anesthesia and post operative hepatic necrosis. Washington DC Government printing office.

Casey, N.D., Chandler, J., Gifford, D., et al., 2005. Microbubble production in an in vitro cardiopulmonary bypass circuit ventilated with xenon. Perfusion 20, 145–150.

Clarke, K.W., 1999. Desflurane and sevoflurane. New volatile anesthetic agents. Vet Clin N Am Small Anim Pract 29, 793–810.

Clarke, K.W., 2008. Options for inhalation anaesthesia. In Practice 30, 513–518.

Clarke, K.W., Song, D.Y., Lee, Y.H., et al., 1996a. Desflurane anaesthesia in the horse; minimum alveolar concentration following induction of anaesthesia with xylazine and ketamine. J Vet Anaesth 23, 56–59.

Clarke, K.W., Song, D.Y., Alibhai, H.I.K., et al., 1996b. Cardiopulmonary effects of desflurane in ponies after induction of anaesthesia with xylazine and ketamine. Vet Rec 139, 180–185.

Constant, I., Seeman, R., Murat, I., 2005. Sevoflurane and epileptiform EEG changes. Paediatr Anaesth 15, 266–274.

De Hert, S.G., Turani, F., Mathur, S., et al., 2005. Cardioprotection with volatile anesthetics: mechanisms and clinical implications. Anesth Analg 100, 1584–1593.

Diana, P., Tullock, W.C., Gorcsan, J., 3rd, et al., 1993. Myocardial ischemia: a comparison between isoflurane and enflurane in coronary artery bypass patients. Anesth Analg 77, 221–226.

Dingley, J., Ivanova-Stoilova, T.M., Grundler, S., et al., 1999. Xenon: recent developments. Anaesthesia 54, 335–346.

Dunlop, C.I., Steffey, E.P., Miller, M.F., et al., 1987. Temporal effects of halothane and isoflurane in laterally recumbent ventilated male horses. Am J Vet Res 48, 1250–1255.

Dunning, M.B., 3rd, Bretscher, L.E., Arain, S.R., et al., 2007. Sevoflurane breakdown produces flammable concentrations of hydrogen. Anesthesiology 106, 144–148.

Ebert, T.J., Muzi, M., 1993. Sympathetic hyperactivity during desflurane anesthesia in healthy volunteers. A comparison with isoflurane. Anesthesiology 79, 444–453.

Ebert, T.J., Harkin, C.P., Muzi, M., 1995. Cardiovascular responses to sevoflurane: a review. Anesth Analg 81, S11–S22.

Eger, E.I., 2nd, 1984. The pharmacology of isoflurane. Br J Anaesth 56 (Suppl 1), 71S–99S.

Eger, E.I., 2nd, 1992. Desflurane animal and human pharmacology: aspects of kinetics, safety, and MAC. Anesth Analg 75, S3–S7; discussion S8–9.

Eger, E.I., 2nd, 1994. New inhaled anesthetics. Anesthesiology 80, 906–922.

Eger, E.I., 2nd, 1995. New drugs in anesthesia. Int Anesthesiol Clin 33, 61–80.

Eger, E.I., 2nd, Johnson, B.H., Weiskopf, R.B., et al., 1988. Minimum alveolar concentration of I-653 and isoflurane in pigs: definition of a supramaximal stimulus. Anesth Analg 67, 1174–1176.

Eger, E.I., 2nd, Xing, Y., Laster, M., et al., 2003. Halothane and isoflurane have additive minimum alveolar concentration (MAC) effects in rats. Anesth Analg 96, 1350–1353.

Elliott, R.H., Strunin, L., 1993. Hepatotoxicity of volatile anaesthetics. Br J Anaesth 70, 339–348.

Fang, Z.X., Eger, E.I., 2nd, Laster, M.J., et al., 1995. Carbon monoxide production from degradation of desflurane, enflurane, isoflurane, halothane, and sevoflurane by soda lime and Baralyme. Anesth Analg 80, 1187–1193.

Fatheree, R.S., Leighton, B.L., 2004. Acute respiratory distress syndrome after an exothermic Baralyme-sevoflurane reaction. Anesthesiology 101, 531–533.

Francis, R.C., Reyle-Hahn, M.S., Hohne, C., et al., 2008. The haemodynamic and catecholamine response to xenon/remifentanil anaesthesia in Beagle dogs. Lab Anim 42, 338–349.

Frink, E.J., Jr., 1995. The hepatic effects of sevoflurane. Anesth Analg 81, S46–S50.

Goto, T., Suwa, K., Uezono, S., et al., 1998. The blood-gas partition coefficient of xenon may be lower than generally accepted. Br J Anaesth 80, 255–256.

Hall, L.W., 1957. Bromochlorotrifluroethane (fluothane); a new volatile anaesthetic agent. Vet Rec 69, 615–618.

Hall, L.W., 1988. Effects of nitrous oxide on respiration during halothane anaesthesia in the dog. Br J Anaesth 60, 207–215.

Hammond, R.A., Alibhai, H.I.K., Walsh, K.P., Clarke, K.W., Holden, D.J., White, R.N., 1994. Desflurane in the dog: minimum alveolar concentration alone and in combination with nitrous oxide. J Vet Anaesth 21, 21–23.

Harris, P.D., Barnes, R., 2008. The uses of helium and xenon in current clinical practice. Anaesthesia 63, 284–293.

Hartman, J.C., Pagel, P.S., Proctor, L.T., et al., 1992. Influence of desflurane, isoflurane and halothane on regional tissue perfusion in dogs. Can J Anaesth 39, 877–887.

Hathout, L., El-Saden, S., 2011. Nitrous oxide-induced B(1)(2) deficiency myelopathy: Perspectives on the clinical biochemistry of vitamin B(1)(2). J Neurol Sci 301, 1–8.

ISSA, 1996. ISSA International Section on Prevention of Occupational Risks in Health Services Safety in the use of anesthetic gases. Consensus paper from the basic German and French documentation. Working document for occupational safety and health specialists ebookbrowse.com/2-consensus-paper-anaesthetic-gases-pdf-d515518 accessed 18/3/13.

Ishiguro, Y., 2001. Cardiovascular effects of xenon. Int Anesthesiol Clin 39, 77–84.

Jevtovic-Todorovic, V., Todorovic, S.M., Mennerick, S., et al., 1998. Nitrous oxide (laughing gas) is an NMDA antagonist, neuroprotectant and neurotoxin. Nat Med 4, 460–463.

Johnston, R.V., Jr, Andrews, J.J., Deyo, D.J., et al., 1994. The effects of carrier gas composition on the performance of the Tec 6 desflurane vaporizer. Anesth Analg 79, 548–552.

Jones, R.M., 1990. Desflurane and sevoflurane: inhalation anaesthetics for this decade? Br J Anaesth 65, 527–536.

Jones, R.M., Nay, P.G., 1994. Desflurane. Anaesth Pharmacol Rev 2, 51–60.

Jordan, B.D., Wright, E.L., 2010. Xenon as an anesthetic agent. AANA J 78, 387–392.

Keller, K.A., Callan, C., Prokocimer, P., et al., 1995. Inhalation toxicity study of a haloalkene degradant of sevoflurane, Compound A (PIFE), in Sprague-Dawley rats. Anesthesiology 83, 1220–1232.

Kenna, J.G., Jones, R.M., 1995. The organ toxicity of inhaled anesthetics. Anesth Analg 81, S51–S66.

Kharasch, E.D., 2008. Adverse drug reactions with halogenated anesthetics. Clin Pharmacol Ther 84, 158–162.

Kharasch, E.D., Schroeder, J.L., Liggitt, H.D., et al., 2006. New insights into the mechanism of methoxyflurane nephrotoxicity and implications for anesthetic development (part 1): Identification of the nephrotoxic metabolic pathway. Anesthesiology 105, 726–736.

Kuratani, N., Oi, Y., 2008. Greater incidence of emergence agitation in children after sevoflurane anesthesia as compared with halothane: a meta-analysis of randomized controlled trials. Anesthesiology 109, 225–232.

Landoni, G., Biondi-Zoccai, G.G., Zangrillo, A., et al., 2007. Desflurane and sevoflurane in cardiac surgery: a meta-analysis of randomized clinical trials. J Cardiothorac Vasc Anesth 21, 502–511.

Leece, E.A., Corletto, F., Brearley, J.C., 2008. A comparison of recovery times and characteristics with sevoflurane and isoflurane anaesthesia in horses undergoing magnetic resonance imaging. Vet Anaesth Analg 35, 383–391.

Lockwood, G., 2002. Expansion of air bubbles in aqueous solutions of nitrous oxide or xenon. Br J Anaesth 89, 282–286.

Lockwood, G.G., Franks, N.P., Downie, N.A., et al., 2006. Feasibility and safety of delivering xenon to patients undergoing coronary artery bypass graft surgery while on cardiopulmonary bypass: phase I study. Anesthesiology 104, 458–465.

Lozano, A.J., Brodbelt, D.C., Borer, K.E., et al., 2009. A comparison of the duration and quality of recovery from isoflurane, sevoflurane and desflurane anaesthesia in dogs undergoing magnetic resonance imaging. Vet Anaesth Analg 36, 220–229.

Lunam, C.A., Cousins, M.J., Hall, P.D., 1985. Guinea-pig model of halothane-associated hepatotoxicity in the absence of enzyme induction and hypoxia. J Pharmacol Exp Ther 232, 802–809.

Lynch, 3rd, C., Baum, J., Tenbrinck, R., 2000. Xenon anesthesia. Anesthesiology 92, 865–868.

Mandal, P.K., Schifilliti, D., Mafrica, F., et al., 2009. Inhaled anesthesia and cognitive performance. Drugs Today 45, 47–54.

Matchett, G.A., Allard, M.W., Martin, R.D., et al., 2009. Neuroprotective effect of volatile anesthetic agents: molecular mechanisms. Neurol Res 31, 128–134.

Matthews, N.S., Hartsfield, S.M., Mercer, D., et al., 1998. Recovery from sevoflurane anesthesia in horses: comparison to isoflurane and effect of postmedication with xylazine. Vet Surg 27, 480–485.

McMurphy, R.M., Hodgson, D.S., 1995. The minimum alveolar concentration of desflurane in cats. Vet Surg 24, 453–455.

Mennerick, S., Jevtovic-Todorovic, V., Todorovic, S.M., et al., 1998. Effect of nitrous oxide on excitatory and inhibitory synaptic transmission in hippocampal cultures. J Neurosci 18, 9716–9726.

Merin, R.G., Bernard, J.M., Doursout, M.F., et al., 1991. Comparison of the effects of isoflurane and desflurane on cardiovascular dynamics and regional blood flow in the chronically instrumented dog. Anesthesiology 74, 568–574.

Mohamadnia, A.R., Hughes, G., Clarke, K.W., 2008. Maintenance of anaesthesia in sheep with isoflurane, desflurane or sevoflurane. Vet Rec 163, 210–215.

Mutoh, T., Nishimura, R., Kim, H.Y., et al., 1997. Cardiopulmonary effects of sevoflurane, compared with halothane, enflurane, and isoflurane, in dogs. Am J Vet Res 58, 885–890.

National Halothane Study, 1969. Edited by Bunker, J.P., Forrest W.H., Mosteller, F., et al., A study of the possible association between halothane anesthesia and postoperative hepatic necrosis. Washington DC Government printing office.

Nickalls, R.W., Mapleson, W.W., 2003. Age-related iso-MAC charts for isoflurane, sevoflurane and desflurane in man. Br J Anaesth 91, 170–174.

Nitahara, K., Sugi, Y., Higa, K., et al., 2007. Neuromuscular effects of sevoflurane in myasthenia gravis patients. Br J Anaesth 98, 337–341.

Peyton, P.J., Chao, I., Weinberg, L., et al., 2011. Nitrous oxide diffusion and the second gas effect on emergence from anesthesia. Anesthesiology 114, 596–602.

Quasha, A.L., Eger, E.I., 2nd, Tinker, J.H., 1980. Determination and applications of MAC. Anesthesiology 53, 315–334.

Sahin, S.H., Cinar, S.O., Paksoy, I., et al., 2011. Comparison between low flow sevoflurane anesthesia and total intravenous anesthesia during intermediate-duration surgery: effects on renal and hepatic toxicity. Hippokratia 15, 69–74.

Sanders, R.D., Maze, M., 2005. Xenon: from stranger to guardian. Curr Opin Anaesth 18, 405–411.

Sanders, R.D., Franks, N.P., Maze, M., 2003. Xenon: no stranger to anaesthesia. Br J Anaesth 91, 709–717.

Schifilliti, D., Grasso, G., Conti, A., et al., 2010. Anaesthetic-related neuroprotection: intravenous or inhalational agents? CNS Drugs 24, 893–907.

Shaughnessy, M.R., Hofmeister, E.H., 2013. A systematic review of sevoflurane and isoflurane minimum alveolar concentration in domestic cats. Vet Anaesth Analg 40, in press.

Smiley, R.M., 1992. An overview of induction and emergence characteristics of desflurane in pediatric, adult, and geriatric patients. Anesth Analg 75, S38–S44; discussion S44–36.

Smith, I., Nathanson, M., White, P.F., 1996. Sevoflurane – a long-awaited volatile anaesthetic. Br J Anaesth 76, 435–445.

Soares, J.H., Brosnan, R.J., Fukushima, F.B., et al., 2012. Solubility of haloether anesthetics in human and animal blood. Anesthesiology 117, 48–55.

Sonner, J.M., Antognini, J.F., Dutton, R.C., et al., 2003. Inhaled anesthetics and immobility: mechanisms, mysteries, and minimum alveolar anesthetic concentration. Anesth Analg 97, 718–740.

Steffey, E.P., 2002. Recent advances in inhalation anesthesia. Vet Clin N Am Equine Pract 18, 159–168.

Steffey, E.P., Hodgson, D.S., Dunlop, C.I., et al., 1987. Cardiopulmonary function during 5 hours of constant-dose isoflurane in laterally recumbent, spontaneously breathing horses. J Vet Pharmacol Ther 10, 290–297.

Steffey, E.P., Mama, K.R., Galey, F.D., et al., 2005a. Effects of sevoflurane dose and mode of ventilation on cardiopulmonary function and blood biochemical variables in horses. Am J Vet Res 66, 606–614.

Steffey, E.P., Woliner, M.J., Puschner, B., et al., 2005b. Effects of desflurane and mode of ventilation on cardiovascular and respiratory functions and clinicopathologic variables in horses. Am J Vet Res 66, 669–677.

Stevens, W.C., 1972. New halogenated anesthetics: enflurane and isoflurane. Calif Med 117, 47.

Van Rompaey, N., Barvais, L., 2011. Clinical application of the cardioprotective effects of volatile anaesthetics: CON – total intravenous anaesthesia or not total intravenous anaesthesia to anaesthetise a cardiac patient? Eur J Anaesthesiol 28, 623–627.

Wade, J.G., Stevens, W.C., 1981. Isoflurane: an anesthetic for the eighties? Anesth Analg 60, 666–682.

Wagner, A.E., Dunlop, C.I., Wertz, E.M., et al., 1995. Hemodynamic responses of horses to anesthesia and surgery, before and after administration of a low dose of endotoxin. Vet Surg 24, 78–85.

Weiskopf, R.B., Moore, M.A., Eger, E.I., 2nd, et al., 1994. Rapid increase in desflurane concentration is associated with greater transient cardiovascular stimulation than with rapid increase in isoflurane concentration in humans. Anesthesiology 80, 1035–1045.

White, P.F., 1992. Studies of desflurane in outpatient anesthesia. Anesth Analg 75, S47–S53; discussion S53–44.

WHO, 2010. World Health Organisation's list of core medicines (WHO, 2010). http://www.who.int/medicines/publications/essentialmedicines/en/index.html.

Wu, J., Previte, J.P., Adler, E., et al., 2004. Spontaneous ignition, explosion, and fire with sevoflurane and barium hydroxide lime. Anesthesiology 101, 534–537.

Yagi, M., Mashimo, T., Kawaguchi, T., et al., 1995. Analgesic and hypnotic effects of subanaesthetic concentrations of xenon in human volunteers: comparison with nitrous oxide. Br J Anaesth 74, 670–673.

Young, W.L., 1992. Effects of desflurane on the central nervous system. Anesth Analg 75, S32–S37.

Zhang, P., Ohara, A., Mashimo, T., et al., 1995. Pulmonary resistance in dogs: a comparison of xenon with nitrous oxide. Can J Anaesth 42, 547–553.

Chapter | 8 |

Relaxation of the skeletal muscles

INTRODUCTION

To relax skeletal muscles, it is necessary to abolish voluntary muscle contractions and modify the slight tension, which is the normal state (the 'tone' or 'tonus' of the muscle). Tone is maintained by many complex mechanisms but, briefly, it can be said that all result in the slow asynchronous discharge of impulses from cells in the ventral horn region of the spinal cord. This discharge gives rise to impulses in the motor neurons, which cause the muscle fibres to contract. Activity of these ventral horn cells is controlled by impulses from the higher centres (cerebrum, cerebellum, or medulla oblongata) exciting the motor neuron direct, or by impulses through the small motor nerve fibre system (the γ-efferents) which activate them indirectly via the stretch reflex arc. Movements controlled by the γ-fibre system are essentially directed towards governing the length of the muscle. In contrast, voluntary movement involving direct activity in the γ-fibres, results in muscle tension of a given magnitude. The small motor nerve fibre system is, like the motor fibres to the skeletal muscles themselves, a cholinergic one and any drug which can affect the neuromuscular junction may also interfere with the effect of the γ-fibres on the muscle spindles, thus reducing the afferent inflow from the muscle spindles to the brainstem. Thus, there is a possibility that a drug, which paralyses the γ-fibres and so reduces muscle spindle proprioceptive inflow to the higher centres, actually contributes to a sleep-like state.

Relaxation using agents which act centrally

Centrally acting drugs, such as guaiphenesin and benzodiazepines, produce muscle relaxation by selectively depressing the transmission of impulses at the internuncial neurons of the spinal cord, brainstem and subcortical regions of the brain, but the relaxation produced by them is seldom profound. Some degree of muscle relaxation can also be produced by the α$_2$-adrenoceptor agonists.

Most anaesthetic agents cause decreased activity of ventral horn cells in the spinal cord, and thus muscle relaxation, although there is variation between agents in the degree of relaxation produced at a given 'plane' of anaesthesia. In general (with a few exceptions such as ether anaesthesia), profound muscle relaxation from general anaesthetic agents is obtained only when doses are such to produce a deep generalized depression of the whole central nervous system with accompanying dose-dependent depression of the cardiovascular and respiratory systems.

Utilizing drugs which have a peripheral action

Local analgesics injected so as to block the transmission of impulses in motor nerves result in profound muscle relaxation. This is demonstrated strikingly by paravertebral nerve block in cattle, and also following the use of epidural analgesia where the motor nerves are blocked as they leave the spinal cord. The major disadvantage is that the motor block may last longer than desired, and can be a problem at recovery in large animals. Combinations of local analgesia and general anaesthesia are used frequently. Peripheral nerve blocks such as brachial plexus, femoral or epidural blocks, provide excellent intraoperative analgesia, prevent wind-up in the dorsal horn cells of the spinal cord and can thus make a marked contribution to postoperative pain control, and have the added advantage of providing excellent muscle relaxation.

Using specific neuromuscular blocking agents

Modern neuromuscular blocking agents (NMBA) act at the neuromuscular junction, and by their use it is possible to produce quickly, and with certainty, any degree of muscle relaxation by neuromuscular block (NMB) without influencing the excitability and functioning of the central nervous and cardiovascular systems. They are commonly called 'muscle relaxants' or simply 'relaxants'. They do not cross the blood–brain barrier and thereby have no direct action on the central nervous system.

In order that the mode of action of NMBAs be understood, it is essential that the phenomena which occur at the neuromuscular junction upon the arrival of an impulse in the motor nerve should be appreciated. The following brief review of neuromuscular transmission is concerned with those aspects that are of importance in anaesthesia. For a more detailed study, reference should be made to the standard texts of physiology, and the reviews cited below.

THEORY OF NEUROMUSCULAR TRANSMISSION

The neuromuscular junction is the most accessible of the synapses in the body to study and over the last 100 years very much has been revealed about it. Broadly, motor nerve endings contain vesicles of acetylcholine that are released as a result of an action potential in the nerve. After release, the acetylcholine diffuses across the synaptic gap (cleft) and interacts with nicotinic acetylcholine receptors (nAChRs) embedded in the postjunctional membrane of the muscle, directly opposite the sites of its release (the end plates), triggering the chain of events leading to muscle contraction. The acetylcholine is immediately broken down by acetylcholinesterase, which is situated in the synaptic cleft. However, within this synaptic transmission system, there are many processes involved which have been further elucidated or which still await explanation. Martyn et al. (2009) have reviewed recent knowledge of clinical relevance.

Release of acetylcholine

Acetylcholine is synthesized in the nerve cytoplasm by choline acetyl-O-transferase and must be pumped into vesicles (each containing a 'quantum') against its concentration gradient. The vesicles are situated close to the junctional surface. An action potential in the motor nerve triggers the opening of voltage-gated Ca^{2+}-channels, calcium enters the nerve terminal, and the increase in intracellular calcium initiates a very rapid series of events terminating in the exocytotic release of quanta of acetylcholine into the synaptic cleft. Electron microscopy shows small protein particles in the active zone of the nerve endings between the vesicles, and it is thought that these are the Ca^{2+} channels. Abnormalities of some of these proteins have been identified as causing loss of function therefore potentially reduced acetylcholine release and muscle weakness. Ca^{2+} does not directly cause the vesicles to release their acetylcholine, but initiates their exocytosis via a complex protein fusion pathway (Jones, 1984; Lang & Jahn, 2008).

The amount of acetylcholine (number of quanta) released is very dependent on the concentration of ionized extracellular calcium, evidence suggesting that it is proportional to the fourth power of the change in Ca^{2+} concentration. Ca^{2+} continues to flow into the nerve terminal until the outflow of potassium returns the membrane potential to normal. The build-up of calcium within the nerve terminal explains the condition of 'post-tetanic potentiation' seen when the degree of effect a non-depolarizing NMBA is tested by stimulating the nerve with high tetanic frequencies (see 'monitoring block' below). Under these conditions, intracellular calcium increases, and remains

higher than normal for some time. A stimulus applied during this time evokes a greater than normal release of acetylcholine which, in turn, antagonizes the non-depolarizing NMB.

A number of clinically relevant factors may interfere with this complex Ca^{2+} and/or protein mechanism. High extracellular concentrations of magnesium inhibit calcium entry into the cell, thus resulting in muscle weakness. Ca^{2+} antagonists, such as verapamil, may act by inhibiting protein combinations. In dogs, a dose of 1 mg/kg of verapamil has been shown to produce a significant interaction with the non-depolarizing agent, pancuronium, which persists long beyond the period of the calcium antagonist's cardiac effects (Jones, 1984). Clostridial toxins exert their effects by damaging the proteins involved in the exocytotic process. Inhalation anaesthetics may be considered to be non-specific calcium antagonists and so potentiate neuromuscular blockade.

Acetylcholinesterase is an enzyme that is secreted by the muscle and is located in large amounts in the synaptic cleft of the end-plate. It hydrolyses acetylcholine (to choline and acetate) very rapidly, thus terminating the muscle contraction. Choline is taken up into the nerve terminal and used to synthesize more acetylcholine.

Effector mechanisms (nicotinic acetylcholine receptors (nAChRs))

Muscle contraction is initiated by acetylcholine released at the neuromuscular junction acting on the nAChRs on the end-plate at the neuromuscular junction. All nicotinic receptors so far isolated and characterized, function as cation channels, the activation of which causes a change in postjunctional membrane potential. Thus, they behave in a similar manner to receptors for other known chemical transmitters and belong to a family of closely related receptors (5-HT3 receptor, $GABA_A$ receptor, glycine receptor and kainate-type glutamate receptor). The common element in this receptor family is that the receptors consist of five glycosylated protein subunits of varying molecular type. Each of the subunits traverses the muscle membrane at the end-plate region and they are arranged to form the walls of an aqueous pore representing the ion channel through which mainly sodium and potassium ions flow to produce the single channel current measurable by the physiologists' patch-clamping technique. The subunits have been designated α, β, γ, δ and ε with further subdivisions given numbers. In the postsynaptic nAChRs in the end-plates of mature skeletal muscle there are two α1, and one each of β, δ and ε. The neurotransmitter acetylcholine must bind to sites on two α subunits for the ion channel to open, produce the single channel current and initiate muscle contraction. Non-depolarizing NMBAs also attach to these sites so, if even one α subunit is occupied, acetylcholine cannot bind to two and open the channel. In fetal muscle, the ε is 'replaced' by a γ (hence termed the γ-subunit). Although some change from fetal to adult receptors occurs before birth, further conversion continues in the neonatal period. Mature receptors are situated at or very close to the neuromuscular junction, but the fetal γ-subunit may be more widely spread over the muscle surface. In clinical cases of immobility (e.g. by burns or denervation), mature receptors revert to the γ-subunit and also become more widely distributed over the muscle surface – this process commences within hours of immobility so can be a factor in many situations, although it may take days to complete. The clinical importance is the different responses of the two types of receptors to NMBAs. The γ-subunits show long opening times. This makes them very sensitive indeed to depolarizing agents, such as suxamethonium, not only to the relaxant effects, but also for the release of potassium. However, they are very resistant to non-depolarizing NMBAs. The changes in these receptor subtypes (and also other variations, for example α7, a further subtype thought to be of importance and currently under investigation) may explain unexpected differences in response to NMBAs of some patients.

Presynaptic nAChRs are present on the nerve terminal and have an influence on normal neuromuscular transmission. Although different types have been identified pharmacologically, their types in relation to action are not as clear as for the postsynaptic receptors. However, one acts as a positive feedback and responds to low concentrations of acetylcholine by facilitating its release at the end-plate while the second group (or effect), which contain α3β2 units, respond to a high concentration of acetylcholine and act in a negative feedback mechanism. This negative feedback, i.e. the increase in acetylcholine in the synaptic cleft leading to a decrease in further acetylcholine release, is thought to be the cause of post-tetanic fade and train of four (TOF) fade (see 'Monitoring' below) with non-depolarizing NMBAs. Suxamethonium does not stimulate the α3β2 receptor and with a single dose of this agent, TOF fade is not seen, although it will occur if there is a Phase II block (see below).

Other influences on the neuromuscular receptor

General anaesthetics, local analgesics and antibiotics are all potential causes of end-plate ion channel block.

A remarkable property known as 'desensitization' is displayed by the acetylcholine receptor of striated muscle and its associated systems. This was first described by Katz & Thesleff in 1957, and appears as the waning of a stimulant effect or development of repolarization (usually partial but under some circumstances complete) despite the continued presence of acetylcholine or some other depolarizing substance at the end-plate. The rate of this repolarization increases with the concentration of the drug and

is faster when the extracellular concentration of Ca^{2+} is high. The extent of desensitization appears to vary between individuals of any one species. Acetylcholine has been shown to change the affinity of the receptor for certain blocking agents in a way which may be connected with the desensitization process.

NEUROMUSCULAR BLOCK

Consideration of the mechanisms of neuromuscular transmission outlined above suggests many ways in which the process may be modified to produce failure or block of transmission. There are two types of NMBAs, the non-depolarizing and the depolarizing, with very differing properties.

Non-depolarizing NMBs (competitive)

Non-depolarizing NMBs are also termed competitive, curare-like or antagonist NMBs. All non-depolarizing NMBAs block transmission by attaching to the nAChRs, where they themselves exert no direct action. However, even by blocking one α site, they prevent the acetylcholine released following motor nerve stimulation competitively from causing depolarization of the postsynaptic membrane. When the reduction in the degree of depolarization is such that a threshold depolarization of the membrane adjacent to the end-plate is not achieved, a neuromuscular block is present. As the effect is 'all or none' for each motor end-plate, what is seen in any particular muscle during this type of block represents a spectrum of these thresholds. For complete suppression of the motor response to occur, even the most resistant synapses must be blocked. In normal neuromuscular transmission, an excess of acetylcholine is produced by motor nerve stimulation. There also exist many more receptors than necessary for the production of a total increase in cation conductance required to trigger an action potential. This results in a substantial 'safety factor' (Jones, 1984). It has been shown that under certain conditions in cat tibialis muscle, four to five times as much acetylcholine is released as is needed for threshold action. Expressed in terms of receptors this means that 75–80% of the receptors must be occluded before the threshold is reached (Cookson & Paton, 1969). The existence of a safety factor means that the action of the drug is far from terminated at the time when transmission is apparently normal. There is likely to be considerable 'subthreshold action' which is only detectable when a tetanic stimulus is applied to the motor nerve or when the relaxant action of some other drug is potentiated.

As discussed above, acetylcholine is normally metabolized very rapidly by the acetylcholinesterase in the synaptic cleft, thus enabling the non-depolarizing NMBA to occupy the receptor. The use of an anticholinesterase, such as neostigmine, slows the metabolism of acetylcholine, increases the number of molecules available in the synaptic cleft, and therefore 'shifts' the competitive balance in favour of acetylcholine for occupancy of the receptors. This is the basis of reversal of NMB with neostigmine. However, it must be remembered that the increase in acetylcholine will also act on the muscarinic receptors causing a number of side effects and, as long as the NMBA remains in the synaptic cleft (time depending on the metabolism of individual NMBA), there will remain a degree of NMB.

Depolarizing NMB (non-competitive)

Suxamethonium (also termed succinylcholine) and decamethonium (now only used for research purposes) are examples of depolarizing NMBAs. Suxamethonium's structure is that of two molecules of acetylcholine. It works first as an agonist, binding to the muscle nAChRs, depolarizing the end-plate, and therefore triggering muscle contraction, which usually manifests as generalized fasciculation. However, in contrast to acetylcholine that has a rapidly terminated action (ms), with suxamethonium the end-plate remains depolarized until the drug is removed from the plasma, by plasma (pseudo) cholinesterases. Relaxation occurs because the membrane remains depolarized and non-responsive to further stimulation (Burns & Paton, 1951). As discussed above, the depolarizing drugs do not affect the $\alpha3\beta2$ receptor so, with a single relatively small dose, tetanic or TOF fade does not occur, or occurs only minimally. The depolarizing NMBA, however, will affect some other nAChRs and muscarinic acetylcholine receptors, with resultant multiple side effects. In this phase (Phase I) of a depolarizing NMB, use of anticholinesterase to increase available acetylcholine will augment the NMB.

The above simplistic description of the depolarizing NMB does not explain the condition known as Phase II (dual) block that occurs if a suxamethonium NMB is continued for longer than a single short acting dose. Lee (2009) has reviewed the practical aspects of this block, but the actual mechanism is not yet fully understood. The condition as it occurs with infusion of suxamethonium is that, following the standard Phase I block when there is minimal tetanic or TOF fade, there is then a period of tachyphylaxis, whereby a much higher dose of suxamethonium appears to be required before reaching the Phase II block. The Phase II block behaves as if it were a non-depolarizing block, there is tetanic and TOF fade, presumed to be through the same presynaptic feedback mechanism that occurs in the standard non-depolarizing NMBA block; in some but not all stages there can be partial (but not total) reversal by the use of anticholinesterase, and the block is massively increased by very small doses of non-depolarizing NMBAs. Once a Phase II block is established, the duration is very prolonged, and it is for

this reason that suxamethonium is no longer used by infusion or incremental doses. However, a Phase II block can occur with a single dose if sufficiently large, and the anaesthetist should be aware of its existence.

PATTERN OF NEUROMUSCULAR BLOCK

Sensitivity of muscles to neuromuscular block

The concept of sensitivity refers to the concentration of drug at the neuromuscular junction needed to produce a specific degree of blockade. Different muscles have different sensitivities to NMB. The standard often quoted order from most sensitive (lowest doses needed) onward is muscles of facial expression, jaw, tail, neck and distal limbs, proximal limbs, laryngeal/pharyngeal, abdominal wall, intercostal, then most resistant, the diaphragm. It is unlikely that this order is true for all animals and all NMBAs. Whilst Sarrafzadeh-Rezaei & Clutton (2009) found that, in anaesthetized dogs, the nasaolabialis muscles were more sensitive to a vecuronium block than the carpal flexor muscles, but also pointed out that all facial muscles do not have the same sensitivity. Clutton (2007), for small animals, disagrees with the classical list in that he places the diaphragm as being more sensitive than the limbs, although dogs may still breathe through actions of the intercostal muscles. There is considerable evidence that, in horses, the limb muscles are far more sensitive, at least to the onset of NMBAs, than are some of the superficial facial muscles often used for monitoring block (Hildebrand et al., 1986; Mosing et al., 2010).

There are several practical aspects to the potential differences in sensitivity. The first is to find a suitable site for monitoring the NMB by nerve stimulation (see 'Monitoring of neuromuscular block', below). If a very sensitive site is chosen, then a full block may be registered there, while the block of the muscles that the surgeon requires is not optimal. More importantly for recovery, monitoring at a very insensitive site might suggest good reversal of NMB when many important muscles are still at least partially paralysed. The other major use made of differences in muscle sensitivities is to attempt to use low dose NMBAs to achieve relaxation of some muscles while still enabling the animal to breathe spontaneously. Currently, this is most used in the dog in order to keep the eye central and still for ocular surgery. Although the dog may continue to breathe, there is likely to be diaphragmatic and costal muscle weakness that will impair ventilation, increase arterial carbon dioxide, and limit any possible ventilatory response to hypoxia. These authors strongly recommend that the dogs are artificially ventilated, if only to obtain the best ventilatory and cardiovascular conditions necessary for good intraocular surgery.

In human anaesthesia, there are many studies investigating the relative sensitivity of nerve/muscle groups which are used for monitoring NMB in relation to the diaphragm or to other muscles in which it is particularly important to avoid postanaesthetic residual block (e.g. the larynx). Similar investigations in veterinary medicine have been limited. Also, there is still little understanding of the mechanisms underlying the cause of differing muscle sensitivities. Among the mechanisms suggested as being responsible for differing responses are:

1. Perfusion

This is important in relation to onset of action, as NMB can only be produced when the drug binds with acetylcholine receptors at the neuromuscular junction (Donati, 1988). For the onset phase, concentration gradients between the plasma and the receptors are large and thus perfusion plays a major part in the development of neuromuscular block. During recovery from block, plasma concentration changes slowly with time, so that the concentration gradient between plasma and receptors on the different muscles is likely to be small. As a result, perfusion plays only a minor role, duration of blockade being determined mainly by plasma concentration and sensitivity of each muscle.

2. Acetylcholine receptor numbers, distribution and type

The motor innervation pattern of muscles, acetylcholinesterase activity and number and density of receptors at end-plate regions may all play a part, but it is not known exactly how these may contribute to muscle sensitivity to neuromuscular blocking drugs.

3. Fibre and end-plate size in the muscle

In goats, there is a direct association between time to spontaneous recovery from vecuronium or suxamethonium blockade and size of fibres in the diaphragm, posterior cricoarytenoideus, thyroarytenoideus and ulnaris lateralis muscles (Ibebunjo & Hall, 1993). This evidence for influence of fibre size is supported by the fact that laryngeal and facial muscles contain very small fibres while larger fibres are found in the diaphragm and still larger ones in peripheral muscles, a rank order identical to the relative sensitivities of these muscles to neuromuscular block (Donati et al., 1990). Subsequent similar work (Ibebunjo et al., 1996) found that recovery was shortest in the laryngeal muscles and longest in the abdominal muscles, and that this correlated directly with fibre size and inversely with end-plate/fibre size ratio. They concluded that, in the goat, recovery from NMB was shortest in muscles composed of small fibres with large end-plates. Incidentally, in this study, there was no difference in relative muscle sensitivity to depolarizing or non-depolarizing NMBAs.

MONITORING OF NEUROMUSCULAR BLOCK

Knowledge of the degree of NMB is necessary to ensure that the block is adequate for the procedures but, more importantly, to monitor recovery and to be as certain as possible that no residual NMB remains once the person/animal regains consciousness and is no longer being ventilated. In human anaesthesia, inadequate reversal of NMB leads, among other side effects, to inadequate ventilation, impaired hypoxic respiratory response, laryngeal weakness and airway obstruction (Fink & Hollmann, 2012). The same problems can be anticipated to occur in veterinary patients. In the authors' previous experience when only long acting NMBAs were available and monitoring techniques were not, in dogs post-block laryngeal weakness could be a serious problem. In horses, ensuring that limb muscles have returned to normal strength is a prerequisite for a good quality recovery.

In many places, in human and veterinary anaesthesia, degree of NMB is assessed subjectively from the responses of the patient. However, the advent of monitoring by the response to peripheral nerve stimulation enables a more objective, and therefore much safer assessment of onset, depth and recovery from NMB.

Peripheral nerve stimulation

Simple peripheral nerve stimulators (Fig. 8.1) are readily available. However, when monitoring NMB by peripheral nerve stimulation, it is necessary consider the following:

- The site of stimulation
- The strength and the pattern of stimulation
- How to assess the muscle contraction. This can be
  - Subjective
  - Quantitative
    - acceleromyography
    - mechanomyography
    - electromyography.

Site of stimulation

The requirement is a superficially placed motor nerve with easy access that innervates a muscle with contraction that can be observed/monitored, and the movement of which will not be detrimental to surgery. It is important to avoid accidental direct stimulation of the muscle. In humans, the site most used is the ulnar nerve to the adductor pollicis, movement of the thumb being observed/measured. As the NMB differs between different muscles, a specific

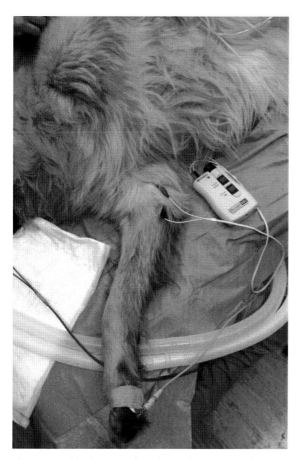

Figure 8.1 This shows a relatively simple nerve stimulator, capable of delivering a range of different stimulation patterns, which is used to monitor neuromuscular block. The needles are placed over the ulnar nerve, approximately 2-4 cm apart. On stimulation, presence or absence of movement of the paw can be seen. The lead on the paw is, in fact, an ECG lead, but the position is where the sensor for acceleromyography would be placed.
Photograph courtesy of Hatim IK Alibhai.

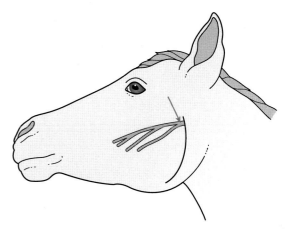

Figure 8.2 One suitable site for stimulation of the facial nerve in the horse.

A number of different nerve/muscle combinations have been employed for assessment of NMB. In horses, the facial nerve (Fig. 8.2) can be palpated on the masseter muscle ventral to the lateral canthus of the eye and, when this is stimulated, produces easily visible contractions of the muscles of the lip and nostrils. The peroneal nerve can be stimulated as it crosses the head of the fibula to produce contractions of the digital extensor muscles (Fig 8.3; see also Fig. 8.7). It is advisable to restrain the hind leg when this nerve is stimulated even if no mechanical recording of the response is proposed. Mosing et al. (2010) describe location of the radial nerve in the non-dependent limb by palpation of the groove between the lateral extensor digitorum and the lateral ulnaris muscles, approximately 4 cm (in Shetland ponies) distal to the lateral tuberosity of the radius. In dogs, muscle responses to electrical stimulation of the ulnar, tibial, peroneal and facial nerves have been reported in many studies. The ulnar nerve is stimulated at its most superficial location on the medial aspect of the elbow and contraction involving the forepaw is assessed visually by palpation or by acceleromyography (see Fig. 8.1). The peroneal nerve is stimulated on the lateral aspect of the stifle and muscle twitch of the hind foot assessed; this site is particularly useful when the head end of the animal is covered, for example during ocular surgery. Peroneal nerve stimulation has been used in the assessment of neuromuscular block in cows, calves, llamas and pigs.

Strength and pattern of stimulation

The observed muscle response following stimulation of a peripheral nerve is only reliable when one electrical stimulus causes the nerve to depolarize, the same number of nerve fibres are stimulated each time, and direct stimulation of muscle fibres is avoided. After a nerve has been

measured result may differ depending on site. This was well demonstrated in a study in Shetland ponies (Mosing et al., 2010) in which the peroneal, the radial and the facial nerves (to the orbicularis orbis muscle) were stimulated, the response being measured by acceleromyography. Following injection of 0.6 mg/kg rocuronium, within the 5-minute measuring period before reversal with sugammadex (see Evoked recovery from NMB below), a full block did not occur in the orbicularis oculi, but did in the limb muscles. This finding is similar to those of previous studies in horses, where muscles stimulated by the peroneal nerve show greater sensitivity to NMBAs than muscles innervated by the facial nerve (Manley et al., 1983; Hildebrand & Arpin, 1988).

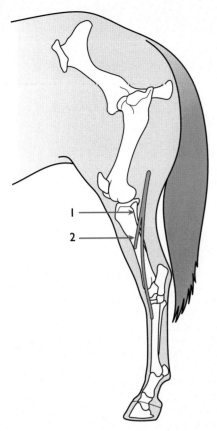

Figure 8.3 Site for stimulation of the peroneal nerve in the horse. The nerve crosses the shaft of the tibia just distal to the head of the fibula and is often palpable at this site in thin-skinned horses.

depolarized to produce an action potential, it is resistant to further stimulation for its refractory period of some 0.5–1.0 ms. Most clinically available peripheral nerve stimulators (see Fig. 8.1) will deliver all of the various stimulation patterns described below. These patterns and their responses have been well illustrated by Viby-Mogensen (2010). A supramaximal stimulus is essential to ensure that all the muscle fibres in the effector muscle contract. With the majority of stimulators, this is achieved at a 'calibration' test prior to administering the NMBA. This generally involves the anaesthetist increasing the current until the maximal muscle contraction is achieved, although some units can self-calibrate. In recent publications on NMB monitoring in horses, currents in the region of 40–60 mA have been employed (Mosing et al., 2010). Supramaximal stimulation can be achieved using surface or needle electrodes; paediatric ECG silver/silver chloride gel electrodes are excellent provided the underlying skin is properly prepared (clipping and cleaning with alcohol). However, in veterinary anaesthesia, needle electrodes are

often preferred, especially in animals with thick skin. It is recommended that the negative electrode of the stimulator is placed distally, and skin temperature (for surface electrodes) should be kept >32°C as hypothermia increases electrical impedance (Fuchs-Buder et al., 2009).

A number of different 'stimulation patterns' are in use, each having advantages/disadvantages under different circumstances. It must be remembered that, as explained earlier (release of acetylcholine), 'fade' following multiple stimulations occurs only with a non-depolarizing or a Phase II block, and is not a feature of a Phase I depolarizing block. This is because at the early stages of recovery, a non-depolarizing block can be partly antagonized by an increase in acetylcholine. The classical theory is that tetanic or multiple stimulations decrease available acetylcholine, probably both by depleting the acetylcholine available for release but also by reducing further acetylcholine release through the negative feedback system. In contrast, a depolarizing block is not antagonized by acetylcholine; hence the absence of fade.

For all patterns, characteristics of the stimulation is usually the same, a monophasic impulse, duration 0.2 ms and rectangular wave form (Fuchs-Buder et al., 2009).

The single twitch

Single twitch stimulation at frequencies of 0.1–1 Hz has been used extensively to investigate effects of NBAs in human subjects. At a stimulus frequency greater than about 0.15 Hz, the response becomes progressively smaller (i.e. fade) owing to the presynaptic 'feedback' effects impairing further release of acetylcholine. Using a single stimulation, a 'control' twitch is needed prior to giving the NMBA for comparison of subsequent twitches.

While repetitive stimuli at a frequency of <0.05 Hz causes fade, there is also a condition known as the 'staircase phenomenon' whereby, in the absence of NMBAs, repetitive stimuli over time potentiate the mechanical response of the muscle, i.e. the twitch size increases, until a point in time where the response appears to stabilize. Both single twitches, 1 Hz every second for 10 minutes, and TOF (see below) pattern, 15-second intervals for 15 minutes, have been shown to cause this, while a tetanic stimulation prior to such stimulation reduced the effect (Kopman et al., 2001). Martin-Flores et al. (2011b) demonstrated that the 'staircase' also occurred in dogs, and that approximately 25 minutes of stimulation was required to obtain an acceptably stable baseline. The clinical importance of this phenomenon is that the anaesthetist must be aware that an increasing 'baseline' of twitch might be occurring throughout the early intraoperative period of monitoring and thus introduce a bias into the subsequent results.

The single twitch is used primarily to assess the speed on onset of NMB. It is of less use for monitoring recovery as it depends on comparison with the pre-NMB twitch, impossible to judge visually and even with measurement, such as acceleromyography, the 'staircase effect' may make the result unreliable.

Train-of-four

Since its description by Ali et al. (1970), the TOF (four pulses at 2.0 Hz) has become the most popular of the methods available to the clinical anaesthetist to monitor competitive NMB. The method involves recording four twitch responses evoked in a muscle by supramaximal stimulation of its motor nerve at a rate of 2 Hz, with an interval of at least 10 seconds (15 seconds is more usually employed) between trains to avoid 'fade' between successive trains of stimuli.

With no NMB, all four twitches should be of equal height. Loss of the fourth response represents 75–80% NMB; loss of twitches 3, 2 and 1 represent 85%, 90% and 98–100% block, respectively. The twitch–height ratio, height (amplitude) of the fourth response (T4) divided by the height of the first (T1) is known as the TOF ratio (Fig. 8.4). With a complete NMB, the TOF ratio will be 0, as T1 will be 0; with complete recovery (or pre-block), the TOF ratio should be 1, i.e. the fourth twitch will be at the same height as the first. In human anaesthesia, it is considered that a TOF ratio of 0.7 means adequate diaphragmatic recovery, but it requires recovery to TOF of 0.9 for return of adequate laryngeal/pharyngeal function, and a TOF of 0.9 is now usually taken as the being acceptable level of recovery from NMB. In veterinary anaesthesia, there is no reason to accept less and, for large animals that require perfect muscle function for recovery, a TOF of 1 would be preferable.

Practically, the major advantage of the TOF is that for normal clinical use it is not necessary to establish a control response before the administration of the NMB. In veterinary anaesthesia, the TOF is now used routinely both clinically and in research studies to assess the recovery from NMB in a large number of species.

Double burst stimulation (DBS)

The DBS consists of two short lasting bursts of tetanus (2–4 pulses at 50 Hz) separated by 0.75 seconds. The interval of 0.75 seconds allows the muscle to relax completely between tetanic bursts, so that response to this pattern of stimulation is two single separated muscle contractions perceived as two twitches. The tetanic bursts fatigue the neuromuscular synapse more than two single twitches so that fade is exaggerated during the second burst. Several different combinations of tetanic stimulation have been used but the pattern known as DBS3,3, or DBS3,2 seem satisfactory (Fig. 8.5). The larger response to DBS means that the first response reappears just before that from TOF stimulation and the second response occurs slightly before the fourth response to TOF (Gill et al., 1990). A fading second response is comparable with TOF ratio <0.6 (Fuchs-Bader et al., 2009). DBS was designed to improve clinical detection of residual curarization because it is easier to compare visually or tactilely the strength of the two contractions to DBS than to compare the strength of the first and fourth contractions with TOF ratio.

Tetanic stimulation and post-tetanic count

Repetitive high frequency stimulation of the motor nerve where the responses to individual stimuli fuse and

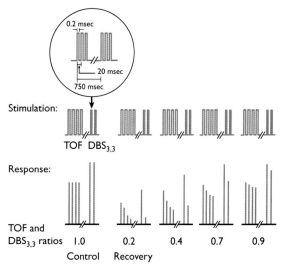

Figure 8.5 Stimulation patterns and muscle response at various degrees of non-depolarizing neuromuscular block. The stimulation pattern shown is a TOF followed by a double burst. At partial recovery, the difference in the degree of 'fade' at partial recovery is more obvious with visual monitoring of movement with the double burst.
From JørgenViby-Mogensen. 2010. Neuromuscular monitoring. In: Miller, R.D., Eriksson, L.I., Fleisher, L.A., et al. (Eds.), Miller's Anesthesia, seventh ed. Churchill Livingstone Elsevier, Philadelphia, with permission.

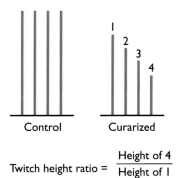

$$\text{Twitch height ratio} = \frac{\text{Height of 4}}{\text{Height of 1}}$$

Figure 8.4 Pattern of responses to TOF stimulation during recovery from non-depolarizing neuromuscular block. Twitch height calculated as percentage inhibition of first response to TOF stimulation.

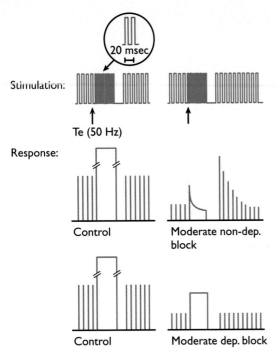

Figure 8.6 Stimulation pattern and evoked responses before and after a moderate neuromuscular block with non-depolarizing and depolarizing NMBAs. The stimulation pattern shown consisted of a series of single stimuli, followed by a 5 second tetanic burst (50 Hz), then a further series of single stimuli. Note the fade in tetanic response with the non-depolarizing block and the subsequent post-tetanic potentiation. With the depolarizing block there is no fade in tetanic response and no post-tetanic potentiation.

From JørgenViby-Mogensen, 2010. Neuromuscular monitoring. In: Miller, R.D., Eriksson, L.I., Fleisher, L.A., et al. (Eds.), Miller's Anesthesia, seventh ed. Churchill Livingstone Elsevier, Philadelphia, with permission.

summate to produce a sustained muscle contraction causes what is known as 'tetany'. The absence or presence of fade due to presynaptic effect of non-depolarizing (but not with a depolarizing – see above) blockade has been used to assess adequacy of recovery in order to judge whether any clinically significant blockade persists (Fig. 8.6). Most usually, a tetanic stimulation of 50 Hz for 5 seconds is employed, after which it may be possible to decide, by visual, tactile or more objective means, whether there is any fade in response to this tetanic stimulation.

A sustained tetanus correlates with a TOF ratio of 0.7 or greater.

As described earlier (release of acetylcholine), as well as the 'fade' during stimulation, in the presence of an NMBA, the transmitter substance released following tetanic stimulation can cause the magnitude of response to a subsequent stimulus to be enhanced. This is termed post-tetanic

facilitation or potentiation (see Fig. 8.6). The effect increases with the duration and frequency of tetanic stimulus and can persist for up to 30 minutes. It can lead to underestimation of neuromuscular block and, to avoid it, it is necessary to delay further tetanic stimulation for at least two minutes (Brull et al., 1991). However, during profound neuromuscular blockade when all responses to single twitch, TOF and tetanic stimulation have been abolished, post-tetanic facilitation following a tetanic burst may allow responses to occur with single twitch stimulation. Post-tetanic count (PTC) is the number of responses to 1 Hz stimulation 3 seconds after a 5 second 50 Hz tetanus (Fuchs-Buder et al., 2009). The number of post-tetanic responses is inversely related to depth of blockade; the smaller the PTC the deeper the neuromuscular block. The major use of this mode of stimulus is to assure that block is total, as the PTC returns before the TOF during recovery from a non-depolarizing block.

Assessment of muscle contraction

Subjectively

Visual or tactile assessment of muscle contraction following peripheral nerve stimulation is the most common method of assessing NMB, both in human and veterinary clinical practice. Although clinically it is adequate to ensure that the NMB is present or that any residual block is only weak, it almost invariably underestimates the degree of residual block in recovery. Some authorities consider that it is inaccurate once the TOF exceeds 0.4, but certainly it cannot distinguish between a TOF of 0.7 (still a clinically relevant degree of NMB) and 1 (Fuchs-Bader et al., 2009). In a study in anaesthetized horses, Martin Flores et al. (2008) compared visual assessment of TOF with acceleromyography, and demonstrated that while both demonstrated onset of block equally, visual assessment suggested that TOF was 1 (i.e. no residual NMB), a median of 12 (range 8–42) minutes before acceleromyography registered a TOF of 0.9. Thus, tactile and visual assessment of twitch is too subjective for research studies into NMB agents or their antagonists, and must also be used with care in situations, such as in horses, where even slight residual block can be dangerous.

Acceleromyography

This involves simple equipment that is practicable to use in clinics. Unfortunately, the units are not cheap, although a recent publication (Langford, 2012) suggests that the accelerometer built into some 'smart phones' can be used to detect the movement. The usual commercially available systems for acceleromyography have the stimulating and measuring (piezo-electrodes) incorporated into one unit. The recording electrodes are placed where the movement resulting from muscle contraction is to occur; for example the hoof for stimulation of the peroneal nerve of the

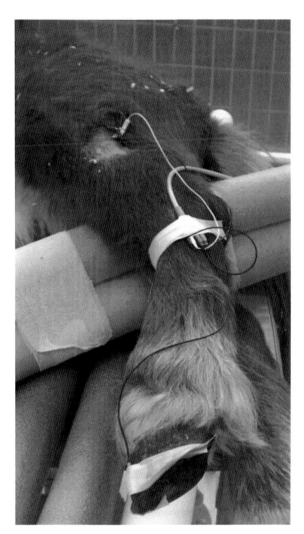

Figure 8.7 This pony's neuromuscular function being monitored by acceleromyography using a commercial system (TOF-Watch®) which incorporates the stimulator and monitor into one unit. Stimulation is of the peroneal nerve. Note that the needles are 'fixed' so that their distance apart will always be constant. The movement sensor is on the coronet of the hoof. *Photograph courtesy of Martina Mosing.*

horses (Fig. 8.7) and the palmar aspect of the paw when the ulnar nerve is stimulated in dogs (see Fig. 8.1). Movement in the stimulated muscle generates a voltage that correlates with acceleration of that muscle. As force = mass × acceleration (Newton's Law), and mass is constant, then acceleration is proportional to the force generated by the muscle. The unit can then calculate and give the size of T1 (which can also be taken as equivalent to the single twitch) and a TOF ratio. The appendage must be free to move, but that movement can be limited by application of a small load.

The use of acceleromyography sounds simple but, unfortunately, a number of potential errors mean that the results are not always identical to those measured by the 'gold standard' of mechanomyography. Although generally adequate for clinical use, where used for research purposes, a number of calibrations and corrections are advised (Fuchs-Buder et al., 2007; Claudius & Viby-Mogensen, 2008). These would include the supramaximal stimulus, avoidance of direct muscle stimulation, pre-block calibration, the use or not of preload etc. The potentiation of the single twitch by the 'staircase effect' discussed above also affects the TOF. It is routine with TOF to apply the train of stimuli every 15 seconds. Prior to the administration of NMBs, the TOF ratio often will then become greater than 1, i.e. the fourth twitch is greater than the first; this is known as 'reverse fade'. While this would be undetectable by subjective assessment of twitch height, it is noted routinely with acceleromyography (although surprisingly, rarely by mechanomyography). Theoretically, this potentiation could result in an overestimation of the size of T4, and therefore overestimation of the TOF ratio (and underestimation of the degree of block). However, changes in T1 are also relevant. Martin-Flores et al. (2011b) studied a group of dogs which had been 'conditioned' or not 'conditioned' by 25 minutes pre-block stimulation. In the 'unconditioned' dogs, the size of T1 in the TOF ratios at full recovery were from 94 to 123% different from the pre-block values, but the TOF ratios remained unchanged. As in clinical practice it may not be practical to stimulate for an adequate time prior to block, the other approach is to recalculate the recovery results in relation to the pre-block TOF, a process termed 'normalization'. For details on the complicated calculations necessary, see Martin-Flores et al. (2011b); normalized TOF ratios are lower than measured ones, so if not 'normalized', a higher TOF ratio is required to ensure adequate reversal of block in clinical circumstances.

Mechanomyography

This is considered the 'gold standard' for monitoring of NMB, but is very impracticable in the clinical setting. The limb or appendage has to be firmly fixed, a load applied, and the force of muscle contraction in response to nerve stimulation is measured with suitable transducers. It is the fixing of the limb that causes the practical problems. There are restraints available for human thumbs but, in veterinary studies, the systems have to be specifically designed. Systems in which the limb is immobilized in a cast have been described for the horses (Hildebrand et al., 1986) and the pig (Clutton et al., 1986) and Clutton et al. (2013) have described a simpler but invasive system for use in experimental pigs. However, mechanomyography remains primarily a research tool for investigating new NMBAs or their reversal, and is not suitable for general clinical use.

Electromyography

With this system, the electrical impulses generated in the muscle in response to nerve stimulation are measured. This involves insertion of three needle electrodes – the active electrode from the belly of the muscle, a reference electrode on the point of origin of the muscle and a ground electrode positioned between the recording and the stimulating electrodes. Although primarily used for research studies, it is not as impracticable to use clinically as is mechanomyography. Its special advantage is that it can be used in muscles such as the diaphragm.

Factors affecting monitoring

Some patient conditions and errors in monitoring techniques other than those discussed above can affect the muscle response observed following stimulation of a motor nerve and can lead to erroneous conclusions being drawn.

Hypothermia

Hypothermia is a common finding during general anaesthesia and may cause the degree of NMB to be overestimated. It is generally accepted that there is a 10% decrease in twitch height per degree C, although the TOF ratio shows only a minimal effect. Reduction in body temperature decreases renal, hepatic and biliary elimination of non-depolarizing drugs and, during hypothermia, reduced doses may be needed to produce any given degree of blockade. Below a body core temperature of 34.5°C (94.1°F) monitoring may become increasingly inaccurate as thermoregulatory vasoconstriction occurs. Reduction of muscle blood flow in hypothermic animals may lead to delay in the onset of the block. Unless allowance is made for this delay, an unduly deep block can result if assessment is too soon after injection of the NMBA and further, unnecessary, doses are administered.

Recognition of paralysis when a nerve stimulator is not used

Simple clinical evaluation of the degree of NMB using such criteria as the respiratory efforts in the anaesthetized animal is not ideal for the reasons discussed above, but is used clinically in many circumstances. The muscular recovery and signs seen will depend to some extent on the species, the anaesthetic agents employed, and on the NMBA employed.

Lack of diaphragmatic activity can be taken to indicate either complete muscle paralysis or a low PaCO$_2$ from artificial ventilation. If an animal can move its limbs in such a way as to be able to maintain itself in sternal recumbency, it usually means that at the most only partial neuromuscular block is present. Short, jerky respiratory efforts would indicate that marked blockade exists. To assess the ability of a partially paralysed animal to breathe, the endotracheal tube may be occluded and the negative pressure generated in the tracheal tube during an attempt at inspiration measured with a simple aneroid manometer (often present as part of a breathing system). An inspiratory pressure of 10–20 cmH$_2$O may indicate that the block is insufficient to produce respiratory inadequacy. Even then, residual paralysis of the muscles of the pharynx and larynx may cause upper airway obstruction after extubation.

NEUROMUSCULAR BLOCKING AGENTS

Requirements of a neuromuscular blocking agent

The ideal NMBA would provide a very rapid onset of paralysis, be short acting, its action easily reversed, be non-cumulative so that it could be given by infusion, be rapidly metabolized but not totally dependent on any single route of elimination, have minimal cardiovascular effects, would not trigger the release of histamine, and would have no other unwanted side effects. No such agent exists, hence the number which have been, or are still in routine use.

In human anaesthesia, the rapid onset is necessary for rapid sequence induction and endotracheal intubation in order to avoid regurgitation and potentially fatal inhalation of gastric content. Histamine release with NMBAs is a major problem in humans, and NMBAs are implicated in a very high percentage of anaphylaxis associated with anaesthesia. Cardiovascular side effects may be the results of this histamine release, or a direct action of the NMBA, most usually at the autonomic system. The need for the ability to extend the block and still have rapid termination of block is equally important.

There are no NMBAs licensed for veterinary use; doses, duration etc. are based on published papers, reviews and the authors' clinical experience. In anaesthesia, NMBAs are always given by the IV route to animals, which are already anaesthetized. In the following section, drugs and doses discussed are all based on IV administration.

Agents which produce depolarizing block

Suxamethonium (succinylcholine)

This agent is the only representative of this group of drugs that is available clinically. It still has the fastest onset and shortest duration of any NMBA. Its structure is of two conjoined acetylcholine molecules and, as discussed above, it first depolarizes the end-plate and, therefore, causes an initial muscle fasciculation (said to be very painful by conscious volunteers) before relaxation occurs. Recovery occurs when the drug is removed from the plasma, this occurring through breakdown by plasma (pseudo) cholinesterase which is now known to be butyrylcholinesterase. Suxamethonium action cannot be reversed. Again, as discussed earlier, at single doses for intubation, the suxamethonium-induced block shows minimal fade to either tetanic or TOF stimulation but, if further or larger doses are given, a Phase II block may occur when 'fade' is present. As suxamethonium is no longer used to produce prolonged NMB, this situation will not be considered further.

Plasma cholinesterase is not present at the muscle end-plates. It is synthesized in the liver, and is lowered in many clinical situations, liver disease, age, etc., but the reduction has to be massive before there is a clinically relevant increase in duration of a suxamethonium NMB. In humans, however, there are many genetic variations of the enzyme, most (but not all) of which make only a little difference to speed of metabolism of suxamethonium. As a result, many studies have looked at methods of detecting the genetic variants, which become clinically very relevant if the gene is homozygous (Lee, 2009). It is probable that different species also have different variants of plasma cholinesterase, and that this might explain the differing sensitivities to suxamethonium. The ability of plasma cholinesterase to hydrolyse butyrylthiocholine has been used to predict sensitivity to suxamethonium in humans, but has not been of value in animals. Faye (1988) has made an extensive study of the role of cholinesterase in the explanation of differing species sensitivity to suxamethonium, and demonstrated massive species differences. Details of the results of this work can be found in previous editions of this book. In her opinion, the affinities of cholinesterase for different substrates are different between species. Faye also considers it is most important that the substrate used for assay is suxamethonium itself. In domestic animals, that low cholinesterase levels may be encountered after exposure to organophosphorus compounds is relevant as these are still used occasionally impregnated in flea collars, or for other means of parasite control.

Suxamethonium stimulates nicotinic and muscarinic receptors throughout the body, leading to a large number of side effects. Anticholinergic premedication will prevent the muscarinic responses. Injection of suxamethonium causes a rise in blood pressure in all animals although, in some species (e.g. the cat), this may be preceded by a fall which can be prevented by the prior administration of atropine. Pulse rate changes are variable, both bradycardia and tachycardia being observed, sometimes in the same animal, but often the heart rate does not change. In horses and dogs, the nicotinic response predominates (Adams & Hall, 1962) – very occasionally a fall in blood pressure with bradycardia is seen, but an increase in both blood pressure and heart rate is the usual response. Cardiac arrhythmias are common.

Suxamethonium has a number of other side effects. It is a very potent trigger of malignant hyperpyrexia, indeed, this syndrome was first recognized as occurring in animals as a result of the use of suxamethonium to intubate anaesthetized pigs (Hall et al., 1966). Following the administration of suxamethonium, there is a rise in serum K, released from the stimulated muscles, possibly contributing to the cardiac arrhythmias. In humans, following an anaesthetic protocol which has included suxamethonium, many patients suffer from myalgia, this is not specifically related to the muscle spasm as it still occurs where prior use of an non-depolarizing NMBA has prevented this from occurring. In birds, suxamethonium produces spastic paralysis of the whole body. Animals susceptible to malignant hyperthermia also respond to suxamethonium with a spastic paralysis.

Dose rates and duration

In humans, following a dose of 1 mg/kg suxamethonium IV, onset of NMB occurs in less than 60 seconds and 90% recovery will take 9–13 minutes (Torda et al., 1997). There are, however, wide species differences in sensitivity. The first published use of depolarizing NMBAs in veterinary patients was by Dr LW Hall (Hall, 1952; Hall & Lehmann, 1953). The following information was gained from his considerable experience. Horses, pigs and cats are relatively resistant, but dogs, sheep and cattle are paralysed by small doses. In horses, 0.1–0.15 mg/kg IV usually cause paralysis of the limb, head and neck muscles without producing diaphragmatic paralysis, this generally lasts for about 4–5 minutes, although limb weakness may persist for some time longer. In cattle and sheep, one-sixth of this quantity (0.02 mg/kg) produces paralysis of the body muscles without diaphragmatic paralysis and this relaxation lasts 6–8 minutes. Pigs require much larger doses; to facilitate endotracheal intubation, the dose required is about 2 mg/kg, which produces complete paralysis for only 2–3 minutes. In cats, 3–5 mg of suxamethonium chloride (total dose) produces 5–6 minutes of paralysis. The dog is comparatively sensitive and doses of 0.3 mg/kg produce total paralysis of 15–20 minutes' duration, a single dose occasionally producing Phase II block.

Apart from its use to facilitate endotracheal intubation in pigs and cats, it seems that today there are no good indications for suxamethonium in veterinary anaesthesia. If it loses its place for human endotracheal intubation to rocuronium/sugammadex (see below), it will almost certainly become unavailable.

Agents which produce non-depolarizing (competitive) block

The numbers of the non-depolarizing NMBAs available demonstrate that the ideal one has yet to be found. Table 8.1 demonstrates the major properties in relation to the requirements in people. Although speed of onset

Table 8.1 Some doses, times of onset and duration of commonly used NMBAs in humans

NMBA	Single dose mg/kg	Onset time in minutes (to % of maximum T1 depression reached; 100% means T1 = zero)	Duration in minutes (to return to % of control T1; 25% means that T1 is 25% of its original control height)
Human			
Pancuronium	0.1	4 (100%)	100 (25%)
Vecuronium	0.1	1.8–2.4 (100%)	44–54 (25%)
Rocuronium	0.6	1.5–1.9 (100%)	32–37 (25%)
Atracurium	0.5 0.5	3.2 (100%) 1.9 (100%)	46 (25%) 69 (95%)
Cisatracurium	0.1 0.1	7.7 (100%) 2.4 (90%)	46 (25%) 45 (25%)
Mivacuarium	0.15 0.15	3.3 (100%) 2.7 (95%)	19 (25%) 10 (5%)

NB: Doses in some animal species may differ – see text. Times are given as guidance, and are approximate, as they would be influenced by relative dose, anaesthetic method, and by method of assessment of NMB. T1 is first stimulus in TOF.
Data obtained mainly from Naguib & Lien (2010) and Craig & Hunter (2009).

(for endotracheal intubation) can be improved by increasing the dose given, this is at the expense of duration, which lengthens accordingly. There are species differences with some of the agents as to doses which are satisfactory, as discussed below and the doses for humans in Table 8.1 are not necessarily suitable for animals.

Structurally the non-depolarizing fall into two categories, the steroidal agents, pancuronium, vecuronium and rocuronium, and the benzylisoquinolinium compounds, mivacurium, atracurium and cisatracurium.

Steroidal Agents

Pancuronium

Pancuronium bromide is an amino steroid non-depolarizing NMBA which works fairly rapidly, but is relatively long acting (see Table 8.1). It has no major undesirable side effects. It is cleared mainly via the kidney so the action is prolonged in renal failure. There is about 20–30% hepatic involvement, but some of the metabolites secreted via the bile have some NMB activity. In liver failure, there may also be a prolonged effect due to an increase in the volume of distribution (Craig & Hunter, 2009).

Pancuronium has been used widely in veterinary anaesthesia since its first introduction. Initially, doses of 0.06 mg/kg were suggested for use in dogs. Gleed & Jones (1982) found that at that dose it took 168 seconds to reach maximal relaxation, and the time to 50% recovery (at which stage they reversed the action with neostigmine) was 31 ± SD 5

minutes. Clutton (2007) suggests a higher dose of 0.1 mg/kg. Hildebrand & Howitt (1984), in a dose-finding study in the horse, required doses of around 0.125 mg/kg for adequate NMB and, indeed, a further increment of 0.03 mg/kg was required to obtain a full NMB of the hind leg. In a retrospective study of clinical use (Hildebrand et al., 1989), it was found that doses of from 0.12 to 0.2 mg/kg had been used, with increments of approximately 0.03–0.05 mg/kg if required to lengthen the NMB, so it would seem that the initial recommendation of 0.06 mg was conservative, although resulting in a more rapid recovery. Clutton (2007) recommends doses of 0.2 mg/kg for pigs but, in contrast, only 0.05 mg/kg were required to obtain a complete block in calves, lasting 43 ± 19 minutes to 50% recovery. At this stage, antagonism with neostigmine (always given with an anticholinergic) was successful.

The prolonged duration of pancuronium means that, in general clinical use, it is not suitable for continuous infusion. It is better to use incremental doses of 25–35% of the original at the time when the NMB has started to become ineffective. In a dose-finding study in pigs, Veres-Nyeki et al. (2012) administered a bolus of 0.1 mg/kg, then an infusion of 0.1 mg/kg/hour, with 'top ups' as required; their overall total dose needed worked out as 0.10–0.21 mg/kg/hour, but they commented on the wide individual variation.

Vecuronium

Vecuronium is a monoquarternary analogue of pancuronium. Due to the instability of the 3-acetyl group in high concentrations in solution, the drug is marketed as a freeze-dried buffered powder with water in a separate ampoule. The powder can be kept on the shelf at room temperature without deterioration. Vecuronium is currently the most specific neuromuscular blocking drug in clinical use and is shorter acting than pancuronium. It shows a low propensity to liberate histamine and possesses a negligible ganglionic blocking action, hence cardiovascular side effects are unlikely to be seen during clinical use. In humans, it is eliminated primarily by biliary excretion but with around 30% eliminated by the urine (Craig & Hunter, 2009).

Vecuronium has been used in a variety of animal species, as single doses, incremental dosing (Jones & Seymour, 1985) or as an infusion. Doses of 0.06 mg/kg give around 10 minutes deep NMB in dogs, and a little longer in the horse. Clutton (2007) recommends 0.05–0.1 mg/kg for dogs and 0.05 mg/kg for cats, while Jones & Seymour (1985) recommend doses of 0.06–0.2 mg/kg in dogs, depending on the duration of block required. Sheep are particularly sensitive (as for many non-depolarizing NMBAs). Martin-Flores et al. (2012c) demonstrated that 0.013 mg/kg (13.2 µg/kg) was an effective ED 95; i.e. effective in 95% of sheep. Clutton & Glasby (1998) used 0.025 mg/kg (25 µg/kg) in a series of sheep and, at this dose, NMB lasted for 40 minutes. In horses, Martin-Flores et al. (2012b) conducted a vecuronium dose–response study, but found great variations between individual animals, these individual variations being confirmed with clinical experience (Martin-Flores et al., 2012a). Testing used the TOF. The lowest dose, 0.025 mg/kg (25 µg/kg), did not cause any T1 depression, and while the highest dose used, 0.1 mg/kg (100 µg/kg), caused an incomplete block, the partial block that was produced was long lasting – up to 2 hours and required reversal with neostigmine.

Usually, it is easy to reverse the NMB from vecuronium with anticholinesterases. However, Martin-Flores et al. (2011a) report a case in a dog where edrophonium failed to reverse NMB more than an hour after administration of 0.1 mg/kg vecuronium. The block was eventually reversed with neostigmine and atropine. There were mitigating factors in that dog was very ill, and had received numerous other agents, including magnesium, which could well have influenced duration of block. Gurney & Mosing (2012) report a case of prolonged NMB in a horse which initially received 0.05 mg/kg vecuronium, but when that failed to provide an effective block, was then given 0.1 mg/kg atracurium; despite several doses of edrophonium it was not until 125 minutes after atracurium administration that the NMB was adequately reversed.

In people, vecuronium can be reversed using sugammadex, but there are as yet no reports of reversal of vecuronium with this agent in veterinary anaesthesia. This may be the reversal treatment of choice in the future.

Rocuronium

Rocuronium, formerly known as Org 9426, a steroidal non-depolarizing NMBA, is a derivative of vecuronium. In humans, onset of block after rocuronium is very rapid (see Table 8.1). Initial animal studies (Muir et al., 1989; Cason et al., 1990) confirmed this, and demonstrated that compared with vecuronium the onset of NMB was very rapid, its duration of action similar and its potency about one-fifth. Rocuronium has minimal cardiovascular effects, however, in anaesthetized cats, it may be considered to have some mild vagolytic activity (Marshall et al., 1994). In cats, more than 50% of the injected dose is eliminated unchanged in the bile and only 9% in the urine (Khuenl-Brady et al., 1990). It does not cause histamine release.

Rocuronium has been used at doses between 0.3 and 0.6 mg/kg in dogs (Auer, 2007) and cats (Auer & Mosing, 2006) and 0.4–0.6 mg/kg in horses (Auer et al., 2007). The time to return of TOF of 0.9 or the T1 of the TOF to 95% of starting value is approximately 20 minutes in the cat, 30 minutes in the dog, but around 60 minutes in the horse. In all species tested, recovery of NM transmission was faster with use of smaller doses. In horses, doses of 0.3 mg/kg were sufficient to keep the eyeball central for 30 minutes for ophthalmic surgery (Auer & Moens, 2011). There appear no reports as yet of doses required in the sheep.

Rocuronium can be reversed by the standard methods using anticholinesterase, but also, very specifically and completely, by the cyclodextrin, sugammadex. Sugammadex will reverse even the deepest NMB induced by rocuronium. In humans the speed of onset of rocuronium is sufficiently rapid to allow endotracheal intubation, so the new ability to reverse rapidly if suddenly needed (e.g. can't intubate can't ventilate scenario) may mean that suxamethonium will no longer be required. In veterinary anaesthesia, the ability for a complete reversal of rocuronium by sugammadex may mean that rocuronium becomes the NMBA of choice for horses.

Benzylisoquinolinium agents

Atracurium

Atracuriumbesylate is a bisquaternaryisoquinoline compound and is available as a mixture of 10 sterioisomers (Amaki et al., 1985). It is eliminated by pH and temperature-dependent Hofmann degradation, as well as by metabolism by non-specific esterases, giving rise to laudanosine and a monoquaternary ester which is further degraded to a second laudanosine molecule and an acrylate ester. None of these degradation products is active at the neuromuscular junction and, although laudanosine crosses the blood–brain barrier and theoretically can lead to excitement reactions, at clinical doses in veterinary anaesthesia such reactions have not been reported. The half-life of the Hofmann degradation process in cats and in people is about 20 minutes (Craig & Hunter, 2009). Coupled with uptake by the liver, kidney and other tissues, the process produces a rapid plasma clearance and an apparent large distribution volume. The Hofmann degradation process does not need an enzyme system and attains a linear relationship between the dose of drug and the rate of metabolism irrespective of the substrate load. The pharmacokinetics in renal failure are unchanged but, in severe liver failure in people, atracurium is slower to reach maximum effect and has a shorter duration of action, due to an increased volume of distribution.

As atracurium at high doses in people causes histamine release, in human anaesthesia, it is usually administered initially at relatively small doses then continued as an infusion for longer periods as required. Veterinary anaesthesia has utilized either this approach or 'top-ups' as necessary. The paralysing dose for the dog is from 0.3 to 0.5 mg/kg and recovery from these doses occurs in about 40 minutes (Jones et al., 1983). For major surgical procedures, Clutton (2007) recommends a loading dose of 0.5 mg/kg for the dog and 0.25 mg/kg for cats, with increments as required of approximately 30% of the original dose. Lower doses (0.1 mg/kg) are usually satisfactory for maintaining a central eye for intraocular surgery. Atracurium has been administered to dogs by continuous infusion of 0.5 mg/kg/hour after a loading dose of 0.5 mg/kg (Jones & Brearley, 1985). Kastrup et al. (2005) demonstrated that the duration of atracurium block is considerably greater with sevoflurane anaesthesia than with total intravenous anaesthesia (TIVA) with propofol. They examined the duration of action of 0.1, 0.2 and 0.3 mg/kg atracurium; under sevoflurane anaesthesia duration of NMB was 40, 46 and 59 minutes respectively, compared to 20, 27 and 40 minutes when anaesthesia was propofol total intravenous anaesthesia.

A single injection of 0.11 mg/kg of atracurium produces paralysis of about 20–30 minutes duration in halothane-anaesthetized horses (Hildebrand et al., 1986). Atracurium has also been administered by infusion to horses under halothane anaesthesia. After a loading dose of 0.05 mg/kg in another investigation, a 95–99% reduction in TOF hoof-twitch response was produced by an infusion of 0.17 ± 0.01 mg/kg/hour (Hildebrand & Hill, 1989).

Cisatracurium

Cisatracurium is one of the 10 isomers of atracurium. It is more potent and causes less histamine release than the parent drug. Its metabolism in people is primarily via Hofmann degradation, although there is a small amount of renal excretion. Onset of action is slower than for atracurium, but recovery times are similar (Craig & Hunter, 2009).

Although cisatracurium has been used in animals in experimental studies, there are as yet few publications looking at dose and effectiveness for veterinary clinical use. Chen et al. (2009) examined the pharmacokinetics in

dogs anaesthetized with pentobarbitone; in vivo terminal half-life was a mean 16.4 ± 2.7 minutes which was considerably shorter than plasma breakdown of the drug in vitro, suggesting a metabolic or renal pathway was also involved in recovery. In clinical use, Adams et al. (2006) examined speed of recovery from NMB in dogs with or without a hepatoportal shunt. They used a loading dose of 0.1 mg/kg, followed by increments of 0.03 mg/kg. NMB lasted from means of 29 (no shunt) to 34 (shunt) minutes and all dogs recovered satisfactorily from anaesthesia and NMB. Jurado et al. (2012) report an accidental overdose of 0.4 mg/kg given over approximately 12 minutes; it resulted in tachycardia and hypertension, which resolved over the next 15–30 minutes.

Mivacurium

Mivacurium, is a benzylisoquinolinediester compound with a potency approximately one-third to one-half that of atracurium. It consists of three sterioisomers of which one is active. Its breakdown products are pharmacologically inactive. Breakdown is by plasma cholinesterase. Low plasma cholinesterase levels are associated with a longer duration of action and a decreased plasma cholinesterase due to hepatic failure results in prolonged activity, although alternative pathways for clearance are available (Savarese et al., 1988).

In humans, mivacurium is fairly slow in onset but is very short acting, making it exceptionally useful for continuous infusion. In veterinary anaesthesia, there are very few reports of its use and, as doses will be very species specific (as they are for suxamethonium), it is impossible to recommend doses for most domestic species. Sheep, however, have active plasma cholinesterase. Clutton & Glasby (1998) successfully used a dose of 0.2 mg/kg, followed (after 15 minutes) by increments of 0.07 mg/kg as required to obtain prolonged block in this species.

Non-depolarizing NMBAs no longer in common use

The NMBA most used in human and veterinary anaesthesia for very many years was *d-tubocurarine chloride* and anaesthetists should have some knowledge of its actions for historical reasons. It first became available in 1944. After IV injection, maximum activity is apparent within 2–3 minutes and lasts for 35–40 minutes in most species of animal. Some 30–40% of the dose is excreted unchanged in the urine within 3–4 hours (Kalow, 1959). It is highly protein bound. An effective dose for NMB of d-tubocurarine chloride given to dogs and cats causes a severe fall in blood pressure and an increase in heart rate. The fall in arterial blood pressure appears to be due to block of impulse transmission across autonomic ganglia – hence tachycardia from vagal block – and/or release of histamine. In pigs, doses of the order of 0.3 mg/kg cause complete relaxation with respiratory paralysis without at the same time causing any marked fall in arterial blood pressure. Doses of 0.22–0.25 mg/kg produce good relaxation with respiratory arrest in anaesthetized horses breathing 0.8–1.0% halothane and no significant hypotension is encountered.

Gallamine triethiodide is eliminated unchanged by the kidneys and so its removal from the plasma is dependent on renal function. It does not cause the degree of histamine release of d-tubocurarine. Gallamine has been used at a dose of 1 mg/kg IV in dogs and cats, this dose resulting in apnoea of 10–20 minutes duration, at 0.5–1 mg/kg in horses and ruminants, and at 4 mg/kg in pigs.

Alcuronium chloride is a diallylnortoxiferine, a derivative of the alkaloid toxiferine obtained from calabash curare. It has been used quite extensively in dogs and horses at 0.1 mg/kg and seemed to have no significant histamine liberating or ganglionic blocking effects. It is relatively long acting and there were problems with its reversal, so it was advised to limit its use to one single injection (Jones et al., 1978).

Pipecuronium bromide is an analogue of pancuronium. In dogs, about 77% of the injected drug is said to be eliminated in the urine with less than 5% being excreted in the bile. One potential advantage of pipecuronium is that it is apparently free from cardiovascular side effects. Its neuromuscular blocking effects in the dog have been investigated (Jones, 1987a,b). It appears to be no longer available.

Factors affecting the action of neuromuscular blocking drugs

Factors such as age, concurrent disease, concurrent administration of other drugs, body temperature, extracellular pH, neuromuscular and other disease and genetic abnormalities may influence response to muscle relaxant drugs, either directly, or indirectly via the pharmacokinetics.

Pharmacokinetics of the NMBAs

All neuromuscular blocking agents contain quaternary ammonium groups making them positively charged at body temperature; they are highly water soluble and relatively insoluble in fat. Their pharmacokinetics can be described by a two- or three-compartment model (see Chapter 3), with a rapid distribution phase, followed by one or two slower elimination phases, consisting of biotransformation and excretion. For most drugs, a two-compartment model is suitable and thus two half-lives can be determined: the half-life of distribution ($t_{1/2\alpha}$) and the half-life of elimination ($t_{1/2\beta}$). The mean residence time (MRT) has been introduced for statistical purposes – the time for 63.2 % of the administered dose to be excreted. The value, known as Css95, is the plasma concentration at which a 95% decrease in muscle contraction occurs. This is particularly important to the anaesthetist because it represents the surgically optimal level of neuromuscular block.

Drug distribution depends on tissue perfusion so that, as mentioned earlier, cardiac output is important in speed of onset, reduction leading to slow and lesser distribution with lengthening of $t_{1/2\alpha}$, a slower onset of action but eventually, a stronger effect, and vice versa if cardiac output is high. Also important is the volume of distribution; the greater this is, the lower the concentration achieved with a set initial IV dose of the drug. Removal of the NMBA from the neuromuscular junction (and, therefore, recovery) depends on the fall in plasma levels, through metabolism and elimination, but also through changes in volume of distribution (Craig & Hunter, 2009). Protein binding is also an important factor in establishing active plasma levels of the NMBA. Thus, any factor that influences cardiac output, muscle blood flow, metabolism, elimination or volume of distribution will affect the speed of onset and of recovery from NMBAs. This explains the range of variations in effects that are seen in clinical practice as age, most anaesthetic agents and disease states will influence one or more of these factors.

Body temperature

The effect of muscle and body temperature on the potency and duration of action of muscle relaxants is difficult to assess; reduction in body temperature will influence regional blood flow and decrease renal, hepatic and biliary elimination of the non-depolarizing NMBAs. Practically, in clinical practice, the requirements of non-depolarizing NMBAs are decreased during moderate hypothermia and delay in onset time of block and unless allowance is made for this, gives rise to the risk of serious overdosing if the drug is being given in incremental doses to assess its effects as administration proceeds.

Administration of other drugs

Any drug which has anticholinesterase properties will prolong the action of suxamethonium or mivacurium and possibly tend to antagonize non-depolarizing neuromuscular blockade. Several antibiotics, especially the aminoglycosides, may produce or enhance non-depolarizing block, possibly by binding calcium to produce hypocalcaemia, or by influencing binding of calcium at presynaptic sites. Antibiotic induced or enhanced competitive block is not invariably antagonized by anticholinesterase drugs or by administration of calcium. General anaesthetics may have a marked effect on neuromuscular block, and this may differ between agents used. Inhalation agents potentiate non-depolarizing relaxants such as pancuronium and atracurium (Kastrup et al., 2005).

Extracellular pH

Hypercapnia augments tubocurarine block and opposes its reversal by neostigmine. Alcuronium and pancuronium block are apparently unaffected by PCO_2, but block due to suxamethonium may be potentiated by acidosis. A number of explanations have been advanced to account for these findings and it seems likely that factors such as protein binding, ionization of the relaxant and ionization of the receptor sites may be important.

Neuromuscular disease

Animals suffering from myasthenia gravis are resistant to depolarizing neuromuscular blockers and are more than normally sensitive to competitive blocking agents, but there are several reports of satisfactory use of atracurium or vecuronium at very low doses in this condition (reviewed by Shilo et al., 2011).

Blood pressure and flow

Recovery from the effects of relaxant drugs is likely to be more rapid if blood flow through the muscle is high and thus maintains a steep concentration gradient between tissues and blood by removing molecules of the agent as soon as they are freed from receptors.

Electrolyte imbalance

A deficiency of calcium, potassium or sodium retards the depolarization of motor end-plates and by thus inhibiting neuromuscular transmission will increase the blocking effects of the non-depolarizing muscle relaxants. In contrast, hyperkalaemia and hypernatraemia render muscles more resistant.

EVOKED RECOVERY FROM NEUROMUSCULAR BLOCK

While it is possible for non-depolarizing NMBAs to be eliminated from the body, thus resulting in termination of action, some agents have a prolonged effect and, even with short acting NMBAs, there is great individual variation in response. Thus, antagonism of non-depolarizing neuromuscular block is usually indicated in routine clinical practice – especially in horses to enable them to stand safely.

The principle underlying use of antagonists to NMBAs is tilting of the balance between the concentration of acetylcholine and the concentration of the drug at the neuromuscular junction in favour of the former. This is most commonly done using drugs that block the acetylcholinesterase at the neuromuscular end-plates and

therefore reduce the breakdown of acetylcholine. With the greater numbers of acetylcholine molecules, there is a greater chance they will occupy the two α sites necessary on the temporarily 'unblocked' receptor (Martyn et al., 2009). There are no effective 'antidotes' to suxamethonium or other agents which act by depolarization, but certain anticholinesterases will reduce the effect of a Phase II block. However, if a Phase II block is not present, prolonged paralysis requiring several hours of ventilatory support may result from anticholinesterase administration.

The commonly used anticholinesterase agents are neostigmine and edrophonium, although pyridostigmine has also been used. The use of these agents in the reversal of neuromuscular blockade in veterinary anaesthesia was well reviewed by Jones (1988). The inhibition of acetylcholinesterase, although it is the main action, is not the only effect of these drugs. Their other actions include a direct stimulation of the receptor as well as a presynaptic effect involving enhancement of acetylcholine release (Deana & Scuka, 1990). Neostigmine and pyridostigmine appear to differ from edrophonium in their effects, the suggestion being that this is caused by differences in their actions on presynaptic receptors (Wachtel, 1990).

Practical aspects of reversal of NMB

There are three general considerations before an anticholinesterase is used to reverse an NMB:

- Anticholinesterases cannot reverse a really deep NMB, and reversal should not be attempted unless there are some signs of recovery (e.g. increase in muscle tone, TOF > 0.4)
- Once all the acetylcholinesterase is blocked, increasing the dose of anticholinesterase will have no further effect on NMB. With neostigmine in humans, this maximal effect occurs around 0.07 mg/kg (Kopman & Eikermann, 2009)
- Muscarinic receptors will also be affected leading to a wide range of unwanted, and sometimes dangerous side effects, such as bradycardia, salivation, defaecation and urination. These are prevented by administration of an anticholinergic prior to or mixed with the anticholinesterase. Atropine has a rapid onset of action so is usually mixed with the anticholinesterase, either neostigmine or edrophonium, while glycopyrrolate's onset may be slower, so it may be preferable to give prior to the fast onset edrophonium.

Reversal agents

Neostigmine

Neostigmine is probably the most widely used anticholinesterase antagonist of non-depolarizing NMBAs in human anaesthesia (Kopman & Eikermann, 2009). The time course of the antagonizing effect is about 7–10 minutes. Atropine or glycopyrrolate may be given first, or may be mixed in the syringe with neostigmine and the mixture given in small repeated doses until full respiratory activity is established or monitoring reveals a satisfactory TOF ratio.

Neostigmine, even if given with full doses of atropine, may cause serious cardiac arrhythmias if there has been gross underventilation during anaesthesia or if CO_2 has been allowed to accumulate at the end of operation with a view to ensuring return of spontaneous respiration. Hypercapnia also increases the neuromuscular block of non-depolarizing agents and so antagonism is likely to be less effective under these conditions. In the absence of facilities for monitoring of neuromuscular block, reliance must be placed on clinical signs to assess when reversal is adequate, as described above (Monitoring neuromuscular block). The atropine–neostigmine mixture should be given in small doses, with a pause between each, until these signs disappear.

Edrophonium

Edrophonium is an effective and reliable antagonist to the non-depolarizing agents. Earlier impressions that its effects were too short lasting were probably due to use of inadequate doses and, with the use of higher doses, the drug is now becoming popular. Doses of edrophonium in excess of 0.5 mg/kg appear similar in effect to that of neostigmine, but the onset of action is considerably shorter (about 1–3 minutes) making it easier to titrate more accurately its administration to full reversal of blockade. For dogs, Clutton (2007) recommends its use at 0.5 mg/kg mixed together with atropine at 0.04 mg/kg.

Sugammadex (Org 25969): a new concept in NMB reversal

Sugammadex is a gamma cyclodextrin that binds very specifically to the aminoglycoside NMBAs, rocuronium and vercuronium, thus preventing them from being effective, reversing the NMB in a manner that does not directly interact with the receptors at the neuromuscular junction (Booij, 2009) and therefore avoiding the unpleasant side effects associated with classical reversal techniques using neostigmine. The property of cyclodextrins to inactivate rocuronium was an 'accidental' discovery when they were being investigated as an alterative solvent – but the investigators recognized the potential – hence this totally new method of reversal of NMB (Bom et al., 2002).

Sugammadex (as Bridion™) first received a licence in Europe in 2008 to reverse, in people, NMB induced by rocuronium or vecuronium, and the product information has been updated in 2012 (EMC, 2012).

Currently (2012), it is not licensed in the USA. The product information states that the dose range is 2–4 mg/kg in humans for routine reversal of either NMBA where some recovery of TOF has already occurred, but doses of 16 mg/kg can be given if immediate reversal of a full blockade of rocuronium is required (there is no similar information given concerning vecuronium). Reversal is very rapid. In the very rare cases of re-curarization, a repeat dose of 4 mg/kg can be given. Following the use of sugammadex, it is advised that rocuronium or vecuronium should not be used for 24 hours or the ensuing neuromuscular block might be unreliable (although this time-lag is probably overcautious). If a new NMB is required in this time, non-steroid types of NMBAs such as cisatracurium can be used without interference.

Although sugammadex effectively reverses both vecuronium and rocuronium, the majority of interest, and therefore of published studies relate to NMB with rocuronium. Rocuronium has a rapid onset block, suitable for endotracheal intubation in people and, therefore, the ability for immediate reversal means that rocuronium/sugammadex could replace suxamethonium for the purpose of intubation. Mirakhur (2009) reviewed the early clinical investigations of sugammadex, many of which were those on which the above licensed dosage regimens were based. These studies demonstrated the very rapid reversal (1–5 minutes), that speed of reversal was increased with increasing doses of sugammadex and that reversal was equally effective after a prolonged NMB by multiple doses of the relaxant. Limited studies in different age groups suggested that age was not a clinically important factor (reversal was slightly longer in the elderly). The anaesthetic technique used did not influence reversal. Major concerns for safety in human anaesthesia relate to possible drug interactions through cyclodextrin binding (some antibiotics, steroids including contraceptives), and to hypersensitivity. In trials in volunteers, one patient developed self-limiting symptoms and was later shown to be hypersensitive to sugammadex by skin tests, and two asthmatic patients had bronchospasm which may or may not have been related to the use of sugammadex (Craig & Hunter, 2009).

Pharmacokinetic studies of sugammadex in humans give a plasma clearance of 120 mL/min, a volume of distribution of 18 L, and a half-life of elimination of 100–136 minutes. Elimination is primarily via the urine. Sugammadex also appears to increase the speed of rocuronium excretion via the urine (although not total speed of rocuronium excretion as the 'captured' rocuronium does not undergo the biliary excretion that would otherwise occur). To date, there have been no clinical concerns in the few patients with renal impairment who have received sugammadex for reversal of rocuronium (Craig & Hunter, 2009).

Since the 'launch' of sugammadex, there have been many published papers and case reports which highlight its use in relation to rapid sequence induction, for reversal if problems intubating, and in cases such as myasthenia gravis where using conventional techniques is problematic. Its price, however, is limiting its use (Fink & Hollmann, 2012), although analyses of cost-benefit in human anaesthesia on the basis of the rapid recovery and reduction in nursing time suggest that this limitation is not as great as at first sight (Chambers et al., 2010; Paton et al., 2010).

Sugammadex in veterinary medicine

Mosing et al. (2012) carried out a cross-over study in eight dogs in which, under isoflurane anaesthesia, NMB was induced with either rocuronium, 0.6 mg/kg, or vecuronium, 0.1 mg/kg. Sugammadex, 8 mg/kg, was administered 5 minutes later. Onset of block was more rapid with rocuronium than vecuronium. Reversal to TOF ratio of 0.9 occurred in less than 2 minutes in each case, demonstrating that sugammadex at this dose could reverse a profound block in dogs. Mosing et al. (2010) also demonstrated that in eight Shetland ponies sugammadex at 4 mg/kg given 5 minutes after rocuronium (0.6 mg/kg) resulted in the return of a TOF ratio of 0.9 within 3.4 (± 1.7) minutes, depending on the nerve stimulated. The potential for complete effective reversal will revolutionize the user of NMB in this species if the cost of reversal should ever become practicable.

USE OF NEUROMUSCULAR BLOCKING DRUGS IN VETERINARY ANAESTHESIA

Indications

The general indications for the use of these drugs in veterinary clinical practice are:

1. To relax skeletal muscles for easier surgical access
   - This is the major reason for use. Not only does relaxant use make surgical access easier, but doing so it minimizes bruising of muscle caused by retractors, thus contributing to postoperative comfort of the animal and to wound healing
   - If used for spinal surgery, the surgeon must be aware of their use; despite the outstanding access they provide, they remove the 'safety muscle twitch' that warns the surgeon that he/she is likely to damage a spinal motor nerve
   - It is used to facilitate eye surgery by ensuring a central position and immobility of the eyeball. In most, but not all species, the extraocular muscles are blocked easily, and only low doses of NMBs are required. At these doses, the animal may be able to breathe spontaneously, but ventilation will still be impaired. The authors of this book consider that in all patients who have received NMBAs, the trachea should be intubated, oxygen administered, and intermittent positive pressure ventilation always should be employed

2. To facilitate control of respiration
   - During intrathoracic surgery but also to 'regularize' inefficient respiration; for example in dogs which are panting

3. To prevent unwanted reflexes
   - Some reflexes may remain during very deep general anaesthesia, for example a head shake during ear surgery

4. To assist in reduction of dislocated joints
   - The effect on the reduction of fractures is not as great since the difficulties of reduction are due primarily to spasm of muscles around the fracture site provoked by haematomas and broken bone fragments

5. To ease the induction of full anaesthesia in animals already unconscious from intravenous narcotic drugs
   - This used to be used in horses following rapid injection of thiopental to induce anaesthesia, but is unnecessary with modern preanaesthetic sedative medication (see Chapter 11)

6. To facilitate the performance of endotracheal intubation and endoscopy
   - In human anaesthesia, a rapidly acting NMBA is employed routinely to enable endotracheal intubation. Most animals can be intubated without the use of these drugs, but they may make endotracheal intubation very much easier in cats and pigs. However, if used for this purpose, a method of ventilation by mask must be available for emergency in case endotracheal intubation should fail.

Essential requirements for use of NMBAs

NMBAs cause paralysis of skeletal muscles with no loss of consciousness, analgesia, or even sedation. Without anaesthesia, any animal which has received one is fully conscious while paralysed, a terrifying situation, even without surgery. If surgery is proceeding, there is the addition of pain and stress. These authors consider that, with the current range of anaesthetic and immobilizing drugs available, there now is *no* situation where an NMBA should be given to a conscious animal.

There are therefore three major essential requirements before an NMBA should be administered: the animal must be unconscious and have adequate analgesia; there must be the ability to ventilate adequately for a sustained period of time; and the anaesthetist should either have experience to recognize when the NMB has waned sufficiently for recovery, or suitable monitors of block available.

Ability to ventilate

To ventilate adequately, it is essential that the trachea has been intubated, the use of a facemask, except in an emergency when intubation attempts fail, is not satisfactory because it is all too easy to inflate the stomach as well as the lungs. Modes of providing intermittent positive pressure ventilation (IPPV) are described in Chapter 9. IPPV should still be given even where such low doses of NMBA have been used that the animal is still making respiratory efforts.

Ensuring unconsciousness and analgesia

Ensuring unconsciousness and analgesia is not easy – in human anaesthesia, awareness during anaesthesia, although rare, remains a problem (Hudetz & Hemmings, 2012). Animals cannot tell us afterwards that they were aware, making it even more imperative that we ensure adequate anaesthesia. During NMB, many of the signs, such as respiratory rate, eyeball position, movement in response to surgery that are normally used to judge the depth of anaesthesia are abolished. It is therefore necessary to ensure that the anaesthetic agents are given at doses that would cause unconsciousness in animals without NMB. Analgesia is judged by autonomic responses to surgery, such as changes in heart rate and arterial blood pressure in response to painful stimuli. Thus, monitoring equipment must also be adequate to assess these parameters at sufficiently short intervals.

In human anaesthesia, the bispectral index (BIS) monitor is used as a supplementary monitor during NMB. Its use has reduced, but not abolished incidences of awareness (Hudetz & Hennings, 2012), and it must be emphasized that one case of awareness is one too many. It is also accepted that, as BIS is based on propofol anaesthesia, the EEG changes are not always comparable with those which occur under inhalation anaesthesia (see Chapters 1 and 7). In dogs, several studies in anaesthetized patients have compared apparent 'depth of anaesthesia' with BIS readings; although the mean (or median) BIS decreases with depth of anaesthesia as would be expected, there were many 'outliers' where a low BIS was associated with a light level of anaesthesia, or vice versa and the authors concluded that the outliers meant that it was not safe to depend on BIS values (or other EEG derived parameters) as the judge of anaesthetic depth in this species (Bleijenberg et al., 2011; Ribeiro et al., 2012).

Prior to the availability of BIS monitors, a number of means were used in human anaesthesia to help assess the adequacy of anaesthesia during NMB. Many were EEG based, such as looking at the effect of evoked auditory potentials on the EEG. These techniques have had experimental use for various purposes in animals, but their success in relation to awareness obviously cannot be assessed. Another technique used in people, which is not applicable to veterinary anaesthesia, is the isolated forearm technique – a tourniquet stops the relaxant reaching one hand, and if awareness is suspected for any reason, the patient is asked to move that hand.

Recovery from NMB

Before administering an NMB, the anaesthetist must be sure that they are able to detect full reversal of NMB, whether by nerve stimulation or clinical judgement as discussed above. In particular, this needs to ensure the restoration of adequate spontaneous respiration. Rate is not necessarily indicative of efficiency and monitoring (e.g. pulse oximetry, tidal volume and/or capnography) is helpful.

Technique of use

In veterinary anaesthesia, NMBAs are used mostly in the dog, cat, and the horse; specific details of the practical use is given in the chapters concerned. However, NMBAs may be required in other species, such as the pig or the sheep, when used for research purposes. The absolute technique will depend on the species, the procedure, and drugs used may also be constrained by the research to be undertaken. Below are generalized suggestions, which can be modified according to species and need.

Use of non-depolarizing NMBAs for surgery

The anaesthetic regimen used must be sufficient to provide adequate anaesthesia, analgesia and unconsciousness throughout the procedure, and should therefore be one with which the anaesthetist is familiar without NMBAs, and whose pharmacokinetic profile in the species concerned is known. It is usual to premedicate fairly heavily with sedatives and analgesics, preferably using those with a long duration of action unless further doses are to be given or infused later in the procedure. An intravenous catheter should be placed. An IV induction with a suitable agent allows rapid endotracheal intubation, although induction with an inhalation agent is possible in small animals. Following endotracheal intubation (essential), the animal is then connected to a suitable anaesthetic breathing system and oxygen together with any other gases (nitrogen, nitrous oxide, fluorinated inhalation anaesthetic agents) administered. The regimen for maintenance of anaesthesia, be it inhalation, total IV infusions, or a mixture of both, can then be commenced and anaesthesia/analgesia stabilized. Inhalation anaesthesia is advised while learning to use NMBAs, as it has the advantage of being easy to ascertain that the animal is receiving an adequate, but hopefully not excessive amount of agent. An inhalation anaesthetic agent monitor provides useful information when using a rebreathing system. Cardiovascular measurements should be made before administration of the NMBA and start of surgery. Minimal monitoring must include some method of measuring pulse rate and rhythm and arterial blood pressure as these parameters will be used to judge if anaesthesia is adequate, and a pulse oximeter to ensure adequate oxygenation. Measurement of end-tidal CO_2 ($ETCO_2$) facilitates adequate application of artificial ventilation.

Before any NMBA is administered, it is essential to confirm that the ventilator is working correctly when attached to the patient. Many anaesthetists have found themselves having to ventilate the patient by hand until the relaxant effects have worn off if they have neglected this precaution!

The NMBA can now be administered; a single starting bolus dose, then increments (approximately 30–40% of initial dose) or an infusion as required. Time (dependent on the agent – see Table 8.1) must be allowed for the block to establish before more NMBA is given. The desired level of block is established easily when TOF monitoring is employed – maintenance of one twitch usually provides good operating conditions, although some surgeons prefer a total block. When an intermittent injection technique is used supplementary doses of NMBAs should not, in general, exceed half the initial dose.

Judgement of depth of anaesthesia is now based on knowledge of how much anaesthetic is being administered coupled with lack of autonomic response (heart rate, blood pressure, pupillary size in some species) to surgery. However, the influence of the anaesthetic related agents being used on these parameters must also be considered; e.g. α_2-agonist or opioid induced bradycardia; atropine causing pupillary dilatation. Also, although usually heart rate increases if anaesthesia is too light, occasionally there is a vaso-vagal response with extreme bradycardia and consequent hypotension. If anaesthesia is exceptionally light, contractions of limb or facial muscles, or small jerky respiratory movements will occur either spontaneously or in response to surgical stimulation may be seen on some occasions.

At the end of surgery, depth of residual block should be assessed, and reversal employed as required. IPPV needs to be continued until spontaneous ventilation is adequate. IPPV can be slowed (but not stopped) to allow arterial carbon dioxide levels to return to 'normal anaesthetized' 40–45 mmHg (5.3–6 kPa) if ventilation has been excessive (a capnography helps with this) but, under anaesthesia, respiration does not increase in response to increased carbon dioxide and, indeed, high levels, coupled with hypoxia, will delay recovery through central depression.

POSTOPERATIVE COMPLICATIONS OF NEUROMUSCULAR BLOCKING AGENTS

Prolonged apnoea

The fear of every anaesthetist when first using NMBAs is that the animal will not breathe at the end of the procedure. If this happens, the animal should be ventilated until the cause of the apnoea can be ascertained and treated. The four most common causes are continual NMB, deep anaesthesia, hypothermia and overventilation.

Continued NMB

Continuing NMB can be identified by peripheral nerve stimulation, but is more difficult to ascertain if this is not available. It is best prevented by the avoidance of excessive doses of NMBAs, mixing NMBAs (Gurney & Mosing, 2012), and by using the newer shorter acting agents. If non-depolarizing agents were used, then the block may be reversed using an anticholinesterase (with an anticholinergic agent – see above), but this will only be effective if there was some return of muscle tone, and there is a maximal dose after which there will be no further effect. There is no antidote to the Phase I block of depolarizing drugs and the only treatment is IPPV until the return of adequate spontaneous breathing.

Deep anaesthesia

Once certain that residual NMB is not the reason for failure to breathe, depth of anaesthesia should be lightened, while still continuing to ventilate the patient. If antagonists (e.g. to opioids, α_2-agonists etc.) are employed, the influence on subsequent postoperative analgesia needs consideration.

Hypothermia

This is one of the commonest causes of prolonged apnoea following the use of non-depolarizing agents. Precautions need to be taken to maintain the body temperature, especially during laparotomy and thoracotomy. This fall is particularly great in small animal patients and there is often difficulty in antagonizing the effects of non-depolarizing drugs in these animals until they are rewarmed.

Overventilation

If the animal has been overventilated, $PaCO_2$ may be sufficiently low to prevent return of spontaneous breathing, and the mode of returning CO_2 to normal (and not above) has been discussed above. In the authors' experience, if other factors (reversal of NMB, light depth of anaesthesia and normothermia) are correct, then the animal will attempt to breathe despite continuing ventilation.

Residual NMB

Animals should not be left in the postoperative period with any residual neuromuscular block. The problems relating to this vary between species, but include respiratory inadequacy, failure to control the airway, post-operative lung infections and, in large animals, problems in regaining their feet.

CENTRALLY ACTING MUSCLE RELAXANTS

Guaifenesin

Guaifenesin (Guaiphenesin, guaicol glycerine ether, GGE or GG) is an agent which, in veterinary medicine, is used, usually in combination with anaesthetics, to give a degree of muscle relaxation. It is thought to exert its effect at the spinal cord by interfering with polysynaptic transmission and, therefore, in contrast with NMBAs, it crosses the blood–brain barrier. It is used primarily in large animals. The doses required, coupled with the fact that concentrated solutions are very irritant, causing damage to the intima of the veins with subsequent (delayed) thrombi formation (Herschl et al., 1992) and has a concentration dependent haemolytic effect, mean that it needs to be used as dilute as possible (preferably no more concentrated than 5%) by IV infusion. A number of stabilized solutions (of varying concentrations depending on the country) are available. A solution in water or 5% dextrose can be made up from the crystals; this is not stabilized and, if spilt, the crystals precipitate out, and are very irritant, including to human skin.

When guaifenesin is given alone by IV infusion, the horse/cow becomes weak, and with sufficiently high doses (around 100 mg/kg) will become recumbent. However, guaifenesin produces no analgesia, nor does it make the animal unconscious and, although the ethical situation is not as for an NMBA, guaifenesin is generally used in combination with an IV anaesthetic agent to ensure that the animal is unconscious. Details of doses and combinations are given in the relevant chapters (11 and 12).

Cattle and horses given guaifenesin, alone or as part of an anaesthetic induction, will breathe spontaneously. Hubbell et al. (1980) investigated its effects in horses and found that at doses which caused recumbency there was a significant fall in arterial blood pressure, a transient but significant fall in PaO_2, but that all other cardiopulmonary parameters, including cardiac output, remained unchanged.

Guaifenesin has been used in other species of animal but its administration is difficult because of the large volumes of solution which must be infused. In humans, it is licensed for oral use in cough medicines as an expectorant, but there are also anecdotal reports of its use in the alleviation of symptoms of fibromyalgia.

Benzodiazepines

Benzodiazepine agents cause muscle relaxation by an action at the spinal cord in a similar manner to that caused by guaifenesin. They are used to good effect for this property in many species and in many anaesthetic combinations. It is considerably easier to administer a small volume of diazepam to a horse than to infuse 500–1000 mL guaifenesin. The benzodiazepine agents most employed in veterinary anaesthesia have been discussed in Chapter 4.

REFERENCES

Adams, A.K., Hall, L.W., 1962. An experimental study of the action of suxamethonium on the circulatory system. Br J Anaesth 34, 445–450.

Adams, W.A., Mark Senior, J., Jones, R.S., et al., 2006. cis-Atracurium in dogs with and without porto-systemic shunts. Vet Anaesth Analg 33, 17–23.

Ali, H.H., Utting, J.E., Gray, C., 1970. Stimulus frequency in the detection of neuromuscular block in humans. Br J Anaesth 42, 967–978.

Amaki, Y., Waud, B.E., Waud, D.R., 1985. Atracurium-receptor kinetics: simple behavior from a mixture. Anesth Analg 64, 777–780.

Auer, U., 2007. Clinical observations on the use of the muscle relaxant rocuronium bromide in the dog. Vet J 173, 422–427.

Auer, U., Moens, Y., 2011. Neuromuscular blockade with rocuronium bromide for ophthalmic surgery in horses. Vet Ophthalmol 14, 244–247.

Auer, U., Mosing, M., 2006. A clinical study of the effects of rocuronium in isoflurane-anaesthetized cats. Vet Anaesth Analg 33, 224–228.

Auer, U., Uray, C., Mosing, M., 2007. Observations on the muscle relaxant rocuronium bromide in the horse – a dose-response study. Vet Anaesth Analg 34, 75–81.

Bleijenberg, E.H., van Oostrom, H., Akkerdaas, L.C., et al., 2011. Bispectral index and the clinically evaluated anaesthetic depth in dogs. Vet Anaesth Analg 38, 536–543.

Bom, A., Bradley, M., Cameron, K., et al., 2002. A novel concept of reversing neuromuscular block: chemical encapsulation of rocuronium bromide by a cyclodextrin-based synthetic host. Angew Chem Int Ed Engl 41, 266–270.

Booij, L.H., 2009. Cyclodextrins and the emergence of sugammadex. Anaesthesia 64 (Suppl 1), 31–37.

Brull, S.J., Connelly, N.R., O'Connor, T.Z., et al., 1991. Effect of tetanus on subsequent neuromuscular monitoring in patients receiving vecuronium. Anesthesiology 74, 64–70.

Burns, B.D., Paton, W.D., 1951. Depolarization of the motor end-plate by decamethonium and acetylcholine. J Physiol 115, 41–73.

Cason, B., Baker, D.G., Hickey, R.F., et al., 1990. Cardiovascular and neuromuscular effects of three steroidal neuromuscular blocking drugs in dogs (ORG 9616, ORG 9426, ORG 9991). Anesth Analg 70, 382–388.

Chambers, D., Paulden, M., Paton, F., et al., 2010. Sugammadex for reversal of neuromuscular block after rapid sequence intubation: a systematic review and economic assessment. Br J Anaesth 105, 568–575.

Chen, C., Yamaguchi, N., Varin, F., 2009. Studies on the pharmacokinetics of cisatracurium in anesthetized dogs: in vitro-in vivo correlations. J Vet Pharmacol Ther 32, 571–576.

Claudius, C., Viby-Mogensen, J., 2008. Acceleromyography for use in scientific and clinical practice: a systematic review of the evidence. Anesthesiology 108, 1117–1140.

Clutton, E., 2007. Surgical relaxation and neuromuscular block. In Practice 29, 574–583.

Clutton, R.E., Glasby, M.A., 1998. A comparison of the neuromuscular and cardiovascular effects of vecuronium, atracurium and mivacurium in sheep. Res Vet Sci 64, 233–237.

Clutton, R.E., Richards, D.L.S., Lee, J.C., 1986. The effects of vecuronium bromide on single-twitch studies in maignant hyperthermia susceptable pigs. Vet Surg 15–461.

Clutton, R.E., Dissanayake, K., Lawson, H., et al., 2013. The construction and evaluation of a device for mechanomyography in anaesthetized Gottingen minipigs. Vet Anaesth Analg 40, 134–141.

Cookson, J.C., Paton, W.D., 1969. Mechanisms of neuromuscular block. A review article. Anaesthesia 24, 395–416.

Craig, R.G., Hunter, J.M., 2009. Neuromuscular blocking drugs and their antagonists in patients with organ disease. Anaesthesia 64 (Suppl 1), 55–65.

Deana, A., Scuka, M., 1990. Time course of neostigmine action on the endplate response. Neurosci Lett 118, 82–84.

Donati, F., 1988. Onset of action of relaxants. Can J Anaesth 35, S52–S58.

Donati, F., Meistelman, C., Plaud, B., 1990. Vecuronium neuromuscular blockade at the diaphragm, the orbicularis oculi, and adductor pollicis muscles. Anesthesiology 73, 870–875.

EMC, 2012. http://www.medicines.org.uk/EMC/medicine/21299/SPC/Bridion+100+mg+ml+solution+for+injection/. Accessed 1/8/2012.

Faye, S., 1988. PhD thesis. University of Leeds, Leeds.

Fink, H., Hollmann, M.W., 2012. Myths and facts in neuromuscular pharmacology. New developments in reversing neuromuscular blockade. Minerva Anestesiol 78, 473–482.

Fuchs-Buder, T., Claudius, C., Skovgaard, L.T., et al., 2007. Good clinical research practice in pharmacodynamic studies of neuromuscular blocking agents II: the Stockholm revision. Acta Anaesthesiol Scand 51, 789–808.

Fuchs-Buder, T., Schreiber, J.U., Meistelman, C., 2009. Monitoring neuromuscular block: an update. Anaesthesia 64 (Suppl 1), 82–89.

Gill, S.S., Donati, F., Bevan, D.R., 1990. Clinical evaluation of double-burst stimulation. Its relationship to train-of-four stimulation. Anaesthesia 45, 543–548.

Gleed, R.D., Jones, R.S., 1982. Observations on the neuromuscular blocking action of gallamine and pancuronium and their reversal by neostigmine. Res Vet Sci 32, 324–326.

Gurney, M., Mosing, M., 2012. Prolonged neuromuscular blockade in a horse following concomitant use of vecuronium and atracurium. Vet Anaesth Analg 39, 119–120.

Hall, L.W., 1952. A report on the clinical use of bis-(β-dimethylaminoethyl) succinate bisethiodide (Brevidil E, M & B 2210) in the dog. Vet Rec 64: 491–492.

Hall, L.W., Lehmann, H., 1953. Response in dogs to relaxants derived from succinic acid and choline. Br Med J 1, 134–136.

Hall, L.W., Woolf, N., Bradley, J.W., et al., 1966. Unusual reaction to suxamethonium chloride. Br Med J 2, 1305.

Herschl, M.A., Trim, C.M., Mahaffey, E.A., 1992. Effects of 5% and 10% guaifenesin infusion on equine vascular endothelium. Vet Surg 21, 494–497.

Hildebrand, S.V., Arpin, D., 1988. Neuromuscular and cardiovascular effects of atracurium administered to healthy horses anesthetized with halothane. Am J Vet Res 49, 1066–1071.

Hildebrand, S.V., Hill, T., 3rd, 1989. Effects of atracurium administered by continuous intravenous infusion in halothane-anesthetized horses. Am J Vet Res 50, 2124–2126.

Hildebrand, S.V., Howitt, G.A., 1984. Dosage requirement of pancuronium in halothane-anesthetized ponies: a comparison of cumulative and single-dose administration. Am J Vet Res 45, 2441–2444.

Hildebrand, S.V., Holland, M., Copland, V.S., et al., 1989. Clinical use of the neuromuscular blocking agents atracurium and pancuronium for equine anesthesia. J Am Vet Med Assoc 195, 212–219.

Hildebrand, S.V., Howitt, G.A., Arpin, D., 1986. Neuromuscular and cardiovascular effects of atracurium in ponies anesthetized with halothane. Am J Vet Res 47, 1096–1100.

Hubbell, J.A., Muir, W.W., Sams, R.A., 1980. Guaifenesin: cardiopulmonary effects and plasma concentrations in horses. Am J Vet Res 41, 1751–1755.

Hudetz, A.G., Hemmings, H.C., Jr, 2012. Anaesthesia awareness: 3 years of progress. Br J Anaesth 108, 180–182.

Ibebunjo, C., Hall, L.W., 1993. Muscle fibre diameter and sensitivity to neuromuscular blocking drugs. Br J Anaesth 71, 732–733.

Ibebunjo, C., Srikant, C.B., Donati, F., 1996. Duration of succinylcholine and vecuronium blockade but not potency correlates with the ratio of endplate size to fibre size in seven muscles in the goat. Can J Anaesth 43, 485–494.

Jones, R.M., 1984. Calcium antagonists. Anaesthesia 39, 747–749.

Jones, R.S., 1987a. Interactions between pipecuronium and suxamethonium in the dog. Res Vet Sci 43, 308–312.

Jones, R.S., 1987b. Observations on the neuromuscular blocking action of pipecuronium in the dog. Res Vet Sci 43, 101–103.

Jones, R.S., 1988. Reversal of nueromuscular block – a review. J Assoc Vet Anaesth 15, 80–88.

Jones, R.S., Brearley, J.C., 1985. Atracurium infusion in the dog. Proceedings of the 2nd International Congress of Veterinary Anaesthesia, Sacramento, pp. 172–173.

Jones, R.S., Seymour, C.J., 1985. Clinical observations on the use of vecuronium as a muscle relaxant in the dog. J Small Anim Pract 26, 213–218.

Jones, R.S., Heckmann, R., Wuersch, W., 1978. Observations on the neuromuscular blocking action of alcuronium in the dog and its reversal by neostigmine. Res Vet Sci 25, 101–102.

Jones, R.S., Hunter, J.M., Utting, J.E., 1983. Neuromuscular blocking action of atracurium in the dog and its reversal by neostigmine. Res Vet Sci 34, 173–176.

Jurado, O.M., Mosing, M., Kutter, A.P., et al., 2012. Cardiovascular effects of cis-atracurium overdose in a dog following misplacement of neuromuscular monitoring electrodes. Vet Anaesth Analg 39, 119–120.

Kalow, W., 1959. The distribution, destruction and elimination of muscle relaxants. Anesthesiology 20, 505–518.

Kastrup, M.R., Marsico, F.F., Ascoli, F.O., et al., 2005. Neuromuscular blocking properties of atracurium during sevoflurane or propofol anaesthesia in dogs. Vet Anaesth Analg 32, 222–227.

Katz, B., Thesleff, S., 1957. A study of the desensitization produced by acetylcholine at the motor end-plate. J Physiol 138, 63–80.

Khuenl-Brady, K., Castagnoli, K.P., Canfell, P.C., et al., 1990. The neuromuscular blocking effects and pharmacokinetics of ORG 9426 and ORG 9616 in the cat. Anesthesiology 72, 669–674.

Kopman, A.F., Eikermann, M., 2009. Antagonism of non-depolarising neuromuscular block: current practice. Anaesthesia 64 (Suppl 1), 22–30.

Kopman, A.F., Kumar, S., Klewicka, M.M., et al., 2001. The staircase phenomenon: implications for monitoring of neuromuscular transmission. Anesthesiology 95, 403–407.

Lang, T., Jahn, R., 2008. Core proteins of the secretory machinery. Handb Exp Pharmacol, 107–127.

Langford, R., 2012. iPhone for monitoring neuromuscular function. Anaesthesia 67, 552–553.

Lee, C., 2009. Goodbye suxamethonium! Anaesthesia 64 (Suppl 1), 73–81.

Manley, S.V., Steffey, E.P., Howitt, G.A., et al., 1983. Cardiovascular and neuromuscular effects of pancuronium bromide in the pony. Am J Vet Res 44, 1349–1353.

Marshall, R.J., Muir, A.W., Sleigh, T., et al., 1994. An overview of the pharmacology of rocuronium bromide in experimental animals. Eur J Anaesthesiol Suppl 9, 9–15.

Martin-Flores, M., Campoy, L., Ludders, J.W., et al., 2008. Comparison between acceleromyography and visual assessment of train-of-four for monitoring neuromuscular blockade in horses undergoing surgery. Vet Anaesth Analg 35, 220–227.

Martin-Flores, M., Boesch, J., Campoy, L., et al., 2011a. Failure to reverse prolonged vecuronium-induced neuromuscular blockade with edrophonium in an anesthetized dog. J Am Anim Hosp Assoc 47, 294–298.

Martin-Flores, M., Lau, E.J., Campoy, L., et al., 2011b. Twitch potentiation: a potential source of error during neuromuscular monitoring with acceleromyography in anesthetized dogs. Vet Anaesth Analg 38, 328–335.

Martin-Flores, M., Campoy, L., Gleed, R.D., 2012a. Further experiences with vercuronium in the horse. Vet Anaesth Analg 39, 218–219.

Martin-Flores, M., Pare, M.D., Adams, W., et al., 2012b. Observations of the potency and duration of vecuronium in isoflurane-anesthetized horses. Vet Anaesth Analg 39, 385–389.

Martin-Flores, M., Pare, M.D., Campoy, L., et al., 2012c. The sensitivity of sheep to vecuronium: an example of the limitations of extrapolation. Can J Anaesth.

Martyn, J.A., Fagerlund, M.J., Eriksson, L.I., 2009. Basic principles of neuromuscular transmission. Anaesthesia 64 (Suppl 1), 1–9.

Mirakhur, R.K., 2009. Sugammadex in clinical practice. Anaesthesia 64 (Suppl 1), 45–54.

Mosing, M., Auer, U., Bardell, D., et al., 2010. Reversal of profound rocuronium block monitored in three muscle groups with sugammadex in ponies. Br J Anaesth 105, 480–486.

Mosing, M., Auer, U., West, E., et al., 2012. Reversal of profound rocuronium or vecuronium-induced neuromuscular block with sugammadex in isoflurane-anaesthetised dogs. Vet J 192, 467–471.

Muir, A.W., Houston, J., Green, K.L., et al., 1989. Effects of a new neuromuscular blocking agent (Org 9426) in anaesthetized cats and pigs and in isolated nerve-muscle preparations. Br J Anaesth 63, 400–410.

Naguib, M., Lien, C., 2010. Pharmacology of muscle relaxants and their antagonists. In: Miller, R.D., Eriksson, L.I., Fleisher, L.A., et al. (Eds.), Miller's Anesthesia, seventh ed. Churchill Livingstone Elsevier, Philadelphia, pp. 859–912.

Paton, F., Paulden, M., Chambers, D., et al., 2010. Sugammadex compared with neostigmine/glycopyrrolate for routine reversal of neuromuscular block: a systematic review and economic evaluation. Br J Anaesth 105, 558–567.

Ribeiro, L.M., Ferreira, D.A., Bras, S., et al., 2012. Correlation between clinical signs of depth of anaesthesia and cerebral state index responses in dogs with different target-controlled infusions of propofol. Vet Anaesth Analg 39, 21–28.

Sarrafzadeh-Rezaei, F., Clutton, R.E., 2009. The effect of volatile anaesthetics on the relative sensitivity of facial and distal thoracic limb muscles to vecuronium in dogs. Vet Anaesth Analg 36, 55–62.

Savarese, J.J., Ali, H.H., Basta, S.J., et al., 1988. The clinical neuromuscular pharmacology of mivacurium chloride (BW B1090U). A short-acting nondepolarizing ester neuromuscular blocking drug. Anesthesiology 68, 723–732.

Shilo, Y., Pypendop, B.H., Barter, L.S., et al., 2011. Thymoma removal in a cat with acquired myasthenia gravis: a case report and literature review of anesthetic techniques. Vet Anaesth Analg 38, 603–613.

Torda, T.A., Graham, G.G., Warwick, N.R., et al., 1997. Pharmacokinetics and pharmacodynamics of suxamethonium. Anaesth Intensive Care 25, 272–278.

Veres-Nyeki, K.O., Rieben, R., Spadavecchia, C., et al., 2012. Pancuronium dose refinement in experimental pigs used in cardiovascular research. Vet Anaesth Analg 39, 529–532.

Viby-Mogensen, J., 2010. Neuromuscular monitoring. In: Miller, R.D., Eriksson, L.I., Fleisher, L.A., et al. (Eds.), Miller's Anesthesia, seventh ed. Churchill Livingstone Elsevier, Philadelphia, pp. 1515–1531.

Wachtel, R.E., 1990. Comparison of anticholinesterases and their effects on acetylcholine-activated ion channels. Anesthesiology 72, 496–503.

Chapter | 9 |

Pulmonary gas exchange: artificial ventilation of the lungs

INTRODUCTION

The techniques used to ventilate the lungs during anaesthesia usually involve endotracheal intubation, then periodic inflation of the lungs. The commonest method used in these circumstances is known as 'intermittent positive pressure ventilation' or IPPV. It is used widely in anaesthesia to counteract anaesthetic-induced respiratory depression, or whenever neuromuscular blocking agents have been used (see Chapter 8). It is also a routine technique in intensive care, but here more sophisticated methods of ventilation are required than for anaesthesia. There are differences between spontaneous breathing and IPPV, and IPPV when the thoracic cage is opened widely at thoracotomy from when it is intact. The anaesthetist must appreciate what these differences are if IPPV is to be correctly managed under all circumstances.

SPONTANEOUS RESPIRATION

In a spontaneously breathing animal, active contraction of the inspiratory muscles lowers the normally subatmospheric intrapleural pressure still further by enlarging the relatively rigid thoracic cavity. The decrease in intrapleural pressure lowers the alveolar pressure (Fig. 9.1) so that a pressure gradient or driving force is set up between the exterior and the alveoli. This overcomes the airway resistance and air flows into the alveoli until, at the end of inspiration, the alveolar pressure becomes equal to the atmospheric pressure. During expiration the pressure gradient is reversed and air flows out of the alveoli.

The transpulmonary pressure is a measure of the elastic forces which tend to collapse the lungs (Fig. 9.1). There is no one single intrapleural pressure; in the ventral parts of the chest it is just sufficient to keep the lungs expanded but because of the influence of gravity acting on the lungs, in the dorsal parts of the chest the intrapleural pressure should be much more below atmospheric. However, it is not at all certain how uniform the pressure on the pleural surface of the lung really is. The hilar forces, the buoyancy

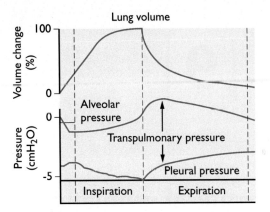

Figure 9.1 Changes in lung volume, pleural and transpulmonary pressures during normal spontaneous breathing (diagrammatic only).

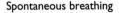

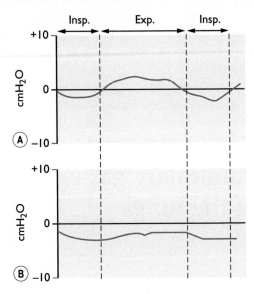

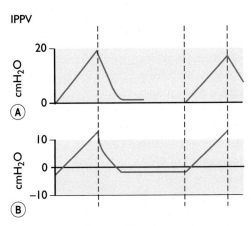

Figure 9.2 Pressure changes (A) at the mouth end of endotracheal tube, (B) in the thoracic oesophagus during spontaneous breathing and IPPV with closed chest (diagrammatic only).

of the lung in the pleural cavity and the different shapes of the lung and chest wall are all possible sources of local pressure differences. Thus, it is customary to measure the intraoesophageal pressure as being representative of the mean intrapleural pressure (Fig. 9.2).

The alveolar pressure changes generate airflow into and out of the lungs against a resistance in a way analogous to that stated by Ohm's Law for electricity, where:

$$R = \frac{E}{R}$$

So that:

$$Resistance = \frac{alveolar\ pressure\ change}{airflow}$$

Airway resistance is largely influenced by the lung volume because the elastic recoil of lung parenchyma exerts traction on the pleural surfaces and walls of airways (holding them patent) when the lungs are inflated above residual volume. As the lungs are further inflated, elastic recoil pressure increases, thus further dilating the airways and decreasing resistance to air flow. This relationship between airway resistance and lung volume is hyperbolic in nature, as shown in Figure 9. 3. Airway resistance also depends on the nature of airflow through the airway. With a clear airway and a low gas flow rate, intrapulmonary flow is largely laminar (streamlined) and airway resistance is also low, but obstruction or a high flow velocity will give rise to turbulence and a greatly increased resistance. Measurement of airway resistance must be made when gas is flowing. During IPPV, when the chest wall is intact, resistance to expansion of the lungs is also offered by the chest wall which then contributes to the total respiratory resistance.

Total respiratory resistance (Rrs) may be estimated by the application of an oscillating airflow to the airways with measurement of the resultant pressure and airflow changes. A technique was developed by Lehane et al. (1980) to measure airway resistance as a function of lung volume during a vital capacity manoeuvre and so to derive specific lower airways conductance, s.Glaw (conductance being the reciprocal of resistance) and the expiratory reserve volume (ERV). The method was modified by Watney et al. (1987, 1988) for use in anaesthetized and paralysed horses and dogs and it was demonstrated that, in ponies, xylazine,

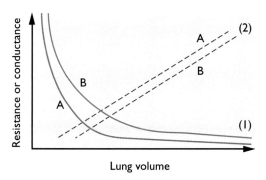

Figure 9.3 Resistance and volume curves together with lower airways conductance curves (Glaw). (1): Resistance curves; (2): (Glaw); (A): normal airway; (B): obstructed airway. *Lehane et al., 1980, by permission of Oxford University Press.*

acepromazine, halothane and enflurane produce bronchodilation and a decrease in ERV while isoflurane appears to increase ERV. In dogs, it was concluded that both bronchoconstriction and changes in lung volume may be responsible for changes in airway resistance seen during hypoxia. During spontaneous breathing, changes in resistance may necessitate a great increase in the work of breathing. The effect of inhalation anaesthetics on total respiratory resistance in conscious horses was studied by Hall & Young (1992) who showed that halothane appeared to have no effect while enflurane and isoflurane seemed to increase it. In contrast in humans, neither isoflurane nor sevoflurane altered résistance, although desflurane at higher concentrations did cause an increase (Nyktari et al, 2011).

Resistance is not the only factor opposing movement of air in and out of the chest; a full analysis includes the effects of compliance and inertance. Adding the compliance and inertance forms the reactance and this can be combined with the resistance in one complex term called the 'impedance'. If the impedance of the respiratory system is known then the resistance and reactance can be determined. A non-invasive method (Michaelson et al., 1975) that does not require patient cooperation has been adapted for use in conscious animals as described by Young and Hall (1989) for horses but it is difficult to use in anaesthetized, intubated animals because the impedance of the tube alone is much greater than that of a non-intubated animal. Small airways contribute little to the total lung resistance; although each one has a large individual resistance, there are large numbers in parallel so that the overall effect is small. This is important because small airway disease (which increases local resistance) is not detected by measurement of total airway resistance until the condition is well advanced.

Anaesthetic apparatus may afford resistance that is considerably higher than that offered by the animal's respiratory tract. However, it is unlikely that moderate expiratory resistance will cause serious problems in spontaneously breathing animals and, indeed, positive end expiratory pressure (PEEP) (see PEEP and CPAP below) has many positive advantages. However, resistance increases the work of breathing, and common sense suggests that apparatus resistance should be kept to a minimum. Purchase (1965a,b) studied the resistance afforded by four closed breathing systems used in horses and cattle and in three, all of which had internal bores of 5 cm, found it to be of the order of 1 cmH$_2$O (0.1 kPa) per 100L/min at flow rates of 600 L/min. The resistance of endotracheal tube connectors was relatively high in comparison with that of the remainder of the apparatus.

During a breathing cycle, mean intrathoracic pressure may be above or below atmospheric pressure as a result of apparatus resistance. For example, if the expiratory flow through a piece of apparatus with a high resistance is great enough to induce turbulence, while the inspiratory rate is low (as it often is in horses) so that during inspiration the flow is laminar, the mean intrathoracic pressure will be above atmospheric. Conversely, if the inspiratory flow rate is greater, there may be a subatmospheric mean intrathoracic pressure. Mean intrathoracic pressures above atmospheric reduce the effect of the thoracoabdominal pump for venous return, with subsequent cardiovascular effects. Large subatmospheric mean intrathoracic pressures may be equally dangerous, perhaps by producing pulmonary oedema, but probably more importantly by reducing lung volume. Trapping of gas in the lungs occurs more readily at low lung volumes and gas trapping produces widespread airway obstruction with serious impairment of respiratory function.

IPPV WHEN THE CHEST WALL IS INTACT

IPPV is applied easily during anaesthesia by rhythmical compression of the reservoir bag of a breathing circuit. This is most simply achieved by manual squeezing, but machines have been designed and built to relieve the anaesthetist of the bag-squeezing duty. If the bag is squeezed as the animal breathes in, the tidal volume may be augmented ('*assisted ventilation*'). The increased ventilation produced results in 'washout' of CO$_2$ and the PaCO$_2$ falls below the threshold for stimulating the respiratory centre so that spontaneous breathing movements cease and the anaesthetist can impose whatever respiratory rhythm is required – '*controlled ventilation*'. A machine provides the most efficient means of ventilating the lungs for prolonged periods, but to use it properly or even to squeeze a bag correctly, it is necessary to understand the principles underlying IPPV and under what circumstances any possible harmful effects may arise.

Compliance has been defined in many ways but the simplest definition is that it is the volume change

197

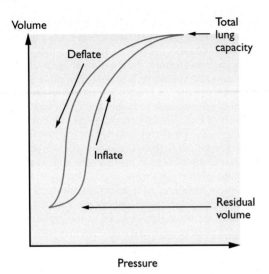

Figure 9.4 Total thoracic compliance curves showing hysteresis. The compliance can be altered by a number of factors: (A) the lung compliance is reduced by lack of surfactant (respiratory distress syndrome), reduction of elastic tissue in the lungs (as in emphysema), and fibrosis or scar tissue; (B) the chest wall compliance is altered by obesity and splinting of the diaphragm by abdominal disorders.

produced by unit pressure change ($\delta V/\delta P$). Compliance shows hysteresis (Fig. 9.4). It is changes in surfactant which seem to be responsible; airway resistance and tissue viscosity play only a small part. Ideally, measurements needed for the calculation necessary to obtain this value should be made when no air is flowing into or out of the lungs (i.e. at the end of inspiration). Compliance measures cannot be compared unless related to a lung volume such as the functional residual capacity (FRC). Unfortunately, measurement of FRC is not a simple procedure and such measurements of compliance as have been made in animals have often omitted this refinement.

As commonly measured, compliance has two components and compliance values can be found for both the lungs themselves and the thoracic cage. When the chest wall is not intact, the total compliance measured approaches that of the lungs alone. It might seem that methods using high airway pressures to inflate the lungs might be safe if, when compliance is reduced, it is the thoracic cage itself which is uncompliant, because alveoli only rupture when overdistended. However, decreased compliance of the lungs themselves is apt to be non-uniform; an airway pressure which produces little ventilation of some regions may overdistend and even rupture alveoli in other regions. During anaesthesia, compliance may be altered by assistants resting their weight on the chest, by the use of retractors and by the degree of muscle relaxation.

Airway resistance has to be overcome to deliver gas to the alveoli at inspiration and to expel it during expiration.

Resistance during anaesthesia is increased by the resistance of apparatus used, such as endotracheal tubes. Animals with pulmonary disease may also have increased airway resistance so that it is necessary to allow a more prolonged expiratory period if the lungs are to deflate to FRC. If this is not done, lung volume will be greater at the start of the next inspiration and there will be a steady increase in FRC until the retractive forces of the lung, which increase with increase in lung volume, become sufficient to empty the lungs to a new FRC in the time available and the inspiratory and expiratory tidal volumes become normally related. While conscious, the animal with expiratory obstruction empties its lungs by active expiratory movements but, when anaesthetized and paralysed or made otherwise apnoeic, expiration may become passive and, consequently, of longer duration. The pattern of IPPV used must make allowance for this, and large tidal volumes should be delivered with long expiratory pauses between each inspiration to allow the chest to return to its original resting position.

The induction of general anaesthesia is usually associated with an increase in resistance due to a decrease in lung volume but this may be countered to some extent by bronchodilation, depending on the agents given.

The most obvious effect of IPPV when the chest is closed is on the circulatory system. During spontaneous breathing, by lowering intrathoracic pressure, inspiration augments the venous return to the heart; in many animals, as can often be seen on the arterial blood pressure trace, there are indications that a increased stroke volume is produced. During IPPV, however, intrathoracic pressure rises during inspiration, blood is dammed back from the thorax, venous return and stroke volume decrease; blood flows freely into the thoracic vessels during the expiratory period. Fortunately, by causing distension of veins this damming back of blood during inspiration produces a reflex increase in venous tone which, in normal animals, appears to compensate for the changed intrathoracic conditions during the inspiratory period and restores the venous return towards normality. Obviously, the extent to which an increase in venous tone can compensate will depend on the degree of venomotor integrity (which can be affected by drugs), the blood volume, the magnitude of the intrathoracic pressure rise and its duration.

The magnitude and duration of the increased pressure within the thorax during the inspiratory phase of IPPV are, therefore, critical and are reflected in the 'mean intrathoracic pressure'. This mean pressure, like the mean arterial blood pressure, is not the simple arithmetical mean between the highest and lowest pressures reached in the system and its calculation is not always easy for the non-mathematician. It is clearly important to keep this mean pressure as low as possible during the respiratory cycle and this can be accomplished in a variety of ways.

1. Short application of positive pressure

The shorter the inspiratory period during IPPV the lower the mean intrathoracic pressure will be for any given applied pressure. Theoretically, it might seem that the peak pressure should never be maintained – expiration should commence as soon as the peak pressure is achieved – or the circulation will suffer. However, the short application of a positive pressure may not result in very good distribution of fresh gas within the lungs. In humans, very short inspiratory periods have the effect of increasing the physiological dead space, while Hall et al. (1968) found a decrease in the physiological dead space/tidal volume ratio in horses ventilated with a ventilator which had a relatively long inspiratory phase. A compromise seems to be necessary here, but exactly what it is likely to be for any one animal of any one species remains pure speculation. It is usually taught that in small animals (dogs, cats, foals, calves, sheep), the inspiratory time should be 1.0–1.5 seconds and in adult horses and cattle 2–3 seconds provided the lungs are healthy.

2. Rapid gas flow rate

If the necessary tidal volume of gas is to be delivered to the lungs in a short inspiratory period, it is clear that the flow rate will need to be high. The rate at which gas can flow into the lungs, however, is largely dictated by the resistance offered by the apparatus used and the airway resistance. The airway resistance to the various lung regions may not be uniform. For example, a bleb of mucus may partially obstruct a small bronchus and greatly increase the resistance to gas flow through it. A high gas flow rate through a neighbouring, unobstructed bronchus may result in overdistension of the alveoli supplied by it in an interval of time so short that the alveoli supplied by the partially obstructed bronchus will not have time for more than minimal expansion. Theoretically, it would seem that under these circumstances alveolar rupture might occur but, in practice, this complication seems rare unless pulmonary contusions exist from auto-trauma.

3. Low expiratory resistance

Any resistance to the airflow created by the passive phase of IPPV will delay the fall in intrathoracic pressure, will result in an increase in mean intrathoracic pressure and possibly in circulatory consequences. However, expiratory resistance can result in more orderly emptying of alveoli and an increase in FRC with consequent widening of the airways that helps to prevent airway collapse. It is now recognized that there are many situations (e.g. in animals with obstructive emphysema) where a higher expiratory resistance is advantageous (see PEEP and CPAP).

4. Subatmospheric pressure during the expiratory phase

If a subatmospheric pressure is applied to the airway during the expiratory phase of IPPV, the inspiratory pressure will be applied from a lower baseline and the pressure gradient necessary to produce the required volume change in the lungs can be achieved with a lower peak pressure. Theoretically, this might be expected to help maintain cardiac output, but changes in arterial blood pressure and cardiac output are proportional to the duration of the increased airway pressure and not necessarily to the peak pressures reached. Consequently, merely decreasing the peak airway pressure may have but little effect if the inspiratory phase is long. Expiratory subatmospheric pressure may also cause airway collapse and air trapping, and is not used in routine ventilation during anaesthesia (although subatmospheric pressures for inspiration are, of course, the basis of the 'iron lung' type ventilators used in human patients with long-term paralysis).

IPPV AFTER OPENING OF THE PLEURAL CAVITY

Collapse of the lung

Normally, distension of the lungs to fill the thoracic cavity is due to the existence of a pressure gradient between the airway and the pleural cavity. The airway pressure is usually atmospheric and the intrapleural pressure subatmospheric due to the outward recoil forces of the chest wall, the lymphatic removal of fluid from the pleural cavity and the limited expansibility of the lungs. This distending force is opposed by what has been termed the 'elasticity' of the lung tissue, although the term 'elasticity' is not strictly applicable because surface tension in the alveoli contributes in a most important manner to the lung retractive force. When the chest is opened and atmospheric pressure allowed to act directly in the pleural cavity, the normal pressure gradient is abolished and the retractive forces cause the lung to collapse (Fig. 9.5).

Paradoxical respiration

The paradox is that during spontaneous breathing following unilateral large openings into the pleural cavity, the lung on the damaged side of the chest becomes smaller on inspiration and larger on expiration. Normally, when the thorax enlarges due to activity of the inspiratory muscles its increased volume comes to be occupied by air which enters via the trachea and blood which enters the right atrium and thin-walled great veins. In the presence of a unilateral open pneumothorax, air enters not only into the lungs via the trachea but also through the chest wall defect into the pleural cavity. The proportion of air entering by each route is largely governed by the relative size of the chest wall defect to the tracheal lumen. When the opening to the hemithorax is large, or when there is

199

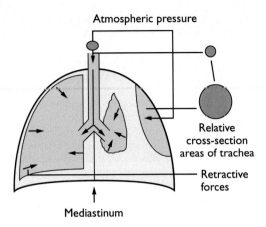

Figure 9.5 Forces responsible for collapse of the lung following unilateral opening of the chest wall during spontaneous breathing. The volume of air entering the pleural cavity at each breath will depend on the relative cross-sectional area of the trachea and the defect in the chest wall.

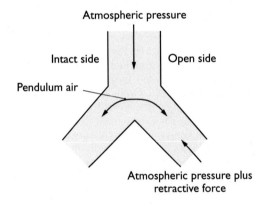

Figure 9.6 Effect of unilateral pneumothorax on intrabronchial pressure.

open pneumothorax breathing spontaneously shuttles air from one lung to the other. This 'pendulum air' produces, in effect, an increase in respiratory dead space, and the animal's respiratory efforts are less effective in producing overall ventilation. It is not seen after bilateral opening of the pleural cavity through a sternotomy. Applying positive pressure to the airway during inspiration abolishes paradoxical respiration.

Mediastinal movement

In any normal animal, the mediastinum is not a rigid partition between the two halves of the chest and, in practice, the behaviour of each half of the chest during respiration is always dependent on the conditions prevailing in the other half. Unilateral pneumothorax can occur in all domestic animals and its presence causes the mediastinum to move towards the intact side during inspiration and the opposite way during expiration. This movement of the mediastinum results in obstruction of the thin-walled great veins and thus impedes the venous return to the heart, but this is not often the major problem as death is usually due to hypoxia. Rigidity of the mediastinum may be encountered in chronic inflammatory pleuritis.

Effects on the circulation

It might be expected that most of the potentially harmful effects of IPPV on the circulatory system would be absent when the pleura is opened widely because an opening in the chest wall should prevent compression of intrathoracic vessels when positive pressure is applied to the airway. There is no evidence to prove if this is the case and, in clinical practice, there will be many other interferences to the circulation (e.g. caused by the surgeon) that will predominate.

POSSIBLE HARMFUL EFFECTS OF IPPV

The effects of IPPV on pulmonary ventilation are, of course, in the main clearly beneficial, and often essential. The potential effects on the circulation have been discussed above. Concern is always voiced that there may be rupture of lung tissue if inspiratory pressures are too high. However, this is no more likely to occur during properly conducted IPPV, particularly if the chest is closed, than during the ordinary activities of life – very high intrapulmonary pressures develop during activities such as coughing, or straining at defaecation or parturition. Care is needed, however, when ventilators are used for, in some, sticking of valves may expose the patient's airway directly to the high pressures at which gases are delivered from the anaesthetic machine to the ventilator. As already

any degree of airway obstruction, the greater volume of air will enter through the hole in the chest wall and the mediastinum will be pushed towards the intact side of the chest. During inspiration, pressure in the bronchi on the open side of the chest will be greater than in the trachea because of the addition of the normal retractive forces of the lung to the atmospheric pressure acting on the pleural surface of the exposed lung (Fig. 9.6). Thus, on inspiration the increased volume on the intact side of the chest is occupied by air from the collapsed lung as well as from the atmosphere. The exposed lung, therefore, becomes smaller. On expiration, the lung on the intact side is discharged partly into the collapsed lung, which becomes larger. In this way, an animal with a unilateral mentioned, uneven inflation of alveoli is a distinct possibility during IPPV but the surrounding tissues seem to provide sufficient support to prevent rupture of the relatively overinflated alveoli.

Any uneven distribution of gas must have the effect of disturbing the normal ventilation/perfusion relationships within the lungs. It appears that these are often upset by anaesthesia itself and, if IPPV produces more uneven gas distribution, it will probably fail to affect any improvement in the alveolar–arterial oxygen tension gradient found during anaesthesia in spite of any improvement in tidal exchange which it may produce. This is most evident in the anaesthetized horse, where IPPV appears to produce very little improvement in the alveolar–arterial oxygen tension (see Chapter 11). Other situations in which the normal relationships between ventilation may be upset occur in all animals where the expansion of one lung or part of a lung is limited by surgical procedures such as 'packing off' and retraction of lung lobes during intrathoracic surgery.

IPPV should remove CO_2 from the animal's lungs and it is possible, over a period of time, to remove either too much or too little causing the animal to suffer from either respiratory alkalosis or acidosis. Respiratory acidosis (hypercapnia) is characterized by sympathetic overactivity, cutaneous vasodilation, a rise in arterial blood pressure and a bounding pulse. Respiratory alkalosis (hypocapnia) may, it has been claimed, lead to cerebral damage from cerebral vasoconstriction because the calibre of the cerebral blood vessels depends on the $PaCO_2$. However, convincing evidence of cerebral damage due to hypocapnia has yet to be produced. However, severe hypocapnia reduces cardiac output in horses (Hall et al., 1968), and can make it difficult to maintain arterial blood pressure at an adequate level.

Administering IPPV via a facemask instead of through an endotracheal tube results in forcing gases down the oesophagus into the stomach, and this mode should only be used in emergency situations. An inflated stomach limits ventilation, and regurgitation of gastric fluid is a distinct possibility. Gas accidentally forced into the stomach should be removed as soon as possible by passing a stomach tube.

PEEP, CPAP AND RECRUITMENT MANOEUVRES

In the above paragraphs, the problems of airway trapping and closure and of the influence of respiratory pressures on the circulation have been outlined. It is now recognized that, in many conditions, particularly in advanced lung disease, the imposition of an expiratory threshold has been shown to have beneficial effects on the PaO_2. Adding such an expiratory resistor during IPPV is known as PEEP

(positive end-expiratory pressure). If airway pressure above atmospheric is maintained throughout the breath it is known as CPAP (continuous positive airway pressure). The two conditions do differ but the terms are often used synonymously.

The respiratory benefits of an expiratory resistor include an overall reduction in airway resistance due to an increase in FRC, movement of the tidal volume above the airway closing volume, a tendency towards re-expansion of any collapsed lung and, possibly, a reduction in total lung water. The net result is that ventilation/perfusion relationships are improved. However, these advantages are, in some circumstances, counterbalanced by circulatory disadvantages due to the inevitable rise in mean intrathoracic pressure.

Both disease and drugs have profound effects on the circulatory response to a rise in mean intrathoracic pressure due to PEEP (or CPAP). In animals with poor lung compliance, much of the applied end-expiratory pressure will be opposed by the excessive pulmonary transmural pressure, thus minimizing the increase in intrathoracic pressure. Thus, the stiffer the lungs, the safer is the application of PEEP or CPAP likely to be. To summarize, PEEP and CPAP may confer respiratory advantages and circulatory disadvantages which interact in a complicated manner rendering it necessary to make direct measurements of the relevant physiological functions to ensure that overall benefit results.

The results of PEEP and CPAP during veterinary anaesthesia have been variable. Colgan et al. (1971) showed that PEEP produced no change in the alveolar–arterial gradient in anaesthetized dogs. Hall and Trim (1975) failed to demonstrate any benefit from PEEP in spontaneously breathing anaesthetized horses, and broadly similar results were obtained by Beadle et al. (1975). In experimental studies in dogs in which anaesthesia was maintained with 1% or 1.5% minimum alveolar concentration (MAC) of sevoflurane (Polis et al., 2001), PEEP of $5 \, cmH_2O$ always reduced shunt and arterial–alveolar gradient but, while cardiac output and arterial blood pressure were unchanged at 1 MAC, at 1.5 MAC, the imposition of PEEP resulted in significant depression of these parameters. In dogs undergoing one lung ventilation for thoracoscopy, 1.5 and $5 \, cmH_2O$ of PEEP improved oxygenation and reduced alveolar–arterial PO_2 differences without altering blood pressures but cardiac output was not measured in this study. Where available, the use of PEEP together with IPPV often is routine in equine anaesthesia.

Recruitment manoeuvres

The technique of 'sighing'– applying a single high tidal volume (which requires a high inspiratory pressure) for one breath to open up a collapsed lung – has been around for a very long time, but was developed with the term *open lung'* in relation to human patients suffering from acute respiratory distress syndrome (ARDS) (Lachmann, 1992; Amato et al., 1995, 1998). The idea is to open the collapsed alveolae with high inspiratory pressures, then to prevent re-collapse by the use of PEEP and this was taken forward to human anaesthesia by Tusman et al. (1999). Moens & Bohm (2011), in a brief editorial review, explain that the two strategies most commonly used in humans (again most usually patients with ARDS) are a single breath at a peak inspiratory pressure (PIP) of 40 cmH$_2$O, the lungs held inflated for 40 seconds, or a series of normally timed inspirations at the PIP of 40 cmH$_2$O with a PEEP of 20 cmH$_2$0. However, in ARDS patients, PIPs of up to 80 cmH$_2$O are sometimes required.

In veterinary anaesthesia, recruitment manoeuvres are most relevant to equine anaesthesia, but many authorities have been concerned that the circulatory effects may be catastrophic, and that high pressures may cause pulmonary damage. Wettstein et al. (2006), in horses under intravenous anaesthesia, used a stepwise manoeuvre, using PEEP and then PIPs of 45, 50 then 55 cmH$_2$O; oxygenation was improved and pulmonary shunt reduced and, although there was a fall in arterial blood pressure and heart rate, cardiac output was unchanged. In horses undergoing anaesthesia for colic, Hopster et al. (2011) used, with success in improving oxygenation, another recruitment modification; one breath with a PIP of 60, one with a PIP of 80, then a third at PIP 60 cmH$_2$O, each held inflated for 10–12 seconds while maintaining PEEP at 10 cmH$_2$0 or higher. Blood pressure and heart rate were only minimally affected, but cardiac output was not measured. To date, fears that the horses might suffer pulmonary damage from these high inflation pressures have not been founded, but numbers are still small.

In summary, PEEP, CPAP and recruitment manoeuvres are used widely in human anaesthesia; PEEP, at least, is used a great deal when ventilating horses, but there is need for more evidence before recommendations can be made for the best, most effective overall, strategies for use in veterinary anaesthetic practice.

MANAGEMENT OF IPPV

Assisted IPPV ventilation can be carried out on any anaesthetized animal but, for full control to be achieved, and the animal not to ventilation 'fight' the imposed ventilation all spontaneous breathing movements have to be abolished. This occurs (1) with neuromuscular block (see Chapter 8); (2) when respiratory centres are severely depressed by relative overdose of anaesthetics or other agents; (3) hyperventilation, by increasing minute volume with assisted ventilation, to lower PaCO$_2$; (4) reflex inhibition of the respiratory centres by regular rhythmical lung inflation. It is believed that if the lungs are slightly overdistended at each inspiration, afferent impulses from pulmonary receptors inhibit the medullary centres.

Manual ventilation

Manual squeezing of the reservoir bag (a procedure often known as 'bagging the animal') can be used to provide IPPV. This should be done gently and rhythmically. Once the desired degree of lung inflation has been produced, the bag should be released and the lungs allowed to empty freely, allowing (as would a ventilator) the expiratory pause to be longer than the time for inflation and the airway pressure to decrease to zero. The rate of lung ventilation should be faster than the normal anaesthetized respiratory rate of the animal and the chest wall movement produced should be more obvious than in normal breathing. Care is needed to avoid overinflation. Most patients can be ventilated with inflation pressures <25 cmH$_2$O and lower pressures may be adequate for small patients. A pressure gauge on the machine and capnography are useful aids for the anaesthetist during this procedure. During thoracotomy, expansion of the lung beyond the limits of the wound indicates that excessive inflation on the lungs is being produced. Manual ventilation is usually carried out for very short periods of time (e.g. following apnoea at anaesthetic induction) but can also be useful to give immediate control; the anaesthetist can alter the rate, rhythm and character of lung inflation to suit the convenience of the surgeon at any particularly critical stage of an operation, and the presence of respiratory obstruction is immediately obvious.

Lung ventilators

There are now a large number of ventilators available commercially for use in veterinary anaesthesia, and a description of all is quite outside the scope of this book. For explanation of their mode of working, the respiratory cycle of a ventilator can be divided into four parts:

1. The inspiratory phase provided by either flow generators or pressure generators. With *flow generators*, the tidal volume delivered to the patient is independent of factors outside the ventilator – if, for example, the patient's airway resistance rises then the inflation pressure increases. The flow is not necessarily constant and is adapted according to the circumstances. *Pressure generators* maintain a constant pressure during the inspiratory phase of the respiratory cycle, often by a weight acting on a concertina bag (e.g. the Manley Ventilator – for many years the 'workhorse' of human and small animal anaesthesia).

2. The changeover from inspiratory to expiratory phase, i.e. the manner in which the ventilator cycles, may be (a) time cycled, in which inspiration is

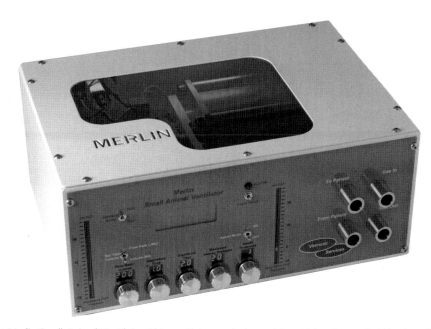

Figure 9.7 The Merlin Small Animal Ventilator. This ventilator works by a piston driving the gas held in the cylinder into the patient. It is microprocessor-controlled, can be pressure, volume, or time cycled and has a tidal volume range 1–800 mL. It also enables assisted ventilation.
Photograph courtesy of Keith Simpson, Vetronic Services, Abbotskerswell, Devon, UK.

terminated after a set time; (b) volume cycled, where inspiration is terminated after a preset volume has been delivered; or (c) pressure cycled, in which case inspiration ceases as soon as a preset pressure is reached. Not all machines conform to this classification in that some show mixed cycling with hybrid cycling mechanisms.

3. In the expiratory phase, the commonest arrangement is to expose the patient's airway to atmospheric pressure.

4. The changeover from the expiratory to the inspiratory phase may be time cycled or patient triggered. In the patient-triggered ventilator, a slight inspiratory effort by the patient triggers the changeover to the inspiratory phase.

The gas to be delivered to the patient may be held in a bellows (that represents the bag) in an airtight surround (bottle) or in a cylinder. With cylinders (e.g. the Merlin ventilator [Fig. 9.7]; and Tafonius, see Chapter 11), the power to drive the piston is electricity. In most ventilators that use bellows, the power to squeeze the bellows is compressed gas, which may be derived from the oxygen source on the machine or from an outside source of compressed gas. Usually control is then by an electrically driven processor (e.g. the Hallowell 2000 [Fig. 9.8] and the Mallard, see Chapter 11). However, ventilator control units can also be time and pressure cycled, requiring no electricity. An example is the Bird Mark 7 (Fig. 9.9).

Ventilator performance in the presence of changed parameters in the patient is extremely complex and anyone contemplating the use of an unfamiliar ventilator is well advised to read any instructions provided by the manufacturer and become thoroughly conversant with its mode of operation before attempting to employ it. As a guide, provided a machine meets the following requirements it should be adequate in most circumstances no matter what its mode of operation or mechanism of cycling may be.

Essential characteristics

All such ventilators should be able to provide a high peak flow so that the inspiratory period is short, with a longer (and adaptable) expiratory pause so that the inspiratory/expiratory ratio can be altered. This would be a minimal requirement. However, other points to consider when making a choice include:

1. Is the ventilator sufficiently versatile for the use required? Are respiratory rates and tidal volumes correct for the species concerned? Tidal volumes for most domestic species need to be in the range of 10 mL/kg but with the ability to use higher volumes if required. Most modern ventilators are very versatile. In systems such as those shown in Figures 9.8 and 9.9, the bellows size may be changed to suit the patient, thus increasing versatility.

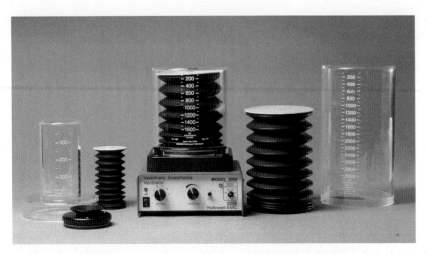

Figure 9.8 The Hallowell 2000 ventilator. It is electronically controlled, time cycled and pressure limited. Interchangeable bellows and housings enable it to deliver accurate tidal volumes of from 20 to 3000 mL at safe working pressures of 10–60 cmH$_2$O with respiratory rates of 6–40 breaths per minute. It can be fitted to all anaesthesia systems with out-of-circuit vaporizers.
Photographs courtesy of Hallowell EMC, 63 Eagle Street, Pittsfield, Massachusetts 01201, USA.

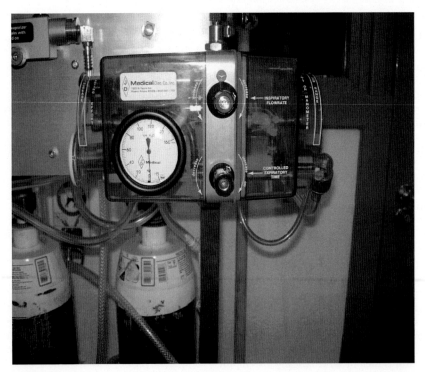

Figure 9.9 The Bird Mark 7 ventilator. This is a versatile unit which can be used for small animal respiratory care, but is also adapted to drive a large animal 'bag in a bottle' type ventilator. The system can be 'patient triggered', so it assists ventilation if the patient breathes in; if there is too long a respiratory pause the 'time cycling' takes over and IPPV occurs. IPPV can be set as preference by increasing the pressure needed to trigger the device.

2. Can it include PEEP (and are you going to want this)?
3. Is it easy to use? When you change one parameter on the 'settings', do others also change? If so, it can make it more difficult to use. Is it easy to clean (including the bellows)? Is it sufficiently quiet?
4. Is there a means of ventilating by hand should the driving force fail? This is particularly important for machines where compression of the bellows is electrically powered. Gas driven machines with electrically powered consoles should have a 'back-up' battery.

For large animal use, a ventilator should be able to deliver a tidal volume up to 20 L, with a cycling rate of between 4 and 15/minute and an inspiratory phase of 2–3 seconds duration. The ventilator should be capable of sustaining pressures of up to 60 cmH$_2$O (6 kPa) in the upper airway during inspiration, although it must be noted that Schatzmann (1988) reported that peak inspiratory pressures above 20 cmH$_2$O lead to overdistension of lung tissue in the apical regions of the horse's lungs and to discharge of unidentified fluid out of the lungs during recovery from anaesthesia. The inspiratory : expiratory ratio should be at least 1 : 2.

Ventilator settings

A survey of the literature reveals wide variations in the recommendations for tidal and minute volumes of respiration when IPPV is used. There are no generally agreed values for the production of adequate levels of ventilation in horses and, even in dogs, where more studies have been done, published figures range from 10 to 20 mL/kg (tidal volume) and from 400 to 600 mL/kg (minute volume), so it is clear that numbers such as these can only be regarded as a very rough guide. In horses and cattle, it is suggested that a tidal volume of 10 mL/kg at a rate of 8–12 breaths per minute, with an inspiratory : expiratory time ratio of 1 : 2 and a peak airway pressure not exceeding 30 cm H$_2$O should provide suitable initial settings for IPPV, although these may need to be modified as anaesthesia proceeds. For both small and large animals, ideally, the end tidal concentration of carbon dioxide should be monitored and ventilation may be adjusted to yield a normal PaCO$_2$.

Weaning from IPPV

It is essential that before any attempt is made to wean the animal off the ventilator the anaesthetist is absolutely certain that any neuromuscular block is fully reversed (see Chapter 8) and that depth of anaesthesia is not that which would inhibit respiration. If both these criteria are confirmed, then spontaneous respiration can be restored by: (1) breaking the rhythm of lung inflation (through ventilating by hand); (2) allowing some accumulation of CO$_2$ by slowing (but not stopping) the ventilation rate; (3) in cases where hypoventilation has been established by the use of centrally acting drugs such a opioids or α$_2$-adrenoceptor agonists, IPPV should be continued until spontaneous breathing is adequate or antagonists have been given.

Other modes of lung ventilation

High frequency lung ventilation

High frequency lung ventilation (HFV) is the term used for ventilation at a very high rate with tidal volumes of less than the anatomical dead space. This can provide adequate gas exchange in the lungs. The means of achieving this are not immediately obvious but there have been many models advanced as explanation (Khoo et al., 1984; Solway et al., 1984; Slutsky & Drazen, 2002). The theoretical advantages of the systems are that, by limiting tidal volume and inflation pressure they may cause less barotrauma, and have less severe circulatory effects compared with conventional IPPV. A definite advantage is that a standard endotracheal tube is not necessary, useful for investigations of the airway, and some of the systems can be used at a tracheostomy making them very suitable for intensive care. The major uses of HFV in humans are for intensive care of neonates, and in patients with ARDS. A full description and analysis of HFV is beyond the remit of this book.

There are a number of types of HFV (Sykes, 1985). The original conventional method is *high frequency positive pressure ventilation (HPPPV)*. In this, intermittent (high frequency – in humans 60–150 breaths/minute) flow of gas is delivered to the endotracheal tube or via a catheter passed down until the tip is just above the carina. Exhalation is passive, so where a catheter has been used, it frees the airway for procedures such as bronchoscopy. In *high frequency jet ventilation (HFJV)*, a high pressure gas source flows into the airway during part of the respiratory cycle, usually 20–35% of the cycle time, through a narrow diameter tube usually at tracheal level. Air is entrained as a result of this. Once again exhalation is passive. In *high frequency oscillatory ventilation (HFOV)*, there is a constant distending airway pressure with oscillations, produced by an electromagnetic valve, at a very high rate (400–2400/minute). This results in very small tidal volumes but gas exchange occurs through enhanced molecular diffusion and coaxial airway flow.

The experimental model of HFV appears to be the dog, and there are very many published papers on the subject. The systems have uses in veterinary anaesthesia, in particular in relation to techniques such as bronchoscopy (Bjorling et al., 1985), but clinical reports are very limited. In an experimental study in dogs, Bednarski & Muir (1989) found that although HFOV was effective in ventilation, cardiac output was reduced to a greater extent than with conventional ventilation. HFJV has been used in a neonatal foal (Bain et al., 1988) and experimentally in adult horses (Dunlop et al., 1985) and HFOV used in three sheep, a foal and a pony (Dodman et al., 1985). Although in all cases ventilation was effective, the lack of more recent reports suggests that HFV is of limited value in veterinary anaesthesia at this time.

Lung ventilation in intensive care

In intensive care, long-term IPPV may be necessary over several days. In addition to choice of assisted or controlled ventilation, PEEP and CPAP, the intensive care unit ventilators may have additional capabilities, such as software providing pressure–volume loops and compliance measurements. IPPV is usually carried out with an air/oxygen mixture (to avoid oxygen toxicity and to minimize alveolar collapse), the inspired O_2 concentration being adjusted to yield an arterial O_2 saturation of over 90% as shown by pulse oximetry. Sedation or low dose total intravenous anaesthesia may be administered to ensure tolerance of the endotracheal tube. A tracheostomy may be needed. Foals may be ventilated via a nasotracheal tube. Humidification of the inspired gases is necessary.

Ventilation in veterinary anaesthesia: the future

There remains a paucity of knowledge as to many ventilatory parameters in anaesthetized domestic animals, whether with spontaneous ventilation or with IPPV and little has been published about non-traditional ventilatory patterns. This is partly due to the fact that the required measurements have been difficult to obtain in the clinical setting. Some anaesthetic monitors now have the option of plethysmography which can be used even in horses (Moens et al., 2009). Other respiratory measurement methods, potentially applicable to clinical patients, are being investigated and validated. For example, Mosing and colleagues have investigated methods of measuring physiological dead space in dogs in a clinical setting (Mosing et al., 2010) and have evaluated volumetric capnography curves in relation to bronchoconstriction in this species (Mosing et al., 2012; Scheffzek et al., 2012). Work at Vienna is investigating the use of respiratory ultrasonic plethysmography in the horse (Russold et al., 2013; Schramel et al., 2012). By the next edition of this book, it may be possible to give more evidence-based recommendations as to the most effective ventilator strategies.

REFERENCES

Amato, M.B., Barbas, C.S., Medeiros, D.M., et al., 1995. Beneficial effects of the 'open lung approach' with low distending pressures in acute respiratory distress syndrome. A prospective randomized study on mechanical ventilation. Am J Resp Crit Care Med 152, 1835–1846.

Amato, M.B., Barbas, C.S., Medeiros, D.M., et al., 1998. Effect of a protective-ventilation strategy on mortality in the acute respiratory distress syndrome. New Engl J Med 338, 347–354.

Bain, F.T., Brock, K.A., Koterba, A.M., 1988. High-frequency jet ventilation in a neonatal foal. J Am Vet Med Assoc 192, 920–922.

Beadle, R.E., Robinson, N.E., Sorensen, P.R., 1975. Cardiopulmonary effects of positive end-expiratory pressure in anesthetized horses. Am J Vet Res 36, 1435–1438.

Bednarski, R.M., Muir, W.W., 3rd, 1989. Hemodynamic effects of high-frequency oscillatory ventilation in halothane-anesthetized dogs. Am J Vet Res 50, 1106–1109.

Bjorling, D.E., Lappin, M.R., Whitfield, J.B., 1985. High-frequency jet ventilation during bronchoscopy in a dog. J Am Vet Med Assoc 187, 1373–1375.

Colgan, F.J., Barrow, R.E., Fanning, G., 1971. Constant positive pressure breathing and cardiorespiratory function. Anesthesiology 34: 145–151.

Dodman, N.H., Lehr, J.L., Spaulding, G.L., 1985. High frequency ventilation in large animals. Proceedings of the 2nd International Congress of Veterinary Anaesthesia, Sacramento, pp. 186–187.

Dunlop, C., Steffey, E.P., Daunt, D., et al., 1985. Experiences with high frequency jet ventilation in conscious horses. Proceedings of the 2nd International Congress of Veterinary Anaesthesia, Sacramento, pp. 190–191.

Hall, L.W., Trim, C.M., 1975. Positive end-expiratory pressure in anaesthetized spontaneously breathing horses. Br J Anaesth 47, 819–824.

Hall, L.W., Young, S.S., 1992. Effect of inhalation anaesthetics on total respiratory resistance in conscious ponies. J Vet Pharmacol Ther 15, 174–179.

Hall, L.W., Gillespie, J.R., Tyler, W.S., 1968. Alveolar–arterial oxygen tension differences in anaesthetized horses. Br J Anaesth 40, 560–568.

Hopster, K., Kastner, S.B., Rohn, K., et al., 2011. Intermittent positive pressure ventilation with constant positive end-expiratory pressure and alveolar recruitment manoeuvre during inhalation anaesthesia in horses undergoing surgery for colic, and its influence on the early recovery period. Vet Anaesth Analg 38, 169–177.

Khoo, M.C., Slutsky, A.S., Drazen, J.M., et al., 1984. Gas mixing during high-frequency ventilation: an improved model. J Appl Physiol: Resp Environ Exercise Physiol 57, 493–506.

Lachmann, B., 1992. Open up the lung and keep the lung open. Intensive Care Med 18, 319–321.

Lehane, J.R., Jordan, C., Jones, J.G., 1980. Influence of halothane and enflurane on respiratory airflow resistance and specific conductance in anaesthetized man. Br J Anaesth 52, 773–781.

Michaelson, E.D., Grassman, E.D., Peters, W.R., 1975. Pulmonary mechanics by spectral analysis of forced random noise. J Clin Invest 56, 1210–1230.

Moens, Y., Bohm, S., 2011. Ventilating horses: moving away from old paradigms. Vet Anaesth Analg 38, 165–168.

Moens, Y.P., Gootjes, P., Ionita, J.C., et al., 2009. In vitro validation of a Pitot-based flow meter for the measurement of respiratory volume and flow in large animal anaesthesia. Vet Anaesth Analg 36, 209–219.

Mosing, M., Iff, I., Hirt, R., et al., 2012. Evaluation of variables to describe the shape of volumetric capnography curves during bronchoconstriction in dogs. Res Vet Sci 93, 386–392.

Mosing, M., Staub, L., Moens, Y., 2010. Comparison of two different methods for physiologic dead space measurements in ventilated dogs in a clinical setting. Vet Anaesth Analg 37, 393–400.

Nyktari, V., Papaioannou, A., Volakakis, N., et al., 2011. Respiratory resistance during anaesthesia with isoflurane, sevoflurane, and desflurane: a randomized clinical trial. Br J Anaesth 107, 454–461.

Polis, I., Gasthuys, F., Laevens, H., et al., 2001. The influence of ventilation mode (spontaneous ventilation, IPPV and PEEP) on cardiopulmonary parameters in sevoflurane anaesthetized dogs. J Vet Med A: Physiol Pathol Clin Med 48, 619–630.

Purchase, I.F.H., 1965a. Function tests on four large animal anaesthetic circuits. Vet Rec 77, 913–919.

Purchase, I.F.H., 1965b. Some respiratory parameters in horses and cattle. Vet Rec 77, 859–860.

Russold, E., Ambrisko, T.D., Schramel, J.P., et al., 2013. Measurement of tidal volume using Respiratory Ultrasonic Plethysmography in anaesthetized, mechanically ventilated horses. Vet Anaesth Analg 40, 48–54.

Schatzmann, U., 1988. Artificial ventilation in the horse. Advances in Veterinary Anaesthesia: Proceedings of the 3rd International Congress of Veterinary Anaesthesia, Brisbane, pp. 29–34.

Scheffzek, S., Mosing, M., Hirt, R., et al., 2012. Volumetric capnography curves as lung function test to confirm bronchoconstriction after carbachol challenge in sedated dogs. Res Vet Sci 93, 1418–1425.

Schramel, J., van den Hoven, R., Moens, Y., 2012. In vitro validation of a new respiratory ultrasonic plethysmograph. Vet Anaesth Analg 39, 366–372.

Slutsky, A.S., Drazen, J.M., 2002. Ventilation with small tidal volumes. New Engl J Med 347, 630–631.

Solway, J., Gavriely, N., Kamm, R.D., et al., 1984. Intra-airway gas mixing during high-frequency ventilation. J Appl Physiol: Resp Environ Exercise Physiol 56, 343–354.

Sykes, M.K., 1985. High frequency ventilation. Thorax 40, 161–165.

Tusman, G., Bohm, S.H., Vazquez de Anda, G.F., et al., 1999. 'Alveolar recruitment strategy' improves arterial oxygenation during general anaesthesia. Br J Anaesth 82, 8–13.

Watney, G.C.G., Jordan, C., Hall, L.W., 1987. Effect of halothane, enflurane and isoflurane on bronchomotor tone in anaesthetized ponies. Br J Anaesth 59, 1022–1026.

Watney, G.C.G., Jordan, C., Hall, L.W., Nolan, A.M., 1988. Effects of xylazine and acepromazine on bronchomotor tone of anaesthetized ponies. Equine Vet J 20, 185–188.

Wettstein, D., Moens, Y., Jaeggin-Schmucker, N., et al., 2006. Effects of an alveolar recruitment maneuver on cardiovascular and respiratory parameters during total intravenous anesthesia in ponies. Am J Vet Res 67, 152–159.

Young, S.S., Hall, L.W., 1989. A rapid, non-invasive method for measuring total respiratory impedance in the horse. Equine Vet J 21, 99–105.

Chapter 10

Apparatus for administration of anaesthetics

ADMINISTRATION OF INTRAVENOUS AGENTS

Agents that are intended to reach the central nervous system (CNS) and produce narcosis or anaesthesia have the most direct route by intravenous (IV) injection.

However, it must be remembered that IV administration results in a more rapid onset and intense effect of drug action than achieved by other routes. Precise control of drug administration is essential and this can be influenced by the size of needle or syringe chosen and the use of syringe pumps and fluid infusion pumps.

Any superficial vein may be used for IV injection and detailed descriptions of the techniques of venepuncture are given in chapters describing anaesthesia in the various species of animal.

Syringes, needles, and catheters

Syringes used in veterinary medicine vary in size from 0.5 mL (insulin syringes) to 60 mL capacity. The nozzles of the syringes may be centred, or eccentrically placed to facilitate percutaneous venepuncture. Hypodermic disposable needles are sharp but the bevels on catheter needles may be shorter to aid placement within the vein. Desensitization of the skin in small animals prior to venepuncture may be achieved by application of a cream containing lidocaine and prilocaine to the skin and covering the area with an occlusive bandage for 30 minutes. In large animals, desensitization is achieved by injection of an intradermal or subcutaneous bleb of 2% lidocaine with a 25 gauge needle.

Administration of supplemental doses of anaesthetic agents to prolong anaesthesia or administration of fluids and antibiotics during anaesthesia requires a venous access. The simplest version is to place a needle in the vein and leave it with the loaded syringe taped to the patient.

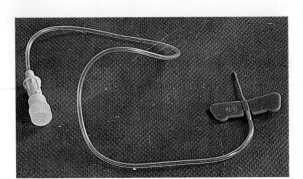

Figure 10.1 'Butterfly' or 'small vein set' or 'infant scalp vein' set. The winged needles aid insertion and subsequent fixation to the patient. The attached plastic tubing allows injection without disturbing the needle.

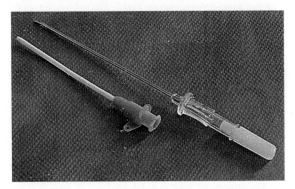

Figure 10.2 Disposable 'catheter over the needle'. The point of the hollow metal needle projects beyond the tapered end of the catheter.

Not uncommonly the needle is displaced from the vein when the animal is moved, resulting in haematoma formation, injection of drugs perivascularly, and failure of ability to inject anaesthetic agents when needed. Improved security is achieved using a needle with wings on the hub and a variable length of extension tubing (Fig. 10.1). These needles are usually restricted to short anaesthetic procedures or specific needs.

A safer practice is to place a catheter in a vein before induction of anaesthesia (Fig. 10.2). The catheters available are purchased in sterile packs and are available in a variety of materials, such as polyvinylchloride, polypropylene, polyethylene, polytetrafluoroethylene (Teflon), and polymerized silicone (silastic). Catheters constructed of polyvinylchloride, polyethylene, and polypropylene are flexible, catheters of silastic or polyurethane have extreme flexibility, and Teflon catheters have minimal flexibility. The catheter materials exhibit varying thrombogenicity, with silastic having none. Many patterns of 'over the

needle' catheters are available. There is some variation on their general shape and some have small handles to aid insertion. Most have plastic needle hubs (flash chamber) or caps through which blood can be seen when the needle enters the vein. Long catheters are chosen for placement in the jugular or saphenous veins.

The choice of catheter size depends on the size of the animal and the purpose for which it is intended. The flow of liquid through a tube is proportional to the driving pressure, which is equal to the pressure difference between the two ends of the tube, and to the internal diameter of the tube, flow being directly proportional to the fourth power of the radius, and inversely proportional to the length of the bore. Flow is also inversely proportional to the viscosity of the fluid, since the more viscous it is the harder it will be to force it through the tube. Thus, for maximum flow of any given liquid at any given pressure, the tube should be short and the diameter large. Furthermore, a small change in diameter has a great effect on flow velocity.

At very high flow rates, the resistance to flow may be disproportionately high. There is a critical flow velocity at which flow changes from linear to turbulent. During turbulence, the driving pressure is largely used up in creating the kinetic energy of the turbulent eddies. The flow no longer depends on the viscosity of the fluid but on its density. The critical velocity at which turbulence occurs depends on the viscosity and density of the fluid and the radius of the tube through which it is flowing. Turbulence will also occur at points in the infusion apparatus where the internal diameter abruptly changes.

The viscosity of blood is greater than that of water, and increases with increased haematocrit (packed cell volume). Viscosity is also increased at low temperatures and the viscosity of blood at 4°C is about 2.5 times as great as at 37°C. Warming blood prior to transfusion will increase flow rate as well as decrease the impact on body temperature.

Skin preparation before insertion of the catheter, securing the catheter, and attentive catheter maintenance are essential to avoid catheter-related blood stream infection. Chlorhexidine is recommended as the best skin antiseptic for providing protection against catheter colonization (Norwood & McAuley, 2005). The catheter should be securely attached to the skin because movement of the catheter in and out of the site of skin insertion increases bacterial contamination. When catheters are to remain in place for an extended time, they should be protected from the environment by sticky pads or bandaging. The catheter site should be checked at least daily for signs of redness, swelling, or discomfort for the animal. Wet or soiled bandages should be changed whenever contamination occurs. Recommendations for changing catheters vary and while some recommend every 72 hours to decrease the risk of phlebitis and catheter-related infections, others suggest a longer retention time is acceptable if the site of catheter insertion appears healthy and daily maintenance is strictly observed. Catheter-associated infection rates of 15–49% have been reported in dogs and cats. A positive culture rate of 24.5% out of 101 central and 50 peripheral catheters in dogs and cats staying a minimum of 48 hours in an ICU unit was recently reported (Marsh-Ng et al., 2007). Since this was a prospective study, careful attention to aseptic technique and bandaging was observed. The three most common bacteria isolated from the catheter tips were not normal skin flora and it was deduced that transmission of bacteria from human hands to the catheter hub or contamination of the catheter cap were most likely causes. There were no differences in contamination rates between the types and location of catheters. Another investigation identified contamination in 23 of 99 (23.2%) of peripheral catheters removed from dogs and cats, most commonly *Staphylococcus aureus* and *S. intermedius* (Jones et al., 2009). None of the usual variables associated with catheter contamination, such as number of attempts at insertion and duration of placement, was associated with contamination and, although the statistical analysis was not conclusive, it appeared that catheters fitted with a Y-connector were 10 times less likely to be contaminated than catheters with a T-connector. The authors postulated that the reason may be that there is a greater distance from the injection port and the catheter when using a Y-connector.

Techniques of catheter insertion differ slightly between species, and are described in the species-specific chapters, but basic principles are described in Box 10.1. In some patients, insertion of the needle and catheter through the skin results in crimping, fraying or expansion of the end of the catheter and, in these cases, a small incision in the skin before insertion may be necessary. When venepuncture is unsuccessful, even when the needle has been only partially withdrawn from the catheter, the needle should not be reinserted into the catheter when still in the patient. If the catheter has been bent, reinsertion of the needle will result in the needle penetrating the side of the catheter and may even shear off the end of the catheter. Safe practice involves removal of the needle and catheter and starting again.

Catheters inserted into jugular veins of dogs, cats, and small farm animals are frequently placed using a modified Seldinger technique that requires inserting a guide wire into the vein to facilitate subsequent insertion of the catheter. Hair is clipped from an area over the jugular vein and the skin is prepared as for surgery. Sterile gloves are worn and a sterile drape with a hole in the centre is applied to isolate the site for catheter insertion. Jugular catheters may have one, two or three lumina for infusion of fluids, drugs and blood sampling (Fig. 10.3). Before inserting the catheter, the proximal and medial lumina should be flushed with heparinized saline and capped to prevent air entrainment. A catheter, or a needle, is inserted into the jugular vein pointing towards the heart. A spring guide wire, with

---

> ### Box 10.1 **Steps for placement of an IV catheter**
>
> - Clip hair and clean skin with 3 alternating applications of chlorhexidine surgical scrub and isopropyl alcohol
> - Topical application or injection of lidocaine (or similar), where applicable
> - Wear sterile surgical gloves when placing a central venous catheter, when catheter placement involves an introducer and Seldinger wire, or when catheter is to remain in place for long-term care
> - Select appropriate catheter size; flushing with heparinized saline is optional
> - Small incision in skin over the vein in some patients with the point of a hypodermic needle (thick-skinned dogs or cats) or scalpel blade (adult cattle)
> - Occlude vein distal to puncture site
> - Hold needle hub for insertion
> - Insert needle and catheter through the skin at an angle of 45° to the skin and into vein
> - Observe blood flow at the hub of the needle, decrease angle of insertion to 30° and introduce needle 0.5 cm further into the vein
> - Hold needle stationary and slide catheter over the needle and deeper into the vein
> - Remove needle and blood should be flowing from catheter
> - When the catheter is above heart level, do not allow aspiration of air
> - Attach catheter cap (or T-port, or 3-way stopcock, or fluid line)
> - Flush with heparinized saline
> - Secure catheter to patient (tape, sutures, glue)

---

or without a flexible J-tip, is threaded through the catheter into the jugular vein and then the catheter is removed while the guide wire is held stationary. A scalpel blade can be used minimally to enlarge the skin incision around the guide wire. A tapered tissue dilator is threaded over the guide wire into the vein using a partial back and forth rotation about its longitudinal axis to enlarge the path through subcutaneous tissue, and then removed. The catheter then is introduced into the jugular vein over the guide wire, which is then removed. The catheter is secured with sutures to the skin. The Seldinger technique using a guide wire can also be used to insert catheters into arteries, and the catheter guide wire can be purchased individually or is packaged as an integral component of the catheter.

Intraosseous needles

An intraosseous (IO) needle is used in animals in which venous catheter placement is particularly difficult, such as

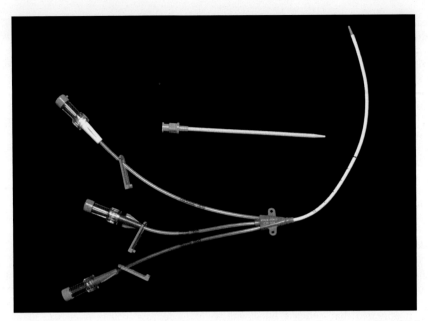

Figure 10.3 A triple lumen catheter that can be inserted percutaneously into a vein using the modified Seldinger technique involving a short catheter, a flexible guide wire (not shown), and a tapered tissue dilator.

very small puppies and kittens and birds, and for emergency resuscitation. This route can be used for administration of crystalloid and colloid solutions, blood, and resuscitation drugs. Speed of infusion is limited. However, administration of fluids may expand the peripheral circulation sufficiently to facilitate subsequent intravenous catheterization. An IO needle should not be inserted through infected skin or into a fractured bone or pneumatic bone in birds. Aseptic technique must be employed to prevent introduction of bacteria and osteomyelitis. In dogs and cats, the sites of needle insertion most commonly used are the trochanteric fossa of the femur, the greater tubercle of the humerus, and the medial surface of the proximal end of the tibia (Fig. 10.4). In birds, the needle is inserted into the proximal end of the ulna. Local infiltration of local anaesthetic solution or general anaesthesia should be administered. Purpose-made IO needles are commercially available. Other options are 22, 20, or 18 gauge spinal needles, hypodermic needles for extremely small patients, and bone marrow needles for large dogs. A stab skin incision with a scalpel blade may be needed to assist insertion of the needle. The needle should be introduced with pressure using a partial back and forth rotation about its longitudinal axis achieved by rolling the needle hub between thumb and forefinger. Loss of resistance may indicate penetration of the cortex. The stilette of the needle is removed and a 3 mL syringe attached. Confirmation of placement is by aspiration of bone marrow into the syringe and then easy injection of heparinized saline with no swelling occurring subcutaneously. A catheter cap or

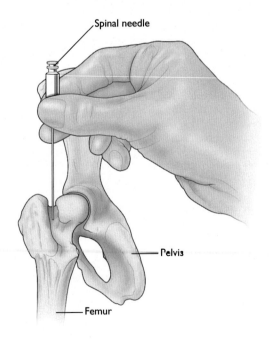

Figure 10.4 Intraosseous (IO) catheterization: anatomical landmarks, viewed from the caudal aspect, and needle approach to the femur of a dog.

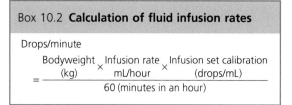

T-port should be attached to the needle. Antibiotic ointment can be smeared at the site of skin insertion and the needle should be secured with tape or sutures. The flow rate of fluid through the needle is not significantly altered by using a large needle size but is dependent on flow through the bone marrow. Pressurizing the source of the fluid doubles the rate of fluid infusion but should be used cautiously. More details about IO infusion have been previously published (Giunti & Otto, 2009).

Vascular access ports

Vascular access ports may be used in patients that need long-term daily intravenous medications, frequent blood sampling, or multiple anaesthetic episodes for radiation therapy. A soft catheter is inserted into a vein, usually the jugular vein, using either a surgical incision and a venotomy or percutaneously using a wire introducer (Seldinger technique). The catheter is connected to a small chamber (port) that is inserted subcutaneously. After the incision is closed, a hypodermic needle can easily penetrate the chamber by percutaneous puncture. There are several publications in the veterinary literature identifying complications of vascular access ports, including seroma formation, catheter blockage, infection, and incision dehiscence, but the complication rate is low (Culp et al., 2010).

Infusion apparatus

Fluid for IV therapy is transferred from plastic bags or bottles, 500 mL up to 10 L, through tubing known as 'administration sets'. Essentially, an administration set consists of a sharp rigid plastic end, that may or may not include an air inlet with its own filter, that is inserted into the outlet of the fluid container, a drip chamber, a filter in sets used for blood products, and a length of tubing that leads to the venous catheter. Most administration sets also have one or more rubber-capped injection sites on the tubing. Some administration sets have two or four bag attachments for fluid loading, prolonged administration, or use in large animals. The inlet to the drip chamber from the fluid bag is available in different diameters to control the number of drops in 1 mL of fluid, for example, paediatric sets deliver 60 drops/mL and adult sets deliver either 15 or 10 drops/mL. The flow rate is controlled by means of a roller clamp and can be calculated from the number of drops that pass through the drip chamber in one minute (Box 10.2). Administration sets that have a 150 mL container 'dosage burette' proximal to the drip chamber can be used to control the fluid volume delivered to small patients. A volume of fluid, for example 20 mL, is let into the burette and the inlet manually closed. The rate of infusion of the fixed volume is adjusted (60 drops/mL) but when the chamber is empty a flap valve closes and shuts off the administration set.

> ### Box 10.2 **Calculation of fluid infusion rates**
>
> Drops/minute
>
> $$= \frac{\substack{\text{Bodyweight} \\ \text{(kg)}} \times \substack{\text{Infusion rate} \\ \text{mL/hour}} \times \substack{\text{Infusion set calibration} \\ \text{(drops/mL)}}}{60 \text{ (minutes in an hour)}}$$

When fluids are administered under the influence of gravity, the speed of infusion depends more on the cross-sectional diameter of the needle or catheter than on the pressure (height of the fluid container above the needle or catheter). Doubling the diameter of the needle or catheter results in a 16-fold increase in the flow rate, whereas a fourfold increase in pressure is required to double the flow rate. In circumstances where the maximum size of the catheter is limited, the flow rate can be increased by pressurizing the system. Bottles can be pressurized by pumping air through the air inlet. This procedure carries a high risk of producing air embolism if the supply of fluid runs out, so it should be used with caution and the infusion should not be left unattended. Pressure can be applied to plastic bags of fluid by manually squeezing them or by placing them within a plastic or fabric bag that can be inflated by pumping in air (pressure infuser). Air embolism can only occur with the latter system if the fluid bag contains air. Air embolism should not occur when fluid is administered by gravity flow through an administration set.

Accurate control of infusion rate is possible using an electronic infusion pump attached to the administration set (Fig. 10.5). These pumps control flow rate in several ways but commonly by applying an intermittent interruption of flow through the infusion line based on the parameters manually entered into the pump. The pumps can be programmed to deliver a set volume per hour and may display the total volume delivered and the volume remaining. Infusion pumps that control flow rate by monitoring the drip chamber are rendered less accurate because they cannot compensate for variations in drop size. Some pumps require use of specially designed administration sets that are substantially more costly than standard administration sets.

Electrically driven syringe drivers (syringe pumps) are useful for accurate administration of small volumes, such as crystalloid or colloid solutions to small patients or anaesthetic agents, such as propofol, fentanyl, or lidocaine (Fig. 10.6). Extension sets between the syringe and the patient can be regular IV extensions with an internal volume of 3 mL/30 cm (12 inches) of line, or microextension sets of 1.7 metres (5 feet) with an internal volume of 0.3 mL. The device may require manual entry of the manufacturer or size of the syringe as well as the volume to be delivered per hour and the volume limit. The cross-sectional diameter of different syringes is preprogrammed in the device to allow accuracy of volume delivery. The

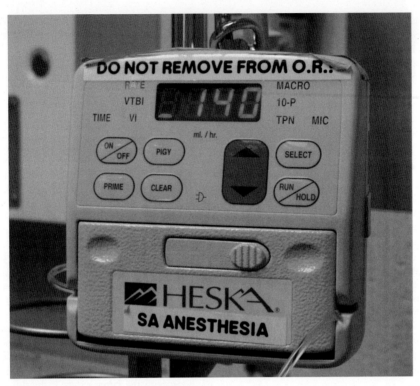

Figure 10.5 Volumetric or constant infusion pump. Devices may warn of the presence of air or occlusion of the infusion line.

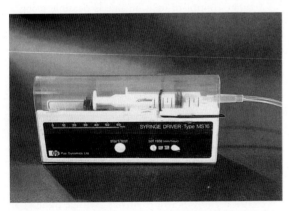

Figure 10.6 Syringe driver (syringe pump). Many types of electrically driven syringe drivers are available. Some must be used with a specified size of syringe, others can be used with a variety of syringe sizes.

barrel of the syringe is stationary and the unit controls the rate of plunger travel to ensure an accurate volume delivery.

Although many infusion pumps have audible alarms that indicate line occlusion, infusion into perivascular tissues may not achieve a high enough pressure to trigger the occlusion alarm. Thus, the site of catheter placement must be regularly checked to confirm that fluid is being delivered intravenously and not subcutaneously or into surrounding bandage or drapes.

The infusion pump rate may be changed manually to adjust administration of anaesthetic agents. A target controlled infusion pump (TCI) is available for administration of propofol where the anaesthetist sets a target blood or effect-site concentration and the computerized infusion device makes the necessary changes to the infusion rate (Chapter 1). This device is expensive and the benefits of TCI over manual control of propofol administration have not yet been confirmed (Leslie et al., 2008). Nonetheless, protocols are being developed for use of this modality in veterinary patients.

ADMINISTRATION OF INHALATION AGENTS

The anaesthesia machine can be complex or simple in appearance (Fig. 10.7). The essential components are the same in all machines: the anaesthesia workstation and a patient delivery circuit through which oxygen (O_2) and anaesthetic gas are delivered to the patient via a mask or tracheal tube.

Anaesthesia workstation

The anaesthesia workstation comprises an O_2 source, a pressure regulator (reducing valve), a flowmeter, and a vaporizer(s). In addition, a pressure gauge measures pressure at the O_2 source, and an emergency 'flush' valve will deliver O_2 directly from the outlet of the regulator to the patient breathing circuit (Fig. 10.8).

Gases and cylinders

There are many different sizes of cylinders (also known as tanks) for different gases. Each cylinder is coded by a letter of the alphabet, and the type of gas by the colour of the cylinder (Table 10.1), although availability of cylinder sizes differs between countries and colour coding of the cylinders is not universal (see later). A new standard governing the colour coding of transportable gas cylinders is in transition in Europe. Designed to improve safety standards, the cylinder shoulders (the curved part at the top of the cylinder) are painted to warn of potential hazards: bright green is an inert gas, light blue is an oxidizing gas, yellow is a toxic gas, red is flammable, and white is oxygen. The product label must always be checked to identify the cylinder contents and the medical gas cylinders have distinctive colouring.

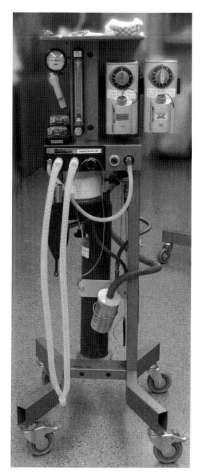

Figure 10.7 Anaesthesia machine for small animals.

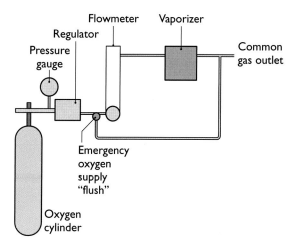

Figure 10.8 Components of an anaesthesia workstation.

Table 10.1 Characteristics of medical oxygen cylinders					
Cylinder code	E[a]	E[b]	F[a]	G[a]	H[b]
Contents (L)	680	625	1360	3400	7100
Approximate dimensions					
mm	865 × 102	660 × 108	930 × 140	1320 × 178	1295 × 235
inch	34 × 4	26 × 4.25	36.6 × 5.5	52 × 7	51 × 9.25
Valve outlet connection	Pin-index	Pin-index	Bullnose	Bullnose	Bullnose
[a]www.bocmedical.co.uk; [b]Airgas South, Inc., Georgia, USA					

Small cylinders are commonly attached to small animal anaesthesia workstations whereas large cylinders must be secured by chains to the wall, supported in a portable cradle, or placed in a room distant from the patient procedures. The cylinder outlets are of several designs but two, the pin-index and bullnose, are commonly used in veterinary medicine. Cylinders with the pin-index system have holes in the head of the cylinder with an arrangement that is specific to each gas. Pins on the yoke that includes the reducing valve and outlet attachment must exactly match the pin-index arrangement on the cylinder, thus making it impossible to connect an incorrect cylinder. The bullnose connections screw into place, are tightened with a wrench, and do not require a sealing washer. The DISS (diameter index safety system) system employs different diameter connections and different screw threads.

Oxygen

Medical grade oxygen cylinders are colour-coded white in Europe and Canada and green in the USA. The cylinders contain compressed oxygen to a pressure of 2000–2200 psi (pounds per square inch) (USA) or 137 bar (UK) when full. Oxygen in the cylinder is in gaseous phase and the cylinder pressure decreases linearly as oxygen is used. Consequently, a half-full cylinder has a pressure of half the full pressure. Observation of the pressure gauge on the cylinder and knowledge of the cylinder capacity permits an easy calculation of the current contents. Veterinary hospitals with high O_2 usage may have a series of several large O_2 (or nitrous oxide) H cylinders that are attached to a manifold and automatically switch from one cylinder to another cylinder as the contents are depleted, or from one series (bank) of cylinders to another.

Liquid oxygen

Bulk oxygen supply in the form of a cylinder of liquid oxygen is often chosen by large hospitals. Liquid oxygen is stored in a cryogenic cylinder that is an insulated, vacuum-jacketed, pressure container equipped with pressure-relief valves and rupture discs to protect the cylinder from increased pressure. The capacity of the cylinder is between 80 and 450 L of liquid oxygen at a pressure of 350 psi and, at 20°C (68°F), the expansion ratio, liquid to gas, is 1 to 860. Strict adherence to safety protocols is essential to avoid personal injury when handling the storage cylinder.

Oxygen generators

Oxygen generators that produce a continuous supply of medical grade 93% O_2 are available for veterinary practice. Convenience, safety, and decreased cost per litre are suggested reasons for using a generator, but it is essential to be certain that O_2 can be generated at a sufficient rate for an emergency situation. Oxygen generators are available in the USA that can generate sufficient O_2 for those practices that have multiple anaesthesia machines and utilize oxygen cages, mechanical ventilators, or offer hyperbaric chamber O_2 therapy.

Nitrous oxide

Nitrous oxide (N_2O) is available in cylinders that are colour-coded blue or, in Europe, with a dark blue shoulder and white body. During the filling process, N_2O is compressed to a liquid so that a full cylinder is approximately one-third liquid and two-thirds gas and exerts a pressure of approximately 760 psi (USA) or 44 bar (UK). As N_2O is used during anaesthesia, liquid is vaporized to replace the lost gas and pressure is maintained constant. Use of a high flow of N_2O may be accompanied by formation of ice crystals on the outside of the cylinder and a slight fall in cylinder pressure; when the cylinder rewarms to room temperature, the cylinder pressure returns to 760 psi or 44 bar if there is any liquid remaining. Consequently, the pressure gauge cannot be used to determine the volume of contents, as all the liquid is not vaporized until the cylinder is approximately 80% used, at which point the pressure reading decreases. Nitrous oxide is also available in different sizes of cylinders.

Air

Compressed medical grade air containing 21% oxygen is available in cylinders for use blended with oxygen for long-term ventilation of dogs and cats in the Intensive Care Unit or for inhalation anaesthesia. In Europe, the colour code of medical grade air is a white and black shoulder with a white body.

Carbon dioxide

Carbon dioxide (CO_2) is available in cylinders colour-coded grey or a grey shoulder with a white body. Currently, CO_2 is more commonly used in veterinary practice independently of the anaesthesia machine to produce pneumoperitoneum during laparoscopy.

Helium–Oxygen

Helium–oxygen (Heliox) 65:35, 70:30, or 80:20 mixtures are available in cylinders for special anaesthesia circumstances, such as anaesthesia or ventilation of people with respiratory distress from airway obstruction where turbulence of airflow in the trachea or bronchi produces resistance to breathing. The density of helium is lower than oxygen and the lighter helium–oxygen mixture tends to maintain laminar flow in the airways, increase flow rate, and decrease work of breathing. The improved airflow in and out of the lungs may support improved blood gases. Use of helium in anaesthesia is not widespread as although there are published case reports in human literature supporting beneficial effects of helium use, studies in larger groups of patients are not conclusive (Harris & Barnes,

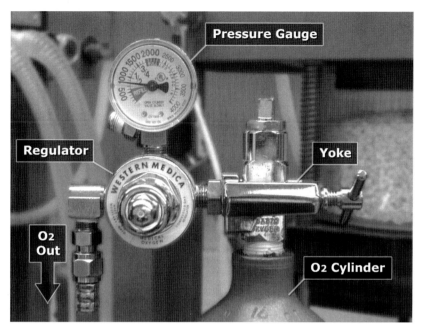

Figure 10.9 A yoke connects an oxygen cylinder to the regulator.

2008; Maggiore et al., 2010). The pressure in a full cylinder is 2000 psi (USA) or 137 bar (UK).

Pressure gauges

Cylinders are connected to pressure gauges that register the pressure of gas within the cylinder from which the anaesthetist may be able to determine the volume of cylinder contents (Fig. 10.9). Pipeline pressure gauges must also be installed close to the locations of use when the gas supply cylinders are situated at a distance.

Regulators

Delivery of pressure as high as in the O_2 cylinder directly to the patient will cause lung damage and, therefore, a regulator (also known as a reducing valve) is necessary to decrease the pressure to a safer workable pressure. The regulator decreases the pressure to 50 psi (4 bar, 350 kPa) and maintains the outlet pressure constant for flows up to 15 L/min. Further, the outlet pressure is maintained as the pressure decreases inside the cylinder. The regulator attachment (yoke) that is placed around a pin-index cylinder head (see Fig. 10.9) or into the outlet of larger cylinders is designed to fit only a cylinder of a specific gas. Where large O_2 cylinders are situated away from the operating room, regulators, similar to those on the simple workstation, reduce the pressure to a working level. Gas is then transported from the remote site through pipes to the hospital rooms where they exit the walls or ceilings. Safety features

to prevent mixing gas supplies are in the form of different sized screw threads for attachment of hoses on the anaesthesia machines or by quick-connect couplings with different configurations. A pressure drop along the pipes generally occurs, consequently, the origin outlet pressure must be adjusted to maintain the pipeline outlet pressure at slightly higher than the workstation regulator outlet pressure. Some large animal mechanical ventilators are unable to function properly if the O_2 pressure decreases.

Flowmeters

Gas flows to the patient breathing circuit are controlled by flowmeters. These are calibrated for each gas in mL/min or L/min as the density and viscosity of each gas determines rate of flow (Fig. 10.10). The calibrations range from 10 mL/min to 10 L/min for small animals and up to 10 or 15 L/min for large animals. The rotameter type of flowmeter consists of a glass tube inside which a rotating bobbin is free to move up and down, allowing gas to flow around it (Fig. 10.11). The tube is tapered with the diameter of the tube gradually increasing from the bottom to the top so that the annular space between the tube and rotameter (orifice) becomes wider as the rotameter rises in the tube, allowing the flow of gas to increase. The rotameter has an upper rim that is of a diameter slightly greater than that of the body, and in which specially shaped channels are cut. The gas flowing through the channels causes the rotameter to spin with the result that it rides on a cushion of gas thereby eliminating errors due to friction

217

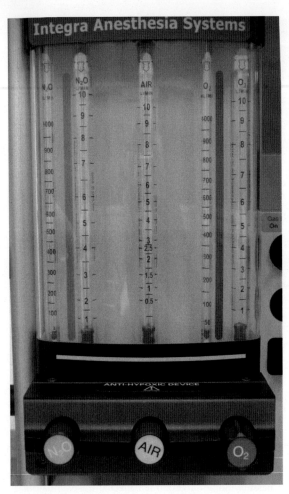

Figure 10.10 Oxygen and nitrous oxide flowmeters each have two tubes on this anaesthesia machine, one is expanded flow 0–1 L/min for accuracy and the other 1–10 L/min. Gas flow is read from the top of the rotameter. The air flowmeter is a single tube.

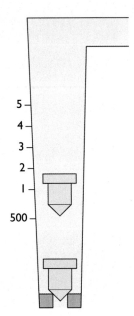

Figure 10.11 Schematic design of a rotameter flowmeter.

between the tube and the bobbin. Flow is read accurately from the top of the rotameter against a scale etched on the outside of the glass tube. Flow is accurate (± 2%) for the calibrated gas if the flowmeter (anaesthesia machine) is absolutely upright.

Ball flowmeters, like the rotameter, are also tapered and are, therefore, variable orifice meters. Flow rate is read from the middle of a ball when there is only one, or when there are two balls, from the point of contact between the two balls.

Vaporizers

Vaporizers for volatile liquid anaesthetic agents consist of a chamber through which O_2 flows and carries anaesthetic

molecules out to the patient. In the early days of anaesthesia, vaporizers were simple and subject to changes in output according to the gas flow, temperature of the liquid, surface area in contact with O_2, and pressure changes generated by artificial ventilation. Simple vaporizers are used today in specific circuits that involve the patient breathing through them (draw-over) such as the Komesaroff or Stephens machines. More commonly, vaporizers have been designed to compensate for extraneous factors (precision vaporizers) and accurately deliver the dialled concentration (Fig. 10.12). The surface area is standardized by use of a wick inside the vaporizer and temperature changes are compensated for by mechanisms that alter either the inflow or outflow of O_2 through the vaporizing chamber. As vaporizers are designed for use in human anaesthesia, the accuracy of the vaporizer is guaranteed only over a very limited temperature range close to 20°C (68°F). The actual specification depends on the make and model but many vaporizers may be unable to compensate for low operating room temperatures of around 17°C (63°F) resulting in low anaesthetic output and inadequate anaesthetic depth. Even more dangerous is the potential for higher than expected concentrations when working at high ambient temperatures. The anaesthetic output decreased progressively during high O_2 flow rates (10 L/min) and to a greater extent from some sevoflurane vaporizers (exceeding 20% of the dial setting) than from isoflurane vaporizers (Ambrisko & Klide, 2011). The output concentration from sevoflurane vaporizers that were only partially filled was similar to that when they were full. Supplying heat by wrapping the vaporizer in a warm cloth

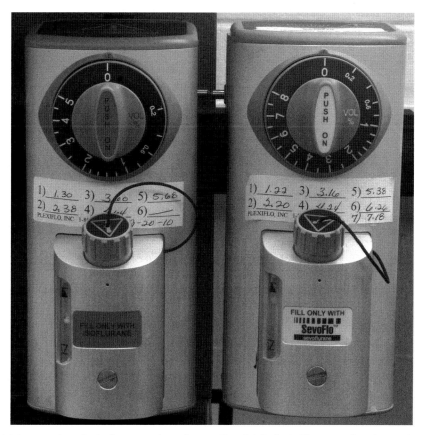

Figure 10.12 Precision vaporizers for isoflurane and sevoflurane. The dials indicate % output of each vaporizer. The handwritten labels below the dials note the actual % delivered at each setting at the time of the last scheduled machine check.

will increase anaesthetic output but can result in an excessive depth of anaesthesia. A check valve on the outlet side of the vaporizer is used to prevent back-pressure from the patient circuit during artificial ventilation altering vaporization and output concentration. The output from precision vaporizers must be measured for accuracy at regular intervals which, in some countries, may be a specific time interval.

The maximum concentration of an anaesthetic agent at a given temperature depends on the vapour pressure of the agent. Isoflurane and sevoflurane have sufficiently different vapour pressures that they must be used in specifically manufactured vaporizers. The vapour pressure of isoflurane is similar to that of halothane, an older agent since discontinued in many countries, and halothane vaporizers can be serviced professionally, cleaned and recalibrated for use with isoflurane.

The fluid level in the vaporizer can be checked through a clear window on the side of the vaporizer. Filling of vaporizers is invariably accompanied by loss of anaesthetic vapour into the room. An inexpensive non-disposable filling spout can be attached to the bottle of isoflurane or sevoflurane and will minimize spilling. New vaporizers have 'keyed' filling ports where the bottle of anaesthetic agent is attached directly to the vaporizer or by using an adapter that is totally closed.

Desflurane is a colourless liquid below a temperature of 22.8 °C. It requires an expensive specialized vaporizer in which the chamber holding the liquid is heated electrically to above boiling point. The vaporizer is a dual gas blender (O_2 and desflurane vapour) with the output from the vaporization chamber pressure regulated to deliver an accurate percentage to the patient circuit. Special care must be taken to follow manufacturer's instructions when filling a desflurane vaporizer as a number of potentially harmful accidents have been reported.

A number of devices, such as the 'Selectatec', are available to enable vaporizers to be easily attached to or removed from the 'back bar' of the workstation, allowing convenient exchange of vaporizers for changing anaesthetic agent, for removal for filling elsewhere, and when a vaporizer has to be sent away for service. Tipping the vaporizer when the dial is not switched off (either when moving the vaporizer or rocking the anaesthesia machine) may result in a surge of high anaesthetic concentration when the vaporizer is first turned on. To avoid accidental overdose, it is advisable to flush the vaporizer and hoses with oxygen before connecting to a patient.

Simple, low internal resistance, draw-over vaporizers for isoflurane or sevoflurane are situated within the circle delivery circuits of the Komesaroff and Stephens anaesthesia machines. The dials of the vaporizers are not calibrated and simply vary the proportion of gas passing through the vaporizers. The outputs of the vaporizers are largely determined by the magnitude of the patient's ventilation that flows through the circuit.

Oxygen flush valve

This valve is situated between the regulator and the flowmeter. Activation causes a flow of oxygen at a pressure of 55 psi (400 kPa) and 60 L/min to the delivery circuit, by-passing the precision vaporizer(s). The flush valve should never be employed for a non-rebreathing circuit with a 0.5 L bag when an animal is attached because of the high risk of rupturing the lungs. With a small animal circle circuit, depending on the duration of flush and the size of the rebreathing bag, use of the flush valve may not be fatal. Two consequences will occur: pressure within the circle increases and the patient's lungs will be inflated; and secondly, O_2 without anaesthetic agent is delivered and thus the circle anaesthetic concentration will decrease. If the depth of anaesthesia is too light, operating the flush valve to fill the reservoir bag will further lighten anaesthesia.

Common gas outlet

The mixture of gases leaves the workstation at the common gas outlet, to which the patient circuit is attached. The outlet configuration and size may differ between machine manufacturers and countries.

Injection vaporization

Injection of liquid isoflurane, sevoflurane or desflurane into a chamber or anaesthesia circuit by-passes the use of conventional vaporizers (Olson et al., 1993; Boller et al., 2005; Hodgson, 2006). The technique involves calculation of priming and maintenance doses based on the desired anaesthetic concentration, volume of the circuit, and the size of the patient, using equations proposed for closed system anaesthesia (Lowe & Ernst, 1981). Vaporization and uptake of anaesthetic agent by the CO_2 absorbent may alter the final anaesthetic percent, consequently, monitoring of anaesthetic gases during liquid injection technique is recommended. This technique is utilized by the Zeus® workstation (Draeger, UK) that employs computer control of the injection of the inhalation agent. A form of disposable vaporizer using liquid anaesthetic

agent is the Anaesthetic Conserving Device, AnaConDa™, so named because very little agent is used. The AnaConDa is a modified heat and moisture exchanger that is connected to the patient at the endotracheal tube. Liquid sevoflurane is supplied continuously from a syringe driver/pump to the patient side of the device, where it is immediately vaporized and delivered to the lungs on inspiration (Soro et al., 2010; Nishiyama et al., 2012). The sevoflurane infusion rate is altered periodically to adjust the depth of anaesthesia.

Magnetic resonance imaging (MRI) compatible machines

The static magnetic field inside the MRI scanner will exert an attractive force on ferromagnetic objects. The degree of attraction depends on the strength of the magnet, the mass of the object, shielding, and the distance to the magnet but can be of sufficient force to generate a projectile effect with potential damage to the magnet, the patient, and to the anaesthetist. It must be remembered that the magnet is continuously on even when no imaging is occurring. Special non-ferrous anaesthesia machines and monitoring equipment are commercially available and must be used for patients in the MRI scanner. An exception may be made if the anaesthesia machine can be located in an adjacent room and either the breathing circuit has really long tubes or a long tube carries O_2 and anaesthetic gas to an MRI compatible circuit (such as the Humphrey ADE) located near the scanner. Equipment may be designated MR conditional, MR safe, or MR unsafe (Farling et al., 2010). MR conditional applies to equipment that has been demonstrated to pose no known hazards with specified conditions of use in an MR environment. The anaesthetist should be familiar with the manufacturers' instructions related to all equipment used in MRI. Monitors should have visual warning alarms as auditory alarms may not be heard. All personnel remaining in the scanning room should wear ear protection.

Delivery (breathing) systems

A breathing circuit is used to deliver O_2 and anaesthetic gas from the workstation to the patient. The circuit may be designed to allow partial or complete rebreathing of exhaled gases after removal of exhaled CO_2. Recycling of gases allows the O_2 inflow to be decreased, even as low as the volume of O_2 needed to supply only metabolic demand of the patient. Low O_2 flows are economical and rebreathing circuits with low O_2 flow maintain humidity of inspired gases and may help to prevent heat loss in patients (Table 10.2). Circuits that have no rebreathing deliver fresh gases to the patient for each breath. The higher O_2 flow required for these circuits results in wastage of significant amounts of volatile anaesthetic gas and increased expense (Table 10.3). Consequently, non-rebreathing circuits are primarily used in small patients such as small cats and dogs, rats, rabbits, small birds, and small wildlife, where required O_2 flow rates are low.

Breathing circuits are available made of heavy-duty materials that are intended for long-term use or made of light plastic materials intended for disposable or semi-disposable use. The 'disposable' circuits are lightweight and less likely to drag on the endotracheal tube and cause accidental extubation. The hoses are available in different lengths and may be manufactured with a colour coding, with the fresh gas being delivered via the blue or green tube. Plastic hoses are transparent and the inside can be observed easily when cleaning. Tubing with a smooth intralumenal wall has better flow characteristics than a wall that is corrugated. Heated hoses are also available in dog and cat sizes.

Rebreathing circuits

All partial or complete rebreathing circuits must have a means of absorbing exhaled CO_2 before delivering the gases back to the patient (Fig. 10.13). The absorber canister consists of one or two transparent plastic canisters filled with granules, short strands, or spheres, of absorbent filled from large containers or airtight foil-lined bags or by insertion of prepackaged disposable cartridges. The granules for an anaesthetic circuit must be of a size that will allow gas to flow through easily but with sufficient surface area exposed to ensure effective absorption. Sometimes efficiency is reduced when the settling of granules forms channels through which the exhaled gases can pass without all CO_2 being removed. Furthermore, some absorbents contain dust that mixes with water formed from the chemical reaction with CO_2 and forms a paste (caking) which may also interfere with absorption by filling spaces between granules. The standard commonly used absorbent is sodalime (such as Sodasorb®) that consists of 80% calcium hydroxide, 2% sodium hydroxide

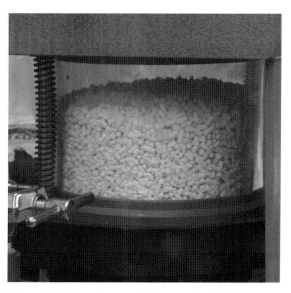

Figure 10.13 A canister containing granules of CO_2 absorbent is an essential component of a rebreathing circuit.

Table 10.2 Rebreathing circuits	
Advantages	**Disadvantages**
Low O_2 inflow 1. decreases volume of waste gases 2. decreases cost 3. retains water vapour and facilitates humidification of inspired gases	Hoses and CO_2 absorbent offer resistance to breathing Deadspace in hoses may be greater than in non-rebreathing circuits Circuit concentration slow to change Inspired concentration may be lower than vaporizer % when low O_2 inflow rates are used

Table 10.3 Non-rebreathing circuits	
Advantages	**Disadvantages**
Minimal resistance to patient's breathing Inspired anaesthetic concentration equals vaporizer setting, facilitating control of depth of anaesthesia Inspired anaesthetic concentration changes within seconds of changing vaporizer % Circuits with small internal volume of connector to endotracheal tube (apparatus deadspace) minimize CO_2 rebreathing No CO_2 absorbent 1. decreases cost 2. no dust 3. no anaesthetic agent breakdown Disposable system can be discarded after bacterial contamination	Inhaled gas is dry and cold, potentiating hypothermia and mucosal dessication High O_2 flow results in relatively more vaporization of anaesthetic gases and that 1. requires increased pollution management 2. increased cost due to wastage of anaesthetic gas and O_2

(NaOH), <1% potassium hydroxide (KOH), and water. However, carbon dioxide absorbents that contain strong bases (NaOH and KOH) promote the formation of Compound A (2-(fluoromethoxy)-1,1,3,3,3-pentafluoro-1-propene) from sevoflurane and also of carbon monoxide (CO) and other toxic compounds from isoflurane and desflurane (Clarke, 2008). Under a set of specific conditions CO can be formed from sevoflurane. Compound A is nephrotoxic in rats but there have been no reports of damage in our domestic species. An absorbent containing barium hydroxide (Baralyme®) was found to have excessive product breakdown particularly when dessicated (Steffey et al., 1997), and has now been withdrawn. Sodalime breakdown is accelerated by use of dry absorbent and by increasing temperatures. Absorption of CO_2 is an exothermic reaction so that the temperature of sodalime increases and, at high temperatures, high concentrations of CO may be produced. Newer absorbents such as Sodasorb® LF (low flow), Amsorb® Plus, and Loflosorb® are available that are 75–85% or more calcium hydroxide and lack strong bases. A number of published investigations have sought to determine differences in CO and Compound A production from different absorbents and comparison of moist versus dessicated absorbents (Stabernack et al., 2000; Versichelen et al., 2001; Kharasch et al., 2002; Yamakage et al., 2009). Only absorbents without both potassium and sodium hydroxide (e.g. Sodasorb® LF, Amsorb® Plus, LoFloSorb®) do not produce compound A.

Carbon dioxide is absorbed by a series of chemical reactions. First, CO_2 and water form carbonic acid, and then the acid reacts with the hydroxide to form carbonate, water, and heat. A pH indicator, ethyl violet, is added to the absorbent to indicate when the absorbent is exhausted. The indicator is colourless at a high pH but, as CO_2 is absorbed, the pH decreases and the indicator changes to a violet colour, resulting in an absorbent colour change from white to violet. Once the absorbent has been exhausted, as indicated by a change in colour, it is no longer functional. Absence of visible colour change in a circuit without a patient attached is no guarantee that the absorbent is unused because the violet colour may fade shortly after disconnection of a patient due to temporal deactivation and deactivation by fluorescent lights.

Rebreathing circuits must have a bag to act as a reservoir of gas (reservoir bag, rebreathing bag) to supply the next inhalation. Bag sizes vary from 250 mL to 40 L and are chosen to match the size of the patient. The bag should be large enough to accommodate a deep breath. Conversely, excessively large bags (1) increase the volume of the circuit and slow rate of change of anaesthetic agent concentration, and (2) obscure assessment of ventilation as small tidal volumes produce small movement in large bags.

Rebreathing circuits must have a spring-loaded adjustable valve ('pop-off' valve) to prevent pressure rising in the circuit when the O_2 inflow exceeds the patient's metabolic oxygen requirement. These valves consist of a simple disc-type valve that can be closed by tightening the screw onto the disc. When this screw is not tightened, the valve is designed to remain closed and prevent leakage of gas from the circuit until the circuit pressure increases to 1–2 cmH_2O, at which point it opens, allows excess gas to exit, and the circuit pressure decrease to 0 cmH_2O. The valve can be screwed down when an increase in circuit pressure, generated by squeezing the reservoir bag, is to be maintained for artificial ventilation of the patient's lungs. If the valve is left closed when the O_2 flow exceeds metabolic oxygen requirement the reservoir bag will exceed its normal capacity and the circuit pressure will no longer return to zero between breaths. This is a life-threatening situation as the increase in intrathoracic pressure decreases return of venous blood to the heart and cardiac output and blood pressure will progressively decrease to zero. Pop-off valves may be adjustable pressure limiting (APL) valves that will automatically discharge when pressure exceeds 60 cmH_2O (adult) or 30 cmH_2O (paediatric). This safety mechanism may avoid pulmonary barotrauma should the circuit pressure abruptly increase following activation of the O_2 flush valve but cardiovascular collapse will occur before these pressures are reached when circuit pressure builds slowly with O_2 inflow from the flowmeter. It is recommended that, if adjustable pressure is a feature, the APL valve be manually set to discharge 5 cmH_2O above the inspiratory pressure needed for a normal lung inflation. Another safety mechanism available is a pop-off valve with an alternative method of closing other than screwing it closed. Either the head of the valve or a button on the exit side of the pop-off valve can be temporarily depressed to occlude gas outflow (Fig. 10.14). This feature can be employed when inflating the patient's lungs to test for an endotracheal tube cuff leak, or when sighing the patient, and can be used during manual artificial ventilation. An additional safety device inserted into the circle circuit will provide a high-pressure audible alert. The device may have an adjustable trigger pressure and be battery powered.

Circle circuit

The components of a circle circuit are arranged in a circle (Fig. 10.15) and two unidirectional valves (one-way valves) ensure that the exhaled gas passes through the CO_2 absorber before returning to the patient (Fig. 10.16). Placement of the reservoir bag in relation to O_2 inlet and CO_2 absorber varies between machine models. One concept is that ideally the reservoir bag should be on the inhalation side of the circuit so that there is least resistance to inhalation, and the CO_2 absorber should be on the exhalation side because the granules offer the most resistance to gas flow. The circle circuit usually has corrugated breathing hoses to decrease the risk of occlusion when bent. Most hoses are corrugated on the inside and tend to create turbulent gas flow. Some hoses are corrugated on

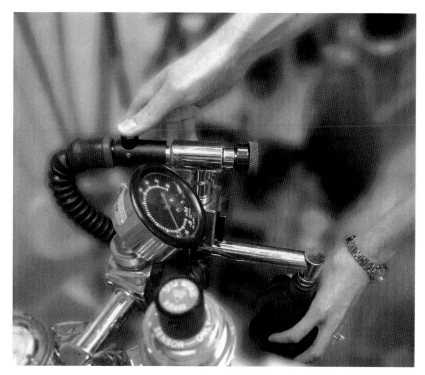

Figure 10.14 The anaesthetist is depressing the 'quick-close' button of the pop-off valve with the thumb of one hand while squeezing the reservoir bag to inflate the dog's lungs with the other hand.

the outside and smooth within the lumen and this feature facilitates increased airflow. Hose diameter varies according to the size of the patient: from 5 cm diameter for horses to 15 mm or 22 mm for small animals to 7 mm for animals <2 kg (Fig. 10.17). The volume of gas within the Y piece connector to the patient constitutes the apparatus deadspace of the circle because it contains exhaled CO_2 that will be breathed in as part of the next inhalation. As the deadspace volume increases in relation to the patient's tidal volume, the greater the impact on $PaCO_2$.

The coaxial circle circuit (Universal-F, UniFlo) is designed with the inspiratory hose positioned within the expiratory hose (Fig. 10.18). Advantages are that the two-hoses-in-one is less cumbersome when positioning the animal and, potentially, the inspired gases are warmed by the warm expired gases in the surrounding hose. A disadvantage is the resistance to breathing is increased as the diameters of the tubes are less than those of conventional parallel systems. These circuits should not be used for animals accommodating an endotracheal tube size with an internal diameter that is larger than the internal diameter of the inspiratory hose.

Oxygen inflow to circle circuits should be no lower than the patient's metabolic oxygen demand, approximately 6 mL/kg/minute for anaesthetized dogs and cats and 3 mL/kg/minute for anaesthetized horses and cattle. If the O_2 flow rate is less than the metabolic O_2 demand of the patient, the reservoir bag will progressively collapse (when O_2 alone is the carrier gas) and when empty, the patient becomes hypoxaemic. A closed system of administration is when O_2 flowing into the circuit exactly equals O_2 used so that there is no excess to leave by the pop-off valve. Note that the pop-off valve does not have to be screwed closed to operate a closed system. A higher flow of O_2 will result in gas leaving through the pop-off valve and this is called a semi-closed system of administration. A semi-closed system of administration can use low, medium or high O_2 flows. Medium and high O_2 flow rates are commonly used early in anaesthesia with precision vaporizers to compensate for the initial high uptake of anaesthetic agent by the patient and the CO_2 absorbent, and dilution by air in the circuit. The vaporizer dial percentage and O_2 flow rate are subsequently decreased for maintenance of anaesthesia. Continued use of high flows increases the amount of liquid anaesthetic agent that is vaporized and the wastage is costly. Low flow rates for small animals are in the range of 10–20 mL/kg/min.

The addition of N_2O automatically requires use of high gas flows because of the risk of the inspired concentration of O_2 decreasing below 30%. Insertion of an oxygen monitor into the inspiratory limb of the circle is recommended for improved safety. Nitrous oxide has low

223

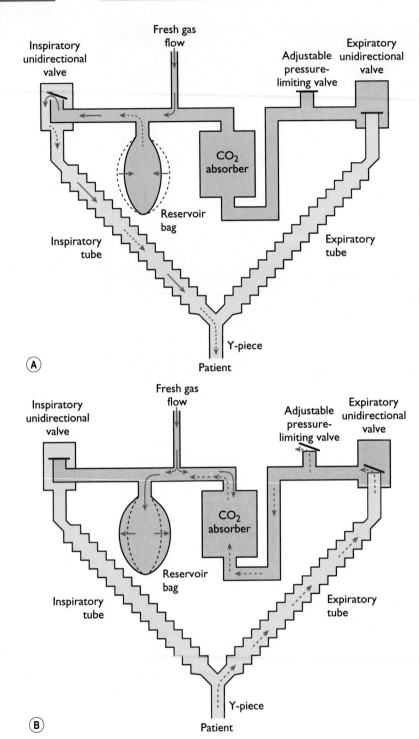

Figure 10.15 (A) Schematic design of a circle rebreathing circuit showing gas movement during spontaneous inhalation. During inhalation, the negative pressure in the inspiratory tubing opens the inspiratory unidirectional valve allowing flow of gas (mixture of fresh gas and exhaled gas with CO_2 removed) from the reservoir bag. FGF = fresh gas flow, APL = adjustable pressure-limiting valve (or pop-off valve), P = patient, → = fresh gas, - - -> = exhaled gas. (B) Schematic design of a circle rebreathing circuit showing gas movement during spontaneous exhalation. During early exhalation, the exhaled gas passes through the expiratory tube, through the expiratory unidirectional valve, through the CO_2 absorber, and into the reservoir bag. Fresh gas continues to flow into the reservoir bag. Towards the end of exhalation, the reservoir bag becomes full, exhaled gas ceases to flow through the absorber, and when the circuit pressure rises above 1–2 cmH_2O pressure, excess gas exits through the APL to the scavenger. FGF = fresh gas flow, APL = adjustable pressure-limiting valve (or pop-off valve), P = patient, → = fresh gas, - - -> = exhaled gas.

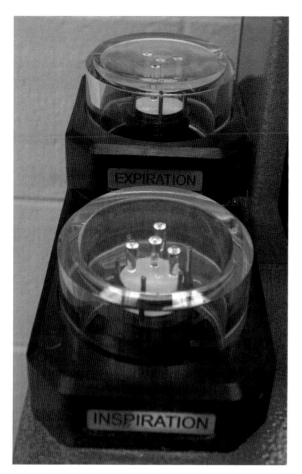

Figure 10.16 Inspiratory and expiratory one-way valves in a rebreathing circuit direct expired gases through the CO_2 absorber.

solubility and equilibrates with the pulmonary blood within several minutes, at which point uptake slows dramatically. Commonly used mixtures O_2:N_2O are 1:1 or 1:2. Supplying a 40:60 mixture of O_2 and N_2O at low flows results in the bulk of the O_2 being absorbed for metabolic needs with little N_2O absorption. As the minutes pass, the proportions of O_2 and N_2O within the circle change from 40:60 towards an ever decreasing concentration of O_2, even to the point of an hypoxic mixture. The recommended gas flows for a small animal circle circuit are O_2 30 mL/kg/min with N_2O added to that flow. For an adult horse connected to a large animal circle, 4 L each of O_2 and N_2O generally will maintain 40–50% O_2 concentration in the circle, however, presence of an O_2 monitor within the circle is a safety factor. Circle systems such as the Komesaroff and Stephens machines have vaporizers placed within the circle circuit. With each recycling of gases around the circle, O_2 containing isoflurane by-passes the vaporizer and joins with an increased concentration of

anaesthetic leaving the vaporizer, and so the inspired isoflurane concentration progressively increases with time. Consequently, a low FGF such as 100 mL/min is commonly used because a higher flow of O_2 would dilute the circle isoflurane concentration. Monitoring the patient for depth of anaesthesia is used to assess the need to adjust the vaporizer. These vaporizer-in-circle (VIC) systems are chosen because they are economical to use and produce less waste anaesthetic gases. Isoflurane and sevoflurane can be used in these machines. One investigation found that the Komesaroff machine did not reliably maintain surgical anaesthesia with sevoflurane in dogs (Laredo et al., 2001) but this finding was not confirmed by Straker et al. (2004) who found the system effective and economical in dogs over 10 kg body weight. Disadvantages included an empty vaporizer and exhausted CO_2 absorbent before the surgery was completed. Artificial ventilation of a patient connected to a system with the vaporizer-in-circle can generate dangerously high anaesthetic concentrations. One investigation of controlled ventilation in dogs connected to a Komesaroff machine documented that increased respiratory rates increased circuit anaesthetic concentrations and that vaporizer settings >2.5/4 produced unnecessarily high anaesthetic concentrations

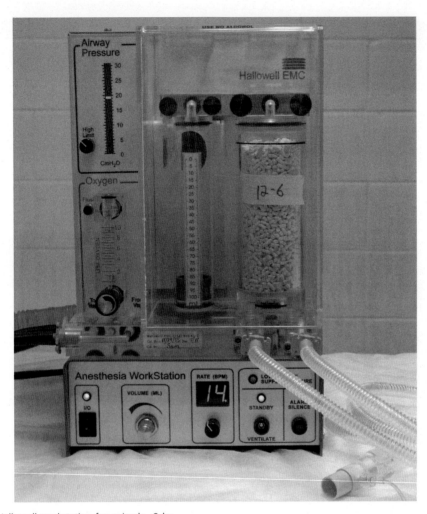

Figure 10.17 Hallowell workstation for animals <2 kg.

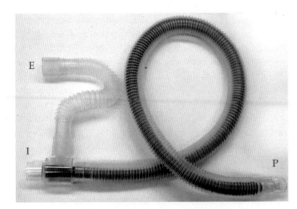

Figure 10.18 Coaxial circle circuit. I = connects to inspiratory valve, E = connects to expiratory valve, P = connects to endotracheal tube. The inner tube is inspiratory.

(Laredo et al., 2009). The transition from induction to maintenance of anaesthesia was made with the vaporizer full-on, then the vaporizer was decreased to 1/4 for isoflurane and 1.5/4 or 2.0/4 for sevoflurane which generally achieved end-tidal anaesthetic concentrations between 1 and 1.2× minimum alveolar concentration (MAC) value. The end-tidal anaesthetic agent concentration measurements also confirmed that deeper anaesthesia was achieved when 14 breaths/min were used compared with 9 breaths/min.

To-and-Fro

In a to-and-fro circuit, the animal's exhaled gases pass through the CO_2 absorbent into a bag and return through the absorbent during inhalation without the use of unidirectional valves (Fig. 10.19). The circuit is cumbersome because the CO_2 absorber is located close to the patient.

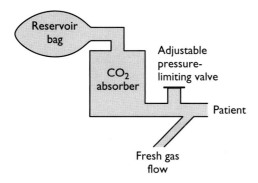

Figure 10.19 To-and-fro rebreathing circuit. FGF = fresh gas flow, APL = adjustable pressure-limiting valve (or pop-off) valve, P = patient.

Inhalation of absorbent dust is more likely to occur with this configuration than in a circle circuit.

Non-rebreathing circuits

Non-rebreathing circuits contain no valves and no CO_2 absorbent to offer resistance to breathing (see Table 10.3). High O_2 flows are used to prevent rebreathing of exhaled CO_2 and provide fresh gas for each breath. A decrease in O_2 flow required to eliminate CO_2 for a given body size can be achieved by rearranging the components of the circuits, thereby increasing feasibility for use in larger animals. Many circuits are available but they are all variations of those originally classified by Mapleson (Fig. 10.20) (Mapleson, 1954).

T-piece

The simplest circuit is the T-piece (Mapleson E) which is commonly used today in its modified form with a reservoir bag attached (Mapleson F, Jackson-Rees) (Fig. 10.21). The T-endotracheal tube adapter can be replaced with an adapter (Norman elbow) that delivers the fresh gas directly to the endotracheal tube and eliminates all circuit deadspace. The constant flow of fresh gas enters close to the endotracheal tube connector and flushes the patient's exhaled gas through a corrugated tube into the reservoir bag and through the exit hole into the waste anaesthetic gas scavenger. The patient inhales fresh gas from the corrugated tube and there is no rebreathing provided that the volume of the tube exceeds one tidal volume of the patient (Fig. 10.22). The fresh gas flow high enough to flush the corrugated tube between breaths must be 2.5 to 3 times the patient's minute volume (MV, breaths per min × tidal volume), or at least 450 mL/kg bodyweight/min. The origin of this FGF calculation has been previously referenced (Hall & Clarke, 1983). The FGF required to prevent CO_2 rebreathing in cats in a more recent investigation was 455 ± 77 mL/kg/min (Holden, 2001). Recent evaluations of respiratory parameters in unsedated young and adult

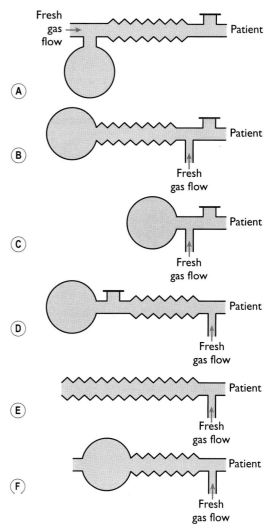

Figure 10.20 The Mapleson classification of patient delivery circuits A to F. FG=fresh gas flow, P=patient.

cats and medium-sized dogs have measured MV as approximately 230 mL/kg/min (Issa & Bitner, 1993; Kirschvink et al., 2006; Fraigne et al., 2008).

The exit hole from the bag into the scavenger may be too small to accommodate O_2 flows higher than 3 L such that pressure builds up in the circuit and interferes with the animal's breathing. Larger animals fair better when attached to a different non-rebreathing circuit that functions with a lower/kg flow rate, such as the Lack circuit, or attached to a paediatric circle circuit.

Bain circuit

The Mapleson D circuit functions similarly to the Mapleson E and F circuits. The Mapleson D incorporates a pop-off valve between the corrugated tube and the reservoir

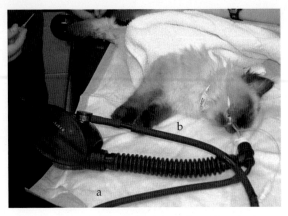

Figure 10.21 A modified T-piece non-rebreathing circuit. Oxygen and anaesthetic agent flow to patient in tube (A) and waste gases leave the circuit in tube (B).

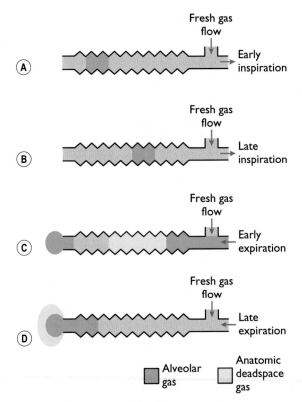

Figure 10.22 Function of the T-piece system in preventing rebreathing when the fresh gas flow exceeds at least twice the patient's minute volume.

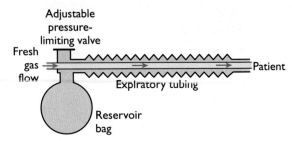

Figure 10.23 Bain circuit (coaxial version) modification of Mapleson D. Note that the bag is on the expiratory limb. The Bain is also available as a parallel system where the inspiratory tubing is a separate, wide-bore corrugated tube. FGF = fresh gas flow, APL = adjustable pressure-limiting valve (or pop-off) valve, P = patient.

(side-by-side) or coaxial, where the inspiratory tube is inside the expiratory tube. The Bain circuit terminates in a block comprising the reservoir bag, the pop-off valve, with or without a pressure gauge, that can be conveniently mounted on the anaesthesia machine. The FGF required to prevent rebreathing has been reported as approximately 260 mL/kg/min (Almubarak et al., 2005). Inspiratory and expiratory resistances are low with this system, but increase with increasing FGF.

Magill and Lack circuits

The Magill circuit (Mapleson A) incorporates a reservoir bag on the inspiratory limb, wide bore corrugated tubing, and a pop-off valve leading to a scavenging system. Rebreathing is prevented by maintaining the FGF slightly in excess of the patient's respiratory minute volume. The animal inhales from the bag and wide bore tubing; the exhaled mixture passes back up the tubing displacing the gas in it back into the bag until it is full. The exhaled gases never reach the bag because the capacity of the tubing is too great and once the bag is distended the increased pressure inside the circuit causes the pop-off valve to open so that the terminal part of expiration (the alveolar gas high in CO_2) passes out of the valve into the scavenger system (Fig. 10.24). During the pause following expiration and before the next inspiration, fresh gas from the workstation pushes the rest of the exhaled gases from the corrugated tube through the pop-off valve.

The Lack circuit is a modification of Mapleson A that has an expiratory tube running from the patient to the pop-off valve (Fig. 10.25). The tubes may be parallel (side-by-side) or coaxial where the expiratory tube runs inside the inspiratory tube (opposite arrangement to the Bain circuit). The FGF required to prevent rebreathing is of the order of 130 mL/kg/min. A smaller version of the parallel form (mini-Lack) is suitable for small patients.

The Maxima circuit is also a modification of Mapleson A with a 15 mm expiratory tube parallel to the 22 mm inspiratory tube and no valve. Evaluation of the circuit

bag. The Bain circuit is a modification in which the corrugated tube has been lengthened and the inspiratory and expiratory gases confined to separate tubes (Fig. 10.23). The reservoir bag and pop-off valve remain on the expiratory side of the circuit. The tubes may be parallel

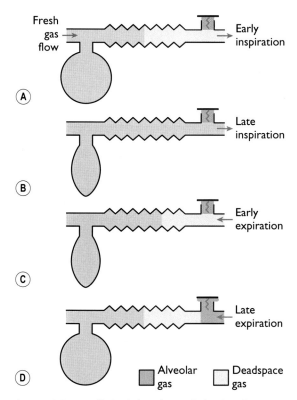

Figure 10.24 Magill circuit (Mapleson A) showing the disposition of fresh gas and exhaled gases (anatomic deadspace and alveolar) during spontaneous breathing.

with anaesthetized adult cats determined that an FGF of 242 mL/kg/min should prevent rebreathing in 95% of cats (Holden, 2001). The author noted that a higher FGF should be used in small cats to ensure accuracy of output of the precision vaporizer.

Hazards of coaxial circuits

In some cases, the internal or external tubing of coaxial circuits is of such a small bore that it imposes excessive resistance to the animals' breathing. In that case, the circuit should not be used when the internal diameter (ID) of the hose is less than the tracheal tube ID size. Also dangerous, the inner tube may become detached from the anaesthesia machine or the patient connector resulting in rebreathing of CO_2. Coaxial systems should be inspected before use and pressure checked.

Humphrey ADE circuit

The Humphrey ADE circuit is so named because it functions as a Mapleson A circuit during spontaneous breathing and as a Mapleson D or E mode during controlled ventilation. The reservoir bag is situated on the inspiratory side of the circuit and, therefore, during spontaneous breathing, gas in

the trachea and large bronchi containing no CO_2 passes back to the bag in the early part of exhalation before the FGF sweeps the remainder of the exhaled gas into the expiratory limb and scavenger. The recommended FGF for this circuit for cats and dogs <7 kg body weight is 70–100 mL/kg/min. The inside surfaces of the hoses are smooth, not corrugated, and that facilitates higher gas flow rates without turbulence (less resistance for large dogs). The FGF becomes uneconomical in larger dogs but then the circuit may be attached to a CO_2 absorber for use as a rebreathing system, and the FGF rate can be decreased accordingly.

Patient devices

Inhalation anaesthetic agents are usually delivered to the patient through a tracheal tube to avoid dilution with air and to limit exposure of personnel to waste anaesthetic gases. Facemasks are used to supply O_2 during induction and recovery from anaesthesia, to administer inhalation agents for induction of anaesthesia in some circumstances in small animals, young large animals, and in pigs, and for maintenance of anaesthesia in very small animals in which tracheal intubation may be difficult.

Facemasks

Facemasks are available in a variety of sizes and shapes (Fig. 10.26). The body or dome of the mask may be opaque or transparent. The rim of the mask that contacts the face may be rigid or a soft cushion, or fitted with a flat rubber seal. The connector is a short 15 mm or 22 mm internal diameter tube that fits into small animal rebreathing or non-rebreathing circuits. A mask should be chosen to be airtight and to conform as best as possible to the shape of the face to minimize deadspace. Care should be taken when using a facemask to avoid damage to the eyes and to avoid obstruction at the nostrils, especially in species that are obligate nasal breathers, such as foals.

Anaesthetic induction chambers

Boxes used for induction of anaesthesia of cats or other small animals are usually made of transparent plastic, so that the animal can be closely observed for movement or abnormal position that might result in airway obstruction. There is an inlet connector for administration of O_2 and inhalation agent and an outlet for connection to the waste anaesthetic gas scavenger. A much higher concentration than required for anaesthesia is administered because the volume of air in the chamber dilutes the inflowing anaesthetic. Therefore, it is important to judge accurately the time for removal of the patient from the chamber otherwise overdosage will occur. After the animal is anaesthetized, the animal is removed and anaesthesia maintained by endotracheal tube or facemask and a standard delivery circuit. Opening the chamber to remove the animal results in considerable room pollution.

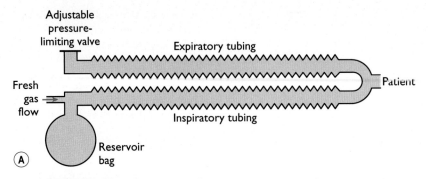

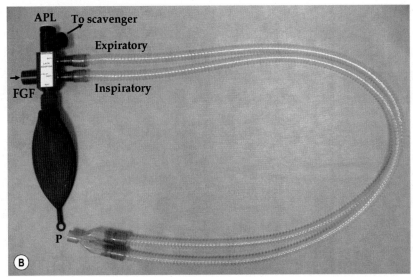

Figure 10.25 (A) and (B) Lack circuit (parallel version) modification of Mapleson A. Note that the bag is on the inspiratory limb. FGF = fresh gas flow, APL = adjustable pressure-limiting valve (or pop-off) valve, P = patient.
Photo courtesy of Dr J Cremer.

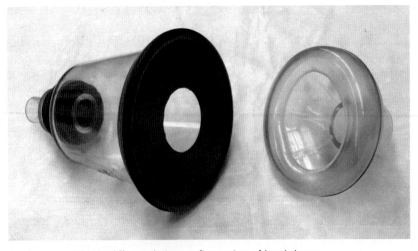

Figure 10.26 Facemasks are available in different designs to fit a variety of head shapes.

Endotracheal intubation

The history of endotracheal intubation in animals is older than that of anaesthesia. In 1542, Vesalius passed a tube into the trachea of an animal and inflated the lungs by means of a bellows to keep the animal alive while the anatomy of its thoracic cavity was demonstrated.

Tracheal tubes may be made of red rubber, polyvinylchloride, or silicone. Red rubber tubes are opaque which makes it difficult to ensure thorough cleaning. They may also kink if the patient's head and neck are flexed. Polyvinylchloride tubes are least expensive, fairly rigid which facilitates intubation, and are less likely to kink. Silicone tubes are soft which makes manipulation of the tube during intubation more difficult. The size of an endotracheal tube is denoted by its internal diameter (ID) in millimetres. The French scale size (three times the outside diameter in millimetres) is used by some manufacturers. The thickness of the wall of the endotracheal tube varies between types of tubes and manufacturers such that two tubes with the same outside diameter may have different lumen sizes. The lengths of the tubes increase with increasing ID. The ID increases by 0.5 mm for endotracheal tubes from 2 to 10 mm, by 1 mm for tubes 10–16 mm, and by 2–5 mm for larger tubes. This wide selection of tubes enables choice of a tube diameter that closely approximates the trachea size of the patient. Use of an endotracheal tube with an ID substantially smaller than that of the trachea results in restriction of airflow and hypoventilation in a spontaneously breathing animal. Excessive length of tube projecting beyond the incisors increases apparatus deadspace and CO_2 rebreathing. The tubes can often be cut short at the circuit end without destroying the cuff inflation tube, in order to accommodate short necks and muzzles in some breeds of dogs and cats. The centimetre marks on the side of the tube inform of how much of the tube is in the patient and may warn of excessive depth of insertion and possible bronchial intubation. The ability to choose the correct endotracheal tube size and length develops with experience, for example, 4.0 or 4.5 mm ID and 12–14 cm measured at the incisors for cats 3–4 kg, and 30 mm ID endotracheal tubes for 500 kg horses.

The standard type endotracheal tube is a tube with a gentle curvature, a hole in the wall of the tube at the bronchial end (Murphy eye), a cuff that can be inflated to provide a seal within the trachea, a connector to the anaesthesia circuit, and centimetre markings along the length of the tube (Fig. 10.27). A one-way valve on the pilot balloon prevents deflation of the tracheal cuff after it has been inflated. The Murphy eye is present to permit airflow should the bevel of the tube become obstructed by contact with the wall of the trachea. When the cuff is inflated, all respired gases must pass through the lumen of the tube avoiding either dilution of inspired gases with room air or pollution of the room with expired gases. A thin layer of

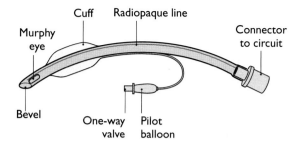

Figure 10.27 Standard endotracheal tube.

lubricant, such as KY gel, on the cuff will facilitate tube insertion.

Tracheal mucosa perfusion pressure is 20–30 mmHg (26–40 cmH_2O) and high endotracheal tube cuff pressure can cause tracheal damage. Distension of the pilot balloon reflects the degree of cuff inflation, however, palpation of the pilot balloon is a fairly inaccurate means of estimating cuff pressure. The usual cuff inflation pressure is achieved by injecting incremental amounts of air into the pilot balloon until no leak of O_2 or anaesthetic gas can be detected by sound of escaping gas or leak detector when the patient's lungs are manually inflated to 25 cmH_2O. Higher cuff pressures up to 35 cmH_2O may be necessary in large dogs, particularly when they are in a position that compromises lung inflation, such as in a prone, head-down position for surgery. Overdistension of the cuff may cause airway obstruction by compressing the lumen of the endotracheal tube (Fig. 10.28). Distension of the cuff may change with time (either increase or decrease) due to diffusion of gases in (nitrous oxide) and out of the cuff and relaxation of the trachea. In large animals, correlation between intracuff pressure and lateral tracheal wall pressure has not been defined and the pilot balloon pressure may be much higher than the 25 cmH_2O circuit pressure required to inflate the lungs. Estimation of adequacy of cuff inflation while avoiding cuff overinflation is difficult in adult horses and cattle, and a pressure gauge can be attached for accurate pressure measurement (Fig. 10.29). One investigation in anaesthetized horses noted that inflation of the endotracheal tube cuff to 80–100 cmH_2O pressure was necessary to prevent leakage around the cuff (Touzot-Jourde et al., 2005). Blind inflation of the cuff generated pressures of 120 cmH_2O. At pressures of 80 and 100 cmH_2O, gross and histological evidence of tracheal epithelial erosion was observed in seven out of 10 horses and the severity of damage was greater at the higher pressure.

Different types of endotracheal tube cuffs have been devised to minimize tracheal mucosa ischaemia and damage. Large volume cuffs may distribute the pressure more evenly and over a wider area of tracheal contact generating a low impact pressure (large volume, low pressure cuffs). Small volume cuffs may result in a smaller area

231

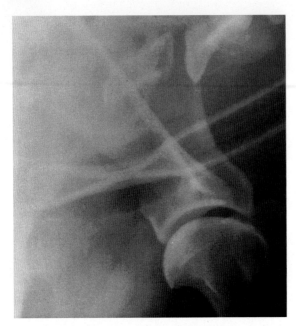

Figure 10.28 Radiograph showing occlusion of an endotracheal tube due to overdistension of the inflatable cuff.

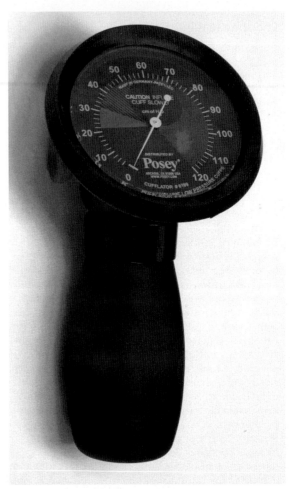

Figure 10.29 A device that attaches to the pilot balloon of an endotracheal tube to measure pressure in the cuff and inflate or deflate the endotracheal tube cuff as needed (Posey® cufflator).

of contact at a greater pressure that, although decreasing the risk of pulmonary aspiration of fluid, increase the risk of mucosal damage (small volume, high pressure cuffs). In the latter tubes, high intracuff pressure may be required to achieve an airtight seal within the trachea.

Some tracheal tubes have cuffs that contain polyurethane foam. Air must be aspirated out of the cuff before tube insertion. Allowing air to enter the cuff results in inflation and a seal. Cuff pressure is not usually monitored with this type of tube because the foam should conform to the trachea and result in a low wall pressure.

Plain endotracheal tubes without cuffs are used for endotracheal intubation of puppies, kittens, rabbits and birds (Fig. 10.30). The tube will not form an airtight seal and leakage is to be expected when controlled ventilation is employed. A Cole tube is a modification of the cuffless endotracheal tube comprising of a narrow distal portion to be inserted into the trachea and a wider proximal portion in the pharynx with the 'shoulders' of the tube forming an airtight seal at the entrance to the larynx. The tube has excellent pressure-flow characteristics and provides less resistance to breathing than a tube of small diameter extending its whole length. Cole tubes are useful for cats and rabbits, although thin-walled cuffed tubes are now available in small sizes.

Endotracheal tubes with a metal spiral within the tube wall (known as guarded tubes) are designed to prevent kinking of the tube even with extreme flexion of the head and neck or bending of the endotracheal tube (see

Fig. 10.30). These tubes are available with or without cuffs and up to 12 mm ID. This type of tube is floppy and a stilette threaded down the centre of the tube will facilitate placement of the tube in the trachea. Care should be taken when using a stilette to ensure that it does not emerge from the end of the endotracheal tube and lacerate the trachea. A potential disadvantage of this type of tube is that if the metal spiral is crimped (during insertion, during surgery, by the dog or cat biting down on it), it will remain kinked and an obstruction to airflow. Further, the thickness of the wall of the tube is greater to accommodate the metal so that a tube must be used with a smaller ID than would be possible using a standard tube.

A tracheotomy tube is a short tube with a right-angled bend for insertion through an incision through the skin over the trachea and through a hole in the trachea.

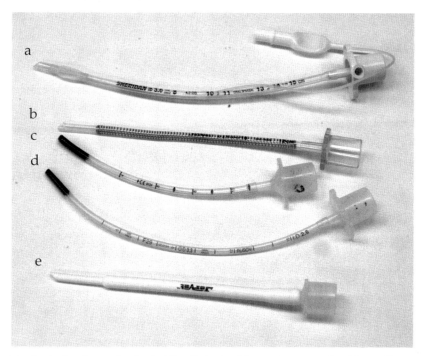

Figure 10.30 Endotracheal tubes for small animals: (A) cuffed tube 3.0 mm ID, 4.2 mm OD; (B) uncuffed metal spiral tube 2.5 mm ID, 4.0 mm OD; (C) uncuffed tube 3.0 mm ID, 4.0 mm OD; (D) uncuffed tube 2.5 mm ID, 3.3 mm OD; (E) Cole tube 2.5 mm ID (the narrow end inserts into the trachea).

Tracheotomy tubes may or may not have a cuff, and may have an internal sleeve that can be removed for cleaning while the major part of the tube remains in the animal.

Endotracheal tubes used for one lung ventilation during thoracotomy in dogs and cats most commonly are single lumen tubes with a bronchial blocker. The bronchial blocker consists of a balloon on the end of a narrow tube that can be inserted under direct endoscopic view into the bronchus of the lung to be collapsed. Inflation of the balloon obstructs airflow into that lung. The endotracheal tube then directs gases to the ventilated lung.

Laser beam contact with a standard endotracheal tube may result in rupture of the tube and ignition of oxygen. Special laser-resistant endotracheal tubes are available for specific laser types. An approved product for laser protection by wrapping a standard endotracheal tube is a two-layered sheet of surgical sponge and adhesive backed silver foil (Dorsch & Dorsch, 2008).

Laryngeal mask airways

Supraglottic airway devices are available in a variety of designs and sizes. The classic laryngeal mask airway (LMA) consists of a tube connected to an elliptical spoon-shaped mask at a 30° angle with an inflatable low pressure cuff that is inserted into the pharynx to cover the epiglottis and entrance to the larynx (Fig 10.31). A supraglottic airway device with a rim that is not inflatable (the i-gel) is also available. Use of the LMA avoids tracheal wall damage that may be associated with endotracheal intubation and is easier to insert than an endotracheal tube in some species. There are numerous publications describing use of LMA in humans, dogs, cats, pigs, rabbits, and rodents. Laryngeal mask airways that are designed for human use are not necessarily a perfect fit in other species so that the device does not always produce an airtight seal. Wiederstein & Moens (2008) achieved successful placement and function of the LMA in 19 out of 30 dogs (63.3%) but a leak at a lung inflation pressure of 10 cmH$_2$O was present in the others. Evidence linking use of the LMA and gastro-oesophageal reflux (GOR, GER) in humans is conflicting, varying from no association to a two- to threefold increase in the incidence of reflux compared with use of an endotracheal tube or a facemask. In contrast to an investigation of the use of a LMA in adult cats (Cassau et al., 2004), kittens anaesthetized with isoflurane experienced a high incidence of gastric reflux and the use of an LMA was associated with an increased occurrence (Sideri et al., 2009). The mechanism of the association is unclear but is presumably related to a decrease in lower oesophageal

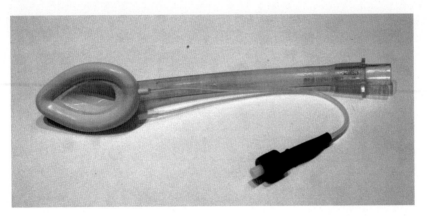

Figure 10.31 Laryngeal mask airway.

sphincter (LOS) pressure. Very young animals have low LOS pressure and it is possible that sustained distension of the pharynx by the inflated LMA may have induced further LOS relaxation (Sideri et al., 2009).

Supraglottic airways marketed for infants are usually too large for the smaller animal species, resulting in failure to seal the airway and subsequent complications of abdominal distension or aspiration of refluxed gastric fluid (Bateman et al., 2005). In 2005, Imai et al. reported on the development of an airway device specifically designed for small laboratory animals. The device was made from silicone moulded from post-mortem anatomy of rabbits, ferrets, rats, and mice, and consisted of a mask to fit over the larynx with an inflatable balloon projection that entered the oesophagus, all connected to a tube with a continuous metal spiral in its wall. The device was tested in rabbits anaesthetized with isoflurane and positive pressure ventilation was accomplished without obvious gas leakage. Crotaz (2010) described re-shaping of the Size 1 igel for rabbits and called the prototype the v-gel. The v-gel is now commercially available in six sizes each for cats and rabbits.

Laryngoscopes

A laryngoscope has detachable blades of different sizes, a light source, and dry electric batteries in the handle (Fig 10.32). A laryngoscope greatly facilitates the process of intubation in many animals by providing sufficient light to view the laryngeal entrance and a blade to depress the tongue; a manoeuvre that moves the epiglottis and exposes the larynx. Tracheal intubation can be accomplished in most dogs with good overhead lighting and horses are intubated (blind) without viewing tube insertion. However, a laryngoscope provides better laryngeal exposure in certain breeds and species, such as brachycephalic dogs, small ruminants, and pigs. A rigid fibreoptic laryngoscope or flexible fibreoptic endoscope is useful for intubation of difficult cases and routinely for intubation of rabbits. The fibreoptic scope is placed inside the

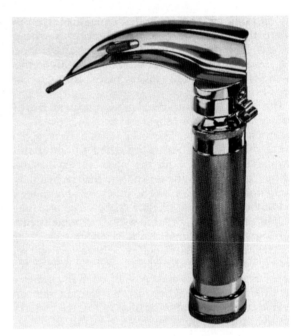

Figure 10.32 Laryngoscope with detachable Macintosh blade – a wide variety of patterns and lengths of blade are available.

endotracheal tube before the scope is used to view the entrance to the larynx, whereupon the endotracheal tube is moved off the scope and advanced into the trachea. Techniques of intubation are described in the species chapters.

Filters and humidity and moisture exchangers

A bacterial biofilm rapidly forms on the inside surface of the endotracheal tube after intubation, and fragments of the biofilm can detach spontaneously. Human and animal studies have shown that anaesthetic circuit or ventilator tubing can be colonized within a few hours. Investigations using endotracheal tubes that are internally coated with bacteriocidal agents in polyurethane have demonstrated absence of bacteria in the endotracheal tube and circle tubing in contrast to colonization with multiple bacterial species when standard endotracheal tubes are used (Berra et al., 2004). The possible origin of the biofilm is leakage of accumulated secretions from above the cuff into the trachea. There are many different types of endotracheal tubes and supraglottic devices for alternatives to airway management. Evidence supporting which ones are most effective at preventing pulmonary aspiration of fluid is confusing despite many research publications because the methods of testing are so variable (Rai & Popat, 2011).

Low volume, high pressure cuffs on endotracheal tubes are more likely to cause tracheal mucosa pressure damage, yet the high volume, low pressure cuffs are more likely to fail to protect against a leak and passage of oral or gastric bacteria into the trachea.

Contamination of the anaesthetic circuit is more likely to occur in rebreathing systems with low FGF than in non- or partial-rebreathing systems. Condensation within the tubes of a rebreathing system may collect bacteria and movement of the tubes during repositioning may result in the bacteria traversing into the patient. Excess contamination of the circuit in human anaesthesia was associated with increased duration of anaesthesia and with the patient coughing, generally at the time of extubation (Rees et al., 2007; Dugani et al., 2010). An investigation of the parallel Lack circuit used for short duration anaesthesia in small animals recovered minimal bacterial growth and the data indicated that bacteria present within the circuit died provided that time was allowed for the circuit to dry out before use on the next patient (Pelligand et al., 2007).

A breathing system filter may prevent bacterial colonization of anaesthetic tubing and protect the patient from bacteria in a previously used circuit, however, clinical investigations have provided evidence of a wide range in filtration performance between commercially available filters (Wilkes, 2011a). A clinical trial in people demonstrated that hydrophobic (pleated) filters perform better than electrostatic filters in preventing transmission of bacteria (Dugani et al., 2010).

Placement of a tracheal tube or supraglottic device bypasses the nasal cavity. Inhalation of dry air may cause impaired mucociliary function in the trachea and even cell damage (Wilkes, 2011a). During anaesthesia, as compared with intensive care, the short periods of low humidity are unlikely to cause severe respiratory dysfunction and, for longer surgeries, sufficient humidity may be provided in a circle circuit with low FGF. The addition of a heat and moisture exchanger (HME) to humidify inspired gases may be advisable for long surgeries involving non-rebreathing systems. Bisinotto et al. (1999) investigated the effect of an HME in anaesthetized artificially ventilated experimental dogs connected to a non-rebreathing circuit with FGF of 5 L/min or a circle circuit with FGF of 1 L/min. Lower relative (37%) and absolute humidity (9 mgH$_2$O/L) was measured in dogs connected to the non-rebreathing circuit with high FGF. The addition of a HME to both circuits increased the humidity of inhaled gas, with relative humidity reaching 90–94% and absolute humidity 22–24 mgH$_2$O/L. These values with the HME are within the recommended lower limit (>20 mgH$_2$O/L) for absolute humidity during anaesthesia. The circle circuit without HME reached an average absolute humidity of 17.8 mgH$_2$O/L after 3 hours. Histological changes were observed in the mucociliary system of the tracheobronchial tree in dogs connected to the non-rebreathing system without HME and these effects were less or absent with HME. Body temperature was not significantly increased when HME was included. In a clinical study of dogs anaesthetized for orthopaedic surgery with isoflurane via a circle, decreases in body temperature were not different when a HME was used (Hofmeister et al., 2011).

Principles and use of these devices have been recently reviewed (Wilkes, 2011a,b). Possible complications to use of these devices are resistance to airflow, obstruction due to accumulation of fluid, increased apparatus deadspace, and altered capnography waveform. The increased deadspace and increase in resistance to airflow may impair CO$_2$ elimination. The recommended lowest patient bodyweight for use of these devices in human anaesthesia is 2.5 kg.

Scavenging waste anaesthetic gases

One of the earliest indications that exposure of operating personnel to waste anaesthetic gases during the process of providing anaesthesia was cause for concern was a publication in 1967 from Russia that documented a high incidence of miscarriages and congenital defects in children of anaesthesiologists. Many surveys were performed, including one published in 1974 that analyzed questionnaires from 40 000 hospital personnel and identified increased risk for spontaneous abortion, cancer, and children with congenital malformations. Nitrous oxide has been shown to be directly teratogenic in experimental animals, causing fetal resorption and skeletal abnormalities in rats. In humans, the most susceptible time of pregnancy for teratogenesis is the first trimester. A meta-analysis of studies in 1985 confirmed increased risk for spontaneous abortion, congenital abnormalities, liver and kidney disease, and cervical cancer. Since there were questions raised relating to collection of data in these studies, it was believed that the argument that waste anaesthetic gases produce adverse effects was not confirmed. A recently published questionnaire-based survey of Australian veterinarians exposed to clinical veterinary work while pregnant identified an increased prevalence for birth defects, most commonly cardiovascular, in female veterinarians compared with the general population (Shirangi et al., 2009). The risk of birth defects was highest in veterinarians who used pesticides at work and who were exposed to radiation and those women who worked long hours per week. There was no significant association between birth defects and maternal exposure to anaesthetic gases. Personal and published experiences leave no doubt that room pollution results in headaches, fatigue and decreased judgement and coordination.

Since the early 1980s, scavenging waste anaesthetic gases has become accepted practice and is endorsed by the European College of Veterinary Anaesthesia and Analgesia and the American College of Veterinary Anesthesia and Analgesia (http://acva.org/docs/Waste_Gas). Current opinion is that there is no increased risk for pregnancy complication from anaesthetic gases when a properly run scavenging system is in operation and that attention is paid to minimize leaks from the anaesthetic circuit. This does not rule out the risk of miscarriage due to stress or long working hours. Sensible precautions for pregnant women include giving up on-call duty and avoiding long periods of standing, avoiding situations where pollution can occur despite use of a scavenging system, such as avoiding anaesthesia administered by facemask and filling of vaporizers, avoiding use of N_2O, and no lifting of heavy dogs or equipment. Some pregnant female personnel choose to wear gas masks when working around anaesthetized patients but these can impair breathing and be added discomfort. Temporary assignment to duties outside the operating room and recovery area, if possible, would remove risk of exposure to inhaled anaesthetic agents. Attention to minimizing waste gas pollution is essential at all times for the health of all personnel, including limiting exposure prior to the diagnosis of pregnancy. Vigilance must be maintained to avoid accidental pollution, such as forgetting to turn on the scavenger suction or leaving the vaporizer and oxygen on after disconnection of a patient.

A scavenging system consists of a means to collect and dispose of anaesthetic gases exiting from the patient delivery circuit. The hoses leading from the breathing system have been 19 mm diameter but new international standards have increased the size to 30 mm. Gases travel in this hose passively. The simplest form of scavenger is a canister containing activated charcoal that will absorb 50 g of halogenated anaesthetic agents, but not nitrous oxide (Fig. 10.33). The canister should be weighed before use, and the date and weight written on the side. The canister should be discarded when the weight has increased by 50 g as, at this point, anaesthetic gases will be escaping into the room. Unfortunately, different brands of commercially available activated charcoal canisters may have different scavenging capacities and anaesthetic agent may pass through the canisters before they reach 50 g weight gain (Smith & Bolon, 2003).

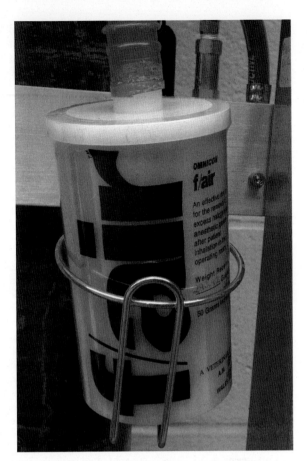

Figure 10.33 Charcoal canister for scavenging waste anaesthetic gas.

A scavenger system that consists of wide-bore tubing can be used passively to transport gas to outside the building. The potential problem with this system is that the patient's breathing is responsible for moving the gas down the tube and the distance of tubing to the outside is likely to offer significant resistance to breathing. Further, debris, insects, or a strong wind may occlude the building outlet.

Many scavenger systems have a means of actively moving air down the tube either by suction or by propulsion. There must be an interface (also known as an air brake) between the patient breathing circuit and the active system for patient safety. Interfaces can be either closed, with a reservoir bag and valves, or open and valveless (Figs 10.34, 10.35). The purpose of the interface is to prevent the suction apparatus from aspirating gas from the patient's breathing circuit and, conversely, to prevent resistance in the scavenger producing back pressure in the circuit and compromising breathing. There should also be a valve or adjustable clamp between the interface and suction unit to control the degree of vacuum applied.

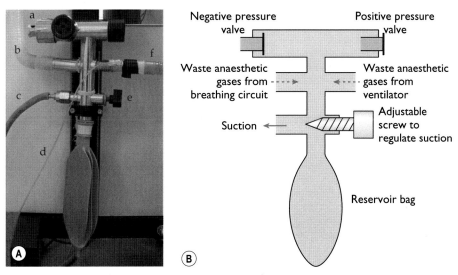

Figure 10.34 (A) Closed interface (air brake) for active scavenging of waste anaesthetic gases. A: Inlet and outlet pressure relief valves; B: exhaust from anaesthetic breathing circuit; C: suction; D: exhaust from anaesthetic gas analyzer; E: adjustable screw for suction; F: exhaust from ventilator bellows. (B) Schematic design of closed interface.

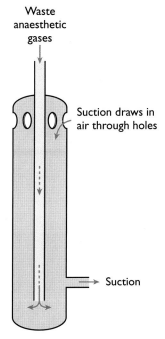

Figure 10.35 Schematic design of an open interface for active scavenging of waste anaesthetic gases.

Current recommendation is that scavenger vacuum hoses be light purple in colour.

The presence of a scavenger system on the anaesthesia machine does not guarantee lack of pollution in the room. Pollution with anaesthetic gases can occur in a variety of

---

Box 10.5 Prevention of room pollution with anaesthetic gases

- Use of scavenging equipment
- Inspection of hoses and bags for holes
- Tightening of connections
- Circuit check before anaesthesia to identify leaks
- Emptying the reservoir bag into the scavenging system at the end of anaesthesia
- Avoiding mask administration of anaesthesia whenever possible
- Scavenging ventilators and gas analysers
- Fill vaporizers at end of day, or in another room
- Using a key-filler system to fill vaporizers
- Turn off flowmeters when not in use
- Turn off N_2O cylinder when not in use

---

situations (Box 10.5). Prevention of pollution involves attention to all the details listed, keeping up with maintenance on the anaesthesia machine and, above all, training new employees in the importance of attention to details and correct operation of the scavenging system.

In many countries, health and safety regulations require monitoring of waste anaesthetic gas concentrations at set intervals, even when scavenging systems are in operation. Even when not required by law, monitoring waste anaesthetic concentrations is a sensible precaution, for example, in practices that perform chamber inductions or maintenance of anaesthesia by facemask because these techniques can result in considerable room pollution. Anaesthetic equipment supply companies have a variety of monitoring aids, including an anaesthetic detection badge or dosimeter which is analogous to a radiation badge, and air monitoring that can be either instantaneous samples from a room that is in use or continuous collection of air sample over 1–8 hours that are then sent to a laboratory for analysis. Different countries have different recommendations for the maximum allowed exposure (http://www.osha.gov//SLTC/wasteanestheticgases) (Barker & Abdelatti, 1997) but no recommendations for sevoflurane or desflurane. The occupational exposure standards (OES) set by the Control of Substances Hazardous to Health (COSHH) regulations for the UK are based on an 8-hour time-weighted average and are 50 ppm for isoflurane, 100 ppm of nitrous oxide. The acceptable values for other European countries are similar for nitrous oxide but less for isoflurane. In the USA, the National Institute of Occupational Safety and Health (NIOSH) has recommended that exposure to halogenated anaesthetic gases should not exceed 2 ppm or 0.5 ppm when breathed in combination with nitrous oxide over a period not to exceed 1 hour. Exposure to nitrous oxide alone should not exceed 25 ppm.

Clinical use of the anaesthesia workstation

The most important function of the anaesthesia workstation is to supply oxygen to the patient. It is essential to ensure that the workstation supply, whether pipeline, cylinder on the machine, or oxygen concentrator, is correctly connected and functional and that the spare cylinder on the anaesthesia machine has sufficient oxygen for back up. When changing an oxygen cylinder, the cylinder should first be turned off using a cylinder wrench (also known as a cylinder key). The O_2 flush lever/button should be depressed to release pressure in the hoses and then the screw of the yoke (depending on the type of connector) loosened to enable the cylinder to be removed. A cylinder should never be left standing upright without secure support because if it falls, cracking the casing, it will resemble a launched missile. It has been recommended in the past that a new cylinder should be partially opened before connection to the anaesthesia machine. This is known as 'venting', the purpose of which is to blow out dust particles that would otherwise become trapped inside the hoses of the anaesthesia machine. Venting has the potential for causing serious personal injury when a jet of oxygen impacts on a person's hands or arms. Furthermore, venting is unnecessary when new cylinders are delivered with plastic or metal covers on the outlets. The new cylinder is lifted into position, the yoke is tightened and the cylinder opened by turning the key or wrench

counterclockwise to check for leaks and to confirm the presence of O_2 in the cylinder. Leakage of O_2 around the yoke of a pin-index cylinder may be corrected by using a new washer (Badcock seal). Although the pin-index and bullnose fittings are different configurations, the principles of cylinder change are the same.

When O_2 is supplied from a remote site through a pipeline to the anaesthesia machine, the pipeline pressure gauge (located in the wall or on the workstation) should be checked for an adequate line pressure of 50-55 psi (350-400 kPa). A staff member should have the daily responsibility of checking the adequacy of O_2 supply and the anaesthetist should ensure that there is a back-up supply of O_2 immediately available.

The flowmeters should be turned on to confirm that O_2 is flowing. When turning off the flowmeter, the knob should be only gently tightened because it consists of a fine point that can easily shear off. The vaporizer should be checked for adequate liquid anaesthetic.

Patient delivery circuits should be examined for cracks and broken parts. The one-way valves should be examined for the presence of the flap valves and their correct positioning. The circuit must be checked for leaks before induction of anaesthesia. For a rebreathing circuit, the pop-off/APL valve should be closed or the exit to the scavenger occluded, a thumb or specific occluder (or a stopper for large animal circle circuits), placed over the endotracheal tube connector and the circuit filled with O_2 from the flowmeter or the emergency O_2 flush (Fig. 10.36). The reservoir bag should be filled to a pressure of 30 cmH$_2$O and, with the flowmeter turned off, should hold that pressure for 10 seconds to determine any leakage of oxygen. The recommendation is that a leak in excess of 100 mL/min at 30 cmH$_2$O pressure is unacceptable. It is important that the flowmeter should be off during the pressure test otherwise the inflow of oxygen will obscure leakage. An alternative technique is to close the pop-off/APL valve and occlude the patient connector, fill the reservoir bag with O_2 and pressurize it to 30 cmH$_2$O while adjusting the O_2 flowmeter so that the pressure can be maintained. The resultant flow on the flowmeter is the magnitude of the circuit leak. Leaks may be detected by application of soapy water over junctions and observation of bubbles when the circuit is pressurized. The pop-off/APL valve should always be opened after a pressure test to avoid an accidental high pressure when first used. A non-rebreathing circuit should also be tested for leaks by occluding patient and expiratory outlets and pressurizing the reservoir bag.

With some absorbents, the indicator in the CO_2 absorbent will change back to its original colour within 15 minutes of cessation of anaesthesia. Consequently, at the end of anaesthesia, the level of used absorbent should be noted or the hourly duration of use should be written on the canister. Exhausted absorbent feels brittle to handle but texture is an imprecise guide. Rate of use of absorbent

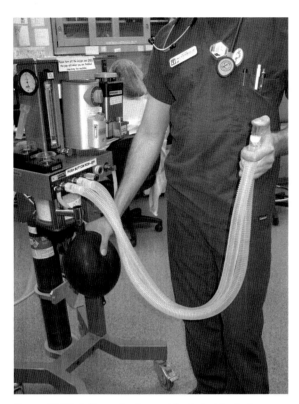

Figure 10.36 Delivery circuits must be tested for leaks before use by checking that pressure can be maintained at 30 cmH$_2$O with <100 mL/min O$_2$ flow.

Table 10.4 Locating a leak in a breathing circuit	
Preanaesthesia check	**During anaesthesia**
Check hoses and bag for holes	Oesophageal intubation
Tighten connections	Leak around endotracheal tube
Leak around CO$_2$ absorber due	cuff
to dust on washers	Scavenger suction too high and
Covers on turret type	opening the pop-off valve
unidirectional valves not	Patient's forceful breathing
tight/cross-threaded	causing gas to exit circuit
Circuit not connected	and not enter reservoir bag
	Prolonged manual ventilation
	causing small holes at the
	neck of the bag
	Iatrogenic pneumothorax

will depend on the commercial product, the capacity of the absorber, the size of the patient, and the flow rate of O$_2$; exhaustion of absorbent occurring most rapidly in a closed system. Loose granules of absorbent should not be changed in the operating room because the process may generate a cloud of dust with some products. Leaks in a circle circuit are often caused by absorbent dust on the washers of the canister and, therefore, the washers should be cleaned before the canister is closed.

Oxygen cylinders should be turned off and pipelines disconnected at the end of the day to prevent continued small leakage during the night. After the cylinders are turned off, the pressure in the lines should be depleted by pressing the oxygen flush valve in order that the next person using the machine is made aware that there is no O$_2$ supply. Ideally, the vaporizer(s) should be filled after the last patient of the day, after personnel have left the room, so that they are less exposed to waste gases.

Troubleshooting the delivery circuits

Patient safety is improved when the anaesthesia machine is checked out before anaesthesia, decreasing the

likelihood for troubleshooting during anaesthesia. Use of checklists decreases the risk of forgetting a vital step. A common problem is collapse of the reservoir bag and that is due to insufficient O$_2$ entering the circuit, due to a leak, or too great a suction from the scavenger. Once it has been determined that there is O$_2$ flowing through the flowmeter, the circuit should be examined (Table 10.4).

Cleaning and sterilizing of anaesthetic equipment

There are two mechanisms involved in the transmission of pathogens by anaesthesia procedures: transmission between patients by the veterinarian, nurse, or assistant, and transfer from contaminated equipment. Veterinary personnel play an important part in transfer of disease and hand hygiene is essential. Hand washing with liquid soap and water should be done between patients and ideally non-sterile gloves worn for routine tasks. An antimicrobial hand rub may be used if there is no visible hand soiling. Anaesthesia equipment can be a vector. Transfer of bacteria easily occurs during induction and maintenance of anaesthesia when the patient is touched for intubation or assessment of depth of anaesthesia and the same hands touch the anaesthesia machine hoses and reservoir bag, vaporizers, and flowmeter knobs. Pre-existing factors, such as old age, diabetes, and renal failure, may be present in patients undergoing surgery that increase the risk for nosocomial infections. Results of one investigation in a human hospital confirmed a high recovery of positive cultures growing pathogenic bacteria taken from the surface of anaesthesia machines, despite the fact that each anaesthesia machine was cleaned at the end of the day (Baillie et al., 2007). A significant decrease in positive cultures was documented when each anaesthesia machine was wiped with a detergent wipe between cases. When animals with infectious disease must be anaesthetized, the anaesthetist should wear a disposable gown, shoe covers, and gloves. The person recording data on the anaesthetic record should not be the same person handling the animal and anaesthesia machine.

Breathing circuits that are reused are potential sources of cross infection between patients. Plastic circuits labelled 'for single use only' in human anaesthesia have an acceptable limited reuse value. However, guidelines established by the Association of Anaesthetists of Great Britain and Ireland in 2008 recommend that a new bacterial/viral breathing circuit filter should be used for every human patient (Gemmell et al., 2008). This is not yet economically feasible for all veterinary patients and it is common in veterinary practice to reuse circuits to the point of dysfunction. Positioning an animal with its head down, or animals that cough during anaesthesia, are likely to induce contamination of the breathing circuit. Breathing circuits used for patients with infectious diseases should either be discarded or thoroughly washed, dried, and sterilized before being used on the next patient. Corrugated hoses should be dry before being reused.

Endotracheal tubes should be thoroughly washed and the lumens cleaned with a soft bristle brush. Protein deposits are particularly difficult to remove from laryngeal mask airways (Clery et al., 2003). Methods of sterilization will depend on the material of the tube. Whatever method is employed, care must be taken that no sterilizing solution remains on the tube or tracheal irritation and damage will result. Ethylene oxide (ETO) is an effective method of sterilization for most tubes but strict adherence to the aeration time specified by the equipment manufacturer is essential to avoid life-threatening tracheal and organ damage from contact with ETO residue (Trim & Simpson, 1982). Several animals suffered tracheal damage on the same day as the patient described in Trim & Simpson (1982), including a cat that required resection of several tracheal rings to restore airway patency. Laryngoscope blades should also be cleaned between patients and the outside of the handle wiped with antiseptic solution.

REFERENCES

Almubarak, A., Clarke, K.W., Jackson, T.L., 2005. Comparison of the Bain system and Uniflow universal anaesthetic breathing systems in spontaneously breathing young pigs. Vet Anaesth Analg 32, 314–321.

Ambrisko, T.D., Klide, A.M., 2011. Accuracy of isoflurane, halothane, and sevoflurane vaporizers during high oxygen flow and at maximum vaporizer setting. Am J Vet Res 72, 751–756.

Baillie, J.K., Sultan, P., Graveling, E., et al., 2007. Contamination of anaesthetic machines with pathogenic organisms. Anaesthesia 62, 1257–1261.

Barker, J.P., Abdelatti, M.O., 1997. Anaesthetic pollution. Anaesthesia 52, 1077–1083.

Bateman, L., Ludders, J.W., Gleed, R.D., et al., 2005. Comparison between facemask and laryngeal mask airway in rabbits during isoflurane anesthesia. Vet Anaesth Analg 32, 280–288.

Berra, L., De Marchi, L., Laquerriere, P., et al., 2004. Endotracheal tubes coated with antiseptics decrease bacterial colonization of the ventilator circuits, lungs, and endotracheal tube. Anesthesiology 100, 1446–1456.

Bisinotto, F.M.B., Braz, J.R.C., Martins, R.H.C., et al., 1999. Tracheobronchial consequences of the use of heat and moisture

exchangers in dogs. Can J Anaesth 46, 897–903.

Boller, M., Moens, Y., Kastner, S.B.N., et al., 2005. Closed system anaesthesia in dogs using liquid sevoflurane injection; evaluation of the square-root-of-time model and the influence of CO2 absorbent. Vet Anaesth Analg 32, 168–177.

Cassu, R.N., Luna, S.P., Teixeira Neto, F.J., 2004. Evaluation of laryngeal mask as an alternative to endotracheal intubation in cats anaesthetized under spontaneous or controlled ventilation. Vet Anaesth Analg 31, 213–221.

Clarke, K.W., 2008. Options for inhalation anaesthesia. In Practice 30, 513–518.

Clery, G., Brimacombe, J., Stone, T., et al., 2003. Routine cleaning and autoclaving does not remove protein deposits from reusable laryngeal mask devices. Anesth Analg 97, 1189–1191.

Crotaz, I.R., 2010. Initial feasibility investigation of the v-gel airway: an anatomically designed supraglottic airway device for use in companion animal veterinary anaesthesia. Vet Anaesth Analg 37, 579–580.

Culp, W.T.N., Mayhew, P.D., Reese, M.S., et al., 2010. Complications associated with use of subcutaneous vascular access ports in cats and dogs

undergoing fractionated radiotherapy: 172 cases (1996–2007). J Am Vet Med Assoc 236, 1322–1327.

Dorsch, J.A., Dorsch, S.E., 2008. Understanding Anesthesia Equipment. Lippincott Williams & Wilkins, Philadelphia.

Dugani, S., Kumar, A., Wilkes, A.R., 2010. Influence of patient factors on the efficacy of breathing system filters at preventing contamination of breathing systems. Anaesthesia 65, 468–472.

Farling, P.A., Flynn, P.A., Darwent, G., et al., 2010. Safety in magnetic resonance units: an update. Anaesthesia 65, 766–770.

Fraigne, J.J., Dunin-Barkowski, W.L., Orem, J.M., 2008. Effect of hypercapnia on sleep and breathing in unanesthetized cats. Sleep 31, 1025–1033.

Gemmell, L., Birks, R., Radford, P., et al., 2008. Infection control in anaesthesia. Anaesthesia 63, 1027–1036.

Giunti, M., Otto, C.M., 2009. Intraosseous catheterization. In: Silverstein, D.C., Hopper, K. (Eds.), Small Animal Critical Care Medicine. Saunders Elsevier, St Louis, pp. 263–267.

Hall, L.W., Clarke, K.W., 1983. Veterinary Anaesthesia. Bailliere Tindall, London.

Harris, P.D., Barnes, R., 2008. The uses of helium and xenon in current clinical practice. Anaesthesia 63, 284–293.

Hodgson, D.S., 2006. An inhaler device using liquid injection of isoflurane for short term anesthesia in piglets. Vet Anaesth Analg 33, 207–213.

Hofmeister, E.H., Brainard, B.M., Braun, C., et al., 2011. Effect of a heat-moisture exchanger on heat loss in isoflurane-anesthetized dogs undergoing single-limb orthopedic procedures. J Am Vet Med Assoc 239, 1561–1565.

Holden, D.J., 2001. A comparison of the 'Maxima' and the modified Ayre's T-piece breathing systems in spontaneously breathing cats. Vet Anaesth Analg 27, 50–53.

Imai, A., Eisele, P.H., Steffey, E.P., 2005. A new airway device for small laboratory animals. Lab Anim 39, 111–115.

Issa, F.G., Bitner, S., 1993. Effect of route of breathing on the ventilatory and arousal responses to hypercapnia in awake and sleeping dogs. J Physiol 465, 615–628.

Jones, I.D., Case, A.M., Stevens, K.B., et al., 2009. Factors contributing to the contamination of peripheral intravenous catheters in dogs and cats. Vet Rec 164, 616–618.

Kharasch, E.D., Powers, K.M., Artru, A.A., 2002. Comparison of Amsorb, sodalime, and Baralyme degradation of volatile anesthetics and formation of carbon monoxide and compound a in swine in vivo. Anesthesiology 96, 173–182.

Kirschvink, N., Leemans, J., Delvaux, F., et al., 2006. Non-invasive assessment of growth, gender and time of day related changes of respiratory pattern in healthy cats by use of barometric whole body plethysmography. Vet J 172, 446–454.

Laredo, F.G., Cantalapiedra, A.G., Agut, A., et al., 2001. The Komesaroff anaesthetic machine for delivering sevoflurane to dogs. Vet Anaesth Analg 28, 161–167.

Laredo, F.G., Belda, E., Escobar, M., 2009. Mechanical ventilation of six dogs anaesthetized with isoflurane or sevoflurane delivered by a Komesaroff anaesthetic machine. Vet Rec 164, 751–754.

Leslie, K., Clavisi, O., Hargrove, J., 2008. Target-controlled infusion versus manually-controlled infusion of propofol for general anaesthesia or sedation in adults. Cochrane Database Syst Rev 3, CD006059.

Lowe, D., Ernst, E.A., 1981. The Quantitative Practice of Anesthesia. Williams & Wilkins, Baltimore.

Maggiore, S.M., Richard, J.-C.M., Abrough, F., et al., 2010. A multicenter, randomized trial of noninvasive ventilation with helium-oxygen mixture in exacerbations of chronic obstructive lung disease. Crit Care Med 38, 1–7.

Mapleson, W.W., 1954. The elimination of rebreathing in various semi-closed anaesthetic systems. Br J Anaesth 26, 323–332.

Marsh-Ng, M.L., Burney, D.P., Garcia, J., 2007. Surveillance of infections associated with intravenous catheters in dogs and cats in an intensive care unit. J Am Anim Hosp Assoc 43, 13–20.

Nishiyama, T., Kohno, Y., Ozaki, M., et al., 2012. Usefulness of an anesthetic conserving device (AnaConDa™) in sevoflurane anesthesia. Minerva Anestesiol 78, 310–314.

Norwood, S., McAuley, C.E., 2005. Vascular catheter-related infections. In: Fink, M.P., Abraham, E., Vincent, J.-L., et al. (Eds.), Textbook of Critical Care. Elsevier Saunders, Philadelphia, pp. 1239–1248.

Olson, K.N., Klein, L.V., Nann, L.E., et al., 1993. Closed-circuit liquid injection isoflurane anesthesia in the horse. Vet Surg 22, 73–78.

Pelligand, L., Hammond, R., Rycroft, A., 2007. An investigation of the bacterial contamination of small animal breathing systems during routine use. Vet Anaesth Analg 34, 190–199.

Rai, M.R., Popat, M.T., 2011. Evaluation of airway equipment: man or manikin? Anaesthesia 66, 1–3.

Rees, L.M., Sheraton, T.E., Modestini, C., et al., 2007. Assessing the efficacy of HME filters at preventing contamination of breathing systems. Anaesthesia 62, 67–71.

Shirangi, A., Fritschi, L., Holman, C.D., et al., 2009. Birth defects in offspring of female veterinarians. J Occup Environ Med 51, 525–533.

Sideri, A.I., Galatos, A.D., Kazakos, G.M., et al., 2009. Gastro-oesophageal reflux during anaesthesia in the kitten: comparison between use of a laryngeal mask airway or an endotracheal tube. Vet Anaesth Analg 36, 547–554.

Smith, J.C., Bolon, B., 2003. Comparison of three commercially available activated charcoal canisters for passive scavenging of waste isoflurane during conventional rodent anesthesia. Contemp Top Lab Anim Sci 42, 10–15.

Soro, M., Badenes, R., Garcia-Perez, M.L., et al., 2010. The accuracy of the anesthetic conserving device (Anaconda©) as an alternative to the classical vaporizer in anesthesia. Anesth Analg 111, 1176–1179.

Stabernack, C.R., Brown, R., Laster, M.J., et al., 2000. Absorbents differ enormously in their capacity to produce compound A and carbon monoxide. Anesth Analg 90, 1428–1435.

Steffey, E.P., Laster, M.J., Ionescu, P., et al., 1997. Dehydration of Baralyme increases Compound A resulting from sevoflurane degradation in a standard anesthetic circuit used to anesthetize swine. Anesth Analg 85, 1382–1386.

Straker, D.J.M., Almubarack, A.I., Alibhai, H.I.K., et al., 2004. A comparison of anaesthesia in dogs with sevoflurane or isoflurane delivered from a Komesaroff vaporizer in-circle system (Abstract). Vet Anaesth Analg 31, 280–281.

Touzot-Jourde, G., Stedman, N.L., Trim, C.M., 2005. Endotracheal intubation in horses: a study of 2 cuff inflation pressures, correlation with liquid aspiration and tracheal wall damage. Vet Anaesth Analg 32, 23–29.

Trim, C.M., Simpson, S.T., 1982. Complication following ethylene oxide sterilization: A case report. J Am Anim Hosp Assoc 18, 507–510.

Versichelen, L.F.M., Bouche, M.-P.L.A., Rolly, G., et al., 2001. Only carbon dioxide absorbents free of both NaOH and KOH do not generate compound A during in vitro closed-system sevoflurane: Evaluation of five absorbents. Anesthesiology 95, 750–755.

Wiederstein, I., Moens, Y.P.S., 2008. Guidelines and criteria for the placement of laryngeal mask airways in dogs. Vet Anaesth Analg 35, 374–382.

Wilkes, A.R., 2011a. Heat and moisture exchangers and breathing system filters: their use in anaesthesia and intensive care. Part 1 – history, principles and efficiency. Anaesthesia 66, 31–39.

Wilkes, A.R., 2011b. Heat and moisture exchangers and breathing system filters: their use in anaesthesia and intensive care. Part 2 – practical use, including problems, and their use with paediatric patients. Anaesthesia 66, 40–51.

Yamakage, M., Takahashi, K., Takahashi, M., et al., 2009. Performance of four carbon dioxide absorbents in experimental and clinical settings. Anaesthesia 64, 287–292.

Section | 2 |

Anaesthesia of the species

Chapter | 11 |

Anaesthesia of the horse

INTRODUCTION

Probably no other species of animal presents as many special problems to the veterinary anaesthetist as the horse. Perioperative (7 day) mortality rate in relation to general anaesthesia in apparently healthy horses is around 1% (Johnston et al., 1995) and has remained constant to that time over at least 30 years (Hall, 1983) despite increasing sophistication of anaesthetic techniques and monitoring. The situation may be improving as a number of more recent surveys have posted lower mortality rates. Of particular note, Bidwell et al. (2007), in a retrospective survey of nearly 18 000 anaesthetics from a referral practice, reported a mortality rate of 0.12 % directly related to anaesthesia, which increased to 0.24 % taking 7-day survival into account. Limited improvement in survival rates results mainly from the longer duration of many surgical procedures that, without the advances that have occurred, would have been impossible to perform. Increased duration of anaesthesia significantly increases the risk.

The veterinary anaesthetist is faced with numerous disturbances of cardiopulmonary and skeletal muscle function in the equine patient associated with general anaesthesia, many of which are only very incompletely understood. Their certain prevention is currently impossible, and measures designed to overcome one problem often only result in exacerbation of another. Developments in the provision of reliable sedation has enabled a wider range of procedures to be carried out under local analgesia than was once considered practicable, but general anaesthesia still remains the only option in many cases.

To the time of Johnston's et al.'s studies (1995), prolonged anaesthesia was usually maintained with inhalation agents and, although in the USA isoflurane was often used, halothane was still the agent in routine use in Europe. Over the past 15 years, new inhalation agents are used, but also a very wide variety of injectable drug combinations have been employed, both on their own as total intravenous anaesthesia (TIVA) and as supplements to inhalation anaesthesia. Some of these combinations have a good evidence base for their use; others have not. Certainly, there is need for a new epidemiological study to see if improvements in mortality and morbidity really have taken place.

There is no ideal method of anaesthesia in the horse – even the two authors do not always agree on which is 'best'. This chapter will attempt to give the reader the background knowledge to understand some of the major causes of the problems that occur, how to avoid or correct them and to assess whether regimens suggested in publications may or may not have a part to play in improving safety. It will then suggest some regimens which have a good evidence base for use and/or that the authors have found useful.

SEDATION OF THE STANDING HORSE

It frequently is necessary to sedate horses to enable procedures to be carried out easily and safely. Horses are not good subjects for sedation for if they experience a feeling of muscle weakness or ataxia they may panic in a violent manner. Historically, the most effective sedative was, for many years, chloral hydrate. Introduction of the mood-altering 'neuroleptic' agents, in particular the phenothiazine, acepromazine, followed in 1969 by xylazine (Clarke & Hall, 1969), and more recently other α_2- adrenoceptor agonists (α_2-agonists) has revolutionized equine sedation and, with the addition of local analgesic techniques, many procedures can now be performed in the standing animal. However, even with modern agents, sedated horses must be handled with caution for they may be aroused by stimulation and when disturbed can respond with a very well aimed kick.

Currently, sedation of the standing horse usually is achieved with combinations of acepromazine, and/or an α_2-agonist plus a small dose of an opioid (see sedative/opioid combinations below).

Phenothiazines

Acepromazine

Acepromazine is the phenothiazine derivative most widely used in horses for both its mood-altering and its sedative actions. Intravenous (IV) doses of 0.03 mg/kg or intramuscular (IM) of 0.05 mg/kg exert a calming effect within 20–30minutes of injection and, although at these dose rates obvious sedation may only be apparent in 60% of horses, they become much easier to handle. Doses may be doubled, but the level of sedation does not always increase, although the duration will. Acepromazine (in paste or tablet forms) also may be given orally at maximally recommended doses of 0.1 mg/kg. Oral availability in horses is high and can be equal to that of the IM route (Hashem & Keller, 1993). Acepromazine is very long acting, and elimination may be further delayed in old or sick animals, particularly in those with even mild liver disease.

Acepromazine at the doses recommended has little effect on ventilation, but causes hypotension through vasodilation (Kerr et al., 1972). Hypovolaemic horses may faint. Tachycardia may result from the fall in arterial blood pressure, but sometimes first degree atrioventicular block is seen. A very small proportion of horses (the authors have seen two such cases) show aberrant reactions, and may become recumbent without any apparent cardiovascular cause; these reactions were more common with other phenothiazine agents. In stallions and geldings, effective sedation with phenothiazine derivatives is associated with protrusion of the flaccid penis or, on very rare occasions, priapism. In either case, physical damage to the penis must be avoided. In a very small proportion of horses, prolonged prolapse occurs. Treatment of this complication is by manual massage, compression bandage and replacement in the prepuce followed by suture of the preputial orifice. It is the opinion of the authors, and of many veterinarians (Driessen et al., 2011) that the low incidence of this complication coupled with the possibility of immediate treatment means that where a phenothiazine agent is the drug of choice its use is not contraindicated in stallions or geldings.

Acepromazine has proved a very safe agent in the horse. The calming and low-level sedative effects it produces make it the agent of choice for interventions such as shoeing, and when used in young animals it appears to assist in training the horse to tolerate many future procedures without sedation. When acepromazine is combined with opioid agents, deep sedation is achieved and such combinations may be used in cases where α_2-agonists would be inappropriate. Acepromazine is an excellent premedicant before general anaesthesia; it calms the horse prior to the insertion of catheters, lengthens the action of the anaesthetic agents, reduces pulmonary 'shunt' fraction (Marntell et al., 2005a) and statistically reduces the overall risk of anaesthesia and surgery (Johnston et al., 1995). Its prolonged duration of action means that it contributes to a quiet recovery.

α_2-adrenoceptor agonists

Three α_2-agonists, xylazine, detomidine and romifidine are marketed for equine sedation and anaesthesia. Two α_2-agonists marketed for small animals have also been used in this species. The general properties of all these agents are described in Chapter 4.

Xylazine

Following the introduction of xylazine, it rapidly gained in popularity because of the reliable sedation produced in horses. Doses of 0.5–1.1 mg/kg IV are followed within 2 minutes by obvious signs of effect. The horse's head is lowered and the eyelids and lower lip droop (Clarke & Hall, 1969; Kerr et al., 1972). Although the horse may sway on its feet, cross its hind legs or knuckle on a foreleg, with xylazine alone, it will remain on its feet and show no panic. Sedation is maximal after about 5 minutes and lasts 30–60 minutes depending on the dose. Doses of 2–3 mg/kg IM give similar effects, maximal sedation being achieved 20 minutes after injection. Xylazine has analgesic properties, particularly in colic (reviewed by England & Clarke, 1996) and, in colic cases, analgesia is associated with the marked reduction in gut movement caused by drugs of this class. Horses sedated with xylazine alone remain very sensitive to touch and the apparently well-sedated horse may, if disturbed, respond with a very sudden and accurate kick.

Investigations into the effects of xylazine in horses have been reviewed (England & Clarke, 1996). There is a transient rise in arterial blood pressures. Mean arterial pressure (MAP) peaks 1–2 minutes after IV injection; the pressure then slowly falls to below resting values and remains depressed for at least one hour (Fig. 11.1). Concurrent with the hypertensive phase, there is profound bradycardia

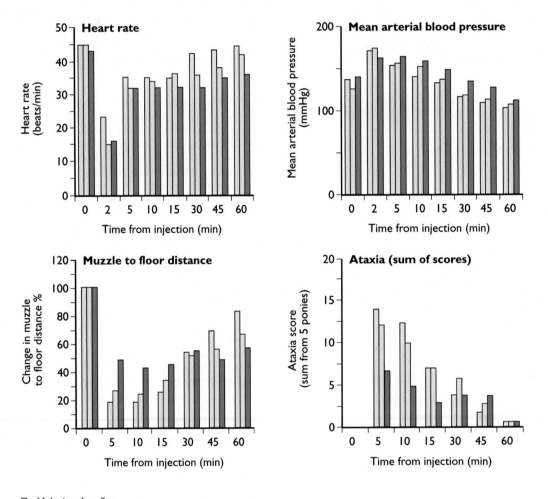

□ Xylazine 1 mg/kg
□ Detomidine 0.02 mg/kg (20 μg/kg)
■ Romifidine 0.08 mg/kg (80 μg/kg)

Figure 11.1 Comparison of some of the sedative and cardiovascular effects of IV doses of xylazine (1 mg/kg), detomidine (20 μg/kg) and romifidine (80 μg/kg). Data from 5 ponies. SE bars are omitted for the sake of clarity
Data as reviewed by England and Clarke.

coupled with both atrioventricular and sinoatrial heart block. Heart block is at its most intense in the first few minutes and, in many cases, disappears as the heart rate increases. Changes in blood pressure are dose dependent in intensity and duration and, following IM injection, changes are similar but less marked. Cardiac output (CO) is significantly reduced, probably because of the bradycardia; IV doses of 1.1 mg/kg cause falls of 20–40% of normal resting values of CO. The changes in MAP result from a balance between peripheral vasoconstriction and the centrally mediated fall in heart rate and CO (see Chapter 4). At doses of up to 1.1 mg/kg, xylazine does not cause severe respiratory depression although there may be a small rise in $PaCO_2$ and a slight decrease in PaO_2. However, some upper airway obstruction may occur; horses may snore if left in the head down position for any length of time. Heavy coated horses may sweat as sedation is waning – most commonly seen if atmospheric temperatures are high. Other side effects are those typical of α_2-agonists (see Chapter 4) and include hyperglycaemia, diuresis, gut stasis and increase in uterine tone; this latter makes it theoretically preferable not to use xylazine in pregnant mares. Changes in insulin production and hyperglycaemia do not appear to be a feature of xylazine action in neonatal foals (Robertson et al., 1990).

When used as a premedicant, xylazine greatly reduces the amount of both injectable and volatile anaesthetic agents subsequently required. In the 30 years since its launch, xylazine has become the 'gold standard' for equine sedation and premedication, particularly in North America. In Europe, until the advent of generic forms and alternative agents forced prices to reduce to a realistic level, its use was limited by much higher pricing.

Detomidine

Detomidine, a very potent α_2-agonist was first used as a sedative and analgesic agent in 1982 and, since its introduction, has gained great popularity for sedation and premedication of all types of horse (Vainio, 1985; Alitalo, 1986; Clarke & Taylor, 1986; Short, 1992). Initially, very high doses (up to 160 µg/kg) of detomidine were recommended but it soon became obvious that maximal sedative effects were obtained with IV doses of 10–20 µg/kg (0.01–0.02 mg/kg) and that higher doses increased the duration rather than depth of sedation. Slightly higher doses appear necessary to provide good analgesia (Hamm et al., 1995). The concentrated but non-irritant form of 10 mg/ml in which detomidine (as Domosedan or Dormosedan, and now generics) is provided makes it very suitable for IM injection, doses approximately twice those given IV being required to produce the same effect.

Detomidine has some effect when injected subcutaneously (SC) and is also absorbed through mucous membranes and there is now a gel form available for this purpose (Gardner et al., 2010; Kaukinen et al., 2011).

When given in food, the effect is less reliable as the drug is extensively metabolized by first pass through the liver. The property of easy absorption across mucous membranes must, for reasons of personal safety, be taken into account when handling the drug.

The type of sedation produced by detomidine is identical to that produced by xylazine; in blind trials comparing IV xylazine (1 mg/kg) IV and detomidine 20 µg/kg IV (England & Clarke, 1996), all parameters assessed and measured except duration of action were identical (see Fig. 11.1). As with xylazine, horses under detomidine sedation are sensitive to touch and may kick. Lower doses of detomidine do not always result in maximal sedation, but may prove useful where a short period of action is required. Detomidine premedication reduces the dose of anaesthetic agents subsequently required.

The cardiovascular properties, bradycardia, peripheral vasoconstriction and changes in arterial blood pressure (see Fig. 11.1) are also as described for xylazine above (Short, 1992). With higher doses, the hypertensive phase is considerably more prolonged (Short et al., 1986). At clinically used doses, respiration is slowed and PaO2 is slightly decreased. Some horses snore. The authors have noted occasional horses (usually but not always those suffering from toxaemic conditions) becoming tachypnoepic for some 10–15minutes after the administration of detomidine and similar reactions have been reported after other α_2-agonists (Bettschart-Wolfensberger et al., 1999; Kendall et al., 2010). The condition appears self-limiting and does not require treatment. Other side effects include reduction in gut motility, hyperglycaemia, sweating and an increase in urination. Doses above 60 µg/kg may cause swelling of the head; this problem can be prevented by propping the head in a normal position. Occasionally urticarial reactions have been noted; these are self-limiting and regress without treatment. Moderate doses of detomidine are claimed to be safe in pregnancy (Jedruch et al., 1989) and many mares have received multiple doses throughout gestation without any maternal or fetal harm resulting.

The actions of detomidine (and of other α_2-adrenoceptor agonists) can be reversed by the specific antagonist, atipamezole. Dose rates from 60 to 200 µg/kg have been used, that required depending on the degree of residual sedation (Nilsfors & Kvart, 1986; Bettschart-Wolfensberger et al., 2001b; Hubbell & Muir, 2006). At the doses of detomidine recommended, it is rare that antagonism is required, but the authors have been grateful of its availability in cases of overdosage of α_2/opioid combinations where a horse has become severely ataxic or even recumbent, and in one case of a massive overdose of detomidine (Di Concetto et al., 2007).

Romifidine

The type of sedation produced by romifidine differs from that produced by the other α_2-agonists; the horse's head does not hang so low, and there is considerably less ataxia (Voetgli, 1988; England & Clarke, 1996), although (Ringer et al., 2013) found no difference from xylazine when comparing the drugs given by constant rate infusion (CRI). Despite the apparent reduced sedation, romifidine at doses of from 40 to 120 μg/kg (0.04–0.12 mg/kg) IV enables a range of clinical procedures to be performed; the effect (and the ataxia) is enhanced by combination with opioids. In clinical practice, romifidine has proved very popular where ataxia is particularly unwelcome, e.g. for shoeing. The pharmacological actions of romifidine other than sedation are similar to all α_2-agonists. Romifidine reduces gut motility, the duration of this effect being dose dependent (Freeman & England, 2001). Self-limiting urticarial reactions may occur occasionally. The degree of analgesia produced by romifidine has been questioned; the results appear to depend on the nociceptive stimulus used (England & Clarke, 1996). Spadavecchia et al. (2005) found good reliable antinociception, Voetgli (1988) that antinociception was not dose related or consistent, and Hamm et al. (1995) claimed there was no analgesic activity. Rohrbach et al. (2009) compared the antinociceptive effects of romfiidine, xylazine and detomidine; all three α_2-agonists provided equal antinociception, although duration was drug dependent. In equine practice, romifidine is widely used for premedication and, as part of anaesthetic combinations, it reduces the dose of anaesthetic agents subsequently used.

Other α_2-agonists

Medetomidine's use has been investigated in horses (Bryant et al., 1991; Bettschart-Wolfensberger et al., 1999). Doses of 5–7 μg/kg (0.005–0.007 mg/kg) IV are sufficient to cause very deep sedation with severe ataxia, and higher doses may result in recumbency. The marked hypnotic properties make the agent unsuitable for routine use as a sedative in horses. However, it appears to be short acting, having a half-life of elimination of 29 minutes (Grimsrud et al., 2012) and its excellent analgesic and muscle relaxant properties mean that it has become quite widely used as a CRI during anaesthesia (see Box 11.1). Bettschart-Wolfensberger et al. (2005) showed that *dexmedetomidine* at 3.5 μg/kg IV in the horse had similar effects as medetomidine.

Practical use of α_2-adrenoceptor agonists

The majority of the sedative, cardiopulmonary and other side effects appear similar with all three α_2-agonists commonly used in horses (see Fig. 11.1). The exceptions are the different manifestation of sedation and less of ataxia with romifidine, and the fact that xylazine appears to have the greatest ecbolic effect, so is not the preferred choice for pregnant mares. Otherwise, the choice will depend on the duration of action required, the route of administration,

and on personal preferences. For example, all three agents provide excellent analgesia in cases of colic, although the bradycardia and lack of gut motility induced must be considered in the subsequent assessment. Before a definitive diagnosis has been made in a colic case, it is preferable to use xylazine or a low dose (up to 15 μg/kg) of detomidine for sedation and analgesia, as high doses may mask signs indicating the requirement for surgery. Following a decision that surgery is required, the longer acting romifidine with its lack of ataxia, may be the most suitable analgesic for transportation. Although there are no scientific studies of combining different α_2-agonists, in practical clinical use, there are many reports of changing from one to another at subsequent dosing; the effects appear to be additive as expected.

α_2-Agonists have marked cardiopulmonary side effects, and it is not surprising that occasional cases of collapse, or even of death have been reported following their use. Some reported cases may have resulted from intracarotid injection, but where there is a delay between injection of the drug and the unexpected event, then such a reaction is probably drug induced. In dogs, xylazine sensitizes the heart to adrenaline-induced arrhythmias but, in horses, such sensitization has not been proved (W.W. Muir, personal communication). However, there are anecdotal reports of collapse in horses which have been given an α_2-agonist when in a high state of excitement. Unfortunately, immediate sedation is necessary in many such situations and, in these cases, sufficient time must be left after drug administration before further stimulation is applied. In such situations, the authors prefer combinations with acepromazine, which may reduce the risk. Clinical reports have suggested that combinations of α_2-agonists and potentiated sulphonamides should be avoided, although any scientific basis for these observations is unproven.

Some veterinarians premedicate horses with an anticholinergic agent (atropine 0.01 mg/kg or glycopyrrolate 0.01 mg/kg) prior to the administration of an α_2-agonist, but use of such combinations is controversial. Anticholinergic drugs will prevent or reverse the bradycardia caused by α_2-agonists and will improve CO but will result in hypertension (Pimenta et al., 2011). Anticholinergic drugs, if used, must be given an adequate time prior to sedation; giving the two drugs together is not a rational choice.

Infusions of α_2-agonists

Where α_2-agonists are being used to provide sedation for surgery, sometimes it is necessary to increase their duration of action. Intermittent dosing, each increment being 25–50% of the original dose administered, is effective, but a constant rate infusion (CRI) provides a more level and controllable plane of sedation. Usually, the agent used is diluted in a saline drip then, following the initial loading dose, is infused to effect. Infusions have been used alone, with opioids (see opioid combinations below) and as an

---

Box 11.1 A summary of some reported α₂-agonist infusions

Xylazine doses are in mg (milligrammes)/kg and mg/kg/h
All other drug doses are given in μg (microgrammes)/kg and μg/kg/h
LD = Loading dose. CRI = continuous rate infusion.

α₂-agonist infused alone.
With no opioid, despite apparent deep sedation, the horse may still respond to stimulus.

Xylazine	LD 0.5 mg/kg	CRI 0.55 mg/kg/h	Authors' experience
Xylazine	LD 1.0 mg/kg	CRI 0.69 mg/kg/h	Ringer et al., 2012b
Detomidine	LD 7.5 ± 1.9 μg/kg	CRI 36 μg/kg/h, for 15 mins, halving dose every 15 minutes.	Wilson et al., 2002 Retrospective clinical study
Romifidine	LD 80 μg/kg	CRI 30 μg/kg/h	Ringer et al., 2012a
Medetomidine	LD 7 μg/kg	CRI 3.5 μg/kg/h	Bettschart-Wolfensberger et al., 1999

α₂-agonist infusions used during general anaesthesia with inhalation agents.
Loading doses taken as that used for an α₂–ketamine anaesthetic induction

Xylazine	CRI 0.50 mg/kg/h	Authors' experience
Detomidine	CRI 10 μg/kg/h	Wagner et al., 1992
	CRI 5.0 μg/kg/h	Schauvliege et al., (2011)
Medetomidine	CRI 3.5 μg/kg/h	Bettschart-Wolfensberger et al., 2001b
Dexmedetomidine	CRI 1.75 μg/kg/h	Gozalo-Marcilla et al., 2013
Romifidine	CRI 40 μg/kg/h	Devisscher et al., 2010

Infusion techniques of α₂-agonists with opioids useful for longer sedation for standing surgery
NB local anaesthesia still used for surgical site

(a) LD Detomidine 10 μg/kg, butorphanol 20 μg/kg CRI detomidine to effect but around 6–12 μg/kg/h	Authors' experience
(b) LD Detomidine 10 μg/kg, buprenorphine 6 μg/kg CRI Detomidine to effect – but around 6–11 μg/kg/h *Need to await the onset of buprenorphine (> 30 mins)*	van Dijk et al., 2003
(c) LD Medetomidine 5 μg/kg after 10 minutes morphine 50 μg/kg – after a further 10 mintues CRI Medetomidine 5 μg/kg/h and morphine 30 μg/kg/h *Satisfactory for laproscopy*	Solano et al., 2009
(d) LD Xylazine 1 mg/kg, butorphanol 18 μg/kg CRI Xylazine 0.69 mg/kg/h, butophanol 25 μg/kg/h *Too high for general clinical use as some horses fell.*	Ringer et al., 2012b
(e) LD Romifidine 80 μg/kg, butorphanol 18 μg/kg CRI Romifidine 40 μg/kg/h, butorphanol 25 μg/kg/h *Too high for general clinical use as some horses fell.*	Ringer et al., 2012a
(f) ACP premed. LD Xylazine 0.5 mg/kg, butorphanol 18 μg/kg CRI Xylazine commenced at 0.65 mg/kg/h but then reduced to 0.4 mg/kg/h, butorphanol 24 μg/kg/h	Benredouane et al., 2011

---

adjunct to general anaesthesia (see PIVA below). Some doses that have been used in these circumstances are summarized in Box 11.1. Of these, the most thorough exploration of suitable dose rates were those of Bettschart-Wolfensberger et al. (1999) for medetomidine and Ringer et al. (2012a,b) for xylazine and romifidine, as in each case a dose that would give a steady level of sedation was elucidated, then the result confirmed with pharmacokinetic studies. However, doses from experimental studies are only a guide in the clinics; sometimes they are inadequate or too high for the individual clinical case, and the infusions should always be given 'to effect'.

α₂-Agonists as analgesics

All α_2-agonists have analgesic properties, those agents that are most specific in their actions (i.e. medetomidine and dexmedetomidine) probably providing the greatest effects. Used as infusions, their use in conscious horses, for example in the postoperative period, is limited by the sedation they induce but, given intraoperatively by infusion as described above to anaesthetized horses, contribute both to analgesia and to hypnosis. For example, a single dose of 0.5 or 1 mg/kg xylazine reduced isoflurane minimum alveolar concentration (MAC) by 25% and 34% respectively (Steffey et al., 2000). A loading dose of 3.5 μg/kg dexmedetomidine followed by a CRI of 1.75 μg/kg/hour reduces the MAC of sevoflurane in horses by over 50% (Gozalo-Marcilla et al., 2013).

The α_2-agonists provide analgesia by central actions, acting at spinal and supraspinal levels. They are therefore very effective when given by the epidural or subarachnoid routes (reviewed by Valverde (2010) and by Natalini (2010)). Details of the extensive investigations carried out into the analgesic and systemic effects in horses of xylazine and detomidine given by this route by R Skarda & Muir are included in the above reviews.

In clinical practice, when α_2-agonists are given epidurally to horses, they are usually combined with local analgesics and/or opioids in order to obtain the optimum onset of action and duration of effect (see epidural analgesia below).

Intrasynovial administration and even local nerve infiltration of α_2-agonists have been claimed to provide analgesia in humans and animals (Valverde, 2010); possible reasons for effectiveness by these routes could be systemic absorption or, in the case of xylazine, the perceived (but not proven) local analgesic effect. Evidence of direct effectiveness by these routes is, as yet, unconvincing.

Sedative and sedative–opioid combinations

In the search for a completely reliable, safe method of producing sedation in standing horses, a number of mixtures of drugs have been used. Appropriate doses of many of these have proved to have a more certain and profound effect than can be regularly obtained from the use of any single drug.

The pharmacological basis for combination of sedatives with opioids has already been discussed (see Chapter 4). Their use in the horse is not new (Martin & Beck, 1956; Klein, 1975) and a very large number of such combinations have been investigated and advocated for use in this species of animal. The addition of opioids, which are often at subanalgesic doses, appears to enhance sedation dramatically and, in particular, diminishes the response to touch, thus reducing the likelihood of provoking well-directed kicks from the horse. The disadvantage, in particular with combinations with α_2-agonists, is that ataxia is also increased and, occasionally, a horse may become recumbent. Opioid 'excitement' reactions, often manifest by 'walking' forward despite attempts of restraint, or by twitching of the superficial muscles of the head, may occur when sedation becomes inadequate and it is irrational to combine a short-acting sedative such as xylazine with opioids with long actions such as buprenorphine or high doses of morphine. Acepromazine has a very long action so problems are less when this is part of the combination. The incidence of opioid-induced excitement occurring can be reduced by administering sedatives first followed by opioids once sedation is apparent, although this is not always practicable and, if the opioid concerned is one which has a delayed onset of action (e.g. buprenorphine), this is neither necessary nor desirable.

Table 11.1 lists some of the sedative/opioid combinations that have been used satisfactorily, but there are many other potential combinations that are likely to be as good. The dose of opioid required is considerably less than that producing analgesia (and with these combinations, local analgesia should still be employed for surgery). In the UK, the combination of IV detomidine (10 μg/kg) or romifidine (40–80 μg/kg) and butorphanol (0.02 mg/kg) has proved very successful, particularly for clipping fractious horses. Caution is needed to prevent cross contamination of the drugs in their multidose bottles; the authors have seen several cases of gross overdosage (the horse becoming very ataxic, or recumbent) where this has occurred.

Acepromazine (0.02–0.05 mg/kg) and α_2-agonists such as xylazine (0.5–1.0 mg/kg), detomidine (10–20 μg/kg) or romifidine (50–100 μg/kg) have often been used together for sedating horses with or without the addition of opioids. The prolonged calming action of acepromazine is useful, particularly if the horse was very excited prior to sedation. Some North American sources have considered that acepromazine and the α_2-agonists should not be used together. The pharmacological reasoning rests on the fact that acepromazine causes hypotension and the α_2-agonist causes bradycardia. However, the maximal bradycardia occurs within 1–2 minutes of injection, and at this time is accompanied by hypertension. If detomidine is given to horses already sedated with acepromazine, there is still a hypertensive response, albeit starting from a lower base (Muir et al., 1979). The authors have administered α_2-agonists to over 4000 horses already sedated with acepromazine with no ill effects (other than an increase in ataxia) and, providing both drugs are given at suitable doses, there is no reason why the combination cannot be used.

Infusions of sedative–opioid combinations

Intravenous infusions of α_2-agonists coupled with opioids are used to provide prolonged sedation for surgery. The

Table 11.1 Some of the sedative/opioid combinations, most of which have been satisfactorily used by the authors; there are many other combinations which are likely to be as satisfactory. All usually intravenous (IV), but can also be given by the intramuscular (IM) route (at the higher end of the scale)

Sedative 1	Sedative 2	Opioid
Acepromazine, 0.05–0.10 mg/kg		Methadone, 0.05–0.10 mg/kg *or* Butorphanol, 0.02–0.04 mg/kg
Acepromazine, 0.02–0.05 mg/kg	Xylazine, 0.5 mg/kg *or* Detomidine, 0.01–0.02 mg/kg (10–20 µg/kg) *or* Romifidine, 0.04–0.1 mg/kg (40–100 µg/kg)	
Acepromazine, 0.02–0.06 mg/kg	Xylazine, 0.5 mg/kg *or* Detomidine, 0.01 mg/kg (10 µg/kg) *or* Romifidine, 0.04–0.08 mg/kg (40–80 µg/kg)	Butorphanol, 0.01–0.02 mg/kg *or* Methadone, 0.05 mg/kg
Xylazine, 0.5–0.6 mg/kg *or* Detomidine, 0.010–0.015 mg/kg (10–15 µg/kg) *or* Romifidine, 0.04–0.08 mg/kg (40–80 µg/kg)		Butorphanol, 0.02–0.05 mg/kg *or* Methadone, 0.05–0.10 mg/kg.
Xylazine 0.7 mg/kg		Morphine 0.3 mg/kg* (hold off feed)

NB. All doses above are in mg/kg (and in µg/kg for detomidine and romifidine). For those used to doses of drugs being quoted as µg/kg; there are 1000 µg in 1 mg. As an example, 0.01 mg/kg detomidine = 10 µg/kg
*Very deep sedation – Morphine may be increased to 0.7 mg/kg (Klein, 1975) but beware of severe respiratory depression.

most usual method is to use a loading dose of α_2-agonist and of opioid at the doses suggested in Table 11.1, then just to infuse the α_2-agonist at the doses discussed above and as shown in Box 11.1, with no further opioid unless the surgery is very prolonged. Such doses of opioid do not provide analgesia and local analgesic blocks are needed for surgery. The danger of higher opioid doses, which might be reached if the opioid is infused, is that the heavily sedated horse becomes recumbent. This did happen in the experimental studies of Ringer et al. (2012a,b). In the clinical situation, infusion doses are given to effect and those given in Box 11.1 can only be a guide.

Benzodiazepines

Diazepam, midazolam, climazolam and zolazepam

The anxiolytic properties of diazepam are not obvious in horses and the drug should not be used on its own as it gives rise to ataxia, sometimes associated with panic, possibly through its muscle relaxing properties (Muir et al., 1982). Another benzodiazepine, climazolam, has been found to have similar properties and the antagonist sarmazenil has been used to reverse its effects. Although not useful as sedatives in adult horses, the benzodiazepine agents can be used in foals which will usually become recumbent following IV 0.1–0.25 mg/kg of diazepam or midazolam (a water-soluble benzodiazepine). The muscle relaxation induced by benzodiazepine agents is useful during anaesthesia, and benzodiazepines such as diazepam, climazolam, midazolam and zolazepam have all been incorporated into anaesthetic regimens used in adult horses.

ANALGESIA

As with all species, the perioperative analgesic requirements in the horse are generally met by non-steroidal analgesics, opioid analgesics and local analgesics. In certain circumstances, α_2-agonists, agents used as anaesthetic agents such as ketamine, and gabapentin, also play a part in the provision of analgesia.

The assessment of analgesic activity is very difficult. Horses respond differently to different types of pain; there may be a violent response such as common (but not invariable) in colic, or the horse may just 'suffer' and stand quietly. A variety of experimental models, such as thermal and mechanical thresholds (Love et al., 2011) or pressure from balloons in the colon, are used to assess antinociception, but response of these to analgesics does not necessarily reflect what will happen in any clinical circumstance.

Wagner (2010) has drawn up a list of equine 'pain behaviours'; the ones relevant to the condition of the horse (e.g. lameness if there is a damaged leg) form the basis for a mode of pain assessment.

One form of analgesia often neglected is to remove the cause; simple treatments such as stabilizing a damaged leg can make a horse seem to be surprisingly comfortable. The reduction of painful swelling by non-steroidal anti-inflammatory analgesics (NSAIDs) almost certainly provides a major contribution to their analgesic actions.

Non-Steroidal Anti-inflammatory Analgesics (NSAIDS)

NSAIDs are widely used in horses for the provision of analgesia for acute pain, for their anti-inflammatory action

Table 11.2 Half-life of elimination and doses of NSAIDs, as per product information, for horse in the UK

	Dose	Half-life of elimination
Carprofen	0.7 mg/kg per 24 h IV, PO for up to 9 days	14–31 h
Meloxicam	0.6 mg/kg per 24 h IV, PO for up to 14 days	3 h
Ketoprofen	2.2 mg/kg per 24 h IV for up to 3-5 days	0.7–1 h
Phenylbutazone	4.4 mg/kg per 12 h for 4 days followed by 2.2 mg/kg each 24–48 h IV, PO	4.5–9 h
Flunixin	1.1 mg/kg per 24 h IV, PO for up to 5 days	1.6–2.1 h
Suxibuzone	6.25 mg/kg every 12 h for 2 days, then ½ dose. Ponies: use ½ horse dose PO only	
Vedaprofen	2 mg/kg loading dose then 1 mg/kg twice a day PO for up to 14 days	
Firocoxib	0.09 mg/kg IV then 0.1 mg/kg PO per 24 h for up to 14 days	30 h
Naproxen*	5 mg/kg IV, then PO 10 mg/kg twice a day for up to 14 days	

NB Licensed doses should not be exceeded. IV: intravenous; PO: by mouth. *Not available for horses in the UK.
Information gained from Compendium Data sheets; from Cunningham and Lees, 1995; McKellar et al., 1991; Kvaternick et al., 2007; Letendre et al., 2008.
NB: The combination 'buscopan-compositum' contains hyoscine and the NSAID metamizole (dipyrone). The dose of metazemole needs to be taken into account with concurrent/subsequent NSAID administration.

in injury and disease, for anti-endotoxaemic actions and for the provision of analgesia in chronic pain. Although they have not been shown to provide any intraoperative analgesia, they are often administered at premedication or intraoperatively so that their analgesic and anti-inflammatory actions will be effective at the time of recovery. A detailed description of the NSAIDs currently available for veterinary use is given in Chapter 5, and some licensed dose rates given there and in Table 11.2.

For many years, phenylbutazone was the NSAID of choice for equine use, and it still remains an inexpensive and very effective agent that may be given by injection in the immediate perioperative period, then orally for continuing postoperative care. Currently, in the UK at least, suxibuzone, a phenylbutazone prodrug, is often used for the follow-up oral administration (see Chapter 5). Although phenylbutazone can cause toxic reactions, these are well known, and can be avoided with correct dosing schedules. However, currently in Europe, phenylbutazone may not be used in food animals and, in many countries, this includes horses. Other older agents used in the horse include meclofenic acid and metamizole (dipyrone). In the last 20 years, the most popular NSAID for use in the horse has been flunixin meglumine, which gives excellent analgesia in a wide variety of circumstances. Several of the newer, very effective and potentially less toxic NSAIDs including carprofen, vedaprofen, ketoprofen and, most recently, the coxib, firocoxib, are now marketed in oral and/or injectable formulations for horses.

The major problem with NSAIDs is their high toxicity and fairly low therapeutic index although, in theory, the newer COX 2 sparing agents and the coxibs (see Chapter 5) should cause fewer problems. The major sites of toxicity of the NSAIDs are the gastrointestinal tract, kidneys, liver and the blood cells. In horses, the gastrointestinal tract appears the organ most affected, overdose of the agent causing stomach ulceration, and also damage to other areas, including the large bowel, leading to diarrhoea. In the horse, renal damage, even in the presence of hypotension, is not common, and NSAIDs are administered before or during anaesthesia without apparent problems. Liver damage due to NSAIDs has been reported in old horses maintained on NSAIDs, and blood dyscrasias have occurred in horses given high doses of phenylbutazone. Many of the injectable preparations are contraindicated for IM use in the horse as they cause local irritation. At least one IV preparation of phenylbutazone can cause severe cardiac arrhythmias if injected too fast (probably because of the solvent, rather than the drug) so, in the absence of evidence to the contrary, it is best that all IV administrations of NSAIDs are given slowly, especially in anaesthetized horses.

The pharmacokinetics of NSAIDs vary greatly between species. In normal horses, the half-lives of some of the commonly used agents are shown in Table 11.2. Breakdown products of some agents are themselves active. Knowledge of the half-life is necessary to assess dosing schedules but efficacy may outlast effective blood levels as, in some cases, the NSAID is concentrated in the inflammatory fluid at the site of injury. Toxic effects, most commonly manifest by diarrhoea, are usually due to cumulation, and are most likely to occur some days into the postoperative period. It is therefore very important not to exceed the data sheet recommendations for doses and frequency of dosing, and to realize that if more than one NSAID is employed, their toxic effects will be additive. Even if the manufacturers guidelines are kept, toxicity may be greater than expected in a sick horse, for example in shocked animals, or in hypoproteinaemia (NSAIDs are highly protein bound). The metabolism of NSAIDs varies greatly between species, even within equids. For example, Sinclair et al. (2006) demonstrated that the pharmacokinetics of meloxicam differed markedly between horses and donkeys.

NSAIDs are widely used as analgesics for colic but the response may be variable – sometimes there is complete relief from pain, even in cases where there is non-viable intestine, while another case with an identical lesion may show no remission of symptoms. NSAIDs prevent the onset of symptoms of endotoxaemia, such as the increase in pulse rate and packed cell volume (PCV). Prevention of these changes coupled with analgesia may prevent recognition of the onset of 'shock' and diagnosis of surgical conditions. Thus, it is better if NSAIDs are not given to horses with colic until there is a definitive diagnosis, and a decision for surgery (or not) is made. When using NSAIDs in the postoperative period in colic cases, consideration must be given to the effect of altered blood protein levels, and of circulation (which may increase half-life) on their pharmacokinetics. It is difficult to distinguish whether diarrhoea following surgery for colic is due to endotoxaemia or is, itself, due to the toxicity of the NSAIDs used.

Opioid analgesics

Opioid analgesics are now widely used in the horse to provide analgesia during and after surgery, as well as in combination with sedative agents for restraint. However, there is some controversy over their use at analgesic doses as to whether their advantages outweigh their disadvantages in this species. The major perceived disadvantage is that in horses the stimulatory effect of opioids dominates the depressive actions, resulting in a dose-related 'excitement' response. Excitement is manifest in various ways from simple muzzle twitching, muscular spasms, ataxia, snatching at food, head pressing, uncontrollable walking through to violent excitement. Tobin & Combie (1982) developed a 'step-counting' method of measuring the walking or locomotor response and obtained dose–response curves very similar to those obtained for analgesia. It is probable that many of these responses primarily are due to stimulation of μ receptors, although the κ agonists, such as butorphanol, do also cause these 'excitement' effects. Stimulation also means that, with very high

doses of opioids (such as the etorphine in Immobilon), the cardiovascular response is tachycardia and arterial hypertension rather than the bradycardia that occurs in the dog. Another perceived disadvantage in horses is that the effects of opioids on gut motility might lead to impacted colic. As for all species, opioids do cause dose-related respiratory depression.

When given during anaesthesia, opioids do not reduce MAC consistently; in any one study MAC will reduce in some animals but increase in others, presumably because of motor stimulation.

Clutton (2010) has presented an analysis of the evidence for and against the use of opioids in horses. The stimulation effects are dose dependent and can be avoided by cautious dosing, but Clutton points out that a problem is that behavioural effects of pain may mimic these stimulation effects, making it difficult to assess over- and underdosage. The excitement effects can be minimized with sedative agents; acepromazine is particularly effective. This efficacy was always thought to be due to dopamine antagonism, but Pascoe & Taylor (2003) showed that specific dopamine antagonists did not reduce the walking response to alfentanil administration. It has always been believed that the presence or absence of stimulation depended on whether or not the horse is in pain at the time of their administration; Clutton (2010) believes this, but agrees that it is unproven. Clutton also concluded that the evidence suggested that the use of opioids at relatively conservative doses did not increase the incidence of postoperative colic, nor did it result in poor quality recovery for anaesthesia. In summary, he concluded that the use of perioperative opioids at the correct doses was beneficial to the horse.

Table 11.3 lists suggested doses for some opioids commonly used perioperatively in the horse. Their pharmacology has been discussed in Chapter 5. Agonists primarily acting at the μ receptor include *morphine, methadone, meperidine (pethidine)* and *fentanyl*. Morphine has been used widely and proved very satisfactory (Clutton, 2010). Meperidine differs from the others in that it has antispasmodic actions on the gut, making it the opioid of choice for treatment of spasmodic colic, although it is very short acting (up to 2 hours). A small but significant number of horses suffer severe anaphylactoid reactions in response to meperidine manifest by severe sweating, shaking, pulmonary oedema and even collapse (Clutton, 1987). Anaphylactoid reactions are less common and less severe, and excitement reactions less likely when meperidine is given by IM injection so this route should be considered the one of choice.

Recently, there has been renewed interest in the use of fentanyl to provide analgesia in horses. Although fentanyl did not provide antinociception to thermal or pressure stimuli (Sanchez et al., 2007), such experimental work does not necessarily mimic clinical pain. Fentanyl patches have been used for analgesia in horses; Taylor & Clarke

Table 11.3 Doses of some opioids used for analgesia

Opioid	Dose and route	Notes
Morphine	0.05–0.1 mg/kg IV or IM Up to 0.3 mg/kg IM*	The higher doses may increase the risk of side effects
Methadone	0.1 mg/kg IV or IM	
Oxymorphone	0.05–0.3 mg/kg IV or IM	
Meperidine (Pethidine)	1–2 mg/kg IM only	Antispasmodic to gut Occasional anaphylactoid reactions – hence IM only.
Butorphanol	0.05–0.1 mg/kg IV or IM	Infusions of 0.013 mg/kg/h (13 µg/kg/h) are used for analgesia** up to a 0.025 mg/kg/h (25 µg/kg/h) in combination with α_2-agonists for sedation***
Buprenorphine	0.006–0.01 mg/kg IV or IM	Slow onset effect (>20 minutes after IV) Do not re-dose before giving time to work Some motor activity in experimental horses****

IM injection minimizes the risk of 'excitement' reactions. Lower doses rates may be used in sedative combinations (see Table 11.1). Doses are in mg/kg by intravenous (IV) and/or intramuscular (IM) injection.
*Clutton (2010). **Sellon et al. (2004); *** Ringer et al. (2012 a,b); **** Love et al. (2012)

(2007) recommend one to three 150 µg patches on a clipped thin skinned area inaccessible to the horse (most usually the neck). Thomasy et al. (2004) used fentanyl patches such that final dosing over 24 hours worked out as from 39 to 110 µg/kg on horses in which pain had not responded to NSAIDs, and found it reduced pain scores (but not lameness). A pharmacokinetic study using patches intended to deliver 60–70 µg/kg showed that peak concentrations were reached at around 12 hours, but uptake was very variable, plasma concentrations never reaching analgesic levels in some individuals (Orsini et al., 2006). It will be interesting, however, to see if a new 'spot on' preparation which has just become available for dogs provides a more stable uptake (Freise et al., 2012; Linton et al., 2012). Evidence to date suggests that, in contrast to most other species, fentanyl does not reduce the MAC of inhalation agents in the horse (Thomasy et al., 2006; Knych et al., 2009); earlier studies suggesting that it could do so were not repeatable.

The advantage of the partial agonist opioid drugs is that they are often less addictive in man and, therefore, in some countries, subject to less control regulations than are pure agonist agents. *Butorphanol* is used widely to provide analgesia in premedication, during surgery, for postoperative analgesia and in sedative/opioid combinations. The licensed dose for analgesia is 0.1 mg/kg IV, but experimental work suggests that this is insufficient for longer effective pain relief (Kalpravidh et al., 1984). All studies of its use in pain-free animals found it to produce behavioural effects – nose twitches, ataxia, shivering, box walking and restlessness at doses of 0.1 mg/kg IV. However, clinically, it has been proved satisfactory (Sellon et al., 2004), infusions of 13 µg/kg/hour providing good analgesia with

minimal side effects in horses, which had just had a coeliotomy. *Buprenorphine*, another partial agonist, gives analgesia for about 8 hours although, even after IV injection, onset of analgesia requires at least 15 minutes. Anecdotal reports suggest that 0.01 mg/kg (10 µg/kg) IM provides good analgesia for several hours. Love et al. (2012) compared the effect of 0.1 mg/kg butorphanol with doses of 5, 7.5 and 10 µg/kg buprenorphine on thermal and mechanical nociceptive thresholds; all buprenorphine doses increased thermal thresholds for more than 7 hours; no severe side effects were noted but, despite premedication with acepromazine, walking behaviour made testing mechanical thresholds difficult following both butorphanol and buprenorphine at any dose. *Pentazocine* is another opioid that has been used in horses in North America. Dose recommendations are very variable, but 0.3–0.5 mg/kg IV appears acceptable.

There are anecdotal reports of the clinical use in horses of *tramadol*, a synthetic analgesic drug thought to be a weak µ agonist. At IV doses of 2 mg/kg it failed to give antinociception in response to thermal stimuli (Dhanjal et al., 2009), but side effects were minimal. By parenteral use, it appears to be very short acting in the horse and oral availability is poor (Stewart et al., 2011). It has been used by the epidural route (see below).

Additional routes of administration of opioid agents

The transdermal use of fentanyl has been described above. Morphine is administered into joints following arthroscopy. This is effective in humans presumably through its action on specific opioid receptors in the synovium. Two recent studies examined the effect of morphine in horses in which a synovitis had been induced with lipopolysaccharide (Lindegaard et al., 2010; van Loon et al., 2010). Intra-articular morphine gave analgesia which was slow in onset but long lasting – there being some effect by 1.5 hours, the effect increasing with time to maximal at 6 hours, and there being excellent analgesia for 224 hours. Combination with local analgesia (ropivicaine) led to effective rapid onset, long-lasting analgesia (Santos et al., 2009).

Opioids are used widely for caudal epidural analgesia, either alone or in combination with α_2-adrenoceptor agonists with or without local analgesia. Their use, and the difference between drugs, has been reviewed by Natalini (2010). Speed of onset and duration of action depend on lipid solubility, hence a very slow onset of action for morphine. Natalini & Robinson (2000) compared the effects of some epidurally administered opioids, using an electrical nociceptive stimulus. Butorphanol did not appear to give effective antinociception. Tramadol and morphine gave complete antinociception; onset and duration of action for tramadol was 30 minutes and 4 hours and for morphine 6 hours and 5 hours respectively. Robinson et al. (1994) found that caudal epidural injection of approximately 0.1 mg/kg morphine in 10 mL of saline resulted in analgesia of at least five dermatomes. Analgesia lasted for 17 hours, but time to maximal analgesic effect was delayed for up to 8 hours. When a higher dose of morphine (approx. 0.2 mg/kg) was used, onset of analgesia was faster (6 hours), lasted longer (19 hours) and spread further (sometimes as far as T9), but the signs of sedation, presumably through systemic absorption of the drug, were greater. In clinical practice, a useful degree of analgesia appears to be present earlier than the experimental evidence would suggest.

As morphine is available in a preparation which does not contain preservatives, and can give very prolonged analgesia, it has become the opioid most used. The dose most commonly used is 0.1 mg/kg. A rare, but serious disadvantage of epidural morphine is pruritus, as horses manifesting this can damage themselves, sometimes quite badly (Burford & Corley, 2006; Kalchofner et al., 2007). In practice, frequently morphine is used in combination with other agents; α_2-agonists and/or local anaesthetics in order to get rapid but long acting pain relief. Some suitable dose regimens are given in Box 11.2.

Other drugs used for analgesia

Gabapentin

Gabapentin is used in people to treat neuropathic pain. In horses, reports of its use to date are anecdotal (Davis et al., 2007). However, a study has examined the pharmacokinetics and the behavioural effects in normal experimental horses of 20 mg/kg IV and by mouth (Terry et al., 2010).

Box 11.2 **Some drugs and drug combinations used by caudal epidural injection**

NB preferably preservative free – otherwise need to be certain that the preparation is not neurotoxic. Many other combinations may be satisfactory.
Volumes are for a 450 kg horse unless otherwise stated. Larger volumes may affect more anterior dermatomes.

Local anaesthetics

Overdose with any will cause ataxia through motor block.
Lidocaine (2%): 5–8 mL: onset 5–20 mins: duration 1–2 h
Mepivicaine (2%): 5–8 mL: onset 10–30 mins: duration 1.5–3 h
Bupivicaine (0.5%): 0.06 mg/kg in 3–4 mL for 300 kg ponies; onset 10 mins; duration 5 h. Variable ataxia.
L-bupivicaine (0.5%): as for racemic bupivacaine above
Ropivicaine 0.1 mg/kg but made up to 10 mL: onset approx. 12 mins: duration 3–4 h. Some slight ataxia.

α_2-agonists

Xylazine: 0.17–0.25 mg/kg: onset 10–20 mins: duration 3–5 h. Mild ataxia.

Detomidine: 20–60 µg/kg: onset 10–15 mins: duration 2–3 h. Systemic side effects.

Opioids

Volumes may be diluted to 10–30 mL
Morphine: 0.1 mg/kg: slow onset (6–8 h): very prolonged duration (12–19 h). Very occasional pruritus.
Tramadol: 1 mg/kg: onset 30 mins: duration 8–12 h

Combinations

Total volume of combination will influence number of dermatomes affected.
Lidocaine 0.22 mg/kg plus xylazine 0.17 mg/kg: onset 5–15 mins: duration 5–6 h
Lidocaine 2%: 5–8 mL plus morphine 0.1 mg/kg: onset 5–15 mins: duration up to 19 h
Xylazine 0.17 mg/kg plus morphine 0.1 mg/kg: onset 10–20 mins: duration up to 19 h
Detomidine 10–30 µg/kg plus morphine 0.1–0.2 mg/kg: onset 20–30 mins: duration 20–24 h

Information obtained from Grubb et al. (1992); Skarda & Muir (1996); Sysel et al. (1996), Robinson & Natalini (2002); Derossi et al. (2005); Natalini (2010); Valverde (2010) and van Loon et al. (2012)

Plasma elimination half-life was 8.5 hours after IV and 7.7 hours after oral administration. Oral bioavailability was only 16%. Behavioural effects were some sedation and an increase in drinking.

Lidocaine

Lidocaine infusions are administered during anaesthesia; their use in this capacity is discussed later (see PIVA below). Lidocaine infusions are used after colic surgery, primarily for their effect in promoting gut motility, but with the hope that they also provide additional analgesia (Doherty, 2009). In conscious horses, Robertson et al, (2005) found that lidocaine infusion resulted in minimal visceral nociception but did have a small effect in reducing response to thermal stimulation.

LOCAL ANALGESIA

Local analgesia can provide total analgesia and often muscle relaxation of the area concerned. While in many animals local techniques to cover a whole limb are employed, in horses, it is necessary to ensure that the horse can stand, so blocks need to be more specific. Many techniques of very specific nerve block are used in horses for purely diagnostic purposes and those and also the methods for producing intrasynovial desensitization will not be considered here. Those to be described here are only the ones which the authors have found useful in operative surgery or for giving pain relief.

EPIDURAL AND INTRATHECAL ANALGESIA

In the last 10–15 years, epidural analgesia in the horse has become used very widely for several purposes, not only in relation to the perioperative period, but for the provision of longer-term pain relief in a number of circumstances. At one time the technique was limited to the use of epidural lidocaine for perineal surgery; increasing the dose of local analgesic solution would lead to motor block and the horse would become recumbent. The combination of low doses of local analgesic and/or α_2-agonist with morphine enables long-acting analgesia to be achieved without ataxia; the use of catheters means that blocks can be 'topped up' or extended to more anterior dermatomes. In the horse, the meninges end in the midsacral region and, although less used, subarachoid injection/catheterization is practicable at this point. Some methods of carrying out the procedures and drugs used have recently been reviewed (Natalini, 2010). For all epidural or spinal blocks, aseptic precautions are essential.

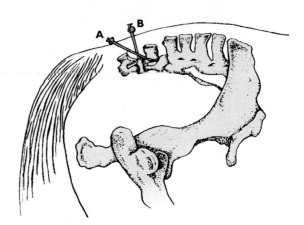

Figure 11.2 Caudal epidural block in the horse. The needle may be inserted at right angles to the skin surface between the first and second caudal vertebrae (B), or it may be introduced further caudally over the cranial border of the second coccygeal vertebra and inclined at an angle of about 30° to the horizontal to advance up the neural canal (A).

Caudal epidural injection and catheterization

The caudal epidural block is performed by entering between the first and second coccygeal vertebrae (Fig. 11.2), the spinal cord and its meninges ending in the midsacral region. The depression between the first and second coccygeal dorsal spinous processes can usually be felt with the finger when the tail is raised, even in the heavy breeds, about 2.5 cm cranial to the commencement of the tail hairs although, in fat animals, it may be impossible to detect any of the sacral or coccygeal dorsal spinous processes. Upward flexion at the sacrococcygeal articulation is seldom discernible; in fact, in many animals this joint is fused. A line drawn over the back joining the two coxofemoral joints crosses the midline at the level of the sacrococcygeal joint. Immediately behind this may be palpated the dorsal spinous process of the first coccygeal bone, and the site for insertion of the needle is the space immediately caudal to this. It may be difficult to locate in well developed or fat animals; 'pumping' the tail may help. Local anaesthetic is injected intradermally at the site. A spinal needle (20 G, 6–10 cm) is inserted in the midline at right angles to the skin (Fig. 11.3A). A 'popping' sensation may be felt as the interarcual ligament is penetrated. The needle is pushed on until it hits the bony floor of the canal, then slightly withdrawn. If a commercial spinal needle with a stylet has been used, then the stylet is withdrawn; air may heard entering as there should be a negative pressure, or if a drop of saline has been placed on the hub, it will be drawn in (hanging drop method). Another test that it is the correct place is the almost complete absence of resistance to injection of a test saline injection

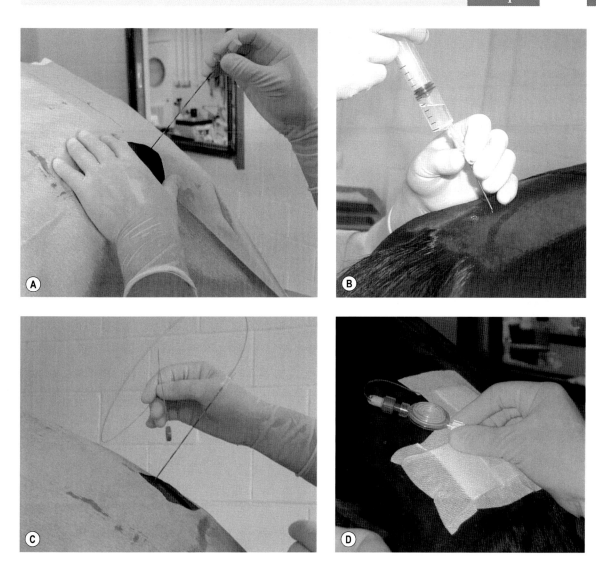

Figure 11.3 Stages of epidural injection and of catheterization (not all from the same horse). (A) After local anaesthetic infiltration of the site of injection, the long spinal needle (or Tuohy needle if catheterizing) is inserted perpendicular to the skin, and advanced into the spinal canal. (B) Checking lack of resistance by injecting saline. (C) Threading a catheter through the needle and (D) the catheter has been sealed with a suitable injection port and is anchored to the skin.
Photographs from Taylor, P.M., Clarke, K.W., 2007. Handbook of Equine Anaesthesia. 2nd edn, Elsevier Ltd, with permission.

(Fig. 11.3B). It is probably preferable not to use air for the test injection as, in dogs, this has been shown to block subsequent spread of radiopaque dye (Iseri et al., 2010).

Catheterization

An epidural catheter is useful for the provision of longer-term analgesia. Very strict aseptic precautions are necessary. Disposable epidural packs are available. The technique is as above, but instead of the epidural needle, a Tuohy needle is employed. The catheter is threaded through this at least 4–6 cm (see Fig. 11.3C) and more depending on

where the block is required. Catheters inserted in the coccygeal region may be advanced at least as far forward as the lumbosacral junction (Sysel et al., 1996). The catheter is then sealed with a suitable injection port and anchored in a way that will keep the site clean (see Fig. 11.3D).

Subarachnoid injection and catheterization

Natalini (2010) describes the technique of intrathecal injection in detail. Strict aseptic precautions are even more important and he advises sedation for the procedure. He suggests that the lumbosacral space is located by palpating the caudal borders of the tuber coxae, the cranial borders of the tuber sacrale and the midline depression between the sixth lumbar and second sacral vertebrae. Local anaesthesia of skin and muscle at the site of injection is required. A spinal needle with stylet is inserted perpendicularly, and advanced until it penetrates the spinal canal. When the stylet is withdrawn, cerebrospinal fluid can be withdrawn. For catheterization, a reinforced epidural catheter is inserted and sealed as described above.

Drugs used by epidural and intrathecal routes

Commonly, three types of drugs are used by the epidural route: local anaesthetics, α_2-adrenoceptor agonists and opioids. The combination of two or all three aims to obtain rapid onset, sufficient analgesia and adequate duration for the procedure in hand. This may be for surgery or may be to provide postoperative or other longer duration analgesia. Ketamine also is occasionally included in combinations but will not be considered further.

Local analgesics give complete and fairly rapid onset analgesia (it can take up to 20 minutes with lidocaine and longer with bupivicaine) but, for anything other than a caudal block (i.e. just sufficient for perineal surgery), there is a danger of motor effects and recumbency. They certainly should be avoided for intrathecal use for this reason. α_2-Agonists work fairly rapidly (within 15 minutes) and, depending on drug and dose, are effective for 2–3 hours. Skarda & Muir (1996) reported that while xylazine (0.25 mg/kg) provided analgesia adequate for perineal surgery and variable bilateral analgesia as far forward as S3 with minimal systemic effects, with epidural detomidine, doses of 60 µg/kg were required, which resulted in variable spread of analgesia sometimes extending to the thoracic region, and systemic effects also occurred. However, when given by the midsacral subarachnoid route, 30 µg/kg detomidine gave good analgesia from the coccyx to the lumbar region with minimal systemic effects. With either of the α_2-agonists, onset of perineal analgesia occurred within 15 minutes. Skarda & Muir (1996) suggested that xylazine was exerting a local anaesthetic effect, hence the low doses required in comparison to those used when the drug is given systemically.

Morphine, as discussed above, gives prolonged analgesia, but has a slow onset.

The combination most commonly used is that of xylazine and lignocaine (Grubb et al., 1992) but many similar combinations have been employed. Opioids have also been combined with local analgesics. Box 11.2 gives some drugs/drug combinations that the authors have found useful and/or have good evidence base. For a more extensive list and combinations suitable for very prolonged analgesia, the reader is referred to Natalini's (2010) extensive review.

Specific Nerve Blocks

Infraorbital nerve block

The infraorbital nerve is the continuation of the maxillary division of the Vth cranial nerve and is entirely sensory. During its course along the infraorbital canal it supplies branches to the upper molar, canine and incisor teeth on that side, and their alveoli and contiguous gum. The nerves supplying the first and second molars (PM1 and 2), the canine and incisors, arise within the canal about 2.5 cm from the infraorbital foramen and pass forwards in the maxilla and premaxilla to the teeth. The nerves to cheek teeth three to six (PM3, Ml, 2 and 3) pass directly from the parent nerve trunk in the upper parts of the canal. After emerging from the foramen the nerve supplies sensory fibres to the upper lip and cheek, the nostrils and lower parts of the face.

The infraorbital nerve may be approached at two sites:

1. At its point of emergence from the infraorbital foramen: the area desensitized will comprise the skin of the lip, nostril and face on that side up to the level of the foramen
2. Within the canal, via the infraorbital foramen when, in addition, the first and second premolars, the canine and incisor teeth with their alveoli and gum, and the skin as high as the level of the inner canthus of the eye, will be influenced (Figs 11.4, 11.5).

The lip of the infraorbital foramen can be detected readily as a bony ridge lying beneath the edge of the flat levator nasolabialis muscle. When it is desired to block the nerve within the canal, it is necessary to pass the needle up the canal about 2.5 cm. To do this, the needle must be inserted through the skin about 2 cm in front of the foramen after reflecting the edge of the levator muscle upwards. An insensitive skin weal is an advantage. For the perineural injection a needle 19 gauge (1.1 mm), 5 cm long, is suitable. The quantity of local analgesic solution required will vary from 4 to 5 mL. For blocking the nerve

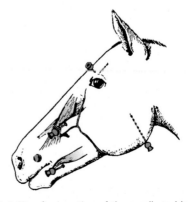

Figure 11.4 Sites for insertion of the needle to block the supraorbital, infraorbital, mental and mandibular nerves.

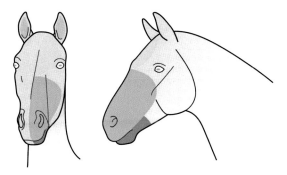

Figure 11.5 Area of skin desensitized after blocking the infraorbital nerve within the canal (mid blue), the supraorbital nerve (light blue) and the mental nerve (darker blue).

at its point of emergence from the canal, the needle is introduced until its point can be felt beneath the bony lip of the foramen. From 4 to 5 mL of 1% mepivacaine is injected, withdrawing the needle slightly as injection proceeds. Loss of sensation should follow in 15–20 minutes and last a further 30–40 minutes if the solution injected contains a vasoconstrictor.

Injections at site 1 may be employed for interferences about the lips and nostrils, such as suturing of wounds, removal of polypi, etc. Extraction of canine or incisor teeth is seldom required in horses and, for extraction of molar teeth, general anaesthesia is usually preferred. For trephining the facial sinuses, local infiltration analgesia offers a good alternative.

Mandibular nerve block

The alveolar branch of the mandibular division of the Vth cranial nerve enters the mandibular foramen on the medial aspect of the vertical ramus of the mandible under cover of the medial pterygoid muscle. It traverses the mandibular canal, giving off dental and alveolar branches on that side, and emerges through the mental foramen. From this point, it is styled the mental nerve. The nerves supplying the canine and incisor teeth arise from the parent trunk within the canal 3–5 cm behind the mental foramen, and pass to the teeth within the bone.

If the mandibular alveolar nerve is injected at its point of entry into the mandibular canal at the mandibular foramen, practically the whole of the lower jaw and all the teeth and alveoli on that side will become desensitized (see Figs 11.4, 11.5).

The technique is difficult and uncertain, for the nerve enters the canal high up on the medial aspect of the vertical ramus. The foramen lies practically opposite the point of intersection of a line passing vertically downwards from the lateral canthus of the eye, and one extending backwards from the tables of the mandibular molar teeth.

A point is selected on the caudal border of the mandible about 3 cm below the temporomandibular articulation. After penetrating the skin, the needle is allowed to lie in the depression between the wing of the atlas and the base of the ear. The needle is advanced as its point is depressed until it passes deep to the medial border of the ramus. It is then advanced further in the direction of the point of intersection of the previously mentioned lines, keeping as close as possible to the medial surface of the mandible but, as the nerve lies medial to the accompanying artery and vein, the needle does not need to follow the bone closely. Following this method, the needle should lie parallel with the nerve for a distance of 3–4 cm. About 5 mL of analgesic solution is injected along this length. German writers describe a modification: the foramen is approached from the ventral border of the ramus, just in front of the angle. The point of the needle must penetrate a distance of 1.0–1.5 cm to reach the foramen.

The chief indications are molar dental interferences in the lower jaw, but most surgeons today prefer to carry out all dental surgery under general anaesthesia and this nerve block will only be used when, for some reason, general anaesthesia is impracticable.

Mental nerve block

Suturing of wounds of the lower lip may be conveniently carried out under mental nerve block. The nerve can be injected as it emerges from the mental foramen and analgesia of the lower lip on that side will ensue (see Figs 11.4, 11.5). Attempts may be made to pass the needle along a canal a distance of 3–5 cm (in which case the canine and incisor teeth will also be desensitized) but this is not easily performed.

The mental foramen is situated on the lateral aspect of the ramus in the middle of the interdental space. It can be palpated after deflecting the pencil-like tendon of the depressor labii inferioris muscle upwards. The nerve may be detected as an emerging thick straw-like structure. From this point, the technique is the same as that outlined for the infraorbital nerve.

Supraorbital nerve block

Suturing of wounds involving only the upper eyelid is easily possible after block of the supraorbital nerve (see Fig. 11.4). The supraorbital (or frontal) nerve is one of the terminal branches of the ophthalmic division of the Vth cranial nerve. It emerges from the orbit accompanied by the artery through the supraorbital foramen in the supraorbital process. It supplies sensory fibres to the upper eyelid and, in part, to the skin of the forehead. The nerve is injected within the supraorbital foramen.

The upper and lower borders of the supraorbital process, close to its junction with the main mass of the frontal bone, is palpable. The foramen is recognized as a pit-like depression midway between the two borders. The skin is prepared and an insensitive weal produced. A needle, 19 gauge (1.1 mm), 2.2 cm long, is passed into the foramen to a depth of 0.5–1.0 cm and 5 ml of analgesic solution injected.

Auriculopalpebral nerve block

The auriculopalpebral nerve is a terminal branch of the facial division of the trigeminal (Vth) cranial nerve innervating the orbicularis oculi muscles. Blocking it prevents voluntary closure of the eyelids but does not in any way desensitize them. In conjunction with topical analgesia of the conjunctiva, it is most useful for examination of the eye, as well as for the removal of foreign bodies from the cornea and other minor eye surgery. It may be blocked by placing 5 ml of 2% mepivacaine solution subfascially at the most dorsal point of the zygomatic arch. A 2.5 cm, 22 gauge (0.7 mm) needle is a convenient size for this injection.

Palmar/plantar nerve block

The nerves confer sensibility to the digit (Fig. 11.6). The medial palmar nerve of the forelimb is one of the terminal branches of the median nerve. At the level of the proximal sesamoid bones, the trunk of the nerve divides into three digital branches, and all three branches are in close relationship with the digital vessels. The dorsal branch in front of the vein distributes cutaneous branches to the front of the digit, and terminates in the coronary cushion. The middle branch, which is small and irregular, descends between the artery and vein. It is generally formed by the union of several smaller branches which cross forwards

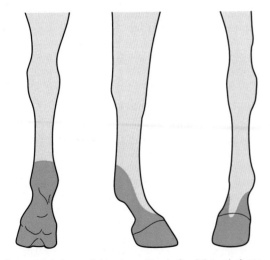

Figure 11.6 Area of skin desensitized after bilateral plantar or palmar nerve block.

over the artery before uniting, and it terminates in the sensitive laminae and the coronary cushion. The palmar branch lies close behind the artery, except at the metacarpophalangeal joint, where the nerve is almost superposed to the artery. It accompanies the digital artery in the hoof, and passes with the palmar branch of that vessel to be distributed to the distal phalanx and sensitive laminae.

The lateral palmar nerve is formed by fusion of the termination of the ulnar nerve with one of the terminal branches of the median. In the metacarpal region it occupies, on the outside of the limb, a position on the flexor tendons analogous to that of the medial palmar nerve on the inside. Unlike the latter nerve, however, it is accompanied by only a single vessel – the lateral palmar vein – which lies in front of it. (A small artery – the lateral palmar metacarpal artery – accompanies the nerve and vein from the carpus to the metacarpophalangeal joint on the lateral aspect of the limb). At the level of the sesamoid bones, it divides into three digital branches exactly as does the medial palmar nerve already described.

In the hind limb, plantar nerves result from bifurcation of the tibial nerve when it gains the back of the tarsus. They accompany the deep digital flexor tendon in the tarsal sheath and, diverging from one another, they descend in the metatarsal region, one at each side of the deep digital flexor tendon. Each is accompanied in the metatarsus by the metatarsal vein of that side, and by a slender artery from the vascular arch at the back of the tarsus. A little below the middle of the metatarsus, the medial nerve detaches a considerable branch that winds obliquely downwards and outwards behind the flexor tendons to join the lateral plantar nerve about the level of the button of the fourth metatarsal bone. At the metatarsophalangeal joint, each nerve, coming into relation with the digital vessels, resolves itself into three branches for the supply of the digit.

In the hind limb, the main artery – the dorsal metatarsal artery – passes to the back of the metatarsus by dipping under the free end of the fourth metatarsal bone, and finally bifurcates above the fetlock, between the two divisions of the suspensory ligament, to form the digital arteries. In the pastern region, the disposition of the nerves and vessels is the same as in the forelimb. Plantar nerve block does not give the same results as palmar block in the forelimb. The skin and deeper tissues on the dorsal aspect of the hind fetlock and pastern are innervated by terminal branches of the fibular nerve. This may be important from a surgical standpoint although less important from a diagnostic point of view (S. Dyson, personal communication, 1991).

Technique for palmar/plantar (abaxial sesamoid) injection

Injection in both fore- and hind limbs is where the nerves course just proximal to the metacarpophalangeal/metatarsophalangeal joint. Although the nerves divide up into three branches at about this point, the injection of 2–3 ml of local analgesic solution medially and laterally still produces complete desensitization of the entire foot (see Fig. 11.6) An advantage of this site is that when the limb is held up and the joint flexed, the nerves and their associated vessels can be palpated so their accurate location is easy.

A strict aseptic technique must be practised and the lateral and medial sites should be clipped and prepared as for an operation. In thin-skinned horses, a 25 gauge (0.5 mm), 2.5 cm long needle is used; disposable needles can usually be introduced through the skin without the horse showing resentment.

After the injections have been completed, the animal is allowed to stand quietly for 10–15 minutes. At the end of this time, the limb is tested for sensation by tapping on the skin with a blunt-ended spike on the end of a short pole. This is a better way of detecting loss of deep sensation than pricking with a needle. Any response to tapping around the coronet and heel indicates failure to block the nerve on that side. One indication of sensation is sufficient to prove this, and successive trials only serve to agitate the animal. It may be necessary to cover the animal's eye to prevent it seeing the approach of the test instrument.

Technique of palmar/plantar metacarpal/ metatarsal injection

An alternative site for blocking the palmar/plantar digital nerves is from 5 to 7 cm proximal to the metacarpophalangeal/metatarsophalangeal joint at the level of the distal enlargements of the second and fourth metacarpal or metatarsal bones. This ensures that the analgesic solution is in contact with the nerve proximal to its point of division. The local analgesic is injected into the groove between the deep digital flexor tendon and the suspensory ligament. The nerve lies deep to the subcutaneous fascia immediately in front of the deep flexor tendon. A 25 gauge (0.5 mm) needle 1.2 cm long is used. The skin over the site is clipped and cleansed. In the great majority of cases, the needle can be inserted without movement on the part of the animal. With the animal standing on the limb, the skin and subcutaneous fascia are tense, and it is easy to penetrate the latter and thus ensure that the subsequent injection is in direct contact with the nerve. If the limb is held raised during insertion of the needle, the flaccidity of the skin may cause the point to enter the subcutaneous connective tissue and the method will fail. If blood escapes from the needle, it should be partially withdrawn, redirected and reinserted. It may be decided, first, to provoke an insensitive skin weal, and then pass the needle through this at the appropriate angle until its point lies beneath the fascia.

When it is intended to block both sides of the limb supplied by these nerves, the opposite side of the leg is similarly dealt with. When dealing with the medial nerve

it is necessary to work around the opposite leg. With the horse standing squarely, the operator passes one hand around the front of the adjacent leg for inserting the needle, while the other is passed behind the limb for holding the syringe on the needle.

The most likely cause of failure is that the solution was injected into the subcutaneous connective tissue, and not beneath the fascia. Fortunately, the skin at the site is now desensitized and a second and deeper injection can be made without restraint.

About 2.5–5.0 ml of 1% mepivacaine or 0.5% bupivacaine solution is commonly injected around each nerve. The average 500 kg horse is given 3 ml over each nerve. In the hind limb, the technique is similar, except that the procedure exposes the operator to a greater risk of injury, especially when dealing with a nervous animal. Thus, not only must the animal be twitched, but the forelimb raised in addition if the operation is to be carried out with the animal standing on the affected limb. Should the operator feel indisposed to make the injection with the hind leg free, it may be raised by an assistant, but the needle must be inserted sufficiently deeply to penetrate the fascia.

Technique of blocking palmar terminal digital nerves

The terminal divisions of the palmar and plantar nerves may be subjected to medial and lateral perineural injection in the pastern region. The site for injection is midway between the fetlock joint and coronet. The palmar or volar border of the first phalanx is located, and the dorsal edge of the (at this point flattened) deep digital flexor tendon is palpated. The nerve lies immediately dorsal to the tendon. About 2 ml of 1% mepivacaine or 0.5% bupivacaine solution is injected SC just proximal to the collateral cartilages. The area desensitized is limited to the palmar or volar part of the foot and heel on that side.

Indications for palmar/plantar block

Palmar/plantar block is commonly used to aid diagnosis of the site of lameness, but it is also very useful to relieve the pain of acutely painful lesions about the foot, and to allow the animal to rest. The practice may be repeated daily for a few days in severe cases. Longest pain relief is obtained by using bupivacaine with a vasoconstrictor such as adrenaline at a concentration of 1 : 200 000.

The nerve blocks allow the painless performance of palmar and plantar neurectomy and of operations about the foot, coronet and heel, such as exposure of a corn or gathered nail track, partial operations for quittor and sandcrack. Even when operations about the foot are performed under general anaesthesia, palmar and plantar blocks can provide analgesia intraoperatively and in the recovery period. The desensitization of the foot which they produce does not seem to be an obstacle to the animal regaining its feet after general anaesthesia or to contribute to ataxia immediately afterwards.

The complete desensitization of the forelimb below the carpus

Simultaneous block of the median, ulnar and musculocutaneous (cutaneous branch) nerves desensitizes the entire manus.

Median nerve

The best site at which to inject the median nerve is the one used for the operation of median neurectomy, i.e. the point on the medial aspect of the limb about 5 cm distal to the elbow joint, where the nerve lies immediately caudal to the radius and cranial to the muscular belly of the internal flexor of the metacarpus, deep to the caudal superficial pectoral muscle and the deep fascia.

With the animal standing squarely, the administrator stoops adjacent to and slightly behind the opposite forelimb. The caudal border of the radius where it meets the distal edge of the caudal superficial pectoral muscle is located with a finger. The point of insertion of the needle is immediately proximal to the finger. A needle, 19 gauge (1.1 mm), 2.5–3.0 cm long, is suitable. It is directed proximally and axially at an angle of 20° to the vertical, to ensure penetration of the pectoral muscle and the deep fascia; 7.5–10.0 ml of local analgesic solution is injected. To facilitate insertion of the needle to the proper depth, it is best first to induce an insensitive skin weal.

The indications for blocking the median nerve alone are limited, for the surface area desensitized is little more than that obtained with medial palmar block (see Figs 11.6 and 11.7).

Ulnar nerve

This nerve may be blocked by injection of 10 ml of local analgesic solution in the centre of the caudal aspect of the limb, about 10 cm proximal to the accessory carpal bone, in the groove between the tendons of the ulnaris lateralis and flexor carpi ulnaris, and beneath the deep fascia.

Musculocutaneous nerve

This nerve is blocked on the medial aspect of the limb where it lies on the surface of the radius halfway between the elbow and carpus, immediately adjacent to the cephalic vein. At this site, it can easily be palpated just cranial to the cephalic vein and blocked by the injection of 10 ml of local analgesic solution.

The complete desensitization of the distal hind limb

The technique of nerve block of the hind limb sometimes works extremely well but is unreliable, especially for

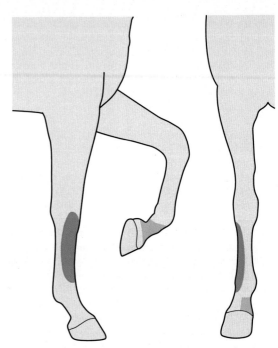

Figure 11.7 Areas of skin desensitization after block of the ulnar (darker blue) and median nerves (light blue) (S. Dyson, personal communication, 1991).

removal of cutaneous sensation. Westhues and Fritsch (1960) described techniques for blocking the tibial and peroneal (fibular) nerves.

Tibial nerve

Injection is made about 1.5 cm above the point of the tarsus, in the groove between the gastrocnemius and the deep digital flexor tendons. Palpation of the nerve at this site is facilitated by holding up the foot and slightly flexing the leg, although the injection is best made with the limb bearing weight. Care must be taken to inject deep to the subcutaneous fascia or only the superficial branch of the nerve will be affected. Some 20 ml of local analgesic solution should be injected at this site through a 2.5 cm, 20 gauge (0.9 mm) needle that has been placed beneath the fascia.

Peroneal (fibular) nerve

The superficial and deep branches of this nerve are best blocked simultaneously in the groove between the tendons of the long and lateral digital extensors about 10 cm proximal to the lateral malleolus of the tibia. First, a 3.75 cm, 22 gauge (0.7 mm) needle is introduced subcutaneously and 10 ml of the local analgesic solution injected through it to block the superficial nerve. The needle must then be inserted another 2–3 cm to penetrate the deep fascia and

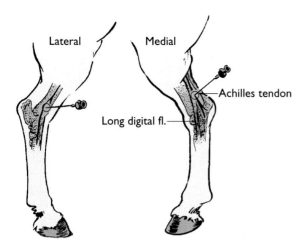

Figure 11.8 Sites for injection about the peroneal nerve on the lateral aspect and the tibial nerve on the medial aspect of the horse's hind limb.

about 1.0–1.5 ml of local analgesic solution injected (Fig. 11.8) around the deep branch.

Saphenous nerve

The deposition of 5 ml of local analgesic solution on the dorsal aspect of the median saphenous vein proximal to the tibiotarsal joint will effectively block the saphenous nerve.

Block of the tibial nerve above the hock, and of the deep peroneal (fibular) nerve, desensitizes the plantar metatarsus, the medial and lateral aspects of the fetlock and whole digit. To produce a complete block distal to the hock, these two nerves must be injected together with the saphenous nerve, the superficial peroneal (fibular) nerve and the caudal cutaneous nerve (a branch of the tibial nerve).

Local analgesia for castration

There are three methods in common use for desensitizing the scrotum, testicle and spermatic cord by injection of local analgesics but, for all of them, it is essential that the animal is properly restrained or sedated if the operator is not to be injured when carrying them out on the standing animal. The animal is placed with its right side against a wall or partition and, if not sedated, a twitch is applied to its upper lip. After preparation of the skin of the scrotum, prepuce and medial aspect of the thighs, the operator stands with his left shoulder pressed lightly against the caudal part of the animal's left chest wall. The neck of the scrotum on the right side is gripped with the left hand and the testicle drawn well down until the skin of the scrotum is tense (Fig. 11.9).

Method 1. A 19 gauge (1.1 mm) needle is quickly thrust into the substance of the testicle to a depth of 3–4 cm and,

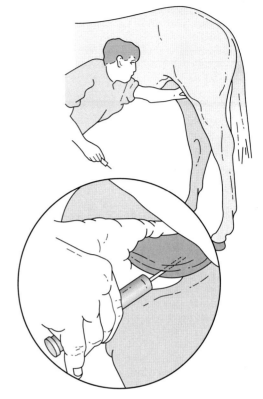

Figure 11.9 Injection into the substance of the testicles after linear infiltration of the scrotal tissues.

depending on the size of the testicles, up to 35 ml of 2% lignocaine injected. When an adequate amount of lignocaine has been injected the testicle feels firm. The procedure is repeated for the left testicle, and local analgesic solution is injected along the median raphe of the scrotum. After about 10 minutes has elapsed castration can be carried out painlessly.

Method 2. The spermatic cord is grasped with the fingers just above the testicle and a 5 cm 19 gauge (1.1 mm) needle thrust into the subcutaneous tissues of that region. The needle is kept stationary to avoid penetration of blood vessels and up to 20 ml of 2% lignocaine injected around each spermatic cord. The scrotal skin is injected along the line of the proposed incisions. This method does not seem as effective as the one described above.

Method 3. A long (12–15 cm) 19 gauge (1.1 mm) needle is thrust through the testicle and directed into the spermatic cord while up to 25 ml 2% lignocaine are being injected. After treatment of both spermatic cords, the scrotal skin is infiltrated. To infiltrate the scrotal skin it is important that the direction of the needle shall be almost parallel to the skin to ensure that its point lies in the subcutaneous connective tissue, for if it enters the dartos or the substance of the testicle itself, difficulty may be experienced in injecting the solution and, what is more important, the skin does not become analgesic. The animal usually moves as the needle is inserted and the operator must be prepared for this.

Some right-handed operators prefer to stand on the right side of the horse, with the left hand holding the scrotum or spermatic cord, so that the left arm is against the stifle and affords some measure of protection against a kick. The person holding the twitch should stand on the same side as the operator.

Paravertebral analgesia

A thoracolumbar paravertebral block of T18, L1 and L2 segmental nerves provides useful anaesthesia of skin, muscles and peritoneum of the paralumbar fossa, and it is an excellent method of analgesia for procedures such as flank laparotomy or for laparoscopy in the standing horse (Moon & Suter, 1993). L3 should not be blocked as, in horses, it provides some innervation to the hind limbs, and its block may cause ataxia.

The basic anatomy of the spinal nerves resembles that of cattle, each nerve bifurcating shortly after leaving the spinal canal, the dorsal branch supplying the skin and superficial tissues, while the ventral branch passes beneath the inter-transverse ligament, and innervates the muscle layers and peritoneum. Thus, as with cattle, it is necessary to block both dorsal and ventral branches of each spinal nerve if adequate analgesia is to be obtained. In cattle, the landmarks for injection are found by palpation of the transverse process of the lumbar vertebrae, but these are almost impossible to locate in horses. However, Moon and Suter (1993) point out that a line from the most caudal portion of the last rib (easily located in almost all horses) and perpendicular to the long axis of the spine passes across the transverse process of L3. Thus, to block the spinal nerve L2, the site chosen is over the transverse process of L3, and approximately 5–6 cm lateral to the midline. A small bleb of local anaesthetic is placed in the skin, then 5 ml of 2% lignocaine (or other suitable local analgesic agent) infiltrated in the muscle. A long spinal needle (e.g. 18 G × 7–15 cm) is then introduced vertically until it impinges on the transverse process; it is withdrawn a little, then redirected slightly cranially, until the inter-transverse ligament between L2 and L3 is penetrated (felt as an increase, then sudden decrease, in resistance). Following aspiration to ensure that the needle is not in a blood vessel, 20 ml of 2% lignocaine is slowly infiltrated, half 2.5 cm below the inter-transverse ligament, and the remainder 2.5 cm above to block the dorsal branch of the nerve. It is easy to enter the peritoneum and this is detected by a loss of resistance (as it penetrates the transverse ligament) and sometimes by hearing air being aspirated through the needle. Should this happen, the needle should be withdrawn to a retroperitoneal position, before the local anaesthetic is deposited. The procedure is repeated to block nerves L1 and T13. The sites for injection are located by measuring 5–6 cm anterior from the previous site (less in ponies), and confirmed by the needle impinging on a transverse process of the vertebrae.

With practice, the technique is simple and reliable, although on occasions analgesia of the ventral area of the paralumbar fossa is inadequate for surgery, and local infiltration become necessary.

GENERAL ANAESTHESIA

General anaesthesia in horses appears beset with more problems than are encountered in any other domestic animal. In particular, cardiopulmonary dysfunction, nerve and ischaemic muscle damage appear more pronounced and can be difficult to avoid. The problems are often interrelated and seem to follow directly from the actions of the anaesthetic agents themselves, or from interference with mechanisms existing in conscious horses to compensate for respiratory or cardiovascular changes induced by recumbency. Other problems relate to the horse's size, its temperament and its tendency to panic. It is necessary to anticipate the problems from the beginning of the anaesthetic protocol in order to take action necessary to avoid or reduce them; hence they will be considered in general at this stage.

Problems relating to size and temperament

When handling horses, the safety not only of the horse, but also of the handlers must be considered, and methods of control used must reflect the temperament of the horse and availability of well-trained personnel. Sedative premedication aids placement of catheters and the smoothness of induction of anaesthesia. The sheer weight and bulk of a large horse makes it difficult to handle, transport or position for surgery without adequate manpower or mechanical aids. Many unconscious horses are transported for short distances (e.g. from the operating table to recovery box) suspended in a net or by their hobbled legs from an overhead hoist. Other methods of moving unconscious horses include trolleys, which may constitute the floor of the anaesthetic induction box and may then become the operating table top.

In clinical practice, anaesthesia in the adult horse is almost always induced by IV agents. Breed is often allied to temperament and must not be ignored in the selection of an anaesthetic technique. Ideally, the horse should regain its feet as rapidly as possible at the first attempt, with minimal ataxia. Unfortunately, this is not easily achieved following prolonged anaesthesia. Although prolonged recumbency is not desirable, it is now appreciated that, in some cases, ultra-fast recoveries may be of poor quality because the horse tries to arise while still disorientated. The best quality recoveries are seen where the drugs given during anaesthesia are eliminated in such a manner that the horse does not try to rise until it is ready. It may be necessary to use sedation to increase the duration of recumbency, and considerable recent research has concentrated on the quality of recovery and how to improve it. Animals which are unused to people may try to rise too soon. Ponies exhibit poor quality recovery as often as do large horses, but it is the heavier animal which is most likely to suffer from serious injury as a result. Other causes of poor quality of recovery from anaesthesia include nerve and muscle damage induced during anaesthesia, and untreated postoperative pain.

DISTURBANCES IN CARDIOPULMONARY FUNCTION

Disturbances of cardiopulmonary function have long been recognized in anaesthetized horses but, in spite of much research, their cause remains uncertain. Because general anaesthesia necessarily involves recumbency, there has been some debate as to the relative importance of the roles of recumbency and of anaesthetic agents in their genesis but, in conscious experimental animals, the cardiopulmonary disturbances produced by lateral recumbency have been found to be minimal (Hall, 1984). However, disturbances, at least of pulmonary function, are more severe following supine rather than lateral recumbency in anaesthetized horses. It is probable that while various postures may magnify effects they do not initiate them.

From the evidence available today, it seems likely that any disturbances resulting from recumbency are minimized in conscious animals by the operation of compensatory mechanisms that fail or become depressed when an anaesthetic is administered. Their failure or depression is manifested in several ways but probably the most important results which affect equine anaesthetic morbidity and mortality are cardiovascular depression, the development of a large alveolar–arterial oxygen tension gradient ($(A–a)PO_2$) and, probably resulting from the first two factors, postanaesthetic myopathy.

Cardiovascular effects

Horses in which anaesthesia is maintained using volatile anaesthetic agents often suffer from hypotension, which may be the result of vasodilation and/or a fall in CO. A number of studies have investigated the effects of volatile anaesthetics alone, i.e. including volatile anaesthetic induction (review by Steffey, 2002; Santos et al., 2005; Steffey et al., 2005a,b). These investigations have demonstrated that all the currently used volatile anaesthetic agents depress the equine heart in a dose-dependent fashion, but there are differences at equipotent concentrations between agents. With halothane, MAP falls mainly as a result of a fall in CO, even at 1 MAC concentrations. Accommodation occurs and, at a given end-tidal concentration, CO and heart rate rise as anaesthesia progresses. The time course of this accommodation is more prolonged (over five or more hours) than would be encountered during normal clinical practice (Steffey et al., 1990). Accommodation is more pronounced in spontaneously breathing animals, probably as a result of hypercapnia. Anaesthesia with isoflurane, sevoflurane or desflurane also results in a dose-related hypotension, mainly arising from vasodilation as, at eqi-MAC values, CO is better maintained than with halothane. However, the degree of hypotension at MAC, in particular in spontaneously breathing horses, is not as great as that seen in many clinical situations With the newer agents, increasing the concentration still results in a dose-related fall in CO.

Such experiments as detailed above provide useful pharmacological information about the volatile anaesthetic agents in horses, but are not typical of normal clinical anaesthetic practice, in which anaesthesia is induced with IV agents. With the IV techniques most commonly employed, the transition to the volatile anaesthetic agent results in marked hypotension; in experimental situations where nothing is done to prevent it, mean arterial blood pressure (MAP) sometimes falls to below 40 mmHg (Gleed & Dobson, 1990; Lee et al., 1998a) even with halothane, although with the newer agents, once again it is better maintained. Surgical stimulation hastens the onset of increased systemic vascular resistance (SVR) (Wagner et al., 1992). The fact that an induction technique itself does not cause cardiovascular depression does not mean that its combination with a volatile agent will not do so. With many total IV techniques, blood pressure is well maintained, but this does not mean that there is no cardiovascular depression.

One factor rarely discussed in relation to anaesthetic-induced cardiovascular depression in horses is the influence of heart rate on CO. Although stroke volume can increase to compensate for bradycardia, there is a limit to the extent to which this can compensate. α_2-Agonists cause bradycardia and CO falls, although not in proportion to heart rate changes suggesting some compensation (Wagner et al., 1991). Many, but certainly not all, treatments that are successful in raising CO under anaesthesia increase, or at least maintain heart rate (Lee et al., 1998a,c). Certainly, this author (KC) considers that the effect of bradycardia in the pathogenesis of low CO in equine anaesthesia has been neglected and deserves further consideration.

Tissue blood flow versus arterial blood pressure

Blood pressure is easy to measure, CO is not, although the development of the lithium dilution technique has started to make it more practicable in the clinical patients. As described above, in clinical practice, although surgical stimulation causes MAP to rise, this is due to vasoconstriction, and CO may fall, probably because of the increased afterload (Wagner et al., 1992). To maintain blood flow, an adequate perfusion pressure must be coupled with good CO. Pink mucous membranes and a rapid capillary refill time indicate good peripheral blood flow. Venous blood oxygen values also give a guide as to the adequacy of perfusion. Although, ideally, mixed venous samples are necessary, in the horse, the oxygen tension of jugular venous blood approximates (Wetmore et al., 1987) and values above 5 kPa (37.5 mmHg) indicate the adequacy of oxygenation and therefore of perfusion of the peripheral tissue. If the horse is being ventilated, end-tidal CO_2 is another indicator of CO.

In clinical practice, a number of different regimens are used to maintain MAP (see Treatment of circulatory depression below). When considering the rationale of these treatments their effect on CO and tissue blood flow needs consideration (see Fig. 11.13 below).

Pulmonary changes

A major problem encountered in equine anaesthesia is that the arterial oxygen tension (PaO_2) is always much lower than might be expected from the inspired oxygen tensions (PiO_2), i.e. there is a large (A–a)PaO_2. A normal (A–a) of about 18 mmHg (2.4 kPa) in standing horses breathing air is doubled in anaesthetized, laterally recumbent animals. Most investigations concerned with (A–a) PO_2 gradients have been carried out under halothane/oxygen anaesthesia, but similar differences have been found during general anaesthesia with other agents. The increased (A–a)PO_2 may be the result of a combination of several factors and these have been, and still are the subject of many investigations.

The PaO_2 depends on the size of the animal and its position during anaesthesia (Hall, 1983), but it is relatively unaffected by the degree of respiratory depression produced by the anaesthetic agent. There has been shown to be no statistically significant difference in (A–a)PO_2 in a series of animals anaesthetized once with spontaneous breathing and on another occasion with IPPV to normocapnia (Hall et al., 1968a,b). The (A–a)PO_2 gradient does not always increase significantly with time (Gillespie et al., 1969) although, in many clinical situations, it appears to do so.

When a horse is disconnected from a breathing circuit containing an O_2-rich mixture of gases and allowed to breathe air, PaO_2 of around 50 mmHg (6.5 kPa) is common. This may represent a blood O_2 saturation of around 90% (Clerbaux et al., 1986) but the steep part of the dissociation curve starts about here and any accident, such as temporary obstruction of the airway, can have very serious consequences. It is not uncommon for cyanosis to be observed in the recovery period if oxygen is not administered, although it must be remembered that cyanosis cannot become apparent if the blood flow to the mucous membranes is inadequate. To improve the situation, O_2 must be insufflated at a minimum rate of 15 L/min. The PaO_2 apparently recovers to normal levels as soon as the animal regains its feet.

Factors other than hypoventilation which may contribute to the large (A–a)PO_2 include diffusion defects in the lungs, right-to-left intrapulmonary vascular shunts, mismatching of ventilation and perfusion in the lungs, atelectasis and a fall in CO without a corresponding fall in tissue oxygen consumption.

Diffusion impairment

There is no evidence that diffusion impairment occurs so this must be regarded as an unlikely cause of hypoxaemia.

Atelectasis

In horses, the (A–a)PO_2 develops very soon after the induction of anaesthesia and thereafter usually but not always remains relatively constant. There is no doubt, however, that atelectasis does occur for total collapse of regions of the dependent lung is commonly seen at autopsy of horses dying while anaesthetized (Fig. 11.10). This collapse is presumably due to compression of the lung by overlying abdominal and thoracic viscera. A totally collapsed lung acts as a venous–arterial shunt and can cause marked arterial hypoxaemia. A shunt of 15% of the total pulmonary blood flow has been found in laterally recumbent horses under halothane anaesthesia, compared with about 5% in the standing animal (Gillespie et al., 1969). Decrease in lung volume short of collapse may not have all that an adverse effect on alveolar ventilation for the alveolar compliance curve predicts that a small alveolus will expand proportionally more for any given change in intra-alveolar pressure.

Radiographic studies (McDonell et al., 1979) and blood samples drawn from pulmonary veins through implanted catheters in conscious and anaesthetized animals in lateral decubitus (Hall et al., 1968a; Hall, 1979) have afforded further confirmation of the impairment of function in the lower lung. Radiographic appearances (Fig. 11.11) are suggestive of a greatly reduced volume of the lower lung in laterally recumbent animals (McDonell et al., 1979; Nyman et al., 1990). When a horse lies on its side, a diffuse radiographic opacity of the lower lung develops within 20 minutes and may be due to alveolar collapse, regional pulmonary congestion and/or interstitial oedema. Spontaneous deep breaths or forced expansion of the lung by compression of an anaesthetic reservoir bag, both of which might be expected to re-expand collapsed alveoli, fail to alter the radiological appearance.

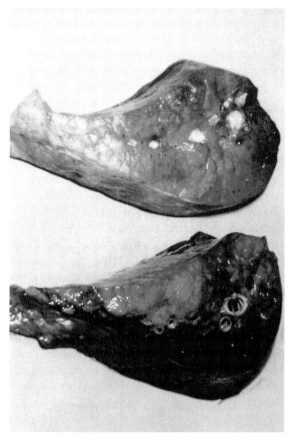

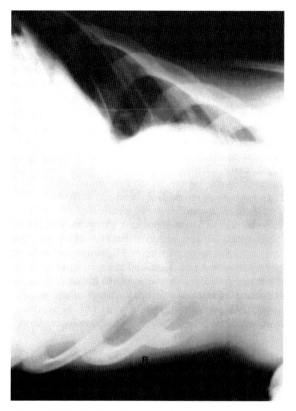

Figure 11.11 Opacity of the lower lung seen in a radiograph taken at full expiration after 20 minutes of halothane anaesthesia in right decubitus.
From McDonell WN, Hall LW, Jeffcott LB (1979), with permission.

Figure 11.10 Slices of the lungs of a Shire horse that died following anaesthesia. The horse had undergone 3 hours of surgery in dorsal decubitus, then been placed in lateral decubitus for recovery. The lung dependent during lateral decubitus (lower picture) shows a large region of total collapse, while the lung which was uppermost in recovery still shows considerable areas of collapse around the hilar region from the period of time in which the horse was in dorsal decubitus.

Venous admixture

It would seem unlikely that total collapse of lung regions resulting in right-to-left vascular shunting accounts for all of the venous admixture which occurs in anaesthetized horses. A substantial amount must be due to the occurrence of gross mismatching of ventilation and perfusion in the lungs. Some indication of this may be obtained from the physiological dead space:tidal volume ratio. In most mammals, this ratio is about 0.3 but, in anaesthetized horses, it is over 0.5 (Hall et al., 1968a,b).

The large physiological dead space:tidal volume ratio partially explains why IPPV is relatively ineffective in decreasing the $(A-a)PO_2$ in horses. The augmented tidal volume resulting from IPPV merely increases ventilation to those regions of the lung which are already overventilated in relation to their perfusion, i.e. those contributing to the physiological deadspace. The increased ventilation will remove carbon dioxide from the lungs and keep the $PaCO_2$ within normal limits but it will not greatly increase the PaO_2.

Effect of cardiac output

CO is usually reduced under anaesthesia but tissue O_2 consumption may remain substantially unchanged. The resulting arterio-mixed venous PaO_2 tension difference, $(A-V)PO_2$, thus increases, and venous blood passing through the anatomical shunt or regions of lung collapse has a greater effect on the $(A-V)PO_2$. As already discussed, reduction in CO does not necessarily relate to MAP. IPPV may reduce CO. Indeed, the oxygen tension in mixed venous blood from the pulmonary artery (PvO_2) is lower when IPPV is used despite a slight increase in PaO_2, presumably because of an increased extraction of oxygen from the blood by the tissue – necessitated by the reduced CO – and hence rate of tissue perfusion. Because

269

right-to-left intrapulmonary shunt increases from the normal 5% in the standing, awake horse to about 15% under halothane anaesthesia (Gillespie et al., 1969), the effect of the shunted blood of lower than normal PO_2 will be to produce noticeable reduction in the mixed PaO_2 of the blood in the left atrium (PaO_2).

Lung volume

The larger the lung the greater the stretch across the airways and the less tendency for closure to occur on expiration. The lung volume at which airway closure starts to occur ('the closing volume') is important for, if airways close, gas trapped distal to the point of closure soon becomes depleted of oxygen and the blood perfusing the region gets through unoxygenated to join the blood from other regions and reduces the mixed PaO_2. Studies strongly suggest that during general anaesthesia the horse's lung volume is reduced to a level at which airway closure may occur and that the reduction in lung volume in the laterally recumbent horse was not equally distributed between the lower and upper lungs (Hall, 1983). In both right and left lateral decubitus, there was a greater reduction in the volume of the lower lung, and pulling the legs together in hobbles reduced lung volume still further.

The effect of airway closure on PaO_2 might be mitigated by collateral ventilation from neighbouring alveoli but,

although anatomical studies indicate that this is possible, it is unlikely to occur in horses. The conclusion was that recumbency rather than anaesthesia was responsible for the reduction of lung volume found in anaesthetized ponies.

Confirmation of serious impairment of expansion of the lowermost lung has been obtained from histological examination of very rapidly frozen lung regions. Also, from the histological appearances, it would seem that a reduction of the tethering effect of lung parenchyma on extra-alveolar vessels might well be responsible for the increased resistance to blood flow in this lung (Hall, 1979).

Preventive methods and/or treatments

A number of strategies have been investigated to attempt to prevent or treat the hypoxaemia, and resultant hypoxia that occurs under anaesthesia. For example, acepromazine premedication has been found to decrease pulmonary shunt (Marntell et al., 2005a). As has been explained above, improving CO and tissue blood flow not only reduces tissue hypoxia, but improves PaO_2 by reducing the effect of the 'shunt'. Some other strategies are as follows and are summarized in Box 11.3.

Box 11.3 **Prevention or treatment of hypoxia under anaesthesia (variable success)**

See text for more detail

Ventilatory strategies

1. Inspired gas (Fi) of 30–50% oxygen (remaining nitrogen or helium)

   Hypothesis is that nitrogen is the 'skeleton of the lung' and prevents alveolar collapse.

   Successful experimentally; variable results clinically. Measure FiO$_2$ and blood gases. Increase FiO$_2$ if partial pressure of arterial oxygen (PaO$_2$) is below 100 mmHg (13.3 kPa).

2. Use of IPPV – no extra strategies

   This reduces hypercarbia but usually fails to improve PaO$_2$. Induces cardiovascular changes.

3. Use of positive-end-expiratory pressures (PEEP)

   Fails with spontaneous breathing, some success with IPPV, but most successful if commenced immediately the horse becomes recumbent.

   PEEP of 5–10 cmH$_2$O now often used with IPPV.

4. Recruitment manoeuvres. Increasing inspired positive pressure for several breaths. Various strategies – see text.

   Controversial; can be very successful but concern over potential pulmonary damage (see text).

Drug-based treatments

1. Premedication with acepromazine reduces pulmonary shunt

2. Beta-agonists:

   a. clenbuterol by injection

   b. salbutamol (albuterol) by inhalation: 2 puffs (during inspiration) of commercial aerosol per 100 kg

   Clenbuterol – too many side effects

   Salbutamol (albuterol) – variable results but appears to do no harm

3. Nitric oxide – pulsed delivery

   Very successful in raising PaO$_2$ and in maintaining the advantages during recovery but not currently practicable as a standard clinical treatment.

Circulatory based treatments

1. Improve cardiac output (choice of anaesthetic and ionotropes).

   Very effective in improving tissue oxygenation by increasing oxygen delivery. In turn, PaO$_2$ will rise as, by raising PvO$_2$ it will reduce the effect of the shunt.

Inspired oxygen concentrations

It has been usual to use oxygen as the carrier gas for the volatile anaesthetic agents but, although counterintuitive, it may be that using such high concentrations of oxygen increases atelectasis. If there is airway trapping, all the oxygen is absorbed, the alveolus becomes collapsed, and it is then difficult to re-inflate. Using nitrogen in the inspired mixture may prevent such collapse. Marntell et al. (2005b) demonstrated that, indeed, high oxygen concentrations increased intrapulmonary shunt. Using a helium/oxygen mixture in a similar manner was even more effective (Staffieri et al., 2009). Many anaesthetists now commence with an inspired oxygen of 40%; if PaO_2 falls, the FiO_2 can be increased. This strategy is only safe to employ if there is the ability to measure both inspired and arterial oxygen.

Ventilatory strategies

It has already been explained that IPPV does not markedly improve the PaO_2, nor reduce the $(A-a)PO_2$ gradient, probably as it only 'over-ventilates' the already expanded alveolae. Another strategy is to increase the expiratory airway pressure to above atmospheric pressure (positive end-expiratory pressure or PEEP) which, in theory, will, by increasing the lung volume to an amount equal to the product of the total compliance and the pressure, decrease the tendency for airways to close and thus raise the PaO_2. As described in Chapter 9, the concern is that this increase in thoracic pressure will lead to a reduction in cardiac output. Imposition of a 10 and 20 cmH_2O expiratory resistance by the insertion of a water trap in the expiratory limb of a circle absorber fails to improve the PaO_2 in horses breathing spontaneously under halothane/oxygen anaesthesia (Hall & Trim, 1975) and, indeed, usually produced immediate respiratory arrest. Broadly similar results were obtained in horses under barbiturate/guaifenesin anaesthesia (Beadle et al., 1975). In contrast, if PEEP of around 10 cmH_2O was initiated immediately the horse became recumbent, it was more effective (Moens & Bohm, 2011). Thus, despite disappointing experimental results many veterinary anaesthetists routinely use IPPV with PEEP.

In Chapter 9, the use of *recruitment manoeuvres* was also discussed. Moens & Bohm review their use in both people and horses. Such manoeuvres have been used in horses previously but usually as one sustained inflation at high positive inspiratory pressure (PIP), and this has often resulted in bradycardia and a fall in CO. However, Wettstein et al. (2006) used a stepwise procedure, using PEEP and then PIPs of 45, 50 then 55 cmH_2O; oxygenation was improved, pulmonary shunt reduced and, although there was a fall in MAP and heart rate, cardiac output was unchanged. In horses undergoing anaesthesia for colic, Hopster et al. (2011) used, with success in improving oxygenation, another recruitment modification; one breath with a PIP of 60, one with PIP 80, then a third at PIP 60 cmH_2O, each held inflated for 10–12 seconds while maintaining PEEP at 10 cmH_2O or higher. Blood pressure and heart rate were only minimally affected, but cardiac output was not measured. There remain concerns over potential pulmonary damage, but it would seem time that recruitment manoeuvres were re-investigated to find the most effective mode.

Pharmacological treatments

Gleed and Dobson (1990) reported that the β_2-agonist clenbuterol (0.8 mg/kg) was effective in increasing PaO_2 in dorsally recumbent halothane anaesthetized horses. Other studies failed to reproduce these results (Dodam et al., 1993; Lee et al., 1998a). In some cases, the injection of clenbuterol is followed by a transient fall in PaO_2, presumably because of the increased O_2 demand associated with the side effects of sweating and tachycardia. However, salbutamol (albuterol), which is available as an aerosol, can be given via the endotracheal tube. The usual dose used for around a 500 kg horse is 10 puffs of the human strength aerosol (each puff is 100 µg) timed at inspiration. Results are again variable, but side effects are rare.

In contrast to the variable results from using β_2-agonists, the pulsed delivery (for a % of the inspiratory time) of nitric oxide (NO) has to date always been successful in improving oxygenation, and this improvement is maintained during recovery after NO administration has ceased (Nyman et al., 2012; Grubb et al., 2013). As yet, this system is not available for routine clinical use but it has potential for the future.

Respiratory stimulants such as doxapram are ineffective at improving oxygenation in anaesthetized horses. At the end of anaesthesia, doxapram can be used to stimulate breathing in cases of refractory apnoea, but will also awake the horse.

Muscle and nerve damage

There used to be an incidence of up to 6.4% of lameness following anaesthesia in the horse (Klein, 1978; Richey et al., 1990), much of which is due to damage to nerves and muscles during recumbency. In the clinical situation, it is not always easy to distinguish between the two syndromes (hence the term 'radial paralysis' was once used to describe the condition now known to be caused by a triceps myopathy; Fig 11.12) and it is probable that it some cases both occur together. Postanaesthetic myopathy is now rare but only because precautions are taken to avoid it.

Postanaesthetic myopathy (rhabdomyolysis)

It is now generally accepted that the common form of postanaesthetic myopathy is due to muscle ischaemia caused by inadequate muscle perfusion (Trim & Mason,

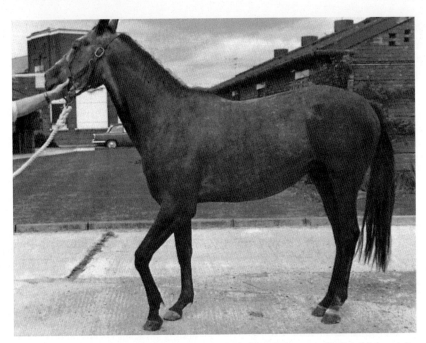

Figure 11.12 Postanaesthetic myopathy shown in the forelimb. Characteristic posture of pain with head thrown back and up when made to walk. In this case, there was hard swelling of the shoulder muscles and triceps. The posture due to pain varies with the muscles involved.

1973; Lindsay et al., 1980, 1989). Clinical surveys (Klein, 1978; Richey et al., 1990) have demonstrated that the incidence of the condition is increased by duration of anaesthesia and by periods of hypotension. In experimental circumstances, it can be induced by prolonged (three plus hours) of hypotensive anaesthesia (Grandy et al., 1987; Lindsay et al., 1989). The failure of perfusion to the muscles is a typical 'compartmental syndrome', i.e. increased pressure within the space limited by the fascial sheath of the muscle compromises the circulation. When intracompartmental muscular pressure increases to the point at which the local circulation fails, the muscle will become ischaemic. Damage will occur at reperfusion and this results in swelling and a further increase in compartmental pressure, thus worsening the situation. The potential for continuing damage at reperfusion explains why horses may appear unaffected when they first rise, the condition becoming apparent over the ensuing hours.

In order to limit the occurrence of myopathy, three factors are necessary:

1. The time of anaesthesia should be kept as short as possible and anaesthetic time should never be wasted
2. Intracompartmental pressure should be reduced to the minimum. The intracompartmental pressure in the triceps muscles of the dependent limb in a horse positioned on a hard surface may reach as high as 50 mmHg; positioning on a soft surface reduces this (Lindsay et al., 1980). However, the weight of a horse or of one of its limbs can compress veins while patent arteries allow blood to flow into muscle capillaries, thus resulting in a rapid increase in intracompartmental pressure to that of arterial pressure (Taylor & Young, 1990) and the total failure of all muscle perfusion; this is probably the reason for myopathy in the non-dependent (or upper) limbs of laterally recumbent horses
3. Blood supply to the muscles should be increased. It has been routine to assume that this means increasing MAP and, certainly, it is necessary to raise this above the 'closing pressure' within the muscle compartment. However, once MAP is above this 'closing pressure', then further improvement in muscle blood flow depends on increasing CO (Lee et al., 1998a,b,c). Positive inotropes such as dobutamine improve CO, MAP and muscle blood flow while vasoconstrictor agents increase MAP but have no action on peripheral perfusion (Fig. 11.13).

The condition described above fails to explain all cases of myopathy and it is probable that the condition is multifactorial. Klein (1978) considered that there were two distinct types of anaesthetic-induced myopathy, the compartmental syndrome and a more generalized form which she considered was more likely to occur in very fit animals;

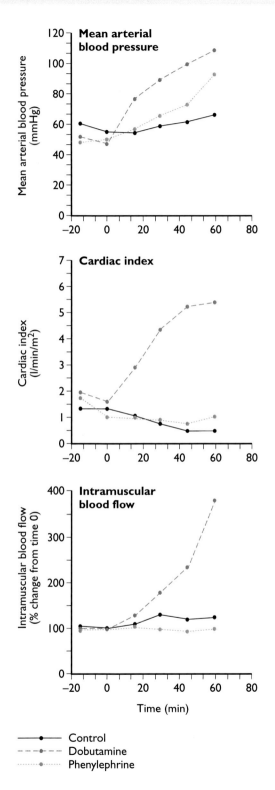

Figure 11.13 Cardiac index, mean arterial blood pressure (MAP) and intramuscular blood flow in the dependent triceps muscle in 6 halothane-anaesthetized ponies. On different occasions, the ponies were given increasing doses of infusions of one of the following: saline (control), phenylephrine or dobutamine. Dobutamine increased MAP, cardiac index and intramuscular blood flow, but while phenylephrine was equally effective in increasing MAP, it failed to improve either cardiac index or intramuscular blood flow.
Adapted from Y.H. Lee et al., 1998c.

the authors have seen two cases of acute generalized rhabdomyolysis occurring in horses 1–2 days after anaesthesia, in which post-mortem findings resembled capture myopathy. The condition has much in common with equine azoturia. It has been postulated that the nutritional status is a factor involved, but no survey has found a significant link. A genetic susceptibility is another possibility. It would appear the generalized condition is sporadic and unpredictable in occurrence.

The treatment for myopathy is mainly symptomatic: analgesia (the condition is very painful), sedation if necessary, prevention of further damage, fluids (to prevent renal damage) and a great deal of tender loving care. As much of the damage occurs at reperfusion, there could be a role for the administration of free radical scavengers but, as yet, there is no evidence as to their efficacy. It is probable that by the time the condition is diagnosed, the damage is already present.

Neuropathy

Nerves may be damaged during the anaesthetic process by the effects of pressure, of stretching, and by ischaemia. Peripheral neuropathies (such as facial nerve damage through pressure from the head collar, Fig 11.14) are easy to diagnose, but other cases (e.g. femoral nerve damage) may be difficult to differentiate from myopathy and, indeed, it is probable that the two conditions frequently occur concurrently. Neuropathy is not painful but, if it involves the motor supply to more than one limb, the horse will be unable to rise. Contused nerves may regain their function once the surrounding swelling has subsided, so symptomatic treatment should be combined with good nursing.

A very occasional but disastrous occurrence following anaesthesia is spinal malacia. The problem has only been reported to occur in young horses positioned on their back for a short procedure. Most, but not all cases have occurred in heavy horses (Brearley et al., 1986; Lam et al., 1995; Trim, 1997). Sometimes the horse fails to regain its feet following anaesthesia, other times it will stand, but an ascending paralysis commences. The condition appears totally painless; many cases have been maintained by good nursing for several days, but the condition always

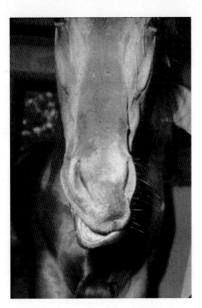

Figure 11.14 Facial nerve paresis resulting from pressure. In this case, the damage resulted from inadequate padding on the operating table but, more typically, it results from pressure exerted by a head collar.

progresses and euthanasia is inevitable. The cause of this condition is unknown.

PREPARATION FOR GENERAL ANAESTHESIA

The preanaesthetic examination and the general principles of preparation prior to anaesthesia described in Chapter 1 are, of course, applicable to horses, but there are some aspects of preanaesthetic preparation of these animals that warrant further consideration.

General considerations

Horses do not vomit, so a totally empty stomach prior to anaesthesia is less important than for small animals. However, most anaesthetists fast horses for around 8–14 hours ('food out at midnight') but leave in water until at least 2 hours prior to anaesthesia, or even until premedication. There is no good evidence to back these recommendations but, particularly in dorsal recumbency, a full stomach will limit ventilation as discussed previously. This becomes obvious when the stomach is very full, for example in some colics. Fasting is not usually employed (or often not practicable) for very short surgery such as normal castration carried out in the field. Over-long starvation is thought to increase the incidence of postoperative impacted colic. If surgery is elective, many authorities like to 'let down' extremely fit horses, reducing their plane of nutrition. Horses brought in from lush grazing develop abdominal distension if not adequately fasted. Just prior to anaesthesia, the horse's mouth should be washed out to prevent food being dislodged from the teeth and pushed into the airway by the endotracheal tube.

Shoes should be removed before anaesthesia, or at least covered with adhesive plaster, to prevent damage to flooring or the animal itself in the recovery period. The horse may receive prophylactic treatment for tetanus. Surgeons may request antibiotics are given prior to the induction of anaesthesia, some of which may influence subsequent events. Gentamicin and other antibiotics of this group will increase the length of action of neuromuscular blocking agents, and are toxic to the kidneys. The IV injection of penicillin causes marked hypotension (through vasodilation) for approximately 40 minutes (Hubbell et al., 1987), and the cardiovascular effects of many other antibiotics are unknown. Although ideally they should be avoided just prior to anaesthesia, current thinking is that high blood levels of antibiotics during surgery prevent infection, and their IV use may be considered essential to the overall success of the case.

In emergencies, the aim of preparation for anaesthesia is to improve the physical status of the horse as much as possible, and to make any preparations which may reduce the risk of the perioperative process. To detail all such preparations is beyond the scope of this chapter. Briefly, orthopaedic cases may need support to the limb to prevent damage at anaesthetic induction, and analgesia and sedation should be chosen to avoid excessive ataxia. Most acute thoracic crises are the result of trauma and horses suffering from chest injuries may be agitated, restless and dyspnoeic, and may require an analgesic both for its sake and to reduce the risk of injury to attendants. Air and/or fluid should be removed from the pleural cavity by the insertion of a chest drain before general anaesthesia is induced. In most emergency cases, hypovolaemia needs to be corrected before induction of anaesthesia. However, where blood loss is acute and the potential for further loss is still present (e.g. haemorrhage from the guttural pouch) such replacement should be limited prior to anaesthetic induction as an increase in blood pressure may result in the commencement of severe and uncontrollable haemorrhage. In such cases, the agents used for sedation and analgesia should have minimal effects (in either direction) on blood pressure. Once the horse has been anaesthetized, blood pressure will almost certainly be reduced, and it may then be necessary to administer rapidly high volumes of fluids. The most common emergency requiring preanaesthetic treatment is the 'colic' (see 'Anaesthesia for horses with colic' below).

Mares nursing foals should not be separated from their offspring in the preanaesthetic period. If it is necessary to operate on the mare, the need for sedation is greatly reduced if anaesthesia is induced in the presence of the foal. Similarly, the presence of a foal's sedated mother contributes to the smooth induction of anaesthesia in the foal.

Ideally, the weight of the horse should be determined by actual weighing, as visual estimation can be very inaccurate. If weighing facilities are not available, the formulae below were validated in over 400 horses at Cambridge University:

$$\text{Weight (lb)} = \frac{\text{Girth}^2 \text{ (inches)} \times \text{length (inches)}}{1320}$$

or

$$\text{Weight (kg)} = \frac{\text{Girth}^2 \text{ (cm)} \times \text{length (cm)}}{10815}$$

Commercially available weigh-tapes base their calculation on the girth measurement only, but still provide a useful estimate of weight, and also are often 'calibrated' to the type of horse (Thoroughbred or Warmblood).

Intravenous techniques

In horses, IV injections are usually made into the jugular vein about half way down the neck. The horse should be handled quietly, as once forcible restraint (such as the twitch) is used, many will tense their neck muscles and obscure the jugular furrow, making the danger of accidental intracarotid injection more likely. The usual aseptic precautions should be taken prior to insertion of a needle or catheter, the size of which depends on personal preference and on what is to be injected. A small fine needle (e.g. 23 G) does not necessarily cause the horse less pain than one of 19 G, but will reduce the damage to the vein which may be important if many such injections are anticipated.

The vein is distended by pressing the thumb into the jugular furrow just below the site of venipuncture (Fig. 11.15A). This tenses the skin and the distended vein is easily palpable. Two methods of placement of a needle may be used. In the first, the point of the needle is directed at an angle of 45° to the vein, slid through the skin, into the vein then advanced up the vein towards the head. This is the author's (KC) personal preference. In the second method, the needle is held at an angle of 90° to the vein, thrust into it, then turned 90° so that it can be advanced up the vessel. A good length of needle (or catheter) should be introduced into the vein otherwise there is a risk that, as the vein subsides on the release of pressure, it will retract away from the needle or that the slightest movement will cause the needle to leave the vessel. Some practitioners leave the pressure on the vein as they inject the drug; this is dangerous as it leaves irritant agents in contact with the lining of the vein, and also means when the pressure is removed, the drug enters the circulation very

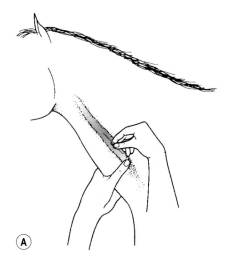

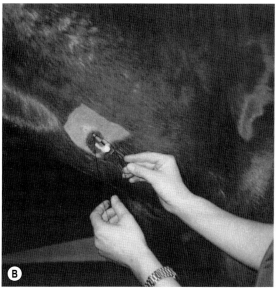

Figure 11.15 Injection into the jugular vein of the horse. (A) The vein is raised by digital pressure on the jugular grove, and the needle inserted at an angel of 45°. (B) A catheter placed towards the head is inserted in a similar manner. For catheterization, aseptic precautions are taken; and a bleb of local anaesthetic, a small hole through the skin, and pre-laying the anchoring sutures are helpful.

rapidly. A free flow of blood indicates that the needle is well placed in the lumen of the vein. If only a few drops of blood fall either (1) the needle is in a perivascular haematoma or (2) the needle is in the vein but its lumen is partially blocked. If red blood spurts, or blood is very free flowing then the needle may be in the carotid artery and should be withdrawn, the fist being placed hard into the jugular furrow over the point of injection and maintained there for at least 5minutes in order to prevent the formation of a haematoma. Unfortunately, intracarotid injection may not be recognized if a small bore needle is employed, but will be if any drug is injected, as a dramatic response is almost immediate. Once the needle is *in situ*, its hub and the syringe should be held and pressed gently and continuously against the animal's neck during any injection so that should the animal move its neck the hand (and needle) will move with the horse and thus overcome any tendency for the needle to be pulled out of the vein.

Catheterization of the jugular vein

Catheters, using over-the needles catheter as described in Chapter 10, are now routine for the administration of IV anaesthetic agents in the horse. Normal antiseptic precautions are taken. It is usually helpful to desensitize the skin by injecting a bleb of local anaesthetic subcutaneously via a very fine needle, or by using an intradermal pressure injector. It is also helpful to make a small 'prick' incision so that the delicate plastic tip of the catheter ensemble is not buckled during its passage through the skin.

Catheters may be placed going up the neck towards the head (see Fig 11.15B), or down towards the heart (Fig. 11.16). To place a catheter up towards the head, the technique is as for the jugular IV injection as described above. Once the catheter ensemble is in the vein, the plastic sheath is advanced into the vein to its maximum length, then secured in position with a partial skin thickness stitch and a stopcock or injection cap attached. The

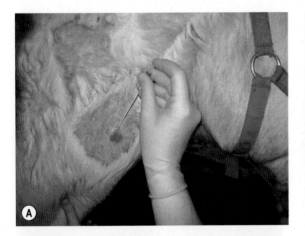
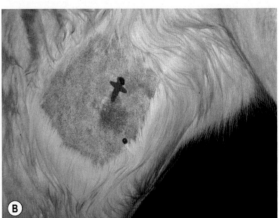
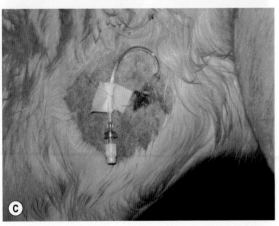

Figure 11.16 This series demonstrates insertion of a jugular catheter towards the heart. (A) The vein is held raised by a thumb in the jugular groove. There is a bleb of local anaesthetic over the insertion site and a pin-prick hole has been made in the skin. The catheter ensemble is inserted through this hole, into the vein and the catheter then slid over the needle into the vein to its full length. (B) Blood can be seen coming out of the catheter as the vein is still raised (this may take a second person) and is maintained so until the catheter is sealed, thus reducing the chance of air embolism. (C) The catheter has been sealed with a valved extension. A sticky-tape 'butterfly' was pre-laid around this extension, and sutured to the skin.
Photographs from Taylor, P.M., Clarke, K.W., 2007. Handbook of Equine Anaesthesia. 2nd edn, Elsevier Ltd, with permission.

catheter may be kept patent by periodically flushing with heparin saline solution (10 IU/mL). Ideally, the skin suture should be laid before venepuncture is attempted so that it may be tied securely around the catheter without risk of displacing this from the vein but, otherwise, the catheter may be fixed in place with a drop of acrylate glue which will hold it while the suture is completed. Catheters placed towards the head are perfectly adequate for anaesthesia unless large volumes of irritant drugs (e.g. guaifenesin) are to be infused.

Where the catheter is to stay in place for some days or where large volumes of fluids are to be infused, slightly longer catheters are placed towards the heart. Several makes of 'over-the needle' catheters of suitable length are available for the purpose and it is now not usual to need to use the 'over the wire' Seldinger technique, although this can be useful where catheterization is difficult. Figure 11.16 describes the process of placing a jugular catheter towards the heart. Care must be taken to avoid air embolism as the tip of the catheter is at a lower pressure than its hub, predisposing to the aspiration of air if the hub is not closed off. A very secure 'cap' to the catheter is essential; it must be impossible for it to be accidentally displaced and a three-way tap is not advisable. There are anecdotal reports of horses being found dead in their box, the catheter open to air. Very little air needs to be aspirated to cause the horse to collapse – the authors have seen one case resulting in collapse where aspiration was heard to occur for less than one second through a 23 G catheter.

The resistance of a catheter to infusion of fluids is governed by Poiseuille's equation; i.e. resistance is proportional to length and inversely proportional to the diameter. Thus, if fast fluid infusion is needed, relatively short wide catheters should be chosen. When catheters are left in place, there is a danger of infection and subsequent thrombophlebitis so full sterile precautions are required for their placement and in subsequent handling of the injection ports.

PREMEDICATION AND CO-INDUCTION

At one time, sedative premedication was given some time prior to induction of anaesthesia. Currently, this may still be so, or the traditional premedicant drugs may be administered either immediately before, or in combination with the anaesthetic induction agents. How, and to some extent which, agents used are a matter of personal preference, but whichever system, or combination of systems are employed, the additive effect of all agents administered should be considered together.

The choice and dose of any premedicant drug will depend on the physical condition and temperament of the horse, the likely duration of the proposed examination or operation and the nature of the anaesthetic technique to be employed. Some anaesthetists favour heavy sedative premedication which decreases the quantities of sedatives and anaesthetics administered later, while others habitually use light premedication and more of the anaesthetic. In the hands of their exponents, both regimens appear to produce similar results.

Anticholinergics

In current practice, anticholinergic drugs are not used in the routine premedication of horses, partly to avoid massive increases in MAP in response to subsequent α_2-agonists. Anticholinergics may be administered if required once the horse is anaesthetized, for example if the surgery is likely to provoke vagal reflexes or should bradycardia develop. Atropine (0.005–0.02 mg/kg) and glycopyrrolate (0.005–0.010 mg/kg) have both been used satisfactorily by IV injection (Singh et al., 1997). Hyoscine (0.1 mg/kg IV) is often used by the surgeons prior to rectal examination and, although this dose is short acting and conservative (Borer & Clarke, 2006), it will increase heart rate for around 15 minutes.

Sedatives

Premedication with sedative agents while the horse is still in its accustomed accommodation greatly improves the process of anaesthetic induction as it keeps the horse calm, reduces apprehension and fear, and makes procedures such as the placement of catheters more pleasant for both horse and anaesthetist.

Acepromazine

In many cases, acepromazine (0.03–0.05 mg/kg IM or 0.03 mg/kg IV) given 30–60 minutes prior to anaesthesia is ideal for premedication; it calms the horse without making it ataxic and its effects usually last throughout the whole perioperative period, and so contributes to a calm recovery. Acepromazine reduces the dose of the parenteral anaesthetics used and reduces MAC of volatile anaesthetic agents (Heard et al., 1986). If α_2-agonists are also used, their effect on MAC overwhelms that of acepromazine but, as their effect wanes usually after 60–90 minutes, the influence of acepromazine premedication becomes obvious; without acepromazine the depth of anaesthesia lightens very suddenly, necessitating a rapid increase in the inspired levels of volatile anaesthetic agents. The use of acepromazine for premedication significantly reduces the overall anaesthetic risk (Johnston et al., 1995).

α_2-Adrenoceptor agonists

Xylazine, detomidine and romifidine are widely used as part of the anaesthetic co-induction process and they reduce markedly the dose of both IV and inhalation anaesthetic agents. However, they may also be used as classic 'premedicants' in which case their residual action must be taken into account when deciding on doses to be used at anaesthetic induction. Doses used IV for premedication are approximately half those used for sedation (i.e. xylazine at 0.5 mg/kg, detomidine at 10 μg/kg and romifidine at 50 μg/kg) so that the horse is able to walk to the anaesthetic induction area. Intramuscular use of these agents is often neglected; 1 mg/kg xylazine or 20 μg/kg detomidine IM give excellent sedation after approximately 20 minutes. If the horse is exceptionally difficult to handle, 40–50 μg/kg detomidine (chosen because of the low volume involved) with or without butorphanol may be given IM, the horse left quietly for at least 20 minutes, after which time, in the authors' experience, IV injection has always become possible, although occasionally only with the aid of a twitch. In such horses, IM injection may be given at any convenient site (the horse often does not anticipate an injection in the pectoral muscles) as swelling at the site of injection rarely occurs after the use of these drugs.

Benzodiazepines

Diazepam and midazolam are used as part of a co-induction process (see below) rather than as classical premedicants.

Analgesics

If not already given, NSAIDs may be administered so that they will be effective by the postoperative period. In the horse (in comparison with the dog), at licensed doses, NSAIDs do not appear to cause renal damage despite intraoperative hypotension.

Opioid analgesics may be used to provide preoperative pain relief if necessary, when full analgesic doses are required, although as discussed earlier, their use is controversial. Opioids can also be used with the α_2-agonist to improve the level of sedation (see Table 11.1). Full doses may be required for difficult horses, although there is a danger the horse may become recumbent. The two drugs are often mixed in the same syringe; this is not recommended by the manufacturers as the necessary tests to ensure chemical stability have not been performed but, with difficult horses, there may only be one opportunity to carry out the injection.

INDUCTION OF ANAESTHESIA

The past 40 years have seen great improvements in equine anaesthesia, but a routine method suitable for every situation has yet to be discovered. The anaesthetist must choose a suitable method with regard to the size, health and temperament of the individual horse, the cost of the procedure and the facilities and staff available.

Facilities for induction

With the exception of occasional emergency situations, anaesthesia should never be induced in horse without there being available the necessary apparatus to resuscitate the horse should it become necessary. Such apparatus includes endotracheal tubes, methods to administer O_2 and apply IPPV, and the drugs likely to be needed should cardiac arrest occur. In the hospital setting, the apparatus needed to administer volatile anaesthetic agents (anaesthetic machine and absorber circuit) will fulfil this role. For field anaesthesia, a portable source of O_2 will be required. IPPV of the lungs can be satisfactorily provided by the use of a stream of oxygen directed into the trachea for the Venturi effect using the 'overide' facility on a demand valve, or using an easily portable to-and-fro circuit.

The cardiopulmonary system of the anaesthetized horse must be monitored continuously throughout anaesthesia, but the degree of sophistication with which this will be done will depend on the facilities available and, in the field, may be limited to those of continuous observation, palpation of the pulse, and possibly the use of a battery operated pulse oximeter. The favoured site for the oximeter probe is across the nasal septum, as it is without hair, usually without pigment, and sufficiently thin. If inhalation agents are being employed, monitoring must be of a high standard and should also include the electrocardiogram and (preferably directly measured) MAP (as described in Chapter 2). A peripheral pulse monitor, end-tidal gases and arterial and venous blood gases are very helpful.

Methods of control at anaesthetic induction

Free fall

In this simplest method of control, one person holds the horse's head as it becomes recumbent. If the horse leans back as anaesthesia takes hold, the handler holds the head down, which steadies the fall and prevents the horse going over backwards (Fig. 11.17). With the type of induction which occurs following use of the dissociative agents, this is less necessary, and the handler simply has to steady the head. If induction is in a padded box, the horse may be placed with its rump to a wall so that the wall takes the weight; this makes induction very smooth, but occasionally results in a hind leg becoming trapped beneath the horse.

The free fall method requires the minimum of staff and is the only practicable method in the field.

Gate method

This method is again simple, and is probably the most widely used in hospital situations. The horse is positioned

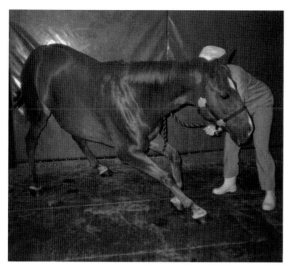

Figure 11.17 Control of a horse during induction of anaesthesia using the 'free-fall' method.

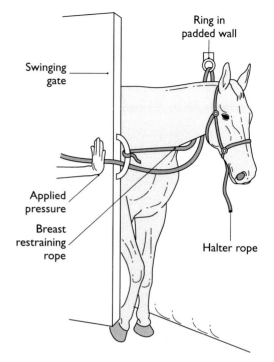

against a wall of the induction box, and restrained there by a gate. A rope, which can easily be released, holds the gate in place and prevents the horse moving forward (Fig. 11.18). When available, several people may press against the gate to support it. As anaesthesia is induced, the rope is released and the gate opened so that the horse may sink to the ground.

A variation of this method manages without the gate, the horse being held against the wall by a number of people. The horse is restrained and its weight supported as it becomes recumbent by head and tail ropes attached to rings in the wall of the induction box.

Tilting table

In this method, the operating table top is tilted to the vertical position; the adequately premedicated or quiet animal is restrained against the table top by straps (Fig. 11.19). As the horse loses consciousness during the induction process it is brought smoothly into lateral recumbency by restoring the table top to its normal horizontal position. The method usually works very well but it is only possible where an adequate number of trained personnel are available, and trouble occurs if the horse panics or a fault develops in the table mechanism at a critical stage of induction. Once the horse is unconscious, padding must be placed underneath it, so the method does not remove the necessity to lift the horse. The horse may be allowed to recover on the horizontal table top and placed on its feet as soon as it is judged able to stand by rotating the top to vertical; or the horse may be transferred to a padded recovery box.

Figure 11.18 Control of a horse during induction of anaesthesia using the 'gate' or 'swinging-door' method. Induction to recumbency is aided by two or three people applying pressure to the gate as the horse sinks towards the floor. An assistant restrains the horse's head and prevents the horse from falling forwards or backwards. The breast control rope which prevents the horse from walking forwards is slackened off as the horse becomes recumbent.

Intravenous regimens for anaesthetic induction

In normal clinical practice, anaesthesia in adult horses is induced with IV agents. The dose of anaesthetic required in the healthy horse will depend on the amount of sedative and opioid analgesic it has received both as premedication and just prior to anaesthetic administration. The number of possible combinations of sedative and anaesthetic agents which are suitable for anaesthetic induction is enormous, and the choice will depend on facilities, the state of the horse, and on personal preference. However, the majority of induction techniques are based on a combination of sedative drugs either with dissociative agents such as ketamine or with hypnotic/anaesthetic agents such as thiopental or alfaxalone. Either method may be also include the use of centrally acting muscle relaxants such as benzodiazepine agents or guaifenesin. The following section and Table 11.4 discuss some combinations which the authors have found satisfactory – there are many others that are equally satisfactory. If the horse is not

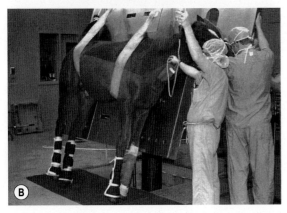

Figure 11.19 Induction of anaesthesia using a tilting table top. The sedated horse is restrained against the table which is rotated to a horizontal position as the animal becomes unconscious and relaxed.

healthy, modifications may have to be made to these protocols. For example, there may be times when the side effects of the α_2-adrenoceptor agonists are contraindicated, and conditions such as toxaemia or hypoproteinaemia reduce the quantity of anaesthetic agent required.

The regimens suggested below involve premedication or co-induction using α_2-agonists. Additional premedication with acepromazine, or the addition of butorphanol (0.01–0.02 mg/kg) does not appear to reduce the doses of agents subsequently needed to induce anaesthesia, although they may influence subsequent maintenance and/or recovery.

Dissociative agents

When the dissociative agents, ketamine or tiletamine, are given on their own to horses, they cause stimulation rather than depression of the central nervous system, with a form of excitement in which there is poor muscle relaxation, tremors and even convulsions. Many drugs have been used in attempts to suppress these most undesirable effects but only the α_2-agonists and the benzodiazepines have proved to be of any real value.

The dissociative anaesthetic agents are not effective in a single brain circulation time, and therefore where sedation with an α_2-adrenoceptor agonist has preceded the IV injection of ketamine, a large horse may take as long as 3 minutes to become recumbent. The method of achieving recumbency is a gradual process; the animal often takes a step or two sideways or backwards, its legs buckle under it, it sinks back on its haunches into sternal recumbency. It then rolls gently over on to its side and may make one or two quite vigorous limb movements before becoming still. Once laterally recumbent, the animal settles much more quickly and the onset of unconsciousness is more rapid when no attempt is made forcibly to restrain the head – if this is done, the horse may even try to rise and can be very difficult to restrain.

Ketamine–α_2-agonist

Ketamine, following premedication with an α_2-agonist produces excellent induction of anaesthesia followed by a spectacularly rapid, but usually very quiet, recovery. Xylazine 1.0–1.1 mg/kg, detomidine 15–20 µg/kg or romifidine 80–100 µg/kg is given IV and then, once maximum sedation has developed (approximately 5 minutes), a bolus of ketamine (2.2–2.5 mg/kg) is injected IV. Lateral recumbency is assumed in 1–3 minutes after the ketamine injection, the longer time occurring with the larger animals. Anaesthesia continues to deepen for 1–2 minutes after the horse becomes recumbent, and even when eye movements cease, relaxation of the jaw muscles is not always good and it may be necessary to prise the mouth open for the passage of an endotracheal tube. Relaxation will occur if more time is allowed.

Relaxation can be improved by the administration of a benzodiazepine agent IV (usually diazepam or midazolam 0.01–0.05 mg/kg), but this is not essential (Muir et al., 1977). Various anaesthetists have advocated giving the benzodiazepine before, mixed with (midazolam only) or after the ketamine injection; this author will not give it before as if anything happens to prevent the rapid follow up of ketamine, the horse becomes weak from the muscle relaxation and is very difficult to control. Benzodiazepines do cause further respiratory depression and should be used with caution in situations where facilities for IPPV are not readily available. If for any clinical reason it is desirable to give a lower dose of α_2-agonist, then the dose rate of the benzodiazepine can be increased to compensate.

The classic signs and stages of anaesthesia are not recognizable; nystagmus and tear formation may be observed and the surest guide to the depth of anaesthesia is the presence or absence of response to surgical stimulation. When no other anaesthetic is given, depending on the degree of surgical stimulation, horses first raise their heads

Table 11.4a Common regimens using dissociative agents (ketamine or tiletamine) suitable for the induction of anaesthesia prior to maintenance with volatile agents, or by TIVA

Premedication* (including drugs given a few minutes before anaesthetic)	Anaesthetic	Maintenance by further IV agents (TIVA) for short duration (20–30 mins) only
Xylazine, 1 mg/kg	Ketamine, 2.2–2.5 mg/kg plus (optional) diazepam 0.01–0.05 mg/kg **Diazepam can be given at same time or immediately following ketamine. Midazolam (0.01–0.03 mg/kg) can replace diazepam in any of the regimens.	Xylazine and ketamine; increments of half original dose- as required*** or 'Triple drip' (see text) or Thiopental 1–2 mg/kg boli as required****
Detomidine 0.015–0.02 mg/kg (15–20 µg/kg)	Ketamine, 2.2–2.5 mg/kg plus (optional) diazepam, 0.01–0.05 mg/kg as above	Ketamine 0.5–1 mg/kg as required ***. After 20–30 minutes may need a further half original dose of detomidine or 'Triple drip' ***** or Thiopental 1–2 mg/kg boli as required****
Romifidine 0.08–0.1 mg/kg (80–100 µg/kg)	Ketamine, 2.2–2.5 mg/kg plus (optional) diazepam, 0.01–0.05 mg/kg as above	Romifidine 25% original dose and ketamine 1 mg/kg as required (Data sheet recommendation)*** or 'Triple drip' or Thiopental 1–2 mg/kg boli as required****
Xylazine, 0.5–1.0 mg/kg or Detomidine, 0.01–0.02 mg/kg (10–20 µg/kg)	Tiletamine, 0.05–1.0 mg/kg IV and Zolazepam, 0.5–1 mg/kg (Tiletamine and zolazepam are supplied as a fixed 50:50 ratio combination)	
Xylazine, 1 mg/kg or Detomidine, 0.01–0.02 mg/kg (10–20 µg/kg) or Romifidine, 0.08 mg/kg (80 µg/kg)	Guaifenesin infused (approximately 15–30 mg/kg) until ataxia, then ketamine, 1.5–2.0 mg/kg	Ketamine 1 mg/kg or Thiopental, 1 mg/kg as required****

All drugs given IV unless otherwise stated. Anaesthesia results from a combination of the effects of the sedative premedicant drugs and of the induction agents. Many combinations other than those listed here can be used safely

*Additional premedication with acepromazine (<0.05 mg/kg) and/or butorphanol 0.02–0.03 mg/kg will not reduce the dose of induction agent required, but may lengthen the duration of action.

**The benzodiazepine is optional but improves relaxation. It is given with (if compatible) or immediately after the ketamine. Midazolam is thought to be more potent than diazepam; being water soluble it can be administered with the ketamine.

***Some veterinarians recommend giving ketamine based 'top ups' at set intervals but no evidence base for safe schedule.

****In some countries, thiopental is no longer available. In the future, propofol or alfaxalone may replace thiopental in these regimens (see text), but it is not yet 'routine' practice.

*****For details of 'triple drip' see Box 11.4 and Table 11.5.

10–30 minutes after the ketamine injection, roll into sternal recumbency some minutes later and stand 5 or 6 minutes after this. Termination of surgical anaesthesia is very abrupt but recovery is remarkably free from excitement and horses usually stand at the first attempt. Once standing there is very little evidence of ataxia.

Ketamine after α_2-agonists appears very safe and, with various adaptations, has become the most standard regimen for use in horses. It is not without disadvantages. The very abrupt end of surgical anaesthesia when no other agents are given can lead to difficulties and, indeed, this rapid 'awakening' may become evident even when anaesthesia is continued with volatile anaesthetic agents, although the problem is less evident with isoflurane or sevoflurane, than it was with halothane, as their uptake is much faster.

Table 11.4b Regimens using hypnotic agents (thiopental) suitable for the induction of anaesthesia prior to maintenance with volatile agents, or by TIVA

Premedication[A] (including drugs given a few minutes before anaesthetic)	Anaesthetic	Maintenance by further IV agents (TIVA) for short duration (20–30 mins) only
Xylazine, 0.5 mg/kg or Detomidine, 0.01 mg/kg (10 μg/kg)	Thiopental, 7–8 mg/kg**	Thiopental, 1 mg/kg as required** Recovery may be prolonged and of poor quality if total thiopentone dose exceeds 12 mg/kg or 'Triple drip'***
Xylazine, 1 mg/kg or Detomidine, 0.015-0.020 mg/kg (15-20 μg/kg) or Romifidine 0.08 mg/kg (80 μg/kg)	Thiopental, 5.5 mg/kg**	As above
Acepromazine, 0.03–0.05 mg/kg IM or IV	Guaifenesin infused (approximately 25–50 mg/kg) until ataxia, then thiopental, 5 mg/kg**	Thiopental, 1 mg/kg** maximal dose as above. Extra guaifenesin may be infused, but maximal doses should not exceed 50 mg/kg, or recovery may be delayed
Xylazine, 0.5–1.0 mg/kg or Detomidine, 0.01 mg/kg (10 μg/kg) or Romifidine, 0.08 mg/kg (80 μg/kg)	Guaifenesin infused (approximately 25–50 mg/kg) until ataxia, then thiopental 5 mg/kg**	As above

*Additional premedication with acepromazine and/or an opioid will not reduce the induction doses required but may lengthen recovery.
**Methohexital (at 50% that of thiopental) can replace thiopental in any of the combinations. In future propofol or alfaxalone may replace thiopental in these regimens but their use is not yet common practice.
***For details of 'triple drip' see Box 4 and Table 11.5.

Other ketamine combinations

Ketamine may also be used with other premedicant agents or in other combinations. Acepromazine premedication alone is inadequate prior to ketamine induction. Many dose schedules, for example utilizing guaifenesin together with α_2-adrenoceptor agonists and ketamine have been recommended, some of which are listed in Table 11.4.

Ketamine/benzodiazepines

Ketamine can be given with benzodiazepine agents alone (i.e. with no α_2-adrenoceptor agonists). In foals, diazepam or midazolam (0.10–0.25 mg/kg IV) followed by ketamine (2.2 mg/kg IV) gives a very satisfactory anaesthesia; usually foals lie down following the benzodiazepine drug. However, in adult horses, the combination is more difficult to employ. Neither agent should be given alone. As both have a variable onset of action, when administered together the quality of induction is very variable depending on which agent takes effect first (Clarke et al., 1997).

One study utilizing midazolam/ketamine found that even after 3 hours of subsequent halothane anaesthesia, recovery was complicated by muscle weakness and, in some cases, it was necessary to antagonize the residual midazolam. The poor quality of induction and recovery with these benzodiazepine/ketamine combinations is unfortunate as during subsequent maintenance with volatile agents, heart rate, MAP and CO are maintained at a considerably higher value than when α_2-adrenoceptor agonists are used in the induction protocol (Luna et al., 1997).

Tiletamine/zolazepam

The idea behind the combination of tiletamine with zolazepam is that there is already a benzodiazepine present to ensure muscle relaxation during subsequent anaesthesia. In the horse, however, this combination has always been used following the administration of an α_2-adrenoceptor agonist. This combination is used after xylazine (Hubbell et al., 1989) or detomidine premedication

(Muir et al., 1999). It produces reasonably safe 'short-term anaesthesia' of a little longer duration than that seen after xylazine/ketamine/diazepam.

Hypnotic/anaesthetic agents

The manner in which a horse becomes recumbent is similar following the injection of any of the hypnotic/anaesthetic agents, and is typified by that with thiopental. Following injection of thiopental, the horse tries to lean backwards and to lift its head, which must be restrained to prevent the horse losing its balance and possibly 'going over backwards'. With restraint, the horse sinks gently to the ground. Premedication with the α_2-adrenoceptor agonists slows the circulation in a dose-dependent manner and the onset of unconsciousness is delayed for 40–120 seconds after completion of the thiopental injection. The horse may make paddling or galloping movements when it first becomes recumbent; these movements disappear within 10–20 seconds as unconsciousness deepens.

Thiopental

Thiopental is a hypnotic/anaesthetic agent which has been commonly employed in equine anaesthesia. The dose required to induce anaesthesia in the horse depends on the amount of sedation present (see Table 11.4). As recovery from an induction dose of thiopental depends on redistribution rather than elimination, reduction in the dose leads to a faster and better quality recovery. Prior to the use of α_2-agonists, a number of combinations were used, and still may be in certain circumstances. Thiopental at 15 mg/kg IV can be given rapidly to unsedated colts for castration; induction is adequate but recovery, although rapid, may be very violent and this method cannot be recommended. Following premedication with acepromazine (0.03–0.05 mg/kg) given at least 30 minutes prior to anaesthesia, thiopental, at a dose of 11 mg/kg IV is a satisfactory induction technique. The horse becomes unconscious and recumbent 25–30 seconds after the thiopental injection and anaesthesia lasts for an adequate time either to enable a short procedure such as castration, or to provide a smooth transition to an inhalation agent. If no maintenance agents are given, the horse regains its feet in approximately 30–40 minutes and, although there may be some ataxia, recovery is usually calm. The dose of thiopental is critical; under dosage through underestimation of weight may lead to excitement during induction and, for this reason, it used to be common practice to follow the injection of thiopental with a small dose (0.1 mg/kg) of succinyl choline, but this agent is now used rarely.

The use of IV α_2-agonists just prior to anaesthetic induction reduces the dose of thiopental required in a dose-dependent manner, and also increases the therapeutic index of the drug, meaning that it is rare for underdosage

to cause excitement. Xylazine 1 mg/kg, or detomidine 20 µg/kg given IV 5 minutes prior to induction reduces the necessary dose of thiopental to about 5.5 mg/kg. Following doses of xylazine of 0.5 mg/kg or detomidine at 10 µg/kg IV, the dose of thiopental required is about 8 mg/kg. Anaesthesia lasts for 15–20 minutes (sufficient to enable castration) and, if no further drugs are administered, the horse will regain its feet after 30–40 minutes. As yet, there is little published information available as to the combination doses of romifidine and thiopental, partly as by the time romifidine was available, thiopental was less used than ketamine. Recovery to standing (in the absence of maintenance agents) occurs in 30–40 minutes, and with less ataxia than when higher doses of thiopental are employed.

Thiopental/guaifenesin

After premedication with acepromazine, and/or α_2-adrenoceptor agonists, guaifenesin (at concentrations of 5–15% depending on the personal preferences of the anaesthetist and the preparations available) is infused into the jugular vein until the horse shows marked ataxia (after approximately 35–50 mg/kg). A bolus IV dose of about 3.5–5 mg/kg of thiopental then produces recumbency and apparent unconsciousness. It is also possible to combine guaifenesin and thiopental solutions for infusion into the jugular vein to produce recumbency but there is much less control over anaesthesia when this is done and profound respiratory depression can be produced. Recovery from these agents alone occurs in 30–40 minutes, but there may be some residual muscle weakness if high doses of guaifenesin are used. Where anaesthesia subsequently is maintained with other agents, the effects of guaifenesin have time to wane.

Propofol

Early studies demonstrated that a rapid injection of propofol (2 mg/kg IV) appears to be just adequate for induction of anaesthesia when given 5 minutes after IV α_2-agonists such as xylazine 0.5 mg/kg, detomidine 15–20 µg/kg, or medetomidine 7 µg/kg (Nolan & Hall, 1985; Bettschart-Wolfensberger et al., 2001b). At these doses of propofol, anaesthesia appears to last for approximately 10 minutes, with recovery to standing within 30 minutes. Without premedication, a dose of 4 mg/kg propofol is necessary to induce anaesthesia and even then horses show some excitement and paddling (Mama et al., 1995; 1996). Brosnan et al. (2011) infused guaifenesin for 3 minutes (approximately 73 mg/kg) before administering propofol at 2.2 mg/kg and found this reduced the side effects and was satisfactory for induction prior to maintenance of anaesthesia with inhalation agents. With the standard 1% preparations of propofol available, it is difficult to inject even 2 mg/kg propofol sufficiently rapidly, which explains some of the poor quality anaesthetic inductions (Bettschart-Wolfensberger et al., 2001b). Muir et al. (2009) used a 10% solution of propofol and investigated doses required for induction with and without xylazine (0.5 mg/kg) premedication. Without xylazine, quality of induction was unacceptable; after xylazine 3–5 mg/kg propofol provided good quality induction.

Propofol is also used by infusion to provide TIVA (see below) and is proving useful for sedation to improve recovery (see below).

Alfaxalone

Following premedication with romifidine 100 µg/kg and butorphanol 50 µg/kg, alfaxalone 1 mg/kg in combination with diazepam 0.02 mg/kg (all IV) provided good quality of anaesthetic induction in ponies, and further boli of alfaxalone 0.2 mg/kg provided adequate anaesthesia for castration (Leece et al., 2009; Kloppel & Leece, 2011). Recovery time to standing was approximately 35 minutes. Keates et al. (2012) found alfaxalone at doses of 1 mg/kg satisfactory following xylazine (0.5 mg/kg) and guaifenesin (35 mg/kg); recovery to standing was 24–47 minutes. The pharmacokinetics of alfaxalone in the horse after this regimen were a plasma half-life of elimination of 33 minutes, clearance of 37 mL/min/kg and volume of distribution of 1.6 L/kg (Goodwin et al., 2011). These values make alfaxalone suitable for infusion. Goodwin et al. (2013) proved this by, following a very similar (but not identical) induction procedure, satisfactorily maintaining anaesthesia with infusions of alfaxalone (2 mg/kg/h) and medetomidine (5 µg/kg/h). Recovery times were a mean (SD) 37 (13.5) minutes. In all these studies, cardiopulmonary parameters were in the ranges expected for equine anaesthesia.

Other induction techniques

The dose of *methohexital* required to induce anaesthesia appears to be half that for thiopental. The non-cumulative pharmacokinetics of methohexitone make it very useful for infusion, and it was used in combination with chloral hydrate sedation to provide anaesthesia of up to an hour's duration, without lengthening recovery.

Etomidate has apparently not been used in horses, and it is probable that current preparations would result in the volume required being too large to be practicable.

Etorphine (Immobilon)

Etorphine has marketing authorization in horses as 'Large Animal Immobilon', a yellow solution containing 2.45 mg etorphine hydrochloride with 10 mg acepromazine maleate per mL. The minimum dose for horses is 0.5 mL of the solution IV per 50 kg body weight. The IM route should only be used in dire emergencies since it results in a period of marked excitement before sedation and anaesthesia ensue. Animals made recumbent with Immobilon are very stiff, with muscle tremors, severe respiratory depression, cyanosis, tachycardia and hypertension. In male animals, priapism is not uncommon. The effects of Immobilon last about 45 minutes. The actions of Immobilon may be antagonized by the injection of Revivon, a blue solution containing 3 mg/mL of diprenorphine hydrochloride. A quantity of Revivon equal to the total volume of Immobilon injected should be given IV as soon as possible after the required period of restraint is complete. Most (but not all) horses regain their feet within a few minutes of this injection. Undesirable hyperexcitability may be associated with the injection of the antagonist and enterohepatic cycling may occur, causing excitement and compulsive walking 6–8 hours after remobilization. An extra half dose of Revivon given subcutaneously at the time of initial reversal may reduce the incidence of this delayed excitement, but should it still occur, a further half dose of Revivon must be given. The product information states that horses must be kept stabled for at least 24 hours after the administration of Immobilon. Donkeys appear particularly susceptible to delayed excitement with Immobilon, and the current product information no longer gives any recommendations for this species. The dangers of etorphine to the life of the anaesthetist have been expressed forcibly in Chapter 18. Any veterinarian using Immobilon should be thoroughly familiar with the latest treatment measures set out in the product information sheet, ensure that adequate supplies of (in date) naloxone are to hand and that another qualified person is present.

Anaesthetic induction with inhalation agents

Although induction of anaesthesia in adult horses with volatile agents of anaesthesia is possible in experimental circumstances, it is not practicable for clinical use with the very limited exception of chloroform by Cox's mask. However, in foals, anaesthesia can be induced with any suitable volatile anaesthetic agent (see Anaesthesia for the Foal below).

MAINTENANCE OF ANAESTHESIA

Endotracheal intubation

In horses, the passage of an endotracheal (ET) tube presents no great problem. Three types of cuffed ET tubes are commercially available; those made of red rubber, of plastic, and of silicone. Prior to insertion, the integrity of the cuff should be confirmed over a period of time to ensure that there is no slow leak. Each anaesthetist has their own 'knack' of inserting the ET tube and the below advice is generalized.

With the anaesthetized horse in lateral recumbency, the head is moderately extended on the neck, the mouth opened, a suitable gag or bite block put in place and the tongue pulled forward. The tube, lubricated on its outside with a suitable lubricant is introduced into the mouth. With red rubber tubes, it helps if the concave side of the curve is directed towards the hard palate. The tube is then advanced, keeping to the midline, until its tip is in the pharynx. It is then rotated so that the concavity of its curve is towards the tongue (Fig. 11.20A) and, at the next inspiration, it is pushed rapidly on into the trachea. The rotation of the tube disengages the palate from the epiglottis. With the straighter shaped silicone tubes, the head needs to be more extended (Fig. 11.20B). It is often easier to insert the tube with its concavity towards the tongue, then to rotate the tube 360° once in the pharynx, once again disengaging the soft palate from the epiglottis. The commonest causes for failure of the tube to enter the trachea are that the alignment of the head and neck is incorrect, that the tube is not in the midline of the orotracheal axis, or that the tip of the tube is sited ventral to the epiglottis: should any of these occur, the tube should be withdrawn to clear the epiglottis, and redirected for a further attempt. Once in the correct position, the tube should advance down the trachea with minimal resistance; force should not be used. Resistance to passing the tube suggests either the endotracheal tube is too large, or that oesophageal intubation has occurred.

Intubation through the mouth permits the use of the largest tube which will comfortably fit the trachea. A 16.0 mm diameter tube is suitable for ponies up to about 150 kg body weight, while a 25–30 mm tube is adequate for most thoroughbreds. Heavy hunters and warmbloods often take surprisingly large tubes.

ET tubes can be passed through the inferior nasal meatus (see Fig. 11.24). Lubrication is essential, and the introduction and removal of nasal tubes entails the risk of damaging the turbinate bones, although with the modern soft silicone tubes this risk is reduced. Despite the limitations, nasal intubation can be very useful in cases where the surgeons require unobstructed access to the mouth. In young foals and in donkeys, the nasal passages are relatively much larger than in adult horses and tubes of adequate size can be introduced through the nostril.

The cuffs of ET tubes are often damaged by contact with the horse's teeth even when a reliable mouth-gag is used to keep the mouth open during intubation and extubation. Red-rubber cuffed tubes are very expensive, but punctured cuffs should not be repaired with home-made patches which may become detached in the airway during anaesthesia. Plastic tubes have met with only partial success; either the plastic is so hard that atraumatic intubation is difficult or, when they reach body temperature, they soften so much that they become obstructed when the head is flexed on the neck. Siliconized latex rubber cuffed tubes are more successful, can be recuffed and, although

the smaller versions for foals, sheep etc. may require an 'introducer' before they can be inserted, those designed for adult horses are sufficiently stiff to enable endotracheal intubation to be performed easily. Static charges on the silicone attracts dust, and it is important that after use and cleaning it is not placed where it will attract such dirt during the induction process.

As the horse has poor laryngeal tone, the cuff of the ET tube must be adequately inflated if IPPV is to be carried out, and a good seal is exceptionally important in cases of colic to prevent inhalation of regurgitated material. Cuffs should therefore be checked for leaks by leaving them inflated for a period of time prior to use.

An uncuffed tube, the 'Cole-pattern tube', has been used in horses but these tubes have to be of the exact size needed for any given animal, and accurately placed in the larynx if they are to provide a gas tight atraumatic seal and acute laryngeal oedema has been reported after their use (Trim, 1984).

Positioning for surgery

Practically the aim in positioning is:

1. To reduce to the minimum possible the pressure at all points in order to enable adequate blood perfusion to muscles and to decrease the chance of a compartmental syndrome occurring
2. To ensure that major veins are not obstructed. If this happens then pressure in the area drained by these veins will increase until it reaches arterial values, after which time there will be no further perfusion to the area
3. To avoid putting anything under tension. Nerves are particularly easily damaged by stretching as well as by direct pressure
4. To allow surgical access.

The first three aims are often at odds with the fourth, necessitating compromise and some sacrifice of surgical convenience for the benefit of the horse.

It is now generally accepted that the best method to reduce pressure on the horse's body is to position it on a soft foam mattress sufficiently deep to allow the horse to sink right in (thus reducing the unit weight at any one point) without 'bottoming' on the hard undersurface. The type of matting used in gymnastics is ideal (Fig. 11.21A) but is difficult to keep clean. Alternatives are air or water mattresses which may be partially inflated under the horse (Figs 11.21B, 11.22). It is very important that air mattresses are not fully inflated – the horse must still be able to sink in or no reduction in pressure is achieved. This is one of the times when compromise from the surgeon is necessary as operating on a horse which is lying on a soggy water or air bed is not conducive to the performance of any delicate surgery.

The edges of tables or overinflated air or water beds can cause pressure points and result in nerve or muscle

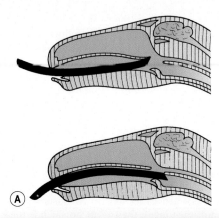

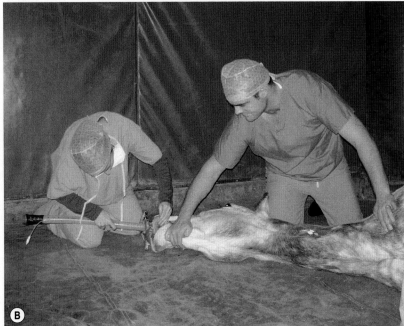

Figure 11.20 The passage of an oral endotracheal tube in a horse. (A) The horse is an 'obligate nose breather'. Tubes passed via the nasal cavity pass easily into trachea. For oral endotracheal intubation, it is necessary to disengage the epiglottis from the soft palate. With red rubber tubes, introduction with the concave cure pointing dorsally will do this; the tube is then turned through 180 degrees and advanced into the trachea. (B) For the straighter silicone tubes, extending the head sufficiently is usually more effective.
Photograph (B) from Taylor, P.M., Clarke, K.W., 2007. Handbook of Equine Anaesthesia. 2nd edn, Elsevier Ltd, with permission.

damage. Operating tables may have such 'edges' in association with sections which slide out, and if so, suitable pads and matting to cover these pressure points are essential.

When horses are positioned in lateral recumbency, the under front leg should be pulled forward, and both upper legs should be supported parallel to the body (see Fig. 11.21). This support reduces pressure on the triceps muscles, brachial vessels and nerves, and also prevents obstruction of the venous drainage of the upper limbs. Supine horses may be supported by a V-shaped back support, often inflatable. The legs may be supported on a hoist or tied to pillars but extending both hind legs, and in particular locking the stifle joints of dorsally recumbent horses, should be avoided unless absolutely essential to the surgery, as it may result in severe hind limb lameness (see Fig 11.22). This lameness is thought to be due to femoral nerve damage, but there may also be a component of gluteal myopathy. If bilateral, the horse will be unable

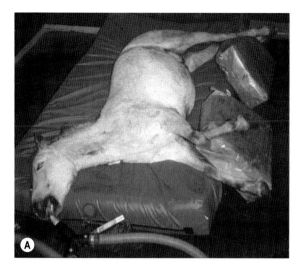

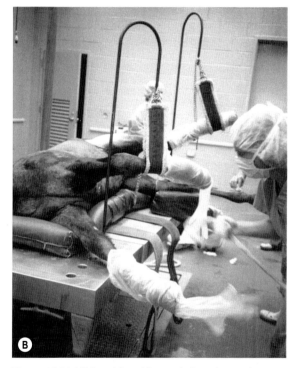

Figure 11.21 Well positioned horses in lateral recumbency. The horses sink into the foam (or 'soggy' air bed) thus reducing pressure at any one point. The upper limbs are supported so that venous drainage is not impaired, and the other forelimb is drawn right forward. While (B) demonstrates positioning with a well-designed operating table, in (A) the same effect is achieved with more primitive facilities.

to rise. The problem is unrelated to weight – the authors have seen it in miniature Shetland ponies, and it can occur after a comparatively short time.

The head is very liable to damage at pressure points and to avoid damage to the masseter muscle, facial nerve and eyes, care must be taken to ensure that the face is not allowed to fall over the edge of the table top or to remain in contact with sharp edges of halters or head collars. Whether in lateral decubitus or supine the head must not be over-extended (this leads to laryngeal paralysis) nor rotated on the neck. If possible, the head should be slightly raised during anaesthesia to ensure good venous drainage and to avoid intense vascular congestion of the nasal passages leading to gross upper respiratory obstruction after extubation. When the anaesthetized horse has to be moved, the head should be supported in a normal position in relation to the neck.

Under field conditions, the facilities may not be available to position the horse as suggested above. However, a horse in lateral recumbency may have adduction of the upper limbs prevented by supporting them on straw bales, and the undermost foreleg may be drawn as far forward as possible to minimize pressure on the brachial vessels and nerves.

Apparatus for administration of oxygen and for ventilation

As stated earlier, even for a short field anaesthetic, there should be the provision for giving oxygen and providing IPPV should respiration fail. In the hospital situation, the apparatus for delivering inhalation anaesthetic agents will provide this, whether or not anaesthetic maintenance is by TIVA or by inhalants. The basic requirements of the machines are as described in detail in Chapter 10. Anaesthetic circuits are either to-and-fro (which are portable and can be very satisfactory) but more usually are circle systems. There are now a number of commercially available large animal machines with circle systems, many of which incorporate a ventilator system. Figure 11.23 shows two relatively sophisticated examples of these, the Tafonius (Fig. 11.23B) also incorporating patient monitoring as well as machine monitoring facilities. However, many simpler systems can be adapted to enable IPPV by the addition of a suitable ventilating unit.

AGENTS FOR THE MAINTENANCE OF ANAESTHESIA

Intravenous agents: total IV anaesthesia (TIVA)

Total IV anaesthesia for short procedures in the field (such as castration) has been used for many years but with

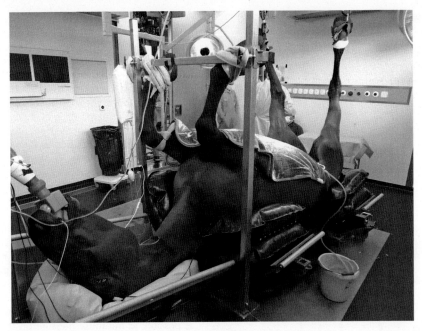

Figure 11.22 A well positioned horse in dorsal recumbency. The air-bed, which holds the horse in position, is not fully inflated – the horse sinks in. The forelimbs tied to the frame keep the position straight. The hind limbs are only partially extended; the stifles are *not* locked. The pad under the head keeps it slightly flexed to ensure that there is no strain on the laryngeal nerves. The bucket collects the urine from the catheterized bladder.
Photograph courtesy of Andrea Schwarz.

modern drugs which are rapidly metabolized and eliminated, TIVA can be used for more prolonged procedures as the duration of recovery is no longer than after anaesthesia with volatile agents.

The use of TIVA does not reduce the need for apparatus or for experienced staff. Most IV anaesthetic techniques cause as much, if not more respiratory depression, than do volatile anaesthetics and, indeed, overdose commonly causes respiratory arrest. Certainly, if it is being used in hospital conditions, it is still necessary to have a means of delivering oxygen to the horse and of providing IPPV if required. MAP is better maintained than with volatile agents, but this does not necessarily mean that there is no cardiovascular depression; CO still may be reduced and peripheral perfusion poor. Adequate cardiopulmonary monitoring is as necessary with IV as with volatile agents.

The current limitations to techniques of TIVA are those of duration and of expense. Many drugs or combinations are long acting and cumulative, so extending length of action with more drug may result in a prolonged and poor quality recovery. The ideal agents for use by infusion (propofol and some of the α_2-agonists) have pharmacokinetics such that neither they nor their active metabolites are cumulative whatever the duration of administration. In a compromise between expense and the ideal agents, the techniques suitable for TIVA can be considered in three categories: those suitable for short procedures such as castration (up to 30 minutes) and which result in a very rapid recovery; those suitable for more prolonged use (up to 1.5–2.0 hours); and those which could be extended indefinitely should the surgery demand. Procedures may last far longer than anticipated and, if necessary, anaesthetists must be prepared to change technique (e.g. to introduce volatile agents, or change to different drug combinations) if required.

TIVA for short procedures (up to 30 minutes)

The techniques for IV induction anaesthesia described above (see Table 11.4) provide adequate anaesthesia for procedures lasting 10–15 minutes and anaesthesia can be 'topped up' with increments of IV drugs for a period of time before cumulation occurs. The most commonly used combinations for short-term anaesthesia are combinations of the α_2-adrenoceptors with ketamine. Anaesthesia is then extended with incremental doses of ketamine, or if available, thiopental.

If no additional agents are given, recovery from ketamine-based methods occurs within 20–25 minutes and is usually very smooth and well controlled. However, recovery can be abrupt, and sometimes the horse may awaken during surgery with little warning so it is essential that a rapid means to deepen anaesthesia is to hand. The duration of surgical anaesthesia can be increased by the

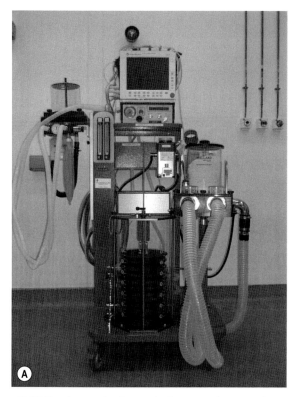 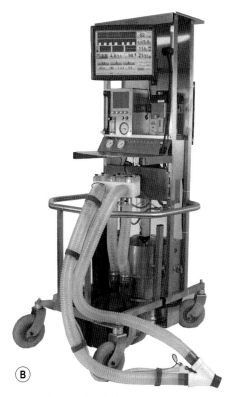

Figure 11.23 Two large animal anaesthetic systems incorporating ventilators. (A) The Mallard. The ventilator is a typical 'bag in a bottle'; air or oxygen compresses the bellows. Regulation is via a microprocessor (on the top of this unit) which enables respiratory parameters, including PEEP, to be set. The horse can breathe spontaneously from the bellows, or a rebreathing bag may be added. This unit has an additional small animal system – very useful for foals.
(Photograph courtesy of Sandra Sanchis.)
(B) Tafonius. This has a cylinder in place of the bellows, and the system is driven (very quietly) by electricity, and is governed by a very sophisticated microprocessor. With spontaneous breathing, the cylinder fills and empties, but resistance is minimal as the motor does the work (via the microprocessor). With IPPV, all respiratory parameters required can be set very accurately. The unit incorporates airway monitoring; the unit pictured had additional patient monitoring, but units without this are available.
Photograph courtesy of Keith Simpson, Vetronic Services Ltd and Stetson Hallowell, Hallowell EMC.

use of local anaesthesia; this technique is particularly suitable for castration (Portier et al., 2009). Choice of the α_2-agonist (xylazine, detomidine or romifidine) utilized prior to ketamine does not influence the quality and duration of anaesthesia, or the speed and quality of recovery (Kerr et al., 1996).

With thiopental-based methods, recovery is slower (30–40 minutes), there is some hind limb weakness, and often more that one attempt to rise is required. Nevertheless, with appropriate premedication rising is usually calm. Although the horse may still move in response to surgery (again, local anaesthesia is a good option to prevent this), it is easy to anticipate, and the abrupt awakenings seen with ketamine do not occur.

Propofol and alfaxalone were discussed in a previous section (IV induction). Alfaxalone either following romifidine/diazepam predication, or following xylazine

and guaifenesin has proved effective in providing anaesthesia for castration.

Agents used to extend the duration of anaesthesia

Any of the methods described below which are suitable for medium-term anaesthesia can be adapted for a shorter duration. However, while CRIs are preferable, in the field, extension of the induction regimen is usually by 'top-up'.

Ketamine

Anaesthesia induced with α_2-agonists/ketamine mixtures may be prolonged with additional ketamine, but there is a danger of undesirable excitatory effects unless the α_2-adrenoceptor induced sedation is still adequate. In clinical practice, incremental doses of half the original dose of both xylazine and ketamine are given as required (see Table 11.4) or at set time intervals. There will be a delay before these agents will be effective, so if the anaesthesia becomes too light, then it may be necessary to give a hypnotic agent (e.g. thiopental) to regain control, as these are effective more rapidly. With detomidine/ketamine combinations only a further dose of ketamine (1 mg/kg) is required initially to extend the duration, although if ketamine increments are to be given more than 30 minutes after anaesthetic induction, it is probably advisable also to administer a small dose of detomidine (approximately 5 µg/kg). With romifidine/ketamine combinations, the product information sheet suggests that incremental doses of 25% of romifidine but 50% of ketamine original doses are needed to extend anaesthesia.

To date, there are no scientific reports as to the use of ketamine (1 mg/kg IV) to lengthen the duration of anaesthesia induced with α_2-adrenoceptor agonist/thiopental, (with or without guaifenesin), although anecdotal reports suggest that the method is practicable.

Barbiturates – thiopental and methohexital

Small doses (0.5–1.0 mg/kg) IV may be given to extend anaesthesia that has been induced with either thiopental or with ketamine. The major advantage of thiopental is that it acts in a circulation time and is ideal to bring an awakening animal quickly back under control. However, overdose may cause apnoea and, as the drug is cumulative, speed and quality of recovery depend on the total dose. Thus, if initial anaesthetic induction was with ketamine, more increments of thiopental may be given than is advisable following induction using thiopental. A total dose of 10 mg/kg still results in a calm recovery in an acceptable time; higher total doses may be safe but will lengthen recovery.

Methohexital (0.5 mg/kg IV) can be given to extend anaesthesia in the situations where increments of thiopental would otherwise be used. However, it is very respiratory depressant and recovery is violent if the horse is not well sedated.

It is probable that propofol or alfaxalone could replace the barbiturate and extend anaesthesia but, at this time, the evidence is not available for any recommendations.

TIVA for medium duration procedures (30–90 minutes)

Anaesthesia which needs to be prolonged for more than 30 minutes is usually achieved by combinations of α_2-agonists, ketamine, and a centrally acting muscle relaxant – guaifenesin or a benzodiazepine (Table 11.5). Ideally, any drug used for infusion to provide long-term anaesthesia should have a short half-life of elimination so that there is no cumulation. Not all these agents have the ideal kinetics, hence their limitations for use beyond 90 minutes (although some extension may be possible at the expense of a more prolonged recovery).

Table 11.5 Some regimens of total intravenous anaesthesia (TIVA) suitable for providing anaesthesia from 30 to 90 minutes duration

Premedication	Anaesthetic	Maintenance
Xylazine, 1 mg/kg or Detomidine, 0.02 mg/kg (20 µg/kg) or Romifidine, 0.08–0.1 mg/kg (80–100 µg/kg)	Ketamine, 2.0–2.2 mg/kg	The 'Triple Drip', a combination of guaifenesin, α_2-adrenoceptor agonist and ketamine infused to effect. For details of how to prepare suitable mixtures, see Box 11.4
Xylazine, 1 mg/kg	Ketamine, 2.0–2.2 mg/kg, midazolam 0.1 mg/kg	Infusion of midazolam (0.002 mg/kg/min), ketamine (0.03 mg/kg/min) and xylazine (0.016 mg/kg/min) (Hubbell et al., 2012) For details of another similar combination, and antagonism of midazolam with flumazenil, see Box 11.4.
Acepromazine, 0.03–0.05 mg/kg IM or IV	Chloral hydrate (10%) infused until ataxia (50–60 mg/kg), then thiopental, 5–6 mg/kg or methohexital, 2.5–3.0 mg/kg	Thiopental, 1 mg/kg (maximal total dose 12 mg/kg) or methohexital, 0.5 mg/kg. If anaesthesia needs to be extended beyond 45 minutes, more chloral hydrate may be required

All agents are given IV unless otherwise stated. Many variations of these combinations can be used safely. Additional premedication with acepromazine (<0.05 mg/kg) may also be used. Additional premedication with an opioid (e.g. butorphanol 0.02–0.03 mg/kg) will not reduce the doses of anaesthetic induction agents.
Regimens including propofol or alfaxalone have not been included here as available concentrations and costs involved mean that they are not practicable for clinical use, but see text for details.
Thiopental, methohexital and chloral hydrate are not available in all countries but information on the combination remains as, where available, it has proved a useful 'field' method when facilities are very limited.

Xylazine and detomidine have adequately rapid kinetics, but residual guaifenesin will cause muscle weakness in recovery, so methods that reduce the dose of this component are preferred. If benzodiazepines are used, then they can be antagonized at the end of surgery – this is expensive. Theoretically, ketamine is not cumulative, but if used by infusion for periods of more than 90 minutes, prolonged and poor quality apparently hallucinatory recoveries have been seen (Bettschart-Wolfensberger et al., 1996). It is postulated that the cause of these poor quality recoveries is the cumulation of the active metabolite, norketamine. The cumulation of norketamine will depend on total dose of ketamine rather than on time, so combinations which can reduce the rate of infusion of ketamine may be used for a longer period.

The ideal agents for anything but short-term anaesthesia is propofol; that will be considered below in the section for prolonged TIVA.

α₂-Agonist/guaifenesin/ketamine – the 'Triple Drip'

The 'Triple Drip' was first used by Greene et al. (1986) who used IV xylazine (1.1 mg/kg) followed by ketamine 2.2 mg/kg for anaesthetic induction, then maintained anaesthesia with an IV infusion of 2.75 mL/kg/h of a guaifenesin/ketamine/xylazine mixture containing 50 mg guaifenesin, 1 mg ketamine and 0.5 mg of xylazine/mL of 5% dextrose in water. This technique, and adaptations of it using different α₂-adrenoceptor agonists are now widely used in operations of up to 90 minutes of duration.

Anaesthetic induction should preferably avoid guaifenesin in order to reduce the total dose of this long-acting agent. There are several recommended combinations for making up the mixture which is then infused to effect (Box 11.4).

Recovery from prolonged infusion of the Triple Drip is not fast (often more than one hour) but is usually calm. Romifidine has been used as the α₂-adrenoceptor agonist component of the combination (McMurphy et al., 2002, Gasthuys, 2011).

α₂-Adrenoceptor agonist/ benzodiazepine/ketamine

The replacement of guaifenesin by a benzodiazepine agent can improve the quality of recovery. The system has been most widely used in Switzerland, where both the benzodiazepine climazolam and its antagonist sarmazenil have been available. Anaesthesia is induced with xylazine and ketamine, then climazolam is given at 0.2 mg/kg IV. Anaesthesia is maintained with an infusion of climazolam 0.4 mg/kg/hr and ketamine 6 mg/kg/h. Infusion ceases at the end of surgery, but the benzodiazepine is not antagonized with sarmazenil (0.04 mg/kg IV) for 20 minutes in order to give time for the ketamine effects to

---

Box 11.4 The 'Triple Drip'

Guaifenesin may be available in plastic bottles as stabilized solutions of 10% or 15%, or as a solid that is made up to the strength required (usually 5%). The more concentrated the solutions the more likely to cause thrombophlebitis.

Guaifenesin is cumulative. Doses totally over 100 mg/kg result in a prolonged and ataxic recovery. It is preferable that the method used to induce anaesthesia does not include guiaphenesin (see Table 11.4).

There are a number of different recipes; all appear to be satisfactory.

10% Guaifenesin (Taylor and Clarke, 2007)

To 500 ml of 10% guaifenesin, add 1000 mg (1 g) of ketamine and *one* of the following: 500 mg of xylazine or 10 mg detomidine or 25 mg romifidine.

Following induction of anaesthesia, the 'Triple Drip is infused to effect. The average rate needed to maintain anaesthesia is 1 mL/kg/h. Higher rates may be needed earlier in procedure and rates should be reduced towards the end of surgery.

5% Guaifenesin (Author (CT)'s preference)

To 1 L (1000 ml) of 5% guaifenesin add 1300 mg of ketamine and 650 mg of xylazine. This recipe has a lower % of guaifenesin and relatively more xylazine and ketamine. Infusion rate is approximately 2 mL/kg/h.

Benzodiazepine-'Triple Drip' (*Auer, 2013)

To 500 mL of saline add 15 mg midazolam, 1000 mg ketamine and 250 mg xylazine or 1.4 mg detomidine. Infusion rate is approximately 1.2 mL/kg/h. 15 minutes after the infusion is stopped, 0.001-0.002 mg/kg (1-2 µg/kg) flumazenil may be given to reverse midazolam. This recipe gives a relatively lower dose of midazolam than that recommended by Hubbell et al. (2012)

*personal communication to KC.

---

have waned (Bettschart-Wolfensberger et al., 1996). A relatively similar protocol was recently reported by Hubbell et al. (2012). Following induction of anaesthesia with xylazine (1 mg/kg), midazolam (0.1 mg/kg) and ketamine (2.2 mg/kg), they infused a combination of midazolam (0.002 mg/kg/min), ketamine (0.03 mg/kg/min) and xylazine (0.016 mg/kg/min) for anaesthesia lasting around 60 minutes. Some horses required additional ketamine boli, but anaesthesia and recovery were satisfactory. A similar combination (Box 11.4) has been used extensively in Switzerland and Austria (Ulrike Auer, personal communication to KC, 2013), both for 'field anaesthesia' or, at approximately half the infusion rate, as an adjunct to inhalation anaesthesia (Mosing, 2007; Ambrisko et al., 2012). At the end of anaesthesia, a period of 15 minutes is allowed for reduction of ketamine effects, then 1–2 µg/kg flumazenil given very slowly IV over 60 seconds. Recovery is usually of good quality.

Chloral hydrate/barbiturate

Chloral hydrate lost favour due to its irritant nature if injected outside the vein and to the fact that if used alone recovery is very slow. However, in combination with the barbiturates, it gives good moderate-term anaesthesia and administration through long IV catheters reduces the risk of perivascular injection. A 10% solution is infused until the horse becomes ataxic (after 40–60 mg/kg have been administered) when thiopental (5 mg/kg) or methohexital (2.5 mg/kg) is injected IV as a bolus. Surgical anaesthesia is maintained by injection of increments of barbiturates (thiopental 1 mg/kg or methohexital 0.5 mg/kg). If anaesthesia is to extend for more than 45 minutes, it may prove necessary to give more chloral hydrate (approximately 10 mg/kg but to effect). If no further chloral hydrate is given, the horse will stand some 50–60 minutes after anaesthetic induction and recovery is usually calm. Cardiopulmonary parameters of this combination have never been investigated, but while anaesthetized, respiration is well maintained, the pulse is strong and mucous membranes are a healthy pink with a fast capillary refill time, all suggesting that there is minimal cardiovascular depression with this combination.

TIVA for long procedures (2 hours and more)

Propofol combinations

The only anaesthetic agent which has undergone sufficient investigation and is sufficiently non-cumulative in the horse to be used for very prolonged anaesthesia is propofol (Nolan et al., 1996). Propofol, however, has several drawbacks: it is a poor analgesic, it produces severe respiratory and moderate cardiovascular depression, and its carrier results in accumulation of triglycerides in blood. In the horse, there are additional disadvantages with existing preparations, large volumes are required and, at such volumes, it becomes very expensive. There must also be some concern as to the dangers of triggering hyperlipaemia in susceptible individuals, although to date, this complication has never occurred. Nevertheless, if TIVA is ever to become practical for anaesthesia of unlimited time in the horse, propofol is the agent most likely to be involved.

In ponies, premedicated with xylazine, Nolan and Hall (1985) required infusion rates of propofol of up to 0.2 mg/kg/min. In a very recent pharmacokinetic study, Boscan et al. (2010) maintained anaesthesia with a propofol infusion of approximately 0.14 mg/kg/min. However, over the past 20 years, a large number of studies have looked at methods to reduce the dose of propofol by providing analgesia and further sedation (Nolan & Hall, 1985; Nolan et al., 1996; Flaherty et al., 1997; Mama et al., 1998; Bettschart-Wolfensberger et al., 2001a; Matthews et al., 1999; Ohta et al., 2004, Umar et al., 2006, 2007). Most combinations utilize α_2-agonists, with or without ketamine. In all studies, the authors commented

on the fact the horse appeared very lightly anaesthetized, yet did not respond to surgery.

Betschart-Wolfensberger (2001a) investigated the use of continuous propofol and medetomidine infusions to provide 4 hours of anaesthesia in ponies. Medetomidine was chosen for its kinetics and its marked analgesic properties. Anaesthesia was induced either with medetomidine/propofol or medetomidine/ketamine and an infusion of medetomidine at 3.5 µg/kg/hour commenced. The minimum propofol infusion required to prevent response to a noxious stimulus ranged from 0.06 to 0.11 mg/kg/min and cardiovascular parameters were well maintained although oxygen supplementation was required to prevent hypoxia. Following 4 hours anaesthesia recovery occurred in approximately 30 minutes, and was of excellent quality. Mama et al. (1998) investigated the use of xylazine infusions of 35 µg/kg/min together with propofol at either 0.15 or 0.25 mg/kg/min for one hour; anaesthetic quality was excellent but, at the higher doses, there was marked hypoxia and recoveries were delayed. Flaherty et al. (1997) maintained anaesthesia in ponies with an infusion of ketamine (40 µg/kg/min) and propofol (0.124 mg/kg/min); anaesthesia was adequate for castration and recovery was smooth. Umar et al. (2007), in horses which had received medetomidine, ketamine and midazolam in the induction regimen, compared propofol TIVA (0.22 mg/kg/min) with a group receiving a CRI of propofol (0.14 mg/kg/min), ketamine (1 mg/kg/h) and medetomidine (1.25 µg/kg/h); both regimens gave adequate anaesthesia but heart rate and resultant CO were reduced in the group where medetomidine had been infused.

These and other propofol combinations have been used successfully in clinical situations but, although the price of propofol has reduced, the regimen is still too expensive for routine clinical use. Likewise, alfaxalone may well be suitable for prolonged TIVA, but as yet would be impracticable in the horse.

ANAESTHETIC MAINTENANCE WITH INHALATION AGENTS

Volatile agents

The four volatile agents suitable for and most used for maintenance of anaesthesia in the horse are isoflurane, sevoflurane, desflurane and, still in use in many parts of the world, halothane. Their main properties relating to uptake and elimination and cardiopulmonary changes have been described in Chapter 7, and will only be briefly revised here.

For all four agents, judgement of depth of anaesthesia is difficult in the horse, especially if an α_2-agonist has been used within the premedication/induction regimen, which it most usually has. Ideally, at least one eye should be rotated slightly forward, and eyes should be moist. Nystagmus may be seen if anaesthesia is very light, but also with ketamine, and if the horse is on the point of death. Decreases in MAP can give an indication of increasing depth of anaesthesia, but modern practice of treating hypotension with positive inotrope agents will counteract this fall and remove this sign. Often, the first sign of inadequate anaesthesia is that the horse starts to move; there may be no warning increase in pulse rate or MAP. It is advisable to have a bolus of rapidly acting IV anaesthetic to hand. Supplementary local anaesthetic nerve blocks, where practicable, reduce the chance of the horse kicking in response to surgical stimulation (Haga et al., 2006). Monitoring of end-tidal anaesthetic agent is very helpful as it provides a measure of the alveolar and therefore the arterial concentration of the anaesthetic and if that should be adequate for the maintenance of anaesthesia.

Halothane

Halothane's advantages in equine anaesthesia are reasonably rapid induction and recovery, minimal excitement during induction or recovery, adequate reflex suppression and sufficient muscle relaxation to allow most surgery to be performed, and ease with which anaesthesia can be controlled. The disadvantages are dose-dependent fall in MAP and CO due to a direct depressant effect of the agent on the myocardium (Hall et al., 1968). There is a marked respiratory acidosis in spontaneously breathing halothane-anaesthetized horses and, while this can be overcome by IPPV, this causes a further fall in CO (Steffey & Howland, 1978). Schatzmann (1982) showed that hypoxaemia causes a respiratory drive in horses anaesthetized with halothane in air, thus demonstrating that hypoxia can overcome halothane-induced respiratory depression.

The MAC value for halothane is about 0.9%. The end-tidal concentration of halothane required for surgery depends on the sedative premedication and anaesthetic induction technique employed, but usually approximate to 0.9–1.1%.

Halothane is a poor analgesic; horses which are apparently well anaesthetized may respond suddenly to surgical stimulation. Many of such responses are spinal reflexes.

Horses normally regain their feet within about 30–40 minutes following the termination of halothane administration after induction with xylazine/ketamine; after acepromazine premedication and thiopental induction, recovery takes about twice as long. Shivering is often seen during recovery; the reason is unknown. Quality of recovery depends on the injectable drugs which have been administered, on the surgery performed and the presence or absence of pain. Horses may take several attempts to rise, and show a measure of incoordination after recovery from halothane, but usually remain calm. However, horses should not be made to walk (e.g. from recovery to loose box or stall) within 10– 15 minutes of standing up.

Isoflurane

Isoflurane has been used for anaesthesia in horses for nearly 30 years (Steffey, 2002). In many ways, it is very similar to halothane, and the signs of depth of anaesthesia in horses and the potential for a sudden response to surgery are identical with both agents. The major differences are that the uptake and elimination of isoflurane are faster than of halothane; although blood pressure falls, it is mainly through vasodilation, and CO is better maintained (Steffey & Howland, 1978; Lee et al., 1998b; Raisis, 2005). Isoflurane is more respiratory depressant than is halothane and it is often necessary to use IPPV on isoflurane-anaesthetized horses as slow respiration prevents uptake of the agent early in anaesthesia. This latter problem could also be caused by the irritant nature of isoflurane on the airways. The MAC of isoflurane is around 1.3–1.4%. Its kinetics mean that induction and changes in depth of anaesthesia are rapid and recovery is impressively quick. However, the quality of recovery can be poor (Rose et al., 1989) and it is usual to administer a further dose of an α_2-agonist or other sedatives (see Anaesthetic Recovery period) at the end of anaesthesia to delay recovery and improve its quality.

In horses, there is no evidence that isoflurane is safer than halothane for anaesthesia; indeed, the multicentre survey of equine deaths associated with anaesthesia directly comparing the two agents showed that while horses anaesthetized with halothane were more likely to die on the table, those with isoflurane were more likely to die afterwards, and that the overall mortality did not differ (Johnston et al., 2004).

Sevoflurane

MAC of sevoflurane in the horse is 2.3% (Aida et al., 1994). Like other volatile anaesthetic agents, sevoflurane causes dose-related depression of respiration, CO and MAP (Aida et al., 1996; Steffey, 2002; Steffey et al., 2005a) but clinically, following anaesthetic induction with injectable agents, the cardiopulmonary depression is similar in extent to that caused by isoflurane (Grosenbaugh & Muir, 1998). Driessen et al. (2006) found that horses anaesthetized with sevoflurane needed less cardiovascular support than those anaesthetized with isoflurane. The speed with which anaesthesia can be deepened means there is rarely a need to give additional injectable anaesthetic agents during anaesthesia. However, the rapidity of uptake is such that care must be taken not to overdose in the early stages of anaesthesia. Recovery from anaesthesia is very fast, but its quality is variable. Without further sedation, the authors have found it to be poor, but if xylazine is administered to horses as soon as sevoflurane is terminated acceptable quality recovery occurs in about 30 minutes, and is often better than following isoflurane anaesthesia (Matthews et al., 1998). Leece et al. (2008) found no difference in either time to or quality of recovery in horses following isoflurane or sevoflurane anaesthesia.

293

Over the past 10 years, sevoflurane has become very popular for use in equine anaesthesia, its major advantage being seen as the ease of maintaining a stable level of anaesthesia, coupled with a rapid recovery.

Desflurane

The few studies that have been performed suggest that desflurane has major advantages for use in horses (Jones et al., 1995; Clarke et al., 1996; Tendillo et al., 1997). The kinetics of desflurane are such that the end-tidal concentration reaches inspired concentrations in a matter of minutes, even in a large horse, and recovery is equally as fast. Consequently, control of anaesthesia is very easy. The MAC of desflurane in the horse is approximately 8%; following IV induction, the horse is connected to the circle circuit which has been primed with 8% desflurane in O_2. In the first 10 minutes the circle system is emptied twice to reduce the contained N_2 concentration but, after this time, the circuit can be run closed – the fresh gas flow rate still containing 8% desflurane, together with enough O_2 to replace that lost by utilization and by leaks from the circuit (usually about 3 L/min in a large horse). The low flow rates used throughout mean that desflurane becomes comparatively inexpensive to use. If anaesthesia is too light, the bag is emptied and refilled with a concentration 1% above the previous level, and depth of anaesthesia changes within a very short space of time. Horses anaesthetized with desflurane rarely react suddenly or violently to surgical stimulation but, occasionally, if anaesthesia is too light, they exhibit muscle tremor and it is sometimes necessary to increase inspired desflurane concentration to as much as 10% to stop this. Recovery from anaesthesia is also very fast – unsedated animals attempt to rise within 6–10 minutes of withdrawal of desflurane and, although they remain calm, are still weak and may fall forward. It is now routine to administer a small dose of IV xylazine (0.1– 0.2 mg/kg,) or xylazine/propofol (Steffey et al., 2009) at the end of anaesthesia, after which horses get to their feet in about 15–20 minutes in a calm and coordinated manner.

The use of desflurane is not without its problems. Cardiopulmonary depression is dose dependent and is similar to that of equipotent doses of isoflurane (Clarke et al., 1996, Steffey et al., 2005b). At alveolar concentrations sufficient for surgery, CO is well maintained, although there is marked hypotension. The rapid kinetics and very fast change in depth of anaesthesia mean that is easy to overdose and, in early work, before it was realized that the initial inspired concentration of desflurane needed to be very little higher than MAC, some horses became very hypotensive (Jones et al., 1995).

The rapid and complete nature of recovery from desflurane means that it is an excellent anaesthetic agent in horses, the major problem being its need for a special vaporizer (see Chapter 9). Anecdotally (Driessen, personal communication to KC, 2012), it is being used

clinically, but as yet there are few peer-reviewed published reports.

Nitrous oxide

The use of N_2O is controversial. Its analgesic properties ensure that less of the volatile agents which lack analgesic properties are required. The disadvantage lies in the potential for causing hypoxia. N_2O will reduce the PiO_2 and particular care needs to be taken when it is used in a rebreathing system. N_2O also passes into the gut spaces, increasing their volume and reducing FRC, thus resulting in a greater fall in PaO_2 than can be explained by the reduction in PiO_2 alone (Lee et al., 1998a). The use of N_2O at the phase of transfer from IV induction to maintenance speeds uptake of the volatile agent by the 'second gas effect'. However, with the rapid kinetics of the volatile agents in use, this effect is no longer necessary. N_2O can provide useful analgesia but, in the horse, it should be used only in situations where it is possible to monitor inspired oxygen concentrations and arterial blood gases.

General points in relation to maintenance of anaesthesia using volatile agents

Practical administration

As illustrated above (see Fig. 11.23), in equine anaesthesia, volatile anaesthetic agents are administered via a circle or to-and-fro absorption system using an out-of circuit vaporizer and, for reasons of economy, they should be used with as low a flow of fresh gas as is practicable. The limitations to the use of minimum flows in the early phase of anaesthesia are: (1) the necessity to remove nitrogen from the animal and the breathing system; and (2) the need to maintain adequate inspired concentrations of volatile agent at a time when it is being taken up by the animal (see Chapter 3). For halothane or isoflurane, at the outset, the anaesthetic system should be primed with O_2 or an air/O_2 mixture and up to 4% of the volatile agent (less in animals with circulatory dysfunction). Following anaesthetic induction, the horse is connected to the system with fresh gas flow of 6–8 L/min (still carrying up to 4% of the anaesthetic agent). The excess of gas is vented via the (scavenged) exhaust valve, thus keeping the inspired anaesthetic agent concentration at an adequate level. The vaporizer setting is reduced in accordance with the clinical needs of the animal. At the end of 10–15 minutes, provided the reservoir bag is filling well, the fresh gas flow can be reduced to about 4 L/min. At these flows rates, with a large horse given halothane, the inspired concentration will be approximately half that of the vaporizer setting; a little higher with isoflurane. The reason for this is that the mass of halothane or isoflurane delivered to the circuit at this low flow rate is insufficient in the first few hours of the anaesthetic period to make up the net losses from the breathing system to the animal's tissues. Reducing the flow rate still further (the minimum needed is that required to keep the reservoir bag filled) will increase the difference between inspired concentrations and the vaporizer setting. If the depth of anaesthesia needs to be altered, the reservoir bag should be emptied and the new concentration of agent given with a high flow of O_2 until the required depth is achieved.

The more insoluble the anaesthetic, the shorter the time required for the tissues to become saturated and therefore the closer is the inspired concentration to the vaporizer setting. As isoflurane is less soluble than halothane, the vaporizer setting and the flow rates can be reduced a little more rapidly; with sevoflurane, these changes occur even faster and, with desflurane, inspired settings are close to those of the vaporizer within minutes, even when very low flow rates are used throughout.

With all volatile anaesthetic agents, difficulty can be experienced in the transition to anaesthesia after induction by an IV technique. When the horse is first connected to the breathing system, respiratory arrest frequently occurs as a result of drug-induced respiratory depression, removal of the hypoxic drive through high PiO_2 (Steffey et al., 1992) and, possibly, the sudden imposition of expiratory resistance. The problem can be overcome by IPPV, but careful monitoring is needed to ensure that overdose does not occur. Attempts to hasten the uptake by the administration of high-inspired concentrations can provoke cardiovascular collapse.

Supplementary analgesia

Ideally, additional analgesia should be provided to horses prior to the start of painful surgery. Local nerve blocks, where practicable, totally reduce response to surgery and may also provide postoperative analgesia. NSAIDs are often given preoperatively or intraoperatively but there is no evidence that their use reduces MAC. The place of opioids is controversial; many anaesthetists consider that butorphanol (0.02–0.04 mg/kg) or morphine (0.1–0.2 mg/kg) improve the quality of anaesthesia and prevent movement in response to surgery but, in some individual animals, even under anaesthesia, their effect is to produce 'excitement' and the dose of volatile anaesthetic needs to be increased to counteract this. Experimental studies have failed to demonstrate an action of opioids on MAC in the horse (reviewed by Clutton, 2010). Once the horse has responded to surgery, a small dose of thiopental (0.5–1 mg/kg) will rapidly regain control, although it may cause a fall in MAP and transient apnoea. Incremental doses of ketamine (0.1–0.2 mg/kg IV) may be given for additional analgesia, but the total dose of increments should preferably not exceed 2 mg/kg, and should not be limited towards the end of anaesthesia. Other options include analgesic infusions and are discussed below (partial IV anaesthesia, or PIVA; also known as supplementary IV anaesthesia).

Partial intravenous anaesthesia (PIVA)

The hypothesis behind PIVA is that volatile anaesthetic agents cause cardiovascular depression; if you can reduce the amount of volatile agent, you will reduce the depression. The problem is that often the infusions also cause cardiovascular depression, and the overall result is no better, and sometimes worse, than with volatile agent alone. Many IV techniques maintain a good MAP, but through vasoconstriction, and CO may well be reduced. A wide variety of combinations has been used; far too many to cover all here. Knowledge of the effects of some infusions has an adequate experimental base, but others and their combinations appears to have been 'trialled' in the clinical situation. The main infusions used are as follows.

Lidocaine

Lidocaine infusions reduce MAC (Doherty & Frazier, 1998; Rezende et al., 2011) and the volatile agent 'sparing' action has been confirmed in all clinical studies. Reported doses used are in the region of a loading dose of 1.3–2 mg/kg given slowly over 10–15 minutes followed by a CRI of 50 µg/kg/min. Lidocaine also improves gut motility, and it therefore is often used during surgery for colic. It is recommended that lidocaine infusions cease 30 minutes prior to stopping the volatile agent in order to improve quality of recovery and reduce ataxia (Valverde et al., 2005). However, CO and other cardiovascular parameters did not differ between horses in which anaesthesia was with sevoflurane alone, or with a lidocaine infusion and sevoflurane such that MAC equivalents were the same in both groups (Wagner et al., 2011). Thus, at least with sevoflurane, lidocaine infusions do not improve the cardiovascular status under inhalation anaesthesia.

α₂-Agonists

Many α_2-agonists have been infused to provide analgesia during both TIVA and inhalation anaesthesia. Doses which have been used are given in Box 11.1. α_2-Agonists consistently reduce MAC (Bettschart-Wolfensberger et al., 2001c; Gonzalo-Marcilla et al., 2012). In many, but not all, clinical studies the isoflurane or sevoflurane-saving properties remained; the exceptions probably relating to the judgement of clinical anaesthetic depth. All studies comment on the good quality of recovery. Arterial blood pressure has always been well maintained. However, α_2-agonists reduce heart rate, and the studies in which CO has been measured, have found that CO in the α_2-agonist group, although satisfactory, is usually less than the comparison group (Ringer et al., 2007). Thus α_2-agonist infusions are useful to maintain a stable level of anaesthesia, to increase blood pressure, to improve recovery, but not to reduce overall cardiovascular depression.

Opioids

As already discussed, opioids do not reduce MAC of inhalation anaesthetic agents in horses. This lack of 'sparing' effect also occurs during clinical anaesthesia. Studies have used butorphanol infusions (loading dose 25 µg/kg, CRI 25 µg/kg/h) or morphine (loading dose 0.15 mg/kg, CRI 0.1 mg/kg/h) in addition to inhalation anaesthesia that was also supplemented by other agents; there was no 'volatile agents sparing effect' but also no differences in cardiovascular parameters nor in recovery quality (Bettschart-Wolfensberger et al., 2011; Villalba et al., 2011).

Ketamine

Muir & Sams (1992) demonstrated that ketamine, infused to produce set target plasma concentrations, reduced halothane MAC. MAC reduction started at plasma values >1 µg/mL and had maximal effect (a 37% reduction) at approximately 10 µg/mL. Cardiac output was increased, with other cardiovascular parameters unchanged. In most clinical studies, ketamine infusions have been combined with other infusions making it difficult to assess the influence of ketamine alone (e.g. Enderle et al., 2008; Villalba et al., 2011; Hubbell et al., 2012). No loading dose is needed as ketamine is used to induce anaesthesia. Infusion doses are then 0.03–0.05 mg/kg/min; with the higher doses reducing infusion rate after 50 minutes.

Treatment of circulatory depression

In the horse, hypotension is common during anaesthesia with volatile agents and, as this parameter is easy to measure, it has usually been routine practice to equate such hypotension with cardiovascular depression. However, it is now realized that, although it is essential that MAP is adequate to perfuse vital organs, once this 'opening' pressure is reached then, as discussed above, perfusion and peripheral blood flow depend on CO. Improving MAP by vasoconstriction may result in a fall in CO, presumably as the result of increased afterload (Wagner et al., 1992; Lee et al., 1998c). The aim of cardiovascular support is, therefore, to increase ABP to an acceptable level (usually taken as a MAP of 65–70 mmHg) by the improvement of CO and blood flow. A number of methods of providing such support have been advocated and investigated in horses anaesthetized with volatile agents. Often the findings concerning efficacy and dosage at different centres do not agree, probably because of differing responses in individual animals. In clinical practice,

more than one of these methods of support may be needed. Few studies have examined such treatments in horses anaesthetized with IV agents, although it is now recognized that cardiovascular support still may be required if good peripheral perfusion is to be maintained.

Increase in circulating fluid volume

It is usual practice to infuse fluids (Hartman's or similar) throughout anaesthesia at a rate of 10 mL/kg/hour. There appears to be no evidence base for this figure, and at this rate it does not prevent the hypotension induced by the volatile anaesthetic agents. In the author's experience, if given for a long period (4 hours plus) to anaesthetized normovolaemic horses, it results in perioperative peripheral oedema. It does, however, maintain an 'open vein' and provide a port for IV drug adminstration.

The hypothesis behind the administration of fluid to the anaesthetized horse is that an increase in the circulating fluid volume to match the increased volume of the dilated vascular bed will restore the venous return. It is difficult to give an adequate bolus to achieve this with electrolytes. The use of hypertonic saline (4 mL/kg) in anaesthetized horses is used frequently. When given prior to anaesthesia and followed by a slower infusion of lactated Ringer it improves blood pressure during anaesthesia (Dyson & Pascoe, 1990). However, Gasthuys et al. (1994) found that when hypertonic saline was given to halothane anaesthetized ponies, the improvement in CO and MAP was significant only at a time point 5 minutes after the cessation of infusion. During the actual infusion of hypertonic saline MAP fell, and these workers suggest that the method is not ideal where hypotension is already severe. Gelatin-based compounds are not suitable as volume expanders in the normovolaemic horse (Taylor, 1998) as the volumes required are too great and, indeed, some ponies developed pulmonary oedema. Hallowell & Corley (2006), in a clinical study in horses undergoing surgery for colic, found that CO under anaesthesia was higher in horses given pentastarch solutions than those given hypertonic saline. An experimental study in which endotoxin was injected into horses failed to confirm the advantage of hetastartch over hypertonic saline (Pantaleon et al., 2006).

Positive inotropes

Many of the sympathomimetic agents are easily oxidized to inactive compounds on exposure to air, and thus should be prepared to the required dilution just prior to use. This property may explain differing results and differing recommendations as to dosage and efficacy. Fortunately, in clinical practice, some changes in potency are acceptable as the drugs are administered to effect by infusion.

The pharmacological action of dopamine, dobutamine and similar agents is to increase heart rate yet, if given too fast to anaesthetized horses, bradycardia or even heart block may occur. This appears to be a vagally-mediated reflex to the improving MAP and, if these drugs are given after treatment with an anticholinergic agent, tachycardia and a rise in MAP occurs with very low doses of the sympathomimetic.

Dopamine

Dopamine is a naturally occurring precursor of noradrenaline which exerts its action at α_1, β_1 and β_2, and dopaminergic adrenoceptors. In horses, infusions of 2.5–5.0 μg/kg/min improve CO while causing vasodilation. Renal perfusion is increased (Trim et al., 1985, 1989) and both CO and ABP improved in horses with endotoxic shock (Trim et al., 1991). Higher doses may cause vasoconstriction via α_1 activity. Signs of overdose are tachycardia and associated arrhythmias, and trembling (Lee et al., 1998c) but these effects cease as soon as the infusion rate is reduced.

Dobutamine

Dobutamine exerts its actions at both α- and β-adrenoceptors (β actions predominating at low doses), but is devoid of action at dopaminergic receptors. In anaesthetized horses, infusions of from 0.5 to 5.0 μg/kg have been found to improve both CO and MAP (Donaldson, 1988; Gasthuys et al., 1991a; Lee et al., 1998c). Overdose of dobutamine causes tachycardia with associated arrhythmias (which may be dangerous in the presence of hypercapnia) but lack of dopaminergic activity means that muscle tremors do not occur.

Dopexamine

Dopexamine is a synthetic catecholamine which has marked activity at β_2-receptors with a lesser action at β_1 and dopaminergic sites. It improves CO through a positive inotropic effect, while causing vasodilation, reducing afterload and improving renal perfusion. Muir (1992a,b) demonstrated in conscious and anaesthetized horses that at doses of 1 μg/kg/min or more, CO and HR increased, while systemic vascular resistance decreased. In conscious horses, ABP changes were minimal but, in anaesthetized animals, dopexamine infusion caused a dose-dependent increase. These advantageous cardiovascular effects in anaesthetized horses have been confirmed by other workers (Young et al., 1997; Lee et al., 1998c) but, in these later studies under halothane anaesthesia, dopexamine was found to cause unacceptable side effects. The initial response to infusion of the drug was a fall in end-tidal anaesthetic agent (presumably because the vasodilation had opened underperfused areas which then took up the halothane) and great difficulty was encountered in keeping the animals unconscious. Higher doses caused sweating, tachycardia and tremor. When infusion was stopped, MAP and heart rate continued to rise, and side effects did not abate for a considerable period of time. The quality of

recovery was poor and, in one study, two horses developed postanaesthetic colic. The cardiovascular effects of dopexamine are ideal for circulatory support, and the side effects almost certainly result from overdosage, but considerably more experimental work is required to elucidate the correct dose before this agent can be recommended for use in clinical practice.

Phenylephrine and methoxamine

Phenylephrine and methoxamine both act as α_2-adrenoceptor agonists, and increase arterial blood pressure by vasoconstriction. An infusion dose of phenylephrine of 0.25–2.00 μg/kg/min in anaesthetized horses raises blood pressure but CO and muscle blood flow fall are unchanged (Lee et al., 1998c). These vasoconstrictor agents should not routinely be used to treat hypotension in anaesthetized horses but may have a role where all other methods have failed.

Norepinephrine

In cases (usually colic cases) which do not respond to the above inotropes, norepinephrine can be infused cautiously to effect (in addition to dobutamine). Doses are 0.05–1.0 μg/kg/min; most horses respond at the lower doses (Brainard – personal communication to CT, 2012). The ECG should be observed continually and the infusion stopped if there are arrhythmias.

Calcium

The use of calcium to counteract anaesthetic-induced cardiovascular depression has been advocated for many years but much of the evidence as to dose and efficacy is anecdotal, and the differing availability of elemental calcium in preparations of different calcium salts sometimes makes comparisons between studies difficult (Gasthuys et al., 1991b). Calcium borogluconate, being readily available in veterinary practice, is a common choice and up to 300 mL of a 40% w/v solution may be given prior to or during anaesthesia by slow IV infusion. Another recommendation is an infusion of 0.25–2.00 mL/kg/min of 10% calcium gluconate (Daunt, 1990). In clinical practice, calcium infusions tend either to be very effective or almost totally ineffective in improving MAP and peripheral blood flow. The rationale of the use of calcium is that plasma calcium levels fall during anaesthesia with volatile agents. Whether calcium has any effect in improving CO depressed by IV agents is not known.

Anticholinergic agents

Glycopyrrolate, atropine, hyoscine

The advantages and disadvantages of the use of anticholinergic agents in equine anaesthesia have been discussed above. However, during anaesthesia with volatile anaesthetic agents, bradycardia may contribute to the fall in CO and this is particularly likely to be the case if α_2-adrenoceptor agonists have been used in the anaesthetic protocol. Atropine (0.005–0.01 mg/kg) or glycopyrrolate (0.005 mg/kg) given IV often do not increase heart rate but, following their use, small doses of dopamine or dobutamine do, with a spectacular effect on CO. Hyoscine 0.1 mg/kg increased heart rate for 10–15 minutes (Borer & Clarke, 2006).

Intermittent positive pressure ventilation (IPPV)

Until the last 15 years, IPPV was used sparingly in anaesthetized horses, partly through concern about induced circulatory changes (see Ventilatory strategies, above), but partly as many people did not have suitable ventilators. While with halothane spontaneous breathing was satisfactory, with the newer agents, respiratory depression is greater and IPPV is now usually employed if the apparatus is available.

When IPPV is employed, it is advisable to retain a degree of hypercarbia, as this helps, at least under halothane anaesthesia, to maintain MAP (Khanna et al., 1995).

Ideally, monitoring of end-tidal CO_2 will enable adjustments to be made to the imposed tidal volume and/or rate of ventilation so that an adequate PaO_2 is maintained with a normal or slightly elevated $PaCO_2$.

Usual settings for the ventilator are to deliver a tidal volume of around 10 mL/kg, at a respiratory frequency between 8 and 10 breaths/min, the airway pressure should be kept as low as is consistent with adequate expansion of the chest wall and the inspiratory time should be between 2 and 3 seconds. The question of the use or otherwise of PEEP has already been discussed. Reduction of respiratory rate to 5–6/minute with the same tidal volumes usually enables spontaneous breathing to return.

Assisted ventilation, in which the horse triggers the ventilator which then delivers a prescribed tidal volume, is a very useful compromise in equine anaesthesia as long as the ventilator has a 'fail safe' mechanism, whereby if the horse does not trigger a breath within a certain time, the ventilator switches to automatic mode.

USE OF MUSCLE RELAXANTS

Centrally acting muscle relaxants

Guaifenesin

The use of guaifenesin as part of the anaesthetic induction technique has been discussed above. Doses of guaifenesin of 5–10 mg/kg may be given to the anaesthetized horse and will produce some relaxation without interfering with respiratory activity but, when given in this way, it causes a

marked fall in MAP, probably through a negative inotropic effect.

Benzodiazepines

Benzodiazepines may also be administered intraoperatively for their muscle relaxant properties. However, when given to horses already anaesthetized with volatile anaesthetic agents, benzodiazepines cause marked respiratory depression.

Neuromuscular blocking agents

For many years, neuromuscular blocking agents (NMBA) have been used sparingly in equine anaesthesia (other than suxamethonium at induction of anaesthesia), the major fear being that residual muscle weakness when the horse tried to rise would adversely affect the quality of recovery. The advent of the short-acting, easily reversed competitive relaxant atracurium, changed this, and neuromuscular blocking agents are now widely used not only to aid abdominal, ophthalmic and thoracic surgery, but in general and orthopaedic surgery to prevent the sudden reflex responses which sometimes occur.

The rules for the use of neuromuscular blocking agents are, as for any species and as explained in Chapter 8: (1) that the facilities which enable immediate and sustained IPPV are available; and (2) that it is possible to be certain that the horse will be unconscious throughout the duration of their effect.

There is a wide variation among individuals in the response to a given dose of neuromuscular blocking agent and in rate of recovery from blockade. Also, some antibiotic agents such as gentamicin greatly reduce the dose of relaxant required. For this reason, no attempt should be made to administer them in fixed doses; they should always be given so as to produce just the desired effect. An incremental dosage regimen enables this to be done; about one-half the anticipated full dose is given initially and further increments of half this initial dose are given at 3–5-minute intervals until the desired degree of relaxation is obtained. Only small doses are needed to suppress unwanted muscle movements during general anaesthesia (e.g. in eye surgery) but large doses will be required to produce the nearly complete blockade demanded by some surgical procedures. In every case, the aim should be to use only a minimum dose and to ensure a complete recovery of neuromuscular function before the termination of anaesthesia. If unwanted muscle tone is returning towards the end of a surgical procedure, it is usually wiser to restore relaxation by a slight deepening of anaesthesia rather than the administration of more neuromuscular blocker.

Monitoring the block

In equine anaesthesia, clinical monitoring of neuromuscular block using a peripheral nerve stimulator as described in Chapter 8 should be considered mandatory. The stimulator is usually used on various branches of the facial, the radial or the superficial peroneal nerves. The reader is referred to Chapter 8 for details and diagrams of nerve stimulation points. The strength of contraction of the relevant muscles is estimated by manual sensing at the muzzle or toe, or better still, by acceleromyography. If this facility is not available, myoneural block may be monitored by careful observation of the breathing and general muscular activity of the anaesthetized horse. Signs of partial blockade include brief, weak inspiratory movements without holding of inspiration, and feeble, unsustained withdrawal responses to painful stimulation. One extremely simple objective test is measurement of airway pressure with a water manometer when the endotracheal tube is occluded before an inspiratory effort. No significant degree of myoneural block is present if the horse can generate a pressure in the occluded airway of more than 25 cm H_2O (2.5 kPa) below atmospheric pressure. If a degree of block is present during anaesthetic recovery, the horse is unable to stiffen the neck or hold up the head when attempting to sit in sternal recumbency, or it may make brief, weak attempts to stand followed by shaking of the limb muscles and collapse.

Neuromuscular blocking drugs

Atracurium

The relatively short duration of action of activity and the lack of cumulative neuromuscular blocking effect make atracurium particularly suitable for use in horses in doses of 0.12–0.20 mg/kg (Hildebrand et al., 1986; Hildebrand & Hill, 1989). The authors recommend an initial dose of 0.1 mg/kg followed, if this does not produce the desired degree of relaxation as indicated by train-of-four stimulation, by doses of 0.01 mg/kg at 2-minute intervals until the block is judged to be adequate (reduction of initial twitch height). Edrophonium 0.5–1.0 mg/kg will antagonize any residual neuromuscular blocking effects at the end of the procedure for which it is given and prior administration of atropine or glycopyrrolate is unnecessary provided the antagonist is injected slowly over more than 1 minute. Atracurium has also been given by continuous infusion at 0.17 mg/kg/h after an initial bolus dose of 0.05 mg/kg (Hildebrand &Hill, 1989). Cardiovascular stability is good but there may be some slowing of heart rate after an initial increase in ABP in response to edrophonium.

Vecuronium

Doses of 0.1 mg/kg produce neuromuscular block of some 20–30 minutes' duration in horses lightly anaesthetized with halothane. However, recent experience has suggested that its action is unreliable in horses. Martin-Flores et al. (2012b) conducted a vecuronium dose–response study in isoflurane anaesthetized horses, but found great variations between individual animals, these individual variations being confirmed with clinical experience (Martin-Flores et al., 2012a). Testing used the TOF. The lowest dose, 0.025 mg/kg (25 µg/kg), did not cause any T1 depression, and while the highest dose used, 0.1 mg/kg (100 µg/kg), caused an incomplete block, the partial block that was produced was long lasting – up to 2 hours, requiring reversal with neostigmine.

Rocuronium

A dose–response study in horses demonstrated that rocuronium at doses of 0.4–0.6 mg/kg IV resulted in a full neuromuscular block; time to return of T1 of the train of four was 38 and 55 minutes respectively (Auer et al., 2007). Doses of 0.3 mg/kg were sufficient for ophthalmic surgery and clinical duration of block was 32 ± 18.6 minutes (Auer & Moens, 2011). Rocuronium NMB can be antagonized by sugammadex (4 mg/kg IV) (Mosing et al., 2010).

Pancuronium bromide

Pancuronium has now been used for many years in horses. During light anaesthesia, doses of 0.06 mg/kg produce complete relaxation with apnoea of about 20 min duration, but it is more usual to give doses of 0.1 mg/kg to be certain of producing apnoea with complete relaxation of respiratory muscles so that IPPV can be performed with the lowest possible airway pressures (Hildebrand & Howitt, 1984).

Suxamethonium chloride

The use of suxamethonium for casting and restraint of horses is considered by the vast majority of veterinary anaesthetists to be an extremely inhumane practice, it is unnecessary and it is unsafe on pharmacological grounds. In the past, suxamethonium (0.1 mg/kg IV) had a place in the provision of short-term muscle relaxation in anaesthetized horses but it has now been replaced by the short-acting competitive blocking agent atracurium.

Termination of neuromuscular block

There is no effective antidote to suxamethonium, but neostigmine is an efficient antidote to the non-depolarizing relaxants. In horses, its use should be preceded by the IV injection of 0.01 mg/kg atropine or glycopyrrolate, and it is then given in incremental doses up to a total dose 0.02 mg/kg. A period of 2–3minutes should be allowed between increments and the effect of each carefully assessed before the next is given. Edrophonium (0.5–1 mg/kg) or neostigmine should be given while IPPV is continued so that there is no danger of hypoxia or hypercapnia because if given to hypoxic or hypercapnic animals neostigmine may cause serious arrhythmias.

ANAESTHETIC RECOVERY PERIOD

General points

Ideally, horses should recover from anaesthesia calmly and quietly, and in as fast a time as possible, but these aims cannot always be achieved. The quality of recovery will depend on a number of factors including the sedative and anaesthetic drugs used throughout the perioperative process, the degree of postoperative pain, the comfort of the horse, its temperament, and limitation to standing caused by surgery or onset of anaesthetic induced myopathy or neuropathy.

In the last 10 years, there have been a large number of publications which have tried to assess quality of recovery, and then apply it to the regimen under study. Assessment of quality of recovery is very subjective, and ease of use tends to go with imprecision (Suthers et al., 2011). Nevertheless, such scoring systems will highlight an excess of unacceptable recoveries.

Simple nursing factors thought to assist in obtaining good quality recoveries are the provision of adequate (but not too sedative) analgesia, and ensuring that the horse has an empty bladder. The recovery box floor needs to be sufficiently soft for comfort, but hard enough for the horse to feel safe when it stands. Most importantly, it should not be slippery. This author (KC) has found the floor surface, Linatex, shown in Figure 11.26 to be successful with these aims. The best size for a recovery box is also contentious – too big and the horse can crash around – too small it gets 'cast'. The recovery box should be quiet and it was always considered that it should be darkened, but Clarke-Price et al. (2008) found that lighting did not influence recovery quality. Positioning is usually at the request of the surgeon but, if the horse has been in dorsal recumbency, placing it left side down allows the larger lung to be uppermost.

Ensuring adequate oxygenation and a patent airway

It is usually routine to deliver oxygen at 15 L/min to the horse once it has been detached from the anaesthetic machine with the intention of reducing the hypoxaemia that otherwise might occur at this time. The oxygen can be simply delivered to the end the ET tube, or while the horse is still intubated, a self-demand valve can be used.

To ensure a patent airway, some anaesthetists leave the ET tube in place until the horse stands but this is not a guarantee; if the gag is displaced, the horse may bite down and obstruct the tube. Horses are obligate nasal breathers, and once the ET tube is removed it is necessary to ensure that the nasal passages are not blocked and oedematous. Nasal congestion occurs when the horse is positioned on the operating table with its head lower than its body. A nasal ET tube (Fig. 11.24) can be placed easily before the

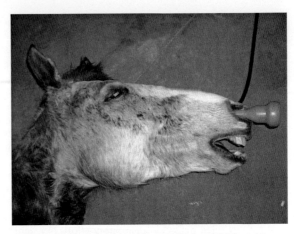

Figure 11.24 A purpose made uncuffed nasal tube with a bulbous end to prevent the danger of inhalation.
From Taylor, P.M., Clarke, K.W., 2007. Handbook of Equine Anaesthesia. 2nd edn, Elsevier Ltd, with permission.

congestion has occurred (i.e. at the start of the procedures). If this was not done, a phenylephrine spray into the nostrils will relieve the congestion.

Sedation

It is important that the horse does not try to rise until it is able to do so. Following prolonged anaesthesia with volatile agents it is now common practice to administer additional sedation (e.g. xylazine at increments of 0.1 mg/kg up to 0.5 mg/kg IV.) in the early recovery period. Most regimens which have used a medetomidine infusion, whether for TIVA or PIVA, have been reported to result in good quality recoveries.

Recently, there have been a number of investigations into suitable combinations of drugs to help ensure a good recovery. Wagner et al. (2012), in a cross-over study, compared recovery from sevoflurane anaesthesia without further sedation with that where xylazine and ketamine were infused for the last 30 minutes of anaesthesia, and a third treatment where infusion of xylazine and propofol was given for the last 15 minutes of anaesthesia. Recoveries were worst with no sedation; recoveries in the propofol groups were superior. However, while Steffey et al. (2009) found that xylazine/propofol infusions after 4 hours of desflurane anaesthesia improved the quality of recovery, it also caused a degree of respiratory depression.

Assisted recovery

Rope-based

A number of rope-based systems have been used so that the horse can be assisted to its feet. All are based on head and tail ropes. Figure 11.25 demonstrates how the rope

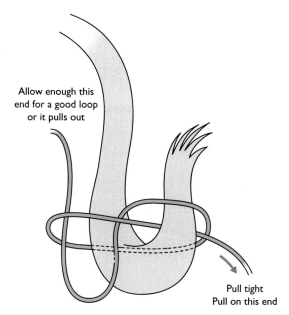

Figure 11.25 A recommended method of tying the tail hitch. *From Taylor, P.M., Clarke, K.W., 2007. Handbook of Equine Anaesthesia. 2nd edn, Elsevier Ltd, with permission.*

Allow enough this end for a good loop or it pulls out

Pull tight
Pull on this end

may be fixed to the tail. When horses are supported by this, it is difficult to understand why the tail does not break; anecdotally it does happen but it would appear to be very rare.

The helpers on the ropes may well be unable to support the weight unaided and if in the recovery box are themselves at risk. A system developed by H. Wilderjans uses a system of blocks and pulleys to give mechanical advantage and also to lead the ropes out of the recovery box. The system uses quick-release systems either from climbing or sailing equipment (Fig. 11.26), and enables the helpers to give support while remaining in safety. Few helpers are needed – one person can handle all the ropes. Its use does not always ensure a perfect recovery, but the fact it is now used in very many clinics shows that it is the most satisfactory of the simple systems developed to date.

Swimming pool

Swimming pools (Fig. 11.27) are the ultimate in recovery systems. Although no doubt superior to all else for recovering horses with fractures, they do need a large experienced team of helpers for their use.

ANAESTHESIA FOR HORSES WITH COLIC

The most common equine emergency case presented to the anaesthetist is that of colic. Most cases of colic presented for surgical treatment have already been treated medically and it is important to consider the drugs used, their route of administration, doses and time of dosing, for they can influence the response to subsequent anaesthesia. Pain is usually indicative of gastric and/or intestinal distension and of acute ischaemia. Its severity may make the horse unmanageable until it becomes utterly exhausted, and pain must be controlled, although this is not always easy. NSAIDs, in particular flunixin, are widely used and can be so effective in reducing both the pain of colic and the signs of toxaemia as to mask the need for surgery. Opioids which are often used include butorphanol, methadone and morphine. Xylazine and detomidine are usually the most effective agents to provide analgesia in colic, but doses should be kept low both to limit their duration of action, and their cardiopulmonary effects in an already stressed horse. The effect of these agents on gut motility is probably unimportant other than related to diagnosis, as it is comparatively short acting. Acepromazine, being an α-adrenergic blocker, will contribute to hypotension in dehydrated or shocked animals and is generally not advised if surgery will be necessary, although doses of up to 0.05 mg/kg are unlikely to do any harm.

The main problem in the preanaesthetic preparation of most colic cases is the replacement of fluids in the dehydrated and shocked animal. Fluid replacement is extremely urgent in surgical cases if any consistent measure of success is to be obtained. Unfortunately, diagnosis is very imprecise, and there is an understandable reluctance on the part of both owners and veterinarians to spend a considerable sum of money and time on cases which may at laparotomy prove to be inoperable. To overcome this reluctance some acceptable routine which does not involve replacement of the major part of the fluid deficit prior to anaesthesia is clearly desirable. Also, it is important to remove the source of any endotoxin (e.g. dead gut) as soon as possible. Our experience indicates that if really vigorous replacement is carried out once the surgeon has confirmed that surgical treatment is possible, a successful outcome is quite as likely as in cases treated before the induction of anaesthesia. Thus, it is possible that 'minimal' preparation can be justified on both surgical and economic grounds but it must be emphasized that for success it must be carried out in a rational manner.

Whenever possible, anaesthesia should not be induced in a colic case until hypovolaemia has been improved and the packed cell volume (PCV) decreased. Tachycardia may persist, due to pain or toxaemia, even after the blood volume has been restored to normal. Hypertonic saline (4 mL/kg IV of 7.5%) followed by large quantities of Ringer's lactate provides an inexpensive method of treating the hypovolaemia rapidly. The starches (e.g. pentastarch) may be more effective in maintaining circulating fluid (Hallowell & Corley, 2006). Other methods include the transfusion of plasma. Acid–base disturbances are seldom a problem in the preoperative period and there is no need

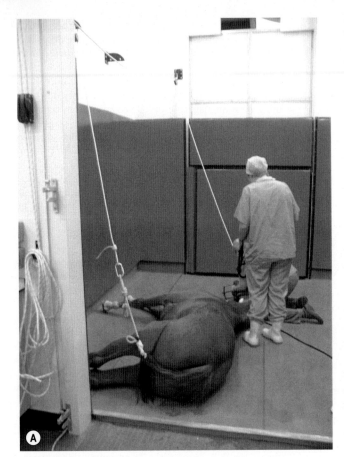
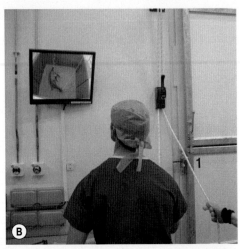
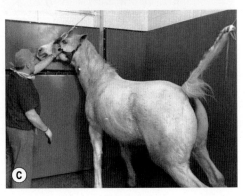

Figure 11.26 Horses can be recovered with head and tail ropes. (A) Head and tail ropes go through pulleys to outside the box. (B) The ropes are tightened to support the horse as it rises – ropes are 'locked' tight using quick release systems (in this case those designed for sailing). (C) Ideally, the horse rises so it is supported by the wall (it does not always work perfectly as shown on the screen in B).
Photograph courtesy of Alan Taylor.

to administer bicarbonate at this stage. The administration of bicarbonate intraoperatively results in a very high PaCO$_2$, and the rapid exhaustion of the carbon dioxide absorbent of the anaesthetic circuit. Even in cases complicated by septic shock, the routine administration of glucocorticoids before operation is of doubtful value. NSAIDs, if not already given, are usually administered both for their analgesic and antitoxaemic effects.

Regardless of whether preoperative fluids are to be given to a colic case, at least one relatively short wide bored reliable IV line must be introduced into the jugular vein. A stomach tube should be passed through one nostril before the horse is anaesthetized and the stomach decompressed. Gastric decompression will minimize the likelihood of regurgitation immediately on induction before ET intubation can be achieved. Whenever possible, the surgical site should be clipped and prepared while the animal is conscious and standing, enabling the time from induction of anaesthesia to opening the abdomen and

relieving intra-abdominal pressure to be kept to the minimum.

The actual method of anaesthesia, within reason, is the anaesthetist's choice – drug doses will need to be adapted to the state of the animal, and familiarity enables this to be done far more safely than any advantage from use of a theoretically safer anaesthetic agent. During anaesthesia, lidocaine infusions (loading dose 1–2 mg/kg over 10–15 minutes, followed by a CRI of 0.05 mg/kg/min) can be given as these are prokinetic and thought to improve gut motility. Blood pressure needs to be supported with fluids and ionotropes; if blood pressure fails to respond to dobutamine infusions, norepinephrine may be given as well. If hypotension is very severe (and MAPs less than 40 mmHg are not uncommon in these animals) then phenylephrine can be used despite the vasoconstriction that it will induce. Often the colic horses are exhausted and will remain recumbent for some time after surgery; no attempt should be made to try to make them rise too soon.

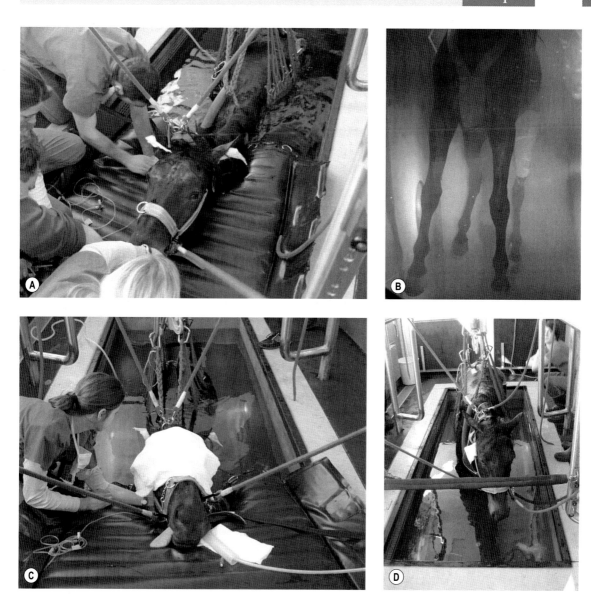

Figure 11.27 Pool recovery. Clockwise (A) The horse is lifted into the pool in slings, and the head supported. (B) At this stage its feet do not touch the ground. (C) It starts to take weight on its feet, the head needs less support; (D) the water is slowly drained out. With this system the floor then rises so the horse can walk out.
Photographs courtesy of Regula Bettschart-Wolfensberger, University of Zurich.

Where there are suitable facilities, assistance to recovery is helpful.

ANAESTHESIA IN THE FOAL

Foals less than 1 week old are 20 times, and 1–4 weeks old 4.3 times more likely to die during or following anaesthesia and surgery than an adult horse (Johnston et al.,

1995). Although this may reflect the fact that many of those requiring surgery at that age have life-threatening illnesses such as ruptured bladder or septicaemia, others are healthy and are anaesthetized for correction of orthopaedic problems, and should not be at special risk.

Foals are born relatively mature compared to many other mammals. Renal function is very mature. Immaturity of liver enzymes may mean that some agents (e.g. NSAIDs) may be more cumulative therefore potentially more toxic (Crisman et al., 1996; Wilcke et al., 1993;

303

1998). However, increased duration of action does not appear to be a major clinically significant problem with the common agents given for general anaesthesia. However, low body fat and low plasma albumin affect pharmacokinetics and initial volume of distribution may differ from adults (see Chapter 3). There is less protein to bind agents such as propofol, so duration of action may be prolonged for these reasons. Lack of fat also means responses to changes in inspired concentrations (increased or decrease) of inhalation agents occur very rapidly. Temperature regulation is poor. Foals may become hypoglycaemic during or after anaesthesia.

The cardiorespiratory system in the newborn has just undergone major functional changes; the lungs may not be fully expanded, and the responses to hypoxia, hypercarbia, hypotension and hypertension are immature. Foals can only increase their cardiac output by increasing heart rate; bradycardia during anaesthesia is life threatening and often does not appear to respond to anticholinergic drugs. The stress of anaesthesia and surgery frequently cause gastric ulcers. The changes with age from neonatal are progressive, so choices of methods of anaesthesia increase accordingly; in general foals over 3–6 months may be anaesthetized as for adults, but large and boisterous foals below this age may require a similar protocol for control.

Practical sedation and anaesthesia of foals

First, the mare and foal should be considered a 'unit' and if possible kept together as long as the foal is conscious to avoid fear. Mares should be sedated, preferably with acepromazine (0.05 mg/kg IV) combined with an α_2-agonist with or without an opioid; doses should be chosen to avoid ataxia. Young foals are left with the mare and do not need to be starved. The condition of 'sick' foals should be assessed (e.g. plasma K^+ in cases of bladder rupture; fluids for toxaemia) and wherever possible stabilized prior to surgery.

Foals are very 'needle-shy' and it is easy to accidentally hit the carotid artery while attempting jugular puncture. Intradermal or subcutaneous local anaesthesia makes jugular catheterization easier, and IM sedation in older foals can be useful.

Young foals may be sedated with diazepam or midazolam, (0.1–0.2 mg/kg IV) with or without opioids; this

often is sufficient to make them lie down. α_2-Agonists are best avoided to reduce bradycardia, but as the foal grows older (and bigger or more boisterous) they may be given at doses in the lower range of those given to adults. Detomidine (up to 20 μg/kg (0.02 mg/kg) if IM) is particularly useful because of the small volume required. Low to moderate doses of acepromazine (0.02–0.05 mg/kg) may also be used for premedication in older foals.

For anaesthesia, in neonatal or sick foals premedication is not necessary. Anaesthesia may be induced using sevoflurane, isoflurane or halothane. This may be administered by mask, remembering that the foal is an obligate nasal breather. An alternative is to pass an endotracheal tube into the trachea via one nostril and administer the anaesthetic through this. Neonatal Thoroughbred foals can accommodate tubes of 7–9 mm internal diameter and in 6-week old foals 11 mm tubes can be passed with ease. Passage of the tube is greatly facilitated by prior preparation of the ventral nasal mucosa with lidocaine ointment or gel and lubrication of the tube with the same preparation. Induction is usually very calm; the foal sinks down. Once orotracheal intubation is accomplished anaesthesia is maintained with the inhalation agent delivered by equipment suitable for the foal's size. Johnston et al.'s (1995) survey suggested that foals were more likely to die if anaesthesia was induced with inhalation agents than with IV drugs, but this may reflect the clinical condition of the foals where this technique was chosen. However, in very young foals anaesthesia also can be induced with diazepam or midazolam (0.2 mg/kg) and ketamine (2.5 mg/kg). Monitoring is as for adult animals. Breathing may be spontaneous but IPPV is usually needed to avoid hypercarbia and acidosis. Heart rate must be kept adequate and a low dose of an anticholinergic (e.g. atropine at 0.005–0.01 mg/kg) may be given. Hypotension should be treated with fluids and dobutamine as for adult horses.

Hypothermia should be prevented by the methods described in small animal chapters. Opioids give analgesia; doses of morphine or methadone at 0.1 mg/g have been used. NSAIDs should be used with caution with dosing less frequently than for adults. Recovery is usually rapid, and young foals can be helped to their feet. As soon as it is safe to do so they should be returned to the mare so that they can suckle. Gastro-protectants such as sucralfate 20 mg/kg orally three times a day are required the day of surgery and some days after.

REFERENCES

Aida, H., Mizuno, Y., Hobo, S., et al., 1994. Determination of the minimum alveolar concentration (MAC) and physical response to sevoflurane inhalation in horses. J Vet Med Sci 56, 1161–1165.

Aida, H., Mizuno, Y., Hobo, S., et al., 1996. Cardiovascular and pulmonary effects of sevoflurane anesthesia in horses. Vet Surg 25, 164–170.

Alitalo, I., 1986. Clinical experiences with Domosedan in horses and cattle. A review. Acta Vet Scand Suppl 82, 193–196.

Ambrisko, T.D., Coppens, P., Kabes, R., et al., 2012. Lithium dilution, pulse power analysis, and continuous thermodilution cardiac output measurements compared with bolus thermodilution in anaesthetized ponies. Br J Anaesth 109, 864–869.

Auer, U., Moens, Y., 2011. Neuromuscular blockade with rocuronium bromide for ophthalmic surgery in horses. Vet Ophthalmol 14, 244–247.

Auer, U., Uray, C., Mosing, M., 2007. Observations on the muscle relaxant rocuronium bromide in the horse – a dose-response study. Vet Anaesth Analg 34, 75–81.

Beadle, R.E., Robinson, N.E., Sorenson, P.R., 1975. Cardiopulmonary effects of positive end-expiratory pressure in anesthetized horses. Am J Vet Res 36, 1435–1438.

Benredouane, K., Ringer, S.K., Fourel, I., et al., 2011. Comparison of xylazine-butorphanol and xylazine-morphine-ketamine infusions in horses undergoing a standing surgery. Vet Rec 169, 364.

Bettschart-Wolfensberger, R., Taylor, P.M., Sear, J.W., et al., 1996. Physiologic effects of anesthesia induced and maintained by intravenous administration of a climazolam-ketamine combination in ponies premedicated with acepromazine and xylazine. Am J Vet Res 57, 1472–1477.

Bettschart-Wolfensberger, R., Clarke, K.W., Vainio, O., et al., 1999. Pharmacokinetics of medetomidine in ponies and elaboration of a medetomidine infusion regime which provides a constant level of sedation. Res Vet Sci 67, 41–46.

Bettschart-Wolfensberger, R., Bowen, M.I., Freeman, S.L., et al., 2001a. Cardiopulmonary effects of prolonged anesthesia via propofol-medetomidine infusion in ponies. Am J Vet Res 62, 1428–1435.

Bettschart-Wolfensberger, R., Freeman, S.L., Jaggin-Schmucker, N., et al., 2001b. Infusion of a combination of propofol and medetomidine for long-term anesthesia in ponies. Am J Vet Res 62, 500–507.

Bettschart-Wolfensberger, R., Jaggin-Schmucker, N., Lendl, C., et al., 2001c. Minimal alveolar concentration of desflurane in combination with an infusion of medetomidine for the anaesthesia of ponies. Vet Rec 148, 264–267.

Bettschart-Wolfensberger, R., Freeman, S.L., Bowen, I.M., et al., 2005. Cardiopulmonary effects and pharmacokinetics of i.v. dexmedetomidine in ponies. Equine Vet J 37, 60–64.

Bettschart-Wolfensberger, R., Dicht, S., Vullo, C., et al., 2011. A clinical study on the effect in horses during medetomidine-isoflurane anaesthesia, of butorphanol constant rate infusion on isoflurane requirements, on cardiopulmonary function and on recovery characteristics. Vet Anaesth Analg 38, 186–194.

Bidwell, L.A., Bramlage, L.R., Rood, W.A., 2007. Equine perioperative fatalities associated with general anaesthesia at a private practice – a retrospective case series. Vet Anaesth Analg 34, 23–30.

Borer, K.E., Clarke, K.W., 2006. The effect of hyoscine on dobutamine requirement in spontaneously breathing horses anaesthetized with halothane. Vet Anaesth Analg 33, 149–157.

Boscan, P., Rezende, M.L., Grimsrud, K., et al., 2010. Pharmacokinetic profile in relation to anaesthesia characteristics after a 5% micellar microemulsion of propofol in the horse. Br J Anaesth 104, 330–337.

Brearley, J.C., Jones, R.S., Kelly, D.F., et al., 1986. Spinal cord degeneration following general anaesthesia in a Shire horse. Equine Vet J 18, 222–224.

Brosnan, R.J., Steffey, E.P., Escobar, A., et al., 2011. Anesthetic induction with guaifenesin and propofol in adult horses. Am J Vet Res 72, 1569–1575.

Bryant, C.E., England, G.C., Clarke, K.W., 1991. Comparison of the sedative effects of medetomidine and xylazine in horses. Vet Rec 129, 421–423.

Burford, J.H., Corley, K.T., 2006. Morphine-associated pruritus after single extradural administration in a horse. Vet Anaesth Analg 33, 193–198.

Clark-Price, S.C., Posner, L.P., Gleed, R.D., 2008. Recovery of horses from general anesthesia in a darkened or illuminated recovery stall. Vet Anaesth Analg 35, 473–479.

Clarke, K.W., Hall, L.W., 1969. 'Xylazine'– a new sedative for horses and cattle. Vet Rec 85, 512–517.

Clarke, K.W., Taylor, P.M., 1986. Detomidine: a new sedative for horses. Equine Vet J 18, 366–370.

Clarke, K.W., Freeman, S., Alibhai, H.I.K., et al., 1997. Cardiopulmonary actions of alpha 2 adrenoceptor agonists administered to ponies during anaesthesia. Proceedings of the 6th International Congress of Veterinary Anaesthesiology, p. 123.

Clarke, K.W., Song, D.Y., Alibhai, H.I., et al., 1996. Cardiopulmonary effects of desflurane in ponies, after induction of anaesthesia with xylazine and ketamine. Vet Rec 139, 180–185.

Clerbaux, T., Serteyn, D., Willems, E., et al., 1986. Determination of the standard oxyhemoglobin dissociation curve in horses. Effects of temperature, pH and diphosphoglycerate. Can J Vet Res 50, 188–192.

Clutton, R.E., 1987. Unexpected responses following intravenous pethidine injection in two horses. Equine Vet J 19, 72–73.

Clutton, R.E., 2010. Opioid analgesia in horses. Vet Clin N Am Equine Pract 26, 493–514.

Cunningham, F.M., Lees, P., 1995. Non-steroidal anti-inflammatory drugs. In: Higgins, A.J., Wright, I.M., (Eds.), Equine Manual. W.B. Saunders, London, pp. 229–237.

Daunt, D.A., 1990. Supportive therapy in the anaesthetized horse. Vet Clin N Am 6, 557–574.

Davis, J.L., Posner, L.P., Elce, Y., 2007. Gabapentin for the treatment of neuropathic pain in a pregnant horse. J Am Vet Med Assoc 231, 755–758.

Derossi, R., Miguel, G.L., Frazílio, F.O., et al., 2005. L-Bupivacaine 0.5% vs. racemic 0.5% bupivacaine for caudal epidural analgesia in horses. J Vet Pharmacol Ther 28, 293–297

Devisscher, L., Schauvliege, S., Dewulf, J., et al., 2010. Romifidine as a constant-rate infusion in isoflurane anaesthetized horses: a clinical study. Vet Anaesth Analg 37, 425–433.

Dhanjal, J.K., Wilson, D.V., Robinson, E., et al., 2009. Intravenous tramadol: effects, nociceptive properties, and pharmacokinetics in horses. Vet Anaesth Analg 36, 581–590.

Di Concetto, S., Michael Archer, R., Sigurdsson, S.F., et al., 2007. Atipamezole in the management of detomidine overdose in a pony. Vet Anaesth Analg 34, 67–69.

Dodam, J.R., Moon, R.E., Olson, N.C., et al., 1993. Effects of clenbuterol hydrochloride on pulmonary gas exchange and hemodynamics in anesthetized horses. Am J Vet Res 54, 776–782.

Doherty, T.J., 2009. Postoperative ileus: pathogenesis and treatment. Vet Clin North Am Equine Pract 25, 351–362.

Doherty, T.J., Frazier, D.L., 1998. Effect of intravenous lidocaine on halothane minimum alveolar concentration in ponies. Equine Vet J 30, 300–303.

Donaldson, L.L., 1988. Retrospective assessment of dobutamine therapy for hypotension in anesthetized horses. Vet Surg 17, 53–57.

Driessen, B., Nann, L., Benton, R., et al., 2006. Differences in need for hemodynamic support in horses anesthetized with sevoflurane as compared to isoflurane. Vet Anaesth Analg 33, 356–367.

Driessen, B., Zarucco, L., Kalir, B., et al., 2011. Contemporary use of acepromazine in the anaesthetic management of male horses and ponies: a retrospective study and opinion poll. Equine Vet J 43, 88–98.

Dyson, D.H., Pascoe, P.J., 1990. Influence of preinduction methoxamine, lactated Ringer solution, or hypertonic saline solution infusion or postinduction dobutamine infusion on anesthetic-induced hypotension in horses. Am J Vet Res 51, 17–21

Enderle, A.K., Levionnois, O.L., Kuhn, M., et al., 2008. Clinical evaluation of ketamine and lidocaine intravenous infusions to reduce isoflurane requirements in horses under general anaesthesia. Vet Anaesth Analg 35, 297–305.

England, G.C., Clarke, K.W., 1996. Alpha 2 adrenoceptor agonists in the horse – a review. Br Vet J 152, 641–657.

Flaherty, D., Reid, J., Welsh, E., et al., 1997. A pharmacodynamic study of propofol or propofol and ketamine infusions in ponies undergoing surgery. Res Vet Sci 62, 179–184.

Freeman, S.L., England, G.C., 2001. Effect of romifidine on gastrointestinal motility, assessed by transrectal ultrasonography. Equine Vet J 33, 570–576.

Freise, K.J., Newbound, G.C., Tudan, C., et al., 2012. Pharmacokinetics and the effect of application site on a novel, long-acting transdermal fentanyl solution in healthy laboratory Beagles. J Vet Pharmacol Ther 35 (Suppl 2), 27–33.

Gardner, R.B., White, G.W., Ramsey, D.S., et al., 2010. Efficacy of sublingual administration of detomidine gel for sedation of horses undergoing veterinary and husbandry procedures under field conditions. J Am Vet Med Assoc 237, 1459–1464.

Gasthuys, F., 2011. How to use the Triple Drip in horses. Abstracts from the European Veterinary Conference Voorjaarsdagen Chapter 6. www.voorjaarsdagen.org/index.php Accessed 5th November 2012.

Gasthuys, F., De Moor, A., Parmentier, D., 1991a. Cardiovascular effects of low dose calcium chloride infusions during halothane anaesthesia in dorsally recumbent ventilated ponies. Zentralbl Vet Reihe A 38, 728–736.

Gasthuys, F., de Moor, A., Parmentier, D., 1991b. Influence of dopamine and dobutamine on the cardiovascular depression during a standard halothane anaesthesia in dorsally recumbent, ventilated ponies. Zentralbl Vet Reihe A 38, 494–500.

Gasthuys, F., Messerman, C., Moor, A.D., 1994. Cardiovascular effects of 7.2% hypertonic saline solution in halothane anaesthetised ponies. J Vet Anaesth 21, 60–65.

Gillespie, J.R., Tyler, W.S., Hall, L.W., 1969. Cardiopulmonary dysfunction in anesthetized, laterally recumbent horses. Am J Vet Res 30, 61–72.

Gleed, R.D., Dobson, A., 1990. Effect of clenbuterol on arterial oxygen tension in the anaesthetised horse. Res Vet Sci 48, 331–337.

Goodwin, W.A., Keates, H.L., Pasloske, K., et al., 2011. The pharmacokinetics and pharmacodynamics of the injectable anaesthetic alfaxalone in the horse. Vet Anaesth Analg 38, 431–438.

Goodwin, W.A., Keates, H.L., Pearson, M., et al., 2013. Alfaxalone and medetomidine intravenous infusion to maintain anaesthesia in colts undergoing field castration. Equine Vet J 45, 315–319.

Gozalo-Marcilla, M., Hopster, K., Gasthuys, F., et al., 2013. Effects of a constant-rate infusion of dexmedetomidine on the minimal alveolar concentration of sevoflurane in ponies. Equine Vet J 45, 204–208.

Grandy, J.L., Steffey, E.P., Hodgson, D.S., et al., 1987. Arterial hypotension and the development of postanesthetic myopathy in halothane-anesthetized horses. Am J Vet Res 48, 192–197.

Greene, S.A., Thurmon, J.C., Tranquilli, W.J., et al., 1986. Cardiopulmonary effects of continuous intravenous infusion of guaifenesin, ketamine, and xylazine in ponies. Am J Vet Res 47, 2364–2367.

Grimsrud, K.N., Mama, K.R., Steffey, E.P., et al., 2012. Pharmacokinetics and pharmacodynamics of intravenous medetomidine in the horse. Vet Anaesth Analg 39, 38–48.

Grosenbaugh, D.A., Muir, W.W., 1998. Cardiorespiratory effects of sevoflurane, isoflurane, and halothane anesthesia in horses. Am J Vet Res 59, 101–106.

Grubb, T., Edner, A., Frendin, J.H., et al., 2013. Oxygenation and plasma endothelin-1 concentrations in healthy horses recovering from isoflurane anaesthesia administered with or without pulse-delivered inhaled nitric oxide. Vet Anaesth Analg doi: 10.1111/j.1467-2995. 2012.00735.x. [Epub ahead of print]

Grubb, T.L., Riebold, T.W., Huber, M.J., 1992. Comparison of lidocaine, xylazine, and xylazine/lidocaine for caudal epidural analgesia in horses. J Am Vet Med Assoc 201, 1187–1190.

Haga, H.A., Lykkjen, S., Revold, T., et al., 2006. Effect of intratesticular injection of lidocaine on cardiovascular responses to castration in isoflurane-anesthetized stallions. Am J Vet Res 67, 403–408.

Hall, L.Q., Senior, J.E., Walker, R.G., 1968a. Sampling of equine pulmonary vein blood. Res Vet Sci 9, 487–488.

Hall, L.W., 1979. Oxygenation of pulmonary vein blood in conscious and anaesthetized ponies. Equine Vet J 11, 71–75.

Hall, L.W., 1983. Equine anaesthesia: discovery and rediscovery. Equine Vet J 15, 190–195.

Hall, L.W., 1984. Cardiovascular and pulmonary effects of recumbency in two conscious ponies. Equine Vet J 16, 89–92.

Hall, L.W., Trim, C.M., 1975. Positive end-expiratory pressure in anaesthetized spontaneously breathing horses. Br J Anaesth 47, 819–824.

Hall, L.W., Gillespie, J.R., Tyler, W.S., 1968. Alveolar-arterial oxygen tension differences in anaesthetized horses. Br J Anaesth 40, 560–568.

Hallowell, G.D., Corley, K.T., 2006. Preoperative administration of hydroxyethyl starch or hypertonic saline to horses with colic. J Vet Int Med 20, 980–986.

Hamm, D., Turchi, P., Jochle, W., 1995. Sedative and analgesic effects of detomidine and romifidine in horses. Vet Rec 136, 324–327.

Hashem, A., Keller, H., 1993. Disposition, bioavailability and clinical efficacy of orally administered acepromazine in the horse. J Vet Pharmacol Ther 16, 359–368.

Heard, D.J., Webb, A.I., Daniels, R.T., 1986. Effect of acepromazine on the anesthetic requirement of halothane in the dog. Am J Vet Res 47, 2113–2115.

Hildebrand, S.V., Howitt, G.A., 1984. Dosage requirement of pancuronium in halothane-anesthetized ponies: a comparison of cumulative and single-dose administration. Am J Vet Res 45, 2441–2444.

Hildebrand, S.V., Hill, 3rd, T., 1989. Effects of atracurium administered by continuous intravenous infusion in halothane-anesthetized horses. Am J Vet Res 50, 2124–2126.

Hildebrand, S.V., Howitt, G.A., Arpin, D., 1986. Neuromuscular and cardiovascular effects of atracurium in ponies anesthetized with halothane. Am J Vet Res 47, 1096–1100.

Hopster, K., Kastner, S.B., Rohn, K., et al., 2011. Intermittent positive pressure ventilation with constant positive end-expiratory pressure and alveolar recruitment manoeuvre during inhalation anaesthesia in horses undergoing surgery for colic, and its influence on the early recovery period. Vet Anaesth Analg 38, 169–177.

Hubbell, J.A., Muir, W.W., 2006. Antagonism of detomidine sedation in the horse using intravenous tolazoline or atipamezole. Equine Vet J 38, 238–241.

Hubbell, J.A., Aarnes, T.K., Lerche, P., et al., 2012. Evaluation of a midazolam-ketamine-xylazine infusion for total intravenous anesthesia in horses. Am J Vet Res 73, 470–475.

Hubbell, J.A., Bednarski, R.M., Muir, W.W., 1989. Xylazine and tiletamine-zolazepam anesthesia in horses. Am J Vet Res 50, 737–742.

Hubbell, J.A., Muir, W.W., Robertson, J.T., et al., 1987. Cardiovascular effects of intravenous sodium penicillin, sodium cefazolin, and sodium citrate in awake and anesthetized horses. Vet Surg 16, 245–250.

Iseri, T., Nishimura, R., Nagahama, S., et al., 2010. Epidural spread of iohexol following the use of air or saline in the 'loss of resistance' test. Vet Anaesth Analg 37, 526–530.

Jedruch, J., Gajewski, Z., Kuussaari, J., 1989. The effect of detomidine hydrochloride on the electrical activity of uterus in pregnant mares. Acta Vet Scand 30, 307–311.

Johnston, G.M., Eastment, J.K., Taylor, P.M., et al., 2004. Is isoflurane safer than halothane in equine anaesthesia? Results from a prospective multicentre randomised controlled trial. Equine Vet J 36, 64–71.

Johnston, G.M., Taylor, P.M., Holmes, M.A., et al., 1995. Confidential enquiry of perioperative equine fatalities (CEPEF-1): preliminary results. Equine Vet J 27, 193–200.

Jones, N.Y., Clarke, K.W., Clegg, P.D., 1995. Desflurane in equine anaesthesia: a preliminary trial. Vet Rec 137, 618–620.

Kalchofner, K., Price, J., Bettschart-Wolfensberger, R., 2007. Pruritus in two horses following epidurally administered morphine. Equine Vet Educ 19, 590–594.

Kalpravidh, M., Lumb, W.V., Wright, M., et al., 1984. Analgesic effects of butorphanol in horses: dose-response studies. Am J Vet Res 45, 211–216.

Kaukinen, H., Aspegren, J., Hyyppa, S., et al., 2011. Bioavailability of detomidine administered sublingually to horses as an oromucosal gel. J Vet Pharmacol Ther 34, 76–81.

Keates, H.L., van Eps, A.W., Pearson, M.R., 2012. Alfaxalone compared with ketamine for induction of anaesthesia in horses following xylazine and guaifenesin. Vet Anaesth Analg 39, 591–598.

Kendall, A., Mosley, C., Brojer, J., 2010. Tachypnea and antipyresis in febrile horses after sedation with alpha-agonists. J Vet Int Med 24, 1008–1011.

Kerr, C.L., McDonell, W.N., Young, S.S., 1996. A comparison of romifidine and xylazine when used with diazepam/ketamine for short duration anesthesia in the horse. Can Vet J 37, 601–609.

Kerr, D.D., Jones, E.W., Holbert, D., et al., 1972. Comparison of the effects of xylazine and acetylpromazine maleate in the horse. Am J Vet Res 33, 777–784.

Khanna, A.K., McDonell, W.N., Dyson, D.H., et al., 1995. Cardiopulmonary effects of hypercapnia during controlled intermittent positive pressure ventilation in the horse. Can J Vet Res 59, 213–221.

Klein, L.V., 1975. Standing sedation in the horse using xylazine and morphine. Proceedings of the 20th World Veterinary Congress 2, 739.

Klein, L., 1978. A review of fifty cases of post-operative myopathy in the horse. Am Assoc Equine Practit 24, 89–94.

Kloppel, H., Leece, E.A., 2011. Comparison of ketamine and alfaxalone for induction and maintenance of anaesthesia in ponies undergoing castration. Vet Anaesth Analg 38, 37–43.

Knych, H.K., Steffey, E.P., Mama, K.R., et al., 2009. Effects of high plasma fentanyl concentrations on minimum alveolar concentration of isoflurane in horses. Am J Vet Res 70, 1193–1200.

Kvaternick, V., Pollmeier, M., Fischer, J., et al., 2007. Pharmacokinetics and metabolism of orally administered firocoxib, a novel second generation coxib, in horses. J Vet Pharmacol Ther 30, 208–217.

Lam, K.H., Smyth, J.B., Clarke, K., et al., 1995. Acute spinal cord degeneration following general anaesthesia in a young pony. Vet Rec 136, 329–330.

Lee, Y.H., Clarke, K.W., Alibhai, H.I., 1998a. The cardiopulmonary effects of clenbuterol when administered to dorsally recumbent halothane-anaesthetised ponies – failure to increase arterial oxygenation. Res Vet Sci 65, 227–232.

Lee, Y.H., Clarke, K.W., Alibhai, H.I., 1998b. Effects on the intramuscular blood flow and cardiopulmonary function of anaesthetised ponies of changing from halothane to isoflurane maintenance and vice versa. Vet Rec 143, 629–633.

Lee, Y.H., Clarke, K.W., Alibhai, H.I., et al., 1998c. Effects of dopamine, dobutamine, dopexamine, phenylephrine, and saline solution on intramuscular blood flow and other cardiopulmonary variables in halothane-anesthetized ponies. Am J Vet Res 59, 1463–1472.

Leece, E.A., Corletto, F., Brearley, J.C., 2008. A comparison of recovery times and characteristics with sevoflurane and isoflurane anaesthesia in horses undergoing magnetic resonance imaging. Vet Anaesth Analg 35, 383–391.

Leece, E.A., Girard, N.M., Maddern, K., 2009. Alfaxalone in cyclodextrin for induction and maintenance of anaesthesia in ponies undergoing field castration. Vet Anaesth Analg 36, 480–484.

Letendre, L.T., Tessman, R.K., McClure, S.R., et al., 2008. Pharmacokinetics of firocoxib after administration of multiple consecutive daily doses to horses. Am J Vet Res 69, 1399–1405.

Lindegaard, C., Thomsen, M.H., Larsen, S., et al., 2010. Analgesic efficacy of intra-articular morphine in experimentally induced radiocarpal synovitis in horses. Vet Anaesth Analg 37, 171–185.

Lindsay, W.A., McDonell, W., Bignell, W., 1980. Equine postanesthetic forelimb lameness: intracompartmental muscle pressure changes and biochemical patterns. Am J Vet Res 41, 1919–1924.

Lindsay, W.A., Robinson, G.M., Brunson, D.B., et al., 1989. Induction of equine postanesthetic myositis after halothane-induced hypotension. Am J Vet Res 50, 404–410.

Linton, D.D., Wilson, M.G., Newbound, G.C., et al., 2012. The effectiveness of a long-acting transdermal fentanyl solution compared to buprenorphine for the control of postoperative pain in dogs in a randomized, multicentered clinical study. J Vet Pharmacol Ther 35 (Suppl 2), 53–64.

Love, E.J., Murrell, J., Whay, H.R., 2011. Thermal and mechanical nociceptive threshold testing in horses: a review. Vet Anaesth Analg 38, 3–14.

Love, E.J., Taylor, P.M., Murrell, J., et al., 2012. Effects of acepromazine, butorphanol and buprenorphine on thermal and mechanical nociceptive

thresholds in horses. Equine Vet J 44, 221–225.

Luna, S.P., Taylor, P.M., Massone, F., 1997. Midazolam and ketamine induction before halothane anaesthesia in ponies: cardiorespiratory, endocrine and metabolic changes. J Vet Pharmacol Ther 20, 153–159.

Mama, K.R., Pascoe, P.J., Steffey, E.P., et al., 1998. Comparison of two techniques for total intravenous anesthesia in horses. Am J Vet Res 59, 1292–1298.

Mama, K.R., Steffey, E.P., Pascoe, P.J., 1995. Evaluation of propofol as a general anesthetic for horses. Vet Surg 24, 188–194.

Mama, K.R., Steffey, E.P., Pascoe, P.J., 1996. Evaluation of propofol for general anesthesia in premedicated horses. Am J Vet Res 57, 512–516.

Martin, J.E., Beck, J.D., 1956. Some effects of chlorpromazine hydrochloride in horses. Am J Vet Res 17, 678–686.

Marntell, S., Nyman, G., Funkquist, P., et al., 2005a. Effects of acepromazine on pulmonary gas exchange and circulation during sedation and dissociative anaesthesia in horses. Vet Anaesth Analg 32, 83–93.

Marntell, S., Nyman, G., Hedenstierna, G., 2005b. High inspired oxygen concentrations increase intrapulmonary shunt in anaesthetized horses. Vet Anaesth Analg 32, 338–347.

Martin-Flores, M., Campoy, L., Gleed, R.D., 2012a. Further experiences with vercuronium in the horse. Vet Anaesth Analg 39, 218–219.

Martin-Flores, M., Pare, M.D., Adams, W., et al., 2012b. Observations of the potency and duration of vecuronium in isoflurane-anesthetized horses. Vet Anaesth Analg 39, 385–389.

Matthews, N.S., Hartsfield, S.M., Hague, B., et al., 1999. Detomidine propofol anesthesia for abdominal surgery in horses. Vet Surg 28, 196–201.

Matthews, N.S., Hartsfield, S.M., Mercer, D., et al., 1998. Recovery from sevoflurane anesthesia in horses: comparison to isoflurane and effect of postmedication with xylazine. Vet Surg 27, 480–485.

McDonell, W.N., Hall, L.W., Jeffcott, L.B., 1979. Radiographic evidence of impaired pulmonary

function in laterally recumbent anaesthetised horses. Equine Vet J 11, 24–32.

McKellar, Q.A., Bogan, J.A., von Fellenberg, R.L., et al., 1991. Pharmacokinetic, biochemical and tolerance studies on carprofen in the horse. Equine Vet J 23, 280–284.

McMurphy, R.M., Young, L.E., Marlin, D.J., et al., 2002. Comparison of the cardiopulmonary effects of anesthesia maintained by continuous infusion of romifidine, guaifenesin, and ketamine with anesthesia maintained by inhalation of halothane in horses. Am J Vet Res 63, 1655–1661.

Moens, Y., Bohm, S., 2011. Ventilating horses: moving away from old paradigms. Vet Anaesth Analg 38, 165–168.

Moon, P.F., Suter, C.M., 1993. Paravertebral thoracolumbar anaesthesia in 10 horses. Equine Vet J 25, 304–308.

Mosing, M., 2007. Klinische Evaluation eines Anästhesieprotokolls mit Ketamin, Midazolam und einem von drei α2-Adrenorezeptoragonisten (Detomidin, Medetomidin, Xylazin) in Kombination mit Isofluran zur Kastration beim Hengst. Pferdeheilkunde 23, 388–397.

Mosing, M., Auer, U., Bardell, D., et al., 2010. Reversal of profound rocuronium block monitored in three muscle groups with sugammadex in ponies. Br J Anaesth 105, 480–486.

Muir, 3rd, W.W., 1992a. Cardiovascular effects of dopexamine HCl in conscious and halothane-anaesthetised horses. Equine Vet J Supplement, 24–29.

Muir, 3rd, W.W., 1992b. Inotropic mechanisms of dopexamine hydrochloride in horses. Am J Vet Res 53, 1343–1346.

Muir, 3rd, W.W., Sams, R., 1992. Effects of ketamine infusion on halothane minimal alveolar concentration in horses. Am J Vet Res 53, 1802–1806.

Muir, 3rd, W.W., Gadawski, J.E., Grosenbaugh, D.A., 1999. Cardiorespiratory effects of a tiletamine/zolazepam-ketamine-detomidine combination in horses. Am J Vet Res 60, 770–774.

Muir, W.W., Lerche, P., Erichson, D., 2009. Anaesthetic and cardiorespiratory effects of propofol at 10% for induction and 1% for maintenance of anaesthesia in horses. Equine Vet J 41, 578–585.

Muir, W.W., Sams, R.A., Huffman, R.H., et al., 1982. Pharmacodynamic and pharmacokinetic properties of diazepam in horses. Am J Vet Res 43, 1756–1762.

Muir, W.W., Skarda, R.T., Milne, D.W., 1977. Evaluation of xylazine and ketamine hydrochloride for anesthesia in horses. Am J Vet Res 38, 195–201.

Muir, W.W., Skarda, R.T., Sheehan, W., 1979. Hemodynamic and respiratory effects of a xylazine-acetylpromazine drug combination in horses. Am J Vet Res 40, 1518–1522.

Natalini, C.C., 2010. Spinal anesthetics and analgesics in the horse. Vet Clin N Am Equine Pract 26, 551–564.

Natalini, C.C., Robinson, E.P., 2000. Evaluation of the analgesic effects of epidurally administered morphine, alfentanil, butorphanol, tramadol, and U50488H in horses. Am J Vet Res 61, 1579–1586.

Nilsfors, L., Kvart, C., 1986. Preliminary report on the cardiorespiratory effects of the antagonist to detomidine, MPV-1248. Acta Vet Scand Suppl 82, 121–129.

Nolan, A., Reid, J., Welsh, E., et al., 1996. Simultaneous infusions of propofol and ketamine in ponies premedicated with detomidine: a pharmacokinetic study. Res Vet Sci 60, 262–266.

Nolan, A.M., Hall, L.W., 1985. Total intravenous anaesthesia in the horse with propofol. Equine Vet J 17, 394–398.

Nyman, G., Funkquist, B., Kvart, C., et al., 1990. Atelectasis causes gas exchange impairment in the anaesthetised horse. Equine Vet J 22, 317–324.

Nyman, G., Grubb, T.L., Heinonen, E., et al., 2012. Pulsed delivery of inhaled nitric oxide counteracts hypoxaemia during 2.5 hours of inhalation anaesthesia in dorsally recumbent horses. Vet Anaesth Analg 39, 480–487.

Ohta, M., Oku, K., Mukai, K., et al., 2004. Propofol-ketamine anesthesia for internal fixation of fractures in racehorses. J Vet Med 66, 1433–1436.

Orsini, J.A., Moate, P.J., Kuersten, K., et al., 2006. Pharmacokinetics of fentanyl delivered transdermally in healthy adult horses – variability among horses and its clinical implications. J Vet Pharmacol Ther 29, 539–546.

Pantaleon, L.G., Furr, M.O., McKenzie, 2nd, H.C., et al., 2006. Cardiovascular and pulmonary effects of hetastarch plus hypertonic saline solutions during experimental endotoxemia in anesthetized horses. J Vet Int Med 20, 1422–1428.

Pascoe, P.J., Taylor, P.M., 2003. Effects of dopamine antagonists on alfentanil-induced locomotor activity in horses. Vet Anaesth Analg 30, 165–171.

Pimenta, E.L., Teixeira Neto, F.J., Sa, P.A., et al., 2011. Comparative study between atropine and hyoscine-N-butylbromide for reversal of detomidine induced bradycardia in horses. Equine Vet J 43, 332–340.

Portier, K.G., Jaillardon, L., Leece, E.A., et al., 2009. Castration of horses under total intravenous anaesthesia: analgesic effects of lidocaine. Vet Anaesth Analg 36, 173–179.

Raisis, A.L., 2005. Skeletal muscle blood flow in anaesthetized horses. Part II: effects of anaesthetics and vasoactive agents. Vet Anaesth Analg 32, 331–337.

Rezende, M.L., Wagner, A.E., Mama, K.R., et al., 2011. Effects of intravenous administration of lidocaine on the minimum alveolar concentration of sevoflurane in horses. Am J Vet Res 72, 446–451.

Richey, M.T., Holland, M.S., McGrath, C.J., et al., 1990. Equine post-anesthetic lameness. A retrospective study. Vet Surg 19, 392–397.

Ringer, S.K., Kalchofner, K., Bollei, J., et al., 2007. A clinical comparison of two anaesthetic protocols using lidocaine or medetomidine in horses. Vet Anaesth Analg 34, 257–268.

Ringer, S.K., Portier, K., Torgerson, P.R., et al., 2013. The effects of a loading dose followed by constant rate infusion of xylazine compared with romifidine on sedation, ataxia and response to stimuli in horses. Vet Anaesth Analg 40, 157–165.

Ringer, S.K., Portier, K.G., Fourel, I., et al., 2012a. Development of a romifidine constant rate infusion with or without butorphanol for standing sedation of horses. Vet Anaesth Analg 39, 12–20.

Ringer, S.K., Portier, K.G., Fourel, I., et al., 2012b. Development of a xylazine constant rate infusion with or without butorphanol for standing sedation of horses. Vet Anaesth Analg 39, 1–11.

Robertson, S.A., Carter, S.W., Donovan, M., et al., 1990. Effects of intravenous xylazine hydrochloride on blood glucose, plasma insulin and rectal temperature in neonatal foals. Equine Vet J 22, 43–47.

Robertson, S.A., Sanchez, L.C., Merritt, A.M., et al., 2005. Effect of systemic lidocaine on visceral and somatic nociception in conscious horses. Equine Vet J 37, 122–127.

Robinson, E.P., Natalini, C.C., 2002. Epidural anesthesia and analgesia in horses. Vet Clin N Am Equine Pract 18, 61–82.

Robinson, E.P., Moncada-Suarex, J.R., Felice, L., 1994. Epidural morphine analgesia in horses. Vet Surg 23, 78.

Rohrbach, H., Korpivaara, T., Schatzmann, U., et al., 2009. Comparison of the effects of the alpha-2 agonists detomidine, romifidine and xylazine on nociceptive withdrawal reflex and temporal summation in horses. Vet Anaesth Analg 36, 384–395.

Rose, R.J., Rose, E.M., Peterson, P.R., 1989. Clinical experiences with isoflurane anaesthesia in foals and adult horses. Am Assoc Equine Practit 34, 555–569.

Sanchez, L.C., Robertson, S.A., Maxwell, L.K., et al., 2007. Effect of fentanyl on visceral and somatic nociception in conscious horses. J Vet Int Med 21, 1067–1075.

Santos, L.C., de Moraes, A.N., Saito, M.E., 2009. Effects of intraarticular ropivacaine and morphine on lipopolysaccharide-induced synovitis in horses. Vet Anaesth Analg 36, 280–286.

Santos, M., Lopez-Sanroman, J., Garcia-Iturralde, P., et al., 2005. Cardiopulmonary effects of desflurane in horses. Vet Anaesth Analg 32, 355–359.

Schatzmann, U., 1982. The respiration of the horse under different anaesthetic medications. Proc Assoc Vet Anaesth 10 (Suppl), 112–118.

Schauvliege, S., Marcilla, M.G., Verryken, K., et al., 2011. Effects of a constant rate infusion of detomidine on cardiovascular function, isoflurane requirements and recovery quality in horses. Vet Anaesth Analg 38, 544–554.

Sellon, D.C., Roberts, M.C., Blikslager, A.T., et al., 2004. Effects of continuous rate intravenous infusion of butorphanol on physiologic and outcome variables in horses after celiotomy. J Vet Int Med 18, 555–563.

Short, C.E., 1992. Alpha 2-agents in animals. Sedation, analgesia and anaesthesia. Veterinary Practice Publishing Company, Santa Barbara, pp. 21–39.

Short, C.E., Matthews, N., Harvey, R., et al., 1986. Cardiovascular and pulmonary function studies of a new sedative/analgetic (detomidine/ Domosedan) for use alone in horses or as a preanesthetic. Acta Vet Scand Suppl 82, 139–155.

Singh, S., McDonell, W., Young, S., et al., 1997. The effect of glycopyrrolate on heart rate and intestinal motility in conscious horses. J Vet Anaesth 24, 14–19.

Sinclair, M.D., Mealey, K.L., Matthews, N.S., et al., 2006. Comparative pharmacokinetics of meloxicam in clinically normal horses and donkeys. Am J Vet Res 67, 1082–1085.

Skarda, R.T., Muir, 3rd, W.W., 1996. Comparison of antinociceptive, cardiovascular, and respiratory effects, head ptosis, and position of pelvic limbs in mares after caudal epidural administration of xylazine and detomidine hydrochloride solution. Am J Vet Res 57, 1338–1345.

Solano, A.M., Valverde, A., Desrochers, A., et al., 2009. Behavioural and cardiorespiratory effects of a constant rate infusion of medetomidine and morphine for sedation during standing laparoscopy in horses. Equine Vet J 41, 153–159.

Spadavecchia, C., Arendt-Nielsen, L., Andersen, O.K., et al., 2005. Effect of romifidine on the nociceptive withdrawal reflex and temporal summation in conscious horses. Am J Vet Res 66, 1992–1998.

Staffieri, F., Bauquier, S.H., Moate, P.J., et al., 2009. Pulmonary gas exchange in anaesthetised horses mechanically ventilated with oxygen or a helium/ oxygen mixture. Equine Vet J 41, 747–752.

Steffey, E.P., 2002. Recent advances in inhalation anesthesia. Vet Clin N Am Equine Pract 18, 159–168.

Steffey, E.P., Howland, Jr., D., 1978. Cardiovascular effects of halothane in the horse. Am J Vet Res 39, 611–615.

Steffey, E.P., Kelly, A.B., Hodgson, D.S., et al., 1990. Effect of body posture on cardiopulmonary function in horses during five hours of constant-dose halothane anesthesia. Am J Vet Res 51, 11–16.

Steffey, E.P., Willits, N., Woliner, M., 1992. Hemodynamic and respiratory responses to variable arterial partial pressure of oxygen in halothane-anesthetized horses during spontaneous and controlled ventilation. Am J Vet Res 53, 1850–1858.

Steffey, E.P., Pascoe, P.J., Woliner, M.J., et al., 2000. Effects of xylazine hydrochloride during isoflurane-induced anesthesia in horses. Am J Vet Res 61, 1225–1231.

Steffey, E.P., Mama, K.R., Galey, F.D., et al., 2005a. Effects of sevoflurane dose and mode of ventilation on cardiopulmonary function and blood biochemical variables in horses. Am J Vet Res 66, 606–614.

Steffey, E.P., Woliner, M.J., Puschner, B., et al., 2005b. Effects of desflurane and mode of ventilation on cardiovascular and respiratory functions and clinicopathologic variables in horses. Am J Vet Res 66, 669–677.

Steffey, E.P., Mama, K.R., Brosnan, R.J., et al., 2009. Effect of administration of propofol and xylazine hydrochloride on recovery of horses after four hours of anesthesia with desflurane. Am J Vet Res 70, 956–963.

Stewart, A.J., Boothe, D.M., Cruz-Espindola, C., et al., 2011. Pharmacokinetics of tramadol and metabolites O-desmethyltramadol and N-desmethyltramadol in adult horses. Am J Vet Res 72, 967–974.

Suthers, J.M., Christley, R.M., Clutton, R.E., 2011. Quantitative and qualitative comparison of three scoring systems for assessing recovery quality after general anaesthesia in horses. Vet Anaesth Analg 38, 352–362.

Sysel, A.M., Pleasant, R.S., Jacobson, J.D., et al., 1996. Efficacy of an epidural combination of morphine and detomidine in alleviating experimentally induced hindlimb lameness in horses. Vet Surg 25, 511–518.

Taylor, P.M., 1998. Endocrine and metabolic responses to plasma volume expansion during halothane anesthesia in ponies. J Vet Pharmacol Ther 21, 485–490.

Taylor, P.M., Clarke, K.W., 2007. A Handbook of Equine Anaesthesia, second ed. Saunders- Elsevier.

Taylor, P.M., Young, S.S., 1990. The effect of limb position on venous and intracompartmental pressure in the forelimb of ponies. J Assoc Vet Anaesth 17, 35–37.

Tendillo, F.J., Mascias, A., Santos, M., et al., 1997. Anesthetic potency of desflurane in the horse: determination of the minimum alveolar concentration. Vet Surg 26, 354–357.

Terry, R.L., McDonnell, S.M., Van Eps, A.W., et al., 2010. Pharmacokinetic profile and behavioral effects of gabapentin in the horse. J Vet Pharmacol Ther 33, 485–494.

Thomasy, S.M., Slovis, N., Maxwell, L.K., et al., 2004. Transdermal fentanyl combined with nonsteroidal anti-inflammatory drugs for analgesia in horses. J Vet Int Med 18, 550–554.

Thomasy, S.M., Steffey, E.P., Mama, K.R., et al., 2006. The effects of i.v. fentanyl administration on the minimum alveolar concentration of isoflurane in horses. Br J Anaesth 97, 232–237.

Tobin, T., Combie, J.D., 1982. Performance testing in horses: a review of the role of simple behavioral models in the design of performance experiments. J Vet Pharmacol Ther 5, 105–118.

Trim, C.M., 1984. Complications associated with the use of the cuffless endotracheal tube in the horse. J Am Vet Med Assoc 185, 541–542.

Trim, C.M., 1997. Postanesthetic hemorrhagic myelopathy or myelomalacia. Veterinary Clin N Am Equine Pract 13, 73–77.

Trim, C.M., Mason, J., 1973. Post-anesthetic forelimb lameness in horses. Equine Vet J 5, 71–76.

Trim, C.M., Moore, J.N., Clark, E.S., 1989. Renal effects of dopamine infusion in conscious horses. Equine Vet J Suppl 124–128.

Trim, C.M., Moore, J.N., White, N.A., 1985. Cardiopulmonary effects of dopamine hydrochloride in anaesthetised horses. Equine Vet J 17, 41–44.

Trim, C.M., Moore, J.N., Hardee, M.M., et al., 1991. Effects of an infusion of dopamine on the cardiopulmonary effects of Escherichia coli endotoxin in anaesthetised horses. Res Vet Sci 50, 54–63.

Umar, M.A., Yamashita, K., Kushiro, T., et al., 2006. Evaluation of total intravenous anesthesia with propofol or ketamine-medetomidine-propofol combination in horses. J Am Vet Med Assoc 228, 1221–1227.

Umar, M.A., Yamashita, K., Kushiro, T., et al., 2007. Evaluation of cardiovascular effects of total intravenous anesthesia with propofol or a combination of ketamine-medetomidine-propofol in horses. Am J Vet Res 68, 121–127.

Vainio, O., 1985. Detomidine, a new sedative and analgesic drug for veterinary use. Pharmacological and clinical studies in laboratory animals, horses and cattle. PhD thesis. University of Helsinki, Helsinki.

Valverde, A., 2010. Alpha-2 agonists as pain therapy in horses. Vet Clin N Am Equine Pract 26, 515–532.

Valverde, A., Gunkelt, C., Doherty, T.J., et al., 2005. Effect of a constant rate infusion of lidocaine on the quality of recovery from sevoflurane or isoflurane general anaesthesia in horses. Equine Vet J 37, 559–564.

van Dijk, P., Lankveld, D.P., Rijkenhuizen, A.B., et al., 2003. Hormonal, metabolic and physiological effects of laparoscopic surgery using a detomidine-buprenorphine combination in standing horses. Vet Anaesth Analg 30, 72–80.

van Loon, J.P., de Grauw, J.C., van Dierendonck, M., et al., 2010. Intra-articular opioid analgesia is effective in reducing pain and inflammation in an equine LPS induced synovitis model. Equine Vet J 42, 412–419.

van Loon, J.P., Menke, E.S., Doornenbal, A., et al., 2012. Antinociceptive effects of low dose lumbosacral epidural ropivacaine in healthy ponies. Vet J 193, 240–245.

Villalba, M., Santiago, I., Gomez de Segura, I.A., 2011. Effects of constant rate infusion of lidocaine and ketamine, with or without morphine, on isoflurane MAC in horses. Equine Vet J 43, 721–726.

Voetgli, K., 1988. Studies on the sedative and analgesic effects of an alpha 2 adrenoceptor agonist (STH 2130) in horses. DVet Med Thesis. University of Berne, Berne.

Wagner, A.E., 2010. Effects of stress on pain in horses and incorporating pain scales for equine practice. Vet Clin N Am Equine Pract 26, 481–492.

Wagner, A.E., Dunlop, C.I., Heath, R.B., et al., 1992. Hemodynamic function during neurectomy in halothane-anesthetized horses with or without constant dose detomidine infusion. Vet Surg 21, 248–255.

Wagner, A.E., Mama, K.R., Steffey, E.P., et al., 2011. Comparison of the cardiovascular effects of equipotent anesthetic doses of sevoflurane alone and sevoflurane plus an intravenous infusion of lidocaine in horses. Am J Vet Res 72, 452–460.

Wagner, A.E., Mama, K.R., Steffey, E.P., et al., 2012. Evaluation of infusions of xylazine with ketamine or propofol to modulate recovery following sevoflurane anesthesia in horses. Am J Vet Res 73, 346–352.

Wagner, A.E., Muir, 3rd, W.W., Hinchcliff, K.W., 1991. Cardiovascular effects of xylazine and detomidine in horses. Am J Vet Res 52, 651–657.

Westhues, M., Fritsch, R., 1960. Die narkose der Tierre. Paul Darey, Berlin.

Wetmore, L.A., Derksen, F.J., Blaze, C.A., et al., 1987. Mixed venous oxygen tension as an estimate of cardiac output in anesthetized horses. Am J Vet Res 48, 971–976.

Wettstein, D., Moens, Y., Jaeggin-Schmucker, N., et al., 2006. Effects of an alveolar recruitment maneuver on cardiovascular and respiratory parameters during total intravenous anesthesia in ponies. Am J Vet Res 67, 152–159.

Wilcke, J.R., Crisman, M.V., Sams, R.A., et al., 1993. Pharmacokinetics of phenylbutazone in neonatal foals. Am J Vet Res 54, 2064–2067.

Wilcke, J.R., Crisman, M.V., Scarratt, W.K., et al., 1998. Pharmacokinetics of ketoprofen in healthy foals less than twenty-four hours old. Am J Vet Res 59, 290–292.

Wilson, D.V., Bohart, G.V., Evans, A.T., et al., 2002. Retrospective analysis of detomidine infusion for standing chemical restraint in 51 horses. Vet Anaesth Analg, 29, 54–57.

Young, L.E., Blissitt, K.J., Clutton, R.E., et al., 1997. Temporal effects of an infusion of dopexamine hydrochloride in horses anesthetized with halothanc. Am J Vet Res 58, 516–523.

Chapter | **12** |

Anaesthesia of cattle

INTRODUCTION

Cattle are by no means good subjects for heavy sedation or general anaesthesia. Regurgitation followed by aspiration of ruminal contents into the lungs can easily occur. Once a ruminant animal is in lateral or dorsal recumbency, the oesophageal opening is submerged in ruminal material, normal eructation cannot occur, and gas accumulates. The degree of bloat depends on the amount of fermentation of the ingesta and on the length of time that gas is allowed to accumulate. Gross distension of the rumen becomes a hazard if anaesthesia or recumbency is prolonged and regurgitation can follow from this. In addition, the weight of the abdominal viscera and their contents prevents the diaphragm from moving freely on inspiration and ventilation becomes shallow, rapid and inefficient for gas exchange within the lungs.

The danger of regurgitation and inhalation of ingesta is always present but the likelihood of it occurring can be minimized by:

1. Withholding all food for 24–48 hours before anaesthesia. Optimum duration for starvation is up for discussion, with some recommending that 24 hours is not only sufficient but also produces the best consistency of rumen contents to minimize regurgitation. A longer period of starvation may result in formation of a more liquid ruminal content which may be regurgitated more easily.
2. Withholding water for 8–12 hours before anaesthesia. The ideal time of withholding water is not documented scientifically, however, hungry cattle will drink water and subsequently regurgitate it during induction of anaesthesia.
3. When the animal is in lateral recumbency during anaesthesia arranging that the occiput is above general body level and that the head slopes so that saliva and any regurgitated material runs freely from the mouth (Fig. 12.1).
4. At the end of anaesthesia, cleaning solid material from the pharynx and leaving the endotracheal tube in the trachea with the cuff inflated until the animal is in sternal recumbency, is swallowing and, most importantly, can withdraw its tongue back into its mouth.

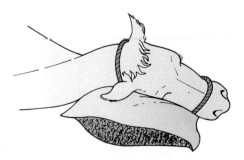

Figure 12.1 Animal's head inclined over a support to allow saliva and any regurgitated ruminal content to drain out of the mouth.

An additional procedure to prevent regurgitation that has been tried but not often used is to pass a modified stomach tube as far down the oesophagus as possible. The tube has a balloon firmly attached to its end that can be inflated to obstruct flow of ingesta from the rumen into the pharynx.

Regurgitation occurs during both light and deep anaesthesia so that it is probable that two mechanisms are involved in the process. During light anaesthesia, ingesta may pass up the oesophagus into the pharynx as a result of an active, but uncontrolled, reflex mechanism. It is then a matter of chance whether or not the protective reflexes, e.g. laryngeal closure, coughing, etc., are active and can or cannot prevent aspiration. Fortunately, laryngeal closure often occurs but, as hypoxia develops, at some point, the animal will take a large breath and any ingesta accumulated in the pharynx will be aspirated. The order in which the reflexes of laryngeal closure, coughing, swallowing, and regurgitation disappear as anaesthesia is deepened differs from one anaesthetic drug combination to another but the relative safety of the various agents is not documented. During deep anaesthesia, on the other hand, regurgitation is a passive process. The striated muscle of the oesophagus loses its tone and any increase in the intraruminal pressure – whether from pressure on the abdominal wall from a rope or belly band or from gas accumulation in the rumen itself – may force ingesta up into the pharynx. The protective reflexes are not active and aspiration may occur easily.

Regurgitation and pulmonary aspiration is a real and serious hazard in sedated or anaesthetized cattle.

Tracheal intubation is not always performed in all sedated or anaesthetized recumbent bovine animals and regurgitation does not always occur. However, some animals will regurgitate, and this has an unreasonably high risk for fatal outcome. Should regurgitation occur during the induction of anaesthesia before endotracheal intubation has been accomplished, the endotracheal tube may be immediately passed into the oesophagus and its cuff inflated so that the regurgitated material passes along the tube and out of the mouth. The trachea can then be intubated with a second tube, taking care to cover the end of the tube to avoid scooping material into its lumen. In actuality, the presence of one endotracheal tube in the pharynx often makes passage of a second tube nearly impossible due to the small size of the bovine pharynx. One option is to intubate the trachea with a stomach tube and attempt to feed the second endotracheal tube over the stomach tube. An alternative is to wait until the flow of ingesta stops, remove the tube from the oesophagus and to rapidly intubate the trachea. However, if the conditions initiating the regurgitation such as ropes tight around the thorax and abdomen have not been removed, or the depth of anaesthesia is light, regurgitation may recommence during the removal of the endotracheal tube from the oesophagus.

Salivation continues as a copious flow throughout general anaesthesia but the loss of saliva is unlikely to produce a significant effect on acid–base status. Antisialagogues are not of much use for they make the secretion more viscid in nature and do not significantly reduce its production. It is important to arrange the head of the anaesthetized animal so that saliva drains from the mouth and does not accumulate in the pharynx. Intubation with a cuffed endotracheal tube will prevent inhalation of saliva.

In two reports involving restraint of unsedated cows or bulls in dorsal or lateral recumbency, a decrease in PaO_2 from an average standing value of 11.4 kPa (86 mmHg) to less than 9.3 kPa (70 mmHg) was measured, with a decrease to below 6.6 kPa (50 mmHg) in some individuals (Semrad et al., 1986; Klein & Fisher, 1988). Arterial PCO_2 remained at or slightly below 5 kPa (38 mmHg). In another investigation of cows from which food was withheld for 18 h, mean PaO_2 in standing animals was 14.5 kPa (109 mmHg) (Wagner et al., 1990). Significant decreases in PaO_2 occurred in both lateral and dorsal positions but only in dorsal recumbency did values decrease to below 9.3 kPa (70 mmHg). These changes indicate that even in unsedated cattle, recumbency creates abnormalities of ventilation and perfusion that are not counterbalanced by normal compensatory mechanisms.

In contrast, when calves 25–53 days of age that had milk replacer withheld for 12 hours were restrained in dorsal recumbency for 95 minutes, the cardiopulmonary changes induced by the change in body position were much less than previously described for adult cattle, perhaps due to the lesser weight of the abdomen on the diaphragm or the caudal vena cava (Meyer et al., 2010). Cardiac output decreased by 15%, O_2 delivery decreased with no change in O_2 extraction ratio, and respiratory rate (RR) and systemic vascular resistances increased. PaO_2 and $PaCO_2$ were unchanged.

Withholding feed before sedation and anaesthesia may reduce pressure on the diaphragm, limit lung collapse and modify the decrease in PaO_2. In a study of fed and non-fed cows anaesthetized with halothane and breathing oxygen, cows fed before anaesthesia had a progressive decrease in PaO_2, reaching hypoxaemic levels after an hour of anaesthesia, whereas cows that were starved before anaesthesia were well oxygenated (Blaze et al., 1988). Severe hypercapnia was measured in both groups with a greater increase measured in the fed cows. Thus, hypoxaemia may develop in recumbent non-starved cattle even when inhaling high O_2 concentrations but supplementation of inspired air with O_2 may prevent hypoxaemia if the cow has been starved first. Respiratory acidosis usually develops in anaesthetized cattle.

Normal values for cardiovascular parameters in unsedated healthy adult cattle are approximately 73 ± 14 beats/ min (mean ± SD) for heart rate, 150 ± 27 mmHg for mean arterial pressure (MAP), and 64 ± 14 mL/kg/min for cardiac output (CO) (Wagner et al., 1990). Withholding feed for 48 h has been determined to cause significant decreases in heart rates in cattle (Rumsey & Bond, 1976; McGuirk et al., 1990). Normal values in calves 2–26 days old have been measured at approximately 112 beats/min, $117–127 \pm 16$ mmHg for systolic arterial pressure (SAP), $77–83 \pm 15$ mmHg for diastolic pressures (DAP), on average 94–98 mmHg for MAP, and on average 150 mL/ kg/min for CO (Kerr et al., 2007). Normal values measured in calves 25–53 days old were on average heart rates 105–125 beats/min, 84–96 mmHg for MAP, and 205 mL/ kg/min for CO (Meyer et al., 2010).

Restraint

The majority of bovine clinical surgery is carried out under local analgesia, frequently in the standing animal. Surgical procedure is made easier by use of appropriate sedation and/or restraining 'crushes' or 'chutes'. Ropes are useful additions for restraining sedated or unsedated cattle and anyone in cattle veterinary practice soon becomes expert at tying quick-release knots, tying bowline knots for rope loops, applying Reuff's method of casting a mature bovine by squeezing with a neck loop and two half-hitches around the body, and assembling figure of eight ties to secure flexed front and hind limbs.

Electroimmobilization

Electrical devices are available in some countries to immobilize cattle by causing muscle tetanus from application of an electrical current between electrodes at the lip and rectum. There are concerns that this technique is neither humane nor analgesic. Holstein cows trained to be led with a halter and enter a set of stocks were observed for behavioural and physiological responses to either immobilization by application of an electric current for 30 s from a commercially available electroimmobilizer or to an intramuscular injection with an 18 gauge needle (Pascoe, 1986). The electrical immobilization was associated with significant aversive behaviour and evidence of distress and the results led the author to believe that electroimmobilization was a strong noxious stimulus that was remembered for several months.

SEDATION AND ANALGESIA

Cattle may not strongly exhibit behavioural signs commonly associated with pain, which may lead to the mistaken perception that bovine animals and young calves do not require analgesia such as is afforded to horses, dogs, and cats. Administration of sedatives and analgesics, including local nerve blocks and non-steroidal anti-inflammatory drugs (NSAIDs), not only fulfills our moral obligation to provide analgesia during surgical procedures but also may increase the safety of the veterinary practitioner during performance of the procedure. These factors must outweigh the economic concern of the cost and increased time involved in administration of analgesic agents to the large numbers of calves that must be castrated and dehorned, and for other disabilities and surgeries. Surveys completed by practitioners who work with cattle indicate an increased awareness by practitioners for the need to provide analgesia in this species (Huxley & Whay, 2006; Hewson et al., 2007; Thomsen et al., 2010; Fajt et al., 2011). Commonly expressed comments were that administration of analgesic drugs makes it safer to work with cattle, that the potency and duration of action of available drugs were considered very important, and that there is a shortage of analgesic drugs available that are both long acting and cost effective. When analgesics were administered, they most commonly were NSAIDs, local anaesthetics, and α_2-adrenergic receptor agonists.

Respondents to the questionnaires were asked to assign pain scores to a variety of disease conditions and surgical procedures and although moderate pain scores were assigned for castration, a high proportion of respondents in North America did not provide analgesia for castration (Fajt et al., 2011). Even when a high pain score was assigned, for example for claw amputation, caesarian section, and umbilical hernia repair, only approximately 60% of practitioners administered NSAIDs for postoperative pain control (Huxley & Whay, 2006; Fajt et al., 2011). Current updates on analgesia practices must include consideration that administration of local anaesthetics and sedatives at the time of the procedure does not guarantee analgesia postoperatively.

Choice of drugs may be influenced by current legislature concerning use of anaesthetic agents in food-producing animals. The licensing of withdrawal periods is done by national agencies so that not only are the kinetics of individual drugs considered but also regional practices and requirements. Human ingestion of drug residues of anaesthetic agents at injection sites has the potential of inducing toxicities or allergic reactions. Requirements of national licensing authorities are not universal. The food safety approach of European agencies specifies a withdrawal period based on a whole-of-life maximal residue limit whereas USA, Canada, and Australia evaluate the risk based on acute exposure (Reeves, 2007).

Many of the anaesthetic agents are administered to cattle as extralabel use, for example ketamine, and some countries offer recommended withdrawal times for meat and milk. In the USA, recommended withdrawal after ketamine is 3 days for meat and 48 hours for milk, however, recent pharmacokinetic measurements after administration of ketamine, 5 mg/kg IV, to lactating Holstein cows indicate that milk withdrawal probably should

be extended to at least 60 hours (Sellers et al., 2010). Persistence of plasma concentrations will be altered by dose administered such that a terminal half-life of approximately 30 minutes was measured following a subanaesthetic dose of ketamine, 0.1 mg/kg IV, given in combination with a sedative dose of xylazine for castration in 4–6 month old Angus calves (Gehring et al., 2008). In Europe, if the drug has a licence for any food animal (including the horse) then withdrawal times for a food animal species for which it does not have a licence are (at the time of writing) 28 days for meat and 7 days for milk. However, any animal that has received certain drugs may never go for human consumption. For example, phenylbutazone in cattle of any age (UK) or cattle >20 months of age (USA) (Davis et al., 2009). In this chapter, information on the pharmacological effects of various agents and their combinations is given in order that informed decisions can be made about their use in all situations. Some of the anaesthetic agents mentioned may be unsuitable in some countries for use in animals for subsequent slaughter.

Knowledge of withdrawal times is important to avoid anaesthetic agent residues in animals and animal products intended for human consumption.

Agents used in bovine species

Xylazine

Xylazine has been used as a sedative in cattle for a long time. The dose rate of xylazine in cattle, 0.02–0.20 mg/kg, with the highest dose intended for IM use, is one-tenth of that used in horses (Table 12.1). Intravenous injection results in deeper sedation than IM administration. Cattle may assume recumbency even at the lowest dose rates, although breed differences in sensitivity to xylazine have been reported. In an investigation comparing Hereford and Holstein cattle, 84% of Herefords spontaneously lay down after xylazine administration, whereas only 22% of Holsteins did so (Raptopoulos & Weaver, 1984). Furthermore, the average duration of recumbency in the Herefords was 90 min compared with 50 min in the Holsteins. Thus, in some situations, the dose rate in Holsteins may be increased to 0.3 mg/kg. Even higher doses may be necessary for free-ranging cows to be immobilized using a dart gun in order to overcome the high circulating catecholamine concentrations induced by excitement. The environmental conditions under which xylazine is administered may influence the response. In a study comparing the effects of xylazine in Holstein heifers under a thermoneutral condition compared with a hot environment (temperature approximately 33°C and relative humidity 63%), the time to standing was increased from 41 min to an average of 107 min during heat stress (Fayed et al., 1989).

Xylazine may cause mild to severe decreases in PaO_2 and moderate increases in $PaCO_2$ in mature cattle (DeMoor

Table 12.1 Dose rates of sedative, analgesic agents, and antagonists

Drug	Dose (mg/kg)	Route	Comments
Xylazine	0.02–0.2	IM, IV	Lowest dose rate for very young calves and standing adults; dose-dependent sedation; recumbency with high dose rate
Detomidine	0.01–0.04	IM, IV	Low dose for standing; high dose for recumbency
Tolazoline	0.5–2.0	IM, IV	Xylazine antagonist; inject slowly if IV; suggest half IM and half IV
Atipamezole	0.025–0.06	IM, IV	Antagonist for xylazine, detomidine, medetomidine; excitement in some cattle; relapse to sedation may occur 1–4 hours after administration
Acepromazine	0.02–0.05	IM, IV	Mild sedation
Butorphanol	0.025–0.05	IM, IV	Adjunct to sedative
Ketamine	0.1–0.4	IM, IV	Adjunct to sedative; low dose for standing

& Desmet, 1971; Raptopoulos & Weaver, 1984). A more detailed discussion of the effects of α_2-agonists on pulmonary function is in the following chapter. Xylazine administration induces bradycardia, decreased MAP and CO, and increased peripheral resistance (Campbell et al., 1979, Rioja et al., 2008). Campbell et al. (1979) also noted second degree atrioventricular heart block in one out of five calves receiving xylazine.

Xylazine has a number of side effects that may have an adverse effect on the animal. It abolishes the swallowing reflex so that regurgitation can result in pulmonary aspiration. The inability of the cow or bull to withdraw its tongue into its mouth and swallow may persist until after the animal regains the standing position. Thus, it is advisable to withhold food and water from cattle before giving xylazine. Gastrointestinal motility is decreased and bloat may develop, while diarrhoea may be observed 12–24 hours after sedation (Hopkins, 1972). Hyperglycaemia may persist for about 10 hours. Increased urine production occurs within 30 minutes of administration and continues for 2 hours (Thurmon et al., 1978). Use of xylazine in animals with urethral obstruction may be responsible for rupture of the urinary bladder or urethra. Xylazine causes contraction of the bovine uterus similar to oxytocin (LeBlanc et al., 1984), and premature birth has been reported after administration to heavily pregnant cows. Administration of xylazine, 0.04 mg/kg IV, to pregnant cows between 219 and 241 days of gestation was followed by a decrease in uterine arterial blood flow by 56% from baseline values associated with an initial 59% reduction in O_2 delivery (Hodgson et al., 2002). The impact on uterine blood flow progressively lessened but was still significant at 45 minutes. Consequently, use of xylazine in pregnant cows in the last trimester of pregnancy is not recommended.

Minor surgical procedures have been performed on cattle sedated with xylazine but local infiltration techniques or nerve blocks should be utilized to ensure sufficient analgesia.

Detomidine

In contrast to xylazine, the dose rates for detomidine in cattle are similar to those used in horses. In Europe, detomidine is licensed for cattle at doses of 0.01–0.04 mg/kg IM or IV, with (at the time of writing) withdrawal times of 12 hours for milk and 2 days for meat. At the higher doses, cattle may lie down. One study (Lin & Riddell, 2003) documented that detomidine, 0.01 mg/kg, IV in Holstein cattle resulted in greater sedation than xylazine, 0.02 mg/kg, during which the cows remained standing. Elimination is mainly by metabolism as there is negligible excretion of the drug in urine. No detomidine was detectable in milk 23 h after dosing and tissue concentrations measured 48 h after dosing were less than 3% of the original dose (Salonen et al., 1989). Detomidine, 0.04 and 0.06 mg/kg, increases electrical activity of the bovine uterus (Vainio, 1988). A lower dose rate of detomidine, 0.02 mg/kg, decreased electrical activity of the uterus and sedation at this dose rate may be safe in the pregnant animal (Vainio, 1988).

The pharmacological effects of detomidine in cattle are very similar to those of xylazine in that it causes bradycardia, hyperglycaemia, and increased urine production. An exception is that detomidine causes a transient increase in blood pressure that is dose dependent in duration, whereas xylazine decreases blood pressure in cattle.

Medetomidine

Deep sedation without recumbency can be obtained with intravenous doses of medetomidine, 0.005 mg/kg, while

0.01 mg/kg produces recumbency and sedation equivalent to that obtained with intravenous doses of 0.1–0.2 mg/kg xylazine (England GCW & Clarke KW, unpublished observations). Duration of sedation of medetomidine, 0.03 mg/kg, IV in calves lasted significantly longer than xylazine, 0.3 mg/kg IV with the mean times to sternal recumbency and to standing after agent administration being 66 and 242 minutes, and 19 and 128 minutes, respectively (Rioja et al., 2008). In a separate experiment, with calves suspended in the upright position, injection of medetomidine, 0.03 mg/kg, IV resulted in hypoxaemia and hypercarbia at 5 and 15 minutes, significant decreases in heart rates and CO, and increases in MAP, systemic vascular resistance, and central venous pressure. Administration of atipamezole, 0.1 mg/kg, IV 20 minutes after medetomidine satisfactorily reversed the sedation and the respiratory and cardiovascular effects, including hypoxaemia. In contrast, atipamezole was not effective in reversing hypoxaemia in sheep when given more than 5 minutes after medetomidine administration. Medetomidine, 0.015 mg/kg, has been administered by epidural injection for analgesia in cows (Lin et al., 1998).

Antagonists of α_2-agonists

As prolonged recumbency causes so many problems in cattle, the availability of α_2-agonist antagonists is of particular value. These antagonists not only cause the animal to awaken, they also antagonize the majority of the side effects of the agonists, including restoring ruminal motility to normal and allowing release of gas from the rumen.

Almost all the α_2-agonist antagonists have been used in cattle sedated with xylazine. Yohimbine, 0.125 mg/kg, with aminopyridine, 0.3 mg/kg, will awaken cattle sedated with 0.2–0.3 mg/kg of xylazine, but will not restore a normal state of consciousness. Tolazoline, 0.5 mg/kg, was documented to be superior to yohimbine for antagonizing xylazine sedation in cattle (Hikasa et al., 1988). Tolazoline at 0.2 mg/kg reverses the suppression of ruminal motility induced by xylazine but higher doses, 0.5–2.0 mg/kg, are required for full reversal of sedation. Xylazine sedation, 0.3 mg/kg, IM in 6-month old Holstein Friesian calves was rapidly reversed within minutes by IV injection of tolazoline 1 and 2 mg/kg, with a more rapid return to normal gait following the larger dose rate (Powell et al., 1998). Care must be taken to administer tolazoline slowly as there are anecdotal reports that intravenous injection has been associated with abrupt adverse haemodynamic changes. In one study, reversal of xylazine sedation in calves with tolazoline caused transient sinus bradycardia and sinus arrest, accompanied by severe systemic arterial hypotension (Lewis et al., 1999). Withholding times are increased after administration of tolazoline. Xylazine is below the limits of detection in meat and organs by 72 hours and in milk by 12 hours whereas the limit of

detection after tolazoline administration was reached in 96 hours for meat and 48 hours for milk, leading to a recommended withholding time (in New Zealand) for tolazoline of 7 days for cattle meat and offal (Delehant et al., 2003).

Atipamezole has been used to reverse sedation induced by administration of α_2-agonist sedatives in cattle with a wide range of dose rates, 0.025–0.2 mg/kg. Atipamezole, 0.025, 0.03, 0.04, and 0.05 mg/kg (25–50 µg/kg), has been used to reverse the effects of xylazine, 0.2–0.3 mg/kg (Thompson et al., 1991; Rioja et al., 2008). Atipamezole, 0.06–0.08 mg/kg, IV effectively reversed within 2 minutes free-ranging cattle immobilized by darting with xylazine, 0.55 mg/kg, or medetomidine, 0.04 mg/kg (Arnemo & Søli, 1993). Of interest, eight out of 26 cows administered high doses of xylazine or medetomidine were in the last 2 months of pregnancy and were observed subsequently to calve normally. Atipamezole has been used at different dose rates to reverse the effects of medetomidine in cattle and calves. In one study (Raekallio et al., 1991), atipamezole, 0.06 mg/kg, given either IV or half IV and half IM to antagonize medetomidine in calves resulted in a rapid smooth recovery to ambulation and, in another (Rioja et al., 2008), atipamezole, 0.1 mg/kg, IV had the same effect. Ranheim et al. (1999) reversed sedation in calves given medetomidine, 0.04 mg/kg, by injecting atipamezole, 0.2 mg/kg, however, the authors' recommendation was that this dose should not be exceeded. Time of administration of atipamezole to standing has been reported from 2 to 12 minutes. Relapse to sedation or recumbency at times varying from 80 minutes to 2 to 3–4 hours after administration of atipamezole have been reported (Arnemo & Søli, 1993; Ranheim et al., 1998, 1999). Atipamezole given to unsedated cattle, or as sedation is waning, may induce a state of excitement, hyperactivity, kicking and bucking.

Acepromazine

Acepromazine may be given in doses of 0.02–0.05 mg/kg IV or 0.1 mg/kg IM to induce mild tranquillization. Acepromazine will decrease the dose rate of subsequently administered anaesthetics and may increase the risk of regurgitation.

Chloral hydrate

Chloral hydrate has been used as a sedative for adult cattle administered orally or by IV injection. To obtain a recumbent, very lightly unconscious adult cow, the drug can be administered by drench or by stomach tube in doses of 30–60 g as a 1 in 20 solution in water. Sedation attains its maximum depth in 10–20 minutes and local analgesics may be injected for nerve blocks while sedation is developing. The degree of sedation is not predictable in an excited animal. Withholding of water to increase thirst may act as an inducement for the animal to drink medicated water. Intravenous injection of chloral hydrate can be given with the cow standing or after casting with ropes. The dose required is between 80 and 90 mg/kg of a 10% solution and the infusion should be stopped before reaching the desired level of sedation because narcosis will continue to deepen after the IV injection is completed. The induction and recovery periods are excitement free. Chloral hydrate should be used cautiously in debilitated cows as rapid IV administration can cause cardiovascular collapse.

Sedative–opioid combinations

Administration of butorphanol to healthy unsedated cows will not predictably induce sedation and may induce behaviour changes including restlessness and bellowing. Butorphanol may provide sedation in cattle that are sick or in pain and may increase the quality of sedation when administered in conjunction with xylazine or detomidine. Reports of use of butorphanol with xylazine in healthy cattle have conflicting results on the degree of contribution of butorphanol to analgesia. Comparisons in adult cows between xylazine, 0.02 mg/kg, detomidine, 0.01 mg/kg, with or without butorphanol, 0.05 mg/kg, all administered IV, revealed no differences in duration or degree of sedation induced by the addition of butorphanol, and that the greatest sedation was observed after detomidine alone (Lin & Riddell, 2003). Sedation was accompanied by impaired swallowing indicated by drooling saliva and, in some cows, lowering of the head; all cows remained standing. A combination of xylazine, 0.02–0.05 mg/kg, butorphanol, 0.025 mg/kg, and ketamine, 0.1–0.4 mg/kg, IM has been used to restrain cattle with the low doses administered for standing restraint and the higher doses when recumbency is desired (Anderson, 2008). The duration of effect is about 45 minutes and tolazoline, 2 mg/kg, IM was recommended when reversal of xylazine was desired. Butorphanol can be detected in the milk for up to 36 hours following administration (Court et al., 1992).

Minimal information is available on the use of μ opioids in cattle. A thermal nociceptive device applying heat to the coronary band of the forefoot of cattle was devised to test multiple IV doses of morphine, 0.1–0.4 mg/kg (Muchado et al., 1998). No conclusion was reached about the analgesic effect except that individual variation was noted and no increased locomotion was observed.

Non-steroidal anti-inflammatory drugs (NSAIDs)

The beneficial effects of NSAIDs in ameliorating signs of post-surgical pain in cattle have been well documented, for example, use of ketoprofen, meloxicam, flunixin, and carprofen have been studied in large groups of calves subjected to castration or dehorning. Not all NSAIDs are licensed for use in cattle in all countries and the veterinarian must adhere to local laws. Use of phenylbutazone in cattle is prohibited.

LOCAL ANALGESIA

A number of local anaesthetic agents (see Chapter 4), with or without the addition of epinephrine, may be used, the choice being influenced by desired duration of action, irritancy, volume, and cost. Lidocaine and mepivacaine are considered to be agents of intermediate duration and bupivacaine and ropivacaine as longer acting. Lidocaine is not approved for use in animals, other than horses, intended for human consumption in EU member countries; in the USA the recommended meat and milk withdrawal time after administration of lidocaine to cattle is 24 hours or one day. However, in adult Holstein cows injected with 100 mL 2% lidocaine (approximately 3.5 mg/kg) in a flank inverted L-block pattern, the last measurable time of lidocaine detection in milk was 32.5 ± 16.2 hours with a mean concentration of 46 ± 30 ng/mL (Sellers et al., 2009). Three of nine cows showed residues at 48 hours with no detectable residues at 60 hours. The authors calculated withdrawal time for meat for safety at 10 times the $t_{1/2b}$, as 4 days and for milk as 3 days for this dose of lidocaine. No lidocaine was detected in serum or milk after caudal epidural administration of lidocaine, 2.2 mg/kg.

Complications following local analgesia include systemic toxicity, infection if aseptic precautions are not followed, and neurological injury. Accidental intravenous or intra-arterial injection should be avoided by syringe aspiration before injection of a local anaesthetic. Recommendations of maximum doses of local anaesthetic have limited evidence base in cattle but clearly depend on the site, volume and speed of administration, and uptake into the systemic circulation. The recommended limit of 6 mg/kg for lidocaine for local infiltration may be valid as obvious sedation and recumbency may be observed when a larger dose has been administered, for example, by repeating paravertebral nerve blocks following initial failure. Cardiovascular collapse will occur when a tourniquet dislodges soon after IV injection of a smaller dose of lidocaine for intravenous regional analgesia. Metabolism of ester-linked local anaesthetics, such as procaine, begins in the blood before the distribution phase and therefore relatively higher doses may be used. The site of injection significantly influences the plasma concentrations, and a hyperdynamic circulation and local vasodilation increase speed of uptake. Epinephrine (1 : 200 000) may be added to local anaesthetics to cause local vasoconstriction and reduce the peak plasma concentrations, such that in many countries the maximum official recommended doses of local anaesthetics in human patients are higher when epinephrine is added (Rosenberg et al., 2004). Rarely, tissue and skin necrosis has been observed in cattle following local infiltration of tissues with lidocaine with epinephrine. Epinephrine included with lidocaine or mepivacaine prolongs the duration of epidural block in the more caudal segments of the spinal cord, but is not of added benefit to the duration of bupivacaine or ropivacaine (Bernards, 2006). The mechanism by which epinephrine increases the duration of epidural lidocaine is not clear but is thought to be partly due to dural vasoconstriction, without an effect on spinal cord blood flow, slowing lidocaine elimination and partly due to an inhibitory effect (hyperpolarization) of sensory and motor neurons.

Neurological injury is rare but might occur following direct trauma from the needle or from introduction of bacteria into the perineural space. Case reports and studies of human patients developing persistent paraesthesias and motor weakness following spinal anaesthesia have occurred more commonly with lidocaine than with other anaesthetics. Lidocaine is known to be neurotoxic and nerve injury after intrathecal or epidural injection may result from pooling of undiluted lidocaine resulting in a prolonged neural contact. Maldistribution of lidocaine after injection may be observed in the patient by detection of failed or uneven analgesia. Efforts at redistributing the lidocaine by altering patient position rather than repeating local anaesthetic administration have been suggested to decrease the risk of neural toxicity (Bernards, 2006). Adjuncts to local anaesthetics may contribute to nerve damage but evidence is conflicting. Addition of epinephrine to preservative-free lidocaine delivered intrathecally (subarachnoid) in rats increased the extent of sensory block over lidocaine alone (Hashimoto et al., 2001). Sensation in the rats' tails was decreased at 4 and 7 days after injection of lidocaine or lidocaine–epinephrine. Subsequent histological examination revealed nerve injury in the rats that received lidocaine that was significantly worse in rats given lidocaine–epinephrine compared with no functional or morphological effects of epinephrine alone. These data raise concern for adverse effects from intrathecal use of lidocaine with epinephrine. In an *in vitro* model of lidocaine-induced toxicity on neuronal cells and astrocytes, epinephrine did not influence the neurotoxicity of lidocaine indicating that epinephrine may act through its vasoconstrictive effects *in vivo* and not by a direct toxic effect (Werdehausen et al., 2011). However, this study evaluated several commonly used adjuncts and determined that the addition of ketamine to lidocaine increased cell toxicity in an additive manner and addition of midazolam increased toxicity to a lesser extent. The mechanism of toxicity of lidocaine and ketamine is the same, namely activation of the mitochondrial pathway of apoptosis (a programmed cell death process).

The techniques described below will describe doses of lidocaine as this, with or without epinephrine, is the agent most commonly employed in cattle. However, for various

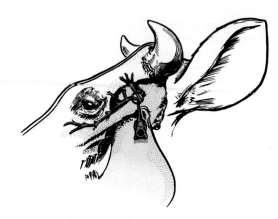

Figure 12.2 Auriculopalpebral nerve block.

legislative reasons (see Chapter 1), procaine is still often used in Europe and, although requiring a slightly longer time for onset of action, appears to be equally satisfactory as lidocaine for procedures where the addition of epinephrine is acceptable.

> *Most clinical surgery in cattle is carried out under local anaesthesia with or without sedation, frequently in the standing animal.*

Techniques

Auriculopalpebral nerve block

The auriculopalpebral nerve is a branch of the facial nerve (VIIth cranial nerve) supplying motor fibres to the orbicularis oculi muscle. The nerve runs from the base of the ear along the facial crest, past and ventral to the eye, giving off its branches on the way. This block is used to prevent eyelid closure during examination or surgery of the eye. It does not provide analgesia to the eye or eyelids and should be used in conjunction with topical analgesia or other nerve blocks for painful procedures.

The needle is inserted in front of the base of the ear at the end of the zygomatic arch until its point lies at the dorsal border of the arch (Fig. 12.2). About 10 mL of 2% lidocaine is injected beneath the fascia at this point.

Cornual nerve block

The horn corium and the skin around its base derive their sensory nerve supply from a branch of the zygomaticotemporal branch of the Vth cranial nerve. The nerve emerges from the orbit and ascends just behind the lateral ridge of the frontal bone (Fig. 12.3). This latter structure can be readily palpated with the fingers. In the upper third of the ridge, the nerve is relatively superficial, being covered only by skin and a thin layer of the frontalis muscle.

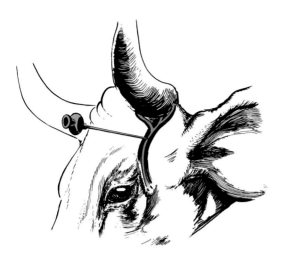

Figure 12.3 Cornual nerve block.

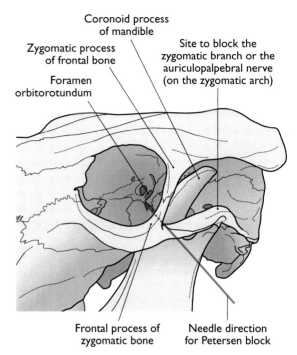

Figure 12.4 Schematic drawing of the Petersen nerve block to block the nerves emerging from the foramen orbitorotundum.

Labels on Figure 12.4:
Coronoid process of mandible
Zygomatic process of frontal bone
Foramen orbitorotundum
Site to block the zygomatic branch or the auriculopalpebral nerve (on the zygomatic arch)
Frontal process of zygomatic bone
Needle direction for Petersen block

The site for injection is the upper third of the temporal ridge, about 2.5 cm below the base of the horn. The needle (18 gauge, 2.5 cm) is inserted so that its point lies 0.7–1.0 cm deep, immediately behind the ridge, and 5 mL of 2% lidocaine solution injected. The needle must not be inserted too deeply otherwise injection will be made beneath the aponeurosis of the temporal muscle and the method will fail. In large animals with well-developed horns, a second injection should be made about 1 cm behind the first to block the posterior division of the nerve. Loss of sensation develops in 10–15 minutes and lasts up to 2 hours. This nerve block has been widely used for the dehorning of adult cattle but the block is not always complete. The infratrochlear nerve, a branch of the Vth cranial nerve, appearing at the dorsal margin of the orbit may also reach the cornual process. Another injection is advisable in adult cattle with well-developed horns caudal to the horn base to block the cutaneous branches of cervical nerves. Thus, a cornual nerve block plus infiltration of lidocaine around the base of the horn is commonly employed.

The legislation relating to dehorning and disbudding of calves differs between countries, for example, in the UK and Sweden, disbudding is not permitted without the use of local anaesthesia ± sedation, whereas in North America, local anaesthesia is not always provided to all calves for dehorning; with the conundrum that fewer calves <6 months of age receive analgesia than calves >6 months of age and beef calves are less likely to receive analgesia than dairy calves (Stafford & Mellor, 2005; Hewson et al., 2007; Fajt et al., 2011). In one survey, cattle producers were less likely than veterinary practitioners to include analgesia when dehorning their calves, indicating a need for client education (Misch et al., 2007).

In the last 15 years, the impact of dehorning and disbudding on cattle has been investigated extensively (Stafford & Mellor, 2005). Local anaesthesia significantly attenuates cortisol response during and immediately after the procedure. Cortisol levels increase some hours after the effects of local anaesthesia have dissipated and, although the plasma cortisol concentrations decrease by 9 hours after dehorning, the calves graze and ruminate less between 24 and 48 hours after dehorning than they do between 48 and 72 hours or compared with animals that were not dehorned. Extension of the duration of analgesia by following the lidocaine injection with bupivacaine may eliminate the cortisol response (delay onset of pain). Administration of an NSAID (e.g. ketoprofen or meloxicam, but not phenylbutazone) with a lidocaine nerve block was documented to provide more effective analgesia and continue pain relief beyond the 2–3 hours provided by lidocaine (Stafford & Mellor, 2005; Stewart et al., 2009; Duffield et al., 2010). Xylazine alone was not effective in eliminating the cortisol response to dehorning.

Petersen eye block

A 22 gauge, 2.5 cm needle is used to infiltrate local analgesic solution subcutaneously, about 5 mL of 2% lidocaine, within the notch formed by the joining of the zygomatic process of the frontal bone and the frontal process of the zygomatic bone cranially, the zygomatic arch ventrally and the coronoid process of the mandible caudally (Fig. 12.4). A 12 or 14 gauge, 2.5 cm needle placed as far rostral and ventral as possible in the desensitized skin of the notch serves as a cannula and an 18 gauge, 10 or 12 cm needle is introduced through it. The long needle is directed in a horizontal and caudal direction until it strikes the coronoid process of the mandible. It is then redirected into the orbit just rostral to the orbitorotundum foramen at a depth of about 8–10 cm from the skin and 10–15 mL of 2% lidocaine solution injected. This blocks the oculomotor, trochlear, abducens nerves and two branches of the trigeminal nerve as they emerge from the foramen orbitorotundum. The needle is withdrawn to the subcutaneous tissue and redirected caudally and laterally to block the zygomatic branch of the auriculopalpebral nerve on the zygomatic arch by the injection of 5–10 mL of the local analgesic solution. The Petersen technique requires more skill to perform than a retrobulbar block but it may be safer.

Peribulbar and retrobulbar block

Retrobulbar injection of the eye is achieved by introduction of a curved needle through the skin about 1 cm lateral to the lateral canthus, or through the conjunctiva. The needle is first directed straight back and away from the eyeball until the point is beyond the globe and then turned inward to penetrate the muscle cone. When no blood is obtained after aspiration, lidocaine is deposited behind the eye.

Peribulbar anaesthesia is produced by inserting the needle in 2 to 4 quadrants of the eye and injecting lidocaine within the orbit but outside the ocular muscles. Injection of a total of 20–30 mL of 2% lidocaine (or its equivalent) for an adult cow or bull will produce corneal analgesia, mydriasis, and proptosis and paralysis of the eyeball. Anaesthesia is produced after spread of the anaesthetic agent; thus a larger volume of lidocaine is required for peribulbar anaesthesia, the onset of block is longer, and the larger volume of solution causes a greater increase in ocular pressure.

Recommendations vary over the use of sharp hypodermic or blunt (e.g. spinal needle) needles for ocular blocks, but penetration of the globe has been reported in human patients with both sharp and blunt needles (Hay, 1991; Wong, 1993). Visual outcome is not a factor when penetration of the globe occurs during nerve block for enucleation. However, bacterial contamination of the orbit is possible.

Potentially adverse effects of both the Petersen block and the retrobulbar block include bradycardia, hypotension, asystole, respiratory depression, apnoea, perforation of the globe and intraorbital or retrobulbar haemorrhage. Symptoms of local anaesthetic spread to the central nervous system vary but respiratory arrest is a usual sign of brainstem anaesthesia. When the block is used for other purposes, care must be taken to ensure that the corneal surface does not become dry because of loss of tear formation for several hours.

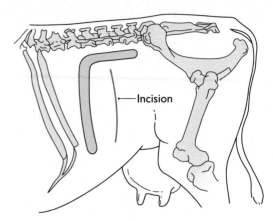

Figure 12.5 The inverted L block used for analgesia for flank coeliotomy involves infiltration of local anaesthetic solution dorsally and cranially to the proposed incision.

Inverted L block

Infiltration of the skin, subcutaneous and deeper tissues in an inverted L shape with 60 mL of 2% lidocaine solution is a commonly used technique to provide analgesia for a flank laparotomy in a standing cow (Fig. 12.5). It is also used in recumbent animals to block the site for a paramedian incision, or repeated in a mirror image to form an inverted U shape and analgesia for a midline incision. Injections must be made both subcutaneously and down to the peritoneum to produce a total block. The block can be achieved by making isolated injections at intervals of about 1 cm, which relies on lateral diffusion of the analgesic solution. Alternatively, a wall of local analgesic solution can be created by inserting a long needle to its depth, and injecting anaesthetic solution in a steady stream as the needle is withdrawn.

Paravertebral nerve block

Paravertebral block involves the perineural injection of local analgesic solution about the spinal nerves as they emerge from the vertebral canal through the intervertebral foramina. This technique is commonly used to provide analgesia for laparotomy. It offers a major advantage over use of local infiltration in that the abdominal wall including the peritoneum is more likely to be uniformly desensitized. Additionally, the abdominal wall is relaxed.

The area of the flank bounded cranially by the last rib, caudally by the angle of the ilium and dorsally by the lumbar transverse processes, is innervated by the thirteenth thoracic and first and second lumbar nerves. The third lumbar nerve, although it does not supply the flank, gives off a cutaneous branch that passes obliquely backwards in front of the ilium. Operations involving the

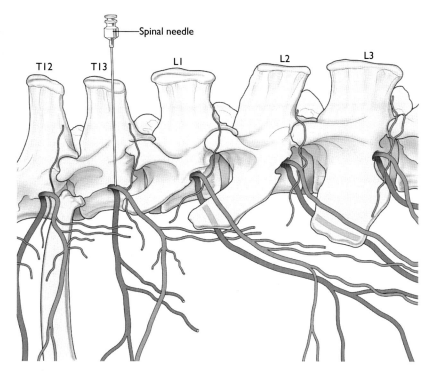

Spinal needle

T12   T13   L1   L2   L3

Figure 12.6 Location of the last two thoracic and first three lumbar segmental nerves. The needle indicates position for paravertebral injection of local anaesthetic to block T13.

abdominal ventral midline will require additional desensitization of the dorsal nerves cranial to the thirteenth. The last thoracic and first lumbar intervertebral foramina in cattle are occasionally double. The last thoracic foramen lies immediately caudal to the head of the last rib and on a level with the base of the transverse process of the first lumbar vertebra (Fig. 12.6). The lumbar foramina are large and are situated between the base of the transverse processes and approximately on the same level. The spinal nerves, after emerging from the foramina, immediately divide into a smaller dorsal and a larger ventral branch. The dorsal branch supplies chiefly the skin and muscles of the loins, but some of its cutaneous branches pass a considerable distance down the flank. The ventral branch passes obliquely ventrally and caudally between the muscles and comprises the main nerve supply to the skin, muscles, and peritoneum of the flank. The ventral branch is also connected with the sympathetic system by a ramus communicans. Paralysis of the nerves at their points of emergence from the intervertebral foramina will provoke desensitization of the whole depth of the flank wall and complete muscular relaxation. Block of the rami communicantes will result in splanchnic vasodilation and potential for hypotension.

The number of nerves to be blocked will depend on the site and extent of the proposed incision. The areas involved by blocking of respective nerves are illustrated in Figure 12.7. Therefore, for rumenotomy, using an incision parallel with and about 7 cm caudal to the last rib, analgesia of the thirteenth thoracic (T13) and first (L1) and second (L2) lumbar nerves is required. The third lumbar nerve (L3) must be blocked for a more caudal incision and for relaxation of the internal oblique muscle. The hair must be clipped from over the injection sites and the skin cleansed with a surgical preparation before insertion of the needle. A number of different techniques for blocking the respective nerves have been described but the most reliable relies on directing the needle towards the cranial border of the transverse process of the vertebra behind the nerve to be blocked. For example, to block the L1, the needle should be directed to strike the cranial border of L2 about 5–6 cm (2 inches) from the animal's midline. At such sites, the cranial borders of the transverse processes are usually in the same cross-sectional plane of the body as the most prominent parts of their lateral borders. Alternatively, the cranial corner of the tip of the transverse process can be used as a landmark whereby vertical insertion of a needle 5–6 cm from the animal's midline will direct the

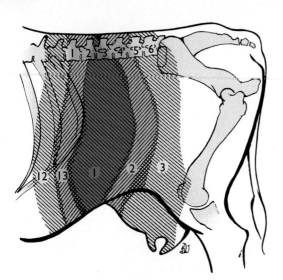

Figure 12.7 Regions of the flank involved after paravertebral block of the respective nerves.

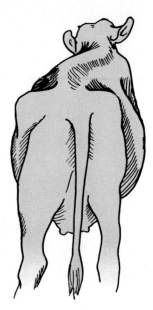

Figure 12.8 Unilateral analgesia with either a paravertebral block or lumbar epidural producing spinal curvature towards the blocked side.

needle to drop off the caudal edge of the previous transverse process. To block the T13, L1, L2, and L3 nerves subcutaneous blebs of local anaesthetic solution should be made in line with the most prominent parts of the extremities of the transverse processes of L2, L3 and L4 at a distance 5–6 cm from the dorsal midline. Location of the transverse process of L1 can be difficult (particularly in well-muscled or obese animals) so another bleb is inserted cranial to L1 a distance equal to that between L1 and L2. A 14 gauge needle is inserted through each skin bleb and the underlying longissimus dorsi muscle infiltrated with 5 mL of 1–2% lidocaine or other local analgesic solution (preferably without epinephrine to avoid necrosis) as it is advanced to a depth of about 4 cm from the skin surface. This infiltration will reduce the cow's movement during the rest of the procedure, but can be omitted. A 14 gauge needle is reintroduced through the first bleb and used as a guide for introducing a longer needle (18 gauge, 10–14 cm) through the longissimus dorsi muscle. The needle is advanced to strike the cranial border of the transverse process and then redirected cranially over the edge of the transverse process and advanced until it is felt to penetrate the intertransverse ligament. Injection of 15 mL 2% lidocaine is made immediately below the ligament and a further 5 mL is injected after the needle is withdrawn to just above the ligament. During final withdrawal of the needle, the skin is pressed downwards to prevent separation of the connective tissue and aspiration of air through the needle. The procedure is repeated at the other sites.

It is important to ensure that the needles are vertical when contact is first made with the cranial border of the transverse processes for, if they are not, redirection over

the edge of the processes may cause their points to lie well away from the course of the nerves. Successful infiltration around the nerves is indicated first by the development of a belt of vasodilation which causes a distinct and appreciable rise in skin temperature. Full analgesia develops in about 10 minutes and when lidocaine with epinephrine 1 : 400 000 is used it persists for about 90 minutes. When a unilateral block is fully developed it produces a curvature of the spine, the convexity of which is towards the analgesic side (Fig. 12.8).

An alternative method of lumbar paravertebral block is to approach the nerves horizontally at the tip of the transverse processes of L1, L2, L3 and L4 to block T13, L1, L2, and L3 nerves. A 14 gauge, 5 cm hypodermic needle is inserted horizontally at the centre of the tip of a transverse process and directed beneath the process as close as possible to the bone. About 10 mL of 2% lidocaine is injected into the area, moving the needle by slightly withdrawing and advancing to achieve a fan-like disposition of the local anaesthetic. The needle is then withdrawn until it is just under the skin and redirected over the top of the transverse process to needle depth, as close as possible to the bone, and an additional 10 mL lidocaine injected in a similar fashion. This technique will not cause sympathetic vasodilation or curvature of the spine.

It is inevitable that partial failure to block these nerves will sometimes occur because the nerves course obliquely and location may be variable with different sizes and conformations of cattle. It should also be remembered that although the flank may be analgesic, signs of discomfort

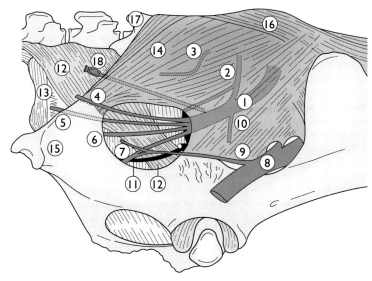

Figure 12.9 Pudendal nerve block. Lateral view of the pelvis with the sacrosciatic ligament enhanced and showing distribution of the sacral spinal nerves. 1: pudendal nerve; 2: middle rectal nerve; 3: caudal rectal nerve; 4, 5: proximal and distal cutaneous branches of pudendal nerve; 6: deep perineal nerve; 7: nerve that becomes the dorsal nerve of the penis; 8: sciatic nerve; 9: branch connecting sciatic nerve with branch of pudendal nerve 7; 10: pelvic nerve; 11: internal pudendal artery; 12: coccygeus muscle; 13: external anal sphincter; 14: broad sacrotuberous ligament; 15: ischial tuber; 16: sacrum; 17: first coccygeal vertebra; 18: needle in position.

may be observed following traction on the mesentery during manipulation of organs.

Pudendal nerve block

A useful nerve block to produce analgesia of the penis for examination and surgical procedures without causing hind limb ataxia is a bilateral pudendal nerve block. The pudendal nerve consists of fibres arising mainly from the ventral branch of the third (2–4) sacral nerve. The nerve passes ventrally and caudally on the medial surface of the broad sacrotuberous ligament to cross the lesser ischiatic foramen where it is accompanied by the internal pudendal artery (Fig. 12.9). The pudendal nerve sends fibres to the caudal cutaneous femoral nerve and provides sensory innervation around the skin of the anus and perineal regional and motor fibres to the penis, vulva, coccygeal and levator ani muscles, and internal and external anal sphincters (Liebich et al., 2009). Between the sacrotuberous ligament and the rectum in the area of approach to the nerve lies the sheet-like coccygeal muscle. The pudendal nerve lies between the ligament and the muscle.

The pudendal nerve is located per rectum with a hand being introduced as far as the wrist and the fingers directed laterally and ventrally to detect the lesser ischiatic foramen. The outline of this foramen may not be clearly identifiable but its position is recognized by the softness and depressability of the pelvic wall. The internal pudendal artery can be palpated 2–3 cm rostral to the cranial dorsal end of the lesser ischiatic foramen. The pudendal nerve can be felt, the size of a straw, dorsal to this point. After clipping and cleaning the skin, the site of insertion of the needle is at the point of deepest depression of the ischiorectal fossa and the needle should be directed rostral and slightly ventral. During the whole procedure a hand is kept in the rectum. When the needle has penetrated to a depth of 5–7 cm, it will be palpable through the rectal wall and its point should be directed to the position of the nerve just described. Lidocaine, 20–25 mL of 2% (or its equivalent), is injected. A further 10–15 mL is injected a little caudal and dorsal to this point to block also the middle rectal nerve that may carry some sympathetic fibres to the penis. A third injection should be made after redirecting the needle a little ventrally just inside the lesser ischiatic foramen where the ventral branch of the pudendal nerve can be palpated distal to its anastomosis with sciatic nerve branches. The onset of penile prolapse may take 30–45 minutes. Another approach to pudendal nerve block is a lateral one. One injection is made over the pudendal nerve just as it passes medial to the dorsorostral quadrant of the lesser sciatic foramen and a second injection is performed between the caudal rectal and pudendal nerves. This latter injection necessitates penetration of the broad sacrotuberous ligament. The site of insertion of the needle is determined by using the cranial tuberosity of the ischial tuber as a fixed point and the length of the broad sacrotuberous ligament as a radius. The distance is used to establish the site on a line drawn parallel to the midline cranial to the fixed point. After clipping, cleaning and disinfecting the skin the site is marked by the SC injection of 2 mL of 2% lidocaine or equivalent drug solution. This injection makes subsequent manipulations less painful and renders the animal more amenable to handling. Either hand is then introduced into the rectum and the lesser ischiatic foramen located. A needle (18 gauge, 12 cm) is introduced through the skin site and directed towards the middle finger held in the foramen until it can be felt to lie alongside the nerve. About 10 mL of the local analgesic solution is injected at this point. The needle is withdrawn 4–5 cm and redirected caudally and dorsally so that it penetrates the broad sacrotuberous ligament at a point about 2.5 cm above and behind the first site of injection. About 5 mL of solution is injected at this point, the needle is withdrawn and the sites massaged to spread the solution in the tissues. Similar injections are carried out on the other side of the animal.

Local analgesia for castration

Handling of calves may provoke a stress response but the procedure of castration may cause acute and chronic pain, exhibited by changed individual and social behaviour. Pain behaviours in cattle include restlessness, altered durations of standing, walking, play activity, and recumbency, or eating and rumination, and other signs such as lameness, short strides, foot stamping, head shaking, and tail wagging. Even though young calves may not exhibit strong signs of discomfort, evidence from studies of neonatal humans and animals supports the conviction that the very young also experience pain.

There are several techniques used for castration of calves, surgical excision, crushing the neck of the scrotum (Burdizzo), or banding (rubber band, elastrator) to produce testicular ischaemia, and each technique may cause different degrees and duration of pain. Castration by surgical excision in calves 2–4 months old was evaluated by use of pedometers, stride length and video recording, and a subjective visual score (VAS) for up to 24 hours (Currah et al., 2009). The calves received either a lidocaine with epinephrine caudal epidural nerve block, 0.6 mg/kg delivered using an 18 gauge, 3.75 cm (1.5 inch) needle inserted at the sacrococcygeal junction, an epidural nerve block and flunixin, 2.2 mg/kg, IV, or saline alone. The results indicate that the calves exhibited behaviours associated with pain after castration, that the calves castrated without analgesia were less mobile after castration and were more likely to be assessed as in more pain by independent observers, and that calves administered flunixin evidenced more analgesia than other calves for 8 hours after castration but that the effect had worn off by 24 hours. Burdizzo castration of 2–7-day-old calves was evaluated by recording behaviours and measuring plasma cortisol concentrations the day before and the day of the procedure (Boesch et al., 2008). Ten mL of either 2% lidocaine, 0.5% bupivacaine, or saline

was infiltrated into the spermatic cord and around the neck of the scrotum 20 minutes before castration. Calves receiving local analgesia struggled significantly less, had lower peak cortisol concentrations, and responded less to palpation of the site after the procedure. The authors concluded that calves <1 week of age perceived and responded to pain of castration, that Burdizzo castration was not completely painless even with local analgesia, and that sensitivity to local palpation increased in the hours following castration, presumably due to inflammation and waning effect of local analgesia.

The impact of castration by the application of bands in 7.5-month-old Angus calves was evaluated for 3 weeks before and for 6 weeks after banding (González et al., 2010). Saliva cortisol concentrations were measured to quantitate the stress of band application and other parameters such as feed intake, average daily gain, feeding behaviour, faecal E. coli concentration, duration of recumbency, and length of stride when walking through a long chute, were used as measurements of the calves' well-being. It was found that caudal epidural xylazine, 0.07 mg/kg, and flunixin meglumine IV administered before banding significantly decreased salivary cortisol concentrations and reduced the time the calves spent lying down on the day of banding. Average daily gain was decreased by castration but not influenced by analgesic medication. However, the animals' responses attributable to pain were greatest in the third and fourth weeks after application of bands. Further research is needed to address chronic pain management for this method of castration.

Governmental laws require that pain from castration must be prevented in calves over 1 month of age in Germany, 2 months in the UK, 9 months in New Zealand, and calves of all ages in Switzerland and Austria (Boesch et al., 2008). Currently used analgesic techniques for calf castrations are local infiltration of the spermatic cord and subcutaneous tissues, caudal epidural nerve block with local anaesthetic or xylazine, and parenteral administration of an NSAID.

Caudal epidural block

The spinal cord and meninges end at the third sacral vertebra in calves and the first sacral vertebra in adult cattle. The diameter of the neural canal as it passes through the sacrum is approximately 1.8 cm in the caudal part and 2 cm in the cranial. In the lumbar regions, the dimensions of the canal are much greater, its width at the last segment being 4 cm. This helps to explain why paralysis of the spinal nerves as far forward as the first sacral is effected with comparatively small quantities of local analgesic solution whereas paralysis of the cranial lumbar nerves necessitates the injection of much larger quantities.

Caudal epidural block is performed by insertion of the needle between the sacrum and first coccygeal vertebra (S5–C1) or between the first and second coccygeal

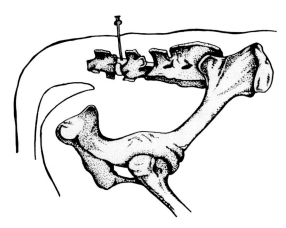

Figure 12.10 Caudal epidural injection made into the first intercoccygeal space.

vertebrae (C1–C2), i.e. beyond the termination of the spinal cord and its meninges (Fig. 12.10). One or more of the following methods may be used:

1. The tail is gripped about 15 cm from its base and raised 'pump-handle' fashion. The first obvious articulation behind the sacrum is the first intercoccygeal space.
2. Standing on one side of the animal and observing the line of the croup, the prominence of the sacrum is seen. Moving the eye back towards the tail, the next prominence to be observed is the spine of the first coccygeal bone. The site for C1–C2 is the depression immediately behind it.
3. The caudal prominence of the tuberosity of the ischium is palpated and the point 10–11 cm in front of it selected. A line drawn directly over the back from this point passes, in a medium-sized animal, through the depression between C1 and C2 spines.

The dimensions of the opening in the dorsal wall of the neural canal in adult cattle are approximately 2 cm transversely, 2.5 cm craniocaudally and about 0.5 cm in depth.

The canal is occupied by six caudal nerves, together with a vein on each side. The aperture between the two vertebral arches is closed by the interarcuate ligament and the space between the spines occupied by connective tissue. Surmounting the spines is a variable amount of fat covered by skin. The floor comprises, about the centre of the space, the intervertebral cartilaginous disc and, in front and behind this, the surface of the vertebral centrum.

An insensitive skin weal can be made with the object of preventing movement during insertion of the injection needle and thus ensuring that the latter is introduced in the correct position and direction. For insertion of the epidural needle, the tail is allowed to hang naturally. The point of the needle (18 gauge, 3.75 cm, 1.5 inch) is applied to the centre of the depression between C1–C2

spines, taking care that it is precisely in the midline. The needle is advanced ventrally and cranially at an angle of 15° with the vertical. If the point of the needle impinges on the floor of the canal, contact with a caudal nerve may cause the animal to move suddenly, and the practitioner should be prepared for this. Assessment of correct placement of the needle can be done using the 'hanging drop' and/or loss of resistance methods. To utilize the 'hanging drop', a drop of saline or local anaesthetic solution can be placed on the hub of the needle. As the needle is advanced into the epidural space negative pressure within the space will suck the liquid into the needle. After insertion of the needle, an empty syringe should be attached to the needle and the syringe plunger aspirated to ensure that the needle is not in a blood vessel. Then a small amount of air or saline or local anaesthetic solution is injected and no resistance to injection should be felt when the needle is in the epidural space. If the needle is introduced too far, crossed the epidural space and penetrated the intervertebral disc, there will be resistance to injection.

Lidocaine, 5 mL of 2%, is commonly used for caudal analgesia in adult cows. Skin analgesia will develop in the tail and croup as far as the mid-sacral region, the anus, vulva and perineum and the posterior aspect of the thighs. Paralysis of motor fibres will cause the anal sphincter to relax and the posterior part of the rectum to balloon. Defaecation will be suspended, stretching of the vulva will produce no response and the vagina will dilate. During parturition straining ceases but uterine contractions are uninfluenced. Motor control of the hind limbs should be retained although mild ataxia may be evident.

The onset of muscular paralysis of the tail occurs from 60 to 90 seconds after injection and is evidence that the injection has been made correctly. Lidocaine analgesia attains its maximum extent over 5–10 minutes, and persists for about an hour after which there is progressive recovery. The block completely disappears by the end of the second hour from the time of injection.

Caudal epidural analgesia can be used to cause relaxation and exposure of the penis in bulls, however, the dose necessary for penile extrusion is very close to that causing motor incoordination of the hind limbs.

Many other drugs are commonly administered into the epidural space at the caudal site. However, it should be remembered that many of the drugs have not undergone safety testing for the potential to cause neurological damage, and that preservatives and solvents present in the formulations may increase the damage. Xylazine, 0.05 mg/kg diluted to 5 mL in 0.9% saline, has been used to provide analgesia of the perineum and to reduce straining during parturition. Xylazine will induce bilateral analgesia of dermatomes supplied by the caudal, caudal rectal, perineal, pudendal, and caudal cutaneous femoral nerves (StJean et al., 1990). Analgesia develops by 12 minutes after administration and persists for 4 hours (Grubb et al., 2002). The tail will be flaccid and mild ataxia may be present. Sufficient xylazine is absorbed to induce mild sedation, decreased ruminal motility (bloat), bradycardia and decreased MAP. These side effects may have a significantly adverse effect in sick animals. The combination of lidocaine, 0.22 mg/kg, with xylazine, 0.05 mg/kg, diluted to 5.7 mL administered to adult cows resulted in the same time of onset as lidocaine and a longer duration (average 5 hours) of analgesia as determined by pin pricks (Grubb et al., 2002). Cutaneous analgesia was more extensive than from lidocaine alone and extended to T13. As with xylazine alone, the combination resulted in mild to moderate sedation and ataxia. A slightly higher dose of xylazine, 0.07 mg/kg in 7.5 mL of 0.9% saline, has been used by caudal epidural injection to provide analgesia for castration in mature bulls (Caulkett et al., 1993). Sedation was evident in these animals and moderate ataxia with recumbency was observed in 14%. Surgery was performed 30 minutes after injection and surgical analgesia was judged to be good in 81% of animals but pain or discomfort during emasculation was apparent in the remaining bulls. Either lidocaine, 0.6 mg/kg, with or without epinephrine, or xylazine, 0.07 mg/kg, injected into the S5–C1 epidural space have been used for analgesia for castration in calves. Epidural administration of ketamine, 0.5 mg/kg in a mean volume of 4 mL, at C1–C2 was found to provide similar duration (approximately 35 minutes) and extent of analgesia without ataxia as lidocaine, 0.2 mg/kg or 50:50 ketamine and lidocaine in 2-year-old heifers (DeRossi et al., 2010). Caudal epidural administration of tramadol, 0.5 mg/kg in mean volume of 5 mL, was compared with lidocaine, 0.22 mg/kg, and 50:50 tramadol and lidocaine in experimental cows in which analgesia was tested with a haemostat clamp (Bigham et al., 2010). Onset of analgesia was longer with tramadol at 14 minutes compared with 4–5 minutes for injections containing lidocaine but duration of analgesia was considerably longer with tramadol at 307 minutes compared with 174 minutes for the tramadol–lidocaine combination or 70 minutes for lidocaine alone. Mild ataxia was observed in the cows receiving lidocaine. The longer duration of analgesia from tramadol warrants investigation of its value for treatment of postoperative pain and of its impact on spinal cord tissue.

Medetomidine, 0.015 mg/kg diluted with 0.9% saline to a volume of 5 mL, has been evaluated for epidural analgesia in cows (Lin et al., 1998). Results of this investigation showed that medetomidine induced analgesia within 10 minutes and lasted 412 ± 156 min (mean $\pm$ SD) – significantly longer than lidocaine, 0.2 mg/kg, which lasted 10–115 min (mean 43 ± 37 min). Systemic effects of absorbed medetomidine included mild to moderate sedation and mild ataxia.

Romifidine, 0.05 mg/kg, and morphine, 0.1 mg/kg, were diluted with 0.9% saline to 30 mL and administered to experimental Holstein Friesian cows through C1–C2 (Fierheller et al., 2004). Analgesia of the flank was tested by application of electrical stimulation. Sedation, including swaying of the hind limbs, lowered head, and recumbency in some animals, developed within 10 minutes and persisted for 6 hours. Analgesia was variable between individuals, peaked at 25 minutes and lasted 12 hours. One cow developed hind limb paresis that may or may not have been related to the epidural injection and was euthanized. The level of analgesia was not tested for surgical incision and the side effects from this romifidine dose were considered to be unacceptable.

Large volumes of anaesthetic agents injected epidurally at S5–C1 or C1–C2 have been used in calves to achieve analgesia sufficiently cranial to allow umbilical hernia repair or flank surgeries (Meyer et al., 2007). A preliminary trial revealed that 0.4 mL/kg of contrast agent (20 mL in a calf weighing 50 kg) will spread cranially to the twelfth thoracic vertebra. Because analgesia at the umbilicus was not adequate following injection of lidocaine alone, subsequent surgeries on clinical patients were performed using xylazine, 0.1 mg/kg, diluted with 2% lidocaine or 2% procaine to a final volume of 0.5–0.6 mL/kg. Such a large volume must be injected slowly (0.5 mL/s) to avoid an increase in CSF pressure and seizures or collapse. A follow-up study investigated the cardiopulmonary effects of dorsal recumbency and high volume caudal epidural in healthy experimental calves (Meyer et al., 2010). Calves that were 25–53 days old and average bodyweight of 58 kg were divided into four groups of seven calves. One group had no treatment and the others received caudal epidural injections of saline, 2% lidocaine 8 mg/kg, or xylazine 0.1 mg/kg diluted to 0.4 mL/kg. The calves were restrained in dorsal recumbency for 95 minutes. No significant differences were measured in calves given saline or lidocaine from calves with no treatment. As expected, xylazine was absorbed from the epidural space and decreased cardiac output by 36%, decreased HR, RR, and O_2 delivery, and increased systemic vascular resistances, $PaCO_2$ and O_2 extraction ratio. The changes were less than changes incurred by IM or IV administration of xylazine. No calf was hypoxic. Motor control of the hind limbs was lost for 4 hours in the lidocaine epidural calves and no signs of toxicity were observed. The authors cautioned that this volume is only suitable for calves of this size. In a similar study (Offinger et al., 2012), epidural analgesia was provided in calves with xylazine, 0.2 mg/kg, and procaine, 12 mg/kg, combined to a total volume of 0.6 mL/kg and injected slowly at the sacrococcygeal junction. Procaine 2%, 0.5 mL/kg was injected circumferentially around the umbilicus to facilitate surgical extirpation and flunixin was administered. HR, MAP, and CO were decreased initially, not dissimilar to xylazine–ketamine–isoflurane anaesthesia, and MAP increased slightly during surgery. Calves were sedated by absorption of xylazine from the epidural space but blood gases were acceptable values. The calves were standing within 3.5 hours of epidural administration.

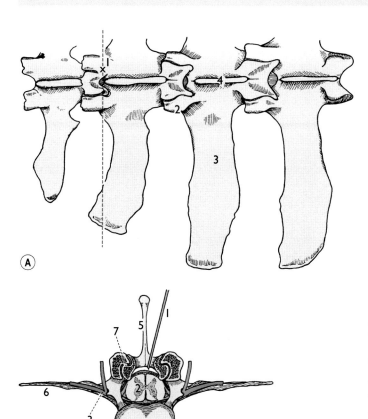

Figure 12.11 Segmental lumbar epidural block. (A) First four lumbar vertebrae viewed from above. 1: Point of insertion of spinal needle through skin; 2: articular process; 3: transverse process; 4: spinous processes. (B) Transverse section through the joints between the articular processes of the 1st and 2nd lumbar vertebrae. The body of the 1st lumbar segment is viewed from its caudal aspect. 1: Needle in position; 2: spinal cord surrounded by meninges; 3: left 1st lumbar nerve; 4: body of 1st lumbar vertebra; 5: spinous process; 6: transverse process; 7: sectioned interlocking articular processes.

Lumbosacral epidural block

When lumbar epidural block is required in adult bovines it is not always possible to produce satisfactory cranial spread from the caudal injection site. Injection of local anaesthetic solution at the lumbosacral junction will cause analgesia but also motor paralysis of the hind limbs and, therefore, is a technique only rarely performed in cows. The technique for producing epidural analgesia by injection at the lumbosacral space in calves is performed similarly to the description given for sheep and goats in the following chapter.

Lumbar epidural block

Bucholz working in the Giessen school in 1948 first described the technique of desensitization of the flank in cattle by epidural injection of local analgesic solution into the vertebral canal in the cranial lumbar region (Hall, 1991). Other reports soon followed from Russia, the UK and the USA employing procaine or lidocaine to produce a belt of analgesia around the animal's trunk without interfering with control of the hind limbs. The technique

is not easy to perform, however, recently there have been several publications describing the technique in more detail to facilitate successful nerve block.

The original technique is described as follows. With the animal standing, the hair is clipped and skin aseptically prepared over the dorsal midline next to the first and second lumbar vertebrae. The site for insertion of the needle is just to the right of the lumbar spinous process on a line 1.5 cm behind the cranial edge of the second lumbar transverse process (Fig. 12.11A). An initial skin weal is made by SC injection of local anaesthetic solution and the skin should be punctured using a 12 or 14 gauge hypodermic needle. The spinal needle (14 gauge, 12 cm) is directed ventrally and medially at an angle of 10–13° to the vertical for a distance of 7.5 cm – at which point the needle enters the neural canal. Resistance to needle insertion will be felt initially before passing through the supraspinous ligament running over the tips of the spinous processes and then again by the interarcuate ligament that lies over the spinal canal. Needle penetration of the interarcuate ligament appears to be painful, even when local anaesthetic has been injected before insertion, and the animal must be adequately restrained. The intervertebral space through which the needle must pass to enter the epidural space is actually an interosseous canal formed by the bases of the spinous process cranially and caudally and by the intervertebral articular processes laterally (Fig. 12.11B). Immediately the needle is felt to penetrate the interarcuate ligament the stilette is withdrawn and if air is heard to enter the needle it is certain that the epidural space has been entered. Alternatively, in the absence of air aspiration and if no fluid flows from the needle, a trial injection is made. If the needle is correctly placed in the epidural space very little pressure will be needed to depress the syringe plunger. If on removing the stilette, CSF fluid flows from the needle, the needle should be withdrawn until flow of fluid ceases and then injection made.

Lee et al. (2004a, 2006) have addressed two important points in this technique. The distance from the skin to the interarcuate ligament varies depending on the breed, size and body condition of the animal. In one report, the distance in adult cattle weighing >400 kg was 8 cm (7–9 cm) and in young animals less than 2 years of age and weighing 276 ± 86 kg was 5.7 cm (5–7.3 cm) (Lee et al., 2006). Once the interarcuate ligament is penetrated, greatest success is achieved if the local anaesthetic solution is deposited below the epidural fat and next to the dura mater. Lee et al. (2006) propose that a Tuohy needle (see Fig. 13.4) (16 gauge, 12 cm) be used, introduced within 0.5 cm of dorsal midline, advanced to just when resistance to insertion is felt at the level of the interarcuate ligament, and that the 'hanging drop' technique be employed to confirm accurate placement. Thus, before penetration of the interarcuate ligament, the stilette is removed and a drop of saline is placed on the needle. The needle is advanced slowly and on penetration of the epidural space, negative pressure sucks the saline into the needle. After about 1 minute the needle is then advanced slowly about 1 cm deeper to penetrate epidural fat and watching the animal closely for flinching or dipping of the back that indicates pressure on the dura and spinal cord. Injection of local anaesthetic solution at this site is likely to be beneath the epidural fat.

The technique just described was tested with lidocaine, xylazine, and xylazine and lidocaine and the combination was found to have the best effect with an average onset time of 11 minutes and five spinal segments blocked (Lee et al., 2004b). Subsequently, the technique was utilized at a bovine referral clinic for analgesia in standing adult cows primarily for omentopexy in treatment of abomasal displacement and for a small number of caesarian sections (Hiraoka et al., 2007). Out of 130 cows, 90 cows were injected with 1 mL xylazine, approximately 0.025 mg/kg, and 3 mL 2% lidocaine, approximately 0.1 mg/kg, and another 18 cows that were in poor condition received 0.5 mL xylazine and 3 mL lidocaine. Local flank infiltration (line block) was resorted to in 22 cows (17%) due to failure to achieve lumbar epidural block. Analgesia was sufficient for surgery in almost all cattle, except for 15 cows that moved and occasionally kicked during surgery and one that required a line block. Light sedation and swaying was observed in some cows and five cows assumed sternal recumbency. Decreasing the xylazine dose to 0.5 mL avoided ataxia and recumbency.

Digital nerve blocks

The nerve supply of the digits of cattle is more complex than in the horse and regional analgesia is more difficult to produce. The skin below the carpus and tarsus is tense and the subcutaneous tissue fibrous, so that precise location of the nerves is not easy.

Analgesia may be produced in the forelimb by injection at the sites indicated in Figure 12.12. The dorsal metacarpal nerve is located by palpation at about the middle of the metacarpus, medial to the extensor tendon. The dorsal branch of the ulnar nerve is blocked about 5 cm above the fetlock on the lateral aspect of the limb, in the groove between the suspensory ligament and the metacarpal bone. At this point, the palmar branch of the ulnar nerve may also be blocked, the two nerves being respectively situated in front of, and behind the suspensory ligament. The axial palmar aspect of the digits may be rendered analgesic by an injection in the midline just above the

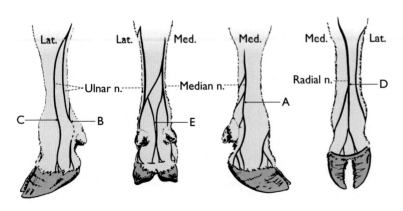

Figure 12.12 Nerve block of the forelimb. To block the whole digit, injections must be made at A, B, C, D, and E. To block the medial digit, inject at A, D, and E. To block the lateral digit, inject at points B, C, D, and E.

fetlock. The injection will reach the lateral branch of the median nerve before it divides, or if it has already divided, its two branches will still be close to each other. The two branches may also be simultaneously blocked on the midline just below the level of the dew claws, i.e. after they have passed from below the fibrous plate of the dew claws. The medial branch of the median nerve is blocked on the medial side of the limb in the groove between the suspensory ligament and the flexor tendons about 5 cm above the fetlock. Blocking the median nerve higher up the limb before it divides is not practical as, at this point, the nerve lies beneath the artery and vein.

An alternative technique that is less precise is to perform a ring block of the limb with local anaesthetic solution in an attempt to block all nerve branches at the same level. This technique should work well in calves.

The hind limb can be blocked to provide loss of sensation below the hock. The peroneal nerve is blocked immediately behind the caudal edge of the lateral condyle of the tibia, over the fibula. The nerve is blocked before it dips down between the extensor pedis and flexor metatarsi muscles to divide into the deep and superficial peroneal nerves. The bony prominence can easily be palpated in most animals and, in some, the nerve itself can be rolled against the bone as it passes superficially, obliquely downwards and cranially, at this point. An 18 or 20 gauge, 2.5 cm, needle is inserted through the skin, the subcutaneous tissue and the aponeurotic sheet of the biceps femoris until its point just touches the bony landmark. Lidocaine, approximately 20 mL of 2% for an adult, is injected at this point. Onset of analgesia is in 20 minutes.

The tibial nerve is blocked about 10–12 cm above the summit of the calcaneus on the medial aspect of the limb, just in front of the gastrocnemius tendon. The gastrocnemius tendon is grasped between the thumb and index finger of one hand while a needle, about 2.5 cm long, is inserted immediately below the thumb until its point can be felt just under the skin by the index finger. About 15 mL of local analgesia solution is injected at this site. A further 5 mL of solution should be injected on the lateral side of the leg to block a small cutaneous nerve. The block takes 15 minutes to develop.

An alternative method for desensitization of the hind limb below the fetlock involves blocking the superficial and deep peroneal nerves separately. The superficial peroneal nerve is blocked in the upper third of the metatarsus where it lies subcutaneously over the midline of the dorsal aspect of the metatarsal bone (Fig. 12.13). The deep peroneal nerve accompanies the dorsal metatarsal vessels in a groove on the cranial aspect of the metatarsal bone under cover of the extensor tendons. Injection is made halfway between the hock and the fetlock. The needle is inserted from the lateral aspect of the bone and the point directed beneath the edge of the tendon.

The plantar metatarsal nerves are blocked on the medial and lateral sides of the limb in the depression between the

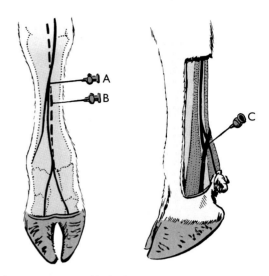

Figure 12.13 Nerve block of the distal part of the hind limb. (A) Injection of the superficial peroneal nerve; (B) injection of the deep peroneal nerve; (C) injection of the plantar metatarsal nerves.

suspensory ligament and the flexor tendons, about 5 cm proximal to the fetlock joint and deep to the superficial fascia (see Fig. 12.13). Five mL of local analgesia solution is injected over each nerve.

Intravenous regional analgesia

Intravenous regional analgesia (IVRA, Bier block) is a simple and commonly used technique to provide analgesia of the limb or digits. It is achieved by injecting local analgesic solution, without epinephrine, into a superficial vein in a limb isolated from the general circulation by a tourniquet. The limb distal to the site of application of the tourniquet becomes analgesic and remains so until the tourniquet is released.

The animal is restrained in lateral recumbency, with or without sedation. The hair over a prominent vein on the relevant limb is clipped and the skin prepared for injection (Fig. 12.14). A tourniquet of rubber tubing or a wide flat rubber band is applied above the carpus or hock, or above the fetlock, to occlude arterial blood flow. The flat tourniquet is preferable as it appears to cause the animals less discomfort than rubber tubing; consequently, they are less likely to be restless. When the tourniquet is to be placed on the hind limb above the hock in an adult animal, rolls of bandage should be placed either side of the limb beneath the tourniquet in the depression between the tibia and the gastrocnemius tendon to ensure occlusion of all blood vessels (Fig. 12.14). An 18–19 gauge needle (for an adult bovine) or butterfly needle is inserted into a vein with its point towards the foot. If the limb is to be

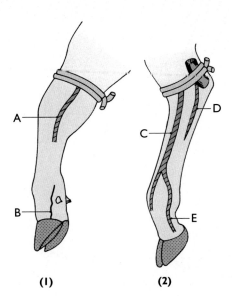

(1)   **(2)**

Figure 12.14 Easily recognized veins of the distal parts of limbs that can be used in placing needles or catheters for intravenous regional analgesia. (1) Medial view of the right foreleg. A: radial vein; B: medial palmar digital vein. (2) Lateral view of the left hind leg. C: lateral branch of lateral saphenous vein; D: lateral plantar vein; E: lateral plantar digital vein.

exsanguinated by application of an Esmarch bandage, the vein may be difficult to locate after application of the bandage; an option is first to place the needle and flush with heparin-saline solution. In adult cattle, 30 mL of 2% lidocaine (without epinephrine to avoid ischaemia) is injected into the vein after first aspirating blood to confirm location of the needle within the lumen of the vessel. Some veterinarians may follow that injection with saline to encourage spread of the local anaesthetic through the limb. Analgesia distal to the tourniquet will develop in 15–20 minutes and persist until the tourniquet is removed. Provided that 10 minutes or more have elapsed since the injection, no adverse effect from the local analgesic solution should be observed when the tourniquet is removed. Analgesia dissipates very rapidly in almost all animals.

Occasionally, the foot is analgesic everywhere except for the skin between the digits. This can be blocked by injection of 5 mL of 2% lidocaine midline on the dorsal aspect of the fetlock and a further 5 mL of solution on the caudal aspect of the fetlock between the dew claws.

The duration of analgesia is limited only by the time it is considered safe to leave a tourniquet in place. Intravenous regional analgesia is safe for up to at least 1.5 hours and this is long enough for most procedures done on the bovine foot.

The volume of lidocaine to be injected for IVRA in calves is 4 mg/kg.

Intranasal local analgesia

Lidocaine, 1.5 mg/kg, sprayed in the ventral nasal meatus and pharynx facilitated rhinotracheobronchoscopy in adult cows (Dadak et al., 2008). Cows treated with lidocaine exhibited quieter behaviour and less swallowing during insertion of the bronchoscope into the trachea. Peak serum concentrations of 1.21 ± 0.73 µg/mL were measured at 2 minutes after administration, decreasing to <150 ng/mL by 60 minutes.

GENERAL ANAESTHESIA

Clearly, choice of technique depends in large part on the circumstances surrounding the need for sedation or anaesthesia. For example, management of a dairy cow for caesarian section is different from management of a beef or feedlot heifer that has not been handled. Sedating a bull for a foot trim or radiographs may be more difficult when done on the farm than when performed in the clinic. Regurgitation during anaesthesia is a real hazard with potential consequence of pulmonary aspiration of ruminal fluid and material, asphyxia, pulmonary abscesses, or pneumonia. Food is customarily withheld from cattle older than 3 months of age before elective anaesthesia for 36 (24–48) hours, water for 8–12 hours, to decrease the volume of the rumen contents. This reduction in gastrointestinal volume has an added benefit of improving oxygenation during recumbency. Animals less than 2 months of age are likely to develop hypoglycaemia if food and milk are withheld for several hours. One recommendation is to prevent the calves from eating solid food for several hours and to withhold milk or milk replacer for 30 to 60 minutes before anaesthesia.

Anaesthetic techniques

Anaesthesia can be induced in the standing animal with only one assistant holding the head during injection, or the cow or bull can be first cast with ropes or strapped to a tilting table and anaesthetized in standing or lateral position. There is a clinically obvious difference in response to anaesthetic drugs between *Bos taurus* breeds and breeds crossed with *Bos indicus*. Dairy breeds in particular are relatively tolerant of the effects of anaesthesia. Breeds such as the Beefmaster, Santa Gertrudis, and Brahman often require a much lower dose of anaesthetic agents.

Premedication is not essential prior to injection of thiopental or thiopental–guaifenesin. Administration of acepromazine or xylazine will decrease the dose rate of induction agent, alter the cardiovascular parameters, and slow recovery from anaesthesia. Premedication with xylazine or detomidine is usual prior to anaesthesia with ketamine, except in young calves in which anaesthesia can be induced with diazepam–ketamine.

Unmaneageable cows and bulls that are confined in a stall but cannot be approached for an IV injection or restrained in a head gate or on a tilting table will have to be given sedative(s) by IM injection achieved by a creative approach appropriate to the situation and facilities, for example, when the bull is walking through a chute immediately prior to exiting into a pen, by lasso and halter of the animal's head that is then pulled tightly against the pen wall, or by administration of drugs by pole syringe. Various drug combinations not routinely used may be appropriate, such as a combination of xylazine-detomidine–low dose ketamine. Once sedated, one to two halters can be applied and the animal's head pulled close to the bars of the stall to facilitate IV injection of additional agents.

Intravenous injection

Use of an indwelling catheter is preferable to avoid perivascular injection of irritant drugs, such as thiopental or guaifenesin, and to facilitate supplemental injections. A 14 gauge, 13 cm long catheter is suitable for insertion in the jugular vein, although a 10 gauge catheter is better for administration of guaifenesin solutions in bulls. The skin of bulls may be 0.5–1.0 cm thick over the jugular vein and insertion of the catheter is easier through a small incision made with a scalpel blade through an intradermal bleb of local analgesic solution. After the catheter needle has penetrated the jugular vein (with the catheter directed towards the heart), both needle and catheter must be advanced until the catheter has also entered the vein. The catheter is advanced about 1 cm over the needle and then both needle and catheter advanced together until the catheter is introduced to its full length (in contrast to usual practice in other species and because catheter support is needed to counter the friction caused by thick skin). The needle is removed and a catheter cap (plug) attached to the catheter. Sutures in the skin are cross-tied around the catheter or white tape attached to the catheter that is then sutured or stapled to the skin. Smaller catheters can be more easily inserted in young calves. A 14 gauge catheter can also be inserted into a cephalic vein in bulls and cows that are restrained in lateral recumbency. When placement of a jugular catheter is not feasible an 18 gauge 7.5 cm catheter can be inserted into an auricular vein for administration of xylazine and ketamine. Once anaesthetized, a jugular vein can be catheterized for fluid administration or infusion of guaifenesin–ketamine for maintenance of anaesthesia.

The tail vein is often used for IV injection of non-irritant low volume agents such as xylazine. However, accidental intra-arterial injection is common and, even after xylazine, there have been reports of sloughing tails. The subcutaneous abdominal (milk) vein should only be used in emergency in female cattle.

Endotracheal intubation

There is a variety of techniques that can be used to facilitate endotracheal intubation in adult cattle. In cattle up to about 300 kg, intubation can be accomplished under direct vision of the larynx using a laryngoscope with a blade suitable for intubating a large dog. The animal is supported in sternal position, the head and neck extended, and the laryngoscope positioned at the corner of the animal's mouth with the tip of the blade on the dorsum of the tongue. The trachea is intubated with an endotracheal tube using a technique similar to that used in dogs and a 10–11 mm internal diameter (ID) tube for most newborn calves up to 18 or 20 mm ID for 300 kg calves. Care must be taken in smaller calves not to use the blade of the laryngoscope as a lever with the incisor teeth acting as a fulcrum.

In large bovine animals, a longer laryngoscope blade will be needed to view the laryngeal opening. A stiff stomach tube or a plastic introducer or a 2 m metal rod with a blunted end is passed through the mouth and into the trachea. The laryngoscope is withdrawn and the endotracheal tube is fed over the tube or introducer and into the trachea, whereupon the tube or introducer is removed. One problem is that the tube may catch on the epiglottis unless it is rotated at the appropriate moment.

Intubation by palpation is a technique commonly employed for cows and bulls. The mouth of the anaesthetized animal must be held open securely using a wedge-shaped gag inserted between the molar teeth or any other gag suitable for ruminants, and the head extended so that the oropharynx and trachea are in a straight line. A 26 mm or 30 mm ID endotracheal tube is used for adult cattle. The anaesthetist grasps the end of the endotracheal tube, guarding the cuff as best as possible, and inserts the arm and tube into the cow's mouth, taking care to remain midline so that the endotracheal tube cuff does not brush against the sharp edges of the molar teeth and tear (Fig. 12.15). The forefinger is used to depress the epiglottis and the free hand is used to advance the endotracheal tube onto the epiglottis. The arm inside the mouth is then advanced a further 5 cm and the forefinger and middle finger are used to spread the arytenoids and open the larynx. The free hand is used to advance the endotracheal tube into the larynx and trachea. If the endotracheal tube catches at the entrance of the larynx, the forefinger should be swept around the tube to free it for insertion. The anaesthetist's arm is removed and the endotracheal tube inserted its full length. The endotracheal tube cuff should be inflated immediately and the tube secured with gauze to the speculum, the halter, or by lengths of gauze or plastic tubing around the head or horns. When there is insufficient room for both the anaesthetist's arm and the

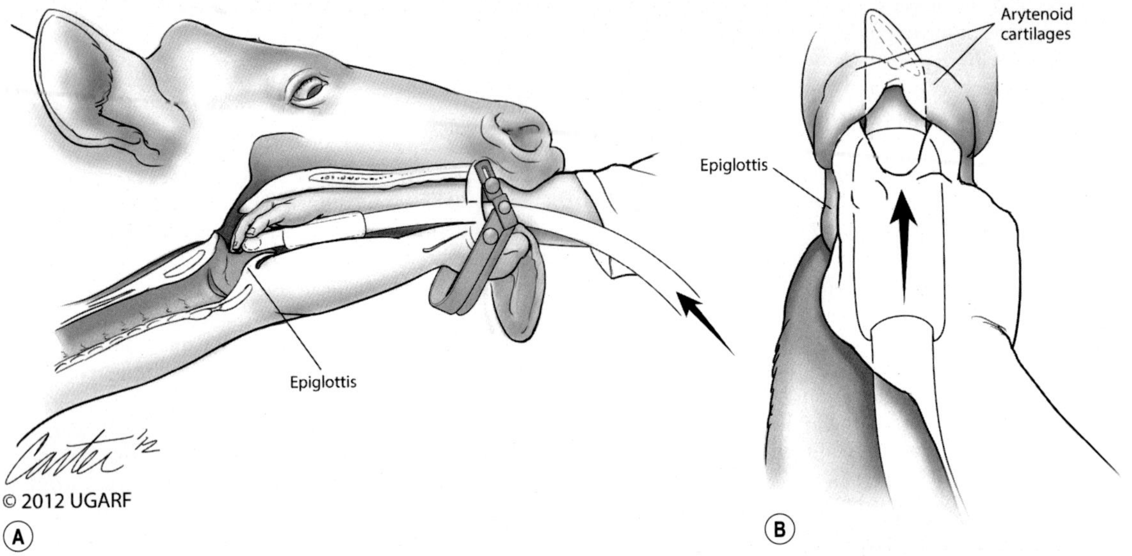

© 2012 UGARF

Ⓐ   Ⓑ

Figure 12.15 Intubation by palpation. The mouth is opened with a speculum wide enough to allow passage of a hand holding the endotracheal tube and the forearm. The epiglottis is depressed with a finger and the tip of the tube advanced onto it. Then two fingers are used to spread the arytenoids so that the endotracheal tube can be pushed into the trachea. © 2000–2012 University of Georgia Research Foundation, Inc. Art by William 'Kip' Carter (University of Georgia), with permission from Wolters Kluwer, Trim, C.M., 1987. Special anesthesia considerations in the ruminant. In: Short, C.E., (Ed.). Principles & Practice of Veterinary Anesthesia. Williams & Wilkins, Baltimore, pp. 285–300.

endotracheal tube, a stomach tube or introducer can be inserted in a manner just described and then the endotracheal tube fed over the tube or introducer and into the trachea after removal of the anaesthetist's arm. Assessment of adequate cuff inflation without overinflation can be difficult in large cattle and use of a pressure measuring device is recommended (see Fig. 10.29).

Endotracheal tubes may be passed 'blind' by the anaesthetist gripping the larynx with one hand and feeding the endotracheal tube into the larynx with the other hand. This is not an easy technique but the success rate of this technique increases with practice.

The lubricant applied to any endotracheal tube used in ruminant animals should never contain a local analgesic drug to avoid desensitization of the mucous membrane of the trachea and larynx after the tube is withdrawn. When the protective cough reflex is absent, foreign material may be inhaled into the bronchial tree.

Injectable anaesthetic agents

Thiopental

Thiopental may be used in adult cattle either alone or after premedication to provide full anaesthesia for operations of short duration or to induce anaesthesia that is then maintained by inhalation agents. In the unpremedicated animal, thiopental, 5% or 10% solution, is injected over 15 seconds into the jugular vein in a dose of 11 mg/kg estimated body weight; if xylazine premedication has been used a dose of 5–6 mg/kg is usually adequate. The animal sinks quietly to the ground within 20–30 seconds of injection and there is a brief period of apnoea. Apnoea seldom lasts for more than 15–20 seconds and artificial respiration is not required. Surgical anaesthesia of about 10 minutes is followed by recovery that is complete within 45 minutes. Recovery is usually quiet and free from excitement. The animal can be propped up and will maintain a position of sternal recumbency about 12–15min after injection of the drug. The period of surgical anaesthesia is brief but adequate for operations of very short duration or for endotracheal intubation prior to maintenance of anaesthesia with an inhalation agent.

Use of thiopental alone may be associated with a higher incidence of regurgitation during induction of anaesthesia than other induction protocols. Overdosage may occur when there is a gross error in estimation of body weight. Underdosage is more frequent and the animal may remain standing, but excitement rarely occurs. Failure to induce anaesthesia may be the result of the injection being made too slowly or because of perivascular injection. Additional thiopental may be injected IV immediately to achieve anaesthesia provided that IV access can be guaranteed. Perivascular injection should be treated by infiltration of the area with 1–2 mg/kg of 2% lidocaine and several hundred mL of 0.9% saline in an attempt to avoid tissue necrosis and abscesses.

Thiopental should not be administered by this rapid injection technique to sick animals or animals with impaired cardiovascular function. Young calves up to 2.5 months of age are not good subjects for thiopental anaesthesia and the use of even small doses for induction of anaesthesia cannot be recommended.

Thiopental–guaifenesin

Approximately 80–100 mg/kg of 5% guaifenesin alone is needed to produce recumbency in cattle. Guaifenesin provides no sedation or anaesthesia and should be combined with at least thiopental or ketamine when used for immobilization. A solution of 2 g thiopental in 50 g guaifenesin is run rapidly into a catheterized vein (perivascular injection of >5% guaifenesin can cause tissue necrosis, abscesses, and skin sloughing) to produce recumbency and muscle relaxation (Table 12.2).

Table 12.2 Dose rates of some anaesthetic agents and combinations (adjustment should be made for body condition and health status)

Drug	Dose	Comments
Adult cattle Thiopental	11 mg/kg IV	Premedication decreases dose rate
Adult cattle Guaifenesin 5% + Thiopental 2.5–5%	50–100 mg/kg IV + 3–4 mg/kg IV	Dose rate decreases >600 kg body weight; premedication decreases dose rate
Calves < 150 kg Xylazine + Ketamine	0.05–0.1 mg/kg IM + 4–6 mg/kg IV or 10 mg/kg IM	Calves <2 months of age may be satisfactorily sedated with lower doses of xylazine
Calves 150–350 kg Xylazine + Ketamine	0.1 mg/kg IM + 4 mg/kg IV or 6 mg/kg IM	20 min duration
Adult cattle Xylazine + Ketamine	0.1 mg/kg IM or IV + 2.2 mg/kg IV	Diazepam or midazolam 0.05 mg/kg can be added to ketamine for induction, 15-20 min duration; for prolongation see below
Prolongation of preceding xylazine–ketamine combination Add 1 g ketamine to 1 L of 5% guaifenesin	Infuse 1.5–2.0 mL/kg/h IV	Tracheal intubation recommended; O$_2$ supplementation recommended; dose rate adjusted to depth required and reduced in very young, old, and large
Calves Add 100 mg xylazine and 1 g ketamine to 1 L of 5% guaifenesin	Induction 0.5 mL/kg and maintenance 2.5 mL/kg/h IV	Tracheal intubation recommended; O$_2$ supplementation recommended
Calves Diazepam (or midazolam) + Ketamine ± Butorphanol	0.25 mg/kg combined in the same syringe with 5 mg/kg IV 0.05–0.1 mg/kg IV, IM	Small increments of this dose rate can be used to induce sedation; full dose can be used for short duration (10–15 min) anaesthesia or tracheal intubation prior to inhalation anaesthesia
Calves Xylazine + Tiletamine–zolazepam	0.1 mg/kg IM + 4 mg/kg IM	O$_2$ supplementation recommended
Calves Propofol	5–6 mg/kg IV 3 mg/kg IV	Unpremedicated calves. When premedicated with xylazine 0.1 mg/kg

The dose rate of guaifenesin 5%–thiopental (50 g:2 g) in unpremedicated cattle up to 500 kg is approximately 2 mL/kg and this rate decreases substantially on a mL/kg basis with increasing body weight, with large bulls seldom requiring more than 1500 mL of the mixture for anaesthesia adequate for endotracheal intubation. Administration of xylazine premedication greatly reduces the dose rate required for anaesthesia. The drugs may also be administered separately, in which case, guaifenesin is first infused IV at 50 mg/kg followed by a bolus injection of 2–4 mg/kg of thiopental and then increments of guaifenesin and thiopental to reach the desired effect.

Guaifenesin–thiopental administration decreases the respiratory tidal volume and blood pressure, and increases respiratory and heart rates.

Pentobarbital

Toosey (1959) found that pentobarbital, 1.9–3.8 mg/kg IV, produced sedation in adult animals which remained standing, but swaying, on their feet. Thirty years later, Valverde et al. (1989) confirmed that 2 mg/kg IV produces reliable sedation in standing adult cattle. These doses produce moderate sedation for 30 minutes and mild sedation for a further 30 minutes. Respiratory rate is significantly decreased but no changes have been measured in arterial blood gases.

There are safer agents than pentobarbital for producing general anaesthesia in cattle and this agent must not be used in calves.

Ketamine

Ketamine alone will not cause seizures in cattle but the quality of anaesthesia obtained by it is poor. Premedication with xylazine before injection of ketamine produces quiet, smooth induction of anaesthesia with good muscle relaxation and a smooth recovery from anaesthesia. In young calves, premedication with xylazine may be substituted with diazepam or midazolam or acepromazine, with or without butorphanol. The dose rate of ketamine is usually higher in calves than in mature animals.

Xylazine is given to adult cattle either IM at 0.1–0.2 mg/kg or IV at 0.05–0.10 mg/kg to produce deep sedation, often with recumbency. Ketamine is then given IV at 2 mg/kg to induce anaesthesia, either immediately after xylazine or up to 10 minutes later. Endotracheal intubation can be performed in some animals soon after the xylazine injection and before ketamine administration. The duration of anaesthesia from xylazine–ketamine is about 15 minutes.

In smaller animals of about 200–350 kg body weight, xylazine, 0.1–0.2 mg/kg, is given IM 5–8 min before ketamine at either 6 mg/kg IM or 4 mg/kg IV. In young calves,

xylazine, 0.1 mg/kg, and ketamine, 10 mg/kg, can be given IM at the same time, or ketamine, 2–6 mg/kg, may be administered IV a few minutes after xylazine. Intramuscular administration of xylazine and ketamine will provide 25–30 minutes of anaesthesia. Anaesthesia can be maintained after any of these combinations by intermittent injections or infusion of guaifenesin–ketamine, 1 g of ketamine in 1 L of 5% guaifenesin, or by inhalation agents.

The combination of diazepam and ketamine will produce less cardiovascular depression in calves than xylazine and ketamine. Diazepam (or midazolam), 0.2–0.25 mg/kg, and ketamine, 5 mg/kg, can be combined and injected intravenously as a bolus or in increments to achieve the desired effect. This combination will provide about 15 min of anaesthesia. Butorphanol, 0.05 mg/kg, can be included with this combination to increase analgesia and muscle relaxation. Anaesthesia may be prolonged by intermittent injections of diazepam and ketamine, or by inhalation agents. Endotracheal intubation and administration of O_2 is advisable.

Medetomidine, 0.02 mg/kg, and ketamine, 0.5 mg/kg, given together IV is a combination that has been described to produce deep sedation lasting 30 min in calves that could be combined with local analgesia for surgery (Raekallio et al., 1991). As might be expected, hypoxaemia developed in the calves in dorsal recumbency. Administration of atipamezole, 0.02–0.06 mg/kg (20–60 µg/kg), produced a rapid smooth recovery. It should be noted that in another study of medetomidine sedation in calves, injection of atipamezole, 0.2 mg/kg (200 µg/kg), to reverse sedation induced transient severe hypotension and even sinus arrest (Ranheim et al., 1998). Therefore, reversal agents should be given cautiously while monitoring the patient closely. Relapse of sedation may occur 90 minutes to 3 hours later.

Ketamine–guaifenesin

Anaesthesia can be induced and maintained by IV infusion of xylazine, guaifenesin and ketamine (GKX). Xylazine, 100 mg and ketamine 1000 mg are added to 1 L of 5% guaifenesin and the mixture infused IV at 1–2 mL/kg in adult cattle. Alternatively, after induction of anaesthesia with xylazine and ketamine, anaesthesia can be maintained by intermittent or continuous infusion of a mixture of guaifenesin–ketamine (1000 mg ketamine added to 1 L of 5% guaifenesin) at approximately 1.5–2 mL/kg/h – there is no need to add xylazine to the maintenance anaesthetic combination for anaesthesia lasting up to an hour because in cattle the duration of effect of xylazine is longer than ketamine. Control of the infusion rate of GK or GKX is best using an infusion pump but counting the drip rate in an administration set with gravity flow from a bag is also a viable alternative. Supplementation with O_2 is advisable to prevent hypoxaemia when general anaesthesia is maintained with guaifenesin–ketamine. Significant hypercarbia is likely to develop with time.

Equivalent quality of anaesthesia between GKX and isoflurane was recorded for experimental abdominal laparoscopy in calves 2–26 days of age (Kerr et al., 2007). Anaesthesia was induced by 0.5 mL/kg of GKX administered IV over 20 seconds (plus a little more in some calves to accomplish endotracheal intubation) and maintained by continuous infusion of GKX at approximately 2.5 mL/kg/h. Anaesthesia was induced and maintained with isoflurane at an end-tidal isoflurane concentration of 1.6% (1.3–1.8%) in another group of calves for comparison. All calves were intubated and artificially ventilated with oxygen. Heart rates were lower and systolic arterial pressures were higher in calves receiving GKX, but cardiac outputs were similar. MAP was lower during the first 15 minutes of isoflurane, presumably because a higher concentration is required for tracheal intubation. In another investigation, administration of xylazine, 0.2 mg/kg, IM in 1-week-old calves decreased cardiac index by 40% but cardiac output gradually increased during infusion of GKX, 1.1 mL/kg/h, IV for maintenance of anaesthesia (Picavet et al., 2004). MAP decreased after the first 30 minutes to 64 ± 6 mmHg. The calves were in lateral recumbency breathing spontaneously at approximately 40 breaths/min and blood gas analysis revealed moderate to severe hypoventilation and some calves were hypoxic. Nasal insufflation of O_2 4 L/min restored SpO_2 from <90% to 97%. At the end of anaesthesia, xylazine was reversed by administration of tolazoline, 0.5 mg/kg, half IV and half IM. Infusion of GKX is a feasible technique for use in the field with the caution that the rate of infusion must be monitored to avoid overdose and O_2 supplementation is advisable. A resuscitator (AMBU) bag can be used to achieve some artificial breaths for a calf. Xylazine, guaifenesin and ketamine are not licensed for use in cattle in most countries and appropriate regulatory agencies should be consulted for withdrawal times.

Tiletamine–zolazepam

The combination of tiletamine–zolazepam (Telazol or Zolatil), 4 mg/kg, and xylazine, 0.1 mg/kg, injected IM in sequence produced anaesthesia within minutes in calves (Thurmon et al., 1989). Analgesia lasted on average 70 min and the calves were able to walk in 130 ± 18 min from the time of the last injection. When higher doses of xylazine were used in another group of calves some became apnoeic. Although not measured in this study, clinical experience has been that calves anaesthetized with tiletamine–zolazepam become hypoxic when placed in dorsal recumbency.

Injection of a combination of detomidine–ketamine–tiletamine–zolazepam (DKTZ) into experimental 8-month-old calves weighing on average 218 kg was evaluated at three dose rates using a pin-prick in the perineal region and an electrical stimulus to the tail base (Re et al., 2011). The drugs were combined by adding 40 mg detomidine and 500 mg ketamine to a vial of lyophilized tiletamine–zolazepam to produce a final solution of 9 mL containing 4.4 mg/mL of detomidine and 55.5 mg/mL of each ketamine and tiletamine–zolazepam, and administered IM at 1.0, 1.3, or 1.5 mL/100 kg. The depression of responses to noxious stimuli were dose dependent with maximum effect between 10 and 20 minutes after administration and a longer duration of depression at the medium (35 minutes) and high dose (55 minutes) rates. Heart rates decreased non-significantly, MAP significantly increased, and respiratory rates remained high. Severe hypoventilation and hypoxaemia were measured by blood gas analysis at 10 minutes after administration with an improvement in some animals noted at the next measurement time of 40 minutes. Recumbency lasted 1 hour after the low dose and 2 hours with the higher dose rates. The authors concluded that DKTZ was effective for immobilization and for minor surgical procedures, with or without local analgesia. Oxygen supplementation should be available.

Propofol

Although propofol is being used for induction of anaesthesia in calves, there are few reports in the scientific literature. Administration of propofol to calves is similar to that in other small species, with an induction dose of 5–6 mg/kg in unpremedicated calves and a reduction in dose rate when premedication is used. Premedication with xylazine, 0.1 mg/kg IM, decreased the propofol dose rate to 3 mg/kg IV in 3–7-month old calves anaesthetized for umbilical hernia repair (Cagnardi et al., 2009). Propofol anaesthesia is short lived but provides good relaxation for endotracheal intubation.

Hypoventilation and hypoxia occur commonly in sedated or anaesthetized cattle.

Inhalation anaesthesia agents

Anaesthesia circuits used for large dogs are suitable for maintaining inhalation anaesthesia in calves up to a body weight of approximately 140 kg or that are intubated with an endotracheal tube of 16 mm internal diameter or less. Calves or cattle that can accommodate an endotracheal tube ≥18 mm ID should be connected to a large animal machine such as is marketed for use in horses.

Endotracheal intubation is generally accomplished after administration of injectable agents. In contrast to its use in other species, xylazine alone has long been a favourite agent to facilitate endotracheal intubation in cattle

(Adetunji et al., 1984). After the animal has become recumbent, orotracheal intubation is accomplished as previously described. Xylazine abolishes the swallowing reflex although coughing usually occurs as the endotracheal tube is inserted. Other common alternatives are diazepam-ketamine IV for calves, xylazine–ketamine IV, IM, or IM followed by IV top-up, or xylazine–guaifenesin–ketamine or guaifenesin–thiopental. Regurgitation during induction of anaesthesia is always a possibility, especially in adult cattle, and management of this event should be pre-planned. A ruminant should never be rolled over before endotracheal intubation is successful.

Mask induction with inhalation anaesthetic agents is possible with little difficulty in calves up to 3 months of age. A small animal circle system can be used to deliver O_2 and anaesthetic initially through a well-fitting mask (mask with a rubber diaphragm). The calf can be unpremedicated or sedated with a combination of diazepam or midazolam, 0.1 mg/kg, butorphanol, 0.05–0.10 mg/kg, and xylazine, 0.02 mg/kg. For induction of anaesthesia with isoflurane or sevoflurane in the standing calf, the mask is applied with the O_2 flowing at 3–4 L/min and after starting the vaporizer setting at zero it is increased by 0.5% increments every few breaths to 4% for isoflurane and 5.5% for sevoflurane. As its legs begin to relax, the calf is allowed to subside to the ground where it is supported in sternal recumbency until the endotracheal tube is inserted and the cuff inflated. The trachea is intubated under direct vision of the larynx using a laryngoscope. The mouth can be held open using lengths of gauze looped around the upper and lower jaws and the tongue pulled to the opposite side of the mouth to the laryngoscope. After intubation, the tube is secured by tying gauze (or other suitable tie) around the tube and around the back of the calf's head or bottom jaw and then the cuff is inflated. Subsequently, the calf can be positioned or lifted onto the operating table. Two similar studies evaluated mask induction with sevoflurane and desflurane in unpremedicated 8–12-week-old Holstein calves. The time from mask induction to tracheal intubation with sevoflurane 7% in O_2 6 L/min was an average of 3.7 minutes and the time to intubation was an average of 2.5 minutes for desflurane delivered as 18% in O_2 6 L/min (Greene et al., 2002; Keegan et al., 2006). Induction with desflurane was free of struggling or breath-holding and it was noted that there was adequate time for intubation.

O_2 flow rates for a small animal circle circuit can be 2–4 L/min initially. The vaporizer setting for isoflurane, sevoflurane, or halothane depends on the CNS depressant effect of the agents used for premedication and induction of anaesthesia, and the relative potency of the agent used, but closely resemble values that would be used for anaesthetizing a large dog. The O_2 flow rate can be reduced to 1 L/min (or less) for maintenance of anaesthesia but the vaporizer setting is usually fairly high, for example 2–3%

isoflurane, because the circuit concentration remains considerably lower. When connecting a cow or bull to a large animal circle circuit, the initial O_2 flow rate should be 8–10 L/min for 15–20 minutes to wash out expired nitrogen and rapidly increase the circuit anaesthetic concentration before reducing the flow to 3 L/min (or similar) for maintenance. An isoflurane vaporizer setting of 3.5% or sevoflurane vaporizer of 4.5% should be sufficient initially. Cantalapiedra et al (2000) measured a mean MAC concentration of 1.14% (sea level) for isoflurane in adult Holstein-Friesian cattle. Cattle tend to breathe fast and shallow, limiting uptake of the inhalation agent. Connecting the patient to a mechanical ventilator, when available, from the beginning of anaesthesia removes the problem of inadequate exposure of pulmonary capillaries to anaesthetic gas for uptake. A respiratory rate of 10 breaths/min and tidal volume of 10 mL/kg should ensure normocarbia. Artificial ventilation will probably be necessary for small calves and values of 12–15 breaths/min and tidal volume of 15 mL/kg are satisfactory in this size patient.

Tracheal intubation is associated with increased circulating catecholamine concentrations and premature ventricular complexes may develop in some animals after intubation, particularly when anaesthesia is not deep and during halothane anaesthesia, an agent that sensitizes the myocardium to catecholamines (Semrad et al., 1986). The prevalence of arrhythmias decreases over 15 minutes.

Nitrous oxide

N_2O/O_2 mixtures are not often used in cattle because of the progressive movement of N_2O into the rumen and intestines resulting in bloat. N_2O is not sufficiently potent to induce or maintain anaesthesia when given on its own and it is usually administered with another inhalation agent.

Adjunct agents

Neuromuscular blocking agents

The fact that in cattle peripheral nerve blocks are easily used to produce skeletal muscle relaxation means that neuromuscular blocking drugs are seldom necessary in clinical anaesthesia. Such further muscle relaxation as may be needed is usually provided by the IV injection of guaifenesin.

In experimental studies, pancuronium (0.1 mg/kg) produces relaxation of 30–40 min duration. Pancuronium, 0.043 mg/kg, produced a 90–99% reduction of hind limb extensor twitch lasting on average 26 minutes (Hildebrand & Howitt, 1984). As in horses, but in contrast to other species of animal, the facial muscles are more resistant to neuromuscular block than are the limb muscles. Monitoring of block should, therefore, be carried out by stimulation of nerves to limb muscles.

Anaesthetic management

Positioning

Correct positioning and padding is important as radial nerve damage may develop in the underneath forelimb in cattle that have been lying in lateral recumbency for more than about 20 minutes. Radial nerve paralysis may develop after any form of general anaesthesia, injectable or inhalational. Padding (e.g. inflated tractor tyre inner tubes, foam pads, air- or water-filled bags) should be inserted under the shoulder and forearm. Position of the limbs in cattle is the same as in anaesthetized horses, but the difference in the anatomy of the shoulders makes it difficult to pull the lower forelimb forward to the same extent. The upper limbs should be elevated into a horizontal position. The head should be positioned with a pad under the poll so that the nose is lower than the crown, allowing saliva and any regurgitated material to drain from the pharynx. Positioning is facilitated when the surgical table has a head board with a downward slope that can be attached. The horns should be protected from breakage. As a safety precaution against excessive movement in cattle that are positioned on an elevated table, the belly bands and halter, although loosened, should remain tied to the table.

> *Attention to positioning of adult cattle during injectable or inhalation anaesthesia may prevent radial nerve paralysis.*

Fluid therapy

For prolonged anaesthesia or major surgery, it is common practice to give 5–10 mL/kg/h of balanced electrolyte solution IV. Calves less than 3 months of age should be given 3–5 mL/kg/h of 5% dextrose in water in addition to 3–7 mL/kg/h balanced electrolyte solution to prevent the development of hypoglycaemia. Hypertonic saline, 2–4 mL/kg, IV over 10–20 minutes may be required for acute blood volume expansion in cases of severe haemorrhage or endotoxic shock.

Monitoring

Monitoring the anaesthetized animal is discussed in Chapter 2 but there are some differences from the general descriptions that should be noted. The bovine eye rotates with increasing depth of anaesthesia into a ventral rather than rostroventral position and only the sclera can be seen; it then rotates back into a central position during deep anaesthesia. The pupil usually constricts to a horizontal slit but some pupillary dilation may occur after ketamine administration. The presence of a palpebral reflex indicates that anaesthesia is light. During ketamine anaesthesia, increased muscle tone may result in a centrally placed eye and strong palpebral reflex.

Respiratory rate may be rapid (20–40 breaths/min) and the depth shallow. Mature bulls and cows breathing spontaneously develop high $PaCO_2$ during inhalation anaesthesia and IPPV is usually necessary to prevent severe hypercapnia. A rate of 10 breaths/min and a tidal volume of 10 mL/kg (5–6 L for an adult cow or bull) will usually maintain a $PaCO_2$ of around 5.3 kPa (40 mmHg). Spontaneously breathing calves usually seriously hypoventilate when supine and IPPV with tidal volumes of 12–15 mL/kg, at rates of 12 breaths/min and an inspiratory pressure of up to 30 mmHg may be necessary to keep the $PaCO_2$ at about 5.3 kPa (40 mmHg). Oxygenation when anaesthesia is being maintained with IV agents can be provided by endotracheal intubation and connection to an anaesthesia machine or a demand valve with an O_2 supply for assisted or controlled ventilation. Insufflation of O_2 at 15 L/min through a small bore tube down an endotracheal tube may prevent hypoxaemia.

Mature bulls and cows usually maintain HRs of 60–80 beats/min during anaesthesia. Tachycardia may develop in response to hypercarbia, hypotension, or light anaesthesia. Bulls and adult cows may develop hypertension during inhalation anaesthesia and systolic pressures of >200 mmHg and diastolic pressures >120 mmHg are not uncommon. Premedication with xylazine results in lower pressures. Values obtained by indirect methods of measurement in adult cattle are often incorrect, but blood pressure is easily and accurately measured by direct means using a 20 or 22 gauge catheter placed in the middle or caudal auricular artery (see Fig 2.18) and connected to a manometer or electrical transducer. Hypotension should be treated in the usual manner, namely, by decreasing the rate of anaesthetic administration, infusing balanced electrolyte solution and administration of dopamine, dobutamine, or ephedrine.

Blood pressure values in calves are similar to those measured in other small ruminant animals. The MAP should be >60 mmHg and values less than this warrant treatment. Cardiovascular values obtained using different monitors and under different study designs may not be directly comparable, but the information may be useful. Mean values in awake calves obtained 30 minutes after isoflurane anaesthesia for instrumentation were HR 111 beats/min, systolic, diastolic, and mean pressures were 123/77 (93) mmHg, respectively, and cardiac index (CI) was 175 mL/kg/min (Kerr et al., 2007). Mean values obtained during subsequent isoflurane anaesthesia without surgery were HR 92 beats/min, blood pressures 87/49(63) mmHg, and CI 134 ml/kg/min. Blood pressures increased after the start of surgery. Similar values were obtained in calves anaesthetized with xylazine–ketamine–isoflurane, with low MAP before the start of surgery and an increase during surgery accompanied by severe hypoventilation and respiratory acidosis (Offinger et al., 2012). In two similar experimental studies, mean values obtained in 8–12-week-old Holstein calves

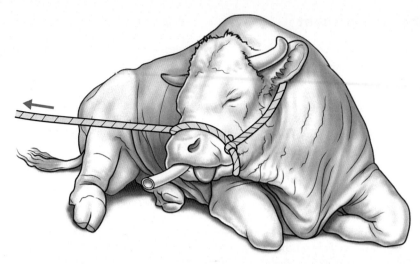

Figure 12.16 Adult cows and bulls must be supported in sternal position as soon as anaesthesia is finished. A halter will help maintain sternal recumbency by bending the animal's head around to face the hind limbs. The animal must be able to pull its tongue back into its mouth before the endotracheal tube is removed.

anaesthetized with an end-tidal concentration of 3.8% sevoflurane and IPPV were HR 72 beats/min, MAP 91 mmHg, and CI 92 mL/kg/min (Greene et al., 2002), and in calves anaesthetized with an end-tidal 9.7% desflurane HR 87 beats/min, MAP 75 mmHg, and CI 124 mL/kg/min (Keegan et al., 2006). The range of values was wide for each measurement. The authors estimated that the sevoflurane and desflurane concentrations were approximately 1.3 MAC. Premedication with acepromazine or xylazine may contribute to low blood pressure. Systolic pressures may be measured non-invasively by oscillometric or Doppler ultrasound technique with the cuff placed above the carpus or on the tail. Blood glucose should be measured at least once during anaesthesia of calves <3 months of age.

Recovery from anaesthesia

Ruminants should be moved into sternal recumbency and propped up in this position as soon as anaesthesia is terminated to allow expulsion of accumulated ruminal gases that impair respiratory function. When an adult cow or bull is confined in a stall for recovery, it can be pushed into a sternal position using support at the shoulder and pulling on a halter. The animal's head is positioned with the head turned towards the hind limbs to the point where the nose may be touching the floor near the hind feet (Fig. 12.16). The halter rope is pulled almost fully caudally to maintain the animal in this position. The mouth speculum can be removed at this time. The

endotracheal tube should not be removed until the animal is swallowing and voluntarily withdraws its tongue into its mouth. This may not occur for some time after coughing and chewing movements return. O_2 administration by insufflation (15 L/min in an adult) down the endotracheal tube, or through a facemask, or by nasal tube, may be necessary when breathing is too shallow. In animals that have been intubated, the tube should be removed with the cuff still partially inflated to withdraw saliva that may have collected above the cuff. If regurgitation occurred during anaesthesia, an attempt should be made to remove any wads of food from the pharynx and to flush the oral and nasal cavities with water before extubation. The animal's nose must be dependent to ensure drainage. The halter can be removed when the animal is judged to be able to maintain sternal recumbency. If the animal assumes lateral recumbency it must be pushed back into sternal position. Mouth breathing in a bovine during recovery from anaesthesia is indicative of hypoxaemia and will occur when some ruminal fluid has been aspirated. Oxygen must be supplied. Antibiotics are administered if aspiration is the cause. Cattle often remain sitting for some time after consciousness has returned and the process of standing is usually much more deliberate than it is in horses. After sevoflurane anaesthesia recovery to standing is often rapid.

Cattle may be allowed to eat and drink within a few hours of recovery to consciousness, the precise time depending, to some extent, on the anaesthetic agents administered. Calves are usually prevented from nursing for an hour. Hypoglycemia should be ruled out if recovery is slow.

REFERENCES

Adetunji, A., Pascoe, P.J., McDonell, W.N., et al., 1984. Retrospective evaluation of xylazine/halothane anesthesia in 125 cattle. Can Vet J 25, 342–346.

Anderson, D.E., 2008. Chemical restraint in cattle: new thoughts for a new era. Proceedings Colorado State University 69th Annual Conference for Veterinarians. Fort Collins, CO, USA.

Arnemo, J.M., Søli, N.E., 1993. Chemical capture of free-ranging cattle: immobilization with xylazine or medetomidine, and reversal with atipamezole. Vet Res Commun 17, 469–477.

Bernards, C.M., 2006. Epidural and spinal anesthesia. In: Barash, P.G., Cullen, B.F., Stoelting, R.K. (Eds.), Clinical Anesthesia, 5th edn. Lippincott Williams & Wilkins, Philadelphia, pp. 691–717.

Bigham, A.S., Habibian, S., Ghasemian, F., et al., 2010. Caudal epidural injection of lidocaine, tramadol, and lidocaine-tramadol for epidural anesthesia in cattle. J Vet Pharmacol Ther 33, 439–443.

Blaze, C.A., LeBlanc, P.H., Robinson, N.E., 1988. Effect of withholding feed on ventilation and the incidence of regurgitation during halothane anesthesia of adult cattle. Am J Vet Res 49, 2126–2129.

Boesch, D., Steiner, A., Gygax, L., et al., 2008. Burdizzo castration of calves less than 1-week old with and without local anaesthesia: Short-term behavioural responses and plasma cortisol levels. Appl Anim Behav Sci 114, 330–345.

Cagnardi, P., Zonca, A., Gallo, M., et al., 2009. Pharmacokinetics of propofol in calves undergoing abdominal surgery. Vet Res Commun 33 (Suppl 1), S177–S179.

Campbell, K.B., Klavano, P.A., Richardson, P., et al., 1979. Hemodynamic effects of xylazine in the calf. Am J Vet Res 40, 1777–1780.

Cantalapiedra, A.G., Villaneuva, B., Pereira, J.L., 2000. Anaesthetic potency of isoflurane in cattle: determination of the minimum alveolar concentration. Vet Anaesth Analg 27, 22–26.

Caulkett, N.A., MacDonald, J.E.D., Cribb, P.N., et al., 1993. Xylazine hydrochloride epidural analgesia: a method of providing sedation and analgesia to facilitate castration of mature bulls. Comp Cont Educ 15, 1155–1159.

Court, M.H., Dodman, N.H., Levine, H.D., et al., 1992. Pharmacokinetics and milk residues of butorphanol in dairy cows after single intravenous administration. J Vet Pharmacol Ther 15, 28–35.

Currah, J.M., Hendrick, S.H., Stookey, J.M., 2009. The behavioral assessment and alleviation of pain associated with castration in beef calves treated with flunixin meglumine and caudal lidocaine epidural anesthesia with epinephrine. Can Vet J 50, 375–382.

Dadak, A.M., Franz, S., Jäger, W., et al., 2008. Pharmacokinetics and clinical efficacy of lidocaine in cattle after intranasal administration during rhinotracheobronchoscopy. J Vet Pharmacol Ther 32, 300–302.

Davis, J.L., Smith, G.W., Baynes, R.E., et al., 2009. Update on drugs prohibited from extralabel use in food animals. J Am Vet Med Assoc 235, 528–534.

Delehant, T.M., Denhart, J.W., Lloyd, W.E., et al., 2003. Pharmacokinetics of xylazine, 2,6-dimethylaniline, and tolazoline in tissues from yearling cattle and milk from mature dairy cows after sedation with xylazine hydrochloride and reversal with tolazoline hydrochloride. Vet Ther 4, 128–134.

DeMoor, A., Desmet, P., 1971. Effect of Rompun on acid-base-equilibrium and arterial O_2 pressure in cattle. Vet Med Rev 2, 163–169.

DeRossi, R., Zanenga, N.F., Alves, O.D., et al., 2010. Effects of caudal epidural ketamine and/or lidocaine on heifers during reproductive procedures: A preliminary study. Vet J 185, 344–346.

Duffield, T.F., Heinrich, A., Millman, S.T., et al., 2010. Reduction in pain response by combined use of local lidocaine anesthesia and systemic ketoprofen in dairy calves dehorned by heat cauterization. Can Vet J 51, 283–288.

Fajt, V.R., Wagner, S.A., Norby, B., 2011. Analgesic drug administration and attitudes about analgesia in cattle among bovine practitioners in the United States. J Am Vet Med Assoc 238, 755–767.

Fayed, A.H., Abdalla, E.B., Anderson, R.R., et al., 1989. Effect of xylazine in heifers under thermoneutral or heat stress conditions. Am J Vet Res 50, 151–153.

Fierheller, E.E., Caulkett, N.A., Bailey, J.V., 2004. A romifidine and morphine combination for epidural analgesia of the flank in cattle. Can Vet J 45, 917–923.

Gehring, R., Coetzee, J.F., Tarus-Sang, J., et al., 2008. Pharmacokinetics of ketamine and its metabolite norketamine administered at a sub-anesthetic dose together with xylazine to calves prior to castration. J Vet Pharmacol Ther 32, 124–128.

González, L.A., Schwartzkopf-Genswein, K.S., Caulkett, N.A., et al., 2010. Pain mitigation after band castration of beef calves and its effect on performance, behavior, Escherichia coli, and salivary cortisol. J Anim Sci 88, 802–810.

Greene, S.A., Keegan, R.D., Valdez, R.A., et al., 2002. Cardiovascular effects of sevoflurane in Holstein calves. Vet Anaesth Analg 29, 59–63.

Grubb, T.L., Riebold, T.W., Crisman, R.O., et al., 2002. Comparison of lidocaine, xylazine, and lidocaine-xylazine for caudal epidural analgesia in cattle. Vet Anaesth Analg 29, 64–68.

Hall, L.W., 1991. Anaesthesia of the ox. In: Hall, L.W., Clarke, K.W. (Eds.), Veterinary Anaesthesia, 9th edn. Ballière Tindall, London, pp. 236–259.

Hashimoto, K., Hampl, K.F., Nakamura, Y., et al., 2001. Epinephrine increases the neurotoxic potential of intrathecally administered lidocaine in the rat. Anesthesiology 94, 876–881.

Hay, A., 1991. Needle penetration of the globe during retrobulbar and peribulbar injections. Ophthalmology 98, 1017–1024.

Hewson, C.J., Dohoo, I.R., Lemke, K.A., et al., 2007. Canadian veterinarians' use of analgesics in cattle, pigs, and horses in 2004 and 2005. Can Vet J 48, 155–164.

Hikasa, Y., Takese, K., Emi, S., et al., 1988. Antagonistic effects of alpha-adrenoceptor blocking agents on reticuloruminal hypomotility induced by xylazine in cattle. Can J Vet Res 52, 411–415.

Hildebrand, S.V., Howitt, G.A., 1984. Neuromuscular and cardiovascular effects of pancuronium bromide in calves anesthetized with halothane. Am J Vet Res 45, 1549–1552.

Hiraoka, M., Miyagawa, T., Kobayashi, H., et al., 2007. Successful introduction of modified dorsolumbar epidural anesthesia in a bovine referral center. J Vet Sci 8, 181–184.

Hodgson, D.S., Dunlop, C.I., Chapman, P.L., et al., 2002. Cardiopulmonary effects of xylazine and acepromazine in pregnant cows in late gestation. Am J Vet Res 63, 1695–1699.

Hopkins, T.J., 1972. The clinical pharmacology of xylazine in cattle. Aust Vet J 48, 109–112.

Huxley, J.N., Whay, H.R., 2006. Current attitudes of cattle practitioners to pain and the use of analgesics in cattle. Vet Rec 159, 662–668.

Keegan, R.D., Greene, S.A., Valdez, R.A., et al., 2006. Cardiovascular effects of desflurane in mechanically ventilated calves. Am J Vet Res 67, 387–391.

Kerr, C.L., Windeyer, C., Bouré, L.P., et al., 2007. Cardiopulmonary effects of administration of a combination solution of xylazine, guaifenesin, and ketamine or inhaled isoflurane in mechanically ventilated calves. Am J Vet Res 68, 1287–1293.

Klein, L., Fisher, N., 1988. Cardiopulmonary effects of restraint in dorsal recumbency on awake cattle. Am J Vet Res 49, 1605–1608.

Leblanc, M.M., Hubbell, J.A.E., Smith, A.C., 1984. The effects of xylazine hydrochloride on intrauterine pressure in the cow. Theriogenology 21, 681–690.

Lee, I., Yamagishi, K., Oboshi, K., et al., 2004a. Comparison of xylazine, lidocaine and the two drugs combined for modified dorsolumbar epidural anaesthesia in cattle. Vet Rec 155, 797–799.

Lee, I., Yamagishi, N., Oboshi, K., et al., 2004b. Eliminating the effect of epidural fat during dorsolumbar epidural analgesia in cattle. Vet Anaesth Analg 31, 86–89.

Lee, I., Yamagishi, N., Oboshi, K., et al., 2006. Practical tips for modified dorsolumbar epidural anesthesia in cattle. J Vet Sci 7, 69–72.

Lewis, C.A., Constable, P.D., Huhn, J.C., et al., 1999. Sedation with xylazine and lumbosacral epidural administration of lidocaine and xylazine for umbilical surgery in calves. J Am Vet Med Assoc 214, 89–95.

Liebich, H.-G., König, H.E., Maierl, J., 2009. Hindlimbs or pelvic limbs (membra pelvina). In: König, H.-E., Liebich, H.-G. (Eds.), Veterinary Anatomy of Domestic Mammals. Schattauer, New York, pp. 215–276.

Lin, H.-C., Riddell, M.G., 2003. Preliminary study of the effects of xylazine or detomidine with or without butorphanol for standing sedation in dairy cattle. Vet Ther 4, 285–291.

Lin, H.C., Trachte, E.A., DeGraves, F.J., et al., 1998. Evaluation of analgesia induced by epidural administration of medetomidine to cows. Am J Vet Res 59, 162–167.

McGuirk, S.M., Bednarski, R.M., Clayton, M.K., 1990. Bradycardia in cattle deprived of food. J Am Vet Med Assoc 196, 894–896.

Meyer, H., Kästner, S.B.R., Beyerbach, M., et al., 2010. Cardiopulmonary effects of dorsal recumbency and high-volume caudal epidural anaesthesia with lidocaine or xylazine in calves. Vet J 186, 316–322.

Meyer, H., Starke, A., Kehler, W., et al., 2007. High caudal epidural analgesia with local anaesthetics or α_2-agonists in calves. J Vet Med A 54, 384–389.

Misch, L.J., Duffield, T.F., Millman, S.T., et al., 2007. An investigation into the practices of dairy producers and veterinarians in dehorning dairy calves in Ontario. Can Vet J 48, 1249–1254.

Muchado, L.C.P., Hurnik, J.F., Ewing, K.K., 1998. A thermal threshold assay to measure the nociceptive response to morphine sulphate in cattle. Can J Vet Res 62, 218–223.

Offinger, J., Meyer, H., Fischer, J., et al., 2012. Comparison of isoflurane inhalation anaesthesia, injection anaesthesia and high volume caudal epidural anaesthesia for umbilical surgery in calves; metabolic, endocrine and cardiopulmonary effects. Vet Anaesth Analg 39, 123–136.

Pascoe, P.J., 1986. Humaneness of an electroimmobilization unit for cattle. Am J Vet Res 47, 2252–2256.

Picavet, M.-T.J.E., Gasthuys, M.R., Laevens, H.H., et al., 2004. Cardiopulmonary effects of combined xylazine-guaiphenesin-ketamine infusion and extradural (inter-coccygeal lidocaine) anaesthesia in calves. Vet Anaesth Analg 31, 11–19.

Powell, J.D., Denhart, J.W., Lloyd, W.E., 1998. Effectiveness of tolazoline in reversing xylazine-induced sedation in calves. J Am Vet Med Assoc 212, 90–92.

Raekallio, M., Kivalo, M., Jalanka, H., et al., 1991. Medetomidine/ketamine sedation in calves and its reversal with atipamezole. J Vet Anaesth 18, 45–47.

Ranheim, B., Arnemo, J.M., Ryeng, K.A., 1999. A pharmacokinetic study including some relevant clinical effect of medetomidine, and atipamezole in lactating dairy cows. J Vet Pharmacol Ther 22, 368–373.

Ranheim, B., Søli, N.E., Ryeng, K.A., et al., 1998. Pharmacokinetics of medetomidine and atipamezole in dairy calves. J Vet Pharmacol Ther 21, 428–432.

Raptopoulos, D., Weaver, B.M., 1984. Observations following intravenous xylazine administration in steers. Vet Rec 114, 567–569.

Re, M., Blanco-Murcia, F.J., Gómez de Segura, I.A., 2011. Chemical restraint and anaesthetic effects of a tiletamine-zolazepam/ketamine/detomidine combination in cattle. Vet J 190, 66–70.

Reeves, P.T., 2007. Residues of veterinary drugs at injection sites. J Vet Pharmacol Ther 30, 1–17.

Rioja, E., Kerr, C.L., Enouri, S.S., et al., 2008. Sedative and cardiopulmonary effects of medetomidine hydrochloride and xylazine hydrochloride and their reversal with atipamezole hydrochloride in calves. Am J Vet Res 69, 319–329.

Rosenberg, P.H., Veering, B.T., Urmey, W.F., 2004. Maximum recommended doses of local anesthetics: a multifactorial concept. Regional Anesth Pain Med 29, 564–575.

Rumsey, T.S., Bond, J., 1976. Cardiorespiratory patterns, rectal temperature, serum electrolytes and packed cell volume in beef cattle deprived of feed and water. J Anim Sci 42, 1227–1238.

Salonen, J.S., Vähä-Vahe, T., Vainio, O., et al., 1989. Single-dose pharmacokinetics of detomidine in the horse and cow. J Vet Pharmacol Ther 12, 65–72.

Sellers, G., Lin, H.C., Riddell, M.G., et al., 2009. Pharmacokinetics of lidocaine in serum and milk of mature Holstein cows. J Vet Pharmacol Ther 32, 446–450.

Sellers, G., Lin, H.C., Riddell, M.G., et al., 2010. Pharmacokinetics of ketamine in plasma and milk of mature Holstein cows. J Vet Pharmacol Ther 33, 480–484.

Semrad, S.D., Trim, C.M., Hardee, G.E., 1986. Hypertension in bulls and steers anesthetized with guaifenesin-thiobarbiturate-halothane combination. Am J Vet Res 47, 1577–1582.

Stafford, K.J., Mellor, D.J., 2005. Dehorning and disbudding stress and its alleviation in calves. Vet J 169, 337–349.

Stewart, M.C., Stookey, J.M., Stafford, K.J., et al., 2009. Effects of local anaesthetic and a nonsteroidal antiinflammatory drug on pain responses of dairy calves to hot-iron dehorning. J Dairy Sci 92, 1512–1519.

StJean, G., Skarda, R.T., Muir, W.W., et al., 1990. Caudal epidural analgesia induced by xylazine administration in cows. Am J Vet Res 51, 1232–1236.

Thompson, J.R., Kersting, K.W., Hsu, W.H., 1991. Antagonistic effect of atipamezole on xylazine-induced sedation, bradycardia, and ruminal atony. Am J Vet Res 52, 1265–1268.

Thomsen, P.T., Gidekull, M., Herskin, M.S., et al., 2010. Scandanavian bovine practitioners' attitudes to the use of analgesics in cattle. Vet Rec 167, 256–258.

Thurmon, J.C., Lin, H.C., Benson, G.J., et al., 1989. Combining telazol and xylazine for anesthesia in calves. Vet Med 84, 824–830.

Thurmon, J.C., Nelson, D.R., Hartsfield, S.M., et al., 1978. Effects of xylazine hydrochloride on urine in cattle. Aust Vet J 54, 178–180.

Toosey, M.B., 1959. The uses of concentrated pentobarbitone sodium solution in bovine practice. Vet Rec 71, 24–27.

Trim, C.M., 1987. Special anesthesia considerations in the ruminant. In: Short, C.E. (Ed.), Principles & Practice of Veterinary Anesthesia. Williams & Wilkins, Baltimore, pp. 285–300.

Valverde, A., Doherty, T.J., Dyson, D.H., et al., 1989. Evaluation of pentobarbital as a drug for standing sedation in cattle. Vet Surg 18, 235–238.

Vainio, O., 1988. Detomidine (letter to the editor). Vet Rec 123, 655.

Wagner, A.E., Muir, W.W., Grospitch, B.J., 1990. Cardiopulmonary effects of position in conscious cattle. Am J Vet Res 51, 7–10.

Werdehausen, R., Braun, S., Hermanns, H., et al., 2011. The influence of adjuvants used in regional anesthesia on lidocaine-induced neurotoxicity in vitro. Regional Anesth Pain Med 36, 436–443.

Wong, D.H.W., 1993. Regional anaesthesia for intraocular surgery. Can J Anaesth 40, 635–657.

Chapter 13

Anaesthesia of sheep, goats, and other herbivores

sedation and general anaesthesia. Tracheal intubation can be technically difficult, particularly in large rams and goats with large curled horns, because extension of the head and neck may be restricted and because the animals' narrow jaws leave little room to view the larynx during insertion of the endotracheal tube. Two factors should be considered in selection of anaesthetic protocols for these ruminants. First, dose rates of some anaesthetic agents differ from those in other species. Secondly, animals that are not used to being handled or isolated may not exhibit signs commonly associated with sickness or pain. If these animals are sick they will have a reduced requirement for anaesthesia and failure to recognize this may result in overdosage.

This chapter describes techniques and drug combinations that can be used to anaesthetize sheep, goats, and camelids in a variety of settings. Local analgesia is useful in these species and details of the techniques are included. The anaesthetic agents listed in this chapter may not be available in all countries and many are not licensed for use in small ruminants. In some countries, ruminants given unapproved drugs cannot be used for food and, in others, some anaesthetic agents have approved withdrawal times. Current information on approved drugs, withdrawal times and extralabel drug use in North America has recently been published (Fajt, 2011). Choice of agents will also depend on whether the animal is intended for food, its health, procedure to be performed, and where the procedure will be performed (e.g. owner's farm, veterinary clinic, or research facility). Some information on methods of anaesthesia of deer, camels, and elephants has been provided in the latter part of the chapter.

Accidental human injection of potent opioids, such as etorphine or carfentanil, α_2-agonist sedatives, such as xylazine, detomidine and romifidine, and dissociative anaesthetics such as ketamine and tiletamine–zolazepam, can have serious consequences and even result in death (Haymerle et al., 2010). Preventative measures, such as wearing gloves and eye protection, particularly when working with darts, should be routine. Naloxone is the recommended antagonist for etorphine (25 ampoules should be available) and naltrexone is an alternative. Atipamezole is not licensed for use in humans at this time.

Sheep and Goats

INTRODUCTION

Anaesthetic management of sheep and goats is usually uncomplicated with the notable exception that regurgitation followed by pulmonary aspiration is always a risk of

LOCAL ANALGESIA

Local analgesia techniques are highly useful in sheep and goat practice because equipment involved is inexpensive, cardiovascular and respiratory depression are less than produced by general anaesthesia, and the risk of regurgitation and aspiration is decreased. The immediate post-surgical recovery time may or may not be shorter than after general anaesthesia, depending on the agents and techniques used. Local anaesthetic agents may induce toxic symptoms when used inappropriately, especially when an excessive volume of local anaesthetic solution is injected. Limiting the initial administration of lidocaine to less than 6 mg/kg and bupivacaine to less than 2 mg/kg has been found to be safe. Bupivacaine is highly cardiotoxic and must never be injected IV. In Europe, at the time of writing (2012), the only agent with a marketing authorization for ruminants as food animals is procaine. In one investigation testing the effects of six local anaesthetic agents in ewes, cardiovascular toxicity in conscious animals was manifested initially as decreased contractility that was followed by seizures and tachycardia, progressing to ventricular tachycardia and, in some individuals, to cardiovascular collapse and death. Seven out of 36 sheep died after receiving slow IV administration of bupivacaine 2.1 mg/kg, levobupivacaine 2.6 mg/kg or ropivacaine 3.2 mg/kg (Copeland et al., 2008). None of the sheep given lidocaine or mepivacaine, 7.4 mg/kg, died. Anaesthetized sheep given these agents developed profound cardiovascular depression and all survived despite plasma concentrations of local anaesthetic twice that achieved in conscious animals.

Ropivacaine was introduced into the human medical market to offer a safer alternative to bupivacaine as the toxicity is lower (Leone et al., 2008). The toxicity of ropivacaine in herbivores has yet to be determined.

Options to extend the duration of epidural or spinal analgesia include addition of an opioid, such as morphine or buprenorphine, or an α_2-adrenoceptor agonist, such as xylazine or dexmedetomidine. Controlled-release of bupivacaine and dexamethasone from polymer micropheres and liposomes is being investigated for prolonged (days) neural blockade (Dräger et al., 1998).

Applications of local anaesthesia

Cornual nerve blocks for dehorning

The cornual branches of the zygomaticotemporal (lacrimal) and infratrochlear nerves provide sensory innervation to the horns. The cornual branch of the lacrimal nerve emerges from the orbit caudal to the frontal process of the zygomatic bone (root of the supraorbital process). The nerve, covered by a thin layer of muscle, divides into several branches that innervate mainly the lateral and caudal parts of the horn. The main trunk of the infratrochlear nerve emerges from the orbit dorsomedially and divides into several branches. The cornual branch soon divides, one division coursing to the dorsal aspect of the base of the horn and ramifying dorsally and dorsomedially. The other division passes to the medial aspect of the base of the horn and gives off branches to the medial and caudomedial parts of it.

The site for producing block of the cornual branch of the lacrimal nerve is caudal to the frontal process of the zygomatic bone (root of the supraorbital process)

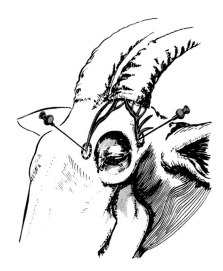

Figure 13.1 Nerve blocks for dehorning of goats. The corneal branches of both the lacrimal and infratrochlear nerves must be blocked. Care must be taken in young animals to ensure attempts to block both nerves do not lead to injection of toxic quantities of local anaesthetic solution.

(Fig. 13.1). The needle should be inserted as close as possible to the caudal ridge of the frontal process of the zygomatic bone to a depth of 1.0–1.5 cm in adult goats. The syringe plunger should be withdrawn before injection to check that the tip of the needle has not penetrated the large blood vessel located at this site. The site for blocking the cornual branch of the infratrochlear nerve is at the dorsomedial margin of the orbit (Fig. 13.1). In some animals, the nerve is palpable by applying thumbnail pressure and moving the skin over this area. The needle should be inserted as close as possible to the margin of the orbit and under the muscle to a depth of about 0.5 cm.

Local analgesic solution such as 2% lidocaine, without epinephrine, should be injected at each site, about 2 mL/site for adult animals or up to a maximum of 6 mg/kg. Care must be taken with young animals not to exceed the toxic dose of lidocaine by limiting the total dose to 4 mg/kg, or inadvertently to inject local anaesthetic intravenously. Cornual nerve blocks are frequently combined with xylazine sedation, such as 0.05 mg/kg for adults and 0.025 mg/kg for kids. A subcutaneous line block with lidocaine may be required on the caudal border of mature horns.

Procaine is marketed in the UK as a 5% solution with epinephrine. In an evaluation of procaine for disbudding 99 dairy goat kids, all kids (median weight 5.3 kg) were injected with a total of 2 mL 5% procaine with epinephrine (12.2–28.6 mg/kg) as subcutaneous horn ring blocks (Pollard, 2008). At least 20 minutes were allowed before start of disbudding and analgesia was satisfactory for the procedure to be performed in the majority of animals. Muscle twitching and lethargy was observed in a few animals after the procedure but the cause was not confirmed.

Alternative analgesic techniques for dehorning include production of light general anaesthesia with diazepam or midazolam and ketamine, or other injectable or inhalation anaesthetic agents. It must be remembered when inhalation anaesthesia is employed, to discontinue oxygen and remove the facemask before application of a hot iron.

Epidural and intrathecal nerve block

High epidural block can be produced by injection of local anaesthetic solution into the epidural space at the lumbosacral junction. Complete analgesia and paralysis can be induced in the hind limbs and abdomen to allow surgery, depending on the volume of local anaesthetic injected (Trim, 1989). The dose rates for different drugs and their times for onset of action are listed in Table 13.1. The dose rates listed are to produce analgesia for flank laparotomy. The dose should be decreased if the animal is old, obese, or pregnant. A lower dose of lidocaine, such as 2% at 1 mL 7 kg, is sufficient for perineal or hind limb surgical procedures, and for caesarian section. The long duration of hind limb paralysis from bupivacaine block for caesarian section interferes with nursing of the newborn and, for that reason, lidocaine with 1:200 000 epinephrine is preferred.

The intention behind inclusion of epinephrine with a local anaesthetic is to increase the intensity of sensory and motor block by decreasing uptake from the epidural space by local vasoconstriction. An added effect would be improved safety because the plasma concentrations of local anaesthetic agent would be lower. Addition of epinephrine has a significant impact on the duration of action of lidocaine, and has been documented to increase uptake of bupivacaine into cerebrospinal fluid (CSF), but has less effect on ropivacaine, presumably because ropivacaine has intrinsic vasoconstrictor properties (Ratajczak-Enselme et al., 2007).

The lumbosacral junction is easy to palpate in thin animals but recognition of landmarks will be necessary to identify the point of needle insertion in muscled or fat animals. Epidural block can be performed with the sheep or goat standing or in lateral recumbency. An imaginary line between the cranial borders of the ilium crosses between the spinous processes of the last lumbar vertebrae (Fig 13.2). The caudal borders of the ilium, where the angle bends to parallel midline, are level with the cranial edge of the sacrum. The point of needle insertion is midline halfway between the spinous process of the seventh lumbar vertebra and the sacrum. If the spinous process of the last lumbar vertebra can be palpated, the next depression caudal to it is the lumbosacral space. This area must be clipped and the skin prepared with a surgical scrub. A spinal needle should be used because it has a stilette to prevent injection of a core of subcutaneous tissue into the epidural space. The notch on the hub of the needle indicates the direction of the bevel and thus the anaesthetist can ensure that injection of local anaesthetic solution is towards the head of the animal.

When epidural nerve block is to be performed on the conscious animal, 1–3 mL 2% lidocaine should be injected subcutaneously with a fine needle at the site intended for insertion of the spinal needle. For lambs, kids, and pygmy goats, a 22 gauge 3.7 cm spinal needle can be used. For adult animals, a sturdier needle, such as a 20 or 18 gauge 6.25 cm spinal needle, is recommended. The needle should be inserted midline perpendicular to the curvature of the hindquarters and perpendicular to the midline sagittal plane of the animal, i.e. not necessarily parallel or perpendicular to the floor or table top (Fig. 13.3). If analgesia of one side or leg is required, the animal should be placed in lateral recumbency with the side to be desensitized underneath for the duration of the injection. Even though bilateral analgesia will develop, hyperbaric solutions such as bupivacaine will travel more cranially on the down side. After injection the spinal needle is withdrawn, the animal should be positioned so that the vertebral column is horizontal. If standing, the goat or sheep should not be allowed to progressively 'dogsit', otherwise analgesia does not fully develop cranially.

Considerable pressure may be needed to introduce the needle through the skin and supraspinous ligament and it may be preferable to puncture the skin first with a larger, sharp hypodermic needle. Once introduced, the spinal needle should be advanced gently for two reasons. First, to be able to appreciate the resistance then penetration of the interarcuate ligament which lies over the epidural space, described as a 'pop', and secondly, to control introduction of the tip of the needle into the epidural space so that movement of the needle can be stopped immediately. Further introduction of the needle will penetrate the spinal cord and the animal, if conscious, will jump and may dislodge the position of the needle. If the tip of the needle strikes bone and the needle does not appear to be

Table 13.1 Epidural analgesia for flank laparotomy in goats

Treatment	Onset (min)	Duration (h)	Standing (h)
Lidocaine 2% with epinephrine, 1 mL/5 kg	25	2	3.5–5.0
Bupivacaine, 0.5% or 0.75%, 1 mL/4 kg	45	4–6	8–12

A lower dose rate, such as 1 mL/7 kg, is sufficient for analgesia of the hind limbs or perineal surgery.

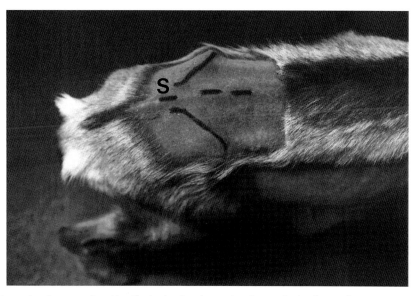

Figure 13.2 Black pen has been used to identify the landmarks used to locate the lumbosacral space in a goat. An imaginary line between the cranial edge of the ilium crosses midline between the spinous processes of the last two lumbar vertebrae. The wings of the ilium angle obliquely towards midline and the sacrum (S).

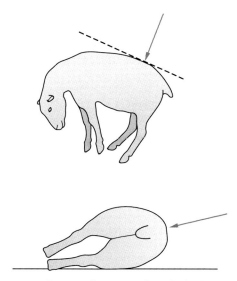

Figure 13.3 Direction of insertion of needle for lumbar epidural injection in sheep in lateral recumbency.

deep enough to be in the epidural space, the needle should be withdrawn until the tip is just under the skin and redirected in a cranial direction. If unsuccessful, the procedure should be repeated with the needle advanced in a caudal direction.

After correct placement of the needle, the stilette should be removed and placed on a sterile surface. A 3 mL syringe

containing a small volume of saline or air (up to 0.5 mL for large sheep/goats) should be attached to the spinal needle and the plunger withdrawn to test for CSF or blood. Attempts at aspiration should reveal only a vacuum and aspiration of air means that the syringe is not tightly attached to the needle. When no CSF or blood is aspirated, a test injection of a small amount of saline or air should be made ('loss of resistance' test). Injection should be easy when the needle is in the epidural space. After confirmation of correct placement of the needle, the 3 mL syringe should be detached and the syringe containing the local anaesthetic solution attached. Injection of the drug should be made over at least 30 seconds. Faster injections result in increased intracranial pressure which, if the animal is conscious, manifests as opisthotonus, nystagmus, and collapse.

Air has been used for many years for the 'loss of resistance' test of placement of a spinal needle in the epidural space. The injected air forms bubbles that interfere with even spread of the local anaesthetic solution, consequently, as small a volume as possible should be used. Use of saline or local anaesthetic solution (being mindful of the total dose injected) instead of air facilitates spread of subsequently injected local anaesthetic solution for nerve block.

A 'hanging drop' technique can be used to locate the epidural space when the animal is standing or positioned in sternal recumbency. The preparation of the skin, landmarks, and insertion of the spinal needle is the same as just described. The spinal needle is advanced until the tip is close to but not penetrating the interarcuate ligament. The stilette is removed and a drop of local anaesthetic solution or saline placed on the hub of the needle. When the needle is advanced through the interarcuate ligament, the drop of liquid will be sucked into the needle. This manoeuvre is used as confirmation of accurate placement of the needle in the epidural space, although failures may occur.

The spinal cord may project into the sacrum in sheep and goats and penetration of the dura will result in aspiration of CSF. Injection into the subarachnoid space of the same volume of local anaesthetic intended for epidural analgesia will result in the block extending further cranially and, potentially, respiratory arrest. Usually, the volume for subarachnoid injection is half the epidural dose. It is fairly common practice after accidental penetration of the subarachnoid space partly to withdraw the spinal needle and redirect it into the epidural space a few millimetres distant from the original insertion. Although initially CSF will leak into the epidural space because of the pressure difference, an experimental study in sheep where dural punctures were made one hour prior to epidural injection of morphine demonstrated that CSF concentrations of morphine were dramatically increased, even when the hole was made with a 25 gauge needle (Swenson et al., 1996). The concern with use of morphine was respiratory depression developing several hours later.

Entry of the needle into a venous sinus should be detected by aspiration of blood, an important manoeuvre as intravenous injection of local anaesthetic agent or morphine will result in cardiovascular depression. The local anaesthetic solution should be warmed when epidural injection is to be made in the conscious animal. Injection of a cold solution will stimulate receptors in the spinal cord and the animal will jerk, possibly dislodging the needle.

Epidural and intrathecal catheters

Catheters can be placed in the epidural or subarachnoid (intrathecal) spaces to facilitate administration of agents for surgical procedures and to continue regional analgesia postoperatively. Spinal catheters are available in a variety of materials and designs. The end of the catheter can be open or it can be closed with lateral holes (eyes) a few millimetres back from the tip. The opposite end can have an attached luer-lok adapter or an adjustable adapter that snaps onto the catheter tubing. Using sterile technique, a Tuohy needle (Fig. 13.4) is inserted at an angle through the skin at the lumbosacral junction until the tip is in the epidural space or advanced deeper to penetrate the meninges, allowing free flow of CSF when the stilette is removed. The catheter is inserted through the needle and advanced approximately 10 cm from the tip of the needle, whereupon the needle is removed carefully without dragging the catheter. An alternative technique is to insert a flexible

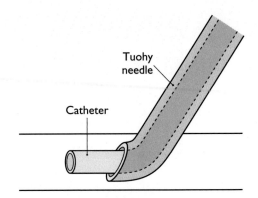

Figure 13.4 Catheter emerging from tip of Tuohy needle. The tip of a Tuohy needle is curved to aid bending of a catheter from the needle into the epidural or subarachnoid space.

guide wire to facilitate advancement of the catheter into the desired space (modified Seldinger technique). The needle is removed and the catheter threaded over the guide wire that is then removed. Extreme care must be taken to secure the catheter to the skin at the site of entry and to ensure sterile injections by covering the skin insertion with bandage and protecting the free catheter end – capped and wrapped in sterile gauze, for example.

Epidural and intrathecal analgesia are not totally without risk. The incidence of complications is probably very low but has not been documented in these species or other large animals (Trim, 2007). Potential complications include spinal haematoma, meningitis, or abscess associated with technique, and pruritus with morphine. Continuous infusions of opioids through intrathecal catheters are frequently used for long-term control of non-cancer pain in humans and there is increasing concern about the development of inflammatory masses adjacent to the tip of the catheters that compress the spinal cord and cause neurological deficits (Yaksh et al., 2002; Follett, 2003; Bedforth & Hardman, 2010). The inflammatory masses that develop in humans commonly do not manifest until after a year of use, however, experimental studies in dogs and sheep have identified inflammation, masses, and functional motor deficits occurring within 28–30 days of continuous infusion of morphine (Coombs et al., 1994; Gradert et al., 2003; Yaksh et al., 2003). The data are confusing at present. Morphine appears to be associated with inflammation, with the degree increasing with increasing dose and concentration and worse with continuous infusion compared with interrupted boluses twice daily. Hydromorphone has been associated with inflammation and, in one study (Johansen et al., 2004), even though inflammation was not greater than caused by saline injections, all the sheep exhibited gait deficits and biting behaviour over the dorsal lumbar area at the site of injection.

Management

Placement of a venous catheter is a sensible precaution when epidural analgesia is to be used for surgery. Epidural injection of local anaesthetic solution causes paralysis of the sympathetic nerves and results in a decrease in blood pressure. Hypotension may develop, especially in hypovolaemic animals, such as for caesarian section, or animals positioned in such a way as to promote pooling of blood in the hind limbs. In these animals, treatment should include expansion of blood volume with intravenous administration of balanced electrolyte solution and injection of ephedrine, 0.06 mg/kg, to induce vasoconstriction. An animal with urethral obstruction given epidural analgesia for perineal urethrostomy or cystotomy may already have a distended urinary bladder at risk for rupture. Nonetheless, administration of fluid intravenously is important to restore blood volume and cardiovascular function. One option is to decrease the size of the bladder by cystocentesis. Alternatively, fluid infusion can begin at the time of epidural administration so that surgical relief of distension can be accomplished before a substantial increase in urine production occurs.

Approximately 50% of human patients experience visceral pain during caesarian section under epidural block with bupivacaine and describe the pain as poorly localized, dull pain, or as a feeling of heaviness or squeezing (Alahuhta et al., 1990). Sheep or goats may respond by movement or vocalization to manipulation of viscera during laparotomy under epidural analgesia with lidocaine or bupivacaine. The animals may be made more comfortable by IV administration of butorphanol, 0.1 mg/kg, diazepam or midazolam, 0.05 mg/kg, or xylazine, 0.02 mg/kg. Disadvantages of adjunct drug administration include respiratory depression, pharyngeal relaxation that may promote regurgitation and pulmonary aspiration, and depression of the lambs or kids delivered by caesarian section.

Sensory block may extend several dermatomes cranial to the level of motor block. Limb movement is possible even when the animal is sufficiently analgesic for surgery. During recovery from epidural block, the ability to move the hind limbs may develop before analgesia is lost, although the ability to stand may not return until long after analgesia is gone.

Respiratory paralysis can occur if local anaesthetic solution travels cranially to the neck. This will occur if too large a volume is injected, e.g. inaccurate calculation of dose. In this event, general anaesthesia must be quickly induced, the trachea intubated and controlled ventilation applied until the animal is able to breathe again.

During recovery from epidural block produced by local anaesthetic solutions, the animal should be allowed to recover quietly. It will be able to maintain sternal recumbency but there is potential for injury to the hind limbs if it makes uncoordinated attempts to rise.

Epidural and intrathecal opioids

Epidural injection of morphine, 0.1 mg/kg, at the lumbosacral junction will produce analgesia without paralysis. Preservative-free solution, 1 mg/mL, will not cause irritation of the meninges. This technique can be used to decrease requirement for inhalation anaesthetic agent and to provide analgesia postoperatively. In one study in goats after stifle surgery, it was observed that goats that were given epidural morphine vocalized less and were less likely to grind their teeth than goats that were not (Pablo, 1993). The duration of pain relief appears to be variable but provided relief for 6 hours after abdominal surgery (Hendrickson et al., 1996).

Intrathecal injection of 2% lidocaine, 2 mg/kg, with buprenorphine, 0.005 mg/kg, in tranquillized adult goats provided sufficient analgesia to perform a 30-minute orthopaedic stifle surgery, and duration of analgesia lasted longer postoperatively than in a comparison group of goats given lidocaine with xylazine, 0.05 mg/kg (Staffieri et al., 2009). The time from subarachnoid injection to start of surgery was on average 13 minutes and the goats were standing in approximately 90–100 minutes. Analgesia lasted for 3 hours after lidocaine–buprenorphine and 2 hours after lidocaine–xylazine, with a waning effect over 24 hours.

Epidural and intrathecal xylazine and dexmedetomidine

Xylazine has been used for epidural or intrathecal analgesia at dose rates ranging from 0.05 to 0.2 mg/kg or higher. Xylazine, 0.05 mg/kg, diluted with saline to 0.1 mL/kg or added to other agents, may be used for epidural analgesia as an adjunct to general anaesthesia for surgery. Systemic effects of sedation and decreased gastrointestinal motility may accompany epidural administration of xylazine in ruminants. A higher dose of xylazine, 0.4 mg/kg, has been injected at the lumbosacral junction of rams to produce analgesia for surgery involving lateral deviation of the penis (Aminkov & Hubenov, 1995). Analgesia extended to T5–T6 within 10 minutes and lasted for 120–140 minutes. Signs of systemic absorption were observed and hind limb motor block lasted an average of 224 minutes. In cattle, administration of atipamezole, 0.025 mg/kg, reversed sedation and flank analgesia after epidural block from xylazine, 0.05 mg/kg, but only epidural administration of atipamezole reversed the ataxia (Lee et al., 2003).

An investigation of epidural and intrathecal administrations of dexmedetomidine, approximate dose 0.0025 mg/kg, in sheep identified the potency of dexmedetomidine in the epidural space to be 10-fold higher than when administered in the intrathecal space (Eisenach et al., 1994). Both routes of administration resulted in rapid decreases in arterial pressure and the mechanism proposed was a direct effect on the spinal cord decreasing sympathetic nervous system outflow.

Caudal epidural nerve block

Injection of 2 (1–4) mL (0.5 mg/kg) of 2% lidocaine solution into the epidural canal through the sacrococcygeal space will provide caudal epidural analgesia for obstetrical procedures involving the vagina, vulva, and perineum. Xylazine, 0.07 mg/kg, may be added to the lidocaine for a prolonged effect up to 36 hours that would be useful in the treatment of vaginal prolapse after lambing (Scott, 1996). A smaller volume of local anaesthetic, 0.75–1.0 mL of 1% lidocaine, will provide analgesia for the docking of lamb's tails. Strict attention must be paid to aseptic technique to avoid complications and several minutes must be allowed for analgesia to develop.

Frequently, the procedure is performed with the animal restrained in a standing position. The wool must be clipped from over the sacrum and the base of the tail and a surgical scrub applied to the skin. The site for needle placement is located by moving the tail up and down and palpating the most cranial point of articulation. A 20 gauge hypodermic needle is inserted midline approximately at a 45° angle to the curvature of the rump so that the tip of the needle enters the vertebral column and may even thread for a few millimetres cranially.

Continuous caudal block can be achieved by placement of an epidural catheter as described in the previous section. Local analgesic solution is injected through the catheter whenever the animal shows signs of returning sensation. Precautions against complications have already been described.

Paravertebral nerve block

In sheep and goats, lumbar paravertebral nerve block is carried out using techniques similar to those employed in cattle. For incisions through the flank, the thirteenth thoracic and first three lumbar nerves are blocked. For each of these nerves, up to 5 mL of 1 or 2% lidocaine is used, divided and injected using a 20 gauge needle above and below the transverse ligament, up to a maximum total dose of 6 mg/kg lidocaine. Onset of analgesia may be as fast as 5 minutes. Duration of analgesia is an hour, or longer when lidocaine with epinephrine is used.

Inverted L block

Flank laparotomy can be performed using local infiltration of lidocaine in an inverted L pattern 2–3 cm cranial and dorsal to the intended skin incision site. Blebs of lidocaine must be injected subcutaneously and deep in the abdominal muscle at approximately 1–1.5 cm intervals along the injection site. The maximum dose of lidocaine to be injected at one time is 6 mg/kg and dilution of a 2% solution to 1% solution may be necessary to provide sufficient volume for injection. The duration of analgesia is about 1.5 hours.

Forelimb digital nerve blocks

Digital nerves are easily blocked with lidocaine at the sites described for cattle. For total analgesia of the metacarpus and digits, lidocaine or lidocaine plus bupivacaine can be infiltrated subcutaneously circumferentially at the carpal–metacarpal junction. Analgesia lasting over 12 hours can be achieved by infiltration of 80% of a combination of lidocaine, 1 mg/kg, and bupivacaine, 0.5 mg/kg, mixed well in the same syringe.

Femoral and sciatic nerve blocks

Recent publications have described use of femoral and sciatic nerve blocks as adjunct analgesic techniques to general anaesthesia in sheep and goats (Adami et al., 2011; Wagner et al., 2011). The nerves were located by insertion of a 22 gauge nerve locator using a pulse width 0.5 ms, frequency 1–2 Hz, and an initial current of 2.0 mA. The sites for needle insertion are first clipped and cleaned with a presurgical preparation. With the animal in lateral recumbency with the surgical leg uppermost, the landmarks for the sciatic nerve are the greater trochanter of the femur and the ischiatic tuberosity. The needle is inserted on an imaginary line between these points at one-third of the distance from the greater trochanter and with the needle at a 60° angle to the skin with the tip of the needle directed towards the greater trochanter. Nerve location is identified when contraction of the quadriceps and extension of the hip and tarsus are observed when the current is reduced to <1.0 mA (generally 0.5 mA).

The femoral nerve is located in the area of the proximal medial thigh. This site can be accessed by abducting the surgical leg 90% and extending it or by turning the animal over into the opposite recumbency. The femoral artery is palpated as proximally as possible and the nerve locator needle inserted cranial to the artery and perpendicular to the skin. Contractions of the quadriceps and extension of the stifle at a current of 0.5 mA identifies the site for injection of bupivacaine.

Bupivacaine (0.5% or 0.75% solution) was injected at 0.5 mg/kg per site. The nerve blocks improved analgesia during surgery (mean anaesthesia time 70–85 minutes), however, the benefit postoperatively was limited to the first 24 hours in one study (Adami et al., 2011) and provided no clear benefit in the other (Wagner et al., 2011). Motor blockade of the limb was present during recovery from anaesthesia, lasting less than 4 hours in the sheep (Wagner et al., 2011) and for longer in the goats in which anxiety and abnormal behaviour were observed (Adami et al., 2011).

Peroneal and tibial nerve blocks

Analgesia of the hind limb below the hock can be achieved by peroneal and tibial nerve blocks. The peroneal nerve is blocked by injection of 5 mL 2% lidocaine (in adult sheep

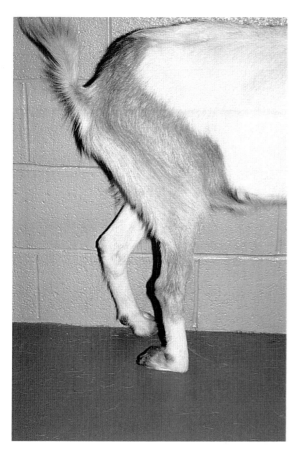

Figure 13.5 Peroneal and tibial nerve blocks produce analgesia distal to the hock. The hock will straighten and the animal will stand on the dorsum of the fetlock.

or goats) where the nerve runs obliquely caudodorsally to cranioventrally approximately 2.5 cm below the lateral condyle of the tibia. The nerve can often be palpated by using thumbnail pressure to move the skin and underlying tissues. Analgesia of the dorsum of the foot is obvious from the animal's stance (Fig. 13.5).

The tibial nerve is blocked by infiltration of 4 mL of 2% lidocaine solution on the medial side of the leg at the hock between the flexor tendons and the gastrocnemius tendon. A further 1 mL is injected at a similar site on the lateral side of the limb to block a small cutaneous nerve, a branch of the common peroneal nerve originating at the middle of the thigh. Onset of analgesia should be within 15 minutes and is accompanied by straightening of the hock (see Fig. 13.5).

Intravenous regional analgesia

Surgery on the limbs can be performed using intravenous regional analgesia (also known as a Bier block). In sheep

and goats, the tourniquet or sphygmomanometer cuff is usually placed on the forelimb above the elbow (taking care not to pinch skin in the axilla) and on the hind limb above the hock (leaving sufficient length of saphenous vein for injection) (Fig. 13.6). The tourniquet must be sufficiently tight to block arterial flow without being excessively tight. The animal is less likely to react adversely to a flat band tourniquet than a round rubber tube. If using a sphygmomanometer cuff, it must be inflated to above systolic blood pressure. Injection of 4 mg/kg lidocaine without epinephrine should be made slowly through a 25 gauge needle in the cephalic or saphenous vein directed towards the foot. Care must be taken to keep the needle immobile within the vein during injection. Blood should be aspirated before injection to confirm needle placement within the vein. Onset of action is in 15–20 minutes. Analgesia will persist as long as the tourniquet is in place but sensation will rapidly return after the tourniquet is removed. The tourniquet should not be released within 10 minutes of the initial injection to allow time for the lidocaine to diffuse into tissues. Thereafter, releasing the tourniquet has no clinical effect on the animal. No long lasting effect has been noted in sheep or goats when the tourniquet has been in place for 2 hours.

Intra-articular local analgesia

The efficacy of intra-articular injection of local anaesthetic solution will depend on the nature of the surgery (because analgesia is limited to intra-articular structures) and the timing of administration. Intra-articular injection of lidocaine, 40 mg, before arthrotomy in adult sheep and another injection of bupivacaine, 10 mg, after joint closure were associated with significantly lower pain scores 3 to 7 hours postoperatively compared with sheep not receiving intra-articular analgesia (Shafford et al., 2004). Intra-articular injection of 0.75 mg/kg of bupivacaine in anaesthetized goats 30 minutes before the start of surgery significantly modified the increases in heart rates and mean arterial pressure (MAP) that occurred in response to stifle manipulation compared with animals injected with saline (Krohm et al., 2011). However, the level of analgesia provided by either pre- or post-surgical injection of bupivacaine was considered insufficient to eliminate the need for systemic analgesia. In experimental animals, 0.5% bupivacaine was found to inhibit synthesis of articular cartilage and cause inflammation whereas exposure to 0.125% bupivacaine was indistinguishable from saline (Webb & Ghosh, 2009). Lesser effects were produced by lidocaine and ropivacaine. Chondrolysis is an uncommon condition in humans that appears to develop after continuous administration of bupivacaine using a 'pain pump' and not from a single injection. The potential for occurrence and significance in other species is yet to be determined.

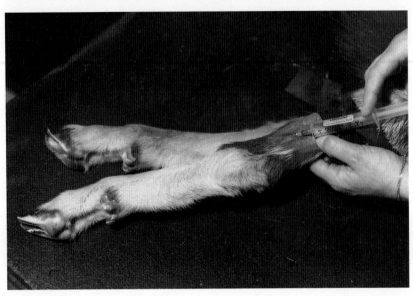

Figure 13.6 Intravenous regional analgesia in the hind limb of a goat. A tourniquet is tied around the limb proximal to the intravenous injection of lidocaine.

Infiltration and topical analgesia

There has been considerable published research on analgesia in sheep for castration, tail docking, and mulesing (surgical removal of folds of perineal skin to minimize risk of fly strike). Analgesia may not be required in some countries for castration of very young ruminants. However, one study measuring EEG in lambs anaesthetized with halothane only for rubber-ring castration, identified a relatively low responsiveness of the cerebral cortex in the first few days of life with a progressive increase over the first 10 days of life (Johnson et al., 2009). The supposition was that this would represent the change in response to a noxious stimulus perceived at different ages. Behaviour changes in 5-, 21-, and 42-day-old lambs after castration and increases in plasma cortisol concentrations are all indicative of considerable pain after castration in the absence of analgesia (Molony et al., 1993). Considerable effort has been expended in the investigation of effective and practical analgesia for mulesing (Paull et al., 2007, Colditz et al., 2009). While not yet defined, significant reduction in indicators of pain associated with mulesing has been produced by use of topical local anaesthetic and injectable carprofen.

Peribulbar injection of lidocaine, approximately 1 mg/kg, or bupivacaine, approximately 0.25 mg/kg, is a useful adjunct to general anaesthesia for eye enucleation. The artery at the medial canthus is easy to lacerate, therefore, insertion of the needle at the lateral canthus and mid-dorsal and ventral edges of the orbit is preferred, and the total volume of local anaesthetic divided between the three sites. Injection is made with a 22 gauge spinal needle

(needle point is less sharp than a hypodermic needle) bent to form a mild curvature to mimic the curvature of the globe within the orbit. It is important to deposit local anaesthetic between the orbit and extraocular muscles and to avoid penetration of the globe. Thus, the needle is inserted adjacent to the edge of the orbit and directed in a curve close to the bone until the tip is deep within the orbit. The syringe must be aspirated before injection to ensure that the needle is not in a blood vessel. The needle should be removed with the same curving action used for insertion, i.e. not in a straight line.

SEDATION

Sedative agents employed in sheep and goats

Different sedatives and sedative opioid combinations, and even low doses of anaesthetic agents such as ketamine, can be chosen to provide the desired characteristics for sedation in a particular situation. Dose rates are listed in Table 13.2. Descriptions and dose rates of drug combinations are in the text.

Acepromazine

Acepromazine, 0.05–0.1 mg/kg, can be used to provide mild tranquilization in sheep and goats. Since acepromazine induces vasodilation, this agent should be used cautiously in animals that are dehydrated or hypovolaemic.

Table 13.2 Anaesthetic agent dose rates for sheep and goats*

Drug	Dose rate	Route	Effect
Acepromazine	0.02–0.1 mg/kg	IM, IV	Tranquillization
Buprenorphine	0.01–0.02 mg/kg	IM	Analgesia
Butorphanol	0.05–0.2 mg/kg	IM, IV	Analgesia
Diazepam	0.1–0.3 mg/kg	IV	Sedation
Fentanyl patch	2 µg/kg	Transdermal	Analgesia
Methadone	0.05–0.2 mg/kg	IM, IV	Analgesia
Midazolam	0.1–0.3 mg/kg	IM, IV	Sedation
Morphine	0.2–0.5 mg/kg	IM	Analgesia
Xylazine	0.02–0.2 mg/kg	IV lower dose, IM larger dose	Sedation
Diazepam or midazolam + ketamine	0.25 mg/kg 5 mg/kg	IV	Induction of general anaesthesia
Xylazine + ketamine or ketamine	0.1 (–0.2) mg/kg 3–5 mg/kg 10 mg/kg	IM IV IM	Premedication and induction of general anaesthesia
Propofol	2–6 mg/kg	IV	Induction of general anaesthesia
Thiopental	5–20 mg/kg	IV	Induction of general anaesthesia
Tiletamine + zolazepam	2–12 mg/kg	IV	Induction of general anaesthesia
Pentobarbital	15–25 mg/kg	IV slowly	Induction of general anaesthesia

Preanaesthetic medication decreases the dose rate of induction and maintenance agents, calms the animal for induction, and provides a more stable anaesthesia.

*Taylor (1998), Abu Serriah et al. (2007), Schauvliege et al. (2006), Ahern et al. (2009), Raske et al. (2010), Krohm et al. (2011), Wagner et al. (2011)

α₂-Agonists

Xylazine, detomidine, medetomidine, dexmedetomidine, or romifidine provide light to heavy sedation according to the drug, dose rate, and route of administration. The dose ranges are different than used in some other species because ruminants are more sensitive to these agents. Variation in the analgesic effects of xylazine has been noted in different breeds of sheep, for example, analgesia after xylazine was less in Welsh mountain sheep than in Clun sheep (Ley et al., 1990). The authors hypothesized that the difference may have been the result of dosing according to body weight rather than body surface area, but other factors such as different body compositions or temperament may have been involved. Animals that are young or sick will require only a low dose to induce sedation. The degree of sedation obtained from an α₂-agonist sedative can be intensified by combination with a benzodiazepine or an opioid or ketamine. α₂-Agonists can be used alone or in combination to provide satisfactory sedation for restraint or they can be used for premedication prior to induction of anaesthesia with other anaesthetic agents.

This group of sedatives induces marked physiological changes. A comparison of IV administration of xylazine, 0.15 mg/kg, detomidine, 0.03 mg/kg, medetomidine, 0.01 mg/kg, and romifidine, 0.05 mg/kg, to sheep maintained in an upright position indicated that all drugs caused a significant decrease in PaO_2 (hypoxaemia) for 45 minutes that outlasted the duration of sedation, despite increased respiratory rates with no significant alteration in $PaCO_2$ (Celly et al., 1997). Thus, hypoxaemia could not be attributed to hypoventilation or to a change in body position. Route of administration may influence pharmacological effects (IM less than IV) as medetomidine, 0.015 mg/kg, injected IV in sheep resulted in respiratory depression and hypoxaemia (Raekallio et al., 1998) whereas medetomidine, 0.03 mg/kg, administered IM induced a significant decrease in PaO_2 but hypoxaemia in only one out of nine sheep (Kästner et al., 2003). The duration of sedation was longer after IM administration, with peak sedation occurring at 30–40 minutes and the time to return of normal behaviour exceeded 6 hours. Investigations of the pulmonary changes induced by xylazine or dexmedetomidine describe diffuse hyperaemia, severe pulmonary capillary congestion progressing to extravasation of red blood cells into alveoli and moderate to severe proteinaceous alveolar oedema at 10 minutes after IV administration (Celly et al., 1999; Kästner et al., 2007). One study design incriminated a hydrostatic cause of the pulmonary oedema associated with a two- to three-fold increase in pulmonary artery pressure (Kästner et al., 2007). Xylazine administration has occasionally been associated with the development of clinical signs of pulmonary oedema in sheep.

Xylazine induces a short-lived decrease in heart rate and a mild decrease in MAP. Detomidine, medetomidine and romifidine induce significant bradycardia with a transient (10 minutes) increase in MAP (Celly et al., 1997). Comparison of the effects of dexmedetomidine, 2 μg/kg, administered IV in sevoflurane-anaesthetized sheep and goats revealed similar changes although there was considerable variation between individual animals in haemodynamic response (Kutter et al., 2006). Cardiac output and heart rate significantly decreased, MAP and systemic vascular resistance (SVR) initially increased followed by a decrease, and MAP and central venous pressure (CVP) increased. Heart rates decreased and CVP increased more in goats than in sheep. Thus, differences in pharmacological effect between individuals are unpredictable and there may be a variation in response between anaesthetized and conscious animals. No doubt the impact of these cardiovascular changes will depend on the dose rate of the agent, concurrent administration of other anaesthetics, and the physical status of the patient. The use and adverse effects of α₂-agonists in sheep have been reviewed (Kästner, 2006).

α₂-Agonist sedatives cause decreased intestinal motility and frequently result in ruminal bloat. Urine production is increased and care must be taken when administering these agents to animals with urethral obstruction. Xylazine is not recommended for use in the last trimester of pregnancy to avoid increasing contractility of the myometrium. Blood glucose increases after administration but to a lesser extent than in cattle.

Antagonists of the effects of α₂-sedatives include tolazoline, up to 2 mg/kg, or doxapram, 0.5 mg/kg, for xylazine, and atipamezole, 25–50 μg/kg, for all the agents. The antagonists can be administered IV (slowly in increments), IM, or half IV and half IM.

Benzodiazepines

Intravenous administration of diazepam, 0.10–0.25 mg/kg, or midazolam, 0.10–0.25 mg/kg, may produce some sedation, ataxia, and analgesia in sheep and goats for 15–30 minutes. The degree of sedation is unpredictable in healthy animals and, in some animals, these agents may induce excitement (Kyles et al., 1995; Raekallio et al., 1998). Midazolam IV or IM and diazepam IV will significantly increase the intensity of sedation when combined with another sedative or opioid. Respiratory depression will be increased and, when combined with medetomidine, haemoglobin O₂ desaturation will be worse (Raekallio et al., 1998). The combination of midazolam, 0.25 mg/kg, and butorphanol, 0.1 mg/kg, IM provides good sedation in sheep for minor procedures such as radiography or cast removal.

Diazepam has been incriminated in the development of pulmonary oedema in a sheep (Stegmann, 2000). A 150% increase in pulmonary vascular resistance was measured in experimental sheep 3 minutes after IV injection of diazepam (Pearl & Rice, 1989). The pulmonary vascular changes have been attributed to propylene glycol induced release of thromboxane A₂ (Quinn et al., 1990).

Flumazenil, 0.01–0.02 mg/kg, can be used to attenuate or reverse sedation and analgesia induced by benzodiazepines (Kyles et al., 1995). Sarmazenil is an antagonist of diazepam and midazolam available in Europe.

Dissociative anaesthetics

A combination of diazepam, 0.25 mg/kg, and ketamine, 5 mg/kg, can be mixed in the same syringe and administered IV in small increments to achieve the desired level of sedation for minor procedures.

Opioids and analgesia

Butorphanol, 0.05–0.20 mg/kg, IM or IV is useful to increase sedation from acepromazine, α₂-agonists, or benzodiazepines. Butorphanol has a rapid onset of action and given 5–10 minutes before diazepam or midazolam and ketamine facilitates a smooth and relaxed induction of anaesthesia. The duration of effect appears to be 1–2 hours. The analgesic effects of butorphanol are not great and vary with the type of stimulus. For example, butorphanol is considered to provide unsatisfactory analgesia for orthopaedic surgery.

A variety of opioids have been administered to sheep and goats to provide analgesia. Meperidine (pethidine), 2–4 mg/kg, IM has been used for many years as an adjunct to anaesthesia in sheep and goats. Methadone, 0.05–0.5 mg/kg, in combination with midazolam, 0.3 mg/kg, IM or IV has been used for premedication to general anaesthesia in sheep and goats (Schauvliege et al., 2006, Adami et al., 2011; Krohm et al., 2011). Morphine is commonly administered at a rate of 0.2–0.5 mg/kg (Wagner et al., 2011). A higher dose of morphine, 2 mg/kg, IV during anaesthesia in experimental goats decreased the isoflurane requirement for claw clamping by 30%, however, the cardiovascular effects were not reported (Doherty et al., 2004).

The value of buprenorphine as an analgesic agent in small ruminants is in question. Clinical experience has shown that, in healthy sheep and goats, buprenorphine, 0.01 mg/kg, IM administered as a premedication agent before induction of anaesthesia appears to cause no sedation and minimal reduction in the isoflurane concentration required to prevent response to a surgical procedure. In contrast, administration of buprenorphine, 0.01 mg/kg, postoperatively appears to alleviate pain as judged by behaviour change, such as muscle relaxation, cessation of teeth grinding, and reversal of increased respiratory and heart rates. Buprenorphine is better given by the IM rather than IV route when administered alone as premedication in healthy animals because IV administration may induce excitement or restlessness. Despite pharmacokinetic studies that have shown that the terminal half-life of buprenorphine in goats and sheep is shorter than in cats and much shorter than in dogs (Ingvast-Larsson et al., 2007), buprenorphine, 0.01 mg/kg, IM is typically administered 45 minutes before anaesthesia and subsequently at 3–6 hour intervals. Buprenorphine given alone to healthy animals may induce agitation, however, tolerance develops after the first injection such that the animals are calmer after the second and subsequent injections (Ingvast-Larsson et al., 2007).

Experimental tests for analgesia are difficult to translate to clinical practice. No antinociceptive activity was detected for approximately 45 minutes in sheep following IV administration of buprenorphine, 0.006 mg/kg (Waterman et al., 1991). Buprenorphine, 0.0015 mg/kg, provided analgesia to the thermal threshold test for 3.5 h but neither this dose nor 0.012 mg/kg produced analgesia to a mechanical threshold test. Pharmacokinetic data confirmed that the drug was rapidly distributed in the body and that there was no correlation between plasma concentration and analgesic activity. In these animals, IV injection of buprenorphine produced excitement exhibited by rapid head movements and the sheep chewing on objects. In another study (Grant et al., 1996), sheep were tested with an electrical current and no analgesia was detected after administration of buprenorphine, 0.005 mg/kg, methadone, 0.6 mg/kg, or flunixin meglumine, 2.2 mg/kg, IM. Analgesia was detected after administration of xylazine, 0.05–0.2 mg/kg, in a dose-dependent manner using the same testing device. Another investigation in sheep compared fentanyl, 2 µg/kg/h applied as transdermal patches 12 hours before anaesthesia with buprenorphine, 0.01 mg/kg, administered at induction and IM every 6 hours to sheep undergoing tibial osteotomy (Ahern et al., 2009). There were no significant differences between the induction doses of thiopental and lidocaine or the isoflurane vaporizer percentages used. The postoperative pain scores for sheep receiving fentanyl were significantly lower than those of sheep receiving buprenorphine, but the scores gave no indication that rescue analgesia was required.

Etorphine and carfentanil are potent opioids that generally are used for immobilization of non-domestic animals.

A study comparing IM administered etorphine or carfentanil, 10, 20, and 40 µg/kg of body weight, in instrumented goats described similar effects for both drugs (Heard et al., 1996). The goats were rapidly immobilized, more quickly with carfentanil (≤ 5 minutes) than with etorphine (5–10 minutes) and etorphine always induced transient struggling. Immobilization was characterized by limb and neck hyperextension with occasional vocalization and bruxation. The goats were partially recovered by an hour after etorphine administration but were unable to stand at 2 hours after carfentanil. Both drugs significantly increased blood pressure and decreased heart rates without changing cardiac outputs. Arterial O_2 content was not decreased and the goats did not regurgitate.

GENERAL ANAESTHESIA

Preparation

Withholding food and water from small ruminants before anaesthesia is not a universal practice. However, many prefer to withhold food for 24 hours and water for 0–12 hours before anaesthesia whenever possible to decrease pressure of the rumen on the diaphragm and aid ventilation, to decrease the severity of bloat, and to decrease the prevalence and volume of regurgitation. Lambs and kids should be prevented from nursing for 30–60 minutes before anaesthesia. When heavy sedation or general anaesthesia is to be administered to an unfasted ruminant, rapid-sequence induction of anaesthesia and intubation of the trachea should be performed.

It is doubtful if atropine has any value as a general premedicant in sheep and goats. The doses necessary to prevent salivation completely (0.2–0.8 mg/kg) produce undesirable tachycardia and ocular effects, while smaller doses merely make the saliva more viscid and hence more difficult to drain from the oropharynx. Furthermore, atropine may decrease intestinal motility in ruminants for hours or days, predisposing them to bloat and delaying return to eating. Bradycardia seldom develops during anaesthesia, except when an α_2-adrenoceptor agonist sedative has been administered. Severe bradycardia can be treated by administration of atropine, 0.02 mg/kg, or glycopyrrolate, 0.005 mg/kg, IV. These dose rates may be inadequate and repeat doses may be required depending on the cause of bradycardia. Atropine up to 0.3 mg/kg has been used to treat bradycardia in sheep sedated with medetomidine (Clarke, personal communication).

Premedication is not essential before induction of general anaesthesia with injectable agents in small ruminants, as excitement at induction is uncommon. However, premedication with an opioid and sedative, either before or at the time of induction of anaesthesia provides muscle relaxation and analgesia, and decreases the dose rate of subsequently administered anaesthetic agents. Administration of an opioid, such as butorphanol, 0.05–0.20 mg/kg, IM or IV or buprenorphine, 0.01 mg/kg, IM will improve muscle relaxation and provide some analgesia. Other opioids, as previously described, may be selected to provide analgesia depending on the procedure to be performed.

Anaesthetic techniques

Intravenous injection

There are many sites available for venepuncture in sheep and goats and the choice depends on the site of the surgical procedure and the personal preference of the anaesthetist. The jugular vein is a common site for placement of a catheter. Adult sheep and goats are restrained standing with their heads bent away from the side of catheter insertion. Smaller animals can be restrained in lateral recumbency. The wool or hair must be clipped and surgical preparation of the skin performed before insertion of a catheter. A subcutaneous bleb of lidocaine at the site of catheter insertion will decrease the likelihood of the animal moving in response to the procedure. The vein should be occluded at the base of the neck, and the catheter (18 or 14 gauge, 7.6–13.3 cm long for mature animals) inserted into the jugular vein directed towards the heart. The catheter should be capped, flushed with heparinized saline, and sutured securely to the skin.

The cephalic vein in the forelimb and the saphenous vein in the hind limb are easily viewed after the wool or hair over them has been clipped. It should be noted that the cephalic vein is more oblique on the limb than in the dog (Fig. 13.7). Sheep can be effectively restrained by lifting them into a sitting upright position (Fig. 13.8). The sheep can be tilted slightly to one side to facilitate access to the saphenous vein and the position conveniently extends the hind limb for catheter placement. Goats are better placed in sternal or lateral recumbency for venepuncture of the cephalic or saphenous veins. A catheter (18 gauge, 5 cm long) can be inserted into either vein, capped, flushed, and secured to the leg with adhesive tape around the catheter and around the leg. A Butterfly needle (21 or 19 gauge) can be used in the cephalic vein.

The ear veins are easily observed after the hair is clipped, especially in goats, and can also be used for intravenous injection.

Endotracheal intubation

After induction of anaesthesia, the sheep or goat should be held in a sternal, head up position until the trachea is intubated and the endotracheal tube cuff inflated to minimize the likelihood of regurgitation and aspiration. If regurgitation occurs during induction of anaesthesia, the animal should be turned into lateral recumbency and the

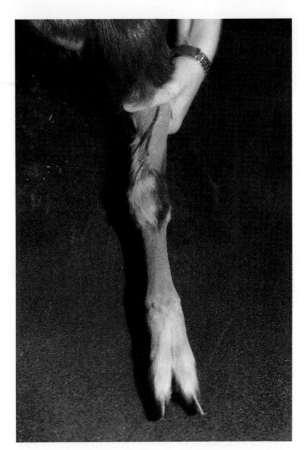

Figure 13.7 The cephalic vein in a goat is short and oblique across the forearm (black pen has been used to identify the location on the left cephalic vein in this animal).

head lowered to allow drainage. Regurgitated rumen material should be quickly scooped out of the mouth before tracheal intubation is attempted.

Endotracheal intubation is best performed under direct vision with the aid of a laryngoscope. Full extension of the head and neck is essential to place the pharynx and trachea in a straight line (Fig. 13.9). Strips of gauze around the upper and lower jaws may be used to hold them open and keep the assistant's fingers out of the anaesthetist's view. The assistant holds the tongue in a gauze square for better grip and draws it out of the mouth through the interdental space. Opening the jaws as widely as possible makes an enormous difference to the ease of insertion of the endotracheal tube into the larynx and trachea. Endotracheal tubes with 11–12 mm internal diameter (ID) are used for many adult sheep and goats, with sizes larger or smaller depending on the breed. A metal or plastic covered stilette inside the endotracheal tube may be used to stiffen it and provide more control over the tip of the tube. The curved shape of 9 mm and 10 mm ID endotracheal tubes commonly used in dogs facilitates insertion into the larynx of smaller animals. A thin film of lubricating jelly should be applied over the cuff of the tube to improve the seal between the tracheal mucosa and cuff after inflation. The laryngoscope blade should be used to depress the dorsum of the tongue and the tip of the blade must be positioned at the base of the tongue and ventral to the epiglottis. Downward pressure on the length of the blade will expose the laryngeal entrance. Care must be taken to avoid damage to the incisor teeth. The tip of the endotracheal tube is placed on the epiglottis and used to flatten it against the tongue before the tube is advanced into the larynx and trachea. Slight resistance may be felt as the tube passes by the vocal cords. A length of gauze, or other type of tie, is tied tightly around the tube behind the incisors and then secured around the back of the head behind the ears, or around the bottom jaw. The cuff is inflated to produce an airtight seal within the trachea when the lungs are inflated to 25–30 cmH$_2$O.

An alternative method of intubation involves inserting a half-metre blunt-ended, thin metal or plastic rod into the trachea under direct vision, removing the laryngoscope, then feeding the endotracheal tube over the rod into the larynx and trachea, whereupon the rod is withdrawn. The tube may have to be rotated 360° as it enters the pharynx in order for the tip to pass over the epiglottis and enter the larynx. Utilizing another method, some anaesthetists are able to pass the endotracheal tube into the trachea blindly. The endotracheal tube (which must have a good curvature to it) is introduced into the mouth

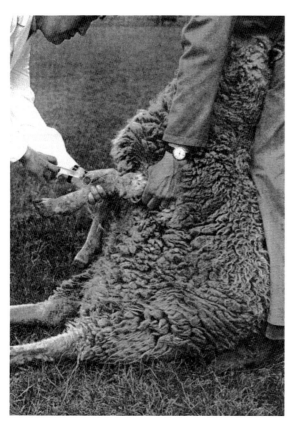

Figure 13.8 Restraint of a sheep for injection into the cephalic vein (or saphenous vein).

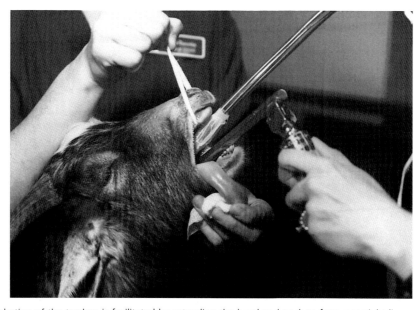

Figure 13.9 Intubation of the trachea is facilitated by extending the head and neck to form a straight line and use of a laryngoscope to view the laryngeal opening. Note that traction on the tongue must not be used to depress the lower jaw.

with one hand and the tip fed into the larynx, which is gripped externally by the anaesthetist's other hand.

Tubes lubricated with an analgesic jelly may also be passed through the nostril. The ventral nasal meatus is relatively large in sheep and goats and, although tubes passed via the nostril must be smaller than those passed through the mouth, reasonably adequately sized ones can be used. If the tube passed up the nostril cannot be passed blindly into the larynx, a laryngoscope is used to view the tip of the tube in the pharynx. The tip of the tube is grasped with forceps and assisted into the laryngeal opening as the tube is advanced through the nostril.

Injectable anaesthetic agents

Major surgery and prolonged diagnostic procedures in sheep and goats are usually performed under inhalation anaesthesia using injectable agents for induction of anaesthesia to facilitate endotracheal intubation. The greatest disadvantage to the use of injectable agents for maintenance of anaesthesia is the high likelihood of hypoxaemia developing. Further, with the exception of propofol, extending anaesthesia time beyond 30 minutes with thiopental or ketamine is often accompanied by prolonged recovery. Thus, total intravenous anaesthesia in sheep and goats most commonly involves a continuous infusion of propofol with endotracheal intubation and the animal breathing oxygen. Preanaesthetic agents including an α_2-agonist sedative or an opioid are commonly included but they also contribute to greater respiratory depression. Administration of oxygen and endotracheal intubation, where appropriate, are sensible precautions during anaesthesia induced by any agent combination.

Each injectable agent has a range of effective dose rates (see Table 13.2). Most commonly, the dose rate must be decreased when drugs administered for premedication result in moderate to severe sedation. Similarly, the dose rates must be decreased, even by 50–70%, in animals with significant disease such as urethral obstruction and azotaemia. Neonatal animals have a decreased requirement for anaesthetic agents compared with adult animals as a result of increased blood–brain permeability, decreased plasma protein binding, and decreased efficiency of drug elimination.

Alfaxalone

The older product of a combination of alphaxalone and alphadalone (Saffan®) that was solubilized in Cremophor EL was injected IV at 3–6 mg/kg to induce anaesthesia lasting approximately 10 minutes. With the recent introduction of the new formulation of alfaxalone in cyclodextrin, no doubt there will soon be many publications concerning the use of this product in small ruminants. Two recent publications from the same institution have described the effects of alphaxalone, 2 mg/kg,

administered IV over 2 minutes in adult sheep. The slow injection of alfaxalone significantly increased heart rates from an average of 73 ± 11 beats/min to 136 ± 30 beats/min at 10 minutes and mean arterial pressure decreased transiently during induction to 74 ± 14 mmHg but soon returned to a value not different from baseline (Andaluz et al., 2012). Respiratory rates and $PaCO_2$ were unchanged, and the decrease in pHa, primarily metabolic, was not clinically significant. PaO_2 values were between 9.6 and 12 kPa (72 and 90 mmHg). The duration of anaesthesia and time to standing were 6.4 ± 4 and 22 ± 11 minutes, respectively (Andaluz et al., 2012). The other publication was directed at evaluating intraocular pressure (IOP) changes associated with induction of anaesthesia with alfaxalone or propofol, 6 mg/kg (Torres et al., 2012). The eyes in both groups were in a rostroventral position, pupils were constricted, and with no change in IOP during the 10 minutes of anaesthesia. The time to standing was similar in both groups and averaged 15–16 minutes.

Alfaxalone was compared with ketamine for induction of anaesthesia in experimental sheep (Walsh et al., 2012). Alfaxalone, 2 mg/kg, with medetomidine, 0.002 mg/kg, and ketamine, 10 mg/kg, with diazepam, 0.5 mg/kg, and were injected IV 'to effect'. Each anaesthetic agent and adjunct was mixed in the same syringe and half injected over 30 seconds, and after 15 seconds half of the remaining dose injected, and so on until the sheep was considered ready for tracheal intubation. Cumulative dose rates were on average 80% of the alphaxalone–medetomidine mixture and 60% of the ketamine–diazepam. The authors commented that anaesthesia with alfaxalone was light, either because the onset time of medetomidine is slower than that of alfaxalone or because drug injection was too slow, since their usual practice is to inject the whole calculated dose over 1 minute. Times from injection to extubation and standing were significantly shorter in the alfaxalone group at 5 min and 9 min compared with 10 min and 22 min after ketamine. Oxygenation was lower in the ketamine group.

Etomidate

Etomidate is utilized for its lack of cardiovascular depression and rapid elimination and is most frequently used in dogs and cats for induction of anaesthesia. There is one report (Clutton & Glasby, 2008) that used etomidate, 0.5 mg/kg, and midazolam, 0.5 mg/kg, IV for induction of anaesthesia in sheep prior to maintenance of anaesthesia with an inhalant agent.

Ketamine

Ketamine when injected alone induces anaesthesia with strong muscle tone and opisthotonus. Previous or concurrent administration of a sedative or opioid provides muscle relaxation to facilitate endotracheal intubation (see Table 13.2). A useful drug combination for induction of anaesthesia is ketamine, 5 mg/kg, and diazepam or midazolam, 0.25 mg/kg, given IV mixed in one syringe or separated. In some animals, one-half to two-thirds of the calculated dose is sufficient to accomplish endotracheal intubation but the remainder of the dose may have to be administered to facilitate a smooth transition to inhalation anaesthesia. The swallowing reflex may be present and concurrent administration of an opioid will improve muscle relaxation and conditions for intubation. For example, butorphanol, 0.05–0.2 mg/kg IM 10 minutes before induction or IV at the time of induction, or hydromorphone, 0.05–0.1 mg/kg IM 15 minutes before induction, or buprenorphine 0.01 mg/kg IM 45 minutes before induction. Other premedication choices before administration of ketamine, 3–5 mg/kg IV, are acepromazine, 0.05 mg/kg IM 45 minutes before induction, or xylazine 0.02–0.1 mg/kg IM or IV 10 minutes before induction. In the case of difficult intubation, additional ketamine, 1–2 mg/kg IV, can be injected in increments as needed.

The combination of ketamine with xylazine is easy to use and produces a longer duration of anaesthesia than diazepam–ketamine. In goats, onset of anaesthesia is approximately 5 minutes after IM xylazine, 0.1 mg/kg, and ketamine, 10–11 mg/kg. If attempts at intubation induce chewing movements, an additional injection of xylazine, 0.1 mg/kg IM, should induce complete relaxation. The duration of surgical anaesthesia is 30–40 minutes. Alternatively, xylazine can be administered IM 5 minutes before induction of anaesthesia by ketamine, 2–4 mg/kg IV. The duration of anaesthesia is shorter after IV compared with IM administration. A disadvantage to the use of xylazine–ketamine to diazepam–ketamine for induction to isoflurane anaesthesia is that the arterial blood pressure is considerably lower with the xylazine combination.

A combination of medetomidine, 0.02 mg/kg, and ketamine, 2 mg/kg has been used to anaesthetize sheep and the effects reversed by injection of atipamezole, 0.125 mg/kg (Laitinen, 1990; Tulamo et al., 1995). In one study, anaesthesia was continued by a further injection of medetomidine, 0.01 mg/kg, and ketamine 1 mg/kg (Tulamo et al., 1995). Administration of atipamezole 45 minutes after induction of anaesthesia resulted in the sheep standing on average 15 minutes later. Hypoxaemia and hypoventilation are consequences of administration of a combination of medetomidine and ketamine (Caulkett et al., 1994; Tulamo et al., 1995). Cardiac arrest at induction has been reported (Tulamo et al., 1995).

Ketamine and guaifenesin (glyceryl guaiacolate, GGE)

Maintenance of anaesthesia with an infusion of guaifenesin and ketamine after induction of anaesthesia with xylazine and ketamine is a common protocol for total intravenous anaesthesia (TIVA) in cattle over 200 kg body weight. Guaifenesin is not often used in sheep and goats because of its cost, but it can be used. In one report (Lin et al., 1993), sheep were anaesthetized by rapid administration of 1.2 mL/kg of a mixture of guaifenesin, 50 mg/mL, ketamine, 1 mg/mL, and xylazine, 0.1 mg/mL, combined in 5% dextrose in water and anaesthesia was maintained by a continuous infusion of 2.6 mL/kg/h. The sheep in this study were intubated, breathing air, and the average PaO_2 was 4.8 kPa (36.4 mmHg). Administration of oxygen during anaesthesia with these agents is advisable to prevent hypoxaemia.

Pentobarbital

Pentobarbital has been used in the past to induce anaesthesia in sheep. Duration of anaesthesia is short – about 15 minutes, in contrast to duration in dogs and cats, because detoxification of pentobarbital in sheep is rapid. The dose rate of pentobarbital without premedication is 20–30 mg/kg administered slowly IV over several minutes. The dose rate for pentobarbital in goats is similar to that in sheep with a variable but longer duration of anaesthesia.

Propofol

Propofol has a licence for clinical use in dogs and cats. Its chief advantage lies in its rapid detoxification and elimination resulting in rapid recovery from anaesthesia, even after multiple supplements. Propofol, 3–7 mg/kg IV, in unpremedicated sheep and goats will induce anaesthesia sufficient for endotracheal intubation (Pablo et al., 1997). The dose needed will depend on the speed of injection, the breed, and the mental state of the animal (i.e. calm or anxious). Premedication of sheep with acepromazine, 0.05 mg/kg, and papaveretum, 0.4 mg/kg (Correia et al., 1996), or detomidine, 0.01 mg/kg, and butorphanol, 0.1 mg/kg, (Carroll et al., 1998), all given IM, or midazolam, 0.3 mg/kg IV in goats, (Dzikiti et al., 2010) decreased the dose of propofol for intubation in their studies to approximately 4 mg/kg.

Anaesthesia can be maintained with an inhalant or maintained by continuous infusion of propofol (TIVA), or both. The cardiopulmonary effects during anaesthesia will reflect the influence of the inhalant and premedication agents. Intubation of the trachea and allowing the animals to breathe oxygen during TIVA is recommended. Apnoea may occur at induction of anaesthesia. Minimal (Dzikiti et al., 2010) or moderate to severe hypoventilation (Lin et al., 1997; Carroll et al., 1998) has been described in sheep and goats during continuous propofol anaesthesia. Blood pressure may be low after induction of anaesthesia with propofol due to decreased myocardial contractility and venodilation. Blood pressure will progressively rise with time and should achieve an acceptable value during TIVA.

The infusion rate of propofol to maintain anaesthesia for a medical or diagnostic procedure or surgery is generally within the range 0.2–0.3 mg/kg/min but depends on the premedication, concurrent infusion of adjunct anaesthetic agents and the intensity of the surgical stimulus. Propofol provides little analgesia and the animals will be less responsive to surgical stimulus when they have received a sedative or sedative and opioid combination. Recovery from anaesthesia is usually smooth and rapid, although evidence of CNS stimulation, exaggerated tail wagging and restlessness, was observed in goats after infusion of propofol and fentanyl, 0.02 mg/kg/h, for TIVA (Dzikiti et al., 2010).

Combination of propofol with ketamine 'ketofol' is an alternative technique for TIVA that has been reported in sheep (Correia et al., 1996). Induction was achieved with propofol, 3 mg/kg, and ketamine, 1 mg/kg. Anaesthesia was maintained for the first 20 minutes with a combined infusion of propofol, 0.3 mg/kg/min, with ketamine, 0.2 mg/kg/min. This infusion rate was subsequently decreased to 0.2 mg/kg/min of propofol and 0.1 mg/kg/min of ketamine. Recovery from anaesthesia was rapid and free from excitement. The theory behind this combination is that since TIVA with ketamine alone in sheep results in excessively prolonged recovery times, reducing the dose rate by including propofol will result in more rapid recovery. Furthermore, ketamine may provide analgesia while propofol does not, and ketamine may induce sympathetic stimulation to offset the cardiovascular depression induced by propofol.

Continuous IV infusion of propofol during isoflurane or sevoflurane anaesthesia will decrease the vaporizer setting according to the agents used for premedication or induction of anaesthesia. In goats anaesthetized with isoflurane only, administration of a bolus dose of propofol, 2 mg/kg, followed by a continuous infusion of propofol at either 0.1 mg/kg/min or 0.2 mg/kg/min decreased isoflurane requirement (minimum alveolar concentration [MAC] value) by 35% and 60%, respectively (Dzikiti et al., 2011a). Ventilation was controlled in this study.

Thiopental

Thiopental has been extensively used to induce anaesthesia in sheep and goats. Onset of action is fast and the drug can be titrated to achieve the desired effect. The dose rate to induce anaesthesia in the unpremedicated animal is wide, 7–20 mg/kg, and the low or high dose does not seem to correlate with any particular patient characteristic, not age nor conformation nor degree of ill health. To avoid overdosage, initially a dose of 5–7 mg/kg of 2.5% thiopental should be injected. Within 30 seconds, the degree of CNS depression can be assessed and further small boluses of drug administered every 20 seconds until the jaws are relaxed for endotracheal intubation. Endotracheal intubation is recommended as regurgitation may occur shortly

after thiopental administration. The duration of anaesthesia is short, at 5–10 minutes, depending on the dose of thiopental administered. Recovery is usually smooth. Preanaesthetic sedation decreases the dose rate proportionately to the degree of sedation.

Tiletamine–zolazepam

Intravenous administration of tiletamine–zolazepam produces longer lasting anaesthesia than diazepam–ketamine. Tiletamine–zolazepam may not provide sufficient analgesia for laparotomy and an additional drug should be included for analgesia. Administration of tiletamine–zolazepam IV alone to sheep at 12 mg/kg resulted in rapid induction of anaesthesia and an average duration of 40 minutes (Lagutchik et al., 1991). Apnoea occurred on induction followed by mild hypoventilation and decreases in oxygenation. Cardiac output decreased significantly by 30%, however, heart rates and mean arterial pressures were not changed. The addition of butorphanol, 0.5 mg/kg, IV injected either 10 minutes before anaesthesia or at the time of induction resulted in greater respiratory depression, hypoxaemia (approximately 10 minutes), and duration of anaesthesia of 30–40 minutes (Howard et al., 1990). Tiletamine–zolazepam at 6.6 mg/kg in combination with butorphanol or ketamine or ketamine and xylazine results in transient or prolonged decrease in arterial blood pressure or hypotension, 30% decrease in cardiac output, and increased pulmonary and systemic vascular resistances (Lagutchik et al., 1991; Lin et al., 1994). Apnoea may occur after induction of anaesthesia and despite minimal change in respiratory rates, mild to moderate hypoventilation is present and hypoxaemia occurs when the animals are breathing air. In one investigation of tiletamine–zolazepam with or without butorphanol (Lin et al., 1994), anaesthesia time was 25–50 minutes, with a longer duration of anaesthesia, 83 ± 27 min (mean and standard deviation), and a protracted recovery, mean 4 hours, when ketamine, 6.6 mg/kg, and xylazine, 0.11 mg/kg, were included.

Inhalation anaesthesia

Inhalation anaesthesia is a popular and reasonably safe technique for providing anaesthesia for surgery and medical diagnostic procedures. Halothane was used universally but is only available now in a few countries. Isoflurane or sevoflurane with O_2 are the most commonly used inhalation anaesthetics in ruminants. They offer advantages over injectable agents of easy control of depth of anaesthesia, O_2 that usually prevents hypoxaemia, facilitation for artificial ventilation, and rapid recovery from anaesthesia. The greatest disadvantages are that the inhalation agents cause respiratory depression and decreased arterial blood pressure such that controlled ventilation and treatment with vasoactive drugs may be necessary.

Tracheal intubation prior to inhalation anaesthesia is commonly accomplished after anaesthesia is first induced with injectable agents. Induction of anaesthesia with the inhalant delivered through a facemask is less desirable in an adult sheep or goat. The longer time for induction allows accumulation of saliva in the pharynx and increases the time before endotracheal intubation, during which regurgitation and aspiration can occur. Induction with an inhalant to achieve endotracheal intubation requires deep anaesthesia, causing decreased arterial pressure. Furthermore, induction using a mask is often physically resented by the adult animal. In contrast, anaesthesia is easily induced in young lambs and kids with isoflurane or sevoflurane via facemask.

Anaesthetic breathing systems that are used for dogs can be used for sheep and goats. The initial vaporizer setting will depend on the anaesthetic agents used for induction of anaesthesia, the potency of the anaesthetic agent (MAC), and the type of breathing system. For example, after induction and intubation in animals anaesthetized with acepromazine and thiopental, or butorphanol or buprenorphine, midazolam and ketamine, and connection to a circle circuit, the vaporizer (precision vaporizer) may be set at 1.5× MAC with an O_2 flow rate of 1–2 L/min. In contrast, after induction of anaesthesia with xylazine or dexmedetomidine and ketamine, or with tiletamine–zolazepam, the CNS depression is greater and the vaporizer setting should be lower, for example, 0.5–1.0× MAC. In either case, as the depth of anaesthesia changes with time and onset of surgery, the vaporizer setting can be adjusted up or down as needed. After about 20 minutes, when the blood anaesthetic concentrations are more stable, O_2 flow can be reduced to 1.0 L/min, or less if desired, to limit wastage of inhalant agent. It should be remembered that a consequence of a low O_2 flow into a circle circuit connected to a large (70 kg) animal is a circuit anaesthetic concentration that may be considerably less than the vaporizer setting, for example, 1% inspired isoflurane with a 1.5% vaporizer setting.

Small lambs and kids may be connected to a nonrebreathing circuit. The inspired anaesthetic concentration is the same as the vaporizer setting and thus during maintenance of anaesthesia should be 1.0–1.5× MAC, depending on the degree of preanaesthetic sedation and administration of adjunct drugs.

Supplementation during anaesthesia with bolus doses of an opioid, or a continuous rate infusion (CRI) of an opioid, lidocaine, or ketamine, or combination of these, will decrease the concentration of inhalation agents required to prevent response to surgical stimuli and thereby decrease the negative impact on arterial pressure. Depending on the agents used, supplements may increase or minimize respiratory depression. Addition of a neuromuscular blocking agent is not common for general veterinary procedures but may be included in research investigations or complicated clinical surgeries.

Potencies of isoflurane, sevoflurane, and desflurane

The concentration required for anaesthesia (MAC) varies according to the species of animal and the testing conditions. Published values for halothane MAC were 0.73–1.09% for sheep and 0.96–1.4% in goats (see Chapter 6). Published MAC values for isoflurane in adult non-pregnant sheep are 1.42 ± 0.19% (Okutomi et al., 2009) and goats 1.29 ± 0.11% and 1.32% (range, 1.29–1.36%) (Hikasa et al., 1998; Dzikiti et al., 2011b). Anaesthetic requirements for inhalants are decreased by pregnancy, and a 21% reduction in isoflurane to 1.02 ± 0.12% was measured in pregnant sheep (Okutomi et al., 2009). MAC was reported to be 50% decreased in newborn lambs compared with adult pregnant sheep (Gregory et al., 1983), however, MAC requirement increased in the first 12 hours of life.

The MAC value reported for sevoflurane in sheep is 1.92 ± 0.17% and a decrease was measured to 1.52 ± 0.15% in pregnant sheep (Okutomi et al., 2009). The MAC value reported for sevoflurane in adult non-pregnant goats is 2.33 ± 0.15% (Hikasa et al., 1998). The MAC value for desflurane in sheep was measured as 9.5% (Lukasik et al., 1998) and 10.5 ± 2.4% for goats (Alibhai, 2001).

The cardiopulmonary effects of isoflurane, sevoflurane, and desflurane have been investigated in sheep and goats (Hikasa et al., 1998, 2000; Mohamadnia et al., 2008; Okutomi et al., 2009). In a light plane of anaesthesia, cardiovascular values remained within acceptable ranges in isoflurane and sevoflurane anaesthetized goats (Hikasa et al., 1998). Increasing depth of anaesthesia resulted in progressive decreases in MAP and systemic vascular resistance and severe increases in $PaCO_2$. Increasing depth of isoflurane or sevoflurane anaesthesia from 1 to 2 MAC in goats during controlled ventilation significantly decreased MAP, systemic vascular resistance, and cardiac index (Hikasa et al., 1998). Changes in cardiovascular parameters in anaesthetized sheep and goats were not different between isoflurane and sevoflurane. Recovery from desflurane and sevoflurane in goats was faster than from isoflurane (Alibhai, 2001). The characteristics and effects of anaesthesia will vary according to which combination of injectable and inhalation agents is used. For example, sheep were anaesthetized with xylazine and ketamine and anaesthesia maintained for orthopaedic surgery with mean end-tidal concentrations of either 1.41% isoflurane, 2.1% sevoflurane, or 7.04% desflurane (Mohamadnia et al., 2008). During recovery, the times of return to swallowing, extubation, and head lift were the same for all three inhalation agents.

An investigation of the effects of isoflurane and sevoflurane anaesthesia in pregnant sheep at 129–143 days of gestation involved measurement of uterine blood flow using an ultrasonic flow meter (Okutomi et al., 2009). No adverse changes were measured during administration of 0.5 or 1.0 MAC of either agent. With increasing depth of anaesthesia, significant decreases in maternal and fetal mean arterial blood pressure (MAP) and increased $PaCO_2$ occurred at 1.5 MAC; at 2.0 MAC, there were significant decreases in maternal and fetal MAP, maternal heart rate (HR), and pHa. Although the decrease in uterine blood flow was not statistically significant, fetal arterial pressure decreased to a greater extent than maternal during deep anaesthesia. Dose related changes in uterine blood flow and maternal HR and MAP and fetal HR and MAP were not different between the two agents at all stages of measurement. Recovery was faster after sevoflurane than isoflurane anaesthesia.

Nitrous oxide

Nitrous oxide (N_2O) can be used as an analgesic adjunct to injectable anaesthesia or used to supplement and decrease the inhalant anaesthetic concentration. A major disadvantage of N_2O is that it rapidly diffuses into the rumen and causes bloat and respiratory compromise. Therefore, N_2O is rarely administered to ruminants

Adjunct agents

Opioids

Remifentanil, 0.75–2.0 μg/kg/min, 100 μg/mL, was infused during halothane anaesthesia in pregnant ewes anaesthetized for fetal surgery (Webster et al., 2005). Controlled ventilation was required to treat hypoventilation and periodically the infusion rate had to be increased in response to surgical stimulus in order to keep the vaporizer setting constant. All sheep were standing within an hour of discontinuation of anaesthesia.

Fentanyl infusions have also been used in sheep to allow lower isoflurane vaporizer settings. In an experimental study in goats (Dzikiti et al., 2011b), a 34% decrease in isoflurane requirement was measured after a fentanyl bolus of 5 μg/kg followed by an infusion of fentanyl, 5 μg/kg/h. Higher dose rates of 15 μg/kg fentanyl bolus with 15 μg/kg/h infusion or 30 μg/kg bolus with 30 μg/kg/h infusion decreased isoflurane requirements by 57% and 74%, respectively. Recovery from anaesthesia was described as good although exaggerated tail wagging (indicative of opioid stimulation) was observed in some goats that received the two higher dose rates. These goats received only isoflurane and fentanyl, consequently, care should be taken to avoid overdose with the higher dose rates of fentanyl when other injectable agents are used for induction of anaesthesia.

Variable plasma concentrations were measured in goats in a pharmacokinetic study of fentanyl administered by transdermal patch (Carroll et al., 1999). However, fentanyl patches, 2 μg/kg/h, applied to the forelimb between carpus and elbow or elbow and shoulder have been used

as part of anaesthetic protocols in sheep with apparent beneficial effect by this author and others (Ahern et al., 2009; Raske et al., 2010). To ensure continued attachment of the patch to the skin, the area must be clipped, prepped as if for a surgical procedure and dried, and an occlusive dressing placed over the patch.

Lidocaine

Lidocaine infusion, 0.025–0.05 mg/kg/min (1.5–3 mg/kg/h) can be used during inhalation anaesthesia to decrease the % of inhalant agent required to prevent movement or autonomic responses to surgical stimulation. In an experimental investigation of lidocaine infusion, 100 μg/hg/min, MAC reduction was much less in anaesthetized goats than in dogs and horses (Doherty et al., 2007). Interestingly, plasma concentrations of lidocaine were lower in the goats than measured in dogs for a given infusion rate.

Ketamine

Ketamine infusions, 1.5 mg/kg/h, in experimental isoflurane-anaesthetized goats decreased isoflurane requirement by 50% in response to a forceps claw clamp (Doherty et al., 2007). Recovery from anaesthesia was rapid and uneventful. In an investigation of sheep undergoing experimental stifle surgery, infusions of ketamine, 0.6 mg/kg/h, and lidocaine, 1.2 mg/kg/h, significantly decreased the isoflurane requirement by approximately 23% when compared with animals not receiving infusions (Raske et al., 2010). Ketamine infusion, 1.2 mg/kg/h IV, produced a decrease in isoflurane requirement in unstimulated experimental sheep anaesthetized with isoflurane but it did not prevent the need to increase markedly the vaporizer setting at the onset of surgical stimulus (Trim, unpublished observations). Concurrent IV infusions of ketamine, 1.2 mg/kg/h, and lidocaine, 3.0 mg/kg/h, with a loading dose of lidocaine, 1 mg/kg, in sheep that had fentanyl transdermal patches, 2 μg/kg, applied 12 hours before anaesthesia, decreased the end-tidal concentration of isoflurane to approximately 60% × MAC and provided satisfactory intraoperative analgesia for minor orthopaedic surgeries (Trim, unpublished observations). Hypoventilation was corrected by controlled ventilation. Recoveries from anaesthesia were good.

Non-steroidal anti-inflammatory agents

Although carprofen, 2–2.2 mg/kg, or flunixin meglumine, 1–1.1 mg/kg, SC do not block the effects of intense pain or cortisol response to pain, these agents provide some relief after surgical procedures as evidenced by amelioration of behaviour (Grant et al., 1996; Paull et al., 2007; Colditz et al., 2009).

Neuromuscular blockade

Administration of atracurium, 0.5 mg/kg, or mivacurium, 0.2 mg/kg, IV as loading doses have been used to achieve neuromuscular blockade in sheep, followed by one-third of the loading dose to prolong blockade when there was evidence of return of neuromuscular transmission (Clutton & Glasby, 2008). This study documented heart rates and MAP changes in response to injections of atropine and edrophonium for reversal of neuromuscular blockade. In contrast to humans and dogs, edrophonium increased, and atropine decreased, these variables. The drug combination that resulted in least autonomic change was atropine, 0.08 mg/kg, with edrophonium, 0.5 mg/kg.

Anaesthetic management

Positioning

A cuffed endotracheal tube should be inserted and the cuff inflated while the animal is in sternal recumbency with the head elevated. After intubation and during anaesthesia, the head and neck should be positioned so that the nose is lower than the pharynx for drainage of saliva and any regurgitated ruminal fluid (Fig. 13.10). Salivation will continue throughout anaesthesia. Saliva ceases to flow only when it is accumulating in the pharynx or because a deep plane of anaesthesia has decreased production.

Fluid therapy

Balanced electrolyte solution, such as lactated or acetated Ringer's solution at 5–10 mL/kg/h should be infused IV when surgery is being performed or when anaesthesia time becomes extended. Animals less than 3 months of age

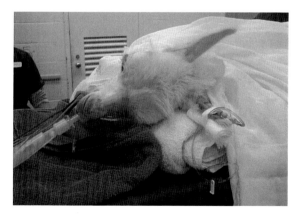

Figure 13.10 The head of this anaesthetized alpaca has been elevated to prevent nasal congestion and the head positioned with the nose lower than the pharynx to facilitate drainage of saliva. A catheter in an ear artery was used for direct measurement of arterial blood pressure. A pulse oximeter probe is clipped to the tongue.

should also receive 5% dextrose in water at 2–5 mL/kg/h. Occasionally, an adult ruminant develops hypoglycaemia, and this should be suspected any time that recovery is more prolonged, or if the animal is more lethargic than expected after recovery from the immediate effects of the anaesthetic agents. The haematocrit and total protein measurements decrease at the onset of inhalant anaesthesia (Hikasa et al., 2000), similar to the effect measured in dogs and presumed due in part to splenic sequestration.

Monitoring

The position of the eyeball during inhalation anaesthesia in goats and sheep is similar to the pattern observed in anaesthetized dogs; the eye rolls rostroventral between light and medium depth anaesthesia, and returns to central position during deep plane of anaesthesia (some variation with different agents). Occasionally, during light anaesthesia, the eye will rotate dorsally ('star gazing'). The palpebral reflex is lost between medium to deep anaesthesia. The pupil should be a narrow slit during an adequate plane of inhalation anaesthesia and dilates in light or deep anaesthesia. The pupil dilates after ketamine administration although, if the dose rate is low, the pupil may close down during inhalation anaesthesia.

An anaesthetic gas analyser may be used to monitor end-expired anaesthetic agent concentration. The highest value that should be allowed is 1.5 times the MAC of the agent. A concentration equal to or substantially less than MAC is often sufficient when premedication has included medetomidine or anaesthesia includes a continuous infusion of opioid, propofol, ketamine, or lidocaine. Older anaesthetic gas analysers utilizing infrared technology were inaccurate with halothane because they detected methane in the ruminant's breath and counted it as halothane. The problem occurs occasionally with isoflurane and is minimal with sevoflurane and desflurane.

Respiratory rates are usually 15–30 breaths/minute. Hypercarbia caused by hypoventilation (primarily decreased tidal volume) is common in anaesthetized sheep and goats. Rumen bloat may develop during anaesthesia despite preoperative fasting, and pressure on the diaphragm impairs ventilation and contributes to increased $PaCO_2$. One consequence of decreased ventilation may be inadequate depth of anaesthesia despite a high vaporizer setting, due to insufficient agent uptake in the lungs. Tachycardia, and sometimes hypertension, may develop as a consequence of the hypercapnia and these parameters should return to normal values after the onset of controlled ventilation. Hypercarbia causes portal vein vasoconstriction that may contribute to hepatic ischaemia (Box 13.1).

Capnography is a non-invasive monitor of ventilation and an end-tidal CO_2 value of >55 mmHg is an indication for the need for artificial ventilation. Tidal volumes of 12–15 mL/kg at 8–12 breaths/minute with peak

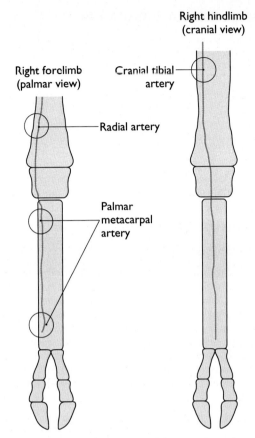

Figure 13.11 Schematic drawing of the arteries on the forelimbs and hind limbs for palpation of pulses and indirect blood pressure measurement.

inspiratory pressures of 18–25 mmHg should maintain arterial CO_2 concentration within normal values. Sheep lungs progressively collapse during general anaesthesia. Periodic artificial lung inflations ('sighing') when the animal is breathing spontaneously may reverse some of the collapse. Controlled ventilation started immediately after induction of anaesthesia may limit lung collapse. Applying positive end-expiratory pressure (PEEP) can also prevent lung collapse. Bloating can often be relieved by passage of a wide bore tube through the mouth and into the rumen, however, the tube is easily blocked by ingesta. Tachycardia as a result of rumen bloat will not disappear until the rumen is decompressed.

Haemoglobin O_2 saturation and pulse rate can be monitored using a pulse oximeter probe on the tongue, lip, or ear. Oxygenation is usually adequate when the inspired gas is O_2 rich. Peripheral arteries that are easily palpated or can be used for non-invasive methods of blood pressure measurement are on the caudomedial side of the forelimb above or below the carpus and on the hind limb on the dorsal surface of the metatarsus (Fig. 13.11). Doppler ultrasound and oscillometric methods are used for non-invasive arterial blood pressure measurement (NIBP) and provide valuable information for management of anaesthesia. It must be remembered that the values obtained may not be accurate for all individuals. Comparison of an oscillometric monitor (Surgivet Advisor) with invasive blood pressure measurement in isoflurane-anaesthetized sheep determined that correlation between the two methods was good but that, in general, NIBP slightly overestimated systolic pressures and underestimated diastolic and mean arterial pressures (Trim et al., 2013). No difference was found between pressures obtained from cuffs on the hind limb or forelimb. Measurement of SAP 80 mmHg or less correlated with hypotension but in some animals a MAP of 60 mmHg resulted in diagnosis of hypotension when there was none.

Invasive measurement of arterial pressure involves catheterization of the auricular arteries located on the outside of the ear (see Chapter 2, Fig. 2.17; Fig. 13.10). When the ear is folded along its natural crease, the median auricular artery can be observed just rostral to the edge of the fold.

A Butterfly needle or 22 or 20 gauge catheter can be inserted for direct measurement of arterial pressure and for collection of blood for pH and blood gas analysis. Some published normal values measured in awake sheep are pHa 7.53 ± 0.01, $PaCO_2$ 3.9 ± 0.1 kPa (29 ± 0.8 mmHg), PaO_2 13.4 ± 0.5 kPa (101 ± 4 mmHg) (Okutomi et al., 2009) and awake goats are pHa 7.48 ± 0.03, $PaCO_2$ 4.8 ± 0.5 kPa (36 ± 3.7 mmHg), PaO_2 10.6 ± 1.3 kPa (80 ± 10 mmHg), and base excess 3.3 ± 4.9 mmol/L (Hikasa et al., 1998).

Heart rates are most frequently between 60 and 120 beats/minute, except that when an α_2-agonist has been administered they are lower. Heart rates less than 55 beats/min should be considered as bradycardia and heart rates greater than 140 beats/min should be investigated for possible abnormal cause. Mean arterial pressure is generally 75–95 mmHg during anaesthesia; less than 65 mmHg is hypotension.

It is not uncommon for the animal's temperature to decrease to 37.2°C (99°F) before anaesthesia after 24 hours without food. Hypothermia may develop during anaesthesia and efforts should be made to prevent heat loss. Sheep and goats require external application of heat when rectal temperature decreases to 35.5°C (96°F) to avoid prolonged recovery. Conversely, anaesthesia in a hot environment may result in hyperthermia. Temperature in clinical patients can be monitored with a thermometer or probe inserted 3–5 cm into the rectum, through the oesophagus into the thorax, or inserted in the nasal meatus. Accuracy of peripheral temperature measurements in comparison with pulmonary artery blood confirmed that rectal temperature accurately reflects core temperature in anaesthetized normovolaemic and hypovolaemic sheep, but is altered in the presence of epidural nerve block (Mansel et al., 2008). Temperature measured in the nose or ear will be lower than core temperature.

Treatment of hypotension

Mean arterial blood pressures less than 65 mmHg should be treated appropriately according to the suspected cause of the hypotension. Anaesthetic agent-induced vasodilation causing a relative hypovolaemia should first be treated by decreasing the vaporizer setting. In some cases, this step might include administration of an adjunct drug to provide additional analgesia while maintaining decreased inhalation agent administration. Circulating blood volume should be expanded with a 10 mL/kg bolus of balanced electrolyte solution and/or infusion of hetastarch, 5–10 mL/kg, over 15 minutes.

Cardiac contractility can be increased by IV infusion of dopamine or dobutamine, 5–7 μg/kg/min of a 100 μg/mL solution in 0.9% saline. Dopamine will elevate blood pressure through vasoconstriction at the higher dose rate. Once the desired MAP is reached, the infusion rate of either agent can be reduced but generally has to be continued to the end of anaesthesia. Ephedrine, 0.06–0.10 mg/kg, injected as a bolus IV may increase blood pressure by causing splenic contraction, vasoconstriction, increased cardiac contractility and increased heart rate. Ephedrine may be used alone or in conjunction with dopamine or dobutamine. The duration of effect from a bolus of ephedrine varies from 10 to 40 minutes. Repeat doses may be administered but are not always as effective as the first (tachyphylaxis).

Blood loss should be estimated by counting blood-soaked gauzes or by estimating the volume of blood in a suction bottle or in a bucket placed under the surgery table. Blood volume of sheep and goats is 60 mL/kg and a significant decrease in cardiac output develops at a loss of 15%. Up to that point, blood loss can be accommodated by infusion of up to 2.5 times the volume of blood lost with crystalloid fluid, with the addition of hetastarch, 5–10 mL/kg, and hypertonic 7.5% saline solution, 2–4 mL/kg, if needed.

Recovery

The animal should be placed in a sternal position at the end of anaesthesia so that gas in the rumen can be voided through the mouth while the endotracheal tube is in place. Regurgitation during anaesthesia should not be a problem when the endotracheal tube is in position and the cuff adequately inflated. If possible, the head should be positioned so that ingesta cannot accumulate in the nasal meatus. Solid rumen material should be removed from the pharynx before the end of anaesthesia. It must be remembered that regurgitation may occur when the animal is waking up. Consequently, the endotracheal tube must not be removed until the animal is chewing, swallowing and, most importantly, can withdraw its tongue back into its mouth; this may be a considerable time after the animal is able to lift up its head. The endotracheal tube must be held to the front of the mouth as the cheek teeth are sharp and easily lacerate the endotracheal tube or the tube connected to the pilot balloon.

Recovery is usually quiet. If the sheep or goat starts to rise too soon, pressure over the back and withers usually maintains the animal in sternal recumbency. Full control of swallowing and gastrointestinal motility may not return for several hours after xylazine or medetomidine administration and feeding must be delayed. Hay or grass and water may be allowed 3 hours after anaesthesia is discontinued with most anaesthetic agents used in these species.

Assessment of pain

Clinical signs of pain can be masked by the animal's anxiety about surroundings, separation from the herd, and proximity of an unknown human. These may have a profound effect on activity, respiratory rates and heart rates. Slow movements and familiarization with an individual will allow the animal to be calm and accept examination. Teeth grinding has been associated with discomfort or pain but can also be a sign of anxiety as it may be observed before anaesthesia. When surgery involves a limb, decreased weight bearing and lameness are obvious signs of discomfort. Reluctance to stand may or may not be an indication of pain, since this behaviour may become modified within several hours as the sheep become accustomed to being handled. Conversely, sheep may be reluctant to lie down and persist in standing with a hunched back. Sheep and goats normally eat voraciously after anaesthesia and the lack of interest in eating is an obvious sign of lack of well-being.

A variety of clinical signs can be monitored in an attempt to determine the degree of postoperative discomfort and a number of pain scoring systems have been published (Table 13.3). Sheep and goats may fail to show clinically obvious signs of pain that more sophisticated techniques may detect. For example, sheep anaesthetized for experimental facial surgery (Abu-Serriah et al., 2007)

Table 13.3 Example of a pain assessment score for sheep following limb surgery

Variable	Score			
	0	1	2	3
Mental assessment	Normal and alert	Slight change or some depression	No score	Signs of depression
Temperature*	Normal			Abnormal
Heart rate*	Normal			Abnormal
Respiratory rate*	Normal		Abnormal	
Recumbency	Normal	No score	No score	Sitting all the time
Ease of standing	Normal, gets up easily	Slightly delayed rising	Requires encouragement to stand	Unwilling or unable to stand
Limb position	Weight bearing	Mostly weight bearing	Occasionally bearing weight	Unable or unwilling to bear weight
Shifting weight	Normal	Mild or occasional	Moderate	Constantly shifting
Relationship to pen partner	Normal – mostly nearby	No score	Spends more time separately	Stays away constantly
Appetite	Interested in eating/cudding	Mildly reduced interest	Moderately reduced interest	Inappetant
Palpation of surgical site	No signs of pain but may lift foot in response to touch	Mild response	Moderate signs of pain, avoidance response	Severe signs of pain, startles away, vocal
Scores				

*Establish reference ranges for species, breed, in the recovery environment to be used. Identify a score that dictates use of rescue analgesia.
(Modified from Ahern et al., 2009)

were given lidocaine infiltration, morphine systemically during surgery, carprofen, and buprenorphine postoperatively for up to 24 hours after surgery. Despite apparent acceptable behaviour, it was determined that the sheep had developed hyperalgesia (exaggerated response to noxious stimuli applied remote from the injury) in the fore limbs and allodynia (increased sensitivity to touch) for 3 days after surgery.

Camelids

INTRODUCTION

Llamas (*Lama glama*) may weigh up to 200 kg and live up to 20 years. Alpacas (*Lama pacos*) commonly weigh 65–80 kg but may weigh up to 100 kg. These animals should be handled with care as llamas can kick, swinging the limb forward and out, and males may bite. Use of side rails is not advised, as a leg can be broken. Some commercial llama chutes incorporate straps, which are passed under the animal's thorax and caudal abdomen to prevent the animal assuming sternal recumbency. Most llamas and alpacas tolerate a halter with a rope lead. Suggestions for manual restraint include holding the haltered head and exerting the full force of your weight on the hind limbs to force the animal into a sternal recumbent submissive position (Jessup & Lance, 1982). This works because the forelimbs are the main weight bearers and the hind limbs cannot be locked up. Tapping behind the knee of the forelimb may help. Weanlings or yearlings should not be tied as they may struggle and injure cervical vertebrae. Aggressive handling or striking an animal will result in fear, distrust and spitting.

LOCAL ANALGESIA

Applications for local anaesthesia

Caudal epidural analgesia

Caudal epidural injection of lidocaine, xylazine, or a combination of these has been evaluated in llamas (Grubb

Table 13.4 Comparison of mean times for onset and duration of epidural analgesia with 2% lidocaine, 0.22 mg/kg, and diluted 10% xylazine, 0.17 mg/kg, in six llamas

Treatment	Onset (min)	Duration (min)
Lidocaine	3	71
Xylazine	21	187
Lidocaine/xylazine	4	326

Grubb et al., 1993.

et al., 1993). Injections were made into the sacrococcygeal space where the epidural space is shallow and easily entered. The procedure was performed with a 20 gauge, 2.5 cm long needle inserted at a 60° angle to the base of the tail. Onset of action was rapid after injection of lidocaine and analgesia lasted longest when a combination of lidocaine and xylazine was used (Table 13.4). Ataxia did not develop, although the llamas tended to lie down. The dose rate of xylazine used in this study was toward the high end of the dose range used in ruminants and from which some systemic effects are to be expected. Mild sedation developed in half the llamas given epidural xylazine, beginning 20 minutes after injection and lasting for 20–30 minutes. The synergistic effect on duration of analgesia caused by combining xylazine with lidocaine is similar to that in horses.

Caudal epidural analgesia has been used during castration of alpacas aged 6 to 18 months (Padula, 2005). The alpacas were manually restrained up against a wall. Epidural injection was made through a 22 gauge, 1.5 inch needle inserted in the first coccygeal space identified as the depression located by manipulating the tail up and down. Three combinations were compared: 1.5 mL of 2% lidocaine, 1 mL 2% lidocaine with IM 20 mg 2% xylazine, and 0.75 mL of a 1 : 1 combination of 2% xylazine and lidocaine. Some animals in each treatment group showed signs of inadequate analgesia of the spermatic cord during application of the emasculators, and supplemental lidocaine infiltration was required.

Local analgesia for castration

A technique for castration in the standing llama has been performed in more than 100 animals without complications (Barrington et al., 1993). Butorphanol, 0.1 mg/kg, IM was administered 15 minutes before applying a surgical scrub to the perineal region. Lidocaine, 2–5 mL of a 2% solution, was injected into each testicle until it became turgid and a further 1–2 mL was deposited subcutaneously at the site of the proposed incision as the needle was withdrawn. The lower dose of lidocaine is recommended for llamas weighing less than 30 kg. These authors noted that llamas given butorphanol are not sedated but also that they do not exhibit the signs of discomfort and restlessness during the procedure that have been observed in animals castrated with only local analgesia.

Caudal epidural analgesia has also been used for castration (see earlier).

Caesarian section

Surgical approach through the left paralumbar fossa with the animals sedated and restrained in right lateral recumbency has been recommended for caesarian section (Anderson, 2009). Sedation can be provided by a low dose of butorphanol and analgesia by lidocaine infiltration as a line block or inverted-L. It was also stated that crias are minimally affected by maternal administration of a low dose of xylazine. In contrast, this author's experience with other ruminants has been that maternal sedation with xylazine results in significant sedation of lambs and calves delivered by caesarian section.

GENERAL ANAESTHESIA

Preparation for anaesthesia

A number of publications are available documenting the reference ranges for haematological and biochemical values in llamas and alpacas (Fowler & Zinkl, 1989; Hajduk, 1992). In comparison with common domestic ruminants, llamas and alpacas may have higher erythrocyte counts ($11–14×10^{12}$/L) and small mean corpuscular volume, with packed cell volumes of 0.25–0.45 L/L (25–45%). Blood glucose concentrations of 108–156 mg/dL were measured in nursing 2–6-month-old llamas compared with 74–154 mg/dL in adult llamas.

Preparation for anaesthesia is the same as for sheep and goats. Bloat, regurgitation, and aspiration can occur in llamas and, therefore, the animals should be fasted for 24 hours and water withheld for 8–12 hours before elective anaesthesia. Crias may take solid food as early as 2 weeks but weaning may not occur until age 4–7 months. Fasting is not usually done in paediatric patients because of the risk for hypoglycaemia except that nursing is prevented for 30–60 minutes before anaesthesia. A rapid induction and intubation sequence with the animal in sternal or upright position until tracheal intubation is accomplished is necessary for emergency procedures in animals that are not fasted.

Severe bradycardia was reported occurring during halothane anaesthesia and there is some preference for premedication with atropine, 0.02 mg/kg (Riebold et al., 1989).

369

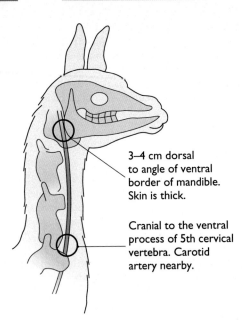

Figure 13.12 Schematic drawing showing the landmarks for jugular vein puncture in llamas.

3–4 cm dorsal to angle of ventral border of mandible. Skin is thick.

Cranial to the ventral process of 5th cervical vertebra. Carotid artery nearby.

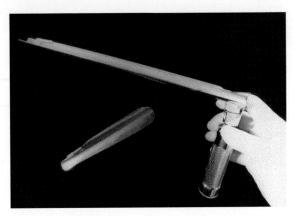

Figure 13.13 The long 35 cm Wisconsin laryngoscope blade is useful for intubation of adult llamas, seen here in comparison with a blade used for intubation of large dogs.

Anaesthetic techniques

Venepuncture

Jugular venepuncture for collection of blood or placement of a catheter is not as easy as in sheep and goats. Two sites are recommended (Fig. 13.12) (Amsel et al., 1987). One site is high in the neck at the level of the mandible. An imaginary line is drawn continuous with the ventral border of the mandible and the point of needle insertion is 3–4 cm dorsal from its angle in an adult animal. Disadvantages to this site are that the overlying skin is very thick, and movement of the head may dislodge a needle or kink a catheter. The second site is lower on the neck where the ventral processes of the fifth cervical vertebra can be palpated. Placing a thumb in the depression just medial to the ventral process can raise the jugular vein. The overlying skin is less thick, facilitating catheter insertion. A disadvantage to the site is that the carotid artery is nearby and can be penetrated. The skin over the selected area should be clipped and aseptically prepared. A bleb of local anaesthetic solution should be injected subcutaneously at the proposed site of insertion and a nick made in the skin with a scalpel blade or the tip of a large hypodermic needle. The insertion of the catheter should be directed towards the heart. Camelid venous blood is significantly brighter red than observed in equine patients and colour should not be the only reason for assessing correct catheter placement (Grint & Dugdale, 2009). Observed pulsatile blood flow through the catheter or needle confirms that the catheter is in the carotid artery and it should be withdrawn.

When the carotid artery has been penetrated, pressure should be immediately applied with a fist for 5 minutes to avoid a large haematoma. A 14 gauge or 16 gauge, 13 cm long catheter is inserted in adult llamas or alpacas. Occasionally, threading the catheter may be hindered by prominent valves in the vein. Other veins, such as an ear vein, cephalic vein, or saphenous vein can be used in depressed, sedated, anaesthetized, or young animals.

Endotracheal intubation

The technique for endotracheal intubation is similar to that in sheep and goats. A clear view of the laryngeal opening in adult llamas is essential and a laryngoscope with a long blade may be helpful (Fig. 13.13). A 10 mm ID tube can be used in a 60 kg llama and a 12 mm in a llama of 100 kg. Endotracheal tubes 10–12 mm ID should be selected for adult alpacas. Intubation is made easier by inserting a metal rod inside the endotracheal tube to stiffen it. The halter should be removed before attempted intubation as it will often limit how wide the jaws can be opened.

Llamas and alpacas are obligate nasal breathers and airway obstruction may occur during anaesthesia in animals that are not intubated due to dorsal displacement of the soft palate, and during recovery from anaesthesia after extubation due to nasal mucosal congestion and oedema. Positioning the head above the body during recumbency will help prevent nasal congestion (see Fig. 13.10).

Orotracheal intubation is satisfactory for most animals. Nasotracheal intubation has been recommended in llamas to provide a clear airway during any phase of anaesthesia (Riebold et al., 1994). A long tube will be needed, such as the 40–55 cm long tubes manufactured for nasotracheal intubation in foals. The internal diameter will be about

2 mm less than the size of tube chosen for orotracheal intubation. The tube should be well lubricated, and lubricant containing phenylephrine can be used to cause vasoconstriction in the nasal mucosa and limit haemorrhage. The tip of the tube is inserted medially and ventrally into the ventral nasal meatus, with the bevel directed laterally to minimize trauma to the conchae. It is important to keep a finger on the tube inside the nares to ensure that the tube remains in the ventral meatus while the tube is advanced slowly and without twisting. If the tube is in the middle meatus it will impact on the ethmoid and cause significant haemorrhage. A further obstruction to intubation in llamas is the large diverticulum, 1 cm wide and 2 cm deep, at the caudodorsal angle of the nasopharynx. If the tip of the tube is level with the pharynx and it cannot be advanced then the tube should be withdrawn several centimetres, redirected and advanced again. The arytenoid cartilages and epiglottis protrude above the soft palate into the nasopharynx. Hyperextension of the head and neck may allow the nasotracheal tube to enter the larynx. Alternatively, a laryngoscope can be inserted into the mouth to view the tip of the tube. While the tube is slowly and gently advanced, its tip is gripped with forceps, or hooked with the hook created on the tip of a malleable stilette, and directed into the larynx.

Anaesthetic agents

Response to an anaesthetic agent or combination may be different between species, and may be different between individuals due to the level of pre-injection excitement or anxiety, and the degree of absorption from an IM site (Table 13.5).

Sedatives

Xylazine is often used as a sedative in doses of 0.4–0.6 mg/kg IV. This dose will provide 30–45 minutes of recumbency. Bradycardia will be induced with little change in blood pressure. Sedation can be reversed by tolazoline but not doxapram. There have been reports of adverse reactions in llamas after administration of tolazoline. Adverse signs in a llama after a large dose of tolazoline included anxiety, convulsions, salivation, tachypnoea, hypotension and diarrhoea (Read et al., 2000). Recommendations for tolazoline administration include maximum dose

Table 13.5 Anaesthetic and adjuncts agents used in healthy camelids			
Drug	**Dose rate**	**Route**	**Comments**
Xylazine	0.25–0.6 mg/kg	IV, IM	Provides sedation lasting 30–45 minutes
Medetomidine	0.01–0.03 mg/kg	IM	Dose-dependent sedation 1–2 hours
Diazepam	0.1–0.25 mg/kg	IV	Mild sedation, no analgesia. Adjunct to opioid or injectable anaesthetic agent
Midazolam	0.1–0.25 mg/kg	IV, IM	Mild sedation, no analgesia. Adjunct to opioid or injectable anaesthetic agent
Butorphanol	0.05–0.2 mg/kg	IV, IM	Mild sedation. Use to augment effects of other sedatives
Morphine	0.25 mg/kg	IM	Sedation and analgesia
Xylazine + ketamine	0.25 mg/kg 2.5 mg/kg	IV IV	Induction of general anaesthesia
Xylazine + ketamine	0.25 mg/kg 5 mg/kg	IV, IM IM	General anaesthesia. Higher doses may be required for alpacas
Xylazine + ketamine with midazolam or diazepam	0.25 mg/kg 2.5 mg/kg 0.1–0.2 mg/kg	IM IV IV	Induction of general anaesthesia. Diazepam or midazolam injected before ketamine or in the same syringe
Guaifenesin + ketamine	0.25–0.5 mL/kg 5% 2.5 mg/kg	IV IV	Induction of anaesthesia following premedication with low dose xylazine or butorphanol
Propofol	2–4 mg/kg	IV	Premedication with low dose xylazine or butorphanol and midazolam. Induction of anaesthesia
Atipamezole	0.125 mg/kg	IV, IM	Reversal of xylazine or medetomidine
Tolazoline	1–2 mg/kg	IM, half IV half IM	Reversal of xylazine. Slow IV injection over minutes, titrate

rate of 2 mg/kg to be given slowly IV or IM. Medetomidine produces dose-dependent light to heavy sedation in llamas, with 0.03 mg/kg IM inducing heavy sedation for 1 to 2 hours. The sedative effects of medetomidine can be reversed by IV atipamezole, 0.125 mg/kg. Midazolam, 0.5 mg/kg, IV or IM has been observed to induce moderate sedation in alpacas (Aarnes et al., 2012). Sedation was induced almost immediately after IV administration and lasted up to 75 minutes. Onset of sedation after IM injection was slower, about 15 minutes, and less intense.

Opioids

In clinical patients, butorphanol, 0.1 mg/kg IV or IM, is a useful adjunct to premedication to increase the degree of sedation and facilitate induction of anaesthesia. The dose should be decreased to 0.05 mg/kg IV for severely ill patients. The contribution of butorphanol to analgesia in camelids has not yet been defined. Butorphanol, 0.1 mg/kg, IM in llamas produced some antinociception to experimental compression over the withers but not at the metacarpus (Carroll et al., 2001). Heart rates were decreased, MAP was unchanged, and rectal temperatures increased. It appears that absorption of butorphanol from IM injection in llamas is rapid and complete, and clearance is greater than in horses and cows but less than in sheep and dogs (Carroll et al., 2001). The volume of distribution of butorphanol at steady state is smaller in llamas and that means that a small dose is needed to achieve a therapeutic concentration. The data support a slightly longer dosing interval for butorphanol in llamas than in dogs. Butorphanol also induces minimal cardiovascular effects in alpacas (Garcia-Pereira et al., 2007). Butorphanol, 0.1 mg/kg, injected IV in isoflurane-anaesthetized alpacas caused vasodilation but no significant effects in heart rates, mean arterial pressures, cardiac outputs, or blood gases.

Investigation of the pharmacokinetic and pharmacodynamic variables of morphine, 0.25 mg/kg IV, and 0.5 mg/kg IM and IV, in llamas identified a large apparent volume of distribution and high systemic clearance (Uhrig et al., 2007). Intramuscular administration prolonged the terminal half-life but had no effect on bioavailablity. Greater sedation and for longer, all ≤2 hours, was achieved with the larger dose. Antinociception was tested using cutaneous electrical stimulation over the metacarpus or brachium, however, reliable analgesia could not be demonstrated for any dose because of high individual variability among the llamas. A dose-dependent increase in rectal temperature was measured, lasting up to 8 hours after administration of the highest dose. Muscle tremors were observed in llamas following administration of 0.5 mg/kg, therefore, the lower dose of morphine, 0.25 mg/kg, was recommended for administration every 4 hours. The authors pointed out that their animals were

healthy and different effects could be obtained in llamas in pain.

Guaifenesin

Guaifenesin, up to 0.5 ml/kg of a 5% solution, is a useful adjunct to anaesthetic induction with ketamine in adult llamas and alpacas. Premedication facilitates the procedure and can consist of a low dose of xylazine, or a combination of diazepam, 0.1 mg/kg, and butorphanol, 0.1 mg/kg, IV. Guaifenesin is most easily injected into the jugular catheter using a 60 ml syringe and a 14 gauge needle. The llama will usually assume sternal recumbency following injection of a half dose of guaifenesin, and ketamine, 2.5 mg/kg, with all or part of the remainder of guaifenesin injected to complete induction of anaesthesia and relaxation sufficient for tracheal intubation. Dose rates of anaesthetic agents must be decreased for animals that are ill, for example, with urethral obstruction, peritonitis, or intestinal obstruction. Xylazine should be avoided in animals with urethral obstruction.

Ketamine

A common anaesthetic combination to provide 30 minutes of anaesthesia in healthy llamas is xylazine, 0.25 mg/kg IV, followed in 10–15 minutes by injection of ketamine, 2.5 mg/kg IV or 5 mg/kg IM. Butorphanol, 0.1 mg/kg IM, can be administered at the same time as the xylazine or 0.05 mg/kg IV, shortly before the ketamine. An alternative combination is xylazine premedication followed by induction of anaesthesia with IV diazepam or midazolam, 0.1–0.2 mg/kg, and ketamine 2.5 mg/kg.

A comparison of xylazine, 0.4 mg/kg, with ketamine, 4 mg/kg, and xylazine 0.8 g/kg, with ketamine, 8 mg/kg, all administered IM to llamas revealed onset time to lateral recumbency of 5–16 minutes, duration of lateral recumbency that was variable for the low dose rates and 69–106 minutes for the high dose rates (DuBois et al., 2004). Hypoxaemia was noted in llamas receiving the high dose rates and was corrected by nasal insufflation of O_2. Tolazoline, 2 mg/kg, IM, shortened the duration of recovery.

Alpacas may require higher dose rates of xylazine and ketamine than llamas. In one investigation of anaesthesia in alpacas induced by combined IM injections of xylazine and ketamine, doses of xylazine, 0.8 mg/kg, and ketamine, 8 mg/kg, induced anaesthesia for an average of 23 (range 0–45) minutes whereas higher doses of xylazine, 1.2 mg/kg, and ketamine, 12 mg/kg, induced anaesthesia for an average of 52 minutes, with the exception of one alpaca that never assumed lateral recumbency (Prado et al., 2008b). Lateral recumbency was assumed on average by 6 minutes in five out of six alpacas in both groups; the unresponsive alpaca was a different animal in each group. Heart rates decreased and mean arterial pressures were maintained at satisfactory values. All animals in the high dose group were hypoxic after induction of anaesthesia and, therefore, facilities to provide oxygen supplementation should be available when using that protocol.

A combination of medetomidine, 10 mg, ketamine, 300 mg, and butorphanol, 30 mg, was administered IM by dart to seven male captive guanaco (*Lama guanicoe*) weighing 112 ± 10.9 kg (Georoff et al., 2010). Mean time to recumbency was 5 minutes (range, 3–12 minutes) and the animals were approached at 20 minutes. Heart rates were between 24 and 52 beats/minutes, mean blood pressure measurements (four animals) 105–182 mmHg, respiratory rates 20 to 44 breaths/minutes, and mean PaO_2 8.76 ± 0.02 kPa (65.9 ± 14.8 mmHg) before oxygen supplementation. Anaesthesia reversal was successfully accomplished by IM atipamezole, 0.45 ± 0.04 mg/kg and naltrexone, 2.7 ± 0.25 mg/kg administered a minimum of 30 minutes after the initial injection of anaesthetic agents.

The combination of ketamine, 5 mg/kg, and midazolam, 0.25 mg/kg, IV is also used for induction of anaesthesia in alpacas prior to inhalation anaesthesia (Vincent et al., 2009). This combination works well following premedication with butorphanol.

Propofol

Propofol, 2.0–3.5 mg/kg IV, can be used for induction of anaesthesia. Anaesthesia may be maintained with an inhalation agent or by continuous infusion of propofol, 0.3–0.4 mg/kg/min. In an investigation of continuous propofol anaesthesia in llamas, MAP remained high and cardiac output was not depressed (Duke et al., 1997). Hypoxaemia did not develop even though the animals were breathing air. Additional analgesia, systemic or local, will be necessary if the procedure is painful.

Alfaxalone

Administration of alfaxalone, 2.1 mg/kg, IV for anaesthesia has been compared with propofol, 3.3 mg/kg, IV and ketamine–diazepam, 4.4 mg/kg–0.22 mg/kg, IV in alpacas (del Alamo et al., 2012). Induction of anaesthesia was good to excellent with all agents. Oxygen supplementation was judged necessary based on SpO_2 <90% or $ETCO_2$ >60 mmHg initially in all but three anaesthetic episodes. Duration of anaesthesia was significantly longer with alfaxalone, mean 34 minutes compared with 19 minutes with propofol and 25 minutes with ketamine–diazepam. Of concern was the poor recovery from alfaxalone anaesthesia that included paddling, twitching, and uncoordinated rolling over. Inclusion of a sedative for premedication or transfer to inhalation anaesthesia is advisable to achieve a better recovery.

Tiletamine–zolazepam

Administration of tiletamine–zolazepam, 2 mg/kg, IM in llamas premedicated 30 minutes before anaesthesia with

IM acepromazine, 0.05 mg/kg, or butorphanol, 0.1 or 0.2 mg/kg, or acepromazine and butorphanol, 0.1 mg/kg, induced lateral recumbency for approximately 90 ± 10 minutes and a time to standing of approximately 100 ± 11 minutes (Prado et al., 2008a). Antinociception, evaluated by lack of movement in response to application of forceps on a digit, developed on average for 14–17 minutes for butorphanol–tiletamine–zolazepam anaesthesia and an average of 35–40 minutes when acepromazine was included for premedication. Respiratory rates and MAP were unchanged whereas blood gas analysis after 5 and 15 minutes of anaesthesia revealed hypoxaemia during all agent combinations.

Administration of xylazine, 0.2 or 0.4 mg/kg, IM with tiletamine–zolazepam, 2 mg/kg, IM to llamas provided antinociception suitable for short procedures for 30 and 51 minutes, respectively (Seddighi et al., 2012). Heart rates decreased significantly and hypoxaemia was present for 15 minutes in some of the llamas receiving xylazine.

Inhalation agents

Maintenance of anaesthesia with isoflurane or sevoflurane is recommended for major surgery. Inhalant agents are administered from a small animal machine with an adult circle circuit, a 5 L bag, and an oxygen flow of 1–2 L/min for adult llamas and alpacas. The MAC for isoflurane in llamas was measured at 1.05 ± 0.17% (sea level equivalent of 1.45% measured at the elevation of Fort Collins, CO, USA) (Mama et al., 1999), and MAC for sevoflurane in llamas was 2.3 ± 0.14% and in alpacas 2.3 ± 0.09% (Grubb et al., 2003). Mean MAC for desflurane in llamas was 8 ± 0.58% and in alpacas 7.8 ± 0.51% (Grubb et al., 2006). Evaluation of six adult llamas anaesthetized with only isoflurane identified a dose-dependent decrease in MAP with increased depth of anaesthesia (Mama et al., 2001). Heart rates progressively increased with time, and that may partly be due to increased $PaCO_2$ in spontaneously breathing animals. Institution of controlled ventilation had no significant effect on the measured cardiovascular parameters, although cardiac output tended to be lower than when the animals were breathing spontaneously.

Mask induction is easy in paediatric patients, particularly after premedication with diazepam or midazolam and butorphanol.

Anaesthetic management

Anaesthetic management is as for sheep and goats described previously in this chapter. The palpebral reflex is usually retained during anaesthesia adequate for surgery. Crinkling of the lower eyelid is an indication of light anaesthesia. Eyelid aperture increases with increasing depth of isoflurane anaesthesia (Mama et al., 2001). Since the eyes are protruberant, care must be taken to avoid corneal scratches by using eye lubricant and closing the

373

eye in contact with a hard surface, and lifting the head any time the animal is moved. Llamas and alpacas breathe spontaneously at 15–25 breaths/minute and appear to ventilate better during anaesthesia than horses or adult cattle. Nonetheless, oxygen should be available for admin istration by mask or nasal tube during total intravenous anaesthesia. Haemoglobin O_2 affinity of camelids is higher than that of humans, dogs, and sheep (see Chapter 2). For example, O_2 content of llama blood at PO_2 6.7 kPa (50 mmHg) is similar to that of sheep blood at 8 kPa (60 mmHg) (Moraga et al., 1996). Despite this advantage, O_2 content is dependent in part on the position of the O_2 dissociation curve and that will be shifted to the right by hypercarbia during anaesthesia, and O_2 delivery is dependent on cardiac output, blood pressure and tissue perfusion, all of which may be decreased during anaesthesia. Parameters for controlled ventilation that will achieve normocarbia are 10–12 breaths/minute at tidal volumes of 15 mL/kg, usually achieved at an inspiratory pressure of 20 cmH$_2$O. When capnography is available, these parameters can be adjusted to maintain ETCO$_2$ at approximately 40 mmHg.

Heart rates are commonly between 60 and 80 beats/min and MAP should be kept above 65 mmHg. Blood pressure can be measured as described for sheep and goats. Balanced electrolyte solutions should be infused at 5–10 mL/kg/h and, in addition in animals <3 months of age, 5% dextrose infused at 3 mL/kg/h. The infusion rate of dextrose should be adjusted based on measurement of blood glucose. A recent report of measurements of blood glucose in alpacas compared results from three point-of-care meters with laboratory measurements (Tennent-Brown et al., 2011). For glucose concentrations between 50 and 200 mg/dL, the limits of agreement were acceptable using whole blood samples for the i-Stat (Abbott Point-of Care Inc., Princeton, NJ, USA) and the AlphaTrak (Abbott Animal Health, Abbott Park, Ill, USA) but only for plasma samples with the Accu-Chek Aviva (Roche Diagnostics, Indianapolis, Ind, USA).

Management of hypotension or decreased peripheral perfusion should include a crystalloid fluid challenge of 10 mL/kg, and/or infusion of hetastarch 5–10 mL/kg over 15 minutes, and/or IV infusion of a catecholamine such as dobutamine, dopamine, or ephedrine. Infusion of dobutamine, 4 µg/kg/min, to alpacas anaesthetized with isoflurane resulted in increased heart rates, MAP, cardiac output, and O_2 delivery to tissues, and no further improvement obtained by increasing the dose rate to 8 µg/kg/min (Vincent et al., 2009). In the same study, norepinephrine, 0.3 and 1 µg/kg/min, IV produced similar effects.

A progressive decrease in body temperature develops during inhalation anaesthesia and efforts should be applied to maintain a normal temperature.

Extubation after anaesthesia should be delayed, as in other ruminants, until the animal can withdraw its tongue into its mouth, and this may occur long after the first swallowing and chewing movements are observed. The animal should be in a sternal head-up position for extubation.

Deer

INTRODUCTION

There are detailed recommendations elsewhere for handling farmed deer, including recommendations for design of deer yards and raceways, deer crushes and chutes, and physical and chemical restraint (Chapman et al., 1987; Fletcher, 1995). Some general guidelines for working with deer include talking to the deer to alert them as to your location and to avoid walking through the middle of a group of deer (Fletcher, 1995). Recommendations are that, except for adult stags, deer are best examined in groups, as they may become frantic when isolated. Deer may become aggressive and kick with their forelimbs, and occasionally bite or kick backward with their hind limbs.

There are considerations of special significance to the anaesthetist. Not only are there differences in responses between farmed deer and wildlife, in that wild deer will require higher doses, but also there are differences between the species in their responses to both physical management and anaesthetic agents. An example given in a concise article on deer handling explains that fallow deer (*Dama dama*), unlike red deer (*Cervus elaphus*), respond favourably to darkened holding pens (Fletcher, 1995). Another author notes that while roe deer (*Capreolus capreolus*) or fallow deer may lie impassive when blindfolded and with their legs tied, the technique is not suitable for muntjac (*Muntiacus reevesi*). Muntjac are small excitable deer that will writhe, struggle and jerk violently against restraint (Chapman et al., 1987). Axis deer (*Axis axis*) are also described as nervous and excitable (Sontakke et al., 2007).

ANAESTHETIC AGENTS

Anaesthetic agents for sedation are frequently administered by darts propelled by a gun or blowpipe, or from a syringe attached to a pole. Injection by hand will require considerable force and a moderately large gauge needle as the skin is tough. Responses to anaesthetic agents may be different between free-ranging and tame deer. Whenever possible food and water should be withheld similar to preanaesthetic preparation for sheep and goats. Respiratory depression and hypoxaemia are common problems during anaesthesia. Monitoring respiratory rates and measurement of haemoglobin O_2 saturation with a pulse oximeter are valuable for detecting inadequate ventilation and oxygenation, although black pigmentation of the mucosa or skin and vasoconstriction from medetomidine may interfere with accurate readings. Administration of O_2 by insufflation through a tube inserted in the nose at 5–10 L/min, a facemask, or anaesthesia machine in the clinic setting will increase arterial oxygenation. Simple devices for non-invasive measurement of blood pressure are available and can be used in a field environment. Direct measurement of arterial pressure can be done with a catheter in an auricular artery. Deer may become hypothermic or hyperthermic during anaesthesia and rectal temperature should always be monitored.

There are several published anaesthetic protocols using a variety of different dose rates. Most of them are directed towards immobilization in the field for short procedures. Deer that are admitted to the clinic for diagnostic or surgical procedures can be intubated and anaesthesia maintained with an inhalation agent. The vaporizer settings are initially low for maintenance of anaesthesia to adjust for the effects of the immobilizing doses of injectable anaesthetic agents. Anaesthetic management is similar to that for sheep and goats and may include continuous infusion(s) of lidocaine, ketamine, or an opioid, local analgesia blocks, or morphine epidural, depending on the location and type of surgical procedure. Medetomidine used for premedication to inhalation anaesthesia appears to persist into the recovery and administration of atipamezole may result in abrupt wakening from sedation. Manual restraint of the deer may be difficult and the environment for recovery should be devoid of projections that might cause injury and must have walls high enough to prevent escape.

Xylazine

The dose rate for xylazine varies between breeds and response to xylazine varies between individuals within a breed. Xylazine alone can be administered IM for sedation in penned red or fallow deer at 0.5–1.5 mg/kg (Fletcher, 1995), 1 mg/kg for wapiti (North American elk; *Cervus canadiensis*), and 2–3 mg/kg for white-tailed deer (*Odocoileus virginianus*) and mule deer (*Odocoileus hemionus*) (Caulkett, 1997). A lower dosage of xylazine, 0.7 mg/kg, was satisfactory for capturing 104 free-ranging mule deer (Jessup et al., 1985). Reversal of sedation is achieved by administration of yohimbine, 0.1–0.2 mg/kg, given half IV and half IM, or tolazoline, 2 mg/kg. More recent publications have recommended tolazoline and atipamezole as more effective antagonists than yohimbine.

Xylazine and ketamine

Xylazine and ketamine have been used to immobilize deer. Dosages of xylazine, 4 mg/kg, and ketamine, 4 mg/kg, administered IM in adult fallow deer induced recumbency in less than 5 minutes (Stewart & English,

1990). Administration of yohimbine 30 minutes later produced satisfactory reversal for release after several minutes. Another recommendation is to mix 400 mg of ketamine with 500 mg of dry xylazine powder and to dose red deer at 1–2 mL, IM and fallow deer up to 3 mL (Fletcher, 1995). Xylazine and ketamine may be administered separately. The deer are sedated first with xylazine administered by dart and ketamine, 1–2 mg/kg, is injected IV when the deer is first approachable (Caulkett, 1997). This decreases the dose of ketamine and there is less chance of CNS excitement occurring when the xylazine sedation is reversed. Additional ketamine may be administered as needed. An investigation of different dose combinations in Axis deer described xylazine, 0.5 mg/kg, and ketamine, 2.5 mg/kg, administered by dart and blowpipe as inducing satisfactory anaesthesia in male deer in 7–8 minutes (Sontakke et al., 2007). The authors preferred xylazine, 1.0 mg/kg, and ketamine, 1.5 mg/kg, for female deer as this combination resulted in longer duration, up to 40 minutes, of anaesthesia. Immobilization was reversed by IV injection of yohimbine, 5–10 mg. All deer survived.

Medetomidine combinations

Medetomidine, 0.06–0.08 mg/kg, IM administered with ketamine, 1–2 mg/kg, IM is a useful combination to sedate deer. The effects of medetomidine can be reversed by injection of atipamezole at a dose rate up to five times the medetomidine dose. Mule deer and mule deer hybrids were immobilized by medetomidine, 0.1 mg/kg, and ketamine, 2.5 mg/kg, IM for 60 minutes followed by reversal with atipamezole, 0.5 mg/kg, injected half IV and half IM (Caulkett et al., 2000). Blood gas analysis revealed hypoxaemia and the authors recommended use of supplemental oxygen with this anaesthetic protocol. Other studies (Mich et al., 2008; Miller et al., 2009) have evaluated in white-tailed deer a combination of butorphanol, azaperone, and medetomidine, at approximate dosages of 0.43 mg/kg, 0.36 mg/kg, 0.14 mg/kg, or 0.34 mg/kg, 0.27 mg/kg, 0.11 mg/kg, or 0.30 mg/kg, 0.16 mg/kg, 0.20 mg/kg, respectively. Results from the third dose rate combination included times to sternal and lateral recumbency on average 8 and 13 minutes, respectively, and an excellent rated quality of induction. Respiration rates were variable and hypoxaemia was identified using pulse oximetry. Immobilization was reversed with naltrexone, tolazoline, and atipamezole. Nasal oxygen supplementation of 3–8 L/min was recommended for animals with respiratory rates <15 breaths/min or SpO_2 <90% at sea level; a lower value at higher altitudes.

Tiletamine–zolazepam

Tiletamine–zolazepam, 1.5 mg/kg, with xylazine, 1.6 mg/kg, IM was compared with tiletamine–zolazepam, 1.0 mg/kg, and medetomidine, 0.099 mg/kg, IM administered to fallow deer by darts delivered by a CO_2-powered rifle (Fernández-Morán et al., 2000). These combinations resulted in recumbent immobilization in most animals on average 6–8 minutes after administration. Respiratory rates were low but hypoxaemia was not detected by pulse oximetry or blood gas analysis. Of the two drug combinations, tiletamine-zolazepam with medetomidine produced a deeper plane of anaesthesia sufficient for minor surgical procedures. White-tailed deer administered tiletamine–zolazepam, 220 mg, approximately 4.5 mg/kg, and xylazine, 110 mg, approximately 4 mg/kg, IM were immobilized to lateral recumbency in 3 minutes (Miller et al., 2004). Evaluation of yohimbine, tolazoline, and atipamezole for reversal of xylazine documented that tolazoline, 200 mg, 4.0 mg/kg, and atipamezole, 11 mg, 0.23 mg/kg, injected half IV and half subcutaneously produced more rapid and effective reversal than yohimbine. A previous investigation of this anaesthetic protocol recorded hypoxaemia in the animals; average SpO_2 85%, range 72–94% (Miller et al., 2003). Captive red deer weighing 90–135 kg were immobilized with xylazine, 1.79 ± 0.29 mg/kg, and tiletamine–zolazepam, 1.79 ± 0.29 mg/kg, administered IM with a dart gun (Auer et al., 2010). Anaesthesia was maintained for surgical implantation of telemetry devices by continuous infusions of ketamine, midazolam, and either xylazine or detomidine. Ketamine, 1000 mg, midazolam, 15 mg, and either xylazine, 250 mg, or detomidine, 1.4 mg, were added to a 500 mL bag of saline and infused with an infusion pump at a rate of 1.2 mL/kg/h for the first 20 minutes followed by a 10% decrease in rate at 10-minute intervals. The deer were intubated and connected to an anaesthesia machine delivering 30–50% inspired O_2. Arterial pressures were satisfactory but capnography and blood gas analysis revealed moderate to severe hypoventilation. Recoveries were excellent after IV administration of 10 mg atipamezole and 1 mg sarmazenil (midazolam antagonist).

Camels

INTRODUCTION

Handling camels can be dangerous and particular caution must be observed during the breeding season when males may be intractable and vicious. Males may press a person to the ground with their neck and body, a crushing effect, or they may bite, causing severe, even fatal, injuries (Ogunbodede & Arotiba, 1997). Domestic camel may sit on command (couched), which avoids the need for casting or the risk of injury with ataxia or falling after administration of anaesthetic agents.

Heart rates in unsedated resting camels are 40–50 beats/min, mean arterial pressures 130–140 mmHg, and respiratory rates 6–16 breaths/min. Haematological and biochemical blood values for camels (*Camelus dromedarius*) have been published (Snow et al., 1988; Nazefi & Maleki, 1998). Measurements made after racing show that, in contrast to dogs and horses, no significant increase in haematocrit occurs after exercise. Although packed cell volume is on average 0.33 L/L (33%), camel erythrocytes have a very high mean corpuscular haemoglobin concentration.

Voluntary regurgitation of rumen contents may occur in agitated camels and withholding of roughage for 48 hours, concentrate for 24 hours, and water for 12 hours before anaesthesia has been recommended.

ANAESTHETIC AGENTS

Satisfactory anaesthesia for tracheal intubation was achieved in six camels (*Camelus dromedarius*) with a mean thiopental dose of 7.25 mg/kg (Singh et al., 1994). Subsequent maintenance with halothane resulted in hypoventilation and a significant decrease in blood pressure. Oxygen supplementation was necessary during recovery from anaesthesia to prevent hypoxaemia. Anaesthesia can also be induced with a mixture of thiopental and guaifenesin prior to inhalation anaesthesia. In camels injected IM with xylazine, 0.25 mg/kg, 30 minutes previously, 1.0–2.3 mL/kg of thiopental–guaifenesin (2 g thiopental in 1 L 5% guaifenesin) given rapidly IV produced sufficient relaxation for intubation (White et al., 1986). Controlled ventilation was employed to treat hypoventilation and MAP was satisfactory.

Xylazine, detomidine, medetomidine, and romifidine can be used for sedation in camels. Analgesia duration is shorter than duration of sedation. Maximal sedation, analgesia and recumbency was achieved with romifidine, 0.125 mg/kg, IV in healthy camels (Marzok & El-Khodery, 2009). Sedation was induced within 3 minutes and lasted an average of 65 minutes; duration of analgesia was an average of 45 minutes. Sedation was accompanied by lowering of the head, pronounced ataxia, and recumbency. Lower doses produced sedation that was less intense and of shorter duration with minimal analgesia. Decreased ruminal contractions, increased blood glucose, and increased urination during recovery were observed. Sedation may be increased, or the dose rate of the α_2-agent decreased, by the addition of butorphanol, 0.05–0.1 mg/kg.

Xylazine, 0.25 mg/kg, has been combined with ketamine, 2.5 mg/kg, IM for sedation and anaesthesia in the dromedary camel (White et al., 1987). Loss of facial expression, drooping of the lower lip, weaving of the head, and drooling of saliva (loss of swallowing reflex) occurs at the onset of sedation. Most camels lay their head and neck on the ground and would assume lateral recumbency if allowed. Anaesthesia can be deepened or maintained by intermittent IV injections of diazepam, 0.05 mg/kg, and ketamine, 2 mg/kg, or by infusion of guaifenesin-ketamine, for TIVA or an inhalation agent. Injectable anaesthetic agents can be administered in low dosage to achieve heavy sedation or in higher dosage to induce general anaesthesia. In either case, analgesia for the procedure (castration, urethrostomy, dental) can be provided by local analgesia.

Intubation of the trachea in adult camels can be done manually using the same techniques that are used in cattle. Intubation may be more easily performed with the camel in sternal rather than lateral position. The head and neck should be fully extended and the anaesthetist's hand with the endotracheal tube introduced until the laryngeal entrance can be palpated. The anaesthetist's fingers hold open the larynx while the tube is advanced forward with the other hand. Male dromedary camels have a dulaa (palatal flap or goola pouch) that extends from the soft palate and must be avoided during intubation. After intubation and lateral recumbency, the camel's head should be elevated with towels or padding to minimize nasal mucosa congestion, and the nose positioned below the pharynx to allow drainage of saliva and regurgitated fluid (Fig. 13.14). Bloat may develop during anaesthesia despite withholding of food and water previously. Supplementation with 15 L/min O_2 is recommended for injectable anaesthesia, into the endotracheal tube during anaesthesia and into the nose for recovery. A pulse oximeter probe can be placed on the tongue to monitor oxygenation and a cuff on the tail for oscillometric measurement of blood pressure. Mean arterial pressure should be approximately 100 mmHg with injectable anaesthetic agents and above 65 mmHg during inhalation anaesthesia. The heart rate

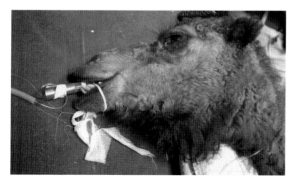

Figure 13.14 The camel's head is elevated (with a towel in this picture) to allow drainage from the pharynx of saliva and regurgitated fluid (which occurred towards the end of the surgical procedure) and to prevent contamination of the right eye. The diameter of the rubber tubing delivering oxygen was too large to be inserted into the endotracheal tube, therefore, one end of venous extension tubing was attached to the rubber tube and the other end (after the adapter was cut off) inserted into the endotracheal tube.

will be slow in the presence of an α_2-agonist. The camel should be moved into sternal position for recovery from anaesthesia and extubation delayed until the tongue appears to be functional. Atipamezole may be used to reverse residual α_2-agonist sedation.

LOCAL ANALGESIA

Nerve blocks of the hind limbs in camels have been described, including the topographical anatomy and technique to block the peroneal, tibial, and plantar nerves (Dudi et al., 1984). Desensitization of the digit can also be achieved using intravenous regional analgesia by injecting 60 mL of 2% lidocaine (without epinephrine) distal to a tourniquet (Purohit et al., 1985).

Xylazine sedation has been combined with a line block with 2% lidocaine to provide satisfactory restraint and analgesia for caesarian section to remove dead calves (Elias, 1991). Epidural analgesia with lidocaine has been combined with sedation for urethrostomy in camels with urethral obstruction. There are anecdotal reports of improved analgesia by inclusion of xylazine or detomidine with the lidocaine for epidural block.

Elephants

INTRODUCTION

Drug administration to free-ranging elephants is by dart gun. Trained elephants are usually relatively quiet and intravenous injection can be made into an ear vein. Accurate estimates of body weight are useful when calculating drug dosages in an attempt to produce consistent anaesthetic effects. Body measurements from 75 Asian elephants (*Elephas maximus*) from 1 to 57 years of age were used to calculate correlations with body weight (Hile et al., 1997). The authors concluded that in Asian elephants the heart girth is the best predictor of weight. Heart girth (cm) was measured just behind the front legs using cotton twine. Weight was predicted using the equation:

$$\text{Weight (kg)} = 18.0 \, (\text{heart girth}) - 3336.$$

Measurement of pad circumference was not a useful predictor of weight.

ANAESTHETIC AGENTS

Medetomidine, 0.003 or 0.005 mg/kg, IM has been used to induce sedation in working Indian elephants

(2000–3000 kg) for producing restraint and performing minor procedures (Sarma et al., 2002). At the higher dose rate, sedation of the elephants was profound with head and ear drooping and severe ataxia, and the animals were unresponsive to verbal commands. Bradycardia and decreased respiratory rates were recorded, however, oxygenation was not measured.

Etorphine has frequently been used to immobilize elephants. Free-ranging African elephants (*Loxodonta africana*) were immobilized by IM injection by darts with 9.5 ± 0.5 mg etorphine (Osofsky, 1997) or 3, 6, or 9 mg of etorphine and 30, 60, or 100 mg of azaperone according to size in juvenile elephants (mean weight 672 kg) (Still et al., 1996). The mean time to recumbency was 9 minutes. Additional etorphine had to be administered IV to maintain immobilization for transportation. All elephants recovered without complication after reversal by IV diprenorphine at approximately three times the dose of etorphine administered. The twenty African elephants that were administered etorphine, 9.5 ± 0.5 mg and 2000 IU hyaluronidase by IM dart (Osofsky, 1997) were immobilized within 5-14 minutes for an average of 30 minutes. Injection of diprenorphine, 24 mg IV with or without an additional half dose administered IM achieved satisfactory reversal. In another report, 10 wild Asian elephants (*Elephas maximus*) were immobilized by IM injection of 3.3 (2.5–4.5) mL of etorphine and acepromazine (LA Immobilon®; etorphine, 2.45 mg/mL, and acepromazine, 10 mg/mL) (Dangolla et al., 2004). The body weight was estimated using the formula: 227 kg/30 cm of visually estimated shoulder height; a distance that tended to be overestimated based on actual measurement made later in the immobilized animals. The authors also commented that the dose rate was greater than previously used in domestic elephants. Time to recumbency was 18 (15–45) minutes and nine elephants assumed lateral recumbency while the tenth required an additional 0.5 ml for complete relaxation. Duration of recumbency was 42 (28–61) minutes. The etorphine was reversed by injection of an equal volume of Revivon® (diprenorphine, 3.26 mg/mL) and the time to standing was 6 (2–12) minutes. Another published report of castration of elephants described IM or IV injection of etorphine, 0.002 mg/kg, to provide satisfactory immobilization for the procedure, with supplements of 1 mg etorphine injected as needed (Foerner et al., 1994).

Elephants are positioned in lateral recumbency during anaesthesia because breathing is severely compromised in the sternal position. Adequacy of ventilation is a feature in larger animals because the anatomical features of elephants oppose collapse of lung. Elephants lack a pleural space and there is a well-developed supportive system of elastic fibres in the lungs and pulmonary vessels. Reported average respiratory rates are 7–9 breaths/min, with a mild to moderate increase in $PaCO_2$. However, a proportion of elephants immobilized with etorphine are reported to be hypoxaemic as determined by pulse oximetry or blood gas analysis. The average PaO_2 of the immobilized elephants in one study, 10.0 ± 1.7 kPa (75 ± 13 mmHg) (Still et al., 1996), was lower than previously reported for recumbent elephants, 11.2 ± 0.4 kPa (84 ± 3 mmHg), or standing unpremedicated elephants, 12.8 ± 0.3 kPa (96 ± 2 mmHg) (Honeyman et al., 1992). The overall mean SpO_2 in 16 immobilized adult elephants was 87.3 ± 2.8% (70–96%) (Osofsky, 1997). In another group of five adult female elephants (3000–3500 kg) immobilized with 10–12 mg of etorphine (Horne et al., 2001), initial PaO_2 values and SpO_2 were 8.4 kPa (63 mmHg), range 5.3–10.2 kPa (40–77 mmHg) and 95 % (75–99 %), respectively. The elephants were intubated with a 35 mm endotracheal tube and controlled ventilation with oxygen achieved using two demand valves in parallel. The demand valves were connected to a single oxygen tank by means of 'Y' assembly and the oxygen cylinder reducing valve was set to an outlet pressure of 60–80 psi (Horne et al., 2001). The outlets of the demand valves were connected to one side of a large animal circle Y-piece while the other side of the Y-piece was plugged with a rubber stopper. The demand valves were activated to achieve inhalation and the stopper removed to allow exhalation. End-tidal CO_2 concentrations were on average 11–13 mmHg lower than measured $PaCO_2$ values during spontaneous or controlled breathing (Horne et al., 2001).

Mean arterial blood pressures measured from a 20 gauge catheter in an auricular artery in two groups of adult African elephants, weighing approximately 3000 or 5000 kg, immobilized with etorphine were 102 mmHg (80–115 mmHg) (Horne et al., 2001) and 186 ± 15 mmHg. A value of 145 ± 3 mmHg for MAP has been reported for standing elephants (Honeyman et al., 1992).

INHALATION ANAESTHESIA

General anaesthesia can be maintained in elephants with inhalation agents when the equipment is available. A standard large animal machine, or two machines in tandem, with a weather balloon replacing the usual rebreathing bag can used for an adult elephant (Heard et al., 1988; Dunlop et al., 1994; Fowler et al., 2000). Induction of immobilization is commonly with etorphine, with or without other agents. Induction of anaesthesia in juvenile (3–5-year-old) African elephants weighing 308 ± 93 kg was achieved with xylazine, 0.1 mg/kg, and ketamine, 0.6 mg/kg, IM followed by IM etorphine, 0.0019 ± 0.00056 mg (Heard et al., 1988). A 198 kg, 3-month-old calf was sedated with xylazine, 0.1 mg/kg, and ketamine, 1.6 mg/kg, IM and subsequently anaesthetized by IV injection of ketamine and diazepam (Abou-Madi et al., 2004). Extraordinary management is required in some cases to ensure safety of the animal and personnel during induction and recovery, in this case, construction of a sling and lift for an elephant with degenerative joint disease (Fowler et al., 2000).

Endotracheal tubes of 18, 22, and 26 mm can be used in elephants weighing 250–304 kg, 204–350 kg, and 280–636 kg, respectively (Heard et al., 1988) and 30–40 mm in adult elephants (Dunlop et al., 1994; Fowler et al., 2000). Wads of food may be present in the oropharynx despite food having been withheld for 24 hours. The trachea can be intubated blindly or by manual palpation of the larynx and guiding the endotracheal tube into the trachea or with the aid of a stomach tube inserted in the trachea. Low vaporizer settings may be adequate to maintain anaesthesia.

Depth of anaesthesia may be monitored using eye signs and respiratory rates. Increases in trunk muscle tone and ear flapping are indicators that the depth of anaesthesia is getting light. An electrocardiogram can be used to monitor heart rate. A non-invasive oscillometric blood pressure cuff can be placed around the tail or a catheter inserted in an ear artery facilitates measurement of blood pressure directly. Balanced electrolyte solution can be administered IV and dobutamine infused to treat hypotension.

The inhalation agent is usually discontinued for up to 30 minutes before a reversal agent, diprenorphine or naltrexone, is injected. Oxygen administration is continued as long as possible.

REFERENCES

Aarnes, T., Fry, P., Hubbell, J., et al., 2012. The pharmacokinetics and pharmacodynamics of midazolam in alpacas. In: Proceedings of the 18th IVEECS Symposium. San Antonio, TX, USA. p. 726.

Abou-Madi, N., Kollias, G.V., Hackett, R.P., et al., 2004. Umbilical herniorrhaphy in a juvenile Asian elephant (Elephas maximus). J Zoo Wildlife Med 35, 221–225.

Abu-Serriah, M., Nolan, A.M., Dolan, S., 2007. Pain assessment following experimental maxillofacial surgical procedure in sheep. Lab Anim 41, 345–352.

Adami, C., Bergadano, A., Bruckmaier, R.M., et al., 2011. Sciatic-femoral nerve block with bupivacaine in goats undergoing elective stifle arthrotomy. Vet J 188, 53–57.

Ahern, B.J., Soma, L.R., Boston, R.C., et al., 2009. Comparison of the analgesic properties of transdermally administered fentanyl and intramuscularly administered buprenorphine during and following experimental orthopedic surgery in sheep. Am J Vet Res 70, 418–422.

Alahuhta, S., Kangas-Saarela, T., Hollmen, A.I., et al., 1990. Visceral pain during caesarian section under spinal and epidural anaesthesia with bupivacaine. Acta Anaesth Scand 34, 95–98.

Alibhai, H.I.K., 2001. Aspects of inhalation anaesthesia in the goat. PhD dissertation. University of London, London.

Aminkov, B.Y., Hubenov, H.D., 1995. The effect of xylazine epidural anaesthesia on blood gas and acid base parameters in rams. Br Vet J 151, 579–585.

Amsel, S.I., Kainer, R.A., Johnson, L.W., 1987. Choosing the best site to perform venipuncture in a llama. Vet Med 82, 535–536.

Andaluz, A., Felez-Ocaña, N., Santos, L., et al., 2012. The effects on cardio-respiratory and acid-base variables of the anaesthetic alfaxalone in a 2-hydroxypropyl-b-cyclodextrin (HPCD) formulation in sheep. Vet J 191, 389–392.

Anderson, D.E., 2009. Uterine torsion and cesarean section in llamas and alpacas. Vet Clin N Am Food Anim Pract 25, 523–538.

Auer, U., Wenger, S., Beigelbock, C., et al., 2010. Total intravenous anesthesia with midazolam, ketamine, and xylazine or detomidine following induction with tiletamine, zolazepam, and xylazine in red deer (Cervus elaphus hippelaphus) undergoing surgery. J Wildlife Dis 46, 1196–1203.

Barrington, G.M., Meyer, T.F., Parish, S.M., 1993. Standing castration of the llama using butorphanol tartrate and local anesthesia. Equine Pract 15, 35–39.

Bedforth, N.M., Hardman, J.G., 2010. The hidden cost of neuraxial anaesthesia (Editorial). Anaesthesia 65, 437–439.

Carroll, G.L., Boothe, D.M., Hartsfield, S.M., et al., 2001. Pharmacokinetics and pharmacodynamics of butorphanol in llamas after intravenous and intramuscular administration. J Am Vet Med Assoc 219, 1263–1267.

Carroll, G.L., Hooper, R.N., Boothe, D.M., et al., 1999. Pharmacokinetics of fentanyl after intravenous and transdermal administration in goats. Am J Vet Res 60, 986–991.

Carroll, G.L., Hooper, R.N., Slater, M.R., et al., 1998. Detomidine-butorphanol-propofol for carotid artery translocation and castration or ovariectomy in goats. Vet Surg 27, 75–82.

Caulkett, N., 1997. Anesthesia for North American cervids. Can Vet J 38, 389–390.

Caulkett, N.A., Cribb, P.H., Duke, T., 1994. Cardiopulmonary effects of medetomidine-ketamine immobilization with atipamezole reversal and carfentanil-xylazine immobilization with naltrexone reversal: a comparative study in domestic sheep (Ovis ovis). J Zoo Wildlife Med 25, 376–389.

Caulkett, N.A., Cribb, P.H., Haigh, J.C., 2000. Comparative cardiopulmonary effects of carfentanil-xylazine and medetomidine-ketamine used for immobilization of mule deer and mule deer/white-tailed deer hybrids. Can J Vet Res 64, 64–68.

Celly, C.S., Atwal, O.S., McDonell, W.N., et al., 1999. Histopathalogic alterations induced in the lungs of sheep by use of alpha2-adrenergic receptor agonists. Am J Vet Res 60, 154–161.

Celly, C.S., McDonell, W.N., Young, S.S., et al., 1997. The comparative hypoxaemic effect of four alpha 2 adrenoceptor agonists (xylazine, romifidine, detomidine and medetomidine) in sheep. J Vet Pharmacol Ther 20, 464–471.

Chapman, N.G., Claydon, K., Claydon, M., et al., 1987. Techniques for the safe and humane capture of free-living muntjac deer (Muntiacus reevesi). Br Vet J 143, 35–43.

Clutton, R.E., Glasby, M.A., 2008. Cardiovascular and autonomic nervous effects of edrophonium and atropine combinations during neuromuscular blockade antagonism in sheep. Vet Anaesth Analg 35, 191–200.

Colditz, I.G., Lloyd, J.B., Paull, D.R., et al., 2009. Effect of the non-steroidal anti-inflammatory drug, carprofen, on weaned sheep following non-surgical mulesing by intradermal injection of cetrimide. Aust Vet J 87, 19–26.

Coombs, D.W., Colburn, R.W., DeLeo, J.A., et al., 1994. Comparative spinal neuropathy of hydromorphone and morphine after 9- and 30-day epidural administration in sheep. Anesth Analg 78, 674–681.

Copeland, S.E., Ladd, L.A., Gu, X.-Q., et al., 2008. The effects of general anesthesia on the central nervous and cardiovascular system toxicity of local anesthetics. Anesth Analg 106, 1429–1439.

Correia, D., Nolan, A.M., Reid, J., 1996. Pharmacokinetics of propofol infusions, either alone or with ketamine, in sheep premedicated with acepromazine and papaveretum. Res Vet Sci 60, 213–217.

Dangolla, A., Silva, I., Kuruwita, V.Y., 2004. Neuroleptanalgesia in wild Asian elephants (Elephas maximus maximus). Vet Anaesth Analg 31, 276–279.

del Alamo, A., Mandsager, R.E., Riebold, T., et al., 2012. Anesthetic evaluation of administration of intravenous alfaxalone in comparison with propofol and ketamine/diazepam in alpacas. In: Proceedings of the 18th IVECCS Symposium. San Antonio, TX, USA. p. 725.

Doherty, T.J., Redua, M.A., Queiroz-Castro, P., et al., 2007. Effect of intravenous lidocaine and ketamine on the minimum alveolar concentration of isoflurane in goats. Vet Anaesth Analg 34, 125–131.

Doherty, T.J., Will, W.A., Rohrbach, B.W., et al., 2004. Efect of morphine and flunixin meglumine on isoflurane minimum alveolar concentration in goats. Vet Anaesth Analg 31, 97–101.

Dräger, C., Benziger, D., Gao, F., et al., 1998. Prolonged intercostal nerve blockade in sheep using controlled-release of bupivacaine and dexamethasone from polymer microspheres. Anesthesiology 89, 969–979.

DuBois, W.R., Prado, T.M., Ko, J.C.H., et al., 2004. A comparison of two intramuscular doses of xylazine-ketamine combination and tolazoline reversal in llamas. Vet Anaesth Analg 31, 90–96.

Dudi, P.R., Chouhan, D.S., Choudhary, R.J., et al., 1984. The study of topographic anatomy and nerve blocks of hindlimb in camels (Camelus dromedarius). Indian Vet J 61, 848–853.

Duke, T., Egger, C.M., Ferguson, J.G., et al., 1997. Cardiopulmonary effects of propofol infusion in llamas. Am J Vet Res 58, 153–156.

Dunlop, C.I., Hodgson, D.S., Cambre, R.C., et al., 1994. Cardiopulmonary effects of three prolonged periods of isoflurane anesthesia in an adult elephant. J Am Vet Med Assoc 205, 1439–1444.

Dzikiti, B.T., Stegmann, F.G., Dzikiti, L.N., et al., 2010. Total intravenous anaesthesia (TIVA) with propofol-fentanyl and propofol-midazolam combinations in spontaneously-breathing goats. Vet Anaesth Analg 37, 519–525.

Dzikiti, B.T., Stegmann, F.G., Cromarty, D., et al., 2011a. Effects of propofol on isoflurane minimum alveolar concentration and cardiovascular function in mechanically ventilated goats. Vet Anaesth Analg 38, 44–53.

Dzikiti, T.B., Stegmann, F.G., Dzikiti, L.N., et al., 2011b. Effects of fentanyl on isoflurane minimum alveolar concentration and cardiovascular function in mechanically ventilated goats. Vet Rec 168, 429.

Eisenach, J.C., Shafer, S.L., Bucklin, B.A., et al., 1994. Pharmacokinetics and pharmacodynamics of intraspinal dexmedetomidine in sheep. Anesthesiology 80, 1349–1359.

Elias, E., 1991. Left ventrolateral cesarian section in three dromedary camels (Camelus dromedarius). Vet Surg 20, 323–325.

Fajt, V.R., 2011. Drug laws and regulations for sheep and goats. Vet Clin N Am Food Anim Pract 27, 1–21.

Fernández-Morán, J., Palomeque, J., Peinada, V.I., 2000. Medetomidine/tiletamine/zolazepam and xylazine/tiletamine/zolazepam combinations for immobilization of fallow deer (Cervus dama). J Zoo Wildlife Med 31, 62–64.

Fletcher, J., 1995. Handling farmed deer. In Practice 17, 30–37.

Foerner, J.J., Houck, R.I., Copeland, J.F., et al., 1994. Surgical castration of the elephant (Elephas maximus and Loxodonta africana). J Zoo Wildlife Med 25, 355–359.

Follett, K.A., 2003. Intrathecal analgesia and catheter-tip inflammatory masses (Editorial). Anesthesiology 99, 5–6.

Fowler, M.E., Zinkl, J.G., 1989. Reference ranges for hematologic and serum biochemical values in llamas. Am J Vet Res 50, 2049–2053.

Fowler, M.E., Steffey, E.P., Galuppo, L., et al., 2000. Facilitation of Asian elephant (Elephas maximus) standing immobilization and anesthesia with a sling. J Zoo Wildlife Med 31, 118–123.

Garcia-Pereira, F.L., Greene, S.A., Keegan, R.D., et al., 2007. Effects of intravenous butorphanol on cardiopulmonary function in isoflurane-anesthetized alpacas. Vet Anaesth Analg 34, 269–274.

Georoff, T.A., James, S.B., Kalk, P., et al., 2010. Evaluation of medetomidine-ketamine-butorphanol anesthesia with atipamezole-naltrexone antagonism in captive male guanacos (Lama guanicoe). J Zoo Wildlife Med 41, 255–262.

Gradert, T.L., Baze, W.B., Satterfield, W.C., et al., 2003. Safety of chronic intrathecal morphine infusion in a sheep model. Anesthesiology 99, 188–198.

Grant, C., Upton, R.N., Kuchel, T.R., 1996. Efficacy of intra-muscular analgesics for acute pain in sheep. Aust Vet J 73, 129–132.

Gregory, G.A., Wade, J.G., Beihl, D.R., et al., 1983. Fetal anesthetic requirement (MAC) for halothane. Anesth Analg 62, 9–14.

Grint, N., Dugdale, A., 2009. Brightness of venous blood in South American camelids: implications for jugular catheterization. Vet Anaesth Analg 36, 63–66.

Grubb, T.L., Riebold, T.W., Huber, M.J., 1993. Evaluation of lidocaine, xylazine, and a combination of lidocaine and xylazine for epidural analgesia in llamas. J Am Vet Med Assoc 203, 1441–1444.

Grubb, T.L., Schlipf, J.W., Riebold, T.W., et al., 2003. Minimum alveolar concentration of sevoflurane in spontaneously breathing llamas and alpacas. J Am Vet Med Assoc 223, 1167–1169.

Grubb, T.L., Schlipf, J.W., Riebold, T.W., et al., 2006. Minimum alveolar concentration of desflurane in llamas and alpacas. Vet Anaesth Analg 33, 351–355.

Hajduk, P., 1992. Haematological reference values for alpacas. Aust Vet J 69, 89–90.

Haymerle, A., Fahlman,, Å., Walzer, C., 2010. Human exposures to immobilising agents: results of an online survey. Vet Rec 167, 327–332.

Heard, D.J., Kollias, G.V., Webb, A.I., et al., 1988. Use of halothane to maintain anesthesia induced with etorphine in juvenile African elephants. J Am Vet Med Assoc 193, 254–256.

Heard, D.J., Nichols, W.W., Buss, D., et al., 1996. Comparative cardiopulmonary effects of intramuscularly administered etorphine and carfentanil in goats. Am J Vet Res 57, 87–96.

Hendrickson, D.A., Kruse-Elliot, K.T., Broadstone, R.V., 1996. A comparison of epidural saline, morphine, and bupivacaine for pain relief after abdominal surgery in goats. Vet Surg 25, 83–87.

Hikasa, Y., Okuyama, K., Kakuta, T., et al., 1998. Anesthetic potency and cardiopulmonary effects of sevoflurane in goats: comparison with isoflurane and halothane. Can J Vet Res 62, 299–306.

Hikasa, Y., Saito, K., Takase, K., et al., 2000. Clinical, cardiopulmonary, hematological and serum biochemical effects of sevoflurane and isoflurane anesthesia in oxygen under spontaneous breathing in sheep. Small Rumin Res 36, 241–249.

Hile, M.E., Hintz, H.F., Erb, H.N., 1997. Predicting body weight from body measurements in Asian elephants (Elephas maximus). J Zoo Wildlife Med 28, 424–427.

Honeyman, V.L., Pettifer, G.R., Dyson, D.H., 1992. Arterial blood pressure and blood gas values in normal standing and laterally recumbent African (Loxodonta africana) and Asian (Elaphus maximus) elephants. J Zoo Wildlife Med 23, 205–210.

Horne, W.A., Tchamba, M.N., Loomis, M.R., 2001. A simple method of providing intermittent positive-pressure ventilation to etorphine-immobilized elephants (Loxodonta africana) in the field. J Zoo Wildlife Med 32, 519–522.

Howard, B.W., Lagutchik, M.S., Januszkiewicz, A.J., et al., 1990. The cardiovascular response of sheep to tiletamine-zolazepam and butorphanol tartrate anesthesia. Vet Surg 19, 461–467.

Ingvast-Larsson, C., Svartberg, K., Hydbring-Sandberg, E., et al., 2007. Clinical pharmacology of buprenorphine in healthy, lactating goats. J Vet Pharmacol Ther 30, 249–256.

Jessup, D.A., Lance, W.R., 1982. What veterinarians should know about South American camelids. Californian Vet 11, 12–18.

Jessup, D.A., Jones, K., Mohr, R., et al., 1985. Yohimbine antagonism to xylazine in free-ranging mule deer and desert bighorn sheep. J Am Vet Med Assoc 187, 1251–1253.

Johansen, M.J., Satterfield, W.C., Baze, W.B., et al., 2004. Continuous intrathecal infusion of hydromorphone: safety in the sheep model and clinical implications. Pain Med 5, 14–25.

Johnson, C.B., Sylvester, S.P., Stafford, K.J., et al., 2009. Effects of age on the electroencephalographic response to castration in lambs anaesthetized with halothane in oxygen from birth to 6 weeks old. Vet Anaesth Analg 36, 273–279.

Kästner, S.B., 2006. α_2-agonists in sheep: a review. Vet Anaesth Analg 33, 79–96.

Kästner, S.B., Ohlerth, S., Pospischil, A., et al., 2007. Dexmedetomidine-induced pulmonary alterations in sheep. Res Vet Sci 83, 217–226.

Kästner, S.B.R., Wapf, P., Feige, K., et al., 2003. Pharmacokinetics and sedative effects of intramuscular medetomidine in domestic sheep. J Vet Pharmacol Ther 26, 271–276.

Krohm, P., Levionnois, O.L., Zilberstein, L., et al., 2011. Antinociceptive activity of pre- versus post-operaative intra-articular bupivacaine in goats undergoing stifle arthrotomy. Vet Anaesth Analg 38, 363–373.

Kutter, A.P., Kastner, S.B., Bettschart-Wolfensberger, R., et al., 2006. Cardiopulmonary effects of dexmedetomidine in goats and sheep anaesthetised with sevoflurane. Vet Rec 159, 624–629.

Kyles, A.E., Waterman, A.E., Livingston, A., 1995. Antinociceptive activity of midazolam in sheep. J Vet Pharmacol Ther 18, 54–60.

Lagutchik, M.S., Januszkiewicz, A.J., Dodd, K.T., et al., 1991. Cardiopulmonary effects of a tiletamine-zolazepam combination in sheep. Am J Vet Res 52, 1441–1447.

Laitinen, O.M., 1990. Clinical observations on medetomidine/ketamine anaesthesia in sheep and it reversal by atipamezole. J Assoc Vet Anaesth 17, 17–19.

Lee, I., Yamagushi, N., Oboshi, K., et al., 2003. Antagonistic effects of intravenous or epidural atipamezole on xylazine-induced dorsolumbar epidural analgesia in cattle. Vet J 166, 194–197.

Leone, S., Di Cianni, S., Casati, A., et al., 2008. Pharmacology, toxicology, and clinical use of new long acting local anesthetics, ropivacaine and levobupivacaine. Acta Biomed 79, 92–105.

Ley, S., Waterman, A.E., Livingston, A., 1990. Variation in the analgesic effects of xylazine in different breeds of sheep. Vet Rec 126, 508.

Lin, H.-C., Purohit, R.C., Rowe, T.A., 1997. Anesthesia in sheep with propofol or with xylazine-ketamine followed by halothane. Vet Surg 26, 247–252.

Lin, H.-C., Tyler, J.W., Welles, E.G., et al., 1993. Effects of anesthesia induced and maintained by continuous intravenous administration of guaifenesin, ketamine, and xylazine in spontaneously breathing sheep. Am J Vet Res 54, 1913–1916.

Lin, H.-C., Wallace, S.S., Tyler, J.W., et al., 1994. Comparison of tiletamine-zolazepam-ketamine and tiletamine-zolazepam-ketamine-xylazine anaesthesia in sheep. Aust Vet J 71, 239–242.

Lukasik, V.M., Nogami, W.M., Morgan, S.E., 1998. Minimum alveolar concentration and cardiovascular effects of desflurane in sheep (abstract). Vet Surg 27, 167.

Mama, K.R., Wagner, A.E., Parker, D.A., et al., 1999. Determination of the minimum alveolar concentration of isoflurane in llamas. Vet Anaesth Analg 28, 121–125.

Mama, K.R., Wagner, A.E., Steffey, E.P., 2001. Circulatory, respiratory and behavioral responses in isoflurane anesthetized llamas. Vet Anaesth Analg 28, 12–17.

Mansel, J.C., Shaw, D.J., Strachan, F.A., et al., 2008. Comparison of peripheral and core temperatures in anaesthetized hypovolaemic sheep. Vet Anaesth Analg 35, 45–51.

Marzok, M., El-Khodery, S., 2009. Sedative and analgesic effects of romifidine in camels (Camelus dromedarius). Vet Anaesth Analg 36, 352–360.

Mich, P.M., Wolfe, L.L., Sirochman, T.M., et al., 2008. Evaluation of intramuscular butorphanol, azaperone, and medetomidine and nasal oxygen insufflation for the chemical immobilization of white-tailed deer, Odocoileus virginianus. J Zoo Wildlife Med 39, 480–487.

Miller, B.F., Muller, L.I., Doherty, T., et al., 2004. Effectiveness of antagonists for tiletamine/zolazepam/xylazine immobilization in female white-tailed deer. J Wildlife Dis 40, 533–537.

Miller, B.F., Muller, L.I., Storms, T.N., et al., 2003. A comparison of carfentanil/xylazine and Telazol®/xylazine for immobilization of white-tailed deer. J Wildlife Dis 39, 851–858.

Miller, B.F., Osborn, D.A., Lance, W.R., et al., 2009. Butorphanol-azaperone-medetomidine for immobilization of captive white-tailed deer. J Wildlife Dis 45, 457–467.

Mohamadnia, A.R., Hughes, G., Clarke, K.W., 2008. Maintenance of anaesthesia in sheep with isoflurane, desflurane or sevoflurane. Vet Rec 163, 210–215.

Molony, V., Kent, J.E., Robertson, I.S., 1993. Behavioural responses of lambs of three ages in the first three hours after three methods of castration and tail docking. Res Vet Sci 55, 236–245.

Moraga, F., Monge, C., Riquelme, R., et al., 1996. Fetal and maternal blood oxygen affinity: A comparative study in llamas and sheep. Comp Biochem Physiol 115A, 111–115.

Nazefi, S., Maleki, K., 1998. Biochemical analysis of serum and cerebrospinal fluid in clinically normal adult camels (Camelus dromedarius). Res Vet Sci 65, 83–84.

Ogunbodede, E.O., Arotiba, J.T., 1997. Camel bite injuries of the orofacial region: report of a case. J Oral Maxillofacial Surg 55, 1174–1176.

Okutomi, T., Whittington, R.A., Stein, D.J., et al., 2009. Comparison of the effects of sevoflurane and isoflurane anesthesia on the maternal-fetal unit in sheep. J Anesth 23, 392–398.

Osofsky, S.A., 1997. A practical anesthesia monitoring protocol for free-ranging adult African elephants (Loxodonta africana). J Wildlife Dis 33, 72–77.

Pablo, L.S., 1993. Epidural morphine in goats after hindlimb orthopedic surgery. Vet Surg 22, 307–310.

Pablo, L.S., Bailey, J.E., Ko, J.C.H., 1997. Median effective dose of propofol required for induction of anesthesia in goats. J Am Vet Med Assoc 211, 86–88.

Padula, A.M., 2005. Clinical evaluation of caudal epidural anaesthesia for the neutering of alpacas. Vet Rec 156, 616–617.

Paull, D.R., Lee, C., Colditz, I.G., et al., 2007. The effect of a topical anaesthetic formulation, systemic flunixin and carprofen, singly or in combination, on cortisol and behavioural responses of Merino lambs to mulesing. Aust Vet J 85, 98–106.

Pearl, R.G., Rice, S.A., 1989. Propylene-glycol-induced pulmonary hypertension in sheep. Pharmacology 39, 383–389.

Pollard, V., 2008. Potential toxicity and efficacy of local anaesthetic when used for disbudding in the goat kid. B Vet Med dissertation. University of London, London.

Prado, T.M., Doherty, T.J., Boggan, E.B., et al., 2008a. Effects of acepromazine and butorphanol on tiletamine zolazepam anesthesia in llamas. Am J Vet Res 69, 182–188.

Prado, T.M., DuBois, W.R., Ko, J.C.H., et al., 2008b. A comparison of two combinations of xylazine-ketamine administered intramuscularly to alpacas and of reversal with tolazoline. Vet Anaesth Analg 35, 201–207.

Purohit, N.R., Chouhan, D.S., Chaudhary, R.J., et al., 1985.

Intravenous regional anaesthesia in camel. Indian J Anim Sci 55, 435–436.

Quinn, D.A., Robinson, D., Hales, C.A., 1990. Intravenous injection of propylene glycol causes pulmonary hypertension in sheep. J Appl Physiol 68, 1415–1420.

Raekallio, M.R., Tulamo, R.-M., Valtamo, T., 1998. Medetomidine-midazolam sedation in sheep. Acta Vet Scand 39, 127–134.

Raske, T.G., Pelkey, S., Wagner, A.E., et al., 2010. Effect of intravenous ketamine and lidocaine on isoflurane requirement in sheep undergoing orthopedic surgery. Lab Anim 39, 76–79.

Ratajczak-Enselme, M., Estebe, J.-P., Rose, F.-X., et al., 2007. Effect of epinephrine on epidural, intrathecal, and plasma pharmacokinetics of ropivacaine and bupivacaine in sheep. Br J Anaesth 99, 881–890.

Read, M.R., Duke, T., Toews, A.R., 2000. Suspected tolazoline toxicosis in a llama. J Am Vet Med Assoc 216, 227–229.

Riebold, T.W., Engel, H.N., Grubb, T.L., et al., 1994. Orotracheal and nasotracheal intubation in llamas. J Am Vet Med Assoc 204, 779–783.

Riebold, T.W., Kaneps, A.J., Schmotzer, W.B., 1989. Anesthesia in the llama. Vet Surg 18, 400–404.

Sarma, B., Pathak, S.C., Sarma, K.K., 2002. Medetomidine – a novel immobilizing agent for the elephant (Elephas maximus). Res Vet Sci 73, 315–317.

Schauvliege, S., Narine, K., Bouchez, S., et al., 2006. Refined anaesthesia for implantation of engineered experimental aortic valves in the pulmonary artery using a right heart bypass in sheep. Lab Anim 40, 341–352.

Scott, P., 1996. Caudal analgesia in sheep. In Practice 18, 383–384.

Seddighi, R., Doherty, T., Elliot, S., et al., 2012. Physiological and antinociceptive effects of xylazine on tiletamine-zolazepam anesthesia in llamas. In: Proceedings of the 18th IVEECS Symposium. San Antonio, TX, USA. p. 733.

Shafford, H.L., Hellyer, P.W., Turner, A.S., 2004. Intra-articular lidocaine plus bupivacaine in sheep undergoing stifle arthrotomy. Vet Anaesth Analg 31, 20–26.

Singh, R., Peshin, P.K., Patil, D.B., et al., 1994. Evaluation of halothane as an anaesthetic in camels (Camelus dromedarius). Zentralbl Veterinarmed 41, 359–368.

Snow, D.H., Billah, A., Ridha, A., 1988. Effects of maximal exercise on the blood composition of the racing camel. Vet Rec 123, 311–312.

Sontakke, S.D., Reddy, A.P., Umapathy, G., et al., 2007. Anesthesia induced by administration of xylazine hydrochloride alone or in combination with ketamine hydrochloride and reversal by administration of yohimbine hydrochloride in captive Axis deer (Axis axis). Am J Vet Res 68, 20–24.

Staffieri, F., Driessen, B., Lacitignola, L., et al., 2009. A comparison of subarachnoid buprenorphine or xylazine as an adjunct for analgesia in goats. Vet Anaesth Analg 36, 502–511.

Stegmann, G.F., 2000. Hypoxaemia and suspected pulmonary oedema in a Dorper ewe after diazepam-ketamine induction of anaesthesia. J S Afr Vet Assoc 71, 64–65.

Stewart, M.C., English, A.W., 1990. The reversal of xylazine/ketamine immobilization of fallow deer with yohimbine. Aust Vet J 67, 315–317.

Still, J., Raath, J.P., Matzner, L., 1996. Respiratory and circulatory parameters of African elephants (Loxodonta africana) anaesthetized with etorphine and azaperone. J S Afr Vet Assoc 67, 123–127.

Swenson, J.D., Wisniewski, M., McJames, S., et al., 1996. The effect of prior dural puncture on cisternal cerebrospinal fluid morphine concentrations in sheep after administration of lumbar epidural morphine. Anesth Analg 83, 523–525.

Taylor, P.M., 1998. Endocrine and metabolic responses to halothane and pentobarbitone anaesthesia in sheep. J Vet Anaesth 25, 24–30.

Tennent-Brown, B.S., Koenig, A., Wiliamson, L.H., et al., 2011. Comparison of three point-of-care blood glucose meters for use in adult and juvenile alpacas. J Am Vet Med Assoc 239, 380–386.

Torres, M.-D., Andaluz, A., García, F., et al., 2012. Effects of an intravenous bolus of alfaxalone versus propofol on intraocular pressure in sheep. Vet Rec 170, 226.

Trim, C.M., 1989. Epidural analgesia with 0.75% bupivacaine for laparotomy in goats. J Am Vet Med Assoc 194, 1292–1296.

Trim, C.M., 2007. The changing face of epidural analgesia (Clinical commentary). Equine Vet Educ 19, 595–596.

Trim, C.M., Hofmeister, E.H., Peroni, J.F., et al., 2013. Evaluation of an oscillometric blood pressure monitor for use in anesthetized sheep. Vet Anaesth Analg DOI:10:1111/vaa.12018.

Tulamo, R.-M., Raekallio, M.R., Ekblad, A., 1995. Cardiovascular effects of medetomidine-ketamine anaesthesia in sheep, with and without 100% oxygen. J Vet Anaesth 22, 9–14.

Uhrig, S.R., Papich, M.G., KuKanich, B., et al., 2007. Pharmacokinetics and pharmacodynamics of morphine in llamas. Am J Vet Res 68, 25–34.

Vincent, C.J., Hawley, A.T., Rozanski, E.A., et al., 2009. Cardiopulmonary effects of dobutamine and norepinephrine infusion in healthy anesthetized alpacas. Am J Vet Res 70, 1236–1242.

Wagner, A.E., Mama, K.R., Ruehlman, D.L., et al., 2011. Evaluation of effects of sciatic and femoral nerve blocks in sheep undergoing stifle surgery. Lab Anim 40, 114–118.

Walsh, V.P., Gieseg, M., Mitcheson, S.L., et al., 2012. A comparison of two different ketamine and diazepam combinations with an alphaxalone and medetomidine combination for induction of anaesthesia in sheep. N Z Vet J 60, 136–141.

Waterman, A.E., Livingston, A., Amin, A., 1991. Further studies on the antinociceptive activity and respiratory effects of buprenorphine in sheep. J Vet Pharmacol Ther 14, 230–234.

Webb, S.T., Ghosh, S., 2009. Intra-articular bupivacaine – potentially chondrotoxic? Br J Anaesth 102, 439–441.

Webster, V.L., Cara, D.M., Walker, R.M., et al., 2005. Description of a technique for anaesthetizing pregnant ewes for fetal surgery. Lab Anim 39, 94–99.

White, R.J., Bali, S., Bark, H., 1987. Xylazine and ketamine anaesthesia in the dromedary camel under field conditions. Vet Rec 120, 110–113.

White, R.J., Bark, H., Bali, S., 1986. Halothane anaesthesia in the dromedary camel. Vet Rec 119, 615–617.

Yaksh, T.L., Hassenbusch, S., Burchiel, K., et al., 2002. Inflammatory masses associated with intrathecal drug infusion: A review of preclinical evidence and human data. Pain Med 3, 300–312.

Yaksh, T.L., Horais, K.A., Tozier, N.A., et al., 2003. Chronically infused intrathecal morphine in dogs. Anesthesiology 99, 174–187.

Chapter | **14** |

Anaesthesia of the pig

INTRODUCTION

Although surgery may be performed on the farm using either local analgesia or general anaesthesia, whenever possible pigs requiring more than minor surgery should be transported to a veterinary clinic having the equipment and personnel needed should complications arise. If the surgery is to be performed using local analgesia, sedation can be added to facilitate restraint. General anaesthesia employed under farm conditions will be dictated by financial concerns, availability of anaesthetic agents, and considerations for the animal such as adequacy of oxygenation. Pigs used in research studies must be anaesthetized using protocols that are appropriate for the particular study. Consequently, these anaesthetic protocols may be simple or complex but always should be selected after careful consideration of analgesia and animal welfare.

Pigs range in size from small newborn piglets to adults weighing 350 kg or more. As a result, the methods of restraint and administration of anaesthetics vary accordingly. While small pigs are easily restrained, large sows and boars may prove both difficult and dangerous. Small pigs can be simply held in arms or restrained on their sides by grasping the undermost legs and leaning on the pig's body. A pig in a pen can be restrained for injection by placing a wooden board between the pig and the person effectively

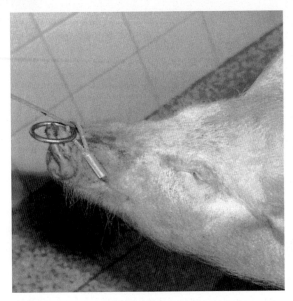

Figure 14.1 Restraint of the pig by a snare applied around the upper jaw.

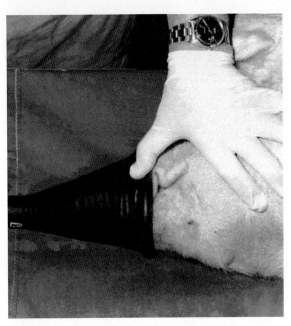

Figure 14.2 Maintaining a clear airway by pushing forward on the vertical ramus of the mandible.

to squeeze the pig against the pen wall or in a corner. Boards used specifically for this purpose should be larger than the pig and may have handles attached on one side to facilitate manipulation of the board. Restraint of large sows and boars is also easy if a weighing crate is available, especially one with a 'head catcher'. Large pigs can be restrained by a rope or wire snare placed around the upper jaw, caudal to the canine teeth (Fig. 14.1). Commercial snares have a metre-long metal handle to facilitate snaring the jaw and controlling the pig once it is caught. In most cases, the pig will try to escape by pulling back against the snare and thus immobilizes itself.

In research studies, a pig may be immobilized by placing it in a webbed sling in sternal position with all four limbs passed through holes in the sling. Although Vietnamese potbellied pigs kept as pets have been handled frequently and are easy to approach, they often resist restraint. The caudal edge of the tusks are razor-sharp and care should be taken to avoid lacerations when handling the jaws of pigs with untrimmed tusks.

Most anaesthetists consider pigs to be good subjects for general anaesthesia, provided due care is exercised. Although they resent restraint, as evidenced by the struggling and loud squeals they produce, they often respond predictably to anaesthetic agents. Recovery from anaesthesia is usually calm, unless the pigs are in pain or disoriented. As they have little body hair, pigs are liable to develop hypothermia when sedated or anaesthetized, or hyperthermia in a hot environment. Pigs tend to be fatter than most other farm animals and this can make accurate IM injections difficult. The shape of the pig's head, together

with the fat in the pharyngeal region (especially in Vietnamese potbellied pigs) coupled with a small larynx and trachea, increases the likelihood of respiratory obstruction in sedated and anaesthetized animals. Results of physiological studies of breathing patterns in non-anaesthetized obese potbellied pigs have identified upper airway syndrome with high inspiratory resistance and progressive limitation of inspiratory airflow. In those studies, mild laryngeal adduction occurred during expiration and a light plane of sleep. During deep sleep, the laryngeal adduction was absent and the pigs became hypoxic and aroused. The authors postulated that the laryngeal adduction identified in the potbellied pigs is a form of autopositive end-expiratory pressure (auto-PEEP) that provides expiratory braking to preserve end-expiratory lung volumes (Tuck et al., 1999, 2001). This effect would be lost during heavy sedation and anaesthesia, thereby resulting in hypoventilation.

Without endotracheal intubation, patency of the airway in pigs is best maintained by keeping the head and neck extended, pushing the lower jaw forward by applying pressure behind the vertical ramus of the mandible (Fig. 14.2), and by pulling the tongue out between the incisor teeth. Salivation, even if not excessive, can contribute to airway obstruction and promote laryngospasm. Consequently, anticholinergics are frequently given before general anaesthesia unless there are specific contraindications.

The anaesthetic agents listed in this chapter may not be available in all countries and many are not licensed for use in pigs. Choice of agents used will also depend on the pig as a food animal or not, its health, the procedure to be performed, and where the procedure will be performed (e.g. owner's farm, veterinary clinic, or research facility). In some countries, pigs given unapproved drugs cannot be used for food.

PORCINE MALIGNANT HYPERTHERMIA

Some breeds (particularly Poland China, Pietrain, and Landrace) and strains of pigs suffer from a biochemical myopathy which manifests itself during general anaesthesia. Malignant hyperthermia (MH) was first reported in Landrace cross pigs following the use of succinylcholine during halothane anaesthesia (Hall et al., 1966). The syndrome bears a close resemblance to a condition described in the early 20th century in pigs with pale, soft, exudative muscle (PSE) and to the Porcine Stress Syndrome. We now know that sudden death may occur in MH-susceptible humans in response to high environmental temperatures, exercise, or stress. Since retrospective studies of several generations of human family trees prior to 1970 identified multiple sudden deaths within families, it is thought that the syndrome had been present but unrecognized; 1970 was the turning point in the history of MH and much research has been published since that time. The MH syndrome is inherited in pigs in an autosomal recessive pattern, while in humans it is autosomal dominant. Only two causative genes have been identified thus far, with mutations of the type 1 ryanodine receptor of skeletal muscle being most commonly involved. All inhalation anaesthetic agents, except nitrous oxide, and the neuromuscular blocking agent, succinylcholine, are triggering agents. Injectable anaesthetic agents do not trigger the syndrome but MH may develop in pigs anaesthetized with injectable agents when the stress of handling and induction of anaesthesia has already initiated muscle metabolism changes. If identified early in pigs anaesthetized with injectable agents, ventilation with oxygen and cooling the pig may abort the syndrome. It is possible that some injectable agents, for example thiopental and alfaxalone, may delay the onset of MH during inhalation anaesthesia (Hall et al., 1972). The MH syndrome does not always occur at the onset of anaesthesia, but may develop at any time during anaesthesia and in the first few hours after anaesthesia.

Individuals suspected of susceptibility to MH can be tested using a muscle biopsy and a laboratory test that measures the degree of contracture induced in muscle fibres exposed to halothane or caffeine (the *in vitro* contracture test or IVCT). Although the test is sensitive, its specificity varies according to European and North American interpretations of the results and some false positives and false negatives are possible (Rosenberg et al., 2007).

Clinical signs

Triggering of the MH syndrome initiates release of calcium from the sarcoplasmic reticulum of skeletal muscle resulting in muscle contracture and increased cellular metabolism with production of heat and lactate (Rosenberg et al., 2007). Increased production of carbon dioxide results in hypercarbia, rapid deep respirations, and increased end-tidal CO_2 concentrations. The carbon dioxide absorber in a rebreathing anaesthetic circuit becomes very hot to touch and the granules rapidly develop intense indicator colour. Release of catecholamines causes an initial increase in blood pressure with tachycardia and multifocal ventricular dysrhythmias. Hyperkalaemia and metabolic acidosis develop and, in some cases, the pH can decrease to less than 6.80. The skin of white pigs becomes blotchy red and white. Signs of advanced MH in most pigs include generalized muscle rigidity with spreading of the digits and a severe and sustained rise in body temperature up to 42.2 °C (108 °F) (Fig. 14.3). Ultimately, the animal becomes hypoxic and without treatment usually dies. In pigs, the signs observed during early development of MH syndrome are likely to be caused by MH, however, in dogs, there are several differential diagnoses that must be considered (see Chapter 2, Table 2.9). Accurate identification of MH relies on the presence of clinical signs and the more signs present the more likely that the patient has MH (Box 14.1).

Treatment of MH

Treatment involves eliminating anaesthetic agent from the anaesthetic circuit, hyperventilation with oxygen to aid elimination of CO_2, aggressive cooling by covering the

---

> Box 14.1 **Clinical signs of malignant hyperthermia syndrome**
>
> - Rapid deep breathing, high end-tidal and arterial CO_2 concentrations
> - Sodalime canister hot and 'blue'
> - Sinus tachycardia, hypertension, ventricular dysrhythmias
> - Muscle rigidity
> - Moderate to severe metabolic acidosis
> - Rapidly increasing body temperature
> - Hyperkalaemia
> - Reversal of MH signs with dantrolene

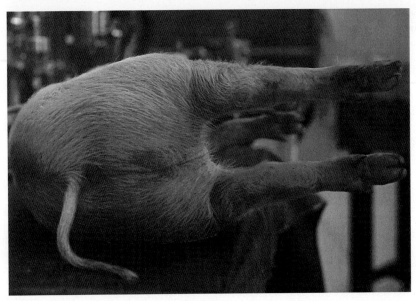

Figure 14.3 Rigidity of the limbs and spreading apart of the digits in a pig developing porcine malignant hyperthermia syndrome.

> ### Box 14.2 **Treatment of malignant hyperthermia syndrome**
>
> - Discontinue inhalation anaesthetic administration, increase oxygen flow
> - Start artificial ventilation and hyperventilate
> - Cool patient with ice water
> - Cold IV fluids
> - Sodium bicarbonate slowly IV, starting with 1.5 mEq/kg
> - Dantrolene IV 2 mg/kg increments up to 10 mg/kg, repeat 1 mg/kg each 6 h for 24 h
> - Change CO_2 absorber granules as necessary

patient with ice, countering metabolic acidosis with injection of sodium bicarbonate and balanced electrolyte solution, and blocking the trigger by administration of dantrolene (Box 14.2). Dantrolene is a hydantoin derivative that was synthesized in 1967 (Krause et al., 2004). It binds to a specific ryanodine protein site and blocks the release of calcium, thereby interrupting the trigger and allowing signs of MH to reverse. Dantrolene is generally administered IV for rapid effect. The oral preparation of dantrolene is less costly. The bioavailability of dantrolene in animals after oral administration is less than decribed for humans. However, when MH susceptibility is suspected, administration of dantrolene orally before

anaesthesia may prevent development of the syndrome. Azumolene, a more water-soluble analogue of dantrolene, has been investigated for treatment of MH but is not recommended due to unacceptable hepatic toxicity reported in humans. Dysrhythmias may be treated as needed but calcium channel blockers should be avoided when dantrolene has been administered. Hyperkalaemia should be treated in the usual recommended way with calcium, sodium bicarbonate, glucose and insulin, and hyperventilation.

SEDATION

The pig's reaction to restraint (struggling and vocalization) is sufficiently vigorous that sedation is widely used to facilitate handling and minor procedures, as well as for restraint prior to local or general anaesthesia. Intramuscular injections can be administered in the neck immediately behind the base of the ear at the level of the second cervical vertebra, or in the triceps, quadriceps, gluteal, or longissimus dorsii muscles. The neck is the preferred site in pigs intended for food to avoid damage in the other muscles. The skin should be clean before injection to avoid production of an abscess. The impact of the site of injection on drug action was evaluated in a study involving IM injection of azaperone, 1 mg/kg, and ketamine, 5 mg/kg (Clutton et al., 1998). Mature gilts were injected using 19 gauge 5 cm needles at four sites: in the neck muscle 5 cm caudal to the base of the ear; in the triceps muscle midway between the point of the shoulder and elbow; in the middle gluteal muscle at the centre of a triangle between midline, tuber coxae and tail-head; and in the quadriceps muscle in the cranial third of an imaginary line connecting patella and tuber ischii The degree of sedation at 16 minutes after injection was not significantly different between the injection sites, although the range of times to recumbency was narrower after injection in the quadriceps muscle. In a separate experiment, the sedative agents were either refrigerated, at room temperature, or warmed, and no differences in response to injection from the pigs were observed.

Agents employed for sedation in pigs

Some of the agents listed in this section may be administered in low or high doses according to whether the desired effect is sedation or anaesthesia (Table 14.1). Commonly, these agents are used in combinations with other agents, and more details may be found in the section on general anaesthesia.

Acepromazine

Phenothiazine derivatives are not as effective in pigs as they are in other species. However, administration of acepromazine, 0.03–0.1 mg/kg IM, renders pigs that are more easily restrained for IV injection, much less likely to dislodge the IV needle by head-shaking, and vocalize less. Acepromazine should be allowed 30 minutes to produce its full effects. Acepromazine has been commonly used with ketamine for anaesthesia in young pigs.

α_2-Agonists

Xylazine is not as an effective sedative as in other species. Recommended dose rates for xylazine are 1–2 mg/kg by IM or IV routes and these will induce a calming effect for about 30 minutes, however, the pigs arouse easily when disturbed and little sedative effect will be apparent. Xylazine induces a transient increase in mean arterial pressure (MAP) and decreased heart rate (HR) for about 15 minutes. Although ineffective when administered alone, xylazine has an additive effect when added to other agents, such as ketamine, butorphanol or midazolam, and increases the degree of sedation.

Table 14.1 Dosages of agents used in sedative and anaesthetic protocols in pigs

Agent	Drug class	Dose (mg/kg)*	Route	Indications
Atropine	Anticholinergic	0.02–0.04	IM, IV	Decrease salivation, treat bradycardia
Glycopyrrolate	Anticholinergic	0.005–0.01	IM, IV	Decrease salivation, treat bradycardia
Acepromazine	Phenothiazine	0.03–0.1	IM, IV	Tranquillizer
Azaperone	Butyrophenone	1–8	IM	Sedative
Diazepam	Benzodiazepine	0.2–0.5	IV	Mild sedative
Droperidol	Butyrophenone	0.3	IM	Sedative
Medetomidine	α_2-agonist	0.005–0.08	IM, IV	Sedative
Midazolam	Benzodiazepine	0.2–0.5	IM, IV	Mild sedative
Xylazine	α_2-agonist	1–2.2	IM, IV	Sedative
Buprenorphine	Opioid	0.01	IM, IV	Analgesia
Butorphanol	Opioid	0.1–0.2	IM, IV	Analgesia
Alfaxalone	Steroid anaesthetic	0.7–3	IV	Anaesthesia
Ketamine	Dissociative anaesthetic	2–20	IM, IV	Sedation or anaesthesia
Metomidate	Hypnotic anaesthetic	3.3	IM, IV	Anaesthesia
Propofol	Hypnotic anaesthetic	1–6	IV	Anaesthesia
Thiopental	Barbiturate	5–12	IV	Anaesthesia
Tiletamine–zolazepam	Dissociative anaesthetic–benzodiazepine	2–5	IM, IV	Sedation or anaesthesia

*Dose depends on the CNS depressant effects of concurrently administered agents, the physical status of the pig, and the desired effect.

Medetomidine produces a dose-dependent sedative effect in pigs that is substantially greater than from xylazine. The effect varies from mild to moderate sedation with medetomidine, 0.005–0.02 mg/kg IM, to heavy sedation produced by medetomidine, 0.08 mg/kg IM. The depth and predictability of sedation can be improved by the addition of butorphanol, 0.2 mg/kg IM, and midazolam, 0.2 mg/kg IM. Medetomidine induces bradycardia and clinical and experimental studies have included atropine, 0.02–0.04 mg/kg IM, or glycopyrrolate, 0.005–0.01 mg/kg IM, to increase heart rates. The addition of atropine to combinations that include (dex)medetomidine is not recommended in dogs because these sedatives induce peripheral vasoconstriction and increased blood pressure and atropine may promote severe hypertension by increasing HR. In pigs, medetomidine has a greater vasoconstrictive effect on the pulmonary circulation and, although increases in pulmonary arterial pressure are not severe when compared with the cardiovascular effects of ketamine or tiletamine, the consequences of these effects should be taken into consideration when anaesthetizing pigs for cardiovascular research or pigs with cardiac disease (Sakaguchi et al., 1996).

When pigs are stressed, their response to anaesthetic agents may be less predictable. In one study, a combination of medetomidine, 0.08 mg/kg, butorphanol, 0.2 mg/kg, and atropine, 0.025 mg/kg, administered to young pigs did not provide sufficient sedation to allow blood sampling in all animals (Ugarte & O'Flaherty, 2005). The addition of ketamine or tiletamine–zolazepam may induce anaesthesia. Dexmedetomidine is twice as potent as medetomidine and, therefore, dose rates for dexmedetomidine are half that used for medetomidine. Administration of medetomidine and dexmedetomidine produce similar cardiovascular effects, including bradycardia, decreased cardiac output, increased systemic vascular resistance and increased MAP.

Azaperone

Azaperone is a licensed and commonly used pig sedative in Europe and is available for use in wildlife in the USA. Azaperone must be given by deep IM injection and the pig should be left undisturbed for 20 minutes for best effect. The dose range is 1–8 mg/kg depending on the effects sought, but it is recommended that a dose of 1 mg/kg is not exceeded for adult boars as higher doses can cause prolapse of the penis.

Azaperone causes vasodilation resulting in a small fall in arterial blood pressure, and some slight respiratory stimulation. Hypothermia may develop in sedated pigs in a cold environment.

Dissociative agents

Ketamine and tiletamine (in combination with zolazepam) can be used to provide sedation. Ketamine, 2–10 mg/kg

IM, combined with acepromazine, or azaperone, or medetomidine, or midazolam may be used to induce relaxation and sedation.

Tiletamine–zolazepam is available as a commercial preparation containing equal parts of each drug and is usually prepared to achieve 500 mg of total drug per ml. Zolazepam is similar to diazepam and is included to provide muscle relaxation. Following IM injection in pigs, the highest plasma concentrations of tiletamine and zolazepam occur within 60 minutes, however, zolazepam is more slowly eliminated than tiletamine (Kumar et al., 2006). Tiletamine–zolazepam, 2–5 mg/kg IM, can be used alone to induce sedation or be combined with xylazine or butorphanol. Recovery can be slow and lethargy and incoordination may persist for several hours.

Droperidol

The butyrophenone compound, droperidol, has been used in pigs and doses of 0.1–0.4 mg/kg give similar sedation to that produced by azaperone. Droperidol, 0.3 mg/kg IM, produced sedation by 15–45 minutes after administration with a duration of 2 hours in young pigs and minimal effect on heart rates and systolic blood pressures (Bustamente and Valverde, 1997). Butyrophenone/analgesic drug mixtures have been used and droperidol, 20 mg/ml, and fentanyl, 0.4 mg/ml, dosed at 1 ml/50 kg IM, produces better sedation than droperidol alone. Sedation develops rapidly and lasts approximately 15 minutes.

Opioids

Opioids administered alone are unlikely to induce sedation in healthy pigs. Butorphanol, 0.2 mg/kg, with xylazine, 1–2 mg/kg, or medetomidine, 0.01–0.02 mg/kg, usually with addition of atropine, 0.02–0.04 mg/kg, is a popular combination for IM administration. The addition of midazolam, 0.2–0.5 mg/kg, to these combinations increases the quality of sedation. Increasing the dose rate for medetomidine results in heavy sedation or anaesthesia. Pet potbellied pigs may be sedated at lower dose rates for medetomidine than is usually used in domestic pigs. Other opioids are used in pigs for analgesia during and after general anaesthesia.

GENERAL ANAESTHESIA

Preparation

Pigs should undergo a physical examination for evidence of ill-health. Clinical patients with abnormalities or suspected systemic disease should be evaluated further using haematological and clinical chemistry laboratory tests. Normal physiological values have been published and reveal that reference values for minipigs may differ from domestic pigs (Hannon et al., 1990; Clark & Coffer, 2008). Potbellied pigs have lower rectal temperatures than domestic pigs (Lord et al., 1999). Other appropriate diagnostics that require patient cooperation, such as radiology and ultrasound, may have to be facilitated by sedation or anaesthesia. Specific patients, such as those with a history of vomiting or recent trauma, may require other precautions for anaesthesia. Rabies is not a common disease in pigs but may occur where rabies is endemic and has been reported in Vietnamese potbellied pigs. Clinical signs of depression and difficulty walking are non-specific for rabies.

Food is generally withheld for 8–12 hours and water for 2 hours before anaesthesia. Although vomiting at induction of anaesthesia or during recovery is uncommon in pigs, it can occur and introduces risk for aspiration, and ventilation is decreased when a full stomach exerts pressure on the diaphragm. Fluid deficits present before anaesthesia should be corrected by fluid therapy. Details of existing drug therapy such as antibiotic food additives, or anthelmintics, should be noted as drug interactions with anaesthetic agents may occur.

Premedication

Salivation may be increased in anxious pigs and by administration of dissociative agents. Laryngospasm is easily induced in pigs and saliva on the arytenoids can be an inciting cause. Atropine, 0.02–0.04 mg/kg, or glycopyrrolate, 0.005–0.01 mg/kg, IM or IV may be included in the premedication to minimize salivation.

Anaesthesia can be induced and maintained with isoflurane or sevoflurane, however, in dogs, use of an inhalant as the sole anaesthetic agent is associated with increased risk of death (Brodbelt et al., 2008). In certain circumstances, use of an inhalant agent alone may be expedient, however, in general, preanaesthetic sedation in pigs is recommended to reduce the subsequent dosages of anaesthetic agents and thereby increase the safety of anaesthetic administration. The degree of sedation required depends, in part, on the anaesthetic technique which is to follow. Agents may be administered IM to induce moderate to severe sedation and anaesthesia induced by titration IV of anaesthetic agents, such as ketamine, ketamine–diazepam (or midazolam), or propofol, or by administration of isoflurane or sevoflurane by facemask. Alternatively, agents may be administered in larger doses IM to induce general anaesthesia sufficient to accomplish endotracheal intubation. Anaesthesia is then maintained with an inhalation agent or injectable agents.

Analgesia

Some anaesthetic agents, like medetomidine, provide some analgesia, while others, such as propofol, thiopental, or isoflurane, provide very little. Analgesia may be provided by several methods, including administration of non-steroidal anti-inflammatory agents (NSAIDs, such as flunixin meglumine, carprofen, meloxicam, or ketoprofen), opioids, and local anaesthetic agents. Keita et al. (2010) reported that meloxicam administered in 5-day-old piglets as a single IM dose, 0.4 mg/kg, 10–30 minutes before castration decreased plasma cortisol concentrations and decreased pain related behaviours 2 and 4 hours after surgery. Butorphanol, 0.2 mg/kg IM or IV, is a frequently administered opioid to pigs in general practice. Advantages of butorphanol include increasing the sedation and analgesia provided by other agent combinations with minimal adverse cardiovascular effects. Disadvantages of butorphanol are that it has a short-lived duration and that the analgesia provided is inadequate for major surgery, particularly orthopaedic surgery. Buprenorphine, 0.01 mg/kg IM or IV, has been used as part of anaesthetic protocols in pigs, with an apparent duration of action of 4 hours. A higher dose rate of buprenorphine, 0.1 mg/kg IM, has been advocated by others (Harvey-Clark et al., 2000; Malavasi et al., 2008). Buprenorphine administration during anaesthesia decreases the concentration of isoflurane required for anaesthesia (Malavasi et al., 2008). Further studies are needed to define optimum dose rate and the extent of analgesia provided by buprenorphine in pigs.

Morphine and meperidine (pethidine) prolong analgesia when administered IM with azaperone and ketamine in pigs (Hoyt et al., 1986). Fentanyl IV infusions, 5–35 μg/kg/h, IV have been included in anaesthetic protocols for research surgery.

Transdermal fentanyl patches, 2 μg/kg/h, have been investigated for use in young growing pigs. Serum fentanyl concentrations were achieved by 12 hours after patch application, but large interindividual differences were measured and no true steady state concentrations were observed (Malavasi et al., 2005). Consequently, the authors recommended that additional agents should be administered to ensure adequate analgesia. Partial patch detachment will change absorption and use of an occlusive dressing over the patch is recommended to improve adhesion. No depression of normal behaviour was noted in healthy pigs after application of a patch. Pigs undergoing abdominal surgery that received both a morphine epidural block and a transdermal fentanyl patch applied at the end of surgery had lower cortisol concentrations at the end of surgery, showed immediate interest in food after anaesthesia recovery, and gained weight in the 2 days following surgery in contrast with pigs receiving no opioids (Malavasi et al., 2006b).

Opioid dependence can develop in pigs. Experimental pigs administered morphine free base daily for 23 days were challenged by an injection of naloxone, 0.02 mg/kg, IM (Risdahl et al., 1992). All the pigs demonstrated behaviour associated with opioid dependence, i.e. 'wet-dog' shakes, crawling and dragging bellies, constant posture changes, increased vocalization, salivation and increased defaecation frequency. A clinical patient, a young 5.9 kg potbellied pig, developed similar signs after discontinuation of transdermal fentanyl after 9 days (Trim & Braun, 2010).

Local analgesic techniques, such as incisional infiltration with bupivacaine, up to 2 mg/kg, will contribute long-term analgesia to an anaesthetic protocol. Other nerve blocks applicable to specific surgeries can be incorporated, such as intercostal nerve blocks and interpleural nerve block for thoracotomy.

Intravenous technique

Injections are made most frequently into auricular veins on the external surface of the ear flap. Pigs are restrained, as previously described, and an assistant applies pressure over the vein as near to the base of the ear as possible. Pressure on the veins can also be achieved using an elastic band applied around the base of the ear. Veins are interleaved with arteries and the sequence from one side of the ear flap to the other is vein-artery-vein-artery-vein (Fig. 14.4). Once the skin has been cleansed and alcohol applied, the veins are usually easily visible (Fig. 14.5).

Venepuncture is performed using a needle or catheter, 23–18 gauge depending on the size of the vein. The veins are shallow and the passage of the needle or catheter should be visible. Backflow of blood from the end of the needle or catheter should be observed but aspiration of blood into a syringe may not be possible. A subcutaneous bleb will be seen after a test injection if the tip of the needle or catheter is perivascular. After correct placement,

the pressure on the vein should be released and a catheter cap attached. The catheter or Butterfly needle should be secured to the skin using adhesive tape, or sutures (through skin only and not cartilage), or glue. Sometimes attachment is easier when a roll of gauze or plastic syringe case is placed on the inside of the ear flap (Fig. 14.6). The needle or catheter should be flushed with heparinized saline.

Other veins that can be used for IV injection are the cephalic vein on the dorsal surface of the forearm, and the femoral vein on the medial surface of the hind limb. Use of long flexible catheters inserted with over-the-needle technique can be used for catheterization of the femoral or subcutaneous abdominal veins (Snook, 2001). Alternative methods employed to locate a vein in difficult catheterizations are ultrasound of peripheral veins and surgical cut-down on the jugular vein.

With experience, it is possible to catheterize the cranial vena cava by a blind technique. Small pigs are restrained on their backs in a V-shaped trough with the neck fully extended, head hanging down, and the forelegs drawn back; large pigs are restrained standing with a nose snare and the head and neck fully extended and, in all cases, with the head, neck and body in a straight line. The skin is clipped and cleaned as for a surgical procedure. A 7.5–10 cm long 10–16 gauge needle, with syringe attached, is pushed through the skin in the depression which can be palpated just lateral to the anterior angle of the sternum and formed by the angle between the first rib and trachea (Fig. 14.7). The needle is directed dorsocaudally towards

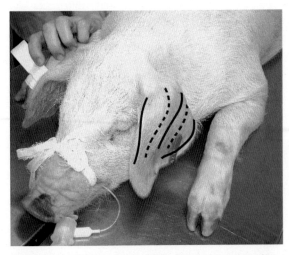

Figure 14.4 Location of veins and arteries on lateral surface of the ear. The solid lines drawn in black pen are veins and the dashed lines represent location of arteries.

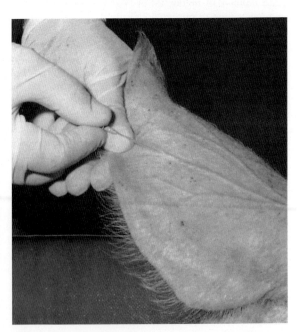

Figure 14.5 Distension of the ear veins by the application of a rubber band around the base of the ear.

blood through it, the needle is completely withdrawn and the catheter secured with skin sutures through adhesive tape applied across the tubing where it exits from the skin puncture. Complications of this procedure include puncture of an artery that is indicated by rapid flow of bright red blood, penetration of the thoracic duct indicated by aspiration of pinkish-white fluid, penetration of the trachea indicated by aspiration of air or blood-tinged froth into the syringe, and damage to the phrenic nerve which is followed by dyspnoea. Haematoma formation after arterial puncture should be limited by immediate removal of the needle and firm pressure with a fist in the sampling site for 5 minutes. Damage to the phrenic nerve is less likely if the needle is inserted from right to left.

Endotracheal intubation

Endotracheal intubation in the pig is not as easy as in most other domestic animals. The shape and size of the head and mouth make use of the laryngoscope and viewing the larynx difficult, especially in brachycephalic breeds. View of the laryngeal opening can be obscured by the large soft palate. Insertion of the endotracheal tube can be obstructed when the tip is caught in the groove between the overlapping cricoid cartilage and the epiglottis or in the adjacent blind sac, the oesophageal diverticulum, located dorsolaterally (Fig. 14.8). The larynx is set at an angle to the trachea, causing difficulty in passing the tube beyond the cricoid ring (Fig. 14.9). Laryngeal spasm is easily provoked so intubation is facilitated by application of lidocaine, 1–2 mg/kg, into the larynx.

The sizes of endotracheal tubes suitable for pigs are small when compared with those used in dogs of a similar body weight. A 6 or 7 mm internal diameter (ID) tube may be the largest which can be passed in a pig weighing about 25 kg; a 9 mm ID tube is suitable for a 50 kg animal; large boars and sows may accommodate tubes of 14–16 mm ID diameter. Endotracheal tube sizes are smaller in potbellied pigs, such that a 90 kg animal can only accommodate a 9–10 mm ID diameter tube. Introduction of the tube may be made easier by the use of a stilette placed inside the endotracheal tube and with the end located at the endotracheal tube adapter bent over to ensure that the tip does not protrude beyond the end of the tube. Forceful intubation can result in pharyngeal or tracheal laceration and the endotracheal tube emerging in the subcutaneous tissues. Trauma to the laryngeal mucosa should be avoided as oedema may cause airway obstruction during recovery from anaesthesia after extubation. Laryngoscope blades used in dogs are suitable in small pigs but longer blades (as described in the ruminant chapter) are necessary in large pigs to expose the larynx to view.

Tracheal intubation can be accomplished with the pig placed in any position, provided that the neck and head are fully extended. With the pig in sternal position, an

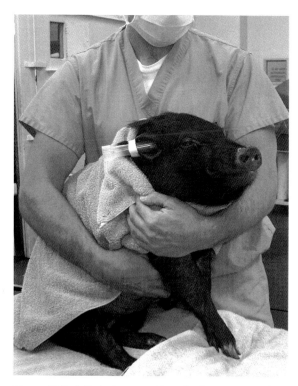

Figure 14.6 Catheter is secured by adhesive tape around the ear and a plastic syringe case that has been inserted into the ear.

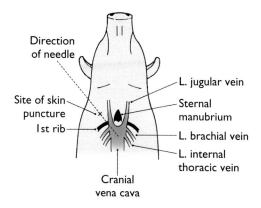

Figure 14.7 Site for the introduction of a needle to penetrate the cranial vena cava. The needle tip is advanced towards an imaginary point midway between the scapulae.

an imaginary point midway between the scapulae and advanced until blood can be freely aspirated through it when a syringe is attached. Sterilized plastic tubing is then threaded through the needle into the cranial vena cava and, after its position has been verified by aspiration of

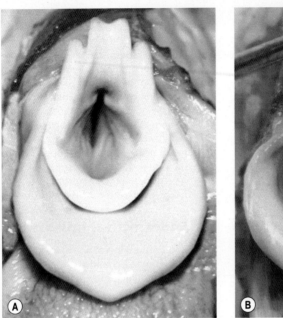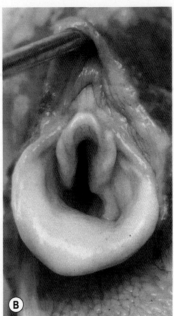

Figure 14.8 (A) Larynx of a 70 kg Large White pig (post-mortem). A 12 mm ID endotracheal tube was the largest tube that could be inserted into the trachea. Note that the entrance to the larynx is larger than the internal diameter of the larynx. (B) Larynx of a 90 kg potbellied sow (post-mortem). The largest endotracheal tube that could be inserted was 9 mm ID. The probe is inserted into the oesophageal diverticulum.

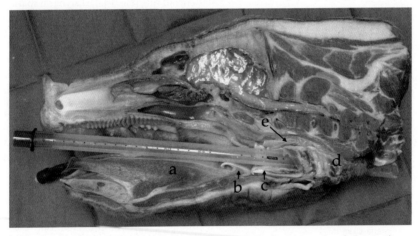

Figure 14.9 Sagittal section of a 43 kg Landrace pig's head to show principal structures in relation to the passage of an endotracheal tube (10 mm ID); a: tongue, b: epiglottis, c: thyroid cartilage, d: trachea, e: oesophagus.

assistant elevates the upper jaw and with the other hand, pulls down on the lower jaw and pulls on the tongue (Fig. 14.10). Gauze strips or lengths of IV administration tubing can be used to open the jaws and a dry gauze assists stabilizing the tongue. The anaesthetist introduces the laryngoscope blade until the tip is between the tongue and the epiglottis, and the tongue is depressed. The soft palate may have to be lifted away from the epiglottis, either with the laryngoscope blade or the tip of the endotracheal tube. The tube is inserted into the larynx under direct vision and is passed between the vocal cords at a level slightly dorsal to the middle of the larynx. If its progress is arrested at the entrance to the trachea, the stilette can be partially withdrawn and the head flexed slightly on the neck, or the

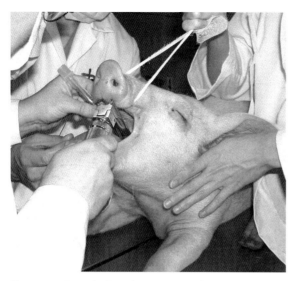

Figure 14.10 Intubation of a pig in sternal position. Note the extension of the head and neck.

endotracheal tube rotated 90–180° about its longitudinal axis. The tube may then be advanced gently into the trachea. An alternative is to introduce a stilette about three times the length of the endotracheal tube through the larynx under direct vision and then to insert the tube over it into the trachea. Placement of the tube in the oesophagus may be recognized by failure of substantial airflow through the tube or absence of misting inside the tube with breathing, breathing sounds or gurgling from the pharynx, evidence of airway obstruction including onset of cyanosis, and failure of carbon dioxide measurement by capnography. In large adult pigs, a speculum made from a length of plastic plumbing pipe covered with duct tape can be inserted between the upper and lower incisors to protect the endotracheal tube.

Placement of a laryngeal mask airway (LMA) is an alternative method for securing the airway (Patil et al., 1997; Fulkerson & Gustafson, 2007; Birkholz et al., 2008). Size 4 has been recommended for 45 kg domestic pigs and size 5 for larger adult miniature pigs. With the cuff deflated and sterile lubricating gel smeared on the outside, while the tongue is immobilized with one hand, the LMA is inserted into the pig's mouth with the other hand and advanced into the pharynx until resistance is felt. The cuff is inflated with up to 30 mL air. In one study comparing the LMA and endotracheal tube in isoflurane-anaesthetized pigs, controlled ventilation was achieved with both airways using tidal volumes of 10–13 mL/kg, respiratory rates 19–25 per minute, and peak inspiratory pressures of 15–23 cm H_2O (Fulkerson & Gustafson, 2007). Adequacy of ventilation was evaluated by observation of chest excursion and

measurements of end-tidal CO_2 35–45 mmHg. No air leakage around the cuff was heard and no gastric distension was observed. Leakage may occur when higher inflation pressures are needed for adequate ventilation.

Injectable anaesthetic agents and combinations

Anaesthesia can be induced by IV injection of diazepam–ketamine, thiopental, or propofol, for short surgical procedures. The degree of relaxation, the dose rates, and the safety of the patient are improved by prior administration of sedative agents. In some cases, agents administered IM for sedation can induce anaesthesia sufficient for endotracheal intubation or short surgical or medical procedures. Total intravenous anaesthesia (TIVA) may be maintained by additional IV supplements of anaesthetic agents and, when appropriate, the inclusion of local analgesia. Hypoxaemia and hypotension may develop during TIVA. These patients should be monitored and oxygen supplementation should be available for treatment of hypoxaemia.

Commonly used premedications for IM administration include butorphanol–atropine–midazolam (BAM), butorphanol–atropine–midazolam–xylazine (BAMX), butorphanol–atropine–midazolam–(dex)medetomidine (BAMM), and tiletamine–zolazepam or azaperone with or without butorphanol. Small pigs may be adequately sedated with acepromazine–butorphanol or midazolam–butorphanol. Dose rates in domestic pigs that have not been previously handled may be much higher than those required for anaesthesia in pet potbellied pigs.

Alfaxalone

Alfaxalone, in its new formulation in cyclodextrin, is licensed for use in dogs and cats in many countries. Induction of anaesthesia with alfaxalone in 60 mixed breed pigs that were premedicated with azaperone IM produced good conditions for endotracheal intubation in 63% of the pigs and some difficulty with jaw tone in 37% of the pigs (Keates, 2003). The gilts, weighing a mean of 116 kg, were premedicated with azaperone, 2.1 mg/kg IM, and anaesthesia was induced with alfaxalone, 0.9 ± 0.2 mg/kg. The mature sows, weighing a mean of 242 kg, were premedicated with azaperone, 1.2 mg/kg, and received alfaxalone, 0.7 ± 0.1 mg/kg, IV. Anaesthesia was maintained with halothane in oxygen. Ventilation was good based on end-tidal CO_2 values. Twitching, most commonly involving the facial or jaw muscles, was observed in one-third of the pigs during recovery from anaesthesia.

Ketamine

Ketamine is a useful agent for induction of anaesthesia in pigs. When used alone, anaesthesia is accompanied by poor muscle relaxation, difficulty in achieving a desired depth of anaesthesia for surgery, and agitation and excessive motor movement in recovery. The addition of sedatives and opioids to ketamine anaesthesia results in a longer duration of action and a quiet recovery. Ketamine may be administered at the time of premedication, for induction of anaesthesia, or both. Many different combinations, and dose rates, have been recommended and the choice may depend of the anaesthetist's preference or availability of agents. The dose rate for IV administration of ketamine for induction of anaesthesia in healthy pigs depends on the degree of preanaesthetic sedation and varies from 10 to 20 mg/kg with light premedication to 1–5 mg/kg following heavy sedation.

A combination of ketamine, 10 or 20 mg/kg, xylazine 2 mg/kg, and midazolam, 0.25 mg/kg, all injected IM produced immobilization in young growing pigs in approximately 2 minutes, duration of 55 minutes (low dose) and 92 minutes (high dose), followed by recovery times of 8–19 minutes (Ajadi et al., 2008). Analgesia was tested by interdigital pinch. No analgesia was present in pigs given the low dose of ketamine but was present for an average of 41 minutes after administration of the higher dose of ketamine. The conclusion was that the high dose of ketamine or other anaesthetic agents must be administered to provide analgesia for surgical procedures when using this drug combination.

In another study, domestic pigs weighing 20 kg were given a combination of atropine, 0.025 mg/kg, medetomidine, 0.08 mg/kg, and butorphanol, 0.2 mg/kg, IM for premedication followed by ketamine, 10 mg/kg, IM 15 minutes later. These agents provided anaesthesia for minor surgical procedures for at least 30 minutes and loss of pedal reflex for a mean of 75 minutes (Sakaguchi et al., 1996). In a separate experiment, administration of atipamezole, 0.24 mg/kg, IM or IV to pigs anaesthetized with atropine–medetomidine–butorphanol–ketamine resulted in arousal within 20 minutes accompanied by ataxia and hind limb weakness. There was no significant difference in mean arousal times and mean walk times between pigs given atipamezole IM or IV.

Guaifenesin–ketamine–xylazine 'Triple Drip'

The combination of ketamine and xylazine in 5% guaifenesin ('Triple Drip') given by IV infusion, although rather expensive, can be used in pigs as in other species of animal to produce and maintain anaesthesia. The solution is usually prepared immediately before use to contain 2 mg of ketamine, 1 mg of xylazine, and 50 mg guaifenesin per mL. Induction of anaesthesia usually needs 0.6–1 mL/kg and anaesthesia is maintained by infusion of approximately 2.2 mL/kg/h, but the rate of infusion must be adjusted to effect as judged by monitoring the usual signs of anaesthesia. Recovery is usually 30–45 minutes following cessation of administration but can be hastened by administration of tolazoline or atipamezole.

Pentobarbital sodium

This drug still has a place for surgery in experimental laboratories. The most satisfactory method of administration of pentobarbital is slow IV injection until the desired degree of CNS depression is obtained. Depths of anaesthesia may be difficult to assess in pigs. Presence or absence of withdrawal to toe pinch may be evidence of anaesthesia. For healthy, unsedated male and female pigs up to 50 kg body weight, the average IV dose of pentobarbital necessary to induce medium depth anaesthesia is about 30 mg/kg. Injection must be made slowly over several minutes and titrated to the onset of muscle relaxation. The dose rate must be reduced for very large pigs and marked variations in susceptibility will be encountered. Administration of other anaesthetic agents allows a decrease in the dose rate of pentobarbital and various combinations have been decribed for anaesthesia in research animals (Liu et al., 2009).

Intratesticular injection of pentobarbital has been used to produce anaesthesia for castration in large pigs. A concentrated solution of pentobarbital sodium (300 mg/mL), such as one commercially available for euthanasia of small animals may be administered at a dose rate of about 45 mg/kg; a very large boar being given 20 mL of solution into each testicle and adequate anaesthesia for castration develops within 10 minutes of injection. The pig must be castrated as soon as it becomes anaesthetized to prevent overdosage by removing the depot of pentobarbital. Safe disposal of the testicles is essential to prevent inadvertent ingestion by dogs that would lead to their death.

Propofol

Propofol has been used to induce anaesthesia in pigs after a variety of preanaesthetic agents. As with other anaesthetics, the dose rate of propofol decreases with increasing sedation. Dose rates 4–5 mg/kg IV have been used in pigs with mild to moderate preanaesthetic sedation (Zaballos et al., 2009) and 1–3 mg/kg IV in pigs with greater sedation. Anaesthesia is generally maintained in clinical patients with inhalation agents. Total intravenous anaesthesia with propofol infusion, 8–13 mg/kg/h, has been reported for experimental studies, in conjunction with continous infusions of fentanyl, 35 μg/kg/h, or remifentanil, 0.5 μg/kg/h (Schoffmann et al., 2009; Zaballos et al., 2009). In another study of TIVA with propofol, 18.5 mg/kg/h, a continuous infusion of dexmedetomidine, 0.2 μg/kg/h, significantly deepened anaesthesia as measured by BIS monitor (Sano et al., 2010). Cardiac output was decreased primarily due to decreased HR, MAP decreased and peripheral vascular resistances were unchanged. Higher dose rates for dexmedetomidine resulted in significant cardiovascular depression.

Tiletamine–zolazepam

In healthy pigs, IM injection of tiletamine–zolazepam induces sedation that is not sufficient to allow endotracheal intubation or a painful procedure. The combination of tiletamine–zolazepam, 4.4 mg/kg, and xylazine, 2.2 mg/kg, IM rapidly induces immobilization sufficient for endotracheal intubation, approximately 20–30 minutes of analgesia, and an acceptable recovery from anaesthesia (Ko et al., 1993, 1995). The addition of ketamine, 2.2 mg/kg, to the combination was found only to prolong analgesia and recumbency times by a few minutes. Tiletamine–zolazepam is available as a powder in multidose vials for reconstitution with 5 mL sterile water that results in a solution containing 250 mg of tiletamine and 250 mg of zolazepam or 100 mg/mL of tiletamine-zolazepam. The powder can be reconstituted with adjunct agents to decrease the final volume for injection (Ko et al., 1995). A mixture of tiletamine–zolazepam–xylazine can be made by adding 2.5 mL of 100 mg/mL xylazine and 2.5 mL of sterile water to 500 mg of powder to produce a solution containing 100 mg/mL of tiletamine–zolazepam and 50 mg/mL of xylazine. To produce a mixture of tiletamine–zolazepam–ketamine–xylazine (TKX), a vial containing 500 mg tiletamine–zolazepam powder should be reconstituted with 2.5 mL of 100 mg/mL ketamine and 2.5 mL of 100 mg/mL xylazine. In each case, the dose rate is 4.4 mg/kg based on the combined concentration of 100 mg/mL tiletamine–zolazepam. Lower dose rates can be used for preanaesthetic sedation followed by induction of anaesthesia by ketamine, 1–2 mg/kg IV, or inhalation agent administered via facemask.

Tiletamine–zolazepam, 4–5 mg/kg, may be combined with medetomidine, 0.05 mg/kg, IM to induce anaesthesia in domestic pigs. Lower dose rates of medetomidine, 0.01 mg/kg, are often sufficient in potbellied pigs.

Thiopental sodium

Anaesthesia can be induced in pigs by thiopental, 5–12 mg/kg, IV depending on premedication, with the larger pigs requiring the smaller dose rate. Thiopental is preferably used as a 2 or 2.5% solution since a 5% solution will cause tissue necrosis if injected outside the vein. Further, use of a more dilute solution of thiopental usually results in administration of a lower total dose of thiopental. Induction of anaesthesia with thiopental sodium is facilitated by preanaesthetic sedation, and lower doses of thiopental are adequate. Apnoea may occur after injection. Duration of anaesthesia is short and may have to be supplemented with inhalation anaesthesia. Supplemental doses of thiopental are cumulative and can result in delay in recovery.

Inhalation anaesthesia

Breathing systems that are used for dogs may be used to administer inhalant anaesthetics to most pigs. Circle circuits designed for equine anaesthesia are more appropriate for very large boars and sows because the circle Y-piece lumen and internal diameters of endotracheal tube adapters of small animal circuits are smaller than their tracheas and impose resistance to air flow. Inhalation agents may be administered via a facemask but endotracheal intubation is preferable as controlled ventilation may be necessary. Large facemasks available for dogs are adequate for small pigs. Masks for large pigs can be constructed from heavy plastic rolled into a cone, and from plastic funnels or plastic containers. Care must be taken so that the mask does not distort or obstruct the nostrils. Adhesive or duct tape can be wrapped around the edge of the mask and the pigs' face to produce an air-tight seal.

Isoflurane and sevoflurane are commonly used to maintain anaesthesia in pigs. Desflurane is used less in clinical practice because of significantly increased expense of the agent and the vaporizer. Nitrous oxide was used extensively in pigs to provide analgesia and decrease the concentration of halothane required for anaesthesia. The improved cardiovascular effects of isoflurane and sevoflurane and the increase in available injectable agents for sedation and analgesia have minimized the need for nitrous oxide.

Drug dosages, mg/kg, for anaesthetic agents are decreased by heavy sedation, old age, obesity, sepsis, severe haemorrhage, and systemic disease.

Isoflurane, sevoflurane

The published values for the minimum alveolar concentration (MAC) for isoflurane in pigs is 1.6–1.9% and for sevoflurane is 2.4–2.66% (Manohar & Parks, 1984; Allaouchiche et al., 2001; Malavasi et al., 2008). The concentration required for anaesthesia will be decreased by prior administration of other anaesthetic agents, for example, induction of anaesthesia with tiletamine–zolazepam-medetomidine decreased isoflurane MAC by 68% (Malavasi et al., 2008). The addition of opioids or the presence of disease will further decrease anaesthetic requirement. For example, in young domestic pigs anaesthetized with sevoflurane, experimental induction of sepsis decreased sevoflurane requirement by 44% (Allaouchiche et al., 2001).

Both isoflurane and sevoflurane induce dose-dependent decreases in cardiac output (CO), stroke volume and MAP in healthy pigs (Manohar & Parks, 1984). Compared with equipotent concentrations of isoflurane, sevoflurane caused a larger decrease in CO but less depression of MAP especially at deeper planes of anaesthesia. Cerebrovascular resistance altered minimally when the pigs were normocarbic, and renal blood flow was unchanged from the conscious state. The more rapid induction and recovery characteristics of sevoflurane give it the advantage over isoflurane for anaesthesia of sick patients and for outpatient anaesthesia.

Desflurane

Different values for desflurane MAC in pigs have been reported; 8.28–10.0% (Manohar & Parks, 1984; Eger et al., 1988), and even as high as 13.8% (Holmstrom et al., 2004). Cardiovascular effects of desflurane in pigs are similar to those in other species, in that increasing desflurane administration to above MAC value results in hypotension but no significant change in heart rates (Martin-Cancho et al., 2006).

Nitrous oxide (N₂O)

Nitrous oxide is not sufficiently potent to induce anaesthesia in pigs but can be used as an adjunct agent to provide analgesia during anaesthesia. One study measured a 21% decrease in isoflurane requirement when 50% inspired N_2O was added, and that the decrease in isoflurane administration was accompanied by a significantly higher MAP compared with measurements recorded during anaesthesia with isoflurane alone (Tranquilli et al., 1985).

When N_2O is part of the anaesthetic protocol, it must be remembered that the pig must breathe oxygen for 5 minutes after N_2O is discontinued to avoid 'diffusion hypoxia'.

Monitoring

Monitoring vital signs is essential for early detection of abnormalities. Common abnormalities during anaesthesia that require treatment are hypoventilation, airway obstruction, hypotension, bradycardia, and hypothermia. Recently, a review of anaesthesia in potbellied pigs identified a high incidence of these abnormalities in a series of clinical patients (Trim & Braun, 2011).

Depth of surgical anaesthesia is assessed by using the position of the eye, rolled rostroventral in the orbit, and the presence or absence of a palpebral reflex, which should be weakly present or just absent. Failure of withdrawal reflex in response to a toe or interdigital pinch is a rough guide for adequacy of anaesthesia. Heart rates and arterial pressures are largely determined by the anaesthetic agents administered, but abrupt increases shortly after an increase in noxious stimulus probably represent signs of inadequate anaesthesia.

Circulation is assessed in similar ways to small animal patients but evaluation of membrane colour and capillary refill time may be complicated by black pigmentation. An oesophageal stethoscope can be used in small pigs but will need to be inserted visually using a laryngoscope. A pulse oximeter can be attached to the tongue, lips, or nose to monitor oxygenation. Arterial blood pressure can be measured non-invasively (NIBP) using the Doppler ultrasound probe placed caudally on a lower extremity with a cuff proximal, or by the oscillometric technique using a

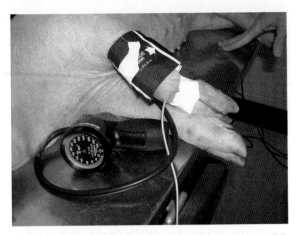

Figure 14.11 Attachment of a Doppler probe on the caudal surface of the forelimb. A cuff is wrapped proximally and connected to a pressure manometer for non-invasive measurement of blood pressure.

single cuff (Fig. 14.11). Accuracy of NIBP measurement in pigs may be influenced by the uneven circumference of a pig's limb interfering with satisfactory placement of the cuff. Systolic arterial pressure measured using Doppler ultrasound may be less than invasive systolic pressure in anaesthetized domestic pigs, whereas diastolic pressure measurements may be similar (Trim, unpublished observations). Data from another investigation indicate that there are no significant differences between systolic pressures measured directly and indirectly in domestic pigs (Hodgkin et al., 1982). Invasive blood pressure measurement is usually made from a catheter inserted in an auricular artery but any artery on the forelimb or hind limb can also be cannulated. Comparison of arterial pressures from auricular and femoral arteries in anaesthetized pigs found no significant differences (Bass et al., 2009). Normal values in awake domestic pigs for heart rate and MAP vary from 103 ± 13 to 114 ± 6 beats/min and 102 ± 9 to 116 ± 16 mmHg, respectively (Tranquilli et al., 1982; Trim & Gilroy, 1985; Hannon et al., 1990; Sakaguchi et al., 1996). Balanced electrolyte solution is infused at 5–10 mL/kg/h. Hypotension, MAP less than 65 mmHg, has many causes during anaesthesia and surgery. Treatment is aimed at the cause and involves decreased anaesthetic agent administration, fluid therapy, and vasoactive drugs (see Chapter 21, Complications). Circulating blood volume in pigs has been reported as 67 mL/kg (Hannon et al., 1990). Anaesthesia impairs the physiological response to haemorrhage and loss of 15% of blood volume in anaesthetized animals (10 mL/kg in pigs) is associated with significant decreases in circulatory function.

Respiratory rates may vary according to the anaesthetic protocol but slow rates less than 10 per minute may indicate hypoventilation. Breathing should be both thoracic and abdominal but visual estimation of depth of breathing is difficult. Rapid shallow breathing during inhalation anaesthesia is frequently accompanied by significant hypercarbia. Adequacy of ventilation is easily monitored non-invasively using end-tidal CO_2 measurement, with values 30–40 mmHg representing normoventilation. Hypoventilation is best treated with controlled ventilation, or lightening the plane of anaesthesia if artificial ventilation is not an option. Artificial ventilation at 10–15 breaths/minute and tidal volumes of 15 mL/kg should achieve normocarbia. Tidal volume/kg should be decreased in obese patients.

Pigs' body temperature frequently mimics ambient temperature, although hypothermia most often develops. Monitoring is important to identify hypo- or hyperthermia. Rectal temperature in normal domestic pigs is 38.5 ± 0.65°C (101.3 ± 1.2°F) (Hannon et al., 1990). Potbellied pigs are reported to have lower rectal temperatures than domestic pigs with a mean value of 37.6 ± 0.8°C (99.7 ± 1.5°F), range 35.1–39.6°C (95.2–103.3°F) (Lord et al., 1999). Potbellied pigs also exhibit diurnal variation in body temperatures, with temperatures in the morning being significantly lower than temperatures in the evening. Prevention of hypothermia during anaesthesia involves application of heat, such as hot water circulating pads or warm air blankets, use of warmed intravenous fluids, and alteration of room temperature, where appropriate.

Postanaesthetic care

It is essential that pigs should be kept warm until they are completely mobile after sedation or general anaesthesia because they are prone to develop hypothermia and recovery will be prolonged.

Close observation after extubation during recovery is necessary so that immediate measures may be taken to relieve any respiratory obstruction. When tracheal intubation was traumatic, dexamethasone, 1 mg/kg, should be injected slowly IV during anaesthesia to decrease laryngeal swelling.

Disorientation and increased activity during recovery may be residual CNS effects of dissociative agents, anxiety, or pain. Administration of midazolam, 0.1–0.2 mg/kg, IV should calm an anxious patient. Rectal temperature should be monitored in active patients as they may develop hyperthermia.

Postoperative pain relief is essential, particularly following all surgical procedures. Provision of analgesia should have been incorporated into the anaesthetic protocol and supplemental doses of opioids may be necessary during recovery. The pigs should be observed as the full effect of opioid develops in case the pigs become reanaesthetized or assume a position that results in airway obstruction.

In research, continuous infusions of medetomidine, 0.02 mg/kg/h, diluted to a convenient volume and infused concurrently with an opioid, have been used to maintain long-term immobility after experimental surgery (Nunes et al., 2007).

Neuromuscular blocking agents

Neuromuscular blocking agents may be used in pigs to provide muscle relaxation for thoracic, abdominal, and orthopaedic surgery, and experimental studies. When using neuromuscular blockade, the pigs must be unconscious and analgesic, and controlled ventilation must be employed. Monitoring equipment should include a method for measuring arterial blood pressure and a peripheral nerve stimulator to monitor neuromuscular blockade. Details on the pharmacology and clinical use of neuromuscular blocking agents are covered in Chapter 8.

Many neuromuscular blocking agents have been used successfully in pig anaesthesia. The depolarizing muscle relaxant suxamethonium (succinylcholine) was primarily used to facilitate endotracheal intubation. The increased availability of anaesthetic agents that induce satisfactory jaw relaxation for intubation has eliminated the need for suxamethonium. The non-depolarizing agents, pancuronium, atracurium, vecuronium, and rocuronium, provide longer durations of paralysis and can be administered as boluses at intervals or as continuous infusions. Initial bolus dose rates are listed (Table. 14.2) (Weiskopf et al., 1990; Herweling et al., 2004; Shi et al., 2008). Neuromuscular blocking agents can also be administered by continuous rate infusions.

Reversal of neuromuscular blockade at the end of anaesthesia involves administration of an acetylcholinesterase inhibitor, such as neostigmine or edrophonium. When using the train-of-four (TOF) pattern of nerve stimulation to monitor neuromuscular function, it is usual to wait

Table 14.2 Neuromuscular blocking agents used in pigs

Agent	Dose rate for initial IV bolus (mg/kg)	Duration of action to 80–95% recovery of digital twitch (min)
Suxamethonium/ succinylcholine	2.0	2–3
Pancuronium	0.06–0.12	25–30
Vecuronium	0.1	17
Atracurium	0.5–0.6	20–60
Rocuronium	1.26	22

399

until at least two twitches are present. Attempt at earlier reversal requires a larger dose of antagonist and increases the risk of adverse effects. When four twitches are apparent, even in the presence of a small degree of fade, a considerably smaller dose rate of anticholinesterase agent is adequate for reversal. It must be remembered that even when the amplitude of extremity twitch has returned to the pre-paralysis value, return of strength of the laryngeal muscles (and therefore, protective reflexes of the airway) will take a longer time. Bradycardia and gastrointestinal stimulation are included in the adverse effects induced by anticholinesterases and generally it is advisable to administer atropine or glycopyrrolate before pharmacological reversal.

LOCAL ANALGESIA

Epidural nerve block

In the pig, the spinal cord ends at the junction of the fifth and sixth lumbar vertebrae and the spinal meninges continue, around the phylum terminale, as far as the middle of the sacrum. At the lumbosacral space, the sac is comparatively small, and it is uncommon that a needle introduced at this point will penetrate into the subarachnoid space. The lumbosacral aperture is large. Its dimensions in the adult are approximately 1.5 cm craniocaudally and 3 cm transversely. The depth of the canal is about 1 cm.

The site for insertion of the needle is located as follows: the cranial border of the ilium on each side is found with the fingers. A line joining them crosses the spinous process of the last lumbar vertebra (Fig. 14.12). The needle can be inserted in the midline immediately behind this spinous process and directed downwards and backwards at an angle of 20° with the vertical, or inserted up to 2.5–4 cm caudal to the spinous process and perpendicular to the pig's back. The depth to which the needle must penetrate in pigs of from 30 to 70 kg will vary from 5 to 9 cm. The landmarks described are readily detected in animals of smaller size but they may be masked by the overlying tissues in larger ones. In large pigs, a point 15 cm cranial to the base of the tail serves as a fairly accurate guide. Provided the needle is introduced in approximately the correct position and direction, the size of the lumbosacral space makes its detection comparatively easy. Alternatively, in large pigs that are standing or in lateral recumbency with the hind limbs placed in a normal standing position, a line perpendicular to the floor passing through the patella will cross midline at the level of the last lumbar spinous process. Needle insertion is 2.5–4 cm caudal to this point and perpendicular to the animal's back. Some animals have straighter hocks than others and adjustment must be made for this difference in anatomy to prevent insertion of the needle too far caudally. Eighteen gauge

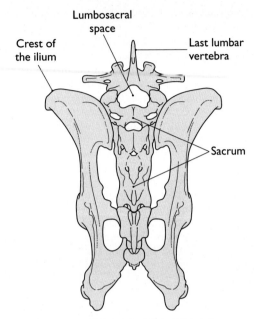

Figure 14.12 Dorsal view of the pig's pelvis. A line connecting the iliac crests crosses the last lumbar vertebra. The lumbosacral space in adult pigs is 2.5–3 cm caudal to this point. The patella can be used as a reliable landmark for location of the iliac crest in larger animals; with the hind legs in a normal standing position, a vertical line through the patella will cross midline on level with the crest of the ilium.

needles are used; 8 cm long for pigs between 30 and 50 kg, 10 cm long for 100 kg pigs, and 15 cm for 200 kg pigs. Spinal needles that have a shorter needle bevel and a stilette are preferable when available.

After preparation of the skin with a surgical scrub, a small volume of lidocaine should be injected with a hypodermic needle as a subcutaneous bleb at the proposed site of needle insertion. Positioning for epidural injection may be determined by patient cooperation facilitated by light or heavy sedation or general anaesthesia. Small pigs may be restrained in sternal position with the hind limbs pulled rostrally, and large pigs may be in lateral position or standing. Insertion of the long needle required to reach the epidural space in large pigs may be facilitated by placement of a 14 gauge 5 cm hypodermic needle through which the 18 gauge 12–15 cm needle is inserted. Insertion of the needle through the interarcuate ligament should be carefully controlled. Rapid penetration may result in the needle touching the spinal cord and sudden movement by the pig that may dislodge needle placement. A syringe should be attached to the needle and aspirated to ensure absence of cerebrospinal fluid (CSF) or blood. A small amount of air, saline, or local anesthetic solution should then be injected to ascertain 'loss of resistance'. Local anaesthetic solution should be injected slowly over at least 30 seconds to avoid an increase in CSF pressure.

Epidural analgesia has been used for the castration of pigs of 40–50 kg, injecting 10 mL of 2% lidocaine solution (5 mg/kg), with or without epinephrine. Complete desensitization of the scrotum, testes and spermatic cord was present in 10 minutes, and there was a partial motor paralysis of the hind limbs. Recovery was complete at the end of the second hour.

Lower dose rates of lidocaine have been recommended at 1 mL of a 2% solution per 7.5 kg (2.7 mg/kg) for pigs weighing up to 50 kg and an additional 1.0 mL for every 10 kg above this in weight. Another suggestion which has proved to be satisfactory is based on occiput–tail base measurement allowing 1.0 mL for the first 40 cm and an additional 1.5 mL for each 10 cm longer length. Epidural analgesia with 20 mL of 2% lidocaine is adequate for caesarian section in sows weighing about 300 kg.

The effects of xylazine and detomidine injected at the lumbosacral space have been evaluated (Lumb & Jones, 1996). Epidural xylazine, 2 mg/kg in 5 mL 0.9% saline, induces sedation, hind limb immobilization, and analgesia extending to the umbilicus within 5 minutes after injection. Duration is up to 2 hours. Detomidine (0.5 mg/kg in 5 mL 0.9% saline) induces sedation but minimal analgesia. Administration of atipamezole, 0.2 mg/kg, reversed the sedation but not the hind limb immobilization or analgesia. In another research study, epidural xylazine, 0.2 mg/kg diluted in saline to 0.5 mL/kg, in isoflurane anaesthetized healthy Landrace–Large White pigs produced analgesia for up to 90 minutes (Tendillo et al., 1995).

Administration of morphine into the epidural space will provide additional analgesia for abdominal or pelvic limb surgery. Preservative-free morphine, 0.1 mg/kg, diluted with saline if necessary to provide a volume of 0.1 mL/kg, will have an expected onset of maximal effect of 40 minutes after injection. Epidural morphine has the advantage of providing analgesia without systemic adverse effects, and the decrease in inhalant agent requirement will result in less respiratory depression. In one study of domestic pigs weighing on average 20 kg and undergoing abdominal surgery, the concentration of isoflurane required to maintain anaesthesia was decreased by 33% in pigs receiving morphine epidural injections compared with pigs without morphine (Malavasi et al., 2006a). The duration of analgesia may last more than 12 hours.

Potential adverse consequences of epidural injection are meningitis or abscess formation as a result of failure of aseptic technique, or neurological deficits as a result of epidural haematoma or trauma. Injection of local anaesthetic solution too rapidly will increase CSF pressure and may result in collapse or seizures. Injection of too large a volume of local anaesthetic solution may result in paralysis of intercostal nerves and impaired ventilation.

Injection of local anaesthetic solution will result in vasodilation of the hind limbs and a decrease in MAP. Hypotension should be treated with IV fluid therapy and ephedrine, 0.1 mg/kg, IV or IM.

Analgesia for castration

Local analgesia can be used to provide analgesia for castration of pigs up to about 5 months of age, but general anaesthesia is more satisfactory for older animals. For intratesticular injection, a needle of suitable size is inserted perpendicularly through the tensed scrotal skin and advanced until its point lies in the middle of the testicle. Between 3 and 15 mL, depending on the size the animal, of 2% lidocaine or 5% procaine are injected, with the majority of drug injected into the testicle and part of the dose injected subcutaneously beneath the scrotal skin as the needle is withdrawn. Both sides are treated in the same manner. The operation may commence about 5 minutes after completion of the injections.

Within Europe, lobby from welfare groups has resulted in some countries (and even supermarket chains) introducing requirements for anaesthesia and analgesia for castration of even the youngest piglets. A number of studies have investigated methods which might be practical for castration of large numbers of pigs on the farm. Most have considered that isoflurane (which has a food animal indication in Europe) by mask is most practical, combined with postoperative analgesia using, for example, meloxicam.

A novel technique for anaesthetizing piglets approximately 1 week old for castration utilizes liquid injection of isoflurane or sevoflurane, oxygen, and a rebreathing inhaler (Hodgson, 2007). Calculation of the liquid volume of isoflurane or sevoflurane to achieve a 1.3× MAC dose utilized the square root of time model and metabolic size to achieve target alveolar concentrations of 1.82% isoflurane or 4.03% sevoflurane. A table of piglet weights and liquid anaesthetic requirement was produced for practical use. This technique is based on total anaesthesia time of less than 5 minutes since rebreathing of carbon dioxide occurs. In one study of 114 piglets, induction time was on average 45 seconds, castration approximately 75 seconds, and recovery about 2 minutes. There were no clinically significant differences between isoflurane and sevoflurane, except that the cost of isoflurane was minimal compared with sevoflurane. The inclusion of general anaesthesia for castration of piglets was accepted by the herdsman of the farrowing house as quiet and stress free.

The use of carbon dioxide to immobilize the pigs, which has been advocated in some countries, has been described as an inappropriate and inadvisable technique by the Association of Veterinary Anaesthetists. Fortunately, the introduction and use of immune-mediated chemical castration will mean that surgery will be no longer necessary.

401

Caesarian section

Sows may be restrained with ropes, lightly sedated, or put under general anaesthesia. Analgesia for a flank laparotomy can be provided by infiltration of lidocaine, up to 4 mg/kg as a 0.5–2% solution, as a line block at the site of incision or a regional block as an inverted-L cranial and dorsal to the incision site. Lidocaine must be infiltrated subcutaneously and deeper into the abdominal muscle down to the peritoneum. Administration of oxygen by mask appears to decrease mortality in exhausted or toxic sows.

Other injectable anaesthetic combinations that have been used for caesarian sections in pigs, including xylazine, 1 mg/kg, and ketamine, 2 mg/kg, IV or light preanaesthetic sedation with a neuroleptanalgesia combination and induction and maintenance of anaesthesia with isoflurane or sevoflurane.

REFERENCES

Ajadi, R.A., Smith, O.F., Makinde, A.F., et al., 2008. Increasing ketamine dose enhances the anaesthetic properties of ketamine-xylazine-midazolam combinations in growing pigs. J S Afr Vet Assoc 79, 205–207.

Allaouchiche, B., Duflo, F., Tournadre, J.P., et al., 2001. Influence of sepsis on sevoflurane minimum alveolar concentration in a porcine model. Br J Anaesth 86, 832–836.

Bass, L.M.E., Yu, D.-Y., Cullen, L.K., 2009. Comparison of femoral and auricular arterial blood pressure monitoring in pigs. Vet Anaesth Analg 36, 457–463.

Birkholz, T., Irouschek, A., Kessler, P., et al., 2008. Feasibility of the laryngeal tube airway for artificial ventilation in pigs and comparison with the laryngeal mask airway. Lab Anim 37, 371–379.

Brodbelt, D.C., Pfeiffer, D.U., Young, L.E., et al., 2008. Results of the confidential enquiry into perioperative small animal fatalities regarding risk factors for anaesthetic-related death in dogs. J Am Vet Med Assoc 233, 1096–1104.

Bustamente, R., Valverde, A., 1997. Determination of a sedative dose and influence of droperidol and midazolam on cardiovascular function in pigs. Can J Vet Res 61, 246–250.

Clark, S.G., Coffer, N., 2008. Normal hematology and hematologic disorders in potbellied pigs. Vet Clin N Am Exot Anim Pract 11, 569–582.

Clutton, R.E., Bracken, J., Ritchie, M., 1998. Effect of muscle injection site and drug temperature on pre-anesthetic sedation in pigs. Vet Rec 142, 718–721.

Eger, E.I., Jr, Johnson, B.H., Weiskopf, B., et al., 1988. Minimum alveolar concentration of I-653 and isoflurane in pigs. Anesth Analg 67, 1174–1177.

Fulkerson, P.J., Gustafson, S.B., 2007. Use of laryngeal mask airway compared to endotracheal tube with positive-pressure ventilation in anesthetized swine. Vet Anaesth Analg 34, 284–288.

Hall, L.W., Trim, C.M., Woolf, C.J., 1972. Further studies of porcine malignant hyperthermia. Br Med J 2, 145–148.

Hall, L.W., Woolf, V., Bradley, J.W.P., et al., 1966. Unusual reaction to suxamethonium chloride. Br Med J 2, 1305.

Hannon, J.P., Bossone, C.A., Wade, C.E., 1990. Normal physiological values for conscious pigs used in biomedical research. Lab Anim Sci 40, 293–298.

Harvey-Clark, C.J., Gilespie, K., Riggs, K.W., 2000. Transdermal fentanyl compared with parenteral buprenorphine in post-surgical pain in swine: a case study. Lab Anim 34, 386–398.

Herweling, A., Latorre, F., Herwig, A., et al., 2004. The hemodynamic effects of ephedrine on the onset time of rocuronium in pigs. Anesth Analg 99, 1703–1707.

Hodgkin, B.C., Burkett, D.E., Smith, E.B., 1982. Noninvasive measurement of systolic and diastolic blood pressure in swine. Am J Physiol 242, H127–H130.

Hodgson, D.R., 2007. Comparison of isoflurane and sevoflurane for short-term anaesthesia in piglets. Vet Anaesth Analg 34, 117–124.

Holmstrom, A., Rosen, I., Akeson, J., 2004. Desflurane results in higher cerebral blood flow than sevoflurane or isoflurane at hypocapnia in pigs. Acta Anaesth Scand 48, 400–404.

Hoyt, R.F., Hayre, M.D., Dodd, K.T., et al., 1986. Long-acting intramuscular anesthetic regimen for swine. Lab Anim Sci 36, 413–416.

Keates, H., 2003. Induction of anaesthesia in pigs using a new alphaxalone formulation. Vet Rec 153, 627–628.

Keita, A., Pagot, E., Prunier, A., et al., 2010. Pre-emptive meloxicam for postoperative analgesia in piglets undergoing surgical castration. Vet Anaesth Analg 37, 367–374.

Ko, J.C.H., Williams, B.L., Rogers, E.R., et al., 1995. Increasing xylazine dose enhanced anesthetic properties of Telazol-xylazine combination in swine. Lab Anim Sci 45, 290–294.

Ko, J.C.H., Williams, B.L., Smith, V.L., et al., 1993. Comparison of Telazol, Telazol-ketamine, Telazol-xylazine, and Telazol-ketamine-xylazine as chemical restraint and anesthetic induction combination in swine. Lab Anim Sci 43, 476–480.

Krause, T., Gerbershagen, M.U., Fiege, M., et al., 2004. Dantrolene – A review of its pharmacology, therapeutic use and new developments. Anaesthesia 59, 364–373.

Kumar, A., Mann, H.J., Remmel, R.P., 2006. Pharmacokinetics of tiletamine and zolazepam (Telazol) in anesthetized pigs. J Vet Pharmacol Ther 29, 587–589.

Liu, D., Shao, Y., Luan, X., et al., 2009. Comparison of ketamine-pentobarbital anesthesia and fentanyl-pentobarbital anesthesia for open-heart surgery in minipigs. Lab Anim 38, 234–239.

Lord, L.K., Wittum, T.E., Anderson, D.E., et al., 1999. Resting rectal temperature of Vietnamese potbellied pigs. J Am Vet Med Assoc 215, 342–344.

Lumb, W.V., Jones, E.W., 1996. Veterinary Anesthesia, third ed. Williams & Wilkins, Baltimore, p. 501.

Malavasi, L.M., Augustsson, H., Jensen-Waern, M., et al., 2005. The effect of transdermal delivery of fentanyl on activity in growing pigs. Acta Vet Scand 46, 149–157.

Malavasi, L.M., Jensen-Waern, M., Augustsson, H., et al., 2008. Changes in minimal alveolar concentration of isoflurane following treatment with medetomidine and tiletamine/zolazepam, epidural morphine or systemic buprenorphine in pigs. Lab Anim 42, 62–70.

Malavasi, L.M., Jensen-Waern, M., Jacobson, M., et al., 2006a. Effects of extradural morphine on end-tidal isoflurane concentration and physiological variables in pigs undergoing abdominal surgery: a clinical study. Vet Anaesth Analg 33, 307–312.

Malavasi, L.M., Nyman, G., Augustsson, H., et al., 2006b. Effects of epidural morphine and transdermal fentanyl analgesia on physiology and behaviour after abdominal surgery in pigs. Lab Anim 40, 16–27.

Manohar, M., Parks, C.M., 1984. Porcine systemic and regional organ blood flow during 1.0 and 1.5 minimum alveolar concentrations of sevoflurane anesthesia without and with 50% nitrous oxide. J Pharm Exper Ther 321, 640–648.

Martin-Cancho, M.F., Lima, J.R., Luis, L., et al., 2006. Bispectral index, spectral edge frequency 95% and median frequency recorded at varying desflurane concentrations in pigs. Res Vet Sci 81, 373–381.

Nunes, S., Berg, L., Raittinen, L.-P., et al., 2007. Deep sedation with dexmedetomidine in a porcine model does not compromise the viability of free microvascular flap as depicted by microdialysis and tissue oxygen tension. Anesth Analg 105, 666–672.

Patil, V.U., Fairbrother, C.R., Dunham, B.M., 1997. Use of the laryngeal mask airway for emergency or elective airway management solutions in pigs. Contemp Top Lab Anim Sci 36, 47–49.

Risdahl, J.M., Chao, C., Murtaugh, M.P., et al., 1992. Acute and chronic morphine administration in swine. Pharmacol Biochem Behav 43, 799–806.

Rosenberg, H., Davis, M., James, D., et al., 2007. Malignant hyperthermia. Orphanet J Rare Dis 2, 21.

Sakaguchi, M., Nishimura, R., Sasaki, N., et al., 1996. Anesthesia induced in pigs by use of a combination of medetomidine, butorphanol, and ketamine and its reversal by administration of atipamezole. Am J Vet Res 57, 529–534.

Sano, H., Doi, M., Mimuro, S., et al., 2010. Evaluation of the hypnotic and hemodynamic effects of dexmedetomidine on propofol-sedated swine. Exp Anim 59, 199–205.

Schoffmann, G., Winter, P., Palme, R., et al., 2009. Haemodynamic changes and stress responses of piglets to surgery during total intravenous anaesthesia with propofol and fentanyl. Lab Anim 43, 243–248.

Shi, Y., Hou, V., Tucker, A., et al., 2008. Changes of extremity and laryngeal muscle electromyographic amplitudes after intravenous administration of vecuronium. Laryngoscope 118, 2156–2160.

Snook, C.S., 2001. Use of the subcutaneous abdominal vein for blood sampling and intravenous catheterization in potbellied pigs. J Am Vet Med Assoc 219, 809–810.

Tendillo, F.J., Pera, A.M., Mascias, A., et al., 1995. Cardiopulmonary and analgesic effects of epidural lidocaine, alfentanil, and xylazine in pigs anesthetized with isoflurane. Vet Surg 24, 73–77.

Tranquilli, W.J., Parks, C.M., Thurmon, J.C., et al., 1982. Organ blood flow and distribution of cardiac output in nonanesthetized swine. Am J Vet Res 43, 895–897.

Tranquilli, W.J., Thurmon, J.C., Benson, G.J., 1985. Anesthetic potency of nitrous oxide in young swine (Sus scrofa). Am J Vet Res 46, 58–60.

Trim, C.M., Braun, C., 2011. Anesthetic agents and complications in Vietnamese potbellied pigs: 32 cases. 1999–2006). J Am Vet Med Assoc 239, 114–121.

Trim, C.M., Gilroy, B.A., 1985. Cardiopulmonary effects of a xylazine and ketamine combination in pigs. Res Vet Sci 38, 30–34.

Tuck, S.A., Dort, J.C., Olson, M.E., et al., 1999. Monitoring respiratory function and sleep in the obese Vietnamese pot-bellied pig. J Appl Physiol 87, 444–451.

Tuck, S.A., Dort, J.C., Remmers, J.E., 2001. Braking of expiratory airflow in obese pigs during wakefulness and sleep. Respir Physiol 128, 241–245.

Ugarte, C.E., O'Flaherty, K., 2005. The use of a medetomidine, butorphanol, and atropine combination to enable blood sampling in young pigs. N Z Vet J 53, 249–252.

Weiskopf, R.B., Eger II, E.I., Holmes, M.A., et al., 1990. Cardiovascular actions of common anesthetic adjuvants during desflurane (I-653) and isoflurane anesthesia in swine. Anesth Analg 71, 144–148.

Zaballos, M., Jimeno, C., Almendral, J., et al., 2009. Cardiac electrophysiologic effects of remifentanil: study in a closed-chest porcine model. Br J Anaesth 103, 191–198.

FURTHER READING

Rosenberg, H., Sambuughin, N., Dirksen, R., 2010. Malignant hyperthermia susceptibility. www.ncbi.nim.nih.gov/bookshelf Last update Jan 19.

Chapter | **15** |

Anaesthesia of the dog

INTRODUCTION

Within the last 10 years, there has been an explosion of new information about different anaesthetic agent combinations that can be used for sedation and anaesthesia in dogs. Anaesthetic protocols can still be straightforward for short anaesthesia for elective procedures but there are more choices for anaesthetic management of increasingly complex and more protracted medical and surgical procedures. Monitoring equipment has become more available for veterinary practice, enabling more precise control of the animal's physiological status and reducing intra- and postanaesthetic complications. There has been a resurgence in the use of nerve blocks in combination with general anaesthesia in concert with increased use of opioids not only to provide analgesia during surgery but with the intention of controlling pain after anaesthesia. This management goal is based on the desire to improve animal welfare but may have added benefits in more rapid recovery, shorter hospitalization time, and improved client satisfaction.

SEDATION AND ANALGESIA

General principles

Selection of a drug or drugs for sedation depends on the purpose for which it is intended and pharmacological details of opioids and sedatives are given in Chapters 4 and 5. Mild behaviour modification can be achieved with a phenothiazine such as acepromazine whereas moderate to heavy sedation is better obtained using an α_2-agonist, such as medetomidine or dexmedetomidine with an opioid, or a neuroleptanalgesic mixture such as acepromazine with morphine or methadone. Intravenous administration produces a more rapid onset and intense effect of a shorter duration than IM administration and, generally, drugs injected IV are at lower dose rates. Dose rates chosen may depend on whether the dog is to be only sedated or whether sedation is to be followed by general anaesthesia. When the drugs are used for premedication to anaesthesia, dose rates are often considerably lower so as to minimize cardiovascular and respiratory depression. Some individuals are sensitive and some resistant to anaesthetic agents and unusual responses should always be recorded in the medical record for valuable information at the dog's next visit.

Many minor procedures can be performed when dogs are sedated and the addition of local anaesthesia allows surgical procedures, depending on the type of nerve block used. Some procedures can be satisfactorily accomplished under only sedation while others are better done with the dog under general anaesthesia, for example dental prophylaxis where general anaesthesia including endotracheal intubation is recommended (American Veterinary Dental Association, 2004). Sedation only for this procedure limits effective cleaning and the absence of an endotracheal tube increases risk of aspiration of water and debris.

Phenothiazines

Acepromazine is a commonly used phenothiazine for sedation in dogs. Use of a 2 mg/mL solution facilitates more accurate dose administration than when a stronger solution is used. When not commercially available, a 2 mg/mL solution can be made by adding 60 mg of acepromazine to a 30 mL bottle of sterile saline, after first removing an equivalent volume of saline. The bottle should be wrapped to protect the solution from the light. The response to acepromazine is not uniform and depends on the animal's temperament, physical condition, and breed. Some giant breeds, for example, the St Bernard, Newfoundland, and Swiss Mountain dog appear sensitive to the drug and may become recumbent and reluctant to move following doses of 0.03 mg/kg. Some dogs of the Boxer breed will 'faint' when given acepromazine and it should be given in only small doses, ± an anticholinergic, or avoided completely in this breed.

The cardiovascular actions of acepromazine are minimal in healthy dogs but are potentiated by hypovolaemia, azotaemia, and old age. The dose rates for acepromazine decrease with increasing size of the animal; for IM administration in small dogs, 0.05–0.1 mg/kg is usually sufficient, for dogs 10–20 kg, 0.05–0.07 mg/kg, for dogs >20 kg, 0.02–0.05 mg/kg, with a maximum dose of 3 mg for most large dogs (Table 15.1). Occasionally, dogs are given 5 mg acepromazine with an opioid to induce profound sedation. Note that these doses are lower than those recommended on the product data sheets but increasing dosage rarely increases the sedative effect. The action of acepromazine is mild mood alteration and may be negligible in aggressive or excited dogs. In general, concurrent administration of an opioid with acepromazine results in significantly greater sedation.

Thirty minutes is usually required after IM injection for appreciable effects to be seen, including calming and protrusion of the third eyelid over the cornea. One investigation found no difference in sedation scores in dogs administered acepromazine, 0.025 mg/kg, and morphine, 0.3 mg/kg, IM at four different sites: the cervical epaxial muscles at the level of C3 and 2–3 cm off midline; the triceps brachii halfway between the elbow and scapula; the middle gluteal muscle injected midway between the greater trochanter of the femur and wing of the ilium; and the quadriceps femoris halfway between the femorotibial joint and the greater trochanter of the femur (Self et al., 2009). The development of sedation at 30 minutes after injection was independent of injection site and the degree of sedation was less at 20 than 30 minutes. Another common site for IM injections in dogs are the epaxial lumbar muscles. Drugs may have incomplete absorption when injected SC but a comparison of IM and SC administration of acepromazine, 0.03 mg/kg, and buprenorphine, 0.02 mg/kg, in clinical patients revealed no difference in sedation assessed after 60 minutes, and no difference in the dose of propofol required for endotracheal intubation (Gurney et al., 2009). Although some effect may be noticed by 5 minutes after IV injection of acepromazine, full effect may not develop for 30 minutes. Oral administration is much less reliable and the tranquillizing effect is greatly influenced by whether the drug is administered with food (poor effect) or on an empty stomach (better effect).

An advantage to including acepromazine for premedication is that it provides some protection against catecholamine-induced ventricular irregular rhythms. Acepromazine should be omitted from premedication when severe blood loss or hypotension is anticipated during surgery as the peripheral α blockade complicates treatment of hypotension. Acepromazine is not recommended for use in brachycephalic breeds or dogs at risk for upper airway obstruction. Acepromazine has been avoided in the past in dogs with a history of seizures but there is recent evidence that administration of acepromazine to dogs with epilepsy has not initiated seizures (Tobias et al., 2006).

Other phenothiazine derivatives that are used include propionyl promazine, promazine, promethazine, methotrimeprazine, and chlorpromazine. The side effects produced by them and the provisions of use are similar to those of acepromazine.

Benzodiazepines

The benzodiazepines, for example, diazepam, midazolam, and climazolam, are frequently used in combinations with opioids, α₂-agonist sedatives, and anaesthetic agents in veterinary practice to augment sedation, decrease dose

Table 15.1 Injectable drugs for sedation, analgesia, or premedication in dogs

Drug	Dose (mg/kg)	Comments
Anticholinergic		
Atropine	0.02–0.04 IM, SC; 0.005–0.02 IV	Duration 30 (IV) – 90 (IM) min
Glycopyrrolate	0.005–0.01 IM; 0.005 IV	Onset 40 min IM; duration 2–3 h
Phenothiazine		
Acepromazine	0.02–0.05 IM,IV; up to 0.1 IM small-medium dogs 0.02–0.05 IM, IV large dogs	Lowest doses for large dogs, max 3 mg for premedication; larger doses used when not followed by anaesthesia; onset IM >30 min
Benzodiazepine		
Diazepam	0.2–0.5 IV	Do not give alone to healthy dogs; poor absorption from IM
Midazolam	0.1–0.5 IM, IV	Do not give alone to healthy dogs
Climazolam	0.5–2.0 IM, IV	In combination with an opioid or anaesthetic agent
α_2-agonist		
Xylazine	0.5–2.0 IM; 0.5–1.0 IV	
Medetomidine*[§]	See product information 0.01–0.05 IM small dogs 0.01–0.02 IM large dogs 0.005–0.020 IV	Dosed on body surface area; dose decreases as size of dog increases; profound sedation; severely decreases dose of anaesthetic agents. Severely decreases subsequent dose rates of anaesthetic agents
Dexmedetomidine*[§]	See product information 0.028–0.040 IM small dogs 0.008–0.014 IM large dogs 0.003–0.010 IM; 0.003–0.005 IV	Dosed on body surface area; dose decreases as size of dog increases; profound sedation; severely decreases dose of anaesthetic agents. Premedication severely decreases dose rates of anaesthetic agents
Romifidine	0.01–0.04	Severely decreases dose of anaesthetic agents
Opioid		
Morphine	0.3–0.5 (range 0.2–1.0) IM, SC	Onset IM 40 min; if IV give over several minutes to avoid hypotension
Meperidine (Pethidine)	2–6 IM, SC	Onset IM 15–20 min; IV contraindicated to avoid hypotension
Methadone (racemic form)	0.1–0.5 IM, SC; 0.1–0.2 IV	Onset IM 10 min
Hydromorphone	0.05–0.2 IM; 0.025–0.1 IV	Onset IM 15 min
Oxymorphone	0.05–0.2 IM; 0.025–0.1 IV	Onset IM 15 min; max initial dose 5 mg
Fentanyl*	0.002–0.010 IM, IV	Onset IM 10 min
Buprenorphine	0.005–0.02 IM, IV	Onset IM, IV >30 min
Butorphanol	0.2–0.4 IM, IV	Onset IM 10 min

*0.010 mg/kg = 10 µg/kg; [§]also refer to manufacturers package insert for sedation doses

rates of other agents, and to block excitatory effects of injectable anaesthetic agents. Benzodiazepines rarely are administered alone to healthy dogs because restlessness, agitation, or even excitement may follow. In contrast, sedation may be induced in geriatric dogs, ill dogs, and dogs with meningitis or seizures. Intravenous administration produces a more intense effect than IM. Diazepam is reserved for IV use as the formulation interferes with IM absorption whereas midazolam is water soluble and administered either IV or IM. The benzodiazepines induce minimal cardiovascular or respiratory effects and have a wide margin of safety. Thus they are good alternative agents to acepromazine in old or sick dogs. Benzodiazepines can be reversed by flumazenil or sarmazenil.

α_2-Agonist sedatives

These sedatives are widely used in veterinary practice for their profound sedation and analgesic properties. They induce significant cardiorespiratory changes (see Chapter 5). The effects include CNS depression, hypnosis and analgesia, decreased cardiac output, increased blood pressure followed by a decrease, and bradycardia. Second degree atrioventricular (AV) heart block develops in some dogs. Since administration of moderate doses of medetomidine and dexmedetomidine decrease cardiac output to 21–40% of the preinjection value (Kuo & Keegan, 2004; Congdon et al., 2011), cautious use and decreased dose rates are recommended for sick dogs and those with cardiac disease. Ventilation and $PaCO_2$ may not significantly change during medetomidine sedation but the respiratory centre sensitivity and response to CO_2 is depressed and some dogs may become hypoxaemic (Kuo & Keegan, 2004; Lerche & Muir, 2004).

Peripheral vasoconstriction increases the difficulty of inserting an IV catheter and interferes with monitoring of patient oxygenation as the gums may be white and a pulse oximeter probe may not be able to detect a signal. Gastrointestinal motility is decreased. Bloody diarrhoea occasionally has occurred up to 24 hours after sedation with medetomidine and dexmedetomidine administered at the higher dose rates, perhaps caused by ischaemia. Decreases in ileal and colonic microvascular blood flows have been measured, presumably resulting from decreased cardiac output and increased systemic vascular resistance (Pypendop & Verstegen, 2000). This group of drugs also causes decreased serum insulin and drug-dependent varying increases in blood glucose concentration, and increased urine output.

The intensity of sedation from injection of these drugs can be influenced by the mental status of the dogs such that sedation is less when the dog is frightened or excited. Sudden arousal from apparently profound sedation with medetomidine may occur and has resulted in serious facial injuries in personnel leaning close to the dog, a reaction that may occur even in previously good-tempered dogs. Concurrent administration of an opioid decreases the likelihood of arousal. The addition of atropine or glycopyrrolate with medetomidine or dexmedetomidine to prevent bradycardia is not recommended because the increased heart rate (HR) may result in extreme hypertension and cardiac dysrhythmias (Ko et al., 2001b; Congdon et al., 2011).

Xylazine

Xylazine was the first α_2-agonist sedative to be widely used in veterinary medicine. Xylazine, 0.5–2.2 mg/kg, IM will produce dose-dependent sedation and will markedly decrease dose rates of other anaesthetic agents administered subsequently. Most dogs will retch or vomit after administration of xylazine as sedation is developing.

There is evidence that xylazine sensitizes the myocardium to catecholamines, although the validity of the test has been questioned. If xylazine increases the prevalence of ventricular dysrhythmias that may explain the increased risk of death occurring during or after anaesthesia in which xylazine was part of the protocol (Dyson et al., 1998).

Medetomidine

Medetomidine is a racemic mixture of two stereoisomers, dextro-medetomidine and levo-medetomidine. It is marketed for small animal practice as 1 mg/mL (1000 µg/mL). Medetomidine provides better sedation and analgesia than xylazine and has a longer duration of action (Tyner et al., 1997). The cardiopulmonary effects of medetomidine are similar to previously described, however, the changes are quantitatively similar for doses ≥5 µg/kg (Pypendop & Verstegen, 1998). Sedation is achieved at 2 µg/kg IV and increasing the dose rate increases the intensity and duration of sedation, from 60 minutes after 5 µg/kg to 120 minutes after 20 µg/kg. Vomiting occurs in about 20% of dogs receiving medetomidine, which is less than xylazine. Medetomidine, 0.01–0.02 mg/kg (10–20 µg/kg), IV significantly decreases serum insulin concentration but plasma glucose concentration remains within the normal physiological range (Burton et al., 1997).

Medetomidine has a steep dose–response curve and doses should, ideally, be calculated on a body surface area (BSA) rather than on body weight. In practice, this means that large dogs require relatively lower doses than smaller dogs. The IM dose rates given to induce profound sedation are up to 750–1000 µg/m^2. The cut-off weight between higher and lower dose rates is 15 kg, so that dogs <15 kg need a higher dose and dogs >15 kg need less. The highest dose rate for a 15 kg dog is roughly equivalent to 0.03–0.04 mg/kg (30–40 µg/kg). The product information sheet contains detailed tables on volume of drug to administer for different weights of dogs. A formula for calculating BSA using kg bodyweight is BSA m^2 = (Bwt kg$^{2/3}$ × 10.1)100 (Pypendop & Verstegen, 2000; Hill & Scott, 2004). The sedative effect is increased in senior dogs and frequently half the dose rate will have the same effect as the full dose in a younger dog.

Dexmedetomidine

The effects and use of dexmedetomidine are similar to those described for medetomidine. The recommended dose rate for inducing mild sedation is 125 µg/m^2, for moderate sedation 375 µg/m^2, and for profound sedation 375–500 µg/m^2. The manufacturer has marketed a solution (0.5 mg/mL, 500 µg/mL) that is half the concentration of small animal medetomidine to facilitate ease of transition from medetomidine to dexmedetomidine so that the volume to be injected is an identical volume for volume substitution. The product information sheet has detailed tables with volume/dose for dogs of varying body weights. In clinical practice, these dose rates must be modified based on evaluation of the individual patient and the required effect.

Romifidine

Romifidine has been administered IM or IV and induces sedation and bradycardia for 2–3 hours. The dogs may vomit before assuming recumbency. Cardiac output is decreased and central venous pressure (CVP) is increased (Pypendop & Verstegen, 2001). Romifidine ≥0.025 mg/kg (25 µg/kg) IV initially increases mean arterial pressure (MAP) followed by a prolonged decrease; MAP is immediately decreased by lower doses. Second degree AV block has been observed. Romifidine at 0.02 mg/kg (20 µg/kg) and 0.04 mg/kg (40 µg/kg) IM has been used alone or in conjunction with a low dose of anticholinergic agent (atropine, 0.01 mg/kg, or glycopyrrolate, 0.001 mg/kg) for sedation and for premedication to inhalation anaesthesia in experimental and clinical dogs (England & Hammond, 1997; Redondo et al., 1999; Lemke, 2001). The dose rate of the induction agent was significantly decreased, thiopental to a mean of 6.5 mg/kg and propofol to 3–4 mg/kg. Administration of an anticholinergic at the doses studied appeared to induce acceptable changes in HR and MAP and may have reduced the incidence of vomiting (Lemke, 2001).

Opioids

When administered alone, few opioids cause significant sedation in healthy dogs. When combined with a sedative or acepromazine, the result can vary from mild to heavy sedation depending on the route of administration, the drug and dose rate used, and the mental and physical status of the animal. Opioids can be used to provide analgesia for animals in pain, as part of an anaesthetic protocol for which a painful medical or surgical procedure is to be performed, and in combination with a sedative to deepen the intensity of sedation (see Table 15.1).

Panting is a side effect of opioid administration that may interfere with the procedure to be performed and may occur in as high as 70% of patients given morphine, oxymorphone, hydromorphone, or fentanyl, lasting from 30 minutes to 3 hours (Dohoo et al., 1986; Cullen et al., 1999). Vomiting is frequently observed after administration of morphine, oxymorphone, and hydromorphone (Box 15.1). Vomition is unlikely to occur after butorphanol, buprenorphine, fentanyl or methadone. Behaviour changes have been reported in a small number of dogs, such as increased whining after administration of

---

> **Box 15.1 Opioids are valuable components of sedation or anaesthetic protocols but anticipate adverse effects**
>
> Vomiting
> Panting
> Respiratory depression when in combination
> Decreased dose requirement for anaesthetic agents
> Acute drop in BP after rapid IV injection during
>   anaesthesia
> Bradycardia, in particular with fentanyl

---

methadone, vocalization after hydromorphone or butorphanol, and temporary aggression to owners or objects for 1 hour to 3 days after acepromazine–oxymorphone or fentanyl–droperidol (Dohoo et al., 1986; Ingvast-Larsson et al., 2010) (Trim, personal observations).

Tramadol

Tramadol is structurally related to codeine and exerts an analgesic effect through weak µ receptor agonist action and blocking of serotonin and norepinephrine uptake in the pain pathways of the spinal cord. Systemic availability is equivalent from IV and IM administration. There are no dosage recommendations for tramadol in dogs but published dose rates are 2 or 3 mg/kg and a redosing interval of 8 hours. Tramadol provides improved postoperative pain control when combined with a non-steroidal anti-inflammatory drug (NSAID). In one study, dogs scheduled for ovariohysterectomy were premedicated with atropine, 0.04 mg/kg, acepromazine, 0.05 mg/kg, and either tramadol, 3 mg/kg, or morphine 0.5 mg/kg, SC before induction of anaesthesia with thiopental and maintenance with halothane (Kongara et al., 2012). Dogs premedicated with acepromazine–tramadol required significantly higher concentrations of halothane for anaesthesia than dogs given acepromazine–morphine. Half of the dogs in each group were given boluses of fentanyl, 1 µg/kg, to treat responses to surgical stimulation. The dogs required additional doses of analgesic agent by one hour after anaesthesia, approximately 4 hours after premedication. This time corresponds to the usual time interval (3–4 hours) for redosing of morphine. In another investigation of postoperative analgesia after maxillectomy or mandibulectomy, tramadol or codeine or ketoprofen, all at 2 mg/kg SC, or combinations of these drugs were administered 30 minutes before the end of surgery (Martins et al., 2010). Tramadol and codeine were repeated at 8-hour intervals for the 24-hour monitoring period. Rescue analgesia was administered to some dogs in every group based on pain scores that included responses to

pressure at the surgical site. Although not statistically significant, mean pain scores were lowest in dogs given ketoprofen with tramadol or codeine. Rescue analgesia denotes
the administration of an analgesic agent during episodes
of pain that are not controlled by a patient's scheduled
analgesic regimen.

Injection of tramadol, 4 mg/kg, IV in experimental dogs
anaesthetized with sevoflurane caused no change in HR or
cardiac output (Itami et al., 2011). Mean arterial pressure
increased for 15 minutes and then returned to pre-
injection value. Measurement of systemic vascular resistance revealed a mild but prolonged vasoconstriction.

Maropitant

Maropitant (Cerenia®) is licensed for use in the USA and
Europe for prevention of motion sickness and acute vomiting in situations such as chemotherapy for dogs ≥16
weeks of age (Sedlacek et al., 2008). It is recommended as
a once-daily administration at 1 mg/kg SC or 2 mg/kg
orally. Absolute bioavailability is much higher after SC
administration than oral, partly due to a hepatic first-pass
effect after oral dosing (Benchaoui et al., 2007). Feeding
status was found to have no significant effect on absorption of the drug. Renal clearance was negligible and no
dosage adjustment was considered necessary for patients
with renal disease.

Maropitant is an antagonist for neurokinin (NK$_1$) receptors for which Substance P is the agonist. These receptors
are present in the dorsal root ganglia and spinal cord
dorsal horn, ascending projections to the brain, and in
some visceral tissues (Boscan et al., 2011). Studies evaluating the analgesic effects of maropitant have yielded conflicting results. Working on the premise that maropitant
may be an effective analgesic for visceral surgery, an experimental study simulated ovariectomy in dogs anaesthetized
with sevoflurane (Boscan et al., 2011). Maropitant, 1 mg/
kg, IV injected over 10 minutes followed by an infusion to
maintain a constant blood concentration was documented
significantly to decrease by 24% the concentration
of sevoflurane required to prevent response to traction
on an ovary. A study recently presented at a national
meeting compared premedication with saline, morphine,
0.5 mg/kg, or maropitant, 1 mg/kg, SC prior to propofol-
isoflurane anaesthesia for ovariohysterectomy (Marquez
et al., 2011). A significantly lower concentration of isoflurane was used for removal of the ovaries and skin closure
in dogs that received maropitant for premedication compared with none; sevoflurane concentrations for dogs
given morphine were intermediate between these groups.
Some dogs panted at the time of intense surgical stimulation, 67%, 38%, and 35% in premedication groups saline,
morphine, or maropitant, respectively. This limited evidence suggests that maropitant provides some analgesia
but investigations are needed to define its role in comparison with the available options.

Sedative–opioid combinations

There are many publications reporting the effects of combinations of a sedative or acepromazine and an opioid,
using different dose rates, routes of administration, and
timing of administrations. In most cases, the combination
results in greater intensity and duration of sedation than
is achieved by the individual drugs. Combinations that
include medetomidine or dexmedetomidine generally
induce the greatest sedation and decreased cardiac output.
Because these α$_2$-sedatives exert such profound sedation
and cardiovascular effects, the dose rates of the opioids
used in combination are often lower than those used in
combination with acepromazine or a benzodiazepine.
Other factors influencing the sedative and cardiovascular
effects of these combinations are the relative dose rates
and route of administration, and the mentation, age and
physical status of the patient. To summarize, advantages
of these combinations include:

- Increased sedation over that achieved by either agent
  alone
- Improved analgesia
- Decreased dose rates of subsequently administered
  injectable and inhalation agents, thus widening their
  safety margins.
- With some combinations and in some patients,
  particularly old patients, sedation may be profound.

NSAIDs

The addition of an NSAID is valuable for management
of perioperative inflammation and analgesia (doses in
Chapter 5). High doses of NSAIDs, hypotension, hypovolaemia, and anaesthetic agents have the potential to alter
renal perfusion and may increase the risk of adverse renal
effects of NSAIDs (KuKanich et al., 2012). Consequently,
general anaesthesia of dogs receiving NSAIDs should
include fluid therapy and appropriate management of circulatory changes to avoid risk of NSAID-induced renal
toxicity. Anaesthesia is not a contraindication to NSAID
administration, nonetheless, some clinicians prefer to
administer the NSAID at the end of anaesthesia when it is
known that the dog is hydrated and not hypotensive. The
effects of NSAIDs in dogs with renal disease have not been
reported but cautious use in these patients is recommended (KuKanich et al., 2012).

Dipyrone (metamizole)

Dipyrone, also known as metamizole, was first produced
commercially in Germany in 1922. The occurrence of
agranulocytosis with some mortality in human patients
led to failure of licensure of dipyrone in several countries,
including the USA, the United Kingdom, Sweden, and
Australia. The incidence of this adverse effect is low
but the potential for the number of cases with widespread
use is disputed. Dipyrone/metamizole is available by

prescription in some countries and over the counter for self-medication in others. In some countries, dipyrone/metamizole has a veterinary licence for use in dogs and horses as an analgesic, antipyretic, antispasmodic, and (weak) anti-inflammatory drug. Inhibition of COX-3 in the brain and spinal cord is a proposed mechanism of action (Chandrasekharan et al., 2002).

Product information for dipyrone 50% in Canada states a dose rate in dogs of 50 mg/kg, to be administered IM or slowly IV at 8–12-hour intervals up to a maximum of 2 days. Several dose rates of metamizole have been evaluated for analgesic efficacy after ovariohysterectomy in dogs anaesthetized with acepromazine, propofol and isoflurane (Imagawa et al., 2011). Dogs given metamizole, 25 or 35 mg/kg IV 10 minutes before the end of surgery had significantly lower pain scores after surgery compared with dogs given tramadol. Four of 20 dogs given metamizole required rescue analgesia. Metamizole was repeated every 8 hours for 2 days. Vomiting in the first 6 hours after anaesthesia was observed in 40% of dogs and this effect was equally distributed through the treatment groups.

Antagonists

Specific antagonist agents are available for benzodiazepines (flumazenil and sarmazenil), α_2-sedatives (atipamezole, and yohimbine and doxapram for xylazine), and opioids (naloxone) (Table 15.2). Flumazenil will reverse the effects of diazepam or midazolam overdose. Butorphanol will almost completely reverse the sedative effects of oxymorphone and hydromorphone (Dyson et al., 1990). Nalbuphine, 0.16 mg/kg, IV partially reversed oxymorphone but appeared to increase sedation when administered after buprenorphine (Jacobson et al., 1994).

GENERAL ANAESTHESIA

None of the currently available anaesthetic agents have all the properties of an ideal agent. In clinical practice, one or more sedative, analgesic, or anaesthetic drugs are given before or during induction of anaesthesia to achieve safer anaesthesia by reducing the dose rates of individual agents. In fact, any of these agents may be suitable for most of our patients and the final choice may be determined by availability, familiarity of use or cost of the drug. However, in some patients, selection of one drug over another may increase safety of anaesthesia.

Preventive analgesia is aimed at attenuating the impact of all factors that stimulate pain pathways in the pre-, intra- and postoperative periods in order to reduce or prevent postsurgical peripheral and central sensitization and chronic pain-related behaviours. Preventive analgesia is demonstrated when postoperative pain and analgesic use are reduced beyond the duration of action of the agent

---

Table 15.2 Antagonists

Drug	Dose (mg/kg)	Comments
Benzodiazepine antagonist		
Flumazenil	0.01 IM, IV	Titrate to effect. Reversing a benzodiazepine–ketamine
Sarmazenil	0.05–0.10 IM, IV	combination will expose ketamine-induced CNS excitement
α_2-agonist antagonist		
Yohimbine	0.11 IV slowly, 0.25–0.5 IM, SC	Antagonist of xylazine
Atipamezole*	Equal volume IM as volume of (dex)medetomidine administered, or less	Antagonist of medetomidine and dexmedetomidine
	0.005–0.020 IV slowly over several min	IV off label use
Opioid antagonist		
Naloxone	0.01–0.02 IM, IV, SC	Antagonizes all opioids
Butorphanol§	0.2–0.3 IM, IV	Partial reversal of analgesia and sedation from µ opioids
Buprenorphine§	0.005–0.01 IM, IV	Decreases analgesia from µ opioids
Analeptic and respiratory stimulant		
Doxapram	0.5–1.0 IM, IV	Stimulates rate and depth of breathing; release of norepinephrine causes generalized arousal

*0.010 mg/kg = 10 µg/kg; §Not specific antagonists and not used in emergencies; used to diminish sedation or signs of dysphoria induced by a µ opioid

used for analgesia (Katz et al., 2011). Although the surgical incision, wound retraction, and manipulation of organs may trigger central sensitization, so also can preanaesthetic noxious input and postoperative inflammatory mediators. Use of opioids alone is not sufficient, hence recommendations for including NSAIDs, nerve blocks, and other agents in the anaesthetic protocol. Patients with presurgical pain may not receive the same pain relief by analgesic therapy because central sensitization is already established. Even in healthy patients, preoperative factors such as genetic predisposition and psychological vulnerability may influence postanaesthetic management.

The intention of preanaesthetic evaluation is to avoid the development of complications. Unfortunately, complications frequently develop in patients not expected to have a problem with anaesthesia. All personnel involved in providing anaesthesia and related medical or surgical procedures should be familiar with the practice's accepted plans for treatment of specific complications and resuscitation procedures. Plans should have been discussed before anaesthesia in a stress-free environment. Key points to a safer anaesthesia are listed (Box 15.2).

Box 15.2 **Key points to improve safety of anaesthesia**

- All dogs that can be handled should have a clinical examination before anaesthesia to identify factors that impact response or choice of agents
- Food should be withheld for 10 hours before anaesthesia, except for paediatric patients
- Allow sufficient time for premedication agents to achieve full effect before induction
- Include analgesic agents for painful procedures
- Develop check lists for specific procedures
- Maintain an anaesthetic record that lists time, dose (mg), and route of all agents administered, record parameters regularly through anaesthesia, add summary
- Dogs given agents to the point of unresponsiveness should be considered to be anaesthetized and not merely heavily sedated
- An indwelling venous catheter or secured indwelling needle is advisable
- Plan to intubate the trachea of all brachycephalic dogs
- A means to supply oxygen and the ability to ventilate should be readily available
- The person assigned to monitoring should have received training
- Attach available monitoring equipment to all anaesthetized dogs
- Continue monitoring into recovery; surveys have identified that currently over half of anaesthetic deaths occur in recovery

---

Preparation for anaesthesia

It is important to be adequately prepared to provide safe general anaesthesia in animals. Preparation includes preanaesthetic evaluation of the ability of the patient to withstand the changes induced by administration of anaesthetic agents and of the potential impact of the procedure on the intra- and postoperative course. Choice of anaesthetic agents and management is based on information derived from the dog's history, physical examination, abnormal values detected in laboratory tests, nature of any current illness, and requirements of the proposed medical or surgical procedure. The significances of many of the conditions that may be discovered during preanaesthetic evaluation are discussed in Chapter 1 and later in this chapter. Some aspects of the preanaesthetic preparation of dogs that deal with routine management are considered here.

Concurrent drug therapy

Previous drug therapy can alter the response of a dog to anaesthesia and surgery so it is essential that details of drug use should be sought from the case history. A full discussion of all possible drug interactions is beyond the scope of this book and reference should be made to textbooks and online sources concerning pharmacology and drug interactions. Interactions that are encountered fairly commonly in canine anaesthesia are described below.

Antibiotics

Chloramphenicol increases the length of action of barbiturate and inhalant agents but this rarely presents a clinical problem. More importantly, antibiotics given rapidly IV during anaesthesia can, in some dogs, cause myocardial depression and induce hypotension (Table 15.3). Antibiotics administered IV should be given slowly over several minutes with a close watch on arterial pressure. Many antibiotics, including the streptomycin group, the polymixins, and tetracyclines, exert an influence at the neuromuscular junction that enhances the effects of non-depolarizing neuromuscular blocking agents. This may induce re-paralysis when these antibiotics are administered at the end of anaesthesia.

Antipsychotic drugs

Three groups of drugs are used to treat aggression, fear or compulsive behaviours in dogs: (1) monoamine oxidase inhibitors (MAOIs), such as selegiline; (2) tricyclic antidepressants (TCAs), such as amitriptyline and clomipramine; and (3) non-tricyclic antidepressants such as fluoxetine and trazadone. Monoamine oxidase inhibitors block the deoxidative deamination of endogenous catecholamines into inactive metabolites, allowing an accumulation of norepinephrine, epinephrine, dopamine, and serotonin. Selegiline HCl is licensed for use in dogs for control of

Table 15.3 Impact of concurrent drug administration on anaesthetic management

Drug	Significance
Antibiotics	IV administration during anaesthesia causes moderate, occasionally severe, decrease in blood pressure in some dogs. Aminoglycoside antibiotics can cause muscle weakness and potentiate neuromuscular block from non-depolarizing relaxants. Chloramphenicol prolongs sleep time from ketamine and inhalant agents
Antipsychotic drugs	Risk of cardiovascular instability Risk of serotonin syndrome
Carbonic anhydrase inhibitors	Induces metabolic acidosis
Cardiovascular drugs	Calcium channel blockers and ACE inhibitors given before anaesthesia may be associated with hypotension
Corticosteroids	Long-term preoperative use may predispose to circulatory collapse, patient may need supplementation
Diuretics	Furosemide (frusemide) decreases serum potassium and may cause muscle weakness and cardiac arrhythmias
Insulin	Risk of hypoglycaemia during and after anaesthesia
Non-steroidal anti-inflammatory drugs	Hypotension during anaesthesia increases risk for toxic effects
Organophosphate anthelmintic/parasiticide	Reduces plasma cholinesterase and prolongs duration of some drugs (suxamethonium/succinylcholine, mivacurium, procaine). Some product information sheets on acepromazine state it should not be given within 1 month of deworming – effects potentiated. May decrease anaesthetic requirement.
Phenobarbital	Chronic use for seizure control associated with decreased hepatic function. Hepatic enzyme induction may increase production of metabolites from halothane to toxic level

clinical signs of cognitive dysfunction syndrome and uncomplicated pituitary dependent hyperadrenocorticism. It is believed to be a MAO-type B inhibitor. Therapeutic effects may be mediated through MAO inhibition and increased dopamine concentrations in the CNS or mediated through its metabolites, amphetamine and methamphetamine. Extreme blood pressure fluctuations have been noted in human patients receiving MAOIs during anaesthesia that included α_2-agonists, and use of meperidine is contraindicated because it may increase neuronal 5-hydroxytryptamine (5-HT). An exaggerated effect after ephedrine administration is described. Little information is available about interactions with anaesthetic agents in dogs but, in one investigation, there were no differences recorded in behaviours or cardiopulmonary measurements following administration of medetomidine, 750 μg/m^2, oxymorphone, 0.1 mg/kg, or butorphanol, 0.4 mg/kg, IV in dogs that were or were not receiving selegiline (Dodam et al., 2004).

Clomipramine is approved for use in dogs to treat canine separation anxiety. Tricyclic antidepressants block uptake of norepinephrine into presynaptic adrenergic nerve terminals, increasing the amount of circulating catecholamines. Neuroleptic drugs, sedatives, atropine, ketamine, and thiopental potentiate the effect of TCAs. These agents do not have to be discontinued before anaesthesia,

but possible drug interactions should be considered. Sympathomimetic drugs such as ephedrine will cause an exaggerated pressor response.

The non-tricyclic antidepressants, such as fluoxetine and trazadone, are used to treat anxiety disorders in dogs and exert a calming effect. Fluoxetine, a selective serotonin reuptake inhibitor (SSRI), and trazadone, a tetracyclic antidepressant and serotonin and norepinephrine reuptake inhibitor (SNRI), have side effects that can lead to complications during anaesthesia. Complications observed in human anaesthesia are increased bleeding, unstable cardiovascular system with hypotension and dysrhythmias, and changed thermoregulation. Recommendations for humans are that fluoxetine be continued up to the time of anaesthesia because of the mental instability that may occur if it is discontinued. *In vitro* studies indicate that fluoxetine significantly enhanced the inhibitory effect of propofol on norepinephrine and serotonin reuptake but had no effect on thiopental or etomidate (Zhao & Sun, 2008). This would suggest that patients receiving fluoxetine might have an altered response to propofol. The duration of trazadone is such that if administered in the evening before anaesthesia, metabolites that can cause adverse effects will be present the following day. A recently reported study of dogs anaesthetized for orthopaedic surgery replaced the acepromazine premedication in half of the dogs with trazodone, 5 mg/kg for dogs >10 kg or 7 mg/kg for dogs ≤10 kg, orally and found no differences in HR and blood pressure during anaesthesia between the groups (Mathews et al., 2011).

Serotonin syndrome is well recognized in humans and is now reported in animals. Ingestion of L-5-hydroxytryptophan, from *Griffonia simplicifolia* seeds used to ease chronic headaches, fibromyalgia, depression and insomnia, was incriminated in 21 dogs exhibiting signs of serotonin toxicity (Gwaltney-Brant et al., 2000). A summary of 189 dogs with serotonin toxicity received in 2002–2004 by the Animal Poison Control Center, Urbana, Ilinois, USA, associated 45 with paroxetine, 59 sertraline, 85 fluoxetine, 4 MAO, and 4 St John's Wort (Mohammad-Zadeh et al., 2008). Signs associated with SSRI administration included lethargy 31%, vomiting 12%, with fewer dogs exhibiting mydriasis, agitation, hyperactivity or depression, tachycardia, tremors and vocalization. There are no clinical data addressing multidrug therapy inducing serotonin toxicity in veterinary patients but the potential for toxicity must increase as more dogs are treated with these agents. Combinations of drugs such as the SSRIs or SNRIs and others with serotonin reuptake inhibitory effect, such as tramadol, are commonly involved. Meperidine, fentanyl and congeners, pentazocine, tramadol, and dextromethorphan are all weak SSRIs and have been implicated in human cases of serotonin syndrome. Tramadol may also be a serotonin releaser. Morphine and its analogues do not cause inhibition of serotonin uptake.

Since the incidence of complications arising from anaesthesia of dogs receiving antipsychotic drugs is not yet determined, anaesthetic considerations should include the behaviour initiating administration of the drug, including herbal supplements, and the pharmacological effect of the drug in addition to usual preanaesthetic evaluation. Recommendations for management of these patients include the possibility of treatment early in the day and on an 'out-patient' basis to minimize stress, and use of dog-appeasing pheromone in the hospital for venous catheterization (Robertson, 2009). Owners should be warned about the possibility of drug interactions. Some dog owners may have to be present for premedication and aggressive dogs should be managed efficiently in a quiet area using experienced personnel to eliminate delays and minimize patient stimulation. The dogs may be reassured by the presence of an item from home in the cage or run. Anaesthetic agents that should be satisfactory are glycopyrrolate, but not atropine, morphine, hydromorphone, oxymorphone, buprenorphine, and butorphanol. Injectable anaesthetic agents should be titrated to individual effect and inhalation anaesthesia can be used for maintenance. Avoidance of α_2-sedatives has been suggested because they cause such major changes in HR and MAP that cardiovascular changes important to the diagnosis of serotonin toxicity may be obscured. Measurement of blood pressure during anaesthesia is advisable.

Symptomatic treatment should be instituted in event of suspected serotonin toxicity, such as cooling if hyperthermic and administration of diazepam to counter seizures. Cyproheptadine is an H1 histamine receptor antagonist with non-specific 5-HT receptor antagonist properties that has been used successfully to treat serotonin syndrome in humans. The recommended dose by Animal Poison Control Center in dogs and cats is 1 mg/kg orally or per rectum every 4–8 hours until clinical symptoms resolve. Chlorpromazine has been used with some success in people.

Barbiturates

Long-term barbiturate therapy for epilepsy will lead to enzyme induction and a decrease in duration of action of similar drugs given for anaesthesia. Administration for years leads to hepatic cirrhosis and decreased hepatic function. The effects of acutely administered phenobarbital (or diazepam) for the seizuring animal will be additive to subsequently administered drugs for anaesthesia.

Cardiovascular drugs

Dogs with cardiac disease are treated with a variety of cardiovascular drugs, some of which decrease vascular resistance. Hypotension may develop during general anaesthesia in dogs receiving these drugs unless the chosen anaesthetic protocols induce minimal vasodilation or myocardial depression. Angiotensin-converting enzyme (ACE) inhibitors, such as captopril, enalapril, or benazapril, in particular, appear to be associated with hypotension that is not easily reversed.

Corticosteroids

Dogs that have been treated with corticosteroid drugs at any time in the 2 months preceding anaesthesia may have reduced ability to respond to stress. For animals that have been on long-term corticosteroid treatment, additional steroid may be advisable in the form of dexamethasone, 0.5–2.0 mg/kg IV, or methylprednisolone, 10–20 mg/kg, or another steroid more appropriate for the individual dog's condition based on knowledge of the history and previous dosing regimen. Further steroid may be needed depending on the severity of the surgical procedure and how the dog recovered from anaesthesia.

Insulin

Diabetic dogs receiving insulin are at risk of developing hypoglycaemia, hypotension, and cerebral damage during anaesthesia. An accepted management for the diabetic dog that must be anaesthetized is given in Table 15.4. The blood glucose level should be maintained between 5.5 and 11.0 mmol/dL (100–200 mg/dL) through frequent measurement of blood glucose concentrations and appropriate IV administration of 5% dextrose in water (D5W) during anaesthesia. Even when preanaesthetic blood

Table 15.4 A protocol for anaesthetic management of a regulated diabetic dog

Sequence of events	Management
Night before surgery	Feed as usual
Morning of the day of surgery	Give one-half of the usual dose of insulin; do not feed
Before anaesthesia	Measure blood glucose; administer dextrose if value is low
During anaesthesia	Administer 5% dextrose in water, 3–5 mL/kg/h, in addition to balanced electrolyte solution; measure blood glucose at the end of anaesthesia, or every 1–2 hours, and adjust dextrose infusion rate according to result
After anaesthesia	Measure blood glucose 2 hours after anaesthesia; adjust treatment according to result; feed and return to insulin therapy as soon as appropriate

Box 15.3 **Management of brachycephalic breeds**

- Anticipate airway obstruction
- Keep under observation after premedication
- Monitor oxygenation before and after anaesthesia
- Wide selection of endotracheal tube sizes
- Controlled ventilation frequently necessary
- Protect against corneal drying and abrasions
- Recover from anaesthesia with head elevated
- Avoid early extubation
- Oxygen in recovery

glucose is high, blood glucose may decrease significantly during the first hour of anaesthesia. Dogs with well-controlled diabetes can experience wide swings in blood glucose for several hours after anaesthesia, and monitoring should be continued until the following day.

Breed characteristics

The breed, age, and conformation have significant impact on choice of drugs and anticipated complications. Breed dispositions for different diseases and traits are extensive and appear to be constantly changing. Variable responses to anaesthetic drugs within breeds have also been reported. Some families of the Boxer breed, for example, are very sensitive to the effects of acepromazine. Several other breeds have been suggested as having increased sensitivity to anaesthetic agents, for example, the Belgian Terveurens and the Siberian Husky. It is very likely, and this hypothesis is supported by experience and anecdotal reports, that there are strains of dogs within many breeds that have a very low tolerance for anaesthetic agents. Consequently, safety is increased when balanced anaesthetic techniques are employed and drugs are administered sequentially and 'to effect'. Information provided by the owner about anaesthetic-related complications with siblings should be incorporated into the anaesthetic plan.

Brachycephalic breeds

Conformation will have an impact on anaesthetic management (Box 15.3). Brachycephalic breeds such as the English Bulldog, French Bulldog, Pug, Boston Terrier, Shi

Tzu, Lhasa Apso, and Pekingese are at risk of airway obstruction because of elongated soft palates, abnormal narrowing of the larynx, everted laryngeal ventricles, narrowing of the space between nasal turbinates, and stenotic nares. Prolonged inspiratory stridor contributes to formation of oedema of the soft palate and laryngeal mucosa and tenacious stringy saliva in the oropharynx. These dogs are also more likely to develop cyanosis during induction of anaesthesia and to vomit in the recovery period. Partial or complete obstruction can occur even during sedation and these dogs should be kept under observation after administration of premedication drugs. Sedated dogs may be hypoxaemic and not exhibit classic signs of hypoxia such as panting or mouth breathing, and routine application of a pulse oximeter probe will identify those patients. Tracheal intubation is more difficult in these breeds and may involve smaller endotracheal tubes than expected based on the body size. The anatomy of the English Bulldog larynx may be distorted such that only an extremely small lumen tube can be inserted.

'Preoxygenation' is advisable to prevent hypoxaemia during induction of anaesthesia and is accomplished by administration of O_2 by facemask for several minutes before and during induction. Acepromazine should be used cautiously, if at all, and propofol, alfaxalone, ketamine, or etomidate are less likely to be associated with prolonged difficulty with breathing during recovery from anaesthesia than thiopental. Opioids are useful agents to provide sedation and analgesia and to decrease the dose of subsequent anaesthetics. One problem with this group is that Bulldogs, Boston Terriers, and Pugs frequently pant during inhalation anaesthesia, necessitating use of controlled ventilation. Brachycephalic dogs often have protuberant eyes and frequent application of ophthalmic lubricant is advisable to prevent corneal drying, and taping the eyelids closed may provide added protection.

Congestion of the nasal mucosa occurring during anaesthesia interferes with airflow after extubation. The patient should be placed in sternal recumbency as soon as

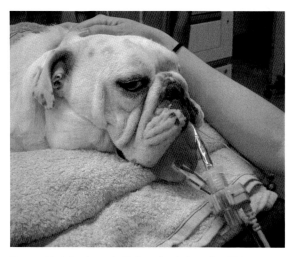

Figure 15.1 Brachycephalic breeds of dogs should be recovered from anaesthesia in a sternal, head-up position to promote decongestion of the nasal mucosa. Oxygenation is monitored with a pulse oximeter clipped to the tongue as in this dog, or on the lip, ear, toe or toe web. This dog is breathing air but a mainstream capnograph is connected to the endotracheal tube.

Table 15.5 Anaesthesia of paediatric and senior/geriatric dogs includes increased risk of these problems

	Paediatric	Senior/Geriatric
Anaesthetic requirement	↓↑*	↓
Ventilation	↓	↓
Blood pressure	↓	↓
Recovery time	↑	↑
Hypothermia	✓	✓
Hypoglycaemia	✓	–

*Decreased in neonate, progressive increase in paediatric

possible at the end of the procedure and the dog's head elevated (Fig. 15.1). Administration of an opioid for recovery of anaesthesia will allow the dog to tolerate the endotracheal tube while exhaling isoflurane or sevoflurane. After extubation, it is important to listen for airflow and not merely rely on chest movement as an indicator of adequate breathing. Opening the dog's mouth, extending the head and neck, and pulling the tongue rostrally may temporarily relieve an obstruction. Oxygenation should be measured using a pulse oximeter and administration of O_2 by mask may be necessary for 10 minutes or longer. Administration of dexamethasone sodium phosphate, 0.5 mg/kg, IV may be advisable after soft palatectomy to minimize postoperative swelling.

Sighthounds

The lean athletic breeds collectively known as 'sighthounds' include Greyhounds, Afghans, Salukis, Borzois, Whippets, Wolfhounds and Deerhounds. Their significance to the anaesthetist is the prolonged recovery from anaesthesia induced by thiopental because of the lack of body fat (and muscle in some breeds), which precludes redistribution and lowering of blood thiopental concentration. Reduced ability to metabolize thiopental and propofol has been documented in greyhounds. For these dogs, propofol yields a vastly improved quality of recovery from anaesthesia. Ketamine is a less satisfactory agent for anaesthesia in these breeds than propofol, unless adequate sedation is provided for recovery, because these dogs may exhibit signs suggestive of dysphoria. Greyhounds are

trained in their racing career not to sit down, and this behaviour must be adjusted for when inserting an IV catheter by accomplishing this in the standing animal or by positioning the animal in lateral recumbency. Many greyhounds will try to stand early after anaesthesia despite significant ataxia.

Age characteristics

Life stage divisions are arbitrary, are affected by both the breed and size of dog, and may be defined differently in various contexts. Guidelines proposed by a panel of experts (Bartges et al., 2012) are similar to those generally applied in veterinary anaesthesiology but provide a more complete definition:

- Neonate, puppy 1–2 weeks of age
- Paediatric, junior dog 2–12 weeks of age
- Adolescent, 3–9 months of age
- Adult, finished growing, socially mature
- Mature, dog is around half life expectancy
- Senior, last 25% of life expectancy
- Geriatric, at life expectancy and beyond.

While individual dogs have problems that influence response to anaesthesia, ageing *per se* has a significant impact on anaesthetic management. A survey of 15 881 deaths of 165 breeds of purebred dogs in the UK has provided information on breed differences in lifespan and provides further evidence that smaller breeds tend to have a longer lifespan than larger dogs (Adams et al., 2010).

Paediatric anaesthesia

Neonatal puppies require small doses of anaesthetic agents. Puppies less than 2 months of age are more likely to develop hypoventilation, hypotension, and hypothermia than young adults (Table 15.5). Oxygen consumption is higher in puppies than in mature animals and respiratory rates are high. Heart rates of around 200 beats/min occur in newborn puppies. Decreased heart rate and decreased preload (blood volume) result in large decreases in cardiac output (Baum & Palmisano, 1997). A small blood loss will cause a greater decrease in cardiac output than in an older animal. The MAP is considerably lower in the first month of life than in mature dogs and the problem for the anaesthetist is how low is too low for blood pressure during anaesthesia? MAP of 55–60 mmHg may be satisfactory during anaesthesia in the first 2 weeks of life provided that peripheral perfusion appears to be adequate as indicated by pink mucous membranes and rapid capillary refill time (CRT). Successful treatment of low pressure can be difficult as the immature heart may not respond satisfactorily to administration of anticholinergic and inotropic agents. The young animal is capable of a significant increase in cardiac output in response to a volume load, but this increase is depressed after the first few weeks of life.

Puppies have immature mechanisms for detoxification. Renal function does not, for example, reach adult function until puppies are 3 months of age (Poffenbarger et al., 1990). Hypoglycaemia may develop during and after anaesthesia. Food should not be withheld for more than a few hours before anaesthesia and the puppy should be fed a few hours after anaesthesia. As prevention against hypoglycaemia, 5% dextrose in water, 3 mL/kg/h, should be infused IV during anaesthesia in addition to balanced electrolyte solution. Hypothermia develops easily in these small patients and will have a significant effect in decreasing blood pressure and metabolic rate, thus prolonging recovery from anaesthesia.

Senior and geriatric dogs

Older dogs have a decreased requirement for anaesthetic agents due to a reduction in the number of neurons and neurotransmitter. The duration of action of drugs may be increased because hepatic and renal function are decreased, resulting in longer recovery from anaesthesia. The prevalence of hypoventilation is higher in senior dogs because chemoreceptor response to high $PaCO_2$ and low PaO_2 is decreased. Hypotension is more likely to develop due to decreased autonomic function with increasing age. Thermoregulation is increasingly impaired and hypothermia develops as a consequence. Pharyngeal and laryngeal reflexes are diminished and aspiration of reflux is more likely to occur than in a younger animal.

Physical examination

The 'preanaesthesia exam' is an important part of the whole process. It is almost impossible to design a safe anaesthetic protocol without observing the temperament of the dog, its physical conformation, auscultating the heart and lungs for abnormalities, assessing any impact of current disease on adequacy of breathing, and ruling out the presence of abnormalities unconnected with the presenting problem.

Auscultation of the thorax

Auscultation of the heart, cardiac rhythm, and lung sounds before anaesthesia is essential to identify abnormalities in animals that exhibit no signs of disease to owners, for example, to detect a patent ductus arteriosus in a young dog scheduled for castration or ovariectomy/ovariohysterectomy. Auscultation of murmurs or abnormal rhythms should be followed up as potential early indicators of cardiomyopathy (Brownlie, 1991). All dogs that have been injured in a road traffic accident or have suffered a fall from a high location should be auscultated for decreased lung sounds indicating lung collapse, pneumothorax, or diaphragmatic hernia. Abnormal ventricular rhythm in these dogs is an indication of traumatic myocarditis, although this clinical sign may not become apparent until 24–36 hours after the trauma. A thoracic radiograph provides valuable information on the integrity of the lungs and diaphragm, and this evaluation is especially important as up to 50% of dogs involved in automobile trauma will have pulmonary contusions.

Overweight and obese dogs

The anaesthetist may either calculate drug dosages based on actual weight, realizing that overweight dogs will receive a higher dose rate than ideal weight dogs, or to calculate the dose rates on ideal weight based on an assessment of body condition. Preferably, anaesthetic drug dosages for an overweight dog should be calculated on its ideal weight since the animal's circulating blood volume is that of a smaller animal and fat contributes little to initial redistribution (Fig. 15.2). Various body condition score (BCS) systems are used to evaluate dogs and cats and it is recommended that all veterinarians within a practice use the same scoring system (Baldwin et al., 2010). The recommended goal for most dogs is 3 out of 5 or 4–5 out of 9. Comparison of methods for estimating body fat in

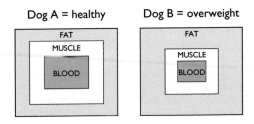

Administration of the same mg/kg dose
in overweight dog = overdosage

Figure 15.2 Schematic representation of the risk for overdosage of overweight dogs with intravenous anaesthetic agents.

dogs revealed that a 9-point scale for assigning a body condition score (BCS) correlated well with dual-energy X-ray absorptiometry (DEXA) which is a non-invasive method for estimating body fat content (Mawbry et al., 2004). This investigation determined that the ideal BCS of 5 corresponded to 11% body fat, and body fat increased by 8.7% for every unit increase in BCS. Ideal bodyweight is calculated by dividing the actual weight by a number based on the BCS, for example, weight of dogs with BCS of 6 = actual weight ÷ 1.087, BCS 7 = weight ÷ 1.174, BCS 8 = weight ÷ 1.261, BCS 9 = weight ÷ 1.348.

An overweight dog is likely to hypoventilate during anaesthesia and assisted or controlled ventilation will probably be necessary. An obese animal breathing air when anaesthetized is likely to become hypoxaemic. Use of a pulse oximeter during preanaesthetic sedation, anaesthesia, and recovery from anaesthesia will warn when O_2 supplementation is needed.

Dogs weighing <5 kg

Death can occur in patients of all ages and health status but complications are more likely to occur in dogs weighing less than 5 kg (Brodbelt et al., 2008). Guessing rather than actually calculating dose rates in mL for these patients may lead to inadvertent overdosage. Use of 1 mL syringes with a 25 gauge needle or insulin syringes increases accuracy of drug administration by controlling the volume in the syringe and minimizing the impact of residual drug in the needle hub. A small mask and selection of endotracheal tube sizes down to 2.0 mm internal diameter (ID) should be available for these small dogs. Surveys have shown that complications are less likely to occur when someone's sole responsibility is to monitor the patient through anaesthesia and recovery, and this is particularly true of small patients. Drape barriers should be placed to lift the drapes and facilitate observation. The volume of fluid administered during anaesthesia must be closely recorded (including volume for flushing catheters and dobutamine or dopamine administration) to avoid over transfusion, as well as the volume of blood loss to avoid hypovolaemia. Heat loss is rapid in small animals and one or more means of supplying warmth should be employed from the start of anaesthesia.

Diagnostic tests

Evaluation of the history and a comprehensive physical examination of a patient prior to anaesthesia may reveal abnormalities that require further elucidation using laboratory tests. Routine testing before a major surgical procedure should be done to provide a baseline for comparison of postoperative tests, although it is likely that tests will have already been run during evaluation of the patients' diseases. With increasing age, hepatocyte numbers decrease, pancreatic enzyme secretion diminishes, nephrons decrease, and glomerular filtration rate decreases

(Hoskins, 1995). These changes predict increased incidence of organ malfunction and are a reason for laboratory measurement of haematological and clinical chemistries of older dogs before anaesthesia even when they are thought to be healthy. The age at which a dog should be considered senior varies with the breed and is reached at 75% of life expectancy, or broadly 9 years old for small and medium dogs and 6 years for giant breeds. Many clinicians require that all dogs over 4 or 5 years of age have blood drawn for a complete blood count (CBC) and clinical chemistries, including but not limited to plasma protein, albumin, blood urea nitrogen and creatinine, liver enzyme tests, glucose, and electrolytes. Considerable controversy exists concerning blood testing of healthy dogs scheduled for elective surgery because when a clinical examination has revealed no abnormalities very few dogs will be found to have a significant laboratory test abnormality (some may have values just outside the accepted normal range) that requires a change in anaesthetic management. Current recommendations proposed by the American Animal Hospital Association is that a minimum database should be routinely run on all mature, senior and geriatric dogs as part of comprehensive wellness care for early detection of disease (Bartges et al., 2012). They also make the point that the laboratory should be aware of specific breed variations of 'normal values'.

Abnormalities in the results of laboratory tests should be noted for the possible modification of the anaesthetic protocol, such as low plasma protein that increases the amount of free and active anaesthetic agent and alters the ability of the dog to maintain a satisfactory blood pressure during anaesthesia. Abnormalities of hepatic or renal function may dictate an adjustment in the selection of anaesthetic agents based on the dog's decreased ability to eliminate the drugs.

Specific blood tests are justified when a dog is in a high-risk population, for example, a Doberman pinscher may suffer from von Willebrand's disease and should be tested for adequate coagulation. Dogs with 30% or less of the normal level of von Willebrand's factor are at risk for haemorrhage during surgery and should be treated with 8-D-arginine vasopressin (DDAVP) or an infusion of fresh plasma or cryoprecipitate before surgery.

Evaluation of the significance of disease

Identification of neurological or cardiac disease, or hepatic or renal malfunction, may have a direct bearing on choice of anaesthetic agents or anaesthetic management as discussed later in this chapter. Some diseases cause derangements of fluid, electrolyte, and metabolic balance and these should be corrected if possible before induction of anaesthesia. Correction of dehydration may not be feasible, but restoration of an adequate circulatory blood volume should be ensured by infusion of appropriate product, such as crystalloid fluid, hypertonic saline, heta-starch, plasma, or blood.

The American Society of Anesthesiologists (ASA) classification of physical status (see Chapter 1) is an objective assessment of a patient's global physiological illness status and should be used to assess prediction for requirement for care, that is, the higher the score the increased requirement for attention to preanaesthetic preparation, choice of anaesthetic protocol, and extent of monitoring during and after anaesthesia. Although the ASA classification reflects the degree of physiological derangement of the patient, specific guidelines are not available for class assignment, consequently, anaesthesiologists may vary in their classifications of some patients. Furthermore, ASA classification does not describe risk of anaesthesia because adverse aspects of the procedure or surgery are not included. For example, consider a relatively physiologically healthy dog that is scheduled to undergo dorsal hemilaminectomy or forelimb amputation, procedures that possess inherent risks for complications including excessive haemorrhage and air embolism. The impact of the procedure on the course of anaesthesia should be considered, for example, surgical procedures in the cranial abdomen or performed with the animal in a prone, head-down position will impair ventilation. Orthopaedic procedures require profound analgesia and may be responsible for significant blood loss. Excision of tumours over the thorax may result in penetration of the pleural cavity. Animals with mast cell tumours are at risk for acute hypotension as a result of histamine release and should be pretreated with an antihistamine such as diphenhydramine, 2 mg/kg. In human medicine, there is a variety of scoring systems for different diseases, for example, the Acute Physiology and Chronic Health Evaluation (APACHE) score, and these scores are adjusted every 5 years to accommodate changes in current management and agents available. Specific illness severity scores are not commonly used at present for clinical veterinary patients but have a place in evaluation of groups of clinical patients included in research investigations of new treatment modalities. Illness severity scores are not designed to be used in isolation to predict outcome for individuals and clinicians should be careful about quoting score results to clients (Hayes et al., 2010). Furthermore, even a disease specific model may be difficult to select for a patient with a primary disease and comorbidities, for example, a patient scheduled for a forelimb amputation and an exploratory laparotomy for splenectomy and liver biopsy.

Food and water restrictions

The times recommended for withholding food before anaesthesia range from 6 to at least 12 hours (most frequently 12 hours), the object being to minimize the volume and acidity of food in the stomach and decrease risk of oesophageal and pulmonary tissue damage from gastric reflux and aspiration. The problem is deciding how long to withhold food since gastric fluid pH decreases with fasting and the longer the fasting period the higher the incidence of gastric reflux. Furthermore, the acidity and volume of gastric fluid not only fluctuate during the day but are also influenced by the type of food eaten before fasting. In one experimental study, dogs were fed different foods and gastric fluid aspirated and tested after induction of anaesthesia. Dogs that were fasted 10 hours before anaesthesia had less volume of fluid in the stomach but greater acidity (mean pH <2.0) compared with dogs fasted only 3 hours (mean pH >2.9) (Savvas et al., 2009). Feeding low-fat or low-protein food with a 10-hour fast resulted in the greatest acidity. The conclusions were that gastric acidity was best controlled by feeding canned food rather than dry food, and for the fasting time to be shorter rather than longer.

The traditional approach has been to recommend 'nothing-by-mouth after midnight'. Currently, a fasting time of 8, 10, or 12 hours has been most frequently published but there is no strong evidence to support any specific time recommendation. Fluid may be gone from the stomach within 60 minutes but dry food may persist for 24 hours. It is not uncommon to observe large quantities of partially digested dry food when dogs vomit after premedication, even when they have been fasted for 10–12 hours. In these cases, it is likely that anxiety created by an unfamiliar environment delayed gastrointestinal transit time. Dogs less than about 16 weeks of age should be fasted only a short time to minimize risk for hypoglycaemia, and not more than 4 hours is the most recent recommendation in the American Animal Hospital Association guidelines for anaesthesia (Bednarski et al., 2011). Minimal fasting also applies to those little dogs at risk for hypoglycaemia such as a 1 kg Yorkshire Terrier or Chihuahua. This author's personal preference for management of a diabetic dog is to fast the patient, reduce the insulin dose by half before anaesthesia and infuse 5% dextrose in water, 3 mL/kg/h, during anaesthesia.

Water should be withheld for 2 hours before anaesthesia, although some clinicians allow water up to the time of premedication.

Gastro-oesophageal reflux

The incidence of gastric fluid entering the oesophagus (gastro-oesophageal reflux, GER, GOR) without reaching the pharynx (silent regurgitation) has been reported in clinical patients as low as 13–17% (Raptopoulos & Galatos, 1995; Favarato et al., 2012), 40–44% (Wilson et al., 2005, 2007), and as high as 50–67% (Raptopoulos & Galatos, 1997; Wilson et al., 2006a,b; Panti et al., 2009; Shaver et al., 2011). Gastric reflux may go unnoticed because the number of dogs in which gastric fluid reaches the pharynx (regurgitation) is small. Investigations of GER/GOR usually involve insertion of a pH electrode through the mouth or nose and into the oesophagus until the tip is just cranial to the cardia. The presence of reflux can be confirmed by oesophagoscopy performed at the end of anaesthesia. While the pH electrode can easily identify sudden decreases in pH due to acid reflux from the stomach, not all cases of reflux of non-acid fluid or alkaline fluid may be identified.

Oesophageal pH in conscious dogs is approximately 8.0. A change in pH to <4.0 is considered to be indicative of acid gastric reflux and pH <2.5 is associated with risk of serious oesophageal mucosal damage and possible stricture formation later. Contact time with oesophageal mucosa may impact on the degree of damage. Measurement of oesophageal pH has defined GER/GOR as occurring at any time from induction to the end of anaesthesia and low oesophageal pH may persist from a few minutes to hours. The position of the dog has and has not been associated with initiation of reflux but intra-abdominal surgery increased the incidence of reflux in one group of patients (Galatos & Raptopoulos, 1995). Oesophageal damage may occur at any point along its length and stricture formation has been described at the thoracic inlet, heart base, and cardia (Wilson & Walshaw, 2004). The primary clinical sign of oesophagitis and stricture was vomiting, often associated with eating, starting on average 3 (0–16) days after anaesthesia. Fortunately, considering the high incidence of GER/GOR in some populations, oesophagitis and stricture formation after anaesthesia are uncommon.

The cause of GER/GOR is largely due to a decrease in lower oesophageal sphincter pressure allowing release of fluid from the stomach. Anaesthetic agents influence sphincter tone to varying degrees. Morphine and acepromazine, meperidine and acepromazine, methadone and acepromazine, and hydromorphone and midazolam were used as premedications in several studies with moderate to high incidences of GER/GOR (Wilson et al., 2005, 2007; Panti et al., 2009, Shaver et al., 2011). Modifying the premedication by eliminating one agent or decreasing dose rate altered the incidence of GER/GOR. Although morphine induces vomiting, the occurrence of vomiting after premedication was found to be unrelated to GER/GOR. A significantly higher incidence of GER/GOR has been recorded when propofol has been used for induction of anaesthesia compared with thiopental (Waterman & Hashim, 1992; Raptopoulos & Galatos, 1997). The lower oesophageal sphincter pressure was found to be decreased during isoflurane anaesthesia compared with halothane (Hashim et al., 1995), whereas another study recorded no statistically significant differences in episodes of acid reflux between halothane (47%), isoflurane (63%), and sevoflurane (60%) (Wilson et al., 2006a).

Altering the gastric acidity before anaesthesia by administration of a histamine H_2 receptor antagonist or proton pump inhibitor (PPI) is not routine practice. The efficacy of these agents differs under different study conditions. Famotidine was found to be less effective than expected when gastric pH was measured using implanted gastric pH telemetry capsules in experimental dogs fed dry food (Tolbert et al., 2011) whereas, in another investigation, both famotidine and omeprazole, but not ranitidine, significantly elevated gastric pH (Bersenas et al., 2005). Omeprazole has been documented to decrease the incidence of GER/GOR in dogs fasted for at least 12 hours and then anaesthetized for orthopaedic surgery (Panti et al., 2009). The dogs received omeprazole, 1 mg/kg, orally at least 4 hours before anaesthesia consisting of acepromazine, methadone, propofol, and isoflurane, with or without epidural nerve block, and the occurrence of acid reflux was decreased from 52% in untreated control dogs to 18%.

The intestinal prokinetic, metoclopramide, increases the lower oesophageal sphincter pressure and has been investigated in management of gastric reflux. Similar to the PPI treatment, metoclopramide will decrease the incidence of GER/GOR but not completely prevent it. In a study of dogs fasted for an average of 17–19 hours before being anaesthetized for orthopaedic surgery, metoclopramide, 1 mg/kg, administered IV before induction of anaesthesia and continued as an infusion of 1 mg/kg/24 hours decreased acid reflux from 63% to 33% (Wilson et al., 2006b). Metoclopramide, at the dosages just described, is the agent that this author uses for dogs that are known to have regurgitated during a previous anaesthetic. Metoclopramide is also added to the anaesthetic management when a dog regurgitates shortly after induction of anaesthesia.

Premedication

Anticholinergics

Anticholinergic drugs are selected after consideration of the needs of individual patients. Atropine or glycopyrrolate may be administered to prevent bradycardia, reduce tracheobronchial secretions, or to prevent salivation that might obstruct the airway or initiate laryngospasm. Glycopyrrolate results in a smaller increase in heart rate after IM administration than atropine and that may be an advantage for dogs in which high heart rates may have adverse effects, e.g. senior and geriatric dogs. Conversely, atropine may be selected when a higher heart rate is required, as in treatment of AV heart block and cardiac arrest. Anticholinergic premedication may be contraindicated in dogs with hypertension or with moderate to severe cardiac disease due to mitral regurgitation, cardiomyopathy, myocardial ischaemia, and traumatic myocarditis as the tachycardia induced may decrease cardiac output, increase the prevalence of ventricular dysrhythmias, and increase myocardial ischaemia by increasing O_2 demand. Dogs with rectal temperatures exceeding 39.7 °C (103.5 °F) should not be given atropine. Concurrent use of an anticholinergic drug with medium to large doses of medetomidine or dexmedetomidine is not recommended.

Atropine may be given IM, IV, or SC. Dose rates commonly used for premedication are 0.04 mg/kg of a 0.5 mg/mL solution IM or SC, or half that dose IV. Onset of action occurs in about 20 minutes after IM injection and lasts about 1.5 hours. Onset of action is within 2 minutes after IV injection in conscious dogs but may take longer in anaesthetized animals with slow circulation, for example with advanced AV heart block or hypotension. A transient slowing of the heart after administration is often observed before the heart rate increases. Higher doses may be used where needed and in the antagonism of neuromuscular block and in cardiopulmonary resuscitation. Glycopyrrolate is administered as 0.01 mg/kg IM and 0.005 mg/kg IV. Onset of action after IM injection is 40 minutes in conscious dogs and the duration of effect on heart rate is 2–4 hours. Onset of action may be faster after IM injection in dogs during inhalation anaesthesia, presumably due to increased muscle blood flow.

Sedative and analgesic premedication

Any of the analgesic and sedative drugs already discussed may be used for premedication. The choice of agent will depend partly on the dog and the reason for anaesthesia and partly on availability and cost. An opioid may provide analgesia during and after anaesthesia, and when administered with a sedative will increase the sedation achieved. Opioids that are μ receptor agonists with a tendency to induce vomition, such as morphine, hydromorphone, and oxymorphone, should be avoided for premedication in dogs that may be adversely affected, such as the presence of neck pain, gastric or intestinal foreign body or obstruction, severe corneal ulcer or ruptured cornea, or at risk for aspiration such as laryngeal paralysis or megaoesophagus. In these circumstances, administration may be withheld until after induction of anaesthesia or another opioid that does not induce vomition, such as fentanyl, methadone or buprenorphine, can be used.

An opioid should be chosen for premedication only after consideration of the desired opioid for intraoperative analgesia and for the immediate recovery from anaesthesia. Some opioid–opioid combinations interact resulting in diminished analgesia. For example, a much higher dose of μ opioid will be necessary when administered after buprenorphine because buprenorphine preferentially occupies μ receptors but provides less analgesia. This was demonstrated in a group of dogs anaesthetized for ovariohysterectomy. All of the dogs were premedicated with acepromazine and half received buprenorphine. A light plane of isoflurane anaesthesia was maintained such that additional opioid was needed to provide analgesia for surgery. Analysis of the data revealed that 2.5 times more sufentanil was needed to treat responses to surgical stimulation in the dogs that had received buprenorphine (Goyenechea Jaramillo et al., 2006). Similarly, premedication with

butorphanol will diminish the analgesic effect of a concurrently administered μ opioid for 1–2 hours.

Administration of butorphanol or buprenorphine after a μ opioid will result in partial reversal (Dyson et al., 1990). For example, consider a dog that has received morphine or hydromorphone and epidural morphine for an orthopaedic procedure. Administration of buprenorphine shortly after the dog regains consciousness will change the dog's behaviour from quiet, relaxed, and comfortable to a dog that is crying, shivering and painful. In certain situations, butorphanol or buprenorphine may be purposely selected for postanaesthetic administration after pre- or intraoperative administration of a μ opioid. For example, a dog that is young and bouncy and must be stretched out on the table for radiography has a μ opioid added to the anaesthetic protocol to achieve a stable and adequate plane of anaesthesia. The dog is expected to have minimal discomfort after anaesthesia and administration of butorphanol facilitates a speedy recovery and an earlier hospital discharge. In another situation, a dog during recovery from anaesthesia exhibits dysphoria ± vocalization that is attributed to the μ opioid administered for postoperative analgesia. After ruling out the possibility that the behaviour of the dog is a consequence of unsatisfactorily treated pain, administration of buprenorphine may result in a calmer patient. As previously mentioned, whining and vocalization may occur in pain-free dogs after administration of methadone or hydromorphone.

Concurrent administration of a sedative and an opioid is a popular choice for premedication. Sedation is much improved by the combination and may dramatically decrease the dose rate of drugs used for induction of anaesthesia and endotracheal intubation. The degree of sedation produced depends on the drugs used and dose rates, further influenced by individual variation. Administration of butorphanol, 0.2–0.4 mg/kg, buprenorphine, 0.01–0.02 mg/kg, morphine 0.5 mg/kg, hydromorphone, 0.05–0.10 mg/kg, or meperidine (pethidine), 3–4 mg/kg, IM alone may induce very little sedation but when combined with acepromazine, 0.02–0.05 mg/kg, the combinations result in moderate to heavy sedation. The choice of opioid may be influenced by the onset time, preferred route of administration, and efficacy. Butorphanol is not a good choice for orthopaedic pain.

Acepromazine IM or IV, 0.02 mg/kg in large dogs and 0.02–0.05 mg/kg in smaller dogs, will calm some dogs sufficiently for venepuncture but have minimal effect in active dogs and here the addition of an opioid is advisable. Acepromazine will not develop a full effect for at least 30 minutes after IM injection. Larger doses of acepromazine do not increase sedation but can contribute to lowering blood pressure during inhalant anaesthesia. Acepromazine contributes to maintenance of a steady plane of anaesthesia and to a smooth recovery from anaesthesia.

The benzodiazepines are not useful drugs to be used alone in healthy dogs as agitation or restlessness may be induced. Combination with an opioid may improve sedation and, for this, IV diazepam is more effective than midazolam. These agents appear to produce more CNS depression in older and sick dogs than in healthy animals. In sick dogs, IV administration of diazepam concurrently with a strong opioid such as oxymorphone or fentanyl may induce such heavy sedation that a miniscule amount of anaesthetic agent is required for endotracheal intubation.

Moderate doses of medetomidine, 0.01–0.02 mg/kg (10–20 µg/kg), or dexmedetomidine, 0.003–0.010 mg/kg (3–10 µg/kg), administered with an opioid produce heavy sedation that seriously decreases the dose of anaesthetic agent needed for induction of anaesthesia. Care must be taken during induction of anaesthesia since these drugs slow circulation time, and sufficient time must be allowed to elapse before administering more anaesthetic agent. The highest dose listed on the manufacturer's package information given IM with butorphanol, 0.2 mg/kg, produces such deep sedation that endotracheal intubation can be accomplished without further drug administration. The cardiovascular effects of this group of drugs are significant and they must be used cautiously in dogs with cardiovascular disease or hypovolaemia.

Transdermal fentanyl

Transdermal fentanyl patches are manufactured for human use. There are two designs of transdermal fentanyl patches: the reservoir, or membrane-controlled system, and the matrix system. A reservoir patch holds the fentanyl in a gel and delivery is determined by a rate-controlling membrane between the reservoir and the skin (Margetts & Sawyer, 2007). The matrix patch incorporates the drug into an adhesive polymer matrix from which fentanyl is continuously released to the skin. The dose of fentanyl delivered depends on the amount of fentanyl in the matrix and the area of the patch applied to the skin, such that one-half of the patch in contact with skin will deliver half of the original dose. Reservoir patches have tighter control on drug delivery but, if the membrane is damaged, there may be a burst of fentanyl into the skin and risk of overdose. Patches are available in different sizes with the dose expressed as µg/h.

Common sites for application are the dorsal cervical area, dorsal or lateral aspects of the thorax, or the caudal abdomen. The hair is clipped without abrading the skin. The area is washed with water and allowed to dry thoroughly. The protective seal is peeled from the patch and the patch held to the skin for 60 seconds to promote adhesion. Generally, an adhesive dressing is placed over the patch for security. Fentanyl forms a depot within the skin, therefore, a large amount of fentanyl is put in the patch to maintain the concentration gradient between patch and skin. Even at the end of 72 hours, matrix fentanyl patches attached to dogs had a mean residual content of 83% (Reed et al., 2011). A dog with a patch must be prevented from dislodging the patch or chewing on it. Extreme sedation was reported in a dog suspected of ingesting a reservoir type patch (Schmiedt & Bjorling, 2007). Fentanyl is an opiate and a controlled substance and a consent form is required in some states in the USA for the dog to be sent home with a patch. Significant toxic and fatal events have developed in children that have ingested fentanyl patches or stuck one on their skin mistaking it for a tattoo or Band-Aid. Owners should be informed of potential risks to people and be given detailed information about disposal. A transdermal patch should be carefully removed using the tips of the fingers or when wearing gloves. The patch should be folded so that the adhesive surfaces stick to each other and wrapped up before disposal in the waste bin. Hands should be washed thoroughly and gloves turned inside out before disposal. Flushing the patch down the toilet (USA) is illegal in UK and Europe.

Analgesic plasma concentrations are achieved by application of patch strength of 4 µg/kg/h (Egger et al., 1998; Robinson et al., 1999; Hofmeister & Egger, 2004; Bellei et al., 2011). There is a dearth of published information on dose rates and plasma concentrations in dogs >40 kg. One 100 µg/h and one 50 µg/patch may be applicable for a 40–50 kg dog and two 100 µg/h patches for larger dogs, or a lower dose rate may be sufficient. The time to effective plasma fentanyl concentrations is 12–24 hours but there is a high degree of variability in individual dogs. When used for premedication, the fentanyl patch should be applied at least 24 hours before surgery. If the patient develops hypothermia during anaesthesia, plasma fentanyl concentrations decrease (Wilson et al., 2006c). When applied at the end of surgery, and even when used as premedication, additional µ opioid will be needed as rescue analgesia in the first 12 hours until plasma fentanyl concentrations increase (Kyles et al., 1998; Robinson et al., 1999; Bellei et al., 2011). Later in recovery, analgesia provided by transdermal fentanyl compares favourably with alternative systemic or epidural opioid administration. The transdermal patch is generally left in place for 72 hours after application. Plasma fentanyl concentration decreases by 5 hours after patch removal.

Potential adverse effects include bradycardia, sedation, and anorexia, and dogs should be monitored for these signs. Mild skin irritation may be observed after the patch is removed and, in some dogs, there may be a delay in hair growth and altered coat colour.

Fentanyl is now available as a liquid-based drug (TD fentanyl solution, not a patch) that contains octyl-salicylate as a skin penetration enhancer and approved for use in dogs (Recuvyra™ TD fentanyl solution). It is applied with an applicator to the skin of dogs between the shoulder blades or to the ventral abdomen as a single dose of 2.7 mg/kg (50 mg/mL, 0.05 mL/kg). Absorption is more rapid from the dorsum resulting in a faster onset of action (Friese et al., 2012b). Mean plasma concentrations of fentanyl were maintained for at least 4 days above the

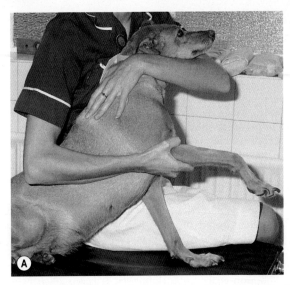
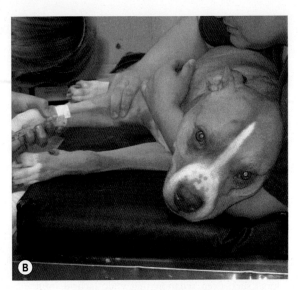

Figure 15.3 (A) Restraint for injection into the cephalic vein. (B) Alternative technique for occluding the cephalic vein for insertion of a catheter.

concentration presumed to provide analgesia (Friese et al., 2012a). In a clinical investigation, 445 dogs anaesthetized for orthopaedic or soft tissue surgery received either TD fentanyl solution applied 2–4 hours before surgery or buprenorphine before surgery and then every 6 hours for 90 hours (Linton et al., 2012). Postoperative analgesia from the two opioid administrations was judged to be similar.

Buprenorphine is also available as a transdermal matrix patch. Pieper et al. (2011) investigating application of a 52.5 µg/h patch in 13 kg Beagles identified onset of thermal antinociception at 36 hours. However, buprenorphine could not be detected in 3/10 dogs. Further information is needed to assess use of buprenorphine patches in dogs.

Intravenous technique

Intravenous injections or placement of indwelling venous catheters in dogs are commonly made into the cephalic vein, but other convenient sites include the lateral saphenous vein, the medial saphenous or femoral vein, the jugular vein and, in anaesthetized animals, the sublingual veins. Whichever site is used, conscious dogs should be handled quietly and forcible restraint reserved for those occasions when it is essential. Muzzles should be of the type with a quick release catch as delay in removal of a muzzle tangled in facial hair in a dog that has vomited during induction of anaesthesia may lead to inhalation of the vomited material.

Haematoma formation after venepuncture should be prevented by application of pressure to the site for an adequate period – usually about a minute. A haematoma

may be painful for the patient and may obscure the vein for several days, preventing subsequent use of the vein. Where a vein has been entered during an unsuccessful attempt at venepuncture, the pressure that was keeping the vein distended should be released and firm pressure applied to the site to stop bleeding before another attempt is made.

If the vein on the right forelimb is to be punctured, an assistant stands on the left side of the animal, passes his or her left arm around the animal's neck and raises its head (Fig. 15.3A). The dog can be in sitting, sternal, or lateral position. The assistant's right hand grips the animal's right forelimb so that the middle, third, and fourth fingers are immediately behind the olecranon and the thumb is around the front side of the limb. Some assistants prefer to place their thumb behind the olecranon and use fingers to occlude the vein (Fig. 15.3B). Pushing on the olecranon extends the limb and applying pressure with the thumb raises the vein. The hand should be rotated so as to pull the cephalic vein slightly lateral, which straightens it and makes it more visible. Venepuncture must be carried out with the usual aseptic precautions, so hair over the vein is clipped and the skin is disinfected. For detailed guidelines for catheter placement see also Chapter 10, Box 10.1.

Venepuncture with a needle and syringe for drug administration is most easily accomplished using a syringe with an eccentrically placed nozzle. This feature allows the syringe to lie closer to the forearm and the needle more or less parallel in the vein such that the needle is more likely to remain in the correct position. Suitable needle sizes depend on the size of the dog and the quantity and viscosity of the fluid to be injected. For most purposes a needle 2.5 cm (1 inch) long and 22 or 23 gauge is satisfactory; a 25 gauge needle can be used for small dogs and a 20 gauge for large dogs.

Two methods of stabilizing the vein prior to needle puncture are employed. In one, the skin over the vein is tautened without flattening the vein by the anaesthetist's free hand grasping the limb distal to the site of venepuncture and gently pulling the skin down. Usually the skin is penetrated in one move and then the vein entered in a second move. Once blood is observed in the needle hub, the needle should always be threaded deeper into the vein before making any injections. The position of the hand holding the skin taut is adjusted slightly to grip the hub of the needle or the syringe between thumb and forefinger while the limb is still held secure in the palm and fingers. In the second method, the thumb of the anaesthetist's free hand is placed just alongside the vein and the skin is not tensed (Fig. 15.4). The vein is stabilized between the needle and the thumb as the needle is advanced through the skin and into the vein. With this method it may be harder to thread the needle up the vein and there is a greater tendency for contamination of the needle by touching the thumb.

The first attempt at needle puncture should be done distally in the limb so that if a haematoma forms further attempts can be made more proximally. In Dachshunds and dogs with similar short, bent forelimbs such as Bulldogs, venepuncture is best attempted where the cephalic vein curves medially on the limb or in the angle where the accessory cephalic and cephalic veins join just proximal to the carpus (Fig. 15.5).

All air should be expressed from the syringe before venepuncture is attempted and there must be sufficient space left in the syringe to allow slight withdrawal of the plunger in order to test whether the needle is within the lumen of the vessel. Blood should enter the syringe when this is done, and no injection must be made if blood does not appear in the syringe or needle hub. Failure to draw blood usually means that either the vein has not been entered, the needle tip has passed through the opposite wall of the vein, or that the needle has become occluded. Failure to aspirate blood into the syringe is also encountered if the assistant has released occlusion pressure on the vein, if the vein is already thrombosed, or when peripheral perfusion is poor as it may be after administration of an α_2-agonist sedative.

The lateral saphenous vein may be used for IV injection or catheter placement at the point where it passes obliquely on the lateral aspect of the hind limb just proximal to the

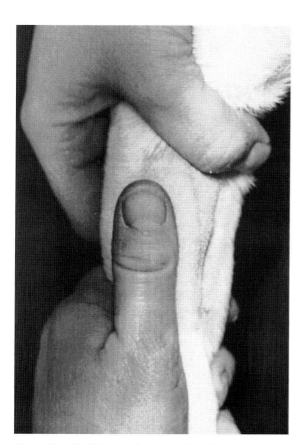

Figure 15.4 Stabilization of the cephalic vein against the thumb.

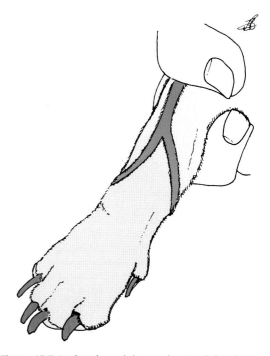

Figure 15.5 In short-legged dogs such as Dachshunds and Bulldogs, often the easiest point for venepuncture is at the junction of the accessory cephalic vein and the cephalic vein.

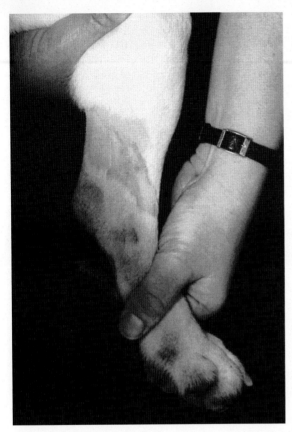

Figure 15.6 The lateral saphenous vein runs obliquely over the lateral surface of the limb from a point caudal on the gastrocnemius muscle to a point craniolaterally on the limb just proximal to the hock.

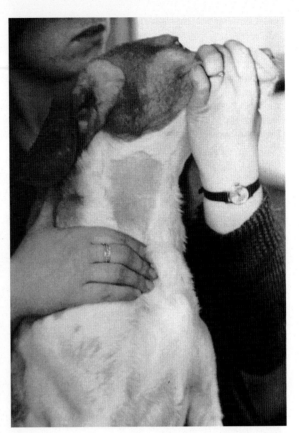

Figure 15.7 Jugular venepuncture in the conscious sitting dog.

hock (Fig. 15.6). The dog may be in sternal position with the leg pulled to one side or restrained in lateral position. Two assistants may be required for an alert dog; one restraining the head and forelimbs and one to raise the vein on the hind limb. There are several ways to accomplish this but one method involves the assistant standing on the opposite side of the animal and placing a hand (right hand for right hind limb and vice versa) on the cranial surface of the stifle, the thumb medially, and the fingers curled around the back of the leg, using pressure on the stifle to hold the leg in extension and fingers to occlude the vein. The person performing venepuncture or catheter placement holds the lower part of the limb, slightly pulling on the skin to tense it over the vein. After insertion of a needle, the hand is rotated to hold the needle hub between thumb and forefinger until the injection is made. The assistant may have to use two hands to immobilize the limb and raise the vein in very large or active dogs (Fig. 15.6). Sometimes the lateral saphenous vein is easier to catheterize in Bulldogs than the cephalic

vein. This breed (and Bloodhounds, Shar pei, etc.) have excessive skin so it is important to avoid short needles or short catheters and to wrap the tape snuggly proximal to the hock to prevent the catheter from sliding out of the vein as the skin moves.

Venepuncture of the jugular vein in the dog can be done with the dog standing or sitting with the head raised (Fig. 15.7). Identifying the jugular vein may be easier with the dog restrained on its side, particularly in smaller or ill patients, and the vein raised by occlusion near the thoracic inlet. A small foam pad, towel, or sandbag placed under the neck of the dog makes the position of the vein more obvious.

Short catheters (18 gauge and 20 gauge, 5 cm (2 inches) long, or 20 gauge or 22 gauge, 2.5 cm (1 inch) long) are commonly inserted into the cephalic or lateral saphenous veins, using the approach just described for venepuncture, prior to induction of anaesthesia for administration of anaesthetic drugs, electrolyte solutions and supportive drugs (see Chapter 10 for examples and insertion technique). Some giant breed dogs may require a 14 gauge or 16 gauge catheter when extensive fluid therapy is required or anticipated. Dogs <1 kg bodyweight may receive a 22 gauge or 24 gauge catheter, or occasionally an intraosseous catheter. The short venous catheters are typically secured with white porous tape attached first around the hub of the catheter and then around the limb. The sequence of taping and protective wrapping is an individual preference but it is essential to ensure that the first piece of tape is firmly stuck on the catheter and adhered to the skin, otherwise the catheter may easily pull out. A variety of catheter caps, T-ports, double T-ports, and extensions are available for attaching to the catheter. A needle on an administration set from a fluid bag may be inserted through the catheter cap/plug but faster flow will be obtained if the cap is removed and the administration set is attached directly to the catheter or T-port. Additionally, contamination is less likely with direct attachment. All connections must be tight or taped together.

Jugular, lateral or medial saphenous veins are used for placement of 'central lines'; long catheters inserted until the tips lie in the cranial or caudal vena cava and that are single, double or triple lumen catheters for multiple therapies and blood sampling (see Fig. 10.3). These catheters are inserted using strictly sterile technique, frequently using a modified Seldinger technique (see Chapter 10), and must be securely wrapped for protection and to prevent contamination.

The sublingual veins are easily accessed in the anaesthetized patient for collection of a small blood sample to measure blood glucose or packed cell volume and total protein. The tongue is pulled over the anaesthetist's finger so that its ventral surface is exposed and the veins are easily visible. It is important to use a small (25 gauge) needle because the vein will bleed freely after the needle is withdrawn. Bleeding will be less if the needle is inserted for a few millimetres under the mucosa before penetrating the vein. Pressure should be applied for a couple of minutes after the needle is removed to avoid a haematoma. Gauze or cotton wool with alcohol should not be used because the alcohol will cause mucosal necrosis. In case of emergency and absence of other adequate venous access, an 18 gauge catheter can be inserted in the lingual vein of a medium or large sized dog for administration of a large volume of electrolyte solution or blood (Fig. 15.8). Tape must not be wrapped tightly around the tongue.

Intraosseous injection

Placement of a catheter in a vein is occasionally difficult in dehydrated animals, especially toy breeds and puppies. The intraosseous route is an acceptable alternative for administration of fluids, blood, and drugs. Absorption is rapid and within one minute for some drugs, such as atropine. Intraosseous injection implies injection into the intramedullary canal of the femur, tibia, or humerus using a Cooke intraosseous needle, a Jamshidi needle or a spinal needle. A 20 gauge, 2.5 cm spinal needle is satisfactory for

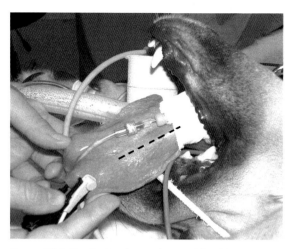

Figure 15.8 Dog in dorsal recumbency with a 22 gauge catheter in the lingual artery for blood pressure measurement. The dashed line is the site of one of the lingual veins that can be catheterized for fluid or blood administration when other veins are not available.

the smallest dogs and is inserted aseptically through the trochanteric fossa of the femur and parallel to the long axis of the bone into the medullary cavity (see Fig. 10.4). The stilette is removed, the needle flushed with heparinized saline, a T-port is attached and flushed again. Bandaging must be secure to prevent the needle from being dislodged as the animal moves about. Potential complications include infection and exceptional care should be taken in maintaining sterility of injections. The needle should be removed after 72 hours.

Vascular port

The vascular port is a subcutaneously implanted system for IV delivery of drugs. It is used when dogs require multiple anaesthetic episodes over a short time, for example for radiation therapy, and the peripheral veins are badly thrombosed. The vascular port consists of two basic parts: an indwelling catheter that is threaded into the jugular vein after surgical dissection in the anaesthetized dog and a rigid puncturable bulb that looks like a volcano and is located subcutaneously in the neck. The bulb has a silicone rubber window that is easily palpated through the skin and allows percutaneous intravenous injections using an appropriate sized needle.

Endotracheal intubation

Cuffed endotracheal tubes for dogs vary from 2.5 mm to 16.0 mm internal diameter (ID). The diameter of the largest tube that can be introduced into the trachea is related to both the size and the breed of the dog with the requirement that the tube selected should be a good approximation of the tracheal lumen diameter but not a 'push' fit. For example, a 14 mm tube can usually be inserted in the trachea of an adult German Shepherd and an 11 or 12 mm tube used for most 25 kg dogs. In contrast, the Bulldog often has an exceptionally small-diameter laryngeal lumen and trachea for its body weight and a selection of smaller tubes should be available at anaesthetic induction of this breed.

The tubes should be checked for length alongside the dog because the tip should not extend beyond the thoracic inlet into the chest. Excess tube extending outside the incisors contributes to dead space and CO_2 breathing and, therefore, some tubes may have to be shortened by cutting off 2–6 cm length with scissors. Thin-walled endotracheal tubes with small volume cuffs should be purchased for use in puppies and very small dogs to allow the largest lumen size possible in their small tracheas. Alternatively, uncuffed or Cole pattern tubes can be used to eliminate the space occupied by the cuff. IPPV and aspiration of foreign material are potential problems with use of uncuffed tubes and should be prevented by packing the pharynx with moistened gauze.

A good light source is needed in the form of bright overhead lighting or a laryngoscope since intubation in dogs is accomplished under direct viewing of the epiglottis and the position of the tube in relation to it. A laryngoscope is advisable for intubation of brachycephalic dogs. It is usual to induce anaesthesia in the dog to a level that is just adequate to allow the dog's mouth to be held open without initiating chewing movements, yawning, or tongue curling. When thiopental, propofol, alfaxalone, or etomidate has been used for induction of anaesthesia and the dog is swallowing when intubation is attempted, the depth of anaesthesia is too light and more drug should be administered. Swallowing during intubation is normal during ketamine anaesthesia.

The dog may be positioned in either sternal or lateral recumbency. In either case, the assistant must hold the dog's head and neck in a straight line with one hand holding the top jaw, thumb and forefinger on either side of the jaw behind the canine teeth and holding the upper lips up and away from the teeth to facilitate the anaesthetist's view (Fig. 15.9). The assistant or the anaesthetist depresses the lower jaw using a finger on the interdental space caudal to the canine tooth. The dog's tongue is pulled rostrally to spread open the larynx and is held either by the assistant or the anaesthetist in such a way as to protect it from laceration by the teeth (Fig. 15.10A). The blade of the laryngoscope is placed flat on the tongue with the tip of the blade depressing the tongue at the base of the epiglottis. In some dogs, the epiglottis may be trapped behind the soft palate and must be released using the tip of the endotracheal tube to push the soft palate dorsally (Fig. 15.10B, C). The lubricated tube should be used to depress the epiglottis onto the tongue and to keep it there

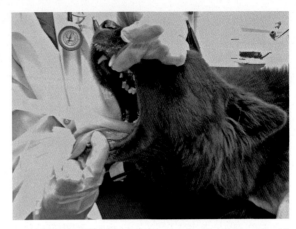

Figure 15.9 Holding the head for tracheal intubation should provide alignment between the pharynx and trachea. The tongue should never be used for leverage to open the mouth.

while the tube itself is advanced in front of the arytenoid cartilages into the trachea (Fig. 15.10D). Frequently, rotating the tube 90° about its longitudinal axis as the tip passes through the larynx allows the tube to be advanced more easily into the trachea. The dog is then moved into lateral recumbency, the anaesthetic circuit connected to the endotracheal tube and the O_2 flowmeter turned on.

The endotracheal tube is positioned within the trachea by gentle palpation at the base of the neck to determine the level of the tip of the tube. This is facilitated by using the other hand to move the endotracheal tube a little within the trachea (Fig. 15.11). Once the tip of the tube is determined to be level with the base of the neck, the tube is further advanced a distance appropriate to the size of the dog (0.5–2.5 cm) to the level of the thoracic inlet. Any markings on the tube level with the incisors are noted for future reference of tube position during that anaesthetic. While the assistant holds the tube in place, the anaesthetist ties a length of gauze or tubing tightly around the tube and then behind the dog's head or around the upper or lower jaw, using a bow or quick release knot (Fig. 15.12). The knot around the tube must be tight to avoid slipping and accidental extubation. The endotracheal tube cuff should be inflated with just enough air to prevent a leak that can be detected when listening for air escaping around the tube during inflation of the lungs by squeezing the reservoir bag to a pressure of 20–25 cmH$_2$O with the 'pop-off' (APL) valve closed. The anaesthetist must remember to release the valve after this procedure. The vaporizer is then turned on.

The process of intubation should be performed gently to avoid trauma to the pharynx and larynx that can cause tissue swelling and damage. Furthermore, any time that the dog's position or location is changed, the endotracheal tube should be briefly disconnected from the breathing circuit to avoid twisting the tube within the trachea and

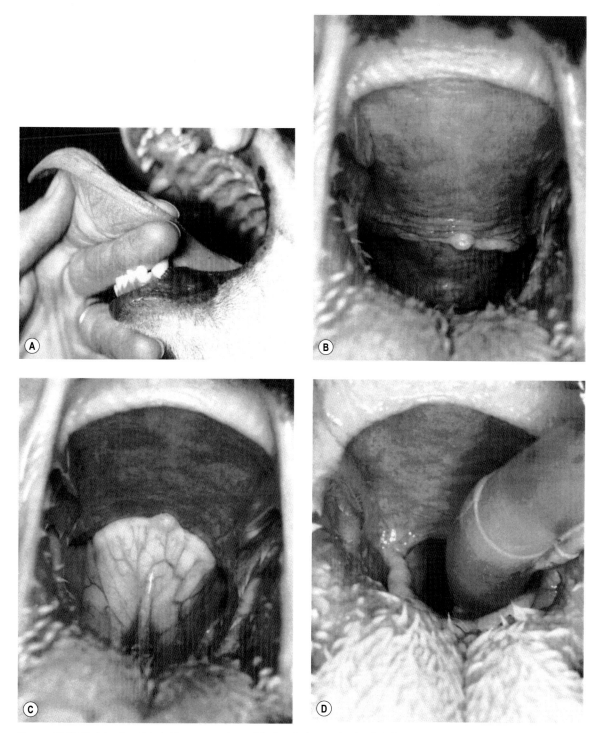

Figure 15.10 Endotracheal intubation as seen by a right-handed anaesthetist. (A) The assistant is holding the upper lips and the anaesthetist is drawing the tongue out of the mouth, protecting its undersurface by placing a finger over the dog's incisor teeth. (B) The epiglottis is almost completely obscured by the soft palate. (C) The soft palate has been lifted by the tip of the tube to allow the tip of the epiglottis to come forward. (D) The tip of the tube has been passed over the epiglottis, through the vocal cords and on towards the sternum.

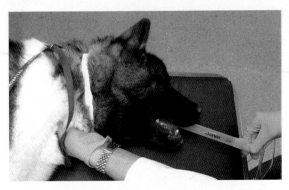

Figure 15.11 Palpating the position of the tip of the endotracheal tube within the trachea at the base of the neck with the thumb on one side of the trachea and fingers on the other. The tube should then be advanced further to place the tip level with the thoracic inlet.

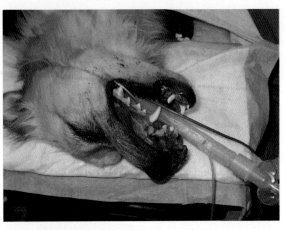

Figure 15.12 The endotracheal tube is secured with tubing (from an old IV administration set) tied around the tube and behind the dog's head. Next to the endotracheal tube is a temperature probe inserted into the oesophagus. Bilateral maxillary nerve blocks were added to the anaesthetic protocol to provide analgesia for repair of trauma to the maxilla.

Table 15.6 Complications occurring during endotracheal intubation

Complication	Clinical signs	Management
Oesophageal intubation	Panting, ± SpO₂<90%, muddy pink/bluish gums, minimal excursion of RB, waking up	To confirm tracheal intubation, look inside dog's mouth to see the ETT passing under the arytenoids, epiglottis should be pressed horizontal by the ETT. Panting may be opioid induced. Oesophageal intubation may obstruct larynx and is seen as chest collapsing on inspiration. Squeezing the RB will inflate abdomen and not the chest
Endobronchial intubation	Panting, may or may not cause hypoxia (SpO₂<90%, muddy pink/bluish gums), minimal excursion of RB, waking up	Observe the cm marks on the side of the ETT as distance inserted may confirm depth, deflate cuff and withdraw ETT a short distance and observe for a decrease in RR and increase in SpO₂
ETT obstruction	Small excursion of RB compared with larger chest movement, presence of hypoxaemia depends on duration of obstruction, resistance felt when artificially inflating lungs	Deflate ETT cuff and partially withdraw tube (overinflation of cuff may compress tube lumen, tip of tube may be against tracheal wall, kinked ETT). Tension pneumothorax will mimic partial ETT obstruction. During surgery, mucus or blood clot may obstruct ETT
Unable to advance ETT	Assuming the tube is not too big, this problem may occur in dogs with tracheal collapse	Rotate the ETT before or during advancement, try a slightly smaller ETT, use a flexible guarded (metal spiral) ETT
Mimics ETT problem	Increased heart rate, decreased SpO₂ as a result of hypotension	Check CRT, femoral pulse, and blood pressure
Unable to extubate	Insert ETT, suspect tube is too large (a 'push fit'), attempts to extubate fail	Move tube in a little further and attempt to aspirate more air from cuff, relax larynx by topical lidocaine and deeper anaesthesia, KY gel in a small syringe and attempt to insert some around the tube. Gentle digital manipulation. Last resort is to cut the tube longitudinally. Don't forget to supply O₂ and continue monitoring during this procedure. Observe for laryngeal mucosa swelling after extubation

ETT = endotracheal tube, RB = Rebreathing bag

tearing tracheal mucosa. The ability to bark may be lost for 1–2 days after anaesthesia when laryngeal swelling occurs as a result of pressure from the tube or friction from being moved around, for example, during dental procedures.

Apnoea may occur following endotracheal intubation in a lightly anaesthetized dog simply as a reflex response to presence of the tube. Management depends on the individual circumstances. For example, if the dog is very light and likely to start chewing on the tube if it does not inhale anaesthetic gas then either some artificial lung inflations or a small dose of injectable anaesthetic agent would be appropriate. In many cases, no artificial ventilation is necessary, as the animal will start breathing when the PCO_2 increases. An exception might be when cyanosis has developed after induction of anaesthesia with propofol in which case two to three lung inflations are needed quickly to restore pink mucous membranes. Other complications may occur as a result of unsatisfactory tube placement, such as oesophageal intubation, endobronchial intubation, and endotracheal tube obstruction. The first step is to look into the dog's mouth and see the tube entering the larynx ventral to the arytenoids. Having confirmed endotracheal intubation, other causes of abnormal clinical signs can be investigated (Table 15.6).

Intubation via pharyngotomy

Tracheal intubation through a pharyngotomy is used when oral surgery requires closure of the jaws for correct alignment, such as repair of bilaterally fractured jaws, or when the endotracheal tube obscures the surgical site, such as during cleft palate repair. Commonly, a tube with a metal spiral in the wall (guarded endotracheal tube) is used so that the surgeon can operate rostrally to the patient and the anaesthesia machine is moved to the side of the patient requiring the endotracheal tube to bend 180° without kinking. The dog is first anaesthetized, orotracheally intubated in the usual way and connected to the anaesthesia machine. The hair is clipped from over the right pharyngeal area just caudal to the angle of the mandible and a surgical scrub applied to the skin. A hand is inserted into the dog's mouth until a finger can palpate the epiglottis, arytenoid cartilages and hyoid apparatus. The finger is then directed towards the lateral wall of the neck at the junction of the intrapharyngeal osteum and laryngopharynx and caudal to the epihyoid bone with enough pressure to create an external bulge (Fig. 15.13A). Large curved forceps are substituted for the finger and a small skin incision is made over the bulge. The underlying tissues are blunt dissected through pharyngeal muscle and mucosa until the forceps can pass through the hole (Fig. 15.13B). The endotracheal tube can be inserted in one of two ways. The existing endotracheal tube can be removed and replaced by a guarded endotracheal tube. The jaws of the instrument are introduced through the pharyngotomy hole into the mouth. The endotracheal tube adapter is removed, if

possible, the tube bent back on itself, and the end grasped by the forceps and withdrawn through the pharyngeal wall followed by the cuff inflation pilot balloon. The adapter is replaced and the endotracheal tube connected to the anaesthesia machine. Alternatively, the forceps can be introduced into the mouth and out through the skin incision (Fig. 15.13B). The tip of the guarded endotracheal tube is grasped and pulled through into the oral cavity and out of the mouth. The tube must then be turned 180° and the tip of the tube grasped by the forceps and advanced into the larynx. Once the tube has entered the larynx, a finger can be introduced to push the tube fully into the trachea and to straighten the tube (Fig. 15.13C). In either case, the guarded endotracheal tube is moved gently until the tip of the tube is at the thoracic inlet. The exterior part of the tube is bent caudally and secured firmly in place before the cuff is inflated in the usual manner (Fig. 15.13D). At the end of anaesthesia, the endotracheal tube is removed while the dog is still anaesthetized and replaced with a clean orotracheal tube for recovery from anaesthesia. The pharyngotomy site is not sutured.

Intravenous agents

Intravenous agents may be administered alone but are usually given after injection of sedatives or opioids. Induction of anaesthesia will then be calmer, fewer adverse side effects of the induction drugs will be observed, their margin of safety will be increased, and recovery may be faster. Some commonly used drug combinations, with dose rates, are given in Table 15.7.

Thiopental

Solutions of thiopental have a high pH and the drug can only be given IV. It should be used as a 2.5% or weaker solution because more concentrated solutions are less easy to titrate to effect, resulting in administration of a higher dose than necessary. A 5% thiopental solution may cause thrombosis of the vein and produces necrosis of overlying tissues and skin if injected perivascularly. Management of even a 2.5% solution into tissues outside the vein should include immediate injection into the area of lidocaine, 2 mg/kg, without epinephrine to precipitate the thiopental into a harmless salt, and a volume of saline appropriate to the size of the dog for dilution of the irritant. Warm compresses should be applied to the leg at intervals over the subsequent 12–24 hours.

The dose of thiopental depends on the condition of the dog, its state of hydration, and especially on previous medication. As a rough guide, the anaesthetist should expect to use up to 12 mg/kg in a dog for induction of anaesthesia. In the healthy but lightly premedicated dog, one half of this, i.e. about 6 mg/kg is given fairly rapidly as a bolus to produce a rapid induction of anaesthesia. If anaesthesia is insufficient to permit endotracheal

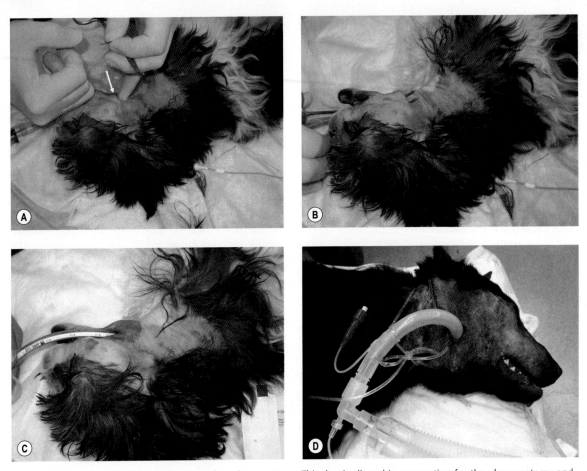

Figure 15.13 Endotracheal intubation through a pharyngotomy. This dog is clipped in preparation for the pharyngotomy and for repair of fractured jaws. (A) Palpation through the mouth to identify the site of skin incision by creating an external bulge (arrow). (B) Introduction of forceps through the mouth and out of the pharyngotomy. (C) The tip of the metal spiral endotracheal tube has been pulled through the pharyngotomy and directed into the trachea. (D) The endotracheal tube, inserted in a different dog, is bent caudally and secured in position with a tie around the neck.

intubation, additional small increments of the remainder should be given at 15–20-second intervals. The whole dose may be needed in a proportion of dogs. A slow administration rate of thiopental significantly decreases the total dose required for anaesthesia but may result in a poorer quality of induction accompanied by involuntary movements (Dugdale et al., 2005). Large dogs require relatively less than small, while geriatric dogs have a reduced anaesthetic requirement. A lower total dose of 5–6 mg/kg of thiopental may be sufficient in dogs with a moderate degree of preanaesthetic sedation from a combination of sedative and opioid, such as acepromazine and morphine, methadone, or hydromorphone. The dose of thiopental required for induction will be greatly decreased to 1–3 mg/kg in dogs that are heavily sedated, for example with medetomidine or dexmedetomidine and butorphanol, or tiletamine–zolazepam. Preanaesthetic

sedation before thiopental is advisable because, like propofol and etomidate, thiopental does not provide analgesia.

Other drugs may be administered IV immediately before thiopental to decrease the dose needed and to enhance the quality of induction. Diazepam or midazolam, 0.1–0.2 mg/kg, or another benzodiazepine may decrease the dose of thiopental required by 15% or more, depending on the physical status of the dog. Potent opioids such as fentanyl, sufentanil, or alfentanil will also substantially decrease the dose of thiopental required for tracheal intubation. Prior or concurrent administration of atropine or glycopyrrolate may be needed to counter bradycardia induced by the opioid. Lidocaine, 1–2 mg/kg, IV can also be administered before thiopental to decrease the dose.

Return to consciousness after thiopental anaesthesia is due to decreased blood concentration from redistribution

Table 15.7 Some examples of drug combinations for anaesthesia with injectable agents*

Premedication	Dose rate (mg/kg)	Induction#	Dose rate (mg/kg IV)
Acepromazine	0.02–0.03 (large dog) IM 0.03–0.1 (small dog) IM	Thiopental	12
Acepromazine + Butorphanol or Meperidine	0.02–0.05 IM 0.3–0.4 IM 3–5 IM	Thiopental	6–10
Acepromazine + Morphine or Hydromorphone or Oxymorphone or Methadone	0.02–0.05 IM 0.2–0.5 IM 0.05–0.10 IM 0.05–0.10 IM 0.1–0.5 IM	Thiopental	4–6
Medetomidine	0.02 IM	Thiopental	1–3
None		Propofol	6–8
Acepromazine or Midazolam + Butorphanol or Hydromorphone or Buprenorphine	0.02–0.05 IM 0.2 IM 0.2–0.4 IM 0.05–0.20 IM 0.01–0.02 IM	Propofol	2–4
Medetomidine or Dexmedetomidine + Butorphanol or Hydromorphone	0.01–0.02 IM 0.003–0.01 IM 0.2 IM 0.05 IM	Propofol	1–2
Fentanyl Diazepam	0.005 IV 0.2 IV	Propofol	1
None or Acepromazine + Hydromorphone or Methadone	 0.02 IV 0.05 IV 0.2 IM	Alfaxalone	2–4
Medetomidine + Butorphanol	0.004 IM 0.1–0.2 IM	Alfaxalone	0.5–1.5
None		Diazepam (5 mg/mL) Ketamine (100 mg/mL)	0.25 5.0 (1 mL/10 kg using a 50:50 mixture)
Sedative and/or opioid		Diazepam (5 mg/mL) Ketamine (100 mg/mL)	0.25 5.0 (1 mL/10 kg using a 50:50 mixture) Inject half first, titrate remainder to effect
Xylazine	1.0 IM, IV	Ketamine	10 IM, IV
Medetomidine or Dexmedetomidine	0.01–0.04 IM 0.003–0.015 IM	Ketamine	2–5 IM, IV
± Opioid		Tiletamine Zolazepam	2–5 IM, IV
Butorphanol or Buprenorphine or Hydromorphone	0.2–0.3 IM, IV 0.01 IM, IV 0.05–0.10 IM, IV	Diazepam Etomidate§	0.2–0.25 1.5 (small dog) 0.5–1.0 (medium to large dog) Up to total 3
None		Fentanyl‡ Diazepam or Midazolam	0.005–0.010 0.25 0.25

*These are only examples as dose rates should be modified appropriately for the breed, the individual, and concurrent disease. Other premedication agents can be used. An anticholinergic drug may be included if appropriate.

#Diazepam or midazolam, 0.2 mg/kg, can be injected IV before thiopental or propofol and will further decrease their dose rates.

§Generally reserved for old dogs or dogs with moderate to severe cardiac disease or compromise.

‡For induction of depressed and ill dogs. These drugs are administered in increments alternately starting with fentanyl.

of the drug into well-perfused organs and muscle. A smoother recovery from thiopental is achieved by ensuring some degree of sedation from other agents. Thiopental is very slowly metabolized in dogs such that 24% of the injected dose is still present in the body after 24 hours. This characteristic has a number of consequences. Administration of multiple doses of thiopental to prolong anaesthesia over 20–30 minutes will result in an unacceptably prolonged recovery, except when very small doses of thiopental are required because of heavy preanaesthetic sedation. Recovery time can be shortened when antagonists can reverse premedicant drugs. Recovery is sufficiently prolonged and accompanied by decreased muscle tone that maintenance of a patent airway can initially be a problem for brachycephalic dogs. Use of a different IV anaesthetic agent produces better results in these breeds. Dogs that are thin or lean or are one of the breeds that constitute 'sighthounds', such as Borzois, Afghans, Greyhounds, have trouble redistributing thiopental because they have no fat and may have little muscle. Blood concentrations remain high for longer, the dogs are slower to regain consciousness and are slow and ataxic to stand. Furthermore, Greyhounds may be deficient in the enzymes required for detoxification of thiopental.

Apnoea occurs in a proportion of dogs after induction of anaesthesia due to depression of the respiratory centres. Only when the $PaCO_2$ accumulates to a higher concentration will spontaneous breathing be stimulated. After a few breaths the $PaCO_2$ decreases below the new set point and breathing ceases. Thus an uneven pattern of breathing may be observed as the dog takes a few breaths and then pauses, and the cycle repeats. Only when the blood thiopental concentration decreases, and respiratory depression is less, will spontaneous breathing become regular. Irregular heart rhythm from occasional premature ventricular complexes (PVCs) may be detected within the first 10 minutes of administration. Treatment for these is rarely needed. However, thiopental sensitizes the myocardium to catecholamines for several hours so that abnormal ventricular rhythm may develop during hypercarbia, hypoxaemia, light anaesthesia, or halothane anaesthesia. A different injectable anaesthetic agent may be a better choice for dogs with myocardial ischaemia or contusions. Thiopental decreases myocardial contractility and venodilation decreases venous return to the heart resulting in a decrease in cardiac output. The heart rate may increase in order to maintain arterial pressure within a normal range.

A striking advantage to use of thiopental for induction of anaesthesia is that depth of inhalation anaesthesia tends to be more even and easy to regulate compared with a ketamine or propofol induction, presumably due to a slower decrease in plasma concentration of injectable agent. Thiopental decreases intracranial pressure (ICP), as does propofol and etomidate, and may be a suitable choice for use in some neurological patients.

Methohexital

Although recovery from a single bolus of methohexital is due mainly to redistribution to the muscles and body fat, the drug is rapidly eliminated from the body by metabolism and excretion so that dogs recover quickly from even large doses. It is advisable to use sedative premedication to smooth induction and recovery because both periods may otherwise be violent. Doses of 4–6 mg/kg IV in a 1% or 2% solution are suitable for the induction of anaesthesia in dogs premedicated with acepromazine. Further small increments given as required may be used to prolong anaesthesia or anaesthesia may be maintained with an inhalant agent. The method of injection is similar to that of thiopental, although a slightly slower rate of initial injection is less likely to result in apnoea. Overdose produces severe respiratory depression, and even anaesthetic doses produce more respiratory depression than equipotent doses of thiopental. Depression of cardiac output with low anaesthetic doses is also greater than after equipotent doses of thiopental (Clarke & Hall, 1975). Cumulation and, therefore, delayed recovery occurs in doses in excess of 10–12 mg/kg.

Because recovery is so rapid and complete, methohexital has been most useful for outpatient anaesthesia and induction of anaesthesia in brachycephalic dogs, thin dogs, and for caesarian section. In current practice, methohexital has been replaced by propofol which provides a rapid recovery without the excitement that can occur with methohexital.

Pentobarbital

Introduction of pentobarbital into veterinary practice in the early 1930s revolutionized anaesthetic techniques. It is no longer used for anaesthesia in clinical practice but may be used in experimental projects.

The approximate dose rate in healthy unpremedicated dogs is 30 mg/kg and this will be reduced by premedication. About one-half to two-thirds of the calculated probable dose is injected rapidly IV in order to ensure that the dog passes quickly through the excitement phase of induction of anaesthesia. Because the onset of action of pentobarbital is much slower than that of thiopental, the remainder of the dose is administered in increments over 3–5 minutes until the desired effect is reached. Loss of the pedal reflex indicates a sufficient depth of anaesthesia for surgery.

When used to control seizures in a patient with neurological disease, pentobarbital must be given over several minutes in small increments to avoid overdosage, as the dose in these patients may be as low as 4 mg/kg.

Ketamine

The dose of ketamine that produces anaesthesia in dogs produces excessive muscle tone and spontaneous muscle activity and is near to that which causes convulsions. Thus, ketamine cannot be recommended as a sole agent for canine anaesthesia. It can be used in combination with various sedative agents to induce anaesthesia for short-term procedures or for induction followed by maintenance of anaesthesia with an inhalation agent. Unless specifically contraindicated, an anticholinergic can be administered for premedication to reduce salivation induced by ketamine.

A common combination used for induction of anaesthesia is diazepam, 0.25 mg/kg, and ketamine, 5 mg/kg, given IV at the same time (equivalent to combining 5 mg/mL of diazepam and 100 mg/mL of ketamine in the same syringe as a 50:50 mixture and dosing at a rate of 1 mL of the mixture per 10 kg of body weight) (see Table 15.7). Midazolam, 0.25 mg/kg, can be substituted for the diazepam but the degree of sedation induced is not as great. Premedication may also include a sedative, opioid, or any combination of these, such as acepromazine, 0.02–0.05 mg/kg, with butorphanol, 0.3–0.4 mg/kg, IM/SC or acepromazine with hydromorphone, 0.1 mg/kg, IM/SC. In which case, approximately one-half of the calculated volume of ketamine–diazepam mixture is administered rapidly initially and the remainder administered in increments as needed. The onset of action is much slower than thiopental or propofol and the signs of anaesthesia differ. The eyelids may be wide open and a brisk palpebral reflex should be present. If the dog shakes its head, then more ketamine is required. Strong jaw tone and a swallowing reflex are normal and are frequently present for endotracheal intubation.

Injection of ketamine, 10 mg/kg, IV to healthy dogs, with or without diazepam, results in increased HR, MAP, CO, and systemic vascular resistance (Haskins et al., 1985, 1986). These positive haemodynamic effects associated with the use of ketamine are attributed to its sympathomimetic activity involving inhibition of neuronal uptake of catecholamines by sympathetic nerve endings (Tsuneyoshi et al., 2004). It must be remembered that these effects may be altered by the presence of hypovolaemia or myocardial ischaemia.

The cardiovascular effects of combinations of ketamine with an α_2-sedative tend to be dominated by the effects of the sedative. Xylazine and ketamine used to be popular for short-term anaesthesia. Xylazine, 1 mg/kg, and ketamine, 10 mg/kg, with atropine, were administered IV or IM, however, the combination is associated with an undesirable incidence of hypoxaemia, occasional respiratory arrest, tachycardia, hypertension, increased left atrial pressure, decreased myocardial contractility, and a 36% decrease in CO (Kolata & Rawlings, 1982). The drugs should be injected in increments because xylazine and ketamine injected rapidly IV cause abrupt severe hypotension of 30–90 seconds duration.

Different dose rates of medetomidine have been paired with ketamine, 3–5 mg/kg, to induce heavy sedation

or anaesthesia or induction to isoflurane anaesthesia. An experimental investigation found that morphine, 0.2 mg/kg, medetomidine, 0.02 mg/kg (20 μg/kg), and ketamine, 5 mg/kg, mixed in the same syringe and administered IM produced good to excellent short-term sedation and mild to moderate analgesia that was judged to be suitable for minor medical and surgical procedures (Ueyema et al., 2008). Tracheal intubation was possible in only half of the dogs but the dogs were unresponsive to toe or tail clamps from 20 minutes after administration to approximately 50 minutes. Cardiovascular changes measured included high MAP at 10 minutes after drug administration followed by a decrease, sinus bradycardia and a 45% decrease in CO for 60 minutes. Injection of atipamezole, 0.1 mg/kg, IM at 60 minutes resulted in return to sternal recumbency within a few minutes. A higher dose of medetomidine, 1000 μg/m², IM followed 10–15 minutes later by ketamine, 3–4 mg/kg, IV produced anaesthesia for 54 ± 31 minutes (mean ± SD) (Hellebrekers & Sap, 1997; Hellebrekers et al., 1998). Some recoveries from medetomidine–ketamine anaesthesia were associated with restlessness and hyperactivity. Premedication with a lower dose of medetomidine, 0.01 mg/kg (10 μg/kg), IM prior to induction of anaesthesia with ketamine, 4 mg/kg, IV allowed rapid intubation but was accompanied by apnoea in 50% of the dogs (Ko et al., 2001a). Although bradycardia <60 beats/minute was present in most dogs, inclusion of atropine was associated with more and varying types of arrhythmias and, therefore, not recommended.

Dexmedetomidine, 0.003–0.005 mg/kg (3–5 μg/kg), IM/IV with a low to moderate dose of an opioid is a useful premedication for induction of anaesthesia with ketamine–diazepam before inhalation anaesthesia. A higher dose rate of dexmedetomidine, 0.015 mg/kg (15 μg/kg), with ketamine, 3 mg/kg, and either butorphanol, buprenorphine, or hydromorphone, combined in the same syringe and injected IM was evaluated for anaesthesia for castration in 30 dogs (Barletta et al., 2011). The dogs assumed lateral recumbency in 4–6 minutes after administration and tracheal intubation was accomplished in all but one dog. Measurements in the first 15 minutes after drug administration revealed that the dogs were moderately to severely hypoventilating despite RR within an acceptable range and 16/30 dogs were hypoxaemic and required O₂ administration. The time from IM injection to skin incision was 20 minutes. Anaesthesia was sufficient for surgery in most dogs but isoflurane at a low vaporizer setting of 0.5–1% was supplied to eight dogs at some point during surgery.

Tiletamine–zolazepam

Tiletamine is available in a premixed combination with zolazepam, a benzodiazepine, under the trade names of Telazol and Zoletil. The drug preparation consists of 500 mg of lyophilized tiletamine–zolazepam (250 mg of tiletamine and 250 mg of zolazepam) that is reconstituted with sterile water. The doses reported are the sum of tiletamine and zolazepam doses so that 4 mg/kg of Telazol is equivalent to 2 mg/kg of tiletamine and 2 mg/kg of zolazepam. Tiletamine–zolazepam, 4 mg/kg, IM with an anticholinergic provides effective sedation for aggressive or dangerous dogs. Sedation is profound but ranges from the dog being just capable of walking to the dog that is almost unconscious and ready for tracheal intubation. Onset of sedation may be within minutes or up to 10 minutes. The dog should be kept under observation after injection in case immediate care is needed to treat apnoea or to move a dog that has assumed a position causing upper airway obstruction. An alternative technique is to provide premedication with other drugs and to use lower doses of tiletamine–zolazepam IV to achieve tracheal intubation prior to inhalation anaesthesia. Restlessness may be observed during recovery due to slow metabolism of tiletamine and the dog may be calmed by administration of diazepam.

Administration of tiletamine–zolazepam results in a dose-dependent duration of anaesthesia, with 6.6 mg/kg IV resulting in an average of 17.5 minutes to arousal and 62.3 minutes to sternal recumbency (Hellyer et al., 1989). A bolus injection IV results in transient decreased myocardial contractility and hypotension at 1 minute followed by increases in HR, MAP, and CO.

Propofol

Propofol, in a white emulsion of glycerol, soybean oil, and egg lecithin, is commonly used in dogs. The carrier vehicle supports bacterial growth and once a bottle is opened the contents may only be used for a maximum of 6 hours before unused drug is discarded. Strict precautions must be taken to avoid contamination when drawing the drug into a syringe and when using that syringe for top-up dosing during anaesthesia. PropoFlo 28 is a preparation containing benzyl alcohol that extends the shelf life of an opened bottle to 28 days. The dose for induction of anaesthesia in unpremedicated dogs is 6–8 mg/kg IV and premedication with acepromazine or an opioid decreases this to about 4 mg/kg (see Table 15.7). The dose rate of propofol will be further decreased by heavy preanaesthetic sedation and particularly by inclusion of medetomidine or dexmedetomidine. Males may require slightly more drug than females (Watkins et al., 1987). Sufficient propofol must be injected initially to by-pass the early excitatory stages of anaesthesia and that is usually about one-third of the calculated dose with the remainder titrated slowly over 60 seconds until the desired effect is produced. Slow drug administration is advisable for several reasons: there is evidence that the cumulative administered dose is less when the drug is injected slowly; that rapid injection of propofol causes an acute transient decrease in blood pressure; and the incidence of apnoea

is less with slow injection. The time of onset of action of propofol is about 15 seconds after injection. Cyanosis of the tongue, due to respiratory depression and an initial decrease in blood pressure, may be noticed. Tracheal intubation, administration of O_2 and two to three artificial ventilations may be necessary to restore pink mucous membranes. Administration of O_2 by facemask before and during propofol administration (preoxygenation) to prevent cyanosis is advisable, particularly in geriatric and sick dogs. Injection of propofol IV may be painful and dogs may vocalize or pull back on their legs. A clinical impression is that this effect is seen more frequently when the catheter has been in place for several hours. No treatment is necessary when sufficient propofol has been given to induce anaesthesia. When the response is observed at the beginning of injection, options are to flush the catheter, inject lidocaine, 0.5 mg/kg, into the catheter and leave it for 30 seconds before injecting propofol, or to inject the propofol into fast flowing IV fluids to achieve dilution. Muscle relaxation is obvious during the onset of anaesthesia and the eyes begin to roll rostroventrally when jaw relaxation is usually sufficient for endotracheal intubation. Twitching of the muzzle, ears, and legs may be observed in some dogs after administration of propofol and lasts about 10 minutes. The twitches are not associated with an inadequate depth of anaesthesia and no attempt should be made to deepen anaesthesia specifically to treat the twitches as they will disappear in time. It is important to palpate a peripheral pulse during or soon after induction of anaesthesia to assess both pressure and rhythm of the pulse. Occasionally, abnormal cardiac rhythms developing within a minute of propofol administration are life threatening. Propofol can be used for induction of anaesthesia followed by maintenance with an inhalation agent or used for total intravenous anaesthesia (see later).

The major advantage to use of propofol over thiopental or ketamine is that elimination is more rapid and recovery is quick (Quandt et al., 1998). Changes in cardiovascular parameters are minimal when propofol is administered to healthy dogs in appropriate dose and speed of injection. It must be remembered that senior and geriatric dogs have a decreased requirement for propofol for induction of anaesthesia, are more prone to apnoea, and recover more slowly than young healthy dogs (Reid & Nolan, 1996). Hypovolaemia also decreases the requirement for propofol and failure to decrease the dose of propofol in these patients will result in a serious immediate decrease in MAP (Ilkiw et al., 1992).

Propofol does not provide analgesia and so premedication with sedatives and opioids is recommended practice. The agents used for premedication will modify the propofol dose requirement (see Table 15.7), the blood pressure, and the duration of recovery from anaesthesia. Systolic blood pressure will be decreased by premedication with acepromazine since acepromazine itself decreases systemic vascular resistance (Smith et al., 1993). The α_2-sedatives dose-dependently markedly decrease the dose rate of propofol, cause bradycardia and sustain blood pressure. Medetomidine, 0.02–0.04 mg/kg (20–40 μg/kg), decreases the induction dose of propofol to 2–4 mg/kg (Vanio, 1991; Hall et al., 1997; Hellebrekers et al., 1998). Romifidine premedication dose-dependently decreased the propofol dose to 1.8–2.5 mg/kg (England et al., 1996).

Propofol may be a good choice for induction of anaesthesia in dogs with seizures, meningitis, brain tumours, or spinal cord disease as it decreases intracranial pressure.

A probable link has been established between the use of propofol and isolated spontaneous cases of pancreatitis in people after anaesthesia (Crawford et al., 2009). The cause has not been confirmed because of the infrequent occurrence and variety of concurrent medications and illnesses. An association between hypertriglyceridaemia and naturally occurring pancreatitis exists in dogs, although it is not known if the hypertriglyceridaemia is a cause of the pancreatitis or an incidental finding (Xenoulis & Steiner, 2010). There are no reports at this time incriminating propofol in the development of postoperative pancreatitis in dogs but it is conceivable that administration of a high dose of propofol might contribute to conditions resulting in pancreatitis in a dog already at risk. Some clinicians avoid the use of propofol in dogs with pancreatitis as a precautionary measure.

There have been verbal reports of individual dogs developing allergic reactions following administration of propofol. It is currently unknown whether dogs with allergies are at increased risk from propofol administration. There are isolated reports of hypersensitivity reactions to propofol in humans that include generalized erythema, urticaria, pruritus, bronchospasm, hypoxaemia, and hypotension (Belsõ et al., 2011; Berasategui, 2011; Murphy et al., 2011a). These reactions have been attributed to propofol itself, but may be responses to the metabisulfite, egg or soybean phosphatides, or egg lecithin content in the propofol formulation (Berasategui, 2011). The package information in some countries lists a history of allergy to egg and soy as a contraindication to the administration of propofol. Currently expressed opinions are that there is no contraindication to use of propofol in egg-allergic or soy-allergic human patients without a history of anaphylaxis (Dewachter et al., 2011; Murphy et al., 2011a). A patient that develops an allergic reaction to propofol may also be allergic to other anaesthetic agents.

Propofol–thiopental

An increase in postsurgical infections has been reported in human and veterinary patients associated with the use of propofol (Heldmann et al., 1999). Combining 1% propofol and 2.5% thiopental at a ratio of 1 : 1 for induction of anaesthesia (mean 2.7 mg/kg propofol and 6.8 mg/kg in unpremedicated dogs) achieved a higher MAP than during propofol alone and a similar recovery (Ko et al.,

1999). This mixture of propofol and thiopental does not support organism growth and maintains bactericidal properties similar to those of thiopental alone (Crowther et al., 1996; Joubert et al., 2005). Mixtures of propofol and thiopental at a ratio less than 1 : 1 do not maintain bactericidal properties.

Propofol–ketamine ('ketofol')

The addition of ketamine to propofol, 'ketofol', has been proposed as a means to add some cardiovascular stimulation and analgesia to propofol anaesthesia. A comparison of induction of anaesthesia with propofol, 4 mg/kg, or with propofol, 2 mg/kg, and ketamine, 2 mg/kg, in dogs premedicated with acepromazine, 0.05 mg/kg, and meperidine (pethidine), 3 mg/kg, and subsequently maintained with halothane and N_2O revealed no significant differences between the two protocols (Lerche et al., 2000). Apnoea after induction was more common in dogs receiving both propofol and ketamine, heart rates were higher, but systolic blood pressures were not different.

Fospropofol

Fospropofol is a phosphate pro-drug for propofol that is converted to propofol within a few minutes after IV injection. Consequently, induction and recovery are slower than from propofol. Fospropofol is being investigated for possible uses.

Etomidate

Etomidate is a clear solution that is water soluble at an acid pH and lipid soluble at physiological pH. Return to consciousness from etomidate is due to redistribution of the drug from brain to tissue. Etomidate is rapidly transformed and results in little hangover or cumulative effect. It is hydrolysed by hepatic enzymes and the clearance rate is five times that of thiopental with a recovery time that is similar to propofol. Etomidate is used only as a single anaesthetizing injection prior to maintenance of anaesthesia with an inhalant agent because a higher dose of the agent causes adrenal suppression. The major advantage to use of etomidate is that it causes no cardiovascular depression and that makes it a good induction drug for dogs with severe cardiac disease, circulatory depression, or old age. Etomidate also decreases intracranial pressure.

Administration of etomidate is similar to that of thiopental. Onset of action is approximately 15 seconds, therefore, up to half of the estimated anaesthetizing dose is injected fairly quickly (5–10 seconds) and the remainder is titrated in increments injected in 10-second intervals. Overdose is obviously undesirable but administration of etomidate too slowly may result in difficulty achieving adequate depth of anaesthesia for tracheal intubation. Premedication with at least an opioid is essential and injection of diazepam or similar agent before etomidate results in a smooth induction of anaesthesia. Etomidate is

437

available in a preparation that contains propylene glycol and, although no evidence of haemolysis has been noted when using these recommended dose rates, some clinicians prefer to inject etomidate into a continuous flow of crystalloid fluid to achieve dilution of the drug. Etomidate is similar to propofol in that in a few dogs twitching of the ears, eyebrows, muzzle, or legs may be observed after induction of anaesthesia. No treatment is necessary as the muscle contractions will abate after about 10 minutes. Also similar to propofol, some dogs may exhibit signs of pain on injection of etomidate.

The dose rates required for etomidate vary according to the size of the dog, with higher doses, 1.5 mg/kg, needed for small dogs and smaller doses, 0.5–1.0 mg/kg, for large dogs. Premedication IM may be with any opioid, for example, butorphanol, buprenorphine, hydromorphone, or oxymorphone, with or without midazolam. Similarly IV premedication with an opioid can be followed by injection of diazepam or midazolam, 0.2 mg/kg, and etomidate. This author has the clinical impression that dogs with patent ductus arteriosus or portosystemic shunts that characteristically have low blood pressure during isoflurane or sevoflurane anaesthesia have better pressure and circulatory characteristics when anaesthesia has been induced with etomidate compared with the other injectable anaesthetic agents. Etomidate is the induction drug of choice for dogs requiring anaesthesia for pacemaker implantation.

The significance of adrenal suppression caused by a single induction dose of etomidate in patients with sepsis is in dispute. A retrospective study of human patients in severe sepsis and septic shock found that use of etomidate did not contribute to mortality and supported the safety of use of etomidate in these patients (Ehrman et al., 2011). Another search of literature bases identified seven studies that evaluated clinical endpoints in septic adult humans receiving etomidate for induction of anaesthesia, discovered that the conclusions were conflicting and thus no firm consensus could be made (Edwin & Walker, 2010). However, a meta-analysis published in 2011 concluded that there is an increased mortality in critically ill patients who receive etomidate (Albert et al., 2011). It has been reported that a single bolus of etomidate in humans induces adrenal inhibition for 48 hours, thus empirical use of steroid supplementation has been recommended (Vinclair et al., 2008). Relative adrenal insufficiency has been identified in some septic dogs and may be associated with hypotension (Burkitt et al., 2007). The concern is that use of etomidate in an anaesthetic protocol for a septic dog will exacerbate the deficiency and adversely impact mortality rate and, therefore, should not be used in these patients. New etomidate products, such as methoxycarbonyl–etomidate (MOC–etomidate) and carboetomidate, cause significantly less adrenocortical depression and are currently being investigated (Sneyd & Rigby-Jones, 2010).

Alfaxalone

The original formulation of alphaxalone and alphadolone in Cremophor EL caused massive histamine release in dogs. Alphaxalone (alfaxalone) has now been reformulated as a clear 1% (w/v) solution in 2-hydroxypropyl-β-cyclodextrin (HPCD). The HPCD increases the solubility of alfaxalone and the formulation no longer causes histamine release. The solution is not irritating to tissues in event of accidental perivascular injection. The recommended dose rate for use with minimal sedation is 2–3 mg/kg, although less will be required to induce anaesthesia in dogs with moderate to heavy sedation (see Table 15.7). Alfaxalone is injected in increments over 60 seconds and dilution of the drug allows more precise titration and less total drug administered (Maddern et al., 2010; Psatha et al., 2011). Induction of anaesthesia is generally good to excellent. Apnoea will occur occasionally after injection of alfaxalone and twitching may be observed. An investigation of alfaxalone administered alone to experimental dogs as a bolus injection, 2 mg/kg, produced no change in CO or systemic vascular resistance (Muir et al., 2008). The duration of anaesthesia was 10 minutes and the dogs assumed sternal position on average 20 minutes after injection. Cardiovascular status was also well maintained at purposefully higher dose of 6 mg/kg in these healthy dogs. Other studies investigating induction of anaesthesia with alfaxalone in dogs without premedication reported either a similar dose, mean 2.6 mg/kg (Maney et al., 2013), or larger, mean 4.2 mg/kg, (Rodríguez et al., 2012). Time to extubation was a mean of 11 minutes with the lower dose and 25 minutes with the higher dose. Alfaxalone administration increased HR and CO with no change in MAP, and some dogs developed hypoxaemia (Rodríguez et al., 2012). Premedication will alter the cardiovascular response to alfaxalone, for example, in experimental dogs given acepromazine, 0.02 mg/kg, and hydromorphone, 0.05 mg/kg, IV before alfaxalone, 2 mg/kg, the average MAP was acceptable but too low in some individuals (Ambros et al., 2008). Hypoventilation may occur depending on the combination of drugs used.

Sedative–opioid combinations

Some combinations are sufficiently potent to induce anaesthesia that is adequate for endotracheal intubation. Combinations of medetomidine or dexmedetomidine with an opioid, with or without a benzodiazepine, will immobilize a healthy dog and a combination of a μ opioid with a benzodiazepine may be sufficient in an old or sick dog. The dogs may initially be responsive to noise and sudden movements, and endotracheal intubation should be performed quietly and gently followed by administration of sufficient inhalation agent to deepen anaesthesia.

(Dex)medetomidine and an opioid

Administration of high doses of medetomidine or dexmedetomidine IM with an opioid, such as butorphanol, 0.1–0.2 mg/kg, or morphine, 0.2–0.5 mg/kg, or hydromorphone, 0.05 mg/kg, or methadone, 0.3 mg/kg, to healthy dogs may induce heavy sedation or even unresponsiveness that allows endotracheal intubation. When followed by administration of an inhalation anaesthetic agent, the vaporizer setting is very low initially, for example 0.5% isoflurane. MAP is usually normal to high and associated with bradycardia. Monitoring with an ECG is advisable as advanced AV heart block can develop, albeit a rare occurrence. SpO_2 should be monitored in recovery after disconnection from the anaesthesia machine as this combination with an inhalation agent can cause significant hypoventilation, resulting in hypoxia when breathing room air.

Fentanyl and diazepam or midazolam

This combination is used for sick dogs where the anaesthetic requirement is likely decreased and where there is a high risk for cardiovascular depression during anaesthesia. The dose rates are fentanyl, 5–10 µg/kg, and diazepam or midazolam, 0.25 mg/kg, and the drugs are drawn into separate syringes. The environment should be quiet and all movements slow. Benzodiazepines may induce CNS stimulation if given alone, consequently, the first drug to be administered is fentanyl, 2 µg/kg, followed soon after by diazepam, 0.1 mg/kg. After about 20 seconds, fentanyl 2 µg/kg and diazepam, 0.1 mg/kg, are injected, and after 20–30 seconds the depth of sedation is assessed by gently attempting to open the jaws. Additional fentanyl, 1–2 µg/kg, up to 10 µg/kg is injected as needed (total fentanyl dose of 6 µg/kg is often sufficient). Some dogs can be intubated while others will require a very small dose of injectable anaesthetic agent or inhalation agent administered through a mask before endotracheal intubation. The dog should not be disturbed until anaesthesia is deepened because it will be easily aroused. The duration of fentanyl is short, about 20 minutes, and therefore either more fentanyl must be administered or a different µ opioid with a longer duration of action administered IM or IV. Fentanyl may be supplemented by bolus injections of fentanyl, 2 µg/kg, at 20-minute intervals or by using a continuous infusion of 6 µg/kg/h.

Fentanyl, 4 µg/kg, and midazolam, 0.2 mg/kg, can be administered IM for premedication to induce light sedation. Induction of anaesthesia can be as just described or with an injectable anaesthetic agent.

Oxymorphone and diazepam or midazolam

Oxymorphone with a benzodiazepine can induce heavy sedation in an old dog or one with a reduced requirement for anaesthetic agents. Oxymorphone, 0.1–0.2 mg/kg, and diazepam, 0.2 mg/kg, are drawn into separate syringes. Through a preplaced IV catheter, oxymorphone

0.05 mg/kg, and diazepam 0.1 mg/kg are injected in sequence, flushing between drugs. These dose rates are repeated after 30 seconds. Further administration of oxymorphone will depend on the patient's response. As described in the previous section, dogs under sedative–opioid sedation are sensitive to noise or handling. After tracheal intubation, the dog must be allowed to breathe inhalant for several minutes before being disturbed and moved into a different position.

Induction of anaesthesia

The aims for induction are for the patient to lose consciousness with minimal stress, to acquire sufficient jaw relaxation for endotracheal intubation (if planned), and to avoid an excessive depth of anaesthesia or cardiovascular depression. Avoidance of complications is key and some recommendations are given in Box 15.4. Each agent has its own characteristics and the previous sections are intended to provide suggestions to obtain the best induction of anaesthesia. Relative anaesthetic overdose, that is, excessive anaesthetic response to average dose rates, may occur in some patients:

1. Failure to adjust and decrease dose rate of anaesthetic induction agents in patients with heavy preanaesthetic sedation, especially those that have received medetomidine, dexmedetomidine, or tiletamine–zolazepam
2. Patients with underlying disease that decreases the requirement for anaesthetic agents, or decreases the

---

Box 15.4 Tips for a safe induction of anaesthesia

- Dehydrated patients should first receive IV fluids to restore blood volume
- Check membranes for hypoxaemia or with a pulse oximeter before induction, especially brachycephalic, old, obese, traumatized, respiratory disease
- Administer O_2 for 2–3 minutes before and during induction to patients at risk for hypoxaemia or hypotension
- Calculate IV anaesthetic agent doses based on ideal weight if overweight, not actual weight
- Assess degree of preanaesthetic sedation, mild, moderate, severe, and adjust anticipated induction dose
- Titrate anaesthetic agents to individual requirement
- Palpate femoral pulse during or immediately after injecting anaesthetic agent
- Hold dogs at risk for regurgitation sternal or upright on hind limbs until trachea is intubated and cuff inflated

ability of the cardiovascular system to compensate for anaesthetic-induced depression. Injection of the 'usual' dose into patients with hypovolaemia results in high blood concentration of anaesthetic. Hypovolemia must be suspected in patients that have had no access to water for several hours, or are likely to be dehydrated (e.g. gastric dilation–volvulus (GDV), intestinal foreign body with vomiting or decreased water intake), or have suffered blood loss (e.g. gastric ulcer, ruptured spleen, fractured humerus, pelvis, or femur). Senior patients have decreased circulating blood volumes compared with young adults, and decreased baroreceptor responsiveness

3. Healthy dogs with an intrinsic predisposition for a low requirement for anaesthetic agents.

Hypoventilation before induction of anaesthesia may result from heavy premedication, also from premedication in English Bulldogs and obese patients, in dogs with spinal cord trauma especially with 'big dog-little dog' syndrome, in dogs with thoracic pathology such as pneumonia, pneumothorax, fractured ribs, or diaphragmatic rupture, and in dogs with abdominal distension particularly GDV, pregnancy, and ascites. These patients should be monitored with a pulse oximeter and be supplied with oxygen during induction of anaesthesia.

Airway obstruction is likely to occur at this time in brachycephalic breeds, and dogs with laryngeal paralysis, oral/nasal tumours, or retro-orbital or pharyngeal abscess. Heavy sedation from premedication should be avoided. Retropharyngeal abscesses can make intubation extremely difficult and anaesthesia should not be started without adequate personnel available to assist if needed. Endotracheal intubation proceeds smoothly for most dogs. Difficulties sometimes occur and their recognition and management are described in the section on endotracheal intubation (see Table 15.6). Apnoea and cyanosis are common features of some anaesthetic agents at the time of first administration, particularly propofol, and the incidence may be decreased by slower administration of the agent during induction. Preoxygenation should prevent haemoglobin desaturation during induction and intubation, and is especially advisable for brachycephalic, old, and sick dogs. Two points to remember are: (1) the tongue and mucous membranes may remain pink in the first few minutes after cardiac arrest; and (2) colour of mucous membranes in hypoxaemic dogs may not be blue but could be dull reddish to pinkish-bluish colour.

Dogs at risk for regurgitation during induction of anaesthesia include animals that have not had food withheld before anaesthesia, emergency anaesthesias, pregnant animals, nervous animals with gastrointestinal stasis, old animals, patients with megaoesophagus, gastrointestinal foreign bodies, or diaphragmatic hernia. These dogs should be held sternal or upright standing on their hind legs during administration of anaesthetic agents and until the endotracheal tube has been inserted, tied in and the cuff inflated. If fluid has been seen in a radiograph of a dog with megaoesophagus, consideration should be given to careful passage of a tube to remove the fluid once the dog has been connected to the anaesthesia machine and a first set of monitored parameters recorded.

Total intravenous anaesthesia (TIVA)

Anaesthesia may be maintained by intermittent or continuous infusion of an injectable anaesthetic agent. Decision of which agent to use is largely determined by the cumulative properties of the agent in that slow elimination will result in a prolonged recovery. Consequently, propofol is the injectable agent most commonly used for TIVA. The dog should be premedicated with agents appropriate to its condition and anaesthesia induced in the normal way with propofol. Propofol is administered continuously thereafter at 12–18 mg/kg/h (0.2–0.3 mg/kg/min). The simplest method is to use a syringe pump with a syringe containing propofol sufficient for the estimated duration of anaesthesia. For short duration anaesthesia, small boluses of propofol can be injected by hand into the IV catheter. Dilution of propofol in a 250 mL or 500 mL bag of lactated Ringer's solution (LRS) can and has been done but tends to be a more expensive method and control of administration is not precise unless the administration set is run through an infusion pump. Propofol without preservative is preferred for TIVA. Intubation of the trachea and administration of oxygen is advisable as some individuals will develop hypoxaemia when breathing air. Controlled ventilation will likely be necessary for prolonged infusions. Joubert (2009), in a detailed review of published investigations of propofol continuous infusions, concluded that most changes in anaesthetic depth were likely to occur in the first hour of administration. Analgesia must be supplied.

An experimental investigation has characterized alfaxalone TIVA. The dogs were premedicated with acepromazine, 0.02 mg/kg, and hydromorphone, 0.05 mg/kg, IV and more than 30 minutes later, anaesthesia was induced with alfaxalone, 2 mg/kg, or propofol, 4 mg/kg, and maintained with alfaxalone, 4.2 mg/kg/h (0.07 mg/kg/min), or propofol, 15 mg/kg/h (0.25 mg/kg/min), respectively, for 2 hours (Ambros et al., 2008). The dogs were intubated and received O_2 via a circle circuit. Induction was judged as smooth in all dogs. RR varied around 6–8 breaths/min but significant hypoventilation was recorded in both groups of dogs. Cardiac output was adequately maintained and, although average MAP stayed above 60 mmHg, some dogs were hypotensive. HR decreased with time with propofol but was better maintained with alfaxalone. The quality of recovery was similar between alfaxalone and propofol and, although not statistically significant, recovery to sternal position was a little earlier after alfaxalone, mean 43 (33–56) minutes compared with propofol, mean 52 (29–84) minutes.

Propofol–fentanyl

For some patients, such as those requiring cranial decompression for cerebral swelling or intracranial haemorrhage after head trauma or for craniotomy for tumour excision, the additional increase in intracranial pressure (ICP) produced by inhalation agents may adversely affect the success of the procedure. TIVA can be employed in conjunction with controlled ventilation to maintain normocarbia in an attempt to avoid an increase in ICP. Maintenance of anaesthesia with continuous infusions of fentanyl and propofol delivered by separate syringe drivers can be used in these patients. Glycopyrrolate for premedication is optional but preferred by this author. HR may slow several hours into the procedure. Repeat dosing of an anticholinergic drug should be avoided if at all possible during craniotomy because the increase in HR and MAP usually causes unwanted bleeding at the operative site. The dog should be premedicated with a μ opioid, such as oxymorphone or hydromorphone, anaesthesia induced with diazepam and propofol, and the trachea intubated and connected to an anaesthesia machine delivering oxygen. Controlled ventilation is instituted at the beginning of anaesthesia to counter respiratory depression induced by propofol and the high dose of fentanyl. Propofol should be infused at 12–18 mg/kg/h (0.2–0.3 mg/kg/min), initially at the higher dose and this can be reduced after 1–2 hours in step-wise fashion. Fentanyl is infused at 24–48 μg/kg/h, starting with the lowest dose and increased if judged necessary. Intensive monitoring using electronic equipment is recommended as warranted by the seriousness of the procedure and relative lack of access of the anaesthetist to the patient. Local anaesthetic solution can be infiltrated at the proposed incision site. Neuromuscular blockade is an option but not necessary for most surgeries. At the end of the procedure, propofol is discontinued but fentanyl is continued at a low dose, 3 μg/kg/h, into recovery or another μ opioid administered as needed. Both propofol and fentanyl are rapidly eliminated when used for short-term procedures, however, half-lives are increased when anaesthesia duration is 4 hours or more and a longer recovery must be expected. Adequacy of ventilation and oxygenation must be monitored during recovery.

Concurrent infusions of propofol and fentanyl can be used for other medical or surgical procedures. A clinical report described a similar protocol for dogs scheduled for a variety of procedures from ovariohysterectomy to cranial cruciate repair (Andreoni & Hughes, 2009). The dogs were premedicated with acepromazine, 0.05 mg/kg, and anaesthesia induced with propofol and maintained with propofol, 12–24 mg/kg/h (0.2–0.4 mg/kg/min), and fentanyl, 30 μg/kg/h. Ventilation was controlled. Time from

discontinuation of anaesthesia to extubation was an average of 33 (range 18–80) minutes.

INHALATION ANAESTHESIA

Many inhalation agents have been used for canine anaesthesia and currently isoflurane and sevoflurane are most commonly used. Nitrous oxide is used selectively in those hospitals that have the equipment for its administration. Desflurane offers the fastest induction and recovery times but is not widely used due to the high cost of the desflurane-specific vaporizer. Halothane is no longer available in some countries.

Inhalation agents are the most commonly used anaesthetic agents to maintain general anaesthesia in dogs, particularly for anaesthesia lasting longer than 20–30 minutes. Anaesthesia with inhalation agents in clinical patients is almost always preceded by administration of injectable agents to induce heavy sedation or general anaesthesia. Inhalation agents are subsequently administered through an endotracheal tube to protect the patient against aspiration of gastric or other fluids, prevent room pollution with anaesthetic gases, and to facilitate use of low O_2 flow thus saving money. Induction of anaesthesia with an inhalant via a mask has potential complications, as described later. The anaesthesia machine must be checked before use as described in Chapter 10.

Inhalation agents

The average concentration of an inhalation agent required for anaesthesia to prevent purposeful movement in response to a noxious stimulus is expressed as the minimum alveolar concentration (MAC), and for details of MAC and inhalant properties see Chapter 7. The published MAC values for inhalation agents in a given species vary due to differences in the experimental design that include the method of determination and variations in animal populations. Published MAC values for isoflurane in dogs range from 1.19% (Credie et al., 2010) to 1.7% (Kulka et al., 2012) and for sevoflurane from 1.75% (Seddighi et al., 2012) to 2.39% (Yamashita et al., 2008). These measurements indicate that sevoflurane is less potent than isoflurane and a higher concentration is needed to maintain anaesthesia. MAC values reported for desflurane were 7.6 % (range 6.9–9.0%) (Pypendop & Ilkiw, 2006) and 10.3% (range 9.8–10.6%) (Hammond et al., 1994). Unfortunately, the wide ranges in values diminish the effectiveness of this measurement for monitoring purposes in clinical patients. Furthermore, the anaesthetic requirement of individual dogs may vary ± 20% from the average MAC. Thus it is not surprising that for the same anaesthetic protocol one dog may require a higher concentration of inhalant than another. In humans, a linear decrease in MAC has been documented from <1 to 82 years of age (Eger, 2001). All the inhalation agents have a common slope and a number of nomograms have been published to aid the anaesthetist in identifying the appropriate MAC (anaesthetic concentration) for a patient of a given age (Nickalls & Mapleson, 2003). These nomograms also provide a calculation for the reduction in MAC provided by inclusion of 50% or 66% N_2O. This information cannot be extrapolated for use in dogs because MAC values are different in the two species. Most MAC studies in dogs are performed in young adults, however, clinical experience supports a decrease in anaesthetic requirement in old dogs. One study measuring MAC during isoflurane anaesthesia in 2–3-year-old and 11-year-old Beagles identified a 20% reduction in MAC in the older dogs, from 1.5% to 1.2% (Magnusson et al., 2000). There is greater variation in human infants <1 year but the general pattern is MAC starting low at birth and increasing to a peak at 3–6 months before progressively decreasing (Mapleson, 1996). One study in 1-month-old Beagles determined a mean MAC for sevoflurane as 2.1 ± 0.2%, a value that is in the middle of the range reported for adult dogs (Morgaz et al., 2009). MAC determinations are done during administration of the inhalation agent only and in clinical practice it is a rare situation in which only one anaesthetic agent is administered. Administration of sedative, analgesic, or anaesthetic drugs before or during anaesthesia decreases the amount of inhalant agent needed for anaesthesia (Yamashita et al., 2008; Ko & Weil. 2009; Credie et al., 2010).

Monitoring anaesthetic administration is part of safe practice. It should be remembered that MAC values are measurements of end-tidal (alveolar) concentrations and that the inspired concentrations will be higher. The vaporizer setting is the same as the inspired concentration for a dog connected to a non-rebreathing circuit, whereas an anaesthetic gas analyser is needed to measure inspired and expired anaesthetic concentrations in a rebreathing circuit. Comparison of these measurements with the MAC value can be an aid to assessing depth of anaesthesia. Although the information may not be a reliable guide to how low the vaporizer can be decreased and still maintain anaesthesia, it may prevent an absolute overdosage since it has been documented that 1.7×MAC is associated with excessive cardiovascular depression (Galloway et al., 2004; Pypendop & Ilkiw, 2006).

Isoflurane, sevoflurane, desflurane, halothane

Increasing concentrations of isoflurane, sevoflurane, desflurane, and halothane cause significant decreases in cardiac index, MAP, and mean pulmonary arterial pressure, a significant increase in CVP, and a decrease or increase in HR (Hoffman et al., 1991; Hysing et al., 1992; Picker et al., 2001). Changes in cardiovascular parameters are similar with isoflurane and sevoflurane (Mutoh et al.,

1997). Heart rates increased during anaesthesia and with increasing depth of anaesthesia when compared with rates when the dogs were conscious (Picker et al., 2001). The greatest increase in HR occurred during desflurane anaesthesia and the least during halothane. The differences between the anaesthetic agents were determined to be due to differences in vagolytic action. Respiratory depression occurs with increasing concentrations of inhalation agents. Although respiratory arrest may occur before cardiac arrest, life-threatening hypotension may develop before a clinically significant decrease in respiratory rate is observed (Galloway et al., 2004; Pypendop & Ilkiw, 2006). Concurrent administration of a μ agonist opioid potentiates respiratory depression with inhalation agents.

Sevoflurane and CO_2 absorbent

Sevoflurane reacts with some CO_2 absorbents (see Chapter 10) and generates several degradation products, of which Compound A is reported to be nephrotoxic. There has been concern that the concentration of Compound A may increase in circle circuits using low O_2 flows. In a clinical trial of sevoflurane in dogs, no evidence of impaired renal function was detected when the O_2 inflow was maintained at 500 mL/min (Branson et al., 2001). Concentrations of Compound A measured in circle circuits administering low-flow (<15 mL/kg/min) O_2 and sevoflurane to dogs were substantially lower than concentrations reported to cause renal toxicity in rats (Muir & Gadawski, 1998).

In rare situations, use of sevoflurane with dry CO_2 absorbent has resulted in spontaneous combustion and fire in the anaesthetic circuit. This might occur during use of absorbent that has been in the circuit canister and unused for a while.

Nitrous oxide (N_2O)

Dogs cannot be anaesthetized with N_2O and O_2 alone. Nitrous oxide is used to provide analgesia either (1) as a supplement to another inhalation agent or (2) as a supplement to injectable agents. A valuable use of N_2O is to speed induction of anaesthesia with halothane by mask utilizing the 'second gas effect'. Isoflurane and sevoflurane induce anaesthesia faster than with halothane such that the inclusion of N_2O may not provide significant benefit to speed of induction (Mutoh et al., 2001). During maintenance of anaesthesia, the addition of N_2O may provide sufficient analgesia to block patient response to intermittent intense surgical stimulation such as traction on ovaries, clamping of the spermatic cord, or the manipulation of a long bone fracture. Several experimental studies have documented a decrease in halothane MAC by inclusion of N_2O. More recently, measurements in dogs anaesthetized for ovariohysterectomy with halothane, isoflurane or sevoflurane revealed that adding 65% N_2O decreased the concentration of all the anaesthetic agents required for surgical anaesthesia; the halothane concentration by 12.4%, isoflurane by 37.1%, and sevoflurane by 21.4% (Duke et al., 2006). In an experimental study in which dogs received only sevoflurane, the addition of 70% N_2O decreased the sevoflurane concentration required to prevent movement by 25% and the concentration to prevent autonomic response to an electrical stimulus by 35%, but with a large variability in % reduction in individual dogs (Seddighi et al., 2012). In another study, the addition of 50% N_2O to desflurane decreased the requirement for desflurane by 23% (Hammond et al., 1994). The intent behind the inclusion of N_2O is that either analgesia is improved without increasing inhalant administration or that inhalant administration can be decreased while providing the same depth of anaesthesia. An increase in MAP may be observed in the latter case (Seddighi et al., 2012).

The percentage of N_2O in the inspired gases should be 50–70% in order to provide the most analgesia. When the O_2 and N_2O flowmeters are set at flow ratios of 1:1 or 1:2, a non-rebreathing system will deliver the desired gas mixture. In contrast, use of a low fresh gas flow into a rebreathing system causes the concentration of N_2O within the circuit to increase and the concentration of O_2 to decrease. To ensure that the percent ratios of O_2 and N_2O remain the same as the flowmeter settings, the O_2 inflow should be set at ≥ 30 mL/kg/min and an equal flow of N_2O added. Flows can be reduced if the inspired O_2 percent is monitored. The increased fresh gas flow into a rebreathing system increases wastage of inhalant agent and, therefore, increases the cost of anaesthesia.

Essential facts to remember about use of N_2O are:

- N_2O will enter any air pocket in the dog and expand its size, thus use of N_2O is contraindicated in animals with pneumothorax, pulmonary blebs or bullae, pneumoperitoneum, or intestinal obstruction with air distension. Movement of N_2O into the air pocket is rapid and elimination is slow
- A condition known as 'diffusion hypoxia' will develop during recovery from anaesthesia when N_2O administration is discontinued and the dog is simultaneously disconnected from the anaesthesia machine. N_2O is poorly soluble in blood and rapidly exits into alveoli in large volumes when administration is discontinued. Room air has 21% O_2 and this becomes diluted by N_2O to a level that cannot sustain arterial oxygenation. To avoid hypoxia, the dog should be given 100% O_2 for at least 5 minutes after N_2O is stopped (remain connected to the anaesthesia machine).

Systems of administration

Factors to take into consideration when choosing a system and a circuit are: (1) avoid increased resistance to breathing imposed by the circuit, for example, the usual sized

CO_2 absorbent canisters impose resistance on small dogs and small diameter hoses do the same for large dogs; (2) systems requiring high O_2 flows are wasteful of inhalation agent and potentially increase pollution; and (3) a circuit with a large apparatus dead space causes significant rebreathing of CO_2 in small dogs. The different types of breathing systems are described in Chapter 10 and a wide variety of circuits with different sizes of hoses are available. As previously stated, the resistance to breathing offered by the CO_2 absorbent and turbulence in large diameter hoses may contribute to hypoventilation in small dogs. The smallest size of animal that should be connected to a circle circuit with large hoses (internal diameter 22 mm) is controversial. Paediatric hoses (internal diameter 15 mm) may be substituted for dogs between 3 and 8 kg bodyweight. An O_2 flow of 1 L/min will facilitate flow of gases around the circle. A much smaller circle is available for dogs, cats, rabbits, birds, that weigh <2 kg (see Fig. 10.19 Hallowell workstation). Scavenging of waste anaesthetic gases is essential. All equipment must undergo a safety check before use.

An important difference between non-rebreathing circuits, such as the T-piece, and rebreathing circuits, such as the circle, is that the inspired concentration of anaesthetic agent can be very different between the systems. The inspired concentration delivered by a non-rebreathing circuit is the same as the vaporizer % and will change within seconds of a change in vaporizer setting. In contrast, the inspired concentration may be the same or substantially lower than the vaporizer setting in a rebreathing circuit with the vaporizer outside the circle. The larger the dog attached to the circle circuit and the lower the fresh gas flow, the greater the impact of exhaled gases on the concentration of anaesthetic in the rebreathing bag. Consider a 30 kg dog connected to a circle circuit with an O_2 inflow of 1 L/min. For every breath that the dog takes, some anaesthetic agent is retained and the exhaled gas has a lower concentration than inspired gas. A dog of this size will exhale approximately 5.4 L/min of gas, a volume that will dilute the concentration entering from the vaporizer. With low-flow anaesthesia, the vaporizer will have to be considerably higher than the desired inspired % in order to maintain anaesthesia. Frequently, high O_2 flow (1–2 L/min) is supplied in the first 15 minutes to deliver sufficient inhalant to effect a smooth transition from injectable to inhalant anaesthesia and to eliminate nitrogen from the circuit, then the flow is decreased to the preferred low O_2 flow.

The minimum O_2 flow into a circle circuit that is safe for the dog is a flow equal to the dog's metabolic O_2 requirement (approximately ≤ 6 mL/kg/min). When this flow rate is used there is no excess O_2 to be discharged through the pressure relief valve, hence the technique is called a closed system of administration. A closed system does not require that the pressure relief valve be closed because the valve is designed to remain closed until the

443

pressure in the circle builds to 2 cmH$_2$O. During low-flow administration, generally considered to be ≤15 mL/kg/min, the O$_2$ inflow exceeds metabolic needs and a small amount of waste gas will enter the scavenging system after each exhalation. Circle circuits that incorporate the vaporizer within the circle are designed for the low-flow system of administration. The dog's breathing draws O$_2$ through the vaporizer and the lower the O$_2$ rate the more quickly the anaesthetic concentration increases. Rebreathing systems that include CO$_2$ absorption are economical because low O$_2$ flows are used and less anaesthetic agent is vaporized. Heat generated by the action of exhaled CO$_2$ on the absorbent and exhaled water vapour are responsible for the dog breathing warm, moist gases that help to maintain body heat and prevent drying damage to the respiratory tract mucosa. Fresh gas inflows for other types of circuits are given in Chapter 10. The vaporizer setting must be adjusted to deliver the estimated anaesthetic requirement and is based on the potency of the inhalation agent, the type of delivery circuit, the physical status of the patient, the characteristics and dose rates of concurrently administered anaesthetic agents, and the nature of the procedure.

Induction using a facemask

Induction of anaesthesia with an inhalation agent via a facemask may be employed in a variety of situations but is also contraindicated in some situations (Table 15.8). Induction and maintenance using an inhalation agent as the sole agent is not advisable. Higher concentrations of inhalant must be used, compared with a balanced anaesthesia, decreasing the safety margin. Sole agent use (induction and maintenance with an inhalation anaesthetic) has been associated with a 5.9-fold increase in the odds of anaesthetic-related death compared with induction of anaesthesia with injectable agents and maintenance with isoflurane (Brodbelt et al., 2008). Endotracheal intubation requires a higher concentration of inhalation agent than is needed for maintenance of anaesthesia. Less cardiovascular depression may be achieved by prior administration of a sedative, opioid, or injectable anaesthetic

and speed of induction is faster. For example, in an experimental study of mask induction in Beagles, with an O$_2$ flow rate 4 L/min and the sevoflurane vaporizer increased by 0.8% increments/15 seconds up to a maximum of 4.8%, time to intubation was an average of 5.8 minutes (Mutoh et al., 2002). Premedication with acepromazine, 0.05 mg/kg, with butorphanol, 0.2 mg/kg, IM or medetomidine, 0.02 mg/kg (20 µg/kg), with midazolam, 0.3 mg/kg, IM decreased the time to intubation to 3.7 ± 0.5 minutes or 2.9 ± 0.6 minutes, respectively.

When induction of anaesthesia with an inhalant and facemask is selected, the procedure should be accomplished calmly and quietly. The dog should be allowed to become accustomed to the facemask while breathing oxygen. The vaporizer setting is increased in 0.5% increments for isoflurane (larger increments for sevoflurane and desflurane) with three to four breaths between increments and the patient monitored closely for signs of increasing depth of anaesthesia (Box 15.5). Attempts to introduce a high concentration of anaesthetic immediately to a conscious dog will result in struggling, breath-holding, and excitement. The release of catecholamines will be counterproductive, as they will increase anaesthetic requirement. It must be remembered that with a non-rebreathing circuit the inspired concentration is the same as the vaporizer setting and the inspired anaesthetic

---

> **Box 15.5 Mask induction 'Dos'**
>
> - Use preanaesthetic sedation
> - Quiet, calm, slow
> - Flush previous gases from circuit
> - Mask with O$_2$ only first
> - Use a close-fitting mask, careful not to rub the eyes
> - Increase vaporizer in 0.5% increments
> - Resist impulse to 'max out' vaporizer
> - Decrease vaporizer setting and dilute circuit concentration before attaching to endotracheal tube

---

Table 15.8 Induction of anaesthesia with isoflurane or sevoflurane via facemask

Advantages	Disadvantages	Contraindications
Rapid elimination/recovery; advantageous for young and old patients Technique results in preoxygenation before tracheal intubation	Generally slower than injectable agents; airway not protected Dog may be frightened; catecholamine release increases anaesthetic requirement Anaesthetic plane for tracheal intubation must be deeper than for maintenance; lowers blood pressure Risk of anaesthetic gas pollution	Airway obstruction impairs uptake, slows induction: brachycephalic breeds, pharyngeal mass, collapsing trachea, pneumonia, diaphragmatic rupture Risk of regurgitation and pulmonary aspiration: full stomach, megaoesophagus, laryngeal paralysis

concentration will change within seconds of a change in the vaporizer setting. The rise in anaesthetic concentration in a rebreathing circuit is slower and thus induction of anaesthesia must be expected to be slower. Increasing the O_2 flowmeter setting for a rebreathing circuit (vaporizer outside the circuit) will increase the rate of concentration rise and speed induction of anaesthesia, as does compressing the rebreathing bag periodically to express dilute anaesthetic gas into the scavenger. For a small dog, induction may be facilitated by using a non-rebreathing circuit during mask administration and then changing to a rebreathing circuit for maintenance of anaesthesia; the objective being to use the non-rebreathing circuit to induce anaesthesia more rapidly and the rebreathing circuit for economy and humidification. The maximum vaporizer setting used during induction should depend on the degree of preanaesthetic sedation, the type of delivery system, and the health of the dog. When a halothane vaporizer is set to above 2.5%, the isoflurane to above 4%, or the sevoflurane to above 5%, the anaesthetist must closely observe the progression of anaesthesia to avoid overdosage. The highest concentration in the circuit should be expressed through the pressure relief valve before attaching the endotracheal tube and the vaporizer setting must be decreased to avoid overdose.

Intraoperative supplements

Additional injectable agents are frequently administered during general anaesthesia to provide or maintain analgesia or to increase the sedative base so that the administration of inhalation agent can be decreased. In the latter case, the usual objective is to find a balance between injectable and inhalation agents that results in the best cardiovascular function. The choice of agent(s) depends on the desired effect and may include bolus injections or continuous infusion (continuous rate infusion, constant rate infusion, CRI) of an opioid, α_2-sedative, benzodiazepine, lidocaine, ketamine, or propofol. The purpose of a CRI is to provide a steady plasma concentration of drug for consistent analgesia or sedation avoiding concentration peaks and troughs that accompany periodic dosing. Nerve blocks are also supplements but are considered in a later section of this chapter. More than one supplement may be included in the anaesthetic protocol, for example, fentanyl or morphine plus lidocaine plus ketamine CRIs for total ear canal ablation, or opioid for premedication plus fentanyl CRI plus lidocaine CRI for forelimb amputation, or opioid for premedication plus top ups plus epidural morphine and bupivacaine for pelvic limb fracture repair. A fentanyl patch should also be considered as a supplement to general anaesthesia when it has been applied at least 12 hours previously. A 75 µg/h patch applied 24 hours before anaesthesia to dogs mean weight 26 kg decreased the concentration required for anaesthesia by 36.6% (Wilson et al., 2006c).

Administration of supplements, opioids, analgesics, CRIs, nerve blocks, may be seen as a nuisance occupying more time, more money, and more worry over risk of overdosage and adverse effects, and all of these concerns are valid. However, the impetus for custom designing anaesthetic protocols is a desire to provide better pain control during and after anaesthesia and to facilitate the dogs' return more quickly to a pain-free state after surgery. Some of the drugs and dose rates of supplements used in dogs are described below and in Table 15.9.

Opioids

Supplementation with additional opioid may become necessary during anaesthesia to avoid increasing the vaporizer setting as the effect of premedication wanes or

Table 15.9 Agents for continuous IV infusion during anaesthesia		
Agent	**Administration**	**Comments**
Fentanyl	2–10 µg/kg/h (with isoflurane or sevoflurane)	Provides analgesia, decreases vaporizer setting, may cause bradycardia and hypoventilation, lowest dose used in recovery
Fentanyl	24–42 µg/kg/h (with propofol anaesthesia 12–18 mg/kg/h)	TIVA for craniotomy, IPPV necessary
Morphine	0.2–0.24 mg/kg/h	Provides analgesia, decreases vaporizer setting, decreases ventilation
Lidocaine	1.5–3.0 mg/kg/h	Provides analgesia, decreases vaporizer setting
Ketamine	0.5 mg/kg/h	Decreases vaporizer setting, analgesia unpredictable
Dexmedetomidine	0.5–1.0 µg/kg/h	Decreases vaporizer setting, supplements opioid analgesia, lower dose often sufficient during anaesthesia and higher dose used in recovery
Propofol	6 mg/kg/h (0.1 mg/kg/min)	Decreases vaporizer setting

to provide analgesia as the surgical stimulus increases. Hydromorphone and methadone, for example, may need to be redosed about 2.5 hours after the initial administration, butorphanol after 1.5 hours, meperidine/pethidine after 1.5–2 hours (not IV), buprenorphine after 3 hours, depending on the initial dose and circumstances. Intravenous injections should be given in increments over at least one minute because bolus injections of opioids sometimes cause an acute decrease in blood pressure.

An opioid may be administered as a CRI, most commonly fentanyl or morphine, but also hydromorphone, sufentanil, or remifentanil. Fentanyl is available as 50 µg/mL in ampoules of different volumes. Where a modest analgesic contribution is required, fentanyl can be administered as a bolus of 2 µg/kg every 20 minutes or as a continuous infusion of 6 µg/kg/h with an increase up to 10 µg/kg/h when considered necessary. A CRI administration is most convenient using a syringe pump and a micro-infusion extension set 1.7 metres (60 inches) long with a small 0.3 mL internal volume attached to the syringe. Bradycardia should be treated with an anticholinergic, such as glycopyrrolate, 0.005 mg/kg IV, and artificial ventilation is usually necessary. A loading dose is not needed if a long-acting opioid, such as hydromorphone, morphine, or methadone was administered for premedication and the fentanyl CRI is started soon after induction of anaesthesia. If an immediate increase in analgesia medication is required during anaesthesia then a loading dose of fentanyl, 2–5 µg/kg, is injected IV over 60 seconds followed immediately by starting the CRI. A decrease in the vaporizer setting is essential as the dose rates of fentanyl are increased, otherwise anaesthetic overdose will occur. In one experimental investigation in isoflurane-anaesthetized dogs, a loading dose of fentanyl, 5 µg/kg, followed by an infusion of fentanyl, 9 µg/kg/h, decreased the requirement for isoflurane by 35% (Ueyama et al., 2009) and, in another, a loading dose of fentanyl, 10 µg/kg, followed by an infusion of fentanyl, 18 µg/kg/h decreased isoflurane requirement by 53% (Hellyer et al., 2001). Concurrent administration of a sedative with fentanyl will achieve a greater effect, for example, injection of diazepam, 0.5 mg/kg, in dogs anaesthetized with isoflurane and a fentanyl CRI resulted in a further 20% decrease in isoflurane requirement (Hellyer et al., 2001). In clinical patients, diazepam, 0.2 mg/kg, IV is usually sufficient to augment a fentanyl CRI during surgery.

A pharmacokinetic investigation of a bolus of fentanyl, 10 µg/kg, IV in conscious dogs identified a rapid decrease in plasma fentanyl concentration for the first 20 minutes and then a more gradual decrease (Sano et al., 2006). When the bolus was followed by an infusion, 10 µg/kg/h, the fentanyl plasma concentrations dipped in the first hour and then increased progressively for 3 hours before levelling out. Total body clearance was significantly lower after a 3-hour infusion than a 1-hour infusion. The fentanyl infusion can be stopped at the end of anaesthesia and

a long-acting opioid administered for recovery, or the infusion can be continued for several hours or overnight, generally at a reduced rate of 2–4 µg/kg/h. The fentanyl infusion rate is titrated down in recovery on an individual basis to find the right degree of sedation that allows the dog to lift its head and safe extubation without airway obstruction.

The lower dose rates just described are to be used in conjunction with inhalation anaesthesia. The reduction in inhalant will depend on the nature of other drugs administered concurrently, for example, administration of lidocaine and ketamine with fentanyl (FLK) decreased the requirement for isoflurane in clinical patients at the time of skin incision by 97% in dogs premedicated with acepromazine and midazolam, induced with propofol and receiving a loading dose (Aguado et al., 2011). High fentanyl dose rates are used when fentanyl is administered with propofol for TIVA (see earlier).

Remifentanil is a synthetic opioid structurally related to fentanyl and sufentanil. Onset of action is rapid and clearance is rapid by enzymatic hydrolysis by esterases and unrelated to liver function. The effects of infusions of remifentanil, 0.1 or 0.15 µg/kg/min, during isoflurane anaesthesia were investigated in dogs undergoing elective orthopaedic procedures (Allweiler et al., 2007). After premedication with acepromazine and meperidine/pethidine, anaesthesia was induced with thiopental. During surgery, isoflurane administration was adjusted based on observation of clinical signs, and was decreased an average of 40–50% by the addition of remifentanil. Bradycardia in some dogs was treated with glycopyrrolate. Recovery to spontaneous ventilation was rapid after discontinuing the remifentanil infusion. Experimental investigations of remifentanil infusions during inhalation anaesthesia have documented dose-dependent decreases in requirement for inhalant (MAC reductions) in dogs (Michelsen et al., 1996; Monteiro et al., 2010b). Infusion rates from 0.15 to 0.90 µg/kg/min allowed step-wise decreases in isoflurane administration from 43 to 71% (Monteiro et al., 2010a). The infusions resulted in the expected bradycardia without any change in MAP. Relevant details are that even the lowest infusion rates were associated with significant decreases in cardiac output and O$_2$ delivery. Increased plasma vasopressin concentrations were measured in these dogs and assumed to be responsible for the peripheral vasoconstriction that maintained MAP. Remifentanil is eliminated rapidly after it is discontinued and, therefore, the onset time of the opioid chosen for recovery must be allowed for to achieve a smooth return to consciousness.

Morphine is administered at a rate of 0.2–0.24 mg/kg/h. Administration is easy and precise if the total dose for 2–3 hours (or anticipated surgery time) is drawn into a syringe and diluted to provide a dose rate of 5 mL/h (or a volume appropriate for the size of the animal) and delivered by syringe pump. An alternative method of administration is to add 10 mg of morphine to a 500 mL bag of

Box 15.6 **MLK for continuous infusion during inhalation anaesthesia**

Formula

500 mL lactated Ringer's or similar
1.6 mL of 15 mg/mL (24 mg) morphine
15 mL of 2% (300 mg) lidocaine
0.6 mL of 100 mg/mL (60 mg) ketamine

Delivery

5 mL/kg/h fluid
Morphine 0.24 mg/kg/h
Lidocaine 3.0 mg/kg/h
Ketamine 0.6 mg/kg/h

Precautions

Decrease vaporizer %
IPPV may be necessary
Use pulse oximeter in recovery

Substitution

Fentanyl for morphine = FLK
Delivery 5 or 10 μg/kg/h

balanced electrolyte solution such as lactated Ringer's solution and the drip delivery adjusted to deliver 10 mL/kg/h. It must be remembered that the bag cannot be used to give a bolus of fluid for cardiovascular support. Another practice for intraoperative supplementation with morphine, lidocaine, and ketamine (MLK) is to add 24 mg of morphine (1.6 mL of 15 mg/mL) to a 500 mL bag of fluid, and also add 15 mL of 2% lidocaine and 0.6 mL of ketamine, 100 mg/mL, and to infuse the mixture IV at 5 mL/kg/h (Box 15.6). This will give the patient morphine, 0.24 mg/kg/h, lidocaine 3 mg/kg/h, and ketamine 0.6 mg/kg/h (different concentrations can be devised to accommodate a fluid rate preference). Combining the drugs into one bag is convenient but removes the preference for adjusting the dose rates of individual drugs according to the patient's responses to anaesthesia and surgery, and an additional bag of fluid will be needed for increased fluid administration. In experimental dogs, a morphine infusion, 0.2 mg/kg/h, decreased the requirement for isoflurane by 48%, and this was not decreased further by the combination of MLK (Muir et al., 2003). A loading dose was not administered and steady state plasma concentrations of morphine were reached by 2 hours of infusion. A similar decrease in isoflurane requirement of 45% was measured in dogs anaesthetized with isoflurane and receiving MLK for ovariohysterectomy or mastectomy (Aguado et al., 2011). These dogs were given a loading dose of MLK over 5 minutes that was equal to the hourly infusion rate. An alternative to a loading dose of MLK is to administer a μ opioid for premedication that can provide analgesia in the earlier part of the anaesthetic period while the plasma concentrations of MLK are increasing. Commonly, dogs given morphine CRI or MLK require assisted or controlled ventilation. The vaporizer setting must be substantially decreased to avoid anaesthetic overdose, and it is advisable after a long anaesthetic to decrease the infusion rate by half for the last 30 minutes of anaesthesia to avoid a prolonged recovery. There are reports of deaths in early recovery after disconnection from the anaesthesia machine involving dogs that have received MLK. It is essential that dogs receiving MLK be monitored for adequacy of ventilation, depth of breathing as well as rate, when disconnected from the anaesthesia machine, and for hypoxia, preferably by using a pulse oximeter.

Lidocaine

Infusion of lidocaine, 0.02–0.08 mg/kg/min, IV has been used for more than 40 years to control abnormal ventricular rhythms in conscious or anaesthetized dogs. More recently, lidocaine infusion has been used intraoperatively to decrease the requirement for inhalation anaesthetic. Lidocaine provides sedation but it is not clear how much analgesia is provided. In a study of a range of lidocaine infusions 0.025–0.100 mg/kg/min, in conscious dogs, no antinociception to electrical stimulation that was different from the saline controls was detected during 12-hour infusions (MacDougall et al., 2009). Lidocaine has anti-inflammatory properties and may exert an effect on the inflammatory component that is associated with surgery. There is limited evidence that intraoperative administration of lidocaine may contribute to the reduction in pain postoperatively in dogs. Lidocaine infusion during anaesthesia for intraocular surgery provided some analgesia postoperatively for 50% of the treated dogs even though plasma lidocaine was undetectable 2 hours after infusion ceased (Smith et al., 2004).

A study evaluated the cardiovascular effects of lidocaine in healthy dogs and dogs with subaortic stenosis anaesthetized with isoflurane (Nunes de Morales et al., 1998). A lidocaine loading dose, 0.4 mg/kg, was injected IV over 10 minutes, and an infusion of 0.12 mg/kg/min in healthy dogs achieved plasma lidocaine concentrations within the therapeutic range with no significant changes in cardiovascular indices. However, a higher infusion dose rate, 0.2 mg/kg/min, produced plasma lidocaine concentrations >7 μg/ml in 50% of the dogs and evidence of impaired myocardial contractility, significantly decreased stroke index and increased CVP and pulmonary artery pressure. The same loading dose and lidocaine infusion of 0.12 mg/kg/min was administered to dogs with subaortic stenosis for control of PVCs and, although these dogs started with a lower cardiac index than the healthy dogs, produced no significant impact on the cardiovascular measurements (Nunes de Morales et al., 1998).

The reduction in inhalation agent requirement from lidocaine administration alone is less than is obtained from an opioid infusion, and is dose dependent. Administration of a loading dose of lidocaine, 2 mg/kg, to anaesthetized experimental dogs and followed by an infusion, 0.05 mg/kg/min, resulted in MAC reductions of 15–29% (Muir et al., 2003; Valverde et al., 2004; Wilson et al., 2008; Matsubara et al., 2009), infusion of lidocaine, 0.1 mg/kg/min, by 29% (Wilson et al., 2008), and infusion of 0.2 mg/kg/min, by 37–43% (Valverde et al., 2004; Wilson et al., 2008; Matsubara et al., 2009). Vomiting in recovery, a presumed sign of lidocaine toxicity, was noted in 75% of dogs receiving the highest dose rate (Matsubara et al., 2009).

Currently, in clinical practice, lidocaine dose rates commonly used are a loading dose, 1–2 mg/kg administered over several minutes followed by an infusion, 0.05 mg/kg/min (3 mg/kg/h). Published evidence supports the use of an infusion, up to 0.1 mg/kg/min, to provide a greater and more consistent contribution to the anaesthetic protocol. Combination with other agents may significantly decrease the concentration of inhalation agent required for anaesthesia. Addition of a lidocaine infusion, 0.05 mg/kg/min, in clinical patients given buprenorphine improved anaesthetic management (Ortega & Cruz, 2011; Columbano et al., 2012) but provided no apparent intraoperative contribution in dogs receiving a fentanyl infusion (Columbano et al., 2012).

Ketamine

Infusion of ketamine, 0.6 mg/kg/h, in experimental dogs decreased the isoflurane requirement by 25% (Muir et al., 2003). It is unknown if the ketamine provides sedation and analgesia. Personal experience suggests that ketamine decreases the anaesthetic requirement by sedation because, although the animal appears to be satisfactorily anaesthetized, an increase in surgical intensity elicits increased HR, MAP and even movement. There is some evidence that low dose ketamine infusion during surgery in humans may decrease central sensitization that leads to secondary hyperalgesia (Stubhaug et al., 1997; De Kock & Lavand'homme, 2007). Central sensitization appears to be reversed some time after surgery in most human patients but may continue in some as chronic pain, and it is not known if decreasing central sensitization reduces the incidence of chronic pain. A similar effect of ketamine in dogs still has to be established.

α₂-Agonist sedatives

Moderate to large doses of medetomidine or dexmedetomidine provide analgesia for approximately 1 hour and may obviate the need for supplementation when used for premedication for short-term anaesthesia. A continuous infusion of dexmedetomidine can be used to provide additional and continuous sedation for longer surgeries. Dexmedetomidine CRI may be a useful adjunct to opioid analgesia and decrease the requirement for inhalation agent during surgery and, if continued after anaesthesia, may promote a smooth recovery in hyperexcitable or frightened dogs. An infusion of dexmedetomidine, 0.5–1.0 µg/kg/h, has been useful during anaesthesia in clinical patients. Options are to discontinue the CRI at the end of surgery, to discontinue the CRI and administer atipamezole IM, or to continue the CRI after anaesthesia at an infusion rate of 1–2 µg/kg/h; all with appropriate opioid or nerve block analgesia. For medium to large dogs, the dexmedetomidine can be diluted with saline to deliver a volume of 1.0 mL/h. Example: a 30 kg dog is scheduled to receive 1 µg/kg/h for 12 hours. Dexmedetomidine, 0.7 mL of 0.5 mg (500 µg)/mL (30 kg × 12 h/500) is added to 11.3 mL saline, mixed well, and delivered at 1 mL/h via a syringe pump.

The sedative, analgesic, and cardiovascular effects of low dose dexmedetomidine infusions have been investigated. The results indicate that a loading dose of dexmedetomidine, 0.5 or 1.0 µg/kg, followed by an infusion, 0.5 or 1.0 µg/kg/h, respectively induce sedation in isoflurane-anaesthetized and conscious dogs (Pascoe et al., 2006; van Oostrom et al., 2011). Sedation but not analgesia was detected using auditory and somatosensory evoked potentials in conscious dogs given dexmedetomidine, 1 µg/kg, and CRI 1 µg/kg/h, but both sedation and analgesia were detected at a higher dose rate, 3 µg/kg/h (van Oostrom et al., 2011). An 18% decrease in isoflurane concentration was measured following administration of dexmedetomidine loading dose, 0.5 µg/kg, and CRI, 0.5 µg/kg/h, using electrical stimulation testing to the fore- and hind limbs (Pascoe et al., 2006). Isoflurane MAC was reduced by approximately 60% during an infusion of 3 µg/kg/h (Pascoe et al., 2006; Uilenreef et al., 2008). Clinical patients were administered dexmedetomidine, 5 µg/kg, and buprenorphine 5 minutes before induction of anaesthesia with propofol and start of a dexmedetomidine CRI and isoflurane for soft tissue or orthopaedic surgery (Uilenreef et al., 2008). The authors compared dexmedetomidine 1, 2, and 3 µg/kg/h and concluded that although HR, MAP, and recoveries were satisfactory, infusion of dexmedetomidine at 1 µg/kg/h was their best choice. In this study, the sedative was antagonized at the end of anaesthesia by atipamezole, 0.0125 mg/kg, IM. In another experimental investigation, administration of a dexmedetomidine loading dose, 1 µg/kg, followed by infusion, 1 µg/kg/h, to dogs anaesthetized with propofol or isoflurane resulted in significant decreases in HR and cardiac output (propofol 44%, isoflurane 33%) (Lin et al., 2008). Oxygen delivery was decreased but remained above the published critical level to meet tissue O_2 demand. The infusion of dexmedetomidine was continued for 22 hours after anaesthesia and plasma concentrations decreased abruptly in the first hour after the infusion was discontinued.

Propofol

An infusion of propofol, 6 mg/kg/h (0.1 mg/kg/min), can be used as a supplement to isoflurane or sevoflurane anaesthesia to smooth the level of anaesthesia and allow a small decrease in the vaporizer setting. Clinical experience has been that the depth of anaesthesia remains more stable and the decrease in inhalation concentration results in an improvement in blood pressure.

Neuromuscular blocking agents

Muscle relaxation can be achieved during anaesthesia by inducing deep general anaesthesia, by incorporation of centrally acting agents, such as diazepam or medetomidine, or by use of peripherally acting agents that induce neuromuscular blockade (see Chapter 8). Neuromuscular blockade provides complete relaxation (paralysis) so that deep general anaesthesia can be avoided with the premise that administration of less inhalant or injectable supplements results in better cardiovascular performance. This may be particularly advantageous for old or ill dogs. Specific surgical procedures for which neuromuscular blocking agents (NMBs, NMBAs, muscle relaxants) are included in the anaesthetic protocol are:

- Ocular surgery to immobilize the eye, ensure the eye remains in a central position in the orbit, and to decrease intraocular pressure (IOP)
- To aid reduction of overriding long bone fractures (may or may not be helpful)
- To abolish thoracic movement during thoracotomy
- To facilitate exposure of deep structures during abdominal surgery or to facilitate closure of the abdominal incision.

Agents used

The non-depolarizing NMBAs most commonly used in clinical practice are pancuronium, atracurium, vecuronium, and rocuronium. Pancuronium is a steroid quaternary ammonium compound and has been in use the longest of these agents. Disadvantages of pancuronium are that its administration may cause tachycardia and a transient increase in blood pressure in some animals and that elimination is through hepatic and renal mechanisms which, when function in a patient is decreased, results in an excessively prolonged duration of action. Dosage should also be reduced in animals with hypoproteinaemia because pancuronium is highly protein bound in the plasma. Vecuronium is a mono-quaternary analogue of pancuronium with only one small structural difference. Vecuronium has no significant adverse cardiovascular

effects, however, most of this drug is excreted in bile and urine unchanged and thus duration of paralysis is prolonged by renal disease. Atracurium has a more rapid onset of action and shorter duration of action. Atracurium has no significant cardiovascular effects, however, in rare cases atracurium causes histamine release, peripheral vasodilation and a small decrease in arterial blood pressure. A major advantage to use of atracurium is that it has two methods of elimination: (1) ester hydrolysis catalysed by non-specific esterases such that normal levels of plasma cholinesterase are not required; and (2) a non-enzymatic process known as the Hoffman reaction, that is independent of liver or kidney function.

Pancuronium is classed as a long-acting NMBA, atracurium, vecuronium, and rocuronium as intermediate acting, and mivacurium, another agent used in people, as a short-acting NMBA. These agents act primarily at the acetylcholine binding sites on the postsynaptic receptors at the neuromuscular junction. At least 75% of receptors must be occupied by an NMBA to begin to decrease neuromuscular function. The binding of the NMBA is competitive with acetylcholine which only lasts for milliseconds in the synaptic cleft before it is destroyed by cholinesterase. If a cholinesterase inhibitor (anticholinesterase) such as edrophonium or neostigmine is administered, acetylcholine is able to accumulate and is able to compete at the receptors, effectively antagonizing the NMBA. Neostigmine also acts at other receptors causing bradycardia and increased gastrointestinal motility. Consequently, atropine or glycopyrrolate is usually administered before or concurrently with the anticholinesterase agent.

Sugammadex (sug/as in hug/ –amma-dex) is a relatively new selective steroidal relaxant binding agent (antagonist) available in some countries. Sugammadex is a modified γ-cyclodextrin constructed of a ring of linked glucose units with a water-soluble exterior and a hydrophobic interior that has a central cavity. Upon contact, rocuronium and, to a lesser extent, vecuronium are bound within the cyclodextrin core preventing binding with an acetylcholine receptor. Sugammadex has the advantages of more complete reversal of the NMDA, no autonomic instability, and no need for concurrent use of an anticholinergic because it does not work through cholinergic mechanisms.

Succinylcholine is a depolarizing NMBA that causes initial muscle fasciculations after injection and before onset of paralysis. Succinylcholine, 0.3–0.4 mg/kg, IV will produce about 20 minutes of paralysis in dogs. Salivation and bradycardia may be induced such that prior administration of an anticholinergic is advisable. There is no reversal agent for succinylcholine but its action usually terminates rapidly and completely. Multiple doses of succinylcholine may be associated with a change in the nature of the neuromuscular block from depolarizing to non-depolarizing (known as Dual or Phase II block) resulting in prolonged paralysis. Identification of Phase II block using a peripheral nerve stimulator permits the use of an anticholinesterase for reversal. Succinylcholine is rarely used today in veterinary practice because the initial muscle contractions may cause hyperkalaemia and cardiac dysrhythmias, particularly in animals with myopathies or severe muscle trauma. Succinylcholine is a specific trigger agent in animals susceptible to Malignant Hyperthermia syndrome.

Artificial ventilation, unconsciousness, and analgesia must be provided when a neuromuscular blocking agent has been administered

Administration

An NMBA weakens or abolishes respiratory muscle function and prevents many of the signs associated with monitoring depth of anaesthesia. Therefore, artificial ventilation, unconsciousness, and analgesia must be provided when an NMBA has been administered. Artificial ventilation (IPPV) should be started before or at the time of injection because onset of complete paralysis may be slow at up to 2 minutes. Not all skeletal muscles are paralysed at the same time due to differential distribution of receptors so that muscles of the head and limbs are paralysed first, followed by the abdominal muscles, intercostal muscles and lastly the diaphragm. Thus, loss of the palpebral reflex and extraocular muscle relaxation allowing the globe to assume a central position occur at a low dose of NMBA. Respiratory muscle function will be decreased and will not be sufficient to ensure normocarbia and IPPV is still needed (Lee et al., 1998). Monitoring depth of anaesthesia can be difficult when breathing, palpebral reflex, and eye position are abolished. Deep anaesthesia increases risk for hypotension and prolonged recovery from anaesthesia. Non-invasive or invasive monitoring of arterial blood pressure is advisable when an NMBA is to be included in the anaesthetic protocol. Insufficient anaesthesia results in awareness, increased sympathetic nervous system stimulation, and increased IOP. One approach is to anaesthetize the dog and achieve a stable plane of anaesthesia before administration of the relaxant. Subsequently, vaporizer settings and oxygen flow rates are used that in the anaesthetist's experience result in adequate depth of anaesthesia. An anaesthetic agent analyser is useful to avoid extremes of anaesthetic depth. In dogs, signs of autonomic stimulation may be observed when anaesthesia or analgesia is inadequate for the procedure:

- Pupillary dilation
- Salivation
- Increased heart rate
- Increased blood pressure
- Tongue twitch
- Small respiratory movements.

Monitoring neuromuscular transmission with a peripheral nerve stimulator provides positive feedback and confidence in decisions for dosing with NMBAs. An inexpensive peripheral nerve stimulator is satisfactory for most clinical cases (see Fig. 8.2) and nerves that can be stimulated are the tibial, peroneal, ulnar, and dorsal buccal branch of the facial nerve. Monitoring neuromuscular transmission provides an assessment of the degree of paralysis that can be used to determine when top-up doses are necessary during anaesthesia. At the end of anaesthesia it is used to assess the need for or response to an anticholinesterase agent and determine a safe time to allow the dog to breathe spontaneously. The peripheral nerve stimulator has two electrodes that can be clipped onto 25 gauge or 22 gauge needles. The needles are inserted through the skin until the tips are close to the nerve. The needles are positioned along the course of the nerve, positive proximal on the limb and negative distal, not touching but <5 cm apart, and not in a muscle belly. The peroneal nerve is located along the craniolateral surface of the tibia and the needles can be inserted either high or low (just proximal to the hock). The tibial nerve is located on the medial surface of the limb, just above the hock and cranial to the gastrocnemius tendon. The unit is turned on and power dialed up until the foot twitches in maximum response to an electrical stimulus. A sequence of four stimuli delivered in quick succession (train-of-four, TOF) provides the most information (see Fig. 8.3). When there is no paralysis, four toe twitches of equal strength should be observed in response to the TOF. No twitches will be observed when complete neuromuscular transmission has been abolished.

Several methods of quantitative monitoring of neuromuscular function have been used. Acceleromyography (AMG) calculates muscle activity using a piezoelectric transducer attached to the stimulated muscle. In the dog, a limb is stabilized in a vacuum pillow leaving just the paw free and the transducer is attached to the paw. Acceleration of the paw generates a voltage proportional to the force of contraction. Thus, the strength of each twitch can be measured and the ratio of the last twitch of a TOF to the first twitch strength can be calculated (TOF ratio). AMG may provide more accurate measures of reversal in recovery when compared with the conventional TOF technique described previously (Brull & Murphy, 2010; Murphy et al., 2011b).

Termination of neuromuscular block

As described in Chapter 8, a variety of factors influence the duration of neuromuscular block. Pancuronium and vecuronium have a prolonged duration of action in dogs with hepatic or renal disease. Other factors that prolong duration are immature organ function in paediatric patients, hypothermia, hypokalaemia, acidosis, and gentamicin. Several studies have confirmed that neuromuscular block is potentiated by inhalation agents in dogs (Kastrup et al., 2005; Nagahama et al., 2006), although no statistical effect of isoflurane or premedication agents was measured in a group of clinical patients (Auer, 2007).

As the effects of neuromuscular block wear off, assuming the anaesthetic depth to be that of light surgical anaesthesia, the dog's eyes, which have been central, start to rotate rostroventrally. Spontaneous respiratory movements may not resume when the dog has been ventilated to a normal $PaCO_2$. When neuromuscular block is being monitored using a peripheral nerve stimulator, toe twitches will be observed in response to an electrical stimulus. Recovery from a non-depolarizing NMBA is accompanied by a fade phenomenon in response to multiple electrical stimuli. When applying the TOF, initially only one of the twitches may be observed. As two, three, and four twitches appear it will be noticed that the fourth twitch is less strong than the first (see Fig. 8.4). The fade is due to occupancy of the presynaptic receptors that normally facilitate release of acetylcholine and indicates a significant presence of NMBA at the neuromuscular junction. Only when all four twitches are observed to be of equal strength is it safe to stop IPPV and allow spontaneous ventilation. A TOF ratio of greater than 0.7 measured using AMG is recommended before extubation. Increased use of AMG in veterinary practice would seem warranted since investigations in human anaesthesia have confirmed that majority of anaesthetists are unable to detect fade at a TOF ratio of >0.4 using subjective visual or tactile assessment of responses to peripheral nerve stimulation (Brull & Murphy, 2010).

Neostigmine and edrophonium are commonly used anticholinesterase antagonists of non-depolarizing neuromuscular block in dogs. The response to reversal agent varies considerably with the degree of block present and should only be attempted when the block begins to wane. When full paralysing doses are given, the time lapse from last administration of vecuronium should be 15 minutes or 40 minutes for pancuronium and atracurium. When TOF twitches are being monitored, at least two twitches and preferably four should be present before attempting to reverse the block. In the absence of this monitoring, decreasing chest compliance, attempts at spontaneous breathing, or rotation of the eye should be observed before attempting to restore normal neuromuscular transmission. Inhalation anaesthesia can be decreased but not stopped during the reversal process so that the patient is still lightly anaesthetized when paralysis is reversed. Furthermore, respiratory acidosis prolongs the action of most non-depolarizing agents and will impair reversal. Artificial ventilation should, therefore, be continued through the reversal process. Monitoring with the peripheral nerve stimulator is continued until the TOF has returned to pre-paralysis strength.

An anticholinergic drug such as atropine, 0.02 mg/kg, or glycopyrrolate, 0.005 mg/kg, should be injected IV 1–2 minutes before administering the anticholinesterase to block the adverse effects of bradycardia, salivation, and increased intestinal motility. Heart rate should be monitored and a repeat dose of an anticholinergic given if bradycardia occurs. The neostigmine is injected IV in small increments until satisfactory reversal is achieved (Table 15.10). Onset of action of neostigmine is slower than edrophonium and may take 5+ minutes. Edrophonium is

Table 15.10 Neuromuscular blocking agents and antagonists in dogs, dose rates and comments for use

Agent	Dose (mg/kg) IV	Comments
Pancuronium	0.06	Abdominal and thoracic surgery
Pancuronium	0.01–0.02	Central eye position for ocular surgery
Atracurium	0.5	Abdominal and thoracic surgery
Atracurium	0.1–0.2	Central eye position for ocular surgery
Vecuronium	0.1	Abdominal and thoracic surgery, ocular surgery
Rocuronium	0.5–0.6	Abdominal and thoracic surgery
Rocuronium	0.1	Central eye position for ocular surgery
Neostigmine	0.05–0.20	Antagonist. Start with 0.25 mg for small dog or 0.5 mg for large dog – repeat in 2–3 min as indicated. Atropine or glycopyrrolate first
Edrophonium	0.25–0.50	Antagonist. Use low dose first. Pretreat with anticholinergic or observe for bradycardia
Sugammadex*	8.0	Antagonist to rocuronium and vecuronium

*Use in dogs not fully investigated

more appropriate for use with intermediate duration NMBAs, rather than pancuronium, and is commonly used to antagonize atracurium. Administration of an anti-cholinesterase may be unnecessary when low doses of relaxant are employed for ocular surgery and only one or two doses given, when the duration of surgery exceeds an hour after the last administration, or when the peripheral nerve stimulator induces a TOF equivalent to pre-paralysis strength.

Residual neuromuscular block may remain even after restoration of apparently normal breathing and the concern is that pharyngeal and laryngeal reflexes may remain weak and airway obstruction or aspiration may occur after tracheal extubation (Kopman & Eikermann, 2009). Residual block is probably present when the dog's eyes remain central with absent palpebral reflexes during a light plane of anaesthesia and the dog must be closely observed during recovery from anaesthesia for evidence of an inability to raise its head and protect the airway. Strong jaw tone may be a better indication of return of muscle function. Peripheral nerve stimulation monitoring is recommended for safe practice.

Sugammadex, 8 mg/kg, injected 5 minutes after rocuronium or vecuronium in anaesthetized dogs returned the T4/T1 ratio to >0.9 in 15–210 seconds (Mosing et al., 2012). No decrease in twitch response or clinical signs of recurarization after anaesthesia were observed in any dog. The authors suggested further studies to define optimal dose rate and safety of sugammadex in dogs.

Dose rates for NMBAs

Whereas a small dose may achieve a centrally placed eye for ocular surgery, a larger dose of agent will be needed for relaxation of thoracic and abdominal muscles (see Table 15.10). An approximate guideline is when the duration of neuromuscular block must be extended beyond one dose, subsequent injections for top up of a small dose used for ocular surgery should equal the first dose but when larger doses have been used for abdominal or thoracic surgery, the top-up doses are one-half the initial dose. However, because of variation in duration of block between dogs, it is better to titrate doses by using information from the peripheral nerve stimulator, either maintaining one twitch only in response to TOF or redosing at the reappearance of one twitch. No increase in IOP was measured in isoflurane-anaesthetized dogs after administration of atracurium, 0.2 mg/kg (McMurphy et al., 2004). Return to first twitch was in 20 minutes although the eye remained in a central position for 45 minutes. In another study in dogs anaesthetized with sevoflurane, atracurium, 0.1–0.3 mg/kg, resulted in a dose-dependent duration of block of 20–35 minutes (Kastrup et al., 2005). These results support clinical experience that anaesthetized dogs administered atracurium,

0.1–0.2 mg/kg, for cataract or corneal surgery will need to be redosed at 20–25-minute intervals to maintain neuromuscular block. Single bolus doses of rocuronium, 0.3 or 0.6 mg/kg, produced neuromuscular blockade of 14 or 22 minutes when administered to dogs given a variety of premedication agents and anaesthesia maintained with either fentanyl–propofol or fentanyl–isoflurane (Auer, 2007). Return to complete recovery was in 23 or 32 minutes, respectively.

A continuous infusion of an NMBA will produce a more consistent blockade. After an initial dose of atracurium, 0.5 mg/kg, blockade can be maintained by an infusion of atracurium, 0.5 mg/kg/h (Jones & Brearley, 1987). Early publications concerning use of vecuronium in dogs described an initial bolus of vecuronium, 0.1 mg/kg, followed by an infusion of 0.1 mg/kg/h (Jones & Young, 1991) and an initial bolus of 0.05 mg/kg with an infusion of 0.054 mg/kg/h (Clutton, 1992). Experimental Beagles anaesthetized with fentanyl–propofol, fentanyl–isoflurane or fentanyl–sevoflurane required vecuronium infusions of 0.2 mg/kg/h for TIVA and 0.1 mg/kg/h for inhalation anaesthesia to maintain AMG TOF count of 1 measured at the ulnar nerve (Nagahama et al., 2006). This study determined that full recovery from paralysis was 50–100% longer after inhalation anaesthesia than TIVA, depending on the end-point TOF ratio of 0.7 or 1.0, suggesting that residual effects of vecuronium may be of concern in dogs.

Rocuronium has been used in clinical patients with a loading dose of 0.5 mg/kg followed by an infusion of 0.2 mg/kg/h lasting 20–146 minutes (Alderson et al., 2007). Atropine and neostigmine were administered for reversal in 10 out of 22 dogs. An increased duration to return of neuromuscular transmission and to adequate spontaneous ventilation was associated with longer infusion durations. The authors suggested that rocuronium infusion rate may need to be decreased with longer anaesthesia times and titrated to individual patient requirements using peripheral nerve stimulator monitoring. A lower dose of rocuronium can be used to cause the eye to assume a central position. Rocuronium, 0.1 mg/kg, injected IV in propofol-anaesthetized dogs caused the globe to rotate to a central position and remain there for 23 ± 11 minutes (Auer et al., 2007). The TOF ratio from the peroneal nerve decreased to 45 ± 21%. The dogs were moderately hypoventilating (ETCO$_2$ 53 ± 5 mmHg) during propofol anaesthesia but the average values were not significantly increased by the administration of rocuronium. Close monitoring of the adequacy of ventilation during a single injection of rocuronium is essential and assisted ventilation is recommended.

Oxygen must always be supplied when an NMBA is administered. Artificial ventilation should be employed when ventilation is decreased and when multiple injections or continuous infusion are administered for longer procedures.

Anaesthetic management

Positioning

Care must be taken when positioning the animal to pad parts of the body that might be subject to pressure ischaemia. Limbs should not be allowed to hang over the side of the table. Whenever possible, heads of brachycephalic dogs should be elevated to minimize nasal congestion. Some positions will compromise abdominal movement and contribute to hypoventilation. A pad under the pelvis of a dog in sternal position may sufficiently elevate the abdomen off the table to allow adequate spontaneous breathing. Consideration should be given to the dog with bad hips when positioning involves extension of the hind limbs. Placing a drape stand in front of the animal may facilitate access to the head for monitoring. A drape stand can be easily created by bending a metal rod into a semicircle, with the diameter of the circle as wide as the operating table, and 15 cm at each end bent at right angles and parallel to the table edges for taping the stand to the operating table. When the instrument table is to be placed over the patient, there should be sufficient space between the table and the patient to allow access for the anaesthetist to check tube connections, pulse oximeter probe, gum colour, catheters etc. The anaesthetist should ensure that the IV injection port is within easy access before the dog is draped. For patients for which access to the IV catheters will be blocked by draping or the surgical team, an administration set for dobutamine or dopamine can be attached close to the catheter and left turned off until required. The dog's eyes should be well lubricated with sterile eye lubricant at the start of anaesthesia and periodically during a long anaesthesia. It should be realized that when dogs with short noses, e.g. Pug, are in dorsal recumbency, the eyes will be immediately ventral to the commissures of the mouth. Regurgitation will result in acid reflux flowing into the corneas causing serious damage.

Monitoring

Recognition of problems during anaesthesia is a combination of intuition, based on observation and evaluation of vital signs compared with normal expected behaviour, and data collected from monitoring equipment. Monitoring equipment is essential because observation, palpation, and measurement of vital signs may not identify a problem or may be insufficient to diagnose the cause of the problem. Recording values at regular intervals on an anaesthetic record provides a clear picture of the progression of anaesthesia, especially when written in graphic form. The anaesthetic record can highlight subtle changes that could otherwise be missed as well as documenting case care and facilitating analysis later (Fig. 15.14). While in hindsight the management of the case in Figure 15.14 should have been different, lessons to be learned include: never accept a catheter that will not deliver a fast fluid flow,

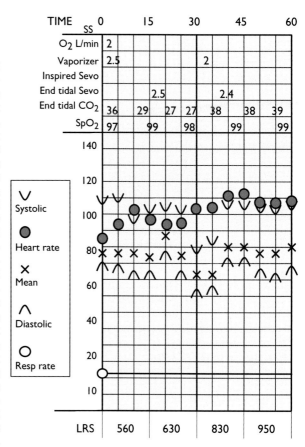

Figure 15.14 This figure is part of the anaesthetic record of a 45 kg Rhodesian Ridgeback anaesthetized with sevoflurane and fentanyl infusion for a forelimb amputation. Changes in more than one parameter on this record indicate that cardiovascular function was decreasing. SS= start of surgery. The fluid flow through the IV catheter was recognized as inadequate and a new catheter was inserted by 20 min after SS. By this time estimated blood loss was 350 mL. Note that the decrease in ETCO$_2$ without a change in IPPV indicated that cardiac output had decreased. Fluid administration was increased by use of a pressure bag around the fluid bag but 10 min later MAP (invasive measurement) also decreased. The vaporizer setting was decreased by 20%. By 20 min after placement of a new catheter, ETCO$_2$ and MAP had returned to pre-hemorrhage values. Total blood loss for the procedure was at least 600 mL as determined by weighing blood-soaked gauzes.

especially for a large dog and when haemorrhage is anticipated during surgery, be observant of changes in monitored values especially when there is no obvious reason, develop an appreciation of the significance of such changes, and blood pressure monitoring can be valuable in the assessment of patient status during anaesthesia. The significance of the degree of haemorrhage was recognized in this case but volume replacement was delayed by lack of venous access. Alternative management at this time should have been an earlier and greater reduction in sevoflurane administration and a request to the surgeons temporarily to cease surgery and employ pressure haemostasis. Administration of a colloid, such as hetastarch, to replace part of the blood loss would have allowed a reduction in the total volume of crystalloid fluid infused and resulted in a better fluid balance. Details about monitoring techniques and interpretations have been described in Chapter 2.

Suggestions for preventing problems during induction of anaesthesia have been given in an earlier section of this chapter (see Box 15.4). Monitoring at this time is directed towards assessment of depth of anaesthesia by using palpebral reflex, eyeball rotation, jaw muscle relaxation (with the exception of ketamine), and absence of gross muscle movement, evaluation of the circulation primarily using heart rate and blood pressure, and identification of inadequate oxygenation by observation of gum colour and use of a pulse oximeter. Not all clinicians agree on whether management of regurgitation should include lavage. The adequacy of inflation of the endotracheal tube cuff should be checked by inflation of the lungs and listening for a leak. A stomach tube may be temporarily inserted to determine the extent and nature of the gastric reflux and to drain as much fluid as possible. The oesophagus may be lavaged with water, but if done, extreme care must be taken to avoid leakage of fluid into the trachea by ensuring cuff inflation and positioning the dog's pharynx lower than its neck. Use of a double lumen tube, one lumen for instilling water and the other for suction, may minimize cranial spread of fluid (Pascoe PJ, personal communication). Metoclopramide administration may be advisable.

During maintenance of anaesthesia in healthy animals, life-threatening abnormalities are most commonly hypoxia during injectable anaesthesia with the dogs breathing air and hypotension during inhalation anaesthesia. Hypoventilation is common but is easily treated with assisted or controlled ventilation. Heart rate can be monitored with multiple items of equipment. Simultaneous comparison of HR (ECG or stethoscope) with pulse rate (palpation or blood pressure monitor) may identify a dysrhythmia. During maintenance of anaesthesia, HR should not decrease below 50 beats/min in dogs, except for animals receiving medetomidine or dexmedetomidine. Higher values are expected in very small and paediatric patients. It is important to look at the gums, not the tongue, when assessing mucous membrane colour. In general, pink mucous membranes indicate good peripheral perfusion and adequate oxygenation. A bright pink colour indicates more vasodilation than a pale pink colour. When vasoconstriction is present, the mucous membranes are pale, even grey or white. Capillary refill time (CRT) provides some information about tissue perfusion. A CRT of 1 second is normal and prolonged time

is the result of low cardiac output and/or low blood pressure.

Palpation of a peripheral arterial pulse is not a reliable guide to arterial pressure. An arterial pulse can often be palpated when pressure is so low that it is life threatening. Changes in strength of the pulse over time may provide an indication of increasing or decreasing pressure. Arterial pressure can be measured by a variety of non-invasive (NIBP) methods or by invasive measurement (Fig. 15.15). Systolic (SAP)/diastolic (DAP) and mean (MAP) pressures for conscious healthy unsedated dogs are 133/75 (94) mmHg and MAP is consistently 90–100 mmHg. Hypotension is confirmed by measurement of MAP <60–65 mmHg or NIBP SAP <80 mmHg (excepting the Doppler ultrasound technique in dogs <5 kg where the NIBP SAP may approximate MAP). Seriously life-threatening pressures are MAP <55 mmHg and DAP <45 mmHg. Unfortunately, NIBP measurements are not always precise and values obtained may differ from actual values by up to 20 mmHg, even when factors that commonly produce errors in measurement are corrected (Box 15.7). Therefore, invasive blood pressure measurements are recommended for dogs at risk for circulatory failure when facilities for measurement are available. Invasive method of pressure measurement involves insertion of a 22 gauge (20–24 gauge) catheter under aseptic conditions into a peripheral artery and connecting it by saline-filled tubing to an electrical pressure transducer and a monitor. Stiff tubing specific for blood pressure monitoring produces the best recording, however, less expensive venous extension tubing is a practical alternative for clinical cases and mean pressures remain accurate. The transducer must

---

Box 15.7 Factors influencing precision of non-invasive blood pressure measurement

Width of the cuff for most monitors should be equal to 40% (40–60) of the circumference of the limb or tail
Falsely high values when:
- Cuff is too small
- Cuff too loose
- Cuff slipped down over carpus or hock
- Cuff is not level with heart (on tail in dorsally or sternally recumbent dog, leg hanging off the table, cuff on forelimb with table in head-down tilt)

Falsely low values when:
- Cuff is too large
- Cuff above heart level*
- Cuff deflated too quickly (Doppler)
- Audible sound too soft (Doppler)

---

*Sometimes reads falsely high when dog is partly dorsal, partly lateral and leg with cuff is stretched up high

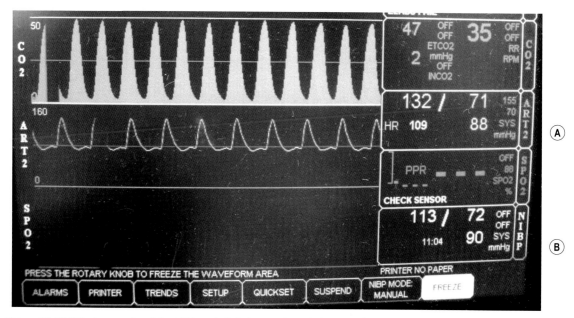

Figure 15.15 This dog was breathing 35 breaths/min but moderately hypoventilating with an end-tidal CO_2 of 47 mmHg. MAP measured by oscillometric technique (B) was the same as obtained by invasive blood pressure measurement (A). Systolic pressures were different.

be placed level with the heart (manubrium, spine or sternum with patient in lateral recumbency; mid-axilla or thoracic inlet with patient in dorsal recumbency) for the pressure to be accurate. The dorsal pedal artery located below the hock on the dorsomedial surface of the metatarsus is the most popular for catheterization because the artery is a reasonable size, the catheter is easily secured, and limited injury will be produced should the procedure result in trauma and haematoma formation (see Fig. 2.16). Catheters can also be placed in the anterior tibial, coccygeal, metacarpal, auricular, lingual, or femoral arteries. Dilute heparin saline (4 units/mL) should be used for multiple flushing of the artery as heparinization of the patient can occur with stronger solutions, especially in tiny dogs. The waveform will provide information on blood flow (area under the curve) and cardiac contractility (steepness of the rising portion of the curve). ECG leads should be attached as standard LA, RA, LL either with clips or with electrodes clipped onto needles inserted through the skin, or sticky electrode pads on the paws and monitored on Lead II. The ECG provides information on heart rate and rhythm. Its main use in anaesthesia is for early recognition of ectopic beats or dysrhythmias that could lead to cardiac arrest. The ECG is not an indicator of blood pressure or tissue perfusion and a normal ECG can be present in the absence of an effective cardiac output or blood pressure.

Inadequate circulation may be present when any of the following are identified:

- Bradycardia
- Tachycardia
- Slow irregular peripheral pulse
- MAP <65 mmHg
- Systolic pressure ≤80 mmHg
- CRT ≥2 seconds
- Weak or non-palpable femoral pulse
- Apnoea or panting
- SpO_2 ≤90%, PaO_2 ≤60 mmHg
- $ETCO_2$ ≤28 mmHg
- Gums bright pink, almost white, or grey
- Dark blood or little oozing at incision site
- Intestinal colour pale pink or white.

Abrupt changes in patient status to include these signs (such as a severe drop in HR, MAP, SpO_2 or $ETCO_2$) may be an indication of severe cardiovascular decompensation and the first step is severely to decrease or cease anaesthetic administration (vaporizer setting) and to alert people in the room. Slower onset or less severe signs may be treated symptomatically but search for the cause is essential. The depth of anaesthesia should be evaluated and adjusted; centrally placed eye, lack of palpebral reflex, partial or complete pupillary dilation are associated with deep anaesthesia. Bradycardia may be induced by some opioids but also may be the result of various causes of hypotension. Sometimes the cause of cardiovascular collapse is suspected because of some event occurring a few minutes earlier, such as a change in body position (see Fig. 2.11), moving a dog with an abdominal mass into dorsal recumbency, following an IV injection of an antibiotic, opioid, sedative or anaesthetic agent, epidural nerve block, surgical exploration of the abdomen, or rapid blood loss. Sometimes an apparent sudden cardiovascular decompensation is actually the culmination of a progressive decrease in cardiovascular function from gradually increasing depth of anaesthesia, haemorrhage without fluid replacement, or progressive hypoventilation.

When monitoring ventilation, it is essential to count RR and estimate depth of the breaths. Fast RR is hyperpnoea and should not be confused with hyperventilation. Arterial PCO_2 may be normal, high or low with a rapid RR. Assisted or controlled ventilation is used to correct hypoventilation.

Other parameters that should be monitored are body temperature and blood glucose concentration in dogs at risk for hypoglycaemia. Hypothermia, 34–35°C (93.2–95°F), will significantly decrease the concentration of isoflurane required for anaesthesia (Wilson et al., 2006c).

Fluid therapy

Crystalloid fluids are commonly administered IV during anaesthesia. Balanced electrolyte solution, such as lactated Ringer's solution, Hartmann's solution, or Normosol-R is usually recommended for all anaesthesia episodes lasting an hour or longer and in very young, old, or sick patients. Fluid loss is increased by evaporation during laparotomy or thoracotomy and for these animals balanced electrolyte solution at 10 mL/kg/h IV is recommended. An infusion rate of 10 mL/kg/h should be halved after 1–2 hours in normovolaemic animals. An infusion rate of 5 mL/kg/h from the beginning of anaesthesia is adequate when a procedure is performed without celiotomy or blood loss. Recommendations for lower fluid infusion rates arise from the concern for fluid retention postoperatively and some discussion about this concern is given in Chapter 21 and in Chapter 2 in the section on monitoring of urine volume. Accurate infusion of the volume of fluid in very small patients is essential and may be accomplished using a paediatric administration set delivering 60 drops/mL (see Box 10.2), by using an infusion pump or syringe driver/pump (see Figs 10.5 & 10.6), or intermittent manual administration of small boluses of fluid from a syringe containing a fixed volume. Restricted fluid administration to 5 mL/kg/h is recommended for some patients in which overload may result in adverse effect, for example, animals with severe mitral insufficiency, cardiomyopathy, or a patent ductus arteriosus. Animals with low plasma protein should receive fluids that will increase oncotic pressure as part of their fluid therapy, such as hetastarch, 5–10 mL/kg administered over 15–30 minutes, or plasma. Patients with low blood glucose or who are at risk for hypoglycaemia (<3 months of age, diabetic, insulinoma) should be given 5% dextrose in water at 3 mL/kg/h. The rate can be increased or decreased according to results obtained from measurement of blood glucose and, at the same time, balanced electrolyte solution should also be infused at 3–7 mL/kg/h.

Cardiovascular support

Oxygen delivery to tissues is determined by blood flow, in turn determined by the cardiac output, arterial blood pressure and diameter of the blood vessels (vasoconstriction or vasodilation), and the amount of oxygen carried in the blood. Thus, tissue hypoxia can occur in the presence of decreased tissue blood flow despite an adequate haemoglobin content and O_2 saturation or in a dog with satisfactory cardiovascular status that is anaemic. Measurement of SpO_2 is not sufficient to ensure adequate tissue oxygenation. Since blood pressure is the product of cardiac output and peripheral vascular resistance, targeting heart rate, cardiac contractility, and pre- and afterload can effectively treat inadequate circulation (Fig. 15.16). A common cause of low blood pressure during anaesthesia is vasodilation induced by the inhalation agent. Decreasing the vaporizer setting may be all that is required to improve blood pressure and, if necessary, supplementing analgesia with injectable drugs. Expansion of blood volume with an additional infusion of crystalloid, 10–20 mL/kg, may improve cardiac output but have little impact on MAP in normovolaemic dogs. Hypotension due to vasodilation from epidural analgesia with a local anaesthetic agent may require in infusion of colloid, such as hetastarch, 5–10 mL/kg, in addition to crystalloid and administration of ephedrine, 0.06 mg/kg, or dopamine, 7 µg/kg/min. Bradycardia may be treated by injection of an anticholinergic or may be corrected when cardiac output and blood pressure are improved by other means. Irregular heart rhythms must be diagnosed using an ECG and treated appropriately (see Chapter 21). In the absence of an obvious cause of decreased venous return, myocardial function may be improved by administration of a catecholamine (Table 15.11). Dopamine and dobutamine are rapidly metabolized and must be administered as continuous infusions after preparing a dilute solution in a bag of saline (Box 15.8). Each practice should have one method of preparing vasoactive drugs to avoid confusion, such as using one size fluid bag and one size infusion set (paediatric 60 drops/mL). In many cases, either dopamine or dobutamine may be the drug of choice since both increase cardiac output. Dobutamine may be preferred in dogs with gastrointestinal hypoperfusion. Dopamine is metabolized to norepinephrine and is the drug of choice for treatment of cardiac arrest and AV heart block. Dopamine, 7 µg/kg/min, was found to be more effective than dobutamine, 6 µg/kg/min, in causing changes in MAP in dogs with moderate blood loss compared with responses in the normovolaemic state (Dyson & Sinclair, 2006). Increasing the dobutamine infusion rate to 10 µg/kg/min increased

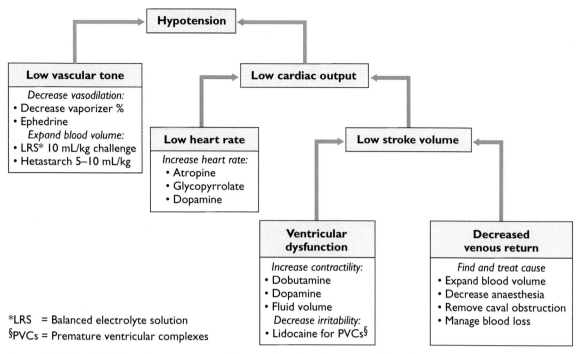

Figure 15.16 Simplified chart for management of hypotension directed at some of the physiological abnormalities that may cause hypotension and listing options for treatment.

arterial pressure, cardiac output and contractility in experimental dogs with severe blood loss during isoflurane anaesthesia (Curtis et al., 1989). Infusion of epinephrine, 0.5 μg/kg/min, after haemorrhage increased cardiovascular function but not as effectively as dobutamine. Dopamine may increase ventricular irritability in patients with traumatic myocarditis, myocardial ischaemia, and cardiomyopathy. The beginning infusion rate of dobutamine is usually 5 μg/kg/min and for dopamine is 7 μg/kg/min and the rate decreased following an appropriate cardiovascular response to MAP 70 mmHg (Table 15.11). Both agents may induce increased heart rates, tachycardia, or PVCs. Occasionally dobutamine slows the HR or initiates second degree AV block. In this situation, the dobutamine infusion rate should be slowed and, if considered appropriate, atropine or glycopyrrolate administered. When low blood pressure persists despite volume expansion and dopamine or dobutamine infusion, a bolus injection of ephedrine, 0.06–0.1 mg/kg, may be an effective stimulant. Ephedrine, 50 mg/mL, is diluted to a concentration of 2.5 mg/mL by mixing 0.5 mL of ephedrine with 9.5 mL of saline. Onset of action may be within a minute but may take up to 5 minutes and the duration of ephedrine is 20–40 minutes. Subsequent injections may have less effect (tachyphylaxis). Ephedrine may cause tachycardia. Ephedrine augments venous return by causing splenic contraction.

Animals in septic shock may have persistent vasodilation and MAP <60 mmHg that is not responsive to fluid resuscitation and administration of dobutamine, dopamine, and ephedrine. Relative adrenal insufficiency occurs in some septic dogs and hypotension has been associated with low plasma cortisol concentrations (Burkitt et al., 2007). Arterial blood pressure may be improved by supplemental administration of hydrocortisone. Use of a vasopressor, such as phenylephrine or norepinephrine that stimulate α₁-receptors or arginine vasopressin that stimulates vasopressin V₁ receptors may be effective treatment. Concerns with use of these vasopressors are: (1) vasoconstriction increases the work of the left ventricle; and (2) vasoconstriction may decrease organ blood flow and induce gastrointestinal ischaemia and renal failure. Thus, these agents are only used after resuscitation has been attempted with fluids and dobutamine, dopamine, and ephedrine administration. Arginine vasopressin is generally recommended for use when phenylephrine or norepinephrine has failed to improve MAP and, in this situation, it is administered at a much lower rate than for treatment of cardiac arrest (see Table 15.11). The mechanisms of vasodilatory septic shock and role of arginine vasopressin have been reviewed (Scroggin & Quandt, 2009).

Decreased preload decreases cardiac output and pressure. Venous return to the heart may be reduced

Table 15.11 Drugs to be used for circulatory support

Drug	Drug class	Dose range	Frequency	Route	Indications
Dobutamine	Catecholamine	3–10 µg/kg/min	Continuous infusion	IV	Hypotension
Dopamine	Catecholamine	5–10 µg/kg/min	Continuous infusion	IV	Hypotension, 3rd degree A V block, cardiac arrest
Ephedrine	Catecholamine	0.06–0.20	Bolus, repeat in 30–40 min	IV	Hypotension
Epinephrine	Catecholamine	0.01–0.015 mg/kg bolus	Repeat in 3 min if heart beat not restored	IV, Intratracheal, Intraosseous	Cardiac arrest
Lidocaine	Antiarrhythmic	1–2 mg/kg	10–15 min	IV	Ventricular premature complexes
Lidocaine	Antiarrhythmic	0.025–0.08 mg/kg/min	Continuous infusion	IV	Ventricular premature complexes
Naloxone	Opioid antagonist	0.02 mg/kg	Bolus, repeat in 20 min if necessary	IV, IM	When opioid present: hypotension unresponsive to other treatment, cardiac arrest
Phenylephrine	Vasopressor	1–4 µg/kg/min	Continuous infusion	IV	Septic shock hypotension unresponsive to other treatment
Norepinephrine	Vasopressor	0.01–1 µg/kg/min	Continuous infusion	IV	Septic shock hypotension unresponsive to other treatment
Vasopressin	Vasopressor	0.05 unit/kg 0.01–0.04 unit /min	Bolus, may repeat once Continuous infusion	IV IV, do not exceed dose	Septic shock hypotension unresponsive to other treatment

Box 15.8 **Preparation of a 100 µg/mL dopamine or dobutamine solution***

$$\frac{\text{Target concentration} \times \text{Total volume}}{\text{Drug concentration}} = \frac{\text{mL of drug to}}{\text{add to total volume}}$$

Example Dopamine

$$\frac{0.1\,\text{mg/mL} \times 500\,\text{mL}}{40\,\text{mg/mL}} = \frac{1.25\,\text{mL to add to}}{500\,\text{mL bag of 0.9\% saline}}$$

Example Dobutamine

$$\frac{0.1\,\text{mg/mL} \times 500\,\text{mL}}{12.5\,\text{mg/mL}} = \frac{4\,\text{mL to add to}}{500\,\text{mL bag of 0.9\% saline}}$$

*Drugs are available in different concentrations; different size bags may be used.

mechanically or be due to a relative or an absolute decrease in blood volume. Increased intra-abdominal pressure, an abdominal mass or gravid uterus, or increased intrathoracic pressure due to increased anaesthetic circuit pressure may mechanically restrict venous return. A change in body position of the dog can result in hypotension. Splanchnic vasodilation initiated by mesenteric traction (mesenteric traction syndrome) or release of catecholamine and vasoactive mediators during manipulation of an intussusception, septic tissue, pancreatic or prostatic abscess, or from a catecholamine-secreting tumour (carcinoid syndrome) also decreases venous return. An absolute decrease in venous return occurs during hypovolaemia and blood loss.

Blood loss should be continuously estimated during anaesthesia. The number of blood soaked gauzes can be counted and multiplied by 6, 8, or 10 mL, depending on the dimensions of the gauze and your estimate of gauze saturation. Blood on the drapes, lap sponges, floor and suction bottle must be added to the total. Comparison of the estimated blood loss with the calculated values of 10%, 15%, and 20% of the patient's blood volume, estimated at 86 mL/kg, provides a guide when assessing the severity of blood loss. Cardiovascular function becomes significantly impaired in healthy animals during anaesthesia at a loss of 15% of their circulating blood volume, with cardiac output decreasing more than blood pressure. Many dogs can tolerate blood loss up to 20% provided they have received fluid therapy. Sick or old dogs, and dogs with cardiac disease may not be able support more than 12–15% blood loss. Further, the speed of blood loss influences the cardiovascular changes and a loss of 5% of blood volume in less than 5 minutes may result in a measurable decrease in blood pressure.

Infusion of balanced electrolyte solution at 2–2.5 times the volume of blood lost will expand blood volume sufficiently to maintain cardiac output. Crystalloid fluid leaves the intravascular space over 60–90 minutes with a high proportion of the load remaining in the interstitial space. To decrease the crystalloid fluid load and avoid oedema, treatment of moderate blood loss should include infusion of a colloid, such as hetastarch 5–20 mL/kg, on a 1 : 1 basis to replace at least part of the blood loss. The impact of blood loss can be tracked with serial measurements of Hct and total protein when IV fluid is administered to maintain normovolaemia. The Hct should not be allowed to decrease below 20% at which point O_2 delivery to tissues becomes compromised. Splenic contraction occurs during recovery from anaesthesia and results in a 3–4% increase in Hct.

Artificial ventilation

Hypoventilation commonly occurs in overweight, senior, and geriatric dogs, following administration of opioids, injectable anaesthetics or high concentrations of inhalation agents, and in dogs during perineal, dorsal hemilaminectomy, or upper abdominal surgeries. Hypoventilation may be the cause of inadequate uptake of inhalation agent and a depth of anaesthesia that is too light for the medical or surgical procedure to be performed. All of these patients will benefit from artificial or controlled ventilation (CV, controlled mandatory ventilation, intermittent positive pressure ventilation, IPPV). IPPV will be required for intrathoracic surgery, during neuromuscular paralysis, in neurological procedures that either include muscle weakness or dictate the need for normal intracranial pressure, and for respiratory or cardiac resuscitation.

Oxygen flow rates into the breathing circuit should not need to be increased at the onset of IPPV. When IPPV is needed to decrease hypercapnia but no change in the depth of anaesthesia is desired, the vaporizer setting should be decreased by 20–25% to adjust for the increase in alveolar ventilation and anaesthetic uptake. When a circle circuit with a vaporizer in the circle is being used, the vaporizer setting should be decreased substantially. In this case, the positive pressure generated in the circuit and the increase in gas flow through the vaporizer can result in a dramatic increase in inspired anaesthetic concentration, with potentially fatal consequences.

Artificial ventilation is achieved by generating a positive pressure at the entrance of the endotracheal tube high enough to force air into the lungs. Positive pressure is generated in a breathing circuit when the outflow through the pop-off valve or exit to the scavenger is closed and the reservoir bag is squeezed. Arterial CO_2 concentrations within normal range can be achieved in healthy dogs with a respiratory rate of 12 breaths/min and tidal volume (breath) of 15 mL/kg, or with a respiratory rate of 20 breaths/min and tidal volume of 11 mL/kg. A fixed RR can be used for all patients regardless of the spontaneous respiratory rate of the dog. Calculation of tidal volume should take into account the body conformation of the patient. Thus, the tidal volume should be calculated based on the ideal weight for an overweight patient and the tidal volume may have to be larger in lean dogs. The target tidal volume is produced in most patients with a peak inspiratory pressure of 15–20 cm H_2O as measured by the pressure gauge on the delivery circuit. Using inspiratory pressure as a guide to the volume delivered may be the only means of measurement but as a guide it can be quite inaccurate. Small thin dogs may require less pressure to inflate the lungs whereas a heavy dog may require a pressure of 25–30 cm H_2O, especially if positioned on the operating table in a prone, head-down tilt for perineal surgery. Maximum inspiratory pressure in dogs with healthy lungs should be 40 cmH_2O, although it should be rarely necessary to reach that value, and a lower maximum value of 20 cmH_2O in dogs with pulmonary disease or trauma. Ventilation strategy for dogs with pulmonary disease should include a tidal volume ≤10 mL/kg with low airway pressure. During manual ventilation, adjusting the amount of squeeze on the reservoir bag can be a combination of observation of peak inspiratory pressure, degree of collapse of the bag, excursion of the thorax, and (if available) measurement of end-tidal CO_2 (ETCO$_2$). Ventilation parameters should be adjusted to achieve ETCO$_2$ values of 30–40 mmHg.

The increase in intrathoracic pressure that occurs during controlled ventilation impedes return of venous blood to the heart and may decrease cardiac output. The longer the inspiratory time the more adverse the cardiac effect. The best technique to avoid excessive depression of cardiac output and blood pressure is to maintain a short inspiratory time and a longer expiratory time. Time of squeezing the bag should be about 1.2 seconds for most patients, so count: Squeeze 1001, release during 1002, pause 1003, pause 1004, squeeze 1001, release during 1002 etc. Pressure in the circuit must drop to zero during expiration. If the pop-off valve is screwed down for artificial ventilation, it will need to be released when the bag is full. It is important to avoid distractions when the pop-off valve is closed because excessive pressure in the circuit can kill a patient. In the event that excess pressure does develop, the anaesthetist must realize that the decrease in coronary blood flow may progress to cardiac arrest several minutes after the pressure in the circuit is released. Use of a pop-off valve with a 'quick-close' button to facilitate artificial ventilation is a safety precaution (see Fig. 10.16).

A ventilator allows the anaesthetist's hands to be free for other tasks and ensures accurate and even breaths. Details about ventilator construction and use are presented in Chapter 9. Some ventilators have a pressure feedback

Table 15.12 Troubleshooting ventilator problems

Complication	Potential causes

Bellows not completely filling	O_2 fails to enter bellows
	   O_2 source to anaesthesia machine failure
	   Ventilator hose not connected to anaesthesia machine
	Leaks present
	   Pop-off (APL) valve open
	   Endotracheal tube cuff needs more air
	   Hose connections need tightening
	   Absorbent dust on canister washers

Irregular bellows movement, spontaneous breathing overriding ventilator setting	Inadequate depth of anaesthesia
	   Vaporizer % high enough?
	   Time interval from last opioid dose?
	   Increase in surgical stimulation?
	Hypoxaemia
	   Note: not all hypoxic animals breathe against the ventilator
	High $PaCO_2$
	   Inadequate ventilator settings
	   Inadequate volume delivery (hose expansion, endotracheal tube cuff leak)
	   Rebreathing CO_2 (high deadspace from adapters, one-way valve stuck open or closed, exhausted CO_2 absorbent)

Ventilator pattern changes	Mechanical obstruction to air flow
	   Surgeon or surgical compression of thorax
	   Kinked or obstructed endotracheal tube
	Decreased driving O_2 pressure
	   O_2 supply to ventilator failing

adapter that must be inserted into the expiratory limb of a circle circuit that triggers an alarm when pressure is too high or too low in the circuit. The control box has settings for RR (frequency) and tidal volume (flow rate), and sometimes inspiratory : expiratory time ratio (set usually at 1 : 2 or 1 : 3) and maximum inspiratory pressure alarm (set at 25–30 cmH$_2$O). These values are usually preset before connecting the dog to the ventilator. Manually delivering several breaths in quick succession to decrease PaCO$_2$ before connection to the ventilator may smooth the transition from spontaneous to controlled ventilation. When the ventilator is turned on, the chest should be observed for movement and the bellows movement for volume delivery, and the pressure gauge on the circuit or bellows for peak pressure. The settings should then be adjusted to fit the individual animal. If the dog was moderately to severely hypoventilating before connection to the ventilator, it may take 5–10 minutes for the PaCO$_2$/end-tidal CO$_2$ to decrease to normal values. The depth of anaesthesia must be monitored and the vaporizer setting adjusted accordingly. When the ventilator is not functioning as expected, the anaesthetist must first check the patient:

- Is the thorax moving in concert with the bellows?
- Auscultate with a stethoscope for air sounds in both sides of the chest
- Is the dog hypoxic – gum colour, SpO$_2$?
- Are the CRT and blood pressures acceptable?

Unsatisfactory IPPV may originate with the ventilator (Table 15.12) and if the problem is serious or not easily identified, consider returning to manual ventilation for safety of the patient while the ventilator problem is corrected. Inadequate volume delivery frequently is the result of small leaks around the endotracheal tube or hose connections, or due to loss of delivery volume from expansion in the hoses to the patient (expansion can be easily observed during inspiration). In the latter case, the volume set on the ventilator must be increased in order for the calculated tidal volume to be delivered to the dog. Significant rebreathing of CO$_2$, and an increase in PaCO$_2$, will occur if one of the one-way (unidirectional valves) is stuck open or closed. The valves become sticky from moisture and absorbent dust and must be cleaned. Partial obstruction of the endotracheal tube can occur if the end of the tube lies on the wall of the trachea or enters a bronchus, or is compressed by retraction during neck surgery, for example, ventral cervical decompression or mass removal. Personnel leaning on the thorax or insertion of retractors for upper abdominal surgery will also limit thoracic expansion.

Postoperative management

The dog should breathe 100% oxygen for about 10 minutes, or shorter or longer as seems appropriate, after

Box 15.9 Predicted scenarios for decreased oxygenation during recovery from anaesthesia

- Heavy sedation with residual inhalation agent
- Long duration anaesthesia, especially with analgesia CRI
- Anaesthesia protocol included NMBA
- Overweight or heavily built dogs
- Senior and geriatric patients
- Brachycephalic breeds
- Head, neck, chest, or abdominal bandages
- Elizabethan collar
- Pharyngotomy tube
- Local swelling from oral/pharyngeal surgery
- Laryngeal paralysis after neck surgery
- Pulmonary disease or thoracic surgery

NMBA = neuromuscular blocking agent

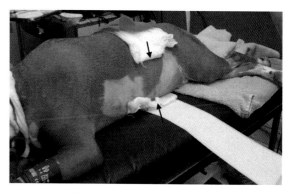

Figure 15.17 This dog was hypoxaemic during recovery from anaesthesia. SpO_2 returned to normal after releasing the pressure on the abdomen and thorax by cutting the abdominal bandage. The distance between the cut ends has been marked by arrows.

discontinuing anaesthetic administration. Hypoxaemia may develop if the animal is disconnected and allowed to breathe room air when still deeply anaesthetized. O_2 should be supplied for at least 5 minutes after N_2O is discontinued to avoid diffusion hypoxia. A pulse oximeter is a valuable monitoring aid during recovery from anaesthesia and a probe can be clipped to the tongue, lip, ear, toe or interdigital web, or a rectal probe can be used (see Fig. 15.1). Patients at increased risk for hypoxaemia include dogs that have received heavy doses of an α_2-sedative, μ opioid, or an infusion of an opioid or opioid combination (Box 15.9). Old, overweight, and ill patients are at greater risk for hypoventilation during and after anaesthesia. Head and neck bandages easily cause external pressure on the pharynx and obstruction after tracheal extubation. One trick to avoid bandaging too tightly is for the assistant to hold the dog's head in a normal partially flexed position as the bandage is applied. It takes experience to apply a thoracic or abdominal bandage to an anaesthetized dog that is not too tight and not too loose. Measurement of SpO_2 when O_2 is discontinued will identify bandages that are too tight. Partial splitting of the bandage will be followed by an increase in haemoglobin saturation (Fig. 15.17). Airway obstruction after tracheal extubation may occur in brachycephalic breeds due to nasal mucosal congestion, any dog from pharyngeal swelling after soft palate or oral surgery, and from pharyngeal/laryngeal compression by a pharyngotomy tube or an Elizabethan collar or a head and neck bandage. It is important to hear or feel air movement through the mouth or nose and not to rely on observation of chest wall movement.

Before the dog regains consciousness, except following laparotomy or some laparoscopies, the urinary bladder should be expressed by abdominal palpation, or

catheterization in males, to avoid soiling of bandages from urination in the cage during recovery. Expressing the bladder is important when the patient has received an epidural that might result in an inability to urinate for several hours. The volume of urine collected should be measured or estimated to assess adequacy of urine flow during anaesthesia. Approximately 1 mL/kg/h of urine should have been produced. When the volume is less, urine output should be monitored after anaesthesia to ensure that urine volume increases when the dog is conscious and regains mobility. Blood should be collected for measurement of Hct and TP concentration from dogs that have suffered blood loss. If the dog has not yet regained consciousness at the time of blood draw, the Hct will increase later by several % due to splenic contraction. It should be remembered that contribution by hetastarch is not recorded by the refractometer. Blood glucose should be measured in diabetic dogs, and in those that are less than 3 months of age or are thin.

Rectal temperature should be measured and heat applied when the temperature is low. The temperature of animals frequently decreases further after the end of surgery when the covering drapes are removed. Warming is highly effective when using a device blowing hot air into pads placed over the animal or overhead radiant heat (hospital infant warmer). Once the patient's temperature has reached 36.4°C (97.5°F) a cage with a heated floor may be sufficient to maintain body temperature. The dog should never be turned side-to-side as a form of stimulation as the change in body position results in an acute drop in blood pressure in some individuals (see Fig. 2.11), and gastric reflux may also be initiated.

When regurgitation has occurred, or when an oral or nasal procedure has been performed, the mouth and pharyngeal area around the epiglottis must be cleaned before extubation and gentle suction of the nasal passages is advisable. Extubation may be done with the dog in sternal position and after the cuff has been only partially deflated in an attempt to squeeze any fluid in the trachea forward into the pharynx.

Tracheal extubation is normally performed when the dog is sufficiently alert to swallow and withdraw its tongue back into the mouth. The tube should be withdrawn between the incisor teeth while the jaws are held apart or the head and neck are overextended to minimize closing power of the lower jaw. Removal of the endotracheal tube through the side of the mouth may result in inadvertent severing of the tube with subsequent inhalation or swallowing of part of the tube. If the tube has been inhaled, the dog must be immediately lightly re-anaesthetized with an injectable agent and O_2 supplied by mask. In big dogs, a smaller endotracheal tube may be inserted inside the broken tube, the cuff inflated, and the tube with the larger piece attached slowly withdrawn. When an endoscope is available it can be used to view directly the piece of the endotracheal tube and facilitate grasping of the tube with fine forceps or biopsy punch. The endoscope can also be used to retrieve pieces of a tube that were swallowed; failing that a gastrotomy must be performed. After retrieval, all pieces of the tube should be fitted together to ensure that no piece has been left behind.

Oxygen supplementation

O_2 therapy should be given to dogs that have trouble adequately oxygenating. Initially, O_2 can be supplied through a facemask attached to the anaesthesia circuit (Fig. 15.18). The simplest method for supplying O_2 for a short time is 'flow-by' oxygen involving a loosely applied facemask supplied with O_2 through a length of tubing from an O_2 cylinder with a regulator and flowmeter (Fig. 15.19). An O_2 chamber, if available, can be used to supply a targeted inspired concentration of 40–60% O_2 and warm the animal at the same time. A disadvantage is that access to the patient is restricted and opening the door or window for examination decreases the cage O_2 concentration. Nasal administration of O_2 may achieve a 40% inspired O_2 concentration and can be a more economical method of administration. One or two nasal tubes are inserted and secured to the dog between the eyes or on the side(s) of the face (Table 15.13, Fig. 15.18). The tubes can be inserted while the dog is still anaesthetized or later using subcutaneous blebs of lidocaine at the sites of suture or staple placement. O_2 is humidified by bubbling through sterile water and insufflated into the patient at 100 mL/kg/min (Fig. 15.20). The oxygen delivery tubing should be secured to a collar or tape around the neck.

Analgesia

Behaviours during recovery from surgery may be obvious or subtle. Thrashing and loudly vocalizing may be

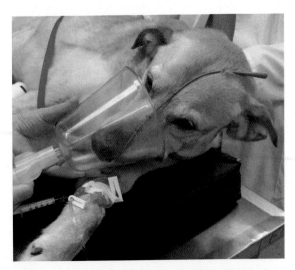

Figure 15.18 Dog recovering from anaesthesia. Oxygen is being supplied via facemask. A nasal tube has been inserted for insufflation of O_2 after the dog is placed in a cage.

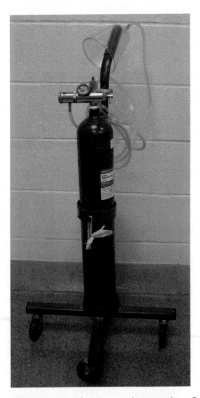

Figure 15.19 Equipment for O_2 supplementation. O_2 cylinder in a portable stand with a combined regulator and flowmeter attached. The O_2 flow rate is dialed in L/min and delivered through tubing and a facemask (mask is resting on the handle of the stand).

Table 15.13 Placement of a nasal O_2 tube

Supplies	Placement
Polyvinyl or rubber feeding tube 5 F or 8 F	Measure tube from medial canthus to nostril
Permanent pen marker	Mark distance with pen
Lubricant gel	Lubricate tube
Suture, haemostat forceps, skin staples	Push nose dorsally, introduce tube dorsally for a few mm, then medially and ventrally Suture or staple at the nares, between the eyes, and on the forehead

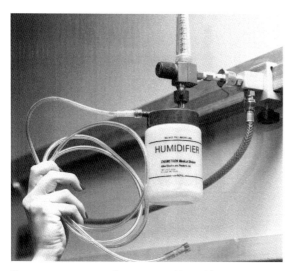

Figure 15.20 Oxygen flowmeter and humidifier containing sterile water for humidification of O_2 delivered by nasal insufflation.

attributable to pain or anxiety or Stage II anaesthesia. Clinical assessment may be difficult, resulting in an incorrect assessment of the degree of pain and subsequent interpretation for treatment. It is important to differentiate the effects of anaesthesia and analgesic drugs from the consequences of surgery. One investigation observed behaviours after anaesthesia and ovariohysterectomy by videotaping the dogs for 24 hours and using hourly observation and interaction to assign sedation and pain scores (Hardie et al., 1997). Control dogs were anaesthetized without surgery. Half of the surgery and control dogs were given oxymorphone 2.5 mg/m², approximately 0.05 mg/kg, IM before anaesthesia and at 6, 12, and 18 hours thereafter. Dogs that were anaesthetized without oxymorphone or surgery spent one-half to three-quarters of their time awake. At all times they actively interacted with the observer, standing up and orienting, tail wagging, door pawing, and by 6 hours trying to escape from the cage. Surgery caused the dogs to spend more time sleeping in lateral recumbency in the first 12 hours, and decreased grooming but increased licking at the incision site. After surgery, the dogs exhibited less of the behaviours described for anaesthesia only. Lip lifting (a warning of aggression) was only seen in the dogs after surgery without oxymorphone. Anaesthesia with oxymorphone caused no changes in waking/sleeping pattern but the dogs spent more time in sternal position and exhibited less greeting behaviour. Thus, a reluctance to rise or a decrease in responsiveness to an observer can be related to opioid administration and unrelated to the presence of pain. The combined effect of surgery and oxymorphone increased the amount of time in lateral recumbency in the first 12 hours and decreased responsiveness to the observer. By 6–12 hours, behaviours returned to normal at a faster rate than in dogs after surgery without oxymorphone. Thus, the quantitative behavioural measurements detected a difference between the surgery groups and found that use of oxymorphone resulted in more rapid return of normal behaviour after ovariohysterectomy. In contrast, the numerical pain scales indicated increased pain in the dogs that had surgery and did not differentiate between administration of pain medication or placebo. This was surprising as the two surgery groups received similar pain scores at a time when they had marked differences in their willingness to move and respond appropriately to the observer. This similarity in pain scores may have been appropriate or may have been due to variation between observers or due to weighting of some of the scaling parameters. For example, a rigid stance (often associated with pain) was common in the dogs that did not have surgery (Hardie et al., 1997). Evaluation is further complicated by the fact that there are individual and breed differences in tolerance for pain.

Various types of pain scoring scales have been described in an attempt to detect severity of pain and provide a guide for analgesia therapy (see Chapter 5). To complete a visual analogue scale (VAS), the patient is observed for a specific behaviour and the observer places a mark on a line on which one end (0) represents no pain and the other end represents the most pain possible, using a scale of 0–10 or 0–100. Use of a numerical rating scale is similar except that a number is assigned to the behaviour where 0 represents normal or preprocedural behaviour and 2 or 3 represents abnormal behaviour (Conzemius et al., 1997; Holton et al., 1998a; Firth & Haldane, 1999). Evaluations of pain scoring techniques have discovered that measurements of some clinical signs, such as HR and RR, do not accurately reflect the severity of postoperative pain. Although combining scores from a variety of observations including activity, mental status, posture, vocalization, is believed to provide a reliable assessment of pain (Firth & Haldane, 1999), scores from different observers may vary considerably (Holton et al., 1998b). Forms for assessment of acute pain designed to be easy to use are the Glasgow

Table 15.14 Examples of IM dose rates of opioids for analgesia in dogs in the early recovery period*

Opioid	Dose rate (mg/kg)	Dosing interval (h)
Morphine	0.2–0.5	4
Meperidine	2–3	2
Hydromorphone	0.05–0.10	4
Oxymorphone	0.05–0.10	4–6
Methadone	0.2–0.5	4
Buprenorphine	0.006–0.02	4–6
Butorphanol	0.2	2

*Dose depends on degree of residual anaesthetic effects

Pain Scale and the Colorado State Acute Pain Scale. These forms can be downloaded as pdf documents by accessing www.google.com and entering Glasgow Pain Scale or Colorado Pain Scale.

Plans for provision of analgesia should have been made before anaesthesia and a multimodal approach should be employed that, whenever possible, includes local nerve blocks. Parenterally administered opioids should be given before consciousness returns. Although this may prolong the time to extubation, with experience, appropriate timing of administration and dose will result in a dog recovering quietly and smoothly from anaesthesia. Examples of opioids for immediate postoperative analgesia are given in Table 15.14 but adjustments should be made for the individual dog's status and anaesthetic protocol. Even when a transdermal fentanyl patch is applied 24 hours before surgery, the analgesia is usually insufficient for the first several hours after anaesthesia and must be supplemented with another μ opioid. A small dose of sedative may be needed to potentiate the effect of the opioid, for example, acepromazine 0.005–0.02 mg/kg IV, or diazepam 0.2 mg/kg IV, or medetomidine 1–2 μg/kg IV, or dexmedetomidine 0.5–1 μg/kg IV. Acepromazine will take several minutes to take effect and before the dog will quieten. Diazepam is a short-lived mild sedative more suited to old patients. Dexmedetomidine is rapidly acting and may induce profound sedation but the effect will wane in 30–45 minutes. A dexmedetomidine infusion, 1 μg/kg/h, IV may contribute to calming an overactive dog. The value of a ketamine infusion, 0.5 mg/kg/h, for analgesia during the recovery period is questionable. Ketamine is not useful as a single agent, however, concurrent infusions of fentanyl and ketamine appear to have a beneficial effect in some dogs compared with fentanyl alone.

Disadvantages of opioid administration include a variable degree of respiratory depression, even hypoxaemia, potential decrease in blood pressure, and decreased effectiveness of the pharyngeal and laryngeal reflexes, with increased risk for aspiration. Both abrupt and progressive development of hypotension may develop after even slow IV administration of an opioid at the end of anaesthesia. Consequently, monitoring should be continued into the recovery period. When an IV infusion of fentanyl or morphine is continued into the recovery period, the infusion may have to be discontinued for a short time if recovery to consciousness and extubation is protracted. The infusion can be restarted when protective pharyngeal/laryngeal reflexes have returned.

Administration of a μ-receptor agonist, such as morphine, hydromorphone or methadone, occasionally results in an apparent dysphoria manifested as restlessness, panting, whining and, occasionally, vocalization. It may be difficult to differentiate between dysphoria and response to pain, however, further administration of an opiate has no calming effect in these dogs. Options are to administer a sedative and wait for the opiate to be metabolized, try a partial reversal with a small dose of naloxone (this is hard to achieve without total reversal of analgesia), or administer a partial agonist such as buprenorphine or butorphanol. With the latter choice, the degree of analgesia will be decreased.

SPECIFIC PATIENT AND PROCEDURE PROBLEMS

Cardiac disease

General recommendations for anaesthesia of dogs with cardiac disease include premedication to present a calm, unstressed animal for induction of anaesthesia and sufficient analgesia during and after surgery. Anaesthetic agents should be chosen based on the pathophysiology of the disease, and low dose rates used initially. Management of cardiovascular function must include maintenance of an adequate blood volume without overload, preoxygenation at induction of anaesthesia and provision of O_2 during anaesthesia to avoid hypoxaemia, cardiovascular support, and assisted or controlled ventilation to prevent moderate to severe hypercarbia. Different forms of cardiac disease require specific management (Table 15.15).

Mitral regurgitation

For dogs with mitral regurgitation, left ventricular preload should be maintained by ensuring normal blood volume. Fluid therapy is initially restricted in dogs with severe mitral insufficiency to 5 mL/kg/h of balanced electrolyte solution but the individual's clinical response to fluid may be used as an estimate of the best level of preload. These dogs with serious comorbid disease may require

Table 15.15 Significance of cardiac disease to anaesthesia

Patient problem	Anaesthetic considerations
Mitral valve insufficiency	Increased risk for hypotension Consider increasing cardiac preload (IV fluids to maintain blood volume), avoid decreasing cardiac contractility, avoid bradycardia, and consider slightly decreasing cardiac afterload (some vasodilation preferable to vasoconstriction).
Cardiomyopathy	Increased risk for hypotension and death Careful choice of anaesthetic agents to avoid decreased cardiac contractility
Ventricular arrhythmias, e.g. automobile trauma, gastric dilatation volvulus, splenic neoplasia	Increased risk for hypotension or ventricular fibrillation and death Consider use of agents that do not sensitize the myocardium to catecholamines, e.g. benzodiazepines, opioids, ketamine, etomidate, alfaxalone, isoflurane, sevoflurane
Patent ductus arteriosus	Increased risk for hypotension before ligation and for pulmonary oedema after ligation. Minimize dose of agents that cause vasodilation and limit intraoperative fluid rate to 6 mL/kg/h

more and other types of fluid to maintain venous return. Heart rate should be normal or slightly elevated as bradycardia decreases cardiac output in the presence of mitral regurgitation. Anticholinergic drugs may be omitted from premedication but may be needed for treatment of bradycardia. Anaesthetic agents should be chosen that maintain myocardial contractility and an infusion of dobutamine may be needed to achieve that goal. A normal or low systemic vascular resistance is preferred because peripheral vasoconstriction increases mitral regurgitation.

Administration of ACE inhibitor medication on the day of anaesthesia is controversial. This author is not alone in believing that omitting one dose is safer for the patient because hypotension that is difficult to reverse develops in some dogs given an ACE inhibitor a few hours before anaesthesia. All other heart medications should be continued. An opioid and benzodiazepine combination is satisfactory for premedication in these patients. Induction of anaesthesia in dogs with severe mitral insufficiency is safely accomplished with diazepam or midazolam and fentanyl and/or etomidate. Xylazine, medetomidine, and dexmedetomidine should be avoided because they induce peripheral vasoconstriction, pulmonary hypertension, and bradycardia. Ketamine, hypercarbia, and hypoxia should be avoided to prevent an increase in pulmonary vascular resistance. Propofol is not an ideal agent for induction of anaesthesia in these patients with severe disease because it decreases myocardial contractility and preload but, if used, the dose must be minimized by first administering an opioid and benzodiazepine. Anaesthesia can be maintained with an inhalation agent and use of analgesic infusions and nerve blocks where appropriate.

Cardiomyopathy

Anaesthesia of these patients should be undertaken with caution and with the realization that life-threatening dysrhythmias or congestive heart failure may develop within 24 hours and up to 5 days after anaesthesia. Choice of anaesthetic protocol should be directed towards avoiding tachycardia, or myocardial depression or hypotension. Fluid restriction, 5 mL/kg/h, is an initial goal, although progression of surgery may alter the patient's requirements.

Ventricular dysrhythmias, myocardial ischaemia, myocardial contusions

Approximately one out of two dogs requiring fracture repair of long bones or pelvis incurred by automobile trauma have radiographic evidence of pulmonary contusions, and by extension, myocardial contusions. Ventricular dysrhythmias that are evidence of myocardial contusion may not appear until approximately 24 hours after the accident. Myocardial ischaemia induced by high intra-abdominal pressure occurring with gastric dilation and volvulus may also manifest as PVCs with or without runs of ventricular tachycardia. Some other clinical conditions, such as neoplasia of the spleen and prostatic abscess, may also be associated with ventricular dysrhythmias. Agents other than thiopental or halothane (because they increase irritability of the myocardium) should be used if possible. Propofol displays both pro- and antiarrhythmic effects (Liu et al., 2011). Occurrences of arrhythmias from propofol in humans are relatively rare and include bradycardia and block of cardiac conduction. In experimental dogs, propofol reduced the arrhythmic dose of epinephrine (ADE) suggesting that it may enhance epinephrine-induced arrhythmias. Personal observations of life-threatening dysrhythmias developed at the time of induction of anaesthesia with propofol in dogs have included ventricular extrasystoles, ventricular tachycardia, atrial fibrillation, and sinoatrial heart block. It is important to remember that anaesthetic agents may depress cardiac contractility to a greater extent in dogs with myocardial ischaemia. Ketamine typically is associated with increased heart rates and high blood pressure that are induced by a centrally mediated release of catecholamines. However, ketamine's negative inotropism is unmasked in dogs with maximal sympathetic nervous system stimulation (anxiety, excitement, pain) or with autonomic blockade or a failing myocardium (ischaemic, contused, acidosis, endotoxaemia). Induction of anaesthesia with ketamine in these patients can result in significant hypotension. Either propofol or ketamine should be administered in small doses and incrementally in patients with the conditions just described.

Lidocaine is the agent most commonly used for treatment of ventricular extrasystoles during anaesthesia because onset of action is rapid. Not all PVCs need to be eliminated. Lidocaine can be administered when PVCs are associated with decreased blood pressure or absent peripheral pulses, are multifocal, or occur in runs of three or more. A loading dose of lidocaine, 1–2 mg/kg, is injected IV followed by an infusion, 1.2–4.8 mg/kg/h (0.02–0.08 mg/kg/min). A single bolus of lidocaine exerts an effect for about 10 minutes. The starting infusion rate is usually 3 mg/kg/h that is then adjusted up or down according to effect. Concurrent administration of lidocaine decreases the inhalation agent requirement and the vaporizer setting must be decreased. In patients with or at risk for PVCs, the loading dose of lidocaine can be given just before the anaesthetic agents administered for induction of anaesthesia. The lidocaine in this case may control myocardial irritability and decrease the dose rate of induction drugs.

Pacemakers

Anaesthesia for transvenous implantation of a pacemaker must exert minimal effect on myocardial contractility and heart rate. Several anaesthetic agent protocols may be satisfactory, most frequently involving premedication with an opioid, induction of anaesthesia with etomidate, and maintenance with isoflurane or sevoflurane. A combination of butorphanol, midazolam, etomidate, and sevoflurane has proven satisfactory for these patients in this author's hands. The dog's neck must be clipped and cleaned and an IV catheter inserted in a cephalic or saphenous vein before drug administration. When external pacing is available, pads are attached for use in the event that the spontaneous ventricular rate fails. Temporary transvenous pacing initiated before the procedure minimizes the risk of hypotension. All equipment and personnel should be assembled before any agent is administered to keep anaesthesia time as short as possible. Dopamine, 7 µg/kg/min, is started first and anaesthetic agents should be administered IV in increments and in sequence. After tracheal intubation is performed and the patient is connected to the anaesthesia circuit and O_2, the vaporizer

should be started at a very low concentration. Useful monitoring includes SpO_2, capnography, NIBP, ECG, and direct arterial pressure. Without pacing, the ventricular rate is usually about 30 beats/min and MAP should be above 70 mmHg. Dopamine will have to be discontinued when the pacemaker is activated.

Patent ductus arteriosus (PDA)

Specific points about PDA physiology that influence anaesthetic management are: (1) MAP is low because the diastolic pressure is low; (2) ligation of the PDA induces pressure changes that acutely increase diastolic pressure; and (3) mature dogs with a PDA are likely to have left atrial and left ventricular enlargement, and pulmonary hypertension and oedema.

Hypotension should be expected during anaesthesia of dogs with a PDA. Consequently, a combination of agents should be chosen to cause the least depression of contractility and least impact on peripheral vascular tone. The drugs should be administered incrementally and in small doses. Intraoperative fluid administration must be limited to 6 mL/kg/h and fluid boluses are not used to treat hypotension. Dobutamine or dopamine, 5–7 µg/kg/min, are used to maintain MAP above 60 mmHg before ligation. Dogs ≤3 months of age should receive 5% dextrose during anaesthesia at 3 mL/kg/h with balanced electrolyte solution at 3 mL/kg/h. Other requirements for management relating to a thoracotomy are discussed in Chapter 20.

Endoscopy

Endoscopy may induce several abnormalities in the patient that must be recognized early by the anaesthetist. Abnormalities include hypoxia, respiratory compromise, regurgitation, accidental tracheal extubation, and response to intense noxious stimulation. Endoscopic procedures require that the anaesthetist be focused on the patient at all times and not be distracted by other duties. Anaesthesia for these patients is equally if not more about monitoring and management than choice of anaesthetic agents.

Bronchoscopy, transtracheal wash (TTW), bronchoalveolar lavage (BAL)

Premedication with atropine or glycopyrrolate is avoided prior to bronchoscopy, TTW, or BAL. An anticholinergic drug will dry respiratory secretions, interfering with sample collection and possibly contributing to small bronchiole plugging. These dogs generally have pulmonary pathology and anaesthesia and the procedure may cause hypoxia, making supplementation with O_2 before induction of anaesthesia and throughout the procedure important. An opioid with a short time of onset and short duration, such as butorphanol, is ideal for these procedures. Anaesthetic management is easier when the endoscope is small enough to be inserted through the lumen of the endotracheal tube. A bronchoscopy adapter allows administration of O_2 and inhalant during bronchoscopy and BAL. The adapter is a plastic elbow connector with the end covered by a rubber plug with a hole in the centre through which the endoscope is inserted forming an airtight seal. Ventilation may have to be assisted if the endoscope is large compared with the endotracheal tube and offers too much resistance to airflow. The endotracheal tube may have to be removed in a very small dog, in which case the dog is anaesthetized first and connected to an anaesthesia circuit breathing anaesthetic agent and O_2 while monitoring equipment is attached. The dog is then extubated while the endoscopy is performed. Gum colour and the SpO_2 must be watched carefully for the onset of hypoxaemia, at which point the endoscope must be removed and the patient given O_2 to breathe. It may be necessary to maintain anaesthesia with small increments of propofol IV. Alternatively, injectable anaesthesia can be planned from the start and a propofol infusion used to maintain anaesthesia. Development of hypoxaemia may be delayed by O_2 insufflation down a thin feeding tube inserted alongside the endoscope or down a side port of the endoscope.

When BAL or TTW are planned, a short sterile endotracheal tube must be used and inserted through the larynx without touching the tip of the tube to the oral mucosa. For TTW, a satisfactory protocol is butorphanol, 0.2 mg/kg, IM for premedication followed by placement of an IV catheter. Propofol is used for anaesthesia and a calculated dose of 4 mg/kg is drawn into a syringe. Anaesthesia is not induced until all personnel and equipment are present. The dog is given O_2 through a mask for several minutes before incremental injections of propofol are injected IV to achieve a light plane of anaesthesia so that the dog's jaws can be opened. Swallowing should be abolished to facilitate introduction of the sterile endotracheal tube, but coughing is permitted. The endotracheal tube cuff is inflated but the tube is not connected to the anaesthesia machine. The sampling tube is then inserted into the endotracheal tube and beyond, followed by instillation of saline and aspiration with coupage. When the sampling tube is connected to a suction unit rather than to a syringe, the degree of suction and the patient must be monitored carefully as it is possible for the suction to cause hypoxia or collapse the dog's lungs. Oxygen should be supplied during recovery from anaesthesia.

Gastroscopy and colonoscopy

Dogs with chronic weight loss and low plasma albumin will have a decreased anaesthetic requirement for injectable anaesthetic agents. When the dog is thin, recovery will be slow from thiopental. During gastroduodenoscopy, the ease of introduction of the endoscope into the duodenum is related to the experience of the operator. However, premedication of dogs with glycopyrrolate and morphine has been documented to increase significantly the number of attempts required to introduce the endoscope into the duodenum successfully (Donaldson et al., 1993). Inflation of the stomach can significantly impair ventilation and cardiovascular function. The anaesthetist must constantly observe the stomach for excessive inflation. Decreases in heart rate, SpO_2, or blood pressure are indications that the stomach must be deflated. Endoscopy for removal of an oesophageal foreign body or for dilation of an oesophageal stricture introduces the potential for pneumothorax. All of the procedures, including placement of oesophageal or gastric feeding tubes, are associated with risk of accidental extubation. The endotracheal tube must be securely tied and kept under observation as scope, hands, and instruments are in and out of the mouth and the endotracheal tube becomes wet and slippery. Movement of the endotracheal tube within the trachea may cause tracheal mucosal damage and the tube must be temporarily disconnected from the circuit when the dog's position is changed.

In contrast to upper gastrointestinal endoscopy, administration of a μ opioid appears to facilitate colonoscopy. Distension of the colon can induce bradycardia, patient response, distension of the stomach, and severe hypoventilation. Occasionally, colonic fluid is forced into the stomach and up into the pharynx. The mouth should always be examined for reflux using a laryngoscope before anaesthesia is discontinued.

Laparoscopy

Choice of anaesthetic agents for laparoscopy will be dependent on the patient and the reason for the procedure. Carbon dioxide insufflated into the abdomen is absorbed into the general circulation and increases $PaCO_2$. Ventilation will be further compromised if the patient is tilted into a head-down position. Controlled ventilation is advisable throughout the procedure. Local infiltration of bupivacaine into the subcutaneous and muscle layers at port sites appears to improve patient comfort postoperatively.

Discussion on thoroscopy is in Chapter 20.

Laryngoscopy

Transnasal laryngoscopy in sedated dogs has been used to identify laryngeal paralysis without the confounding influence of general anaesthesia (Radlinsky et al., 2004). Butorphanol, 0.2 mg/kg, and midazolam, 0.2 mg/kg, are injected IV through a preplaced catheter. A small amount of lidocaine is instilled into a nostril with the dog's nose elevated. The endoscope is then gently inserted and passed to the pharynx for observation of laryngeal movement. The tip of the endoscope is moved lightly to touch the larynx and the resultant response noted.

Oral examination to confirm laryngeal paralysis involves induction of light general anaesthesia. Active arytenoid movements are necessary to avoid misdiagnosis of laryngeal paralysis. Thiopental has been evaluated as the anaesthetic agent that preserves arytenoid motion best (Jackson et al., 2004). Propofol may induce apnoea and weak arytenoid motion, and acepromazine premedication and diazepam–ketamine significantly decrease the ability to assess laryngeal function accurately. Ketamine should not be used to assess laryngeal function for laryngeal paralysis. Doxapram, 0.5–1.0 mg/kg, IV can be administered to dogs during oral examination of laryngeal function to increase rate and depth of breathing. Injection of doxapram, 1.0–2.2 mg/kg has been documented to increase significantly the area of the rima glottidis during propofol anaesthesia and has been recommended as an aid in the diagnosis of laryngeal dysfunction (Miller et al., 2002; Tobias et al., 2004).

Table 15.16 Problems and consequences for anaesthesia for exploratory laparotomy

Problems that may be present before anaesthesia	Problems to be managed during anaesthesia
CNS depression	Gastric reflux, aspiration pneumonia
Myocardial ischaemia	Decreased anaesthetic requirement
Autonomic system overdrive	Increased risk of overdose
Hypovolaemia	Pain
Abdominal distension	
Full stomach	Hypotension, dysrhythmias
Sepsis, endotoxaemia	Reflex bradycardia
	Hypoventilation
	Decreased urine output
	Hypothermia
	± blood transfusion

Rhinoscopy

Rhinoscopy and video otoscopy share a common consideration in that deep anaesthesia or profound analgesia is necessary to prevent patient response to the procedure. Premedication with a μ opioid is preferable over use of butorphanol. Acepromazine is usually avoided for rhinoscopy because the vasodilation it causes may potentiate blood loss initiated by biopsy. Lidocaine may be instilled through the nares to minimize response to insertion of the scope, however, introduction of the endoscope through the mouth and retroflexion behind the soft palate is often a stimulus for the dog to jerk and twist its head. Bilateral maxillary nerve blocks with lidocaine, approximately 1 mg/kg each side, significantly decrease patient response to this procedure (Cremer et al., 2013).

During rhinoscopy, the dog's head should be positioned with the nose down during the procedure for drainage of blood and the pharynx should be packed with gauze. The pharynx must be cleaned before discontinuing anaesthesia and the packing gauze removed. The endotracheal tube should left in place for as long as possible and removed with the cuff still partially inflated.

Urinary bladder

Cystoscopy appears to be painful for the patients both during and after anaesthesia and anaesthetic management must provide adequate analgesia. A morphine epidural may provide long-term analgesia for a dog with substantial tissue trauma after cystoscopy.

Exploratory laparotomy

Dogs and cats with abdominal disease that present as high anaesthetic risks include gastric dilation-volvulus (GDV), splenectomy, intestinal volvulus, intestinal perforation, traumatic abdominal crush or perforation, protein losing enteropathy, pancreatitis, biliary calculi or mucocoele, exploratory for neoplasia, and urinary tract rupture. These patients should be managed before anaesthesia to bring physiological parameters to as close to normal as possible. These patients are prime candidates for hypotension and decreased peripheral perfusion during anaesthesia if they are hypovolaemic and hypoproteinaemic. Blood volume and colloid osmotic pressure should be normalized before anaesthesia and some animals that are anaemic or have been bleeding may need a blood transfusion. Dogs with GDV or a splenic mass are likely to have PVCs and runs of ventricular tachycardia.

It is imperative to practice defensive anaesthesia for these high-risk patients and evaluate the problems before anaesthesia, anticipate the complications, and make contingency plans (Table 15.16). Two IV catheters will be needed when multiple drug or fluid administrations are anticipated. Arterial blood pressure, HR, gum colour, and CRT should be measured preoperatively to assess the patients' cardiovascular status. Measurement of central venous pressure when a jugular catheter is available (tip must be within the thorax) will provide an additional guide to fluid replacement. Dosage of emergency drugs should be calculated before anaesthesia. This will shorten time to treatment of an abnormality and removes the risk of inadvertent inaccurate drug administration. A prepared bag of dopamine or dobutamine should be present in the surgery room.

Dogs that are obviously depressed, or are septicaemic or endotoxaemic, will have a reduced requirement for anaesthetic agents and may need very little drug for endotracheal intubation and maintenance of anaesthesia. Dogs with an intra-abdominal mass are at risk for hypotension from aortocaval compression when they are turned into dorsal position. Preparation of the surgical site should be done with the dogs in an oblique position to delay onset of hypotension that may occur in dorsal recumbency. Balanced electrolyte solutions are used for basic fluid therapy during anaesthesia. Dogs that are hypoglycaemic or have liver disease should receive 5% dextrose at 3 mL/kg/h and the rate adjusted based on measurements of blood glucose. Cardiovascular support with any or all of the following may be necessary in these patients: dobutamine, dopamine, ephedrine, hetastarch, and hypertonic saline IV. Adequacy of ventilation and oxygenation should be monitored during anaesthesia and in recovery. Controlled ventilation may be necessary. Manipulation of ischaemic tissue during surgery, some neoplasms, or mesenteric traction may release catecholamines or other vasoactive products that abruptly cause hypotension. Reperfusion injury may develop in some organs that have been ischaemic when blood supply is restored during surgery. Deferoxamine, 30 mg/kg, IM which inhibits production of hydroxyl radicals, given before anaesthesia may increase survival rate of dogs with GDV (Lantz et al., 1992).

Regurgitation may occur in some of these animals and the pharynx must be cleaned before recovery from anaesthesia.

Gastric dilation-volvulus

Abdominal distension resulting from gastric distension decreases cardiac output up to 90% from normal and the decrease in coronary blood flow causes myocardial ischaemia. These changes have been documented in both clinical and experimental dogs. The increased serum concentrations of markers of myocardial cell injury in clinical patients with GDV have been correlated with the severity of ECG abnormalities and outcome. PVCs may first manifest within 36 hours after the onset of the disease and are clinical evidence of myocardial damage. A retrospective study identified cardiac dysrhythmias in 51% of 166 dogs with GDV, and the majority of patients developed these during anaesthesia (Beck et al., 2006). The presence of preoperative dysrhythmias has been associated with increased mortality. High intra-abdominal pressure (IAP) measured in GDV also significantly decreases blood flow to the intestinal tract, leading to intestinal ischaemia and translocation of bacteria, and decreased hepatic and renal blood flows. Gastric decompression before anaesthesia is important to improve ventilation and cardiovascular function, although IAP will still be higher than normal after decompression. Lidocaine may improve MAP during anaesthesia by controlling the frequency of PVCs and ventricular tachycardia, however, use of lidocaine may not decrease mortality (Buber et al., 2007).

Hypovolaemia and dehydration are frequently present in dogs with GDV on admission to the hospital. Hypotension occurring *at any time* during hospitalization has been correlated with increased risk for death in dogs with GDV, as are the presence of sepsis, disseminated intravascular

coagulation (DIC), and peritonitis (Beck et al., 2006). Re-expansion of plasma volume before anaesthesia is advisable to decrease the severity of cardiovascular depression at induction. Treatment with hypertonic 7.5% saline solution (HSS) or HSS-dextran at 4–5 mL/kg in addition to LRS will restore arterial blood pressure and peripheral perfusion more rapidly than treatment with LRS alone (Schertel et al., 1997). 7.5% HSS has been reported to have several other beneficial effects in other species, including modulation of systemic inflammation and increasing urine output and intestinal motility postoperatively. HSS can be given rapidly over 10–15 min if considered necessary. Hetastarch, 10–20 mL/kg given IV over 30 min can also be used to expand blood volume and improve cardiac output. Not all dogs with GDV are in shock and preoperative treatment should be modified accordingly.

Increased IAP is partly alleviated by bulging of the diaphragm into the thorax. Ventilation is compromised and hypoxaemia is more likely to develop during administration of anaesthetic agents. Preoxygenation during induction of anaesthesia is advisable. A variety of anaesthetic combinations are satisfactory for anaesthesia of these patients, and a frequently used combination for induction of anaesthesia before inhalation anaesthesia is fentanyl–diazepam or midazolam. μ Opioids that induce vomiting should not be administered before anaesthesia as this may increase the risk for aspiration pneumonia and potentially the associated increase in abdominal pressure may result in gastric rupture. A continuous infusion of lidocaine ± fentanyl will contribute to a stable heart rhythm and provide sedation and analgesia.

Peritonitis

Dogs with peritonitis requiring surgical intervention include cases of external trauma, gastric or intestinal perforation, intestinal strangulation and intussusception, pancreatitis, pancreatic abscess, and pancreatic neoplasia, or prostatic abscess. These patients may be septicaemic or endotoxaemic in addition to having abnormalities of fluid balance. Requirement for anaesthetic drugs may be severely decreased. Several anaesthetic agent combinations are satisfactory for anaesthesia of these patients provided that the agents are administered in small increments and titrated to effect. Circulating blood volume must be restored with balanced electrolyte and HSS, hetastarch, or plasma as needed. Circulatory support with dobutamine infusion is frequently necessary. Excessive PVCs and ventricular tachycardia are treated with an infusion of lidocaine. During surgery, manipulation of ischaemic tissue, or sometimes traction on the mesentery, can be followed by an acute severe decrease in blood pressure. A patient recovered with an 'open abdomen' at the first surgery usually requires higher anaesthetic dose rates when re-anaesthetized 2 days later.

Table 15.17 Significance of hepatic disease to anaesthesia

Patient problem	Anaesthetic considerations
Decreased hepatic function	Increased risk for excessive bleeding, hypoglycaemia, prolonged recovery from anaesthesia Consider checking coagulation profile before anaesthesia (may need fresh plasma), monitoring blood glucose and giving 5% dextrose in water 3 mL/kg/h as part of fluid therapy, using anaesthetic agents that are easily eliminated or antagonized During anaesthesia, avoid further hepatic damage by preventing hypotension and hypercarbia
Portosystemic shunt	Increased risk for hypotension, hypoglycaemia, and hypothermia Benzodiazepines contraindicated with encephalopathy; use agents with minimal cardiovascular depressant effects and that can be antagonized or do not depend on hepatic function for elimination During anaesthesia, give 5% dextrose in water 3 mL/kg/h as part of fluid therapy and treat hypotension with dopamine or dobutamine ±hetastarch 5 mL/kg.
Bile duct calculi	Increased risk for surgical procedure to cause hypoventilation and hypotension (mechanical obstruction of venous return) Contraction of bile ducts may be initiated by opiates, impact of partial agonists under debate

Biliary system

Dogs with gall bladder mucocoeles are older, lethargic, anorexic, and may have concurrent pancreatitis or bile peritonitis. These dogs are sick and may have other problems such as cardiac disease. In a retrospective review of 60 dogs undergoing extra hepatic biliary surgery, 43 (72%) survived. The presence of septic bile peritonitis, elevated serum creatinine concentration, prolonged partial thromboplastin times, and lower MAP were significantly associated with mortality (Mehler et al., 2004). Dogs with distension of the gall bladder or bile duct obstruction (calculi) should not be given μ-receptor opioids for premedication because they will cause constriction of the bile duct and possible rupture. Butorphanol and buprenorphine are less likely to cause biliary constriction. Decreased hepatic function can result in prolonged recovery from anaesthesia. Propofol or etomidate may therefore be good choices for induction of anaesthesia in these patients. Maintenance of anaesthesia with isoflurane or sevoflurane is satisfactory. Cardiovascular support with fluids and vasoactive substances will be necessary in these patients.

Hepatic disease

Administration of anaesthesia to dogs with decreased hepatic function must circumvent two possible consequences: (1) recovery from anaesthesia will be slow if the anaesthetic agents used must be detoxified by the liver; and (2) further damage can occur during anaesthesia from hepatic hypoxia as a consequence of arterial hypoxaemia or hypotension or splanchnic vasoconstriction induced by hypercapnia. Dogs with moderate to severe hepatic disease may have disorders of clotting and tests of coagulation should be performed before surgery. Hypoglycaemia is also a potential complication and 5% dextrose in water

should be infused during anaesthesia with balanced electrolyte solution, or directed by intraoperative measurements of blood glucose. Surgical problems relating to the liver, such as portosystemic shunt and bile duct calculi, have other specific anaesthetic considerations (Table 15.17).

Neurological disease

Dogs with neurological disease range from being relatively healthy to comatose. The procedure performed may pose no specific threat, for example, electromyography and nerve biopsy, or may introduce risks of impaired ventilation, haemorrhage, air embolism or severe noxious stimulus, such as dorsal or ventral spinal decompression, and frequently limits access of the anaesthetist to the patient. Cerebellar herniation is a rare complication of cerebrospinal fluid (CSF) collection with generally fatal outcome. Anaesthesia must be managed to prevent increased intracranial and spinal cord pressure for CSF collection, spinal decompression, imaging procedures for dogs with intracranial masses, and craniotomy. Factors that increase intracranial pressure (ICP) are listed in Table 15.18. Anything that increases intracranial volume, notably vasodilation from drugs or increased $PaCO_2$, or increased jugular venous pressure from obstruction or the head in a dependent position, increases ICP. Anaesthetic management should avoid use of ketamine for induction of anaesthesia and monitor and support ventilation to avoid hypercarbia. Thiopental, propofol, etomidate, the benzodiazepines, and opioids decrease ICP. Inhalation agents decrease cerebral metabolic rate but increase ICP by cerebral vasodilation. Their effect may not be significant in most dogs provided that normocarbia is maintained. Inhalation agents are usually avoided in dogs with cerebral trauma and those undergoing craniotomy. Anaesthetic agent dose

Table 15.18 Impact of anaesthetic management on neurological disease

Factors that increase ICP	Factors that decrease or normalize ICP
Hypoxia	SpO$_2$ >90%
Hypercarbia	Normocarbia
Hypertension	Avoiding hypotension or hypertension
Inhalation anaesthetics: halothane, isoflurane, sevoflurane	Anaesthetic agents: thiopental, propofol, etomidate, benzodiazepines, (opioids minimal effect)
Ketamine	Head elevated above heart level
Head-down position	Administration of mannitol

ICP = intracranial pressure

requirement is not usually different from normal for most neurological procedures but dogs with meningitis may require little more than diazepam for endotracheal intubation.

Dorsal hemilaminectomy and ventral cervical decompression

Increased ICP and spinal cord pressure should be avoided in these patients. Artificial ventilation has advantages of maintaining a low spinal pressure and may prevent air embolism that can occur following laceration of a large vein. Positioning a dog for hemilaminectomy should include pads under the head to keep it level with the spine. A long endotracheal tube with a Murphy eye should be selected for dogs anaesthetized for ventral cervical decompression and the tip of the tube inserted as far as the thoracic inlet. If the tube is only inserted to mid-neck, retractors used to expose the surgical site may compress the trachea and occlude the end of the tube. When this happens, the dog's breathing movements will become more exaggerated due to increased PaCO$_2$ whereas movement of the reservoir bag is less. If the dog is connected to a ventilator, irregular movements of the bellows will be seen. If capnography is in use, ETCO$_2$ may decrease or even disappear and the capnograph waveform will change. Blood loss is occasionally severe with these surgical procedures but more frequently occurs as a smaller volume in a short period of time. A check of the suction bottle for blood volume before saline flushing solution is added will aid assessment of blood loss. Balanced electrolyte solution should be infused initially at a rate of 2 : 1 blood loss but substituted with colloid on a 1 : 1 basis when 10% of blood volume is lost.

These surgical procedures may elicit signs during and after anaesthesia that indicate moderate to severe pain. A μ opioid should be included in the anaesthetic protocol for analgesia. Some dogs have increased HR and MAP values in response to surgery despite high concentrations of the inhalant anaesthetic and supplemental opioid and diazepam. Continuous infusion of morphine or fentanyl, with or without ketamine, will modify the patient's response, with return of HR and MAP to normal and allowing a decrease in vaporizer setting. Instillation of preservative-free morphine, 0.1 mg/kg, on an absorbable gelatin sponge placed on the spinal cord at the end of surgery may improve postoperative pain relief. In a study of 12 dogs that underwent hemilaminectomy, the time to administration of rescue analgesia in dogs that had received topical morphine (14 hours in 4/6 dogs) was significantly longer when compared with control dogs (mean of 5 hours but as early as 2 hours in 2 dogs) (Wehrenberg et al., 2009).

Myelography, computed tomography

The anaesthetic protocol should be directed at preventing an increase in ICP. Controlled ventilation assists in lowering ICP and that may facilitate spinal needle placement and injection of contrast agent. Blood pressure should be monitored frequently as injection of radiographic contrast agents may induce hypotension or, more rarely, anaphylaxis. Seizures may occur during recovery from anaesthesia after myelography. Manifestations of an allergic reaction, swelling of lips and eyelids or reddening of the skin, may be observed during recovery after IV injection of contrast agents.

Craniotomy

The anaesthetic protocol using fentanyl and propofol has been described in the section on TIVA. Ideally, two catheters should be placed, one for fluids and one for drug administration. Monitoring equipment is valuable because access to the patient will be obscured by surgical drapes and the need to minimize disturbance of the procedure. Administration of an anticholinergic IV during surgery is likely abruptly to increase HR and bleeding at the operative site and should be avoided if possible; glycopyrrolate IM is less likely to induce this effect.

Ocular surgery

The anaesthetic protocol for young healthy dogs scheduled for eyelid surgery should be chosen based on evaluation of the patient and provide sufficient analgesia to prevent discomfort and rubbing after anaesthesia. The eye is heavily innervated with sensory and pain fibres and any surgery involving the globe will be painful and, in fact, pain may be part of the presenting problem with corneal ulcers, lacerations, and glaucoma. Any procedure involving pressure or traction on the eyeball may induce an oculocardiac reflex resulting in bradycardia, and this is more common in dogs with deep set eyes, such as a

German Shepherd, than dogs with protuberant eyes. Administration of atropine or glycopyrrolate, unless specifically contraindicated, is recommended for premedication before surgeries likely to induce an oculocardiac reflex. A retrobulbar nerve block is recommended before enucleation to provide analgesia and to block the oculocardiac reflex.

An increase in intraocular pressure (IOP) must be avoided when it will have an adverse impact on the outcome. Administration of glycopyrrolate, 0.01 mg/kg, IM can be used for premedication, if preferred, as it does not change pupil diameter or increase IOP (Frischmeyer et al., 1993). Induction of anaesthesia with thiopental or etomidate should not increase IOP. Ketamine, ketamine–diazepam, and propofol have been documented to cause clinically significant increases in IOP in dogs, although the effect of propofol was blunted by prior injection of diazepam (Hofmeister et al., 2006a,b). In these studies, endotracheal intubation produced further increases in IOP (mean 5–8 mmHg) that were not statistically significant. The effect of intubation was minimally attenuated by topical application of lidocaine, 2 mg/kg, on the larynx but not prevented by IV injection of lidocaine. Increases in IOP after intubation could have serious consequences in dogs with a penetrated or near ruptured cornea. Modification of the anaesthetic protocol to minimize adverse effects of tracheal intubation should include adequate preanaesthetic medication, sufficient depth of anaesthesia to prevent coughing, and topical application of lidocaine on the larynx may be advisable. Modest but statistically significant increases in IOP above preanaesthesia measurements were recorded during sevoflurane or desflurane anaesthesia with neuromuscular blockade (Almeida et al., 2004). Hypertension and hypercarbia will increase IOP and should be avoided.

Intraocular surgery, e.g. cataract extraction and corneal graft, generally requires the globe to be positioned centrally in the orbit. Since rostroventral rotation of the eye is a feature of inhalation anaesthesia, administration of an NMBA is common practice with the added benefit of decreasing the incidence of oculocardiac reflex. Access for intraocular surgery may be compromised by pupillary constriction. Miosis has been observed following administration of μ opioids, specifically morphine and oxymorphone. Hydromorphone, 0.04–0.08 mg/kg, and acepromazine, 0.04 mg/kg, caused significant miosis in 16 of 17 dogs at 10 and 25 minutes after IM administration (Stephan et al., 2003). An α_2-agonist, medetomidine, 1500 μg/m^2 administered IV to induce deep sedation decreased pupil size by about one half in all 14 dogs in the study (Verbruggen et al., 2000). No significant changes in IOP were measured in either study. Full dilation of the pupil with ocular medications before opioid administration may block miosis. In a small number of experimental dogs anaesthetized for intraocular surgery, there was no detectable difference in pupil size after treatment with

tropicamide and following administration of morphine, 0.15 mg/kg bolus and infusion of 0.1 mg/kg/h (Smith et al., 2004). Analgesia supplements for intraocular surgery are intracameral lidocaine or an IV infusion of lidocaine, 1 mg/kg bolus + infusion of 1.5–3.0 mg/kg/h (Smith et al., 2004). Administration of an opioid during anaesthesia at the end of surgery for recovery is advisable as neither lidocaine technique produces analgesia in all dogs. Hypotension developing during anaesthesia should be treated by infusion of dobutamine and not fluid boluses to avoid increasing IOP. Catecholamines added to flush solution for phacoemulsification are rapidly absorbed and cause increases in heart rate and blood pressure to varying extents.

Orthopaedic surgery

Anaesthesia for dogs undergoing elective orthopaedic surgery is more straightforward than for dogs requiring surgery after a traumatic accident, and some of the problems of the latter group of dogs are discussed in the later section on trauma. Prolonged anaesthesia, significant blood loss, provision of analgesia, and hypothermia are common problems for anaesthetic management. Analgesia for surgery on the forelimb can include, in addition to parenteral administration of opioid and NSAID, continuous infusion of opioid and lidocaine, paravertebral or brachial plexus nerve block, and digital nerve blocks or intravenous regional anaesthesia (IVRA) for the foot. Analgesia for surgery of the hind limbs and pelvis can include parenteral opioid and NSAID, and epidural nerve block, sciatic and femoral nerve blocks, or intra-articular block, and for the foot, peroneal and tibial or digital nerve blocks or IVRA.

Renal disease

Anaesthesia and surgery decrease urine formation. Dogs with chronic renal disease are at risk for acute renal failure after anaesthesia. For some dogs, fluid therapy should be started at least an hour, and preferably several hours, before anaesthesia to induce diuresis and should be continued after anaesthesia (Table 15.19). Anaesthetic agents should be chosen to ensure a rapid recovery from anaesthesia, IV fluid should be administered during anaesthesia, and physiological abnormalities, such as hypotension and hypercarbia, prevented.

Acute renal failure from urethral obstruction or urinary bladder or ureter rupture include problems of hypovolaemia, azotaemia, and metabolic acidosis, all of which result in decreased anaesthetic requirement and increased risk of hypotension and dysrhythmias. The patients' abnormalities should be corrected before anaesthesia whenever possible. Anaesthetic agents should be administered at markedly decreased rates.

Table 15.19 Significance of renal disease to anaesthesia

Patient problem	Anaesthetic considerations
Chronic renal disease	Increased risk for prolonged recovery from anaesthesia and further deterioration of renal function after anaesthesia. Use a combination of anaesthetic agents to facilitate low dose rates and rapid elimination. Consider initiating diuresis with IV balanced electrolyte infusion before induction of anaesthesia, prevent hypotension during anaesthesia, monitor urine production, continue IV fluids into recovery period
Urethral obstruction, ruptured ureter, urinary bladder or urethra	Increased risk for anaesthetic overdose, hypoventilation, hypotension, and prolonged recovery from anaesthesia. Provide medical treatment before anaesthesia to expand blood volume and decrease serum potassium to <6.5 mmol/L (cystocentesis or abdominal drainage may be necessary). Administer anaesthetic agents in small increments to avoid overdosage and monitor cardiac rhythm and blood pressure during anaesthesia

Trauma

Hit-by-car (HBC, RTA), high-rise syndrome (fell from a great height)

Head trauma must be suspected in animals with obvious skin lacerations on the head, with jaw or cranial fractures, bruising or ecchymoses on the whites of the eyes, or bleeding from the nose. Bleeding within the cranium (subdural haematoma) may be present and anaesthetic management must prevent an increase in ICP in these cases. Auscultation of the thorax is essential to evaluate heart rhythm and confirm air sounds on both sides of the chest. Thoracic radiographs are needed to identify pneumothorax, rib fractures, pulmonary blebs (see Fig. 21.2) and bullae, pulmonary contusions, and diaphragmatic rupture. A significant amount of blood may be sequestered around a fractured humerus, femur, or pelvis. The haematocrit measured at admission to the hospital may not accurately reflect the magnitude of blood loss until fluid therapy has restored normovolaemia. Analgesia must be provided even when anaesthesia for repair is not scheduled until the following day. Opioids form a large part of this preoperative treatment and choices may include administration of buprenorphine or a μ opioid, application of a transdermal fentanyl patch, or infusion of fentanyl and ketamine. Ideally, pain management should be chosen that would be compatible with the subsequent anaesthetic protocol.

Trauma patients may have a full stomach and are at high risk for regurgitation and pulmonary aspiration of fluid or food if anaesthesia must be performed within a few hours of admission to the clinic. The owner may be able to confirm the last feeding time or a radiograph can be taken to determine presence/absence of food in the stomach.

The anaesthetic protocol should be chosen after pre-anaesthetic evaluation of the patients' problems. The detection of PVCs is evidence of myocardial trauma and management should include avoidance of conditions that aggravate myocardial irritability such as hypercarbia, hypoxaemia, hypotension, and catecholamine release. Administration of lidocaine may be indicated.

Radiographic evidence of pulmonary contusions, bleb or bulla adds the risk of pneumothorax developing during anaesthesia. Care must be taken when inflating the lungs and peak inspiratory pressure should be limited to <20 cmH$_2$O.

Big dog-little dog

A major concern when preparing to anaesthetize a dog that has been attacked by a larger animal is that the severity of organ damage may not be immediately apparent. Crushing injury to the head or cervical spine may result in increased ICP or spinal cord damage leading to hypoventilation and hypoxaemia. Subsequent administration of anaesthetic agents may result in severe respiratory depression. Observation of the character of chest wall movement during breathing and evaluation of SpO$_2$ with a pulse oximeter before anaesthesia may identify patients in or at risk for ventilatory failure. Puncture wounds of the skin may overlie torn muscles and penetration of the thoracic or abdominal cavities. Facilities and means for artificial ventilation must always be present for these cases. Crushing and shaking of the dog's body may have created severe destruction of underlying organs. Hypotension and circulatory collapse are likely sequels to general anaesthesia. Anaesthetic agents that cause minimal cardiovascular depression should be administered in small increments and dose rates for crystalloid and colloid fluids, and vasoactive agents should be calculated before anaesthesia.

LOCAL ANALGESIA

Local analgesia is most frequently used as an adjunct to heavy sedation or general anaesthesia in the treatment of perioperative pain. Techniques for performing these blocks are described in this section. Electrical nerve stimulators or ultrasound imaging can be used to identify accurately the location of the nerves to be blocked (Fig. 15.21).

473

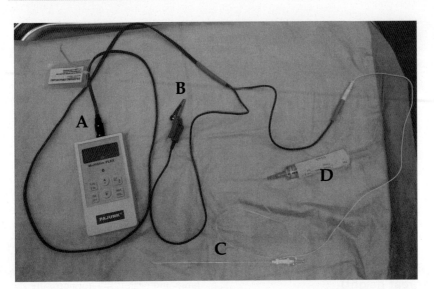

Figure 15.21 Nerve stimulator locator. (A) Stimulator supplying electrical current; (B) ground lead; (C) needle supplied in a sterile pack delivers stimulation to nerve and is connected to syringe (D) containing local anaesthetic solution.

The duration of some nerve blocks can be extended by insertion of catheters that allow intermittent or continuous administration of additional local anaesthetic solution or opioid. New formulations of anaesthetic agents are being developed that provide slow release of injected agents, such as liposome-encapsulated lidocaine, bupivacaine, mepivacaine, and hydromorphone. Liposomes are microscopic lipid vesicles that carry the drug within a central aqueous compartment surrounded by lipid (Wiles & Nathanson, 2010).

It is important to avoid injecting doses of local anaesthetic agent that exceed the recommended maximum total doses. A maximum total dose of lidocaine recommended for dogs is 10 mg/kg and 3 mg/kg for bupivacaine. The toxic dose of lidocaine, as determined by the onset of muscle tremors in conscious dogs, is a mean of 11 mg/kg (Lemo et al., 2007). The CNS signs of toxicity developed before significant decreases in blood pressure. Administration of bupivacaine or ropivacaine to the point of seizures was achieved with doses of 4.3 mg/kg bupivacaine and 4.9 mg/kg of ropivacaine (Feldman et al., 1991). Bupivacaine is highly cardiotoxic when injected IV. Initial treatment of local anaesthetic toxicity is directed towards correction of hypotension or cardiopulmonary resuscitation in the event of a cardiac arrest. When resuscitation is unsuccessful, IV administration of a lipid emulsion (ILE) that is used for parenteral nutrition may decrease the adverse effects (see Chapter 21).

Auriculopalpebral nerve block

The nerve runs caudal to the mandibular joint at the base of the ear and, after giving off the cranial auricular branch,

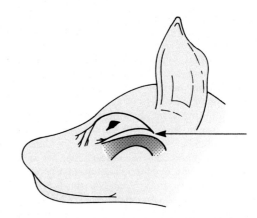

Figure 15.22 Auriculopalpebral (palpebral branch) nerve block. The nerve is blocked where the zygomatic ridge dips medially.

proceeds as the temporal branch along the dorsal border of the zygomatic arch towards the orbit. Before reaching the orbit, the nerve divides into two branches that pass medially and laterally to supply the orbicularis muscle.

The needle is introduced through the skin and fascia over the midpoint of the caudal third of the zygomatic arch (just where the arch can be felt to dip sharply medially) and 2% lidocaine, up to 1 mg/kg, is injected (Fig. 15.22). The blocking of this branch of the facial nerve does not produce any analgesia. Paralysis of the orbicularis muscle facilitates examination and procedures involving the eyeball and helps to prevent squeezing of the eye. Adequate lubrication of the cornea is necessary because the blink reflex is lost.

Brachial plexus block

Block of the brachial plexus will provide analgesia distal to the elbow. Injection can be made with the anaesthetized dog in lateral recumbency using a 22 gauge 3.75 cm, 6.25 cm, or 8.75 cm long spinal needle, according to the size of the dog. Bupivacaine, 2.5 mg/kg, should provide at least 6 hours of analgesia with an onset time of 10–40 minutes. Alternatively, lidocaine, 6 mg/kg, can be used for a shorter duration of action – approximately 2 hours. The brachial plexus originates from the ventral branches of the sixth, seventh, and eighth cervical and the first and second thoracic spinal nerves that form three cords that run for a short distance before segregating into the nerves of the thoracic limb. Local anaesthetic solution must be spread over a wide area to block all the nerves. Bupivacaine can be used as a 0.5% solution or diluted with saline by 25% to produce a larger volume for injection and increase the spread of anaesthetic. Greater dilution than this impairs the quality of nerve block.

A successful block is consistently obtained using the following technique. An area rostral to the cranial border of the scapula, between the point of the shoulder and over the caudal cervical vertebrae should be clipped and the skin prepared as for surgery. An assistant should lift the leg and the attached scapula horizontally to create a gap between the scapula and the thoracic wall. The anaesthetist, wearing sterile gloves, should insert the point of the needle halfway between the point of the shoulder and the transverse process of the sixth cervical vertebra, where the cranial border of the scapula is concave (scapular notch) (Fig. 15.23). The needle is then advanced gently and without resistance to insertion on a path medial to the scapula and parallel to the dog's back as far as the first or second rib. The bupivacaine, 2.5 mg/kg, can be drawn up by the anaesthetist using a sterile syringe after donning sterile gloves or the bupivacaine can be drawn up separately from the procedure and labeled, but can only be handled by the anaesthetist after the spinal needle is in its correct position (Fig. 15.24). The aim is to divide the total volume of bupivacaine into small blebs that will coalesce along the line of needle insertion. Aspiration before injection of local anaesthetic is essential to ensure that the tip of the needle is not in a blood vessel. After injection of a small amount of anaesthetic solution, the needle is withdrawn a short distance, the syringe is aspirated and, if no blood appears, another small volume of local anaesthetic injected. The process is repeated until the last of the anaesthetic is deposited just before the needle exits the skin. Brachial plexus block can also be performed using an electrical needle locator technique and with ultrasound guidance. The anatomy of the area is described later in this chapter, however, use of ultrasound is best learned with the aid of video teaching modules or a continuing education programme.

Some complications may occur as a consequence of this procedure. Large blood vessels pass through the area for injection and needle puncture may create a haematoma. Further, the local anaesthetic solution may be injected intravascularly, the needle may enter the thorax and permit entry of air into the pleural cavity, the brachial plexus may be damaged, causing neuritis or permanent paralysis, or infection may be introduced into the axilla. However, complications are rare if due care is exercised and the technique may be regarded as a relatively safe procedure,

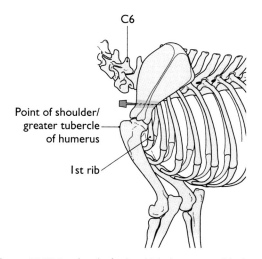

Figure 15.23 Landmarks for brachial plexus nerve block.

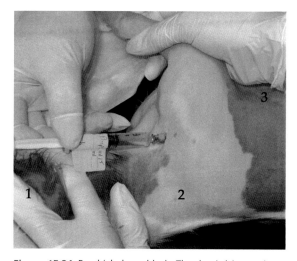

Figure 15.24 Brachial plexus block. The dog is lying on its left side and, for orientation, 1: dog's head; 2: spine; 3: sternum. The assistant is elevating the right forelimb and scapula. The anaesthetist has inserted the spinal needle to its full depth, removed the stilette, and attached a syringe containing bupivacaine.

and of particular value for intraoperative and postoperative analgesia for surgical procedures distal to the elbow.

Other regional techniques that involve the brachial plexus nerves are the paravertebral nerve blocks and the RUMM blocks.

Digital nerve blocks

Nerve blocks for surgery on the metacarpus and digits can be performed at one of three levels depending on the site of the procedure: above the carpus; midmetacarpal level; or at the level of the proximal phalanges. Local anaesthetic solution can be infiltrated subcutaneously just proximal to the distal extremity of the radius at three sites: on the dorsomedial aspect to block branches of the radial nerve; on the palmar surface of the limb at the caudomedial aspect to block branches of the radial and median nerves; and the caudolateral aspect to block branches of the ulnar nerve. A ring block is also an option provided that good coverage is possible without exceeding the maximum total dose rate of local anaesthetic. Blockade of the hind paw can be achieved by peroneal and tibial nerve blocks. The digits of fore- and hind limbs may be blocked by infiltration of local anaesthetic solution on the dorsal and palmar/plantar aspects of the foot at the level of the metacarpal or metatarsal bones (Fig. 15.25). A ring block can

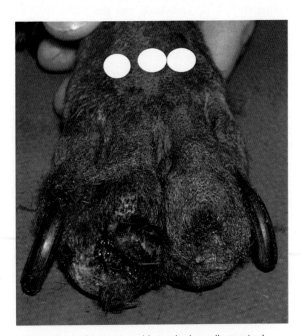

Figure 15.25 This 10-year-old standard poodle required anaesthesia for amputation of two digits. A light plane of general anaesthesia was augmented by infiltration of bupivacaine subcutaneously between the metatarsal bones at three sites on the dorsal surface (white dots) and three sites on the plantar surface proximal to the metatarsal pad.

be performed at the proximal end of the third phalanx for more distal surgery.

Epidural and intrathecal block

Epidural block with lidocaine, bupivacaine, or ropivacaine can provide analgesia for major surgery of the hind limbs and pelvis in sedated or anaesthetized dogs (Heath et al., 1989). Opioids, morphine, oxymorphone, fentanyl, and buprenorphine have been used in the epidural space to provide analgesia during and after surgery. Opioid analgesia is not sufficient to be the entire source for surgery and will not block acute pain in most animals in the immediate recovery period. Analgesia from lumbosacral epidural injection of opioids will provide some analgesia for thoracotomy but is not effective analgesia for forelimb surgery. Combinations of local anaesthetic and opioid have been found to be synergistic and epidural administration of medetomidine or ketamine may contribute to analgesia. Epidural block is contraindicated if the dog has a coagulopathy or skin damage or infection over the lumbosacral area. Hair is slow to grow in the clipped area and may not return fully for a year.

> *Epidural injection is contraindicated with skin infection, local tissue damage, or coagulopathy*
> *Hair is slow to grow back*

Technique

Details of epidural nerve block have been discussed in Chapters 5 and 13. The spinal cord ends in the dog at the junction of the sixth and seventh lumbar vertebrae, and the meninges continue to the middle of the sacrum. Not infrequently a needle inserted at the lumbosacral space penetrates the dura and CSF is aspirated. The volume for injection into the subarachnoid space (intrathecal) is much less than the volume for epidural injection.

The epidural injection may be performed in the conscious or anaesthetized dog in lateral or sternal recumbency. In lateral recumbency, the hind limbs may be held perpendicular to the body or pulled forwards. When the dog has a dislocated hip or pelvis fracture, the hair over the area must be clipped wider to facilitate sterile palpation of the unaffected side in order accurately to determine landmarks. Alternatively, location of the lumbosacral space in these patients may be easier with the dog positioned with the abnormal side down. A satisfactory epidural block may be obtained independent of the side of recumbency. However, cranial spread of fluid injected into the epidural space is greater on the dependent side (Gorgi et al., 2006), therefore, a more extensive block may be obtained if injection is performed with the side scheduled for operation next to the table. For epidural injection in sternal recumbency, the dog's body is squarely positioned with the hocks pulled forward so that the

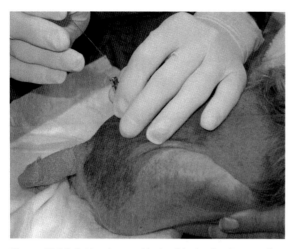

Figure 15.26 Epidural nerve block with the dog in sternal position and the hind limbs pulled cranially. Note that the spinal needle is held immobile using a thumb and forefinger on the hub and the hand is resting on the dog's back.

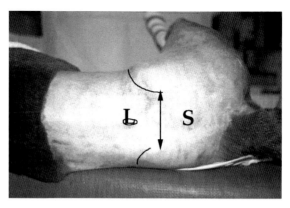

Figure 15.27 Site for epidural injection. This dog is anaesthetized and clipped for orthopaedic surgery. An imaginary line between the caudal dorsal iliac spines crosses midline at the lumbosacral space. An imaginary line between the iliac crests crosses midline between the spinous processes of the last two lumbar vertebrae.

hind limbs are in extension and the spine is curved (Fig. 15.26). The hair should be clipped over a sufficient area to observe the landmarks for injection and to maintain sterility. The skin should be given a surgical scrub. The site for needle insertion is located by identifying the caudal dorsal iliac spines of the pelvis (Fig. 15.27). If the dog is lean, these landmarks are the most prominent dorsal part of the pelvis. An imaginary line joining the caudal dorsal iliac spines crosses midline at the lumbosacral junction that can be palpated as a depression between them. The caudal dorsal iliac spines are difficult to palpate in heavily muscled or fat dogs and dogs with rounded hindquarters. The cranial borders of the pelvis, the iliac crests, can usually be palpated and an imaginary line at this point crosses midline between the last two lumbar vertebrae. The spinous process of the last lumbar vertebra is palpated and the lumbosacral space is identified as a depression immediately caudal. When the lumbosacral depression cannot be palpated, the space between the last two (L6 and L7) lumbar vertebrae can be identified as just described, then the space between the L5 and L6 vertebrae is identified by palpating cranially, the distance between the L5–L6 and L6–L7 spaces is measured, and the same distance caudally from the L6–L7 interspinal space identifies the site for needle insertion.

In conscious dogs, an insensitive skin weal is made with a fine needle and a bleb of local anaesthetic. A 22 or 21 gauge spinal needle, 3.75 cm for small dogs and 6.25 cm for large dogs, is inserted midline perpendicular to the skin and curvature of the rump (Fig. 15.28). Penetration of different layers between the skin and the

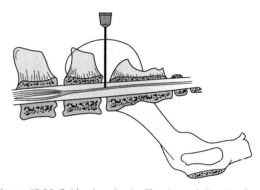

Figure 15.28 Epidural analgesia. The site and direction for insertion of the needle.

epidural space imparts a distinct 'popping' sensation to the fingers as the needle encounters increased tissue resistance. The interspinous ligament just beneath the skin can be difficult to penetrate and offer the first pop. The needle should be advanced gently and penetration of the ligamentum flavum over the epidural space may offer resistance to the tip of the needle and then a pop and loss of resistance is appreciated as the needle enters the epidural space. Sometimes the hand holding the needle is observed to travel faster for a short distance. Should bone rather than ligament be encountered, it indicates that insertion site of the needle was incorrect and that the needle has struck an articular process or the roof of the first sacral vertebra. If this occurs, the needle is slightly withdrawn and a search made for the space by redirecting it a little caudally, cranially, or laterally. Part of the success in performing epidural analgesia is developing knowledge of the approximate depth between the skin and the epidural space, as failure of block is frequently because the needle has not been inserted to a sufficient depth and not through the interarcuate ligament. The hub of the needle should be held securely with thumb and forefinger as the stilette is removed, so that the tip of the needle remains in position. A 3 mL syringe containing 0.25–0.50 mL of air or saline should be attached and when no cerebrospinal fluid (CSF) or blood can be aspirated into the syringe (a vacuum should be encountered), injection of air or fluid should offer no resistance ('loss of resistance', LOR). Confirmation of correct placement is made by ensuring that the needle is midline, that it is sufficiently deep (needle should be supported securely by surrounding tissues when the tip is in the epidural space), that a slight resistance then penetration 'pop' is appreciated during traverse of the interarcuate ligament, and there is no resistance to injection of the air or saline. If CSF or blood is aspirated into the syringe, the syringe should be disconnected, the stilette reinserted, and the tip of the spinal needle repositioned. Injection of the anaesthetic solution should be made over at least 30 seconds to avoid an increase in intracranial pressure. Some clinicians recommend that the injection should be given over 1–3 minutes. The injectate should be warmed before performing epidural analgesia in the conscious dog to avoid movement in response to the cold solution. After the injection has been made, the needle should be withdrawn while using the other hand to apply pressure to the skin at the site of needle insertion. This will prevent air entering the subcutaneous tissues and perhaps limit leakage of fluid from the epidural site into the needle track.

Confirmation of needle placement in the epidural space

The 'loss of resistance' technique just described is a commonly used method in clinical veterinary practice for identifying the epidural space. As the spinal needle penetrates the skin, muscle, and ligamentum flavum, pressure increases within the needle. The pressure decreases on entering the epidural space. Subsequent injection with saline or air is translated to a characteristic tactile sensation of 'loss of resistance'. Injection of air results in small bubbles within the epidural space and may result in a patchy block (Dalens et al., 1987) or limit cranial spread of analgesic solution (Iseri et al., 2010). Consequently, the smallest amount of air possible or sterile saline or a little local anaesthetic solution should be used for testing. Bubbles in the epidural space may compress the spinal cord (Iseri et al., 2010). Some clinicians no longer use air for the LOR test for this reason. A 'hanging drop' technique has been advocated as a useful technique to determine placement of the needle in the epidural space but

must be performed with the dog in sternal position. The spinal needle is advanced until the tip is close but not in the epidural space. The stilette is removed and a drop of local anaesthetic solution or saline placed on the hub of the needle. The needle is advanced through the ligamentum flavum at which point the bleb of solution will be sucked into the needle as confirmation of accurate placement. These techniques do not always accurately identify the epidural space and occasionally produce a false positive result. A 6.8% failure rate was estimated in one retrospective study of epidural analgesia in canine and feline surgical patients (Troncy et al., 2002). Radiological imaging is sometimes used for confirmation of epidural needle or catheter placement in experimental studies, but this is time consuming and expensive. Ultrasound is another modality that has been used to confirm needle position but appropriate training is necessary to ensure accuracy. Nerve stimulation of the spinal cord using an electrically insulated spinal needle at 0.3 mA at 0.1 milliseconds in conjunction with loss of resistance may increase the success rate for correct needle placement (Garcia-Pereira et al., 2010). Using saline instead of air for the LOR test with nerve stimulation may improve electrical conductance. Connection of the spinal needle to a pressure transducer and detection of pressure waves caused by arterial pulsations transmitted to the CSF may confirm epidural placement (de Medicis et al., 2005; Lennox et al., 2006; Iff et al., 2007). A combination of LOR test and observation of epidural pressure waves in one clinical study involving 98 dogs resulted in 77% successful epidural blocks (Iff & Moens, 2010). Epidural pressure waves were only observed after injection of the anaesthetic drugs in one-third of the dogs. The absence of pulsatile waveform does not confirm misplacement and other testing modalities are recommended (Wilson, 2007). Correct placement may be confirmed when transient jugular vein compression results in a distinct rise in CSF and epidural pressures (Chilvers et al., 2007).

Epidural catheter

A catheter can be introduced into the epidural space through a correctly placed Tuohy needle (Fig. 15.29). Details are discussed in Chapter 13. This technique is useful for continuing administration of analgesic agents postoperatively.

> *Use of an epidural does not preclude the need for additional analgesia postoperatively in some dogs*

Drugs used in the epidural space

The generally recommended dose of 2% lidocaine or 0.5% bupivacaine required to produce analgesia up to L1 dermatome after injection into the epidural space at the lumbosacral junction is 0.2–0.22 mL/kg (1 mL per 4.5 kg body weight). There has been discussion as to the

Lidocaine 2% with or without 1:200 000 epinephrine will produce analgesia in 15 minutes and last 1.5–2.0 hours. In conscious dogs with an indwelling epidural catheter previously placed at the lumbosacral space to deliver bupivacaine 0.5% 0.14 mL/kg and 0.22 mL/kg, average onset time to desensitization of the perineum was 3–5 minutes and onset of hind limb desensitization was about 20 minutes (Duke et al., 2000). The average duration of block of the perineum and hind limbs was 2.3 hours whereas analgesia of the flank was of considerably shorter duration. In the same study, injection of ropivacaine resulted in loss of sensation at the perineum in 7–20 minutes and the average durations of analgesia at the perineum and hind feet were between 115 and 140 minutes. Thus, there were no significant differences between the two agents using 0.5% solutions and injected volumes of 0.14 and 0.22 mL/kg. Injection of bupivacaine or ropivacaine using a 0.75% concentration and 0.22 mL/kg produced longer durations of analgesia and potentiated the duration of analgesia in the more proximal dermatomes up to T13–L1 (flank and caudal rib). Injections of 0.22 mL/kg produced a higher success rate (>80%) of block than 0.14 mL/kg at all concentrations. No clinically significant effects on the mean cardiopulmonary measurements were detected but MAP decreased below baseline in some dogs. Hypotension following epidural injection of local anaesthetic agents can be a significant adverse problem (see following section).

An opioid can be used alone in the epidural space or injected in combination with a local anaesthetic to intensify the analgesia for the operative period and to extend analgesia for longer postoperatively. Morphine, 0.1 mg/kg in a total volume of 0.10–0.25 mL/kg as a preservative-free solution, is the opioid used most frequently for epidural injection in veterinary medicine. This dose rate for morphine is recommended by the authors and is commonly reported by others (Valverde et al., 1989, 1991; Branson et al., 1993; Pascoe & Dyson, 1993; Hendrix et al., 1996; Robinson et al., 1999; Smith & Yu, 2001; Fowler et al., 2003; Pacharinsak et al., 2003). The onset of analgesia from epidural morphine is about 45 minutes and lasts 6–12 hours (Branson et al., 1993), an average of 19.6 hours (Troncy et al., 2002), or as long as 23 hours (Bonath & Saleh, 1985). Morphine preparations containing phenol or formaldehyde should not be used whereas the preservative chlorbutanol has not been shown to be neurotoxic (Du Pen et al., 1987). Analgesia from morphine may extend as far forward as the forelimb (Valverde et al., 1989). The addition of bupivacaine to morphine for epidural analgesia in dogs for orthopaedic surgery has been reported to increase the effectiveness of analgesia in a prospective study (Kona-Boun et al., 2006).

Oxymorphone is another opioid that when injected into the epidural space lasts significantly longer than an IM or IV injection, significantly decreases the concentration of inhalation agent required for anaesthesia, and

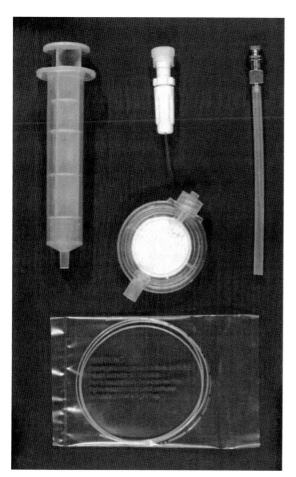

Figure 15.29 Epidural sets are available for the introduction of a catheter into a dog's epidural space. This set contains a 10 mL syringe, 19 gauge Tuohy needle graduated 10–45 mm × 5 mm, open-ended catheter marked at 20–100 mm × 10 mm from tip, loss-of-resistance device, flat filter and Luer Lock connector.

acceptable dose for epidural injection in giant breeds of dogs and some clinicians have recommended a limit for a maximum injected volume of 6 mL, 8 mL, or 10 mL for fear of excessive cranial migration of local anaesthetic solution resulting in respiratory muscle paralysis. Nonetheless, volumes of 0.24 mL/kg have been injected into the epidural space of dogs without complications (Valverde, 2008). The calculated dose should be decreased in pregnant and obese animals. The dose can be calculated on the animal's non-pregnant or ideal weight and further decreased due to a reduction in epidural space from distended blood vessels or excess fat, respectively. Conversely, epidural block may not extend as far cranially as expected in dogs that have experienced serious weight loss.

analgesia persists for hours into the recovery period. The duration of analgesia after epidural injection of oxymorphone, 0.05 mg/kg, was 7.6 hours after hind limb orthopaedic surgery (Vesal et al., 1996) and 10 hours after thoracotomy (Popilskis et al., 1991). Epidural administration of oxymorphone, 0.1 mg/kg with 0.75% bupivacaine added to a total volume of 0.2 mL/kg, provided postoperative analgesia for 24 hours after orthopaedic surgery (Torske et al., 1998).

Buprenorphine, 0.005–0.01 mg/kg, alone or with bupivacaine and diluted to 0.1–0.2 mL/kg can be administered by epidural injection. In a clinical study of dogs anaesthetized approximately 3 hours for cranial cruciate surgery, epidural injection of buprenorphine, 0.004 mg/kg, was compared with morphine, 0.1 mg/kg, both diluted with sterile saline to 0.2 mL/kg (Smith & Yu, 2001). There were no differences in postoperative pain scores between the two agents, although 50% of dogs in each group required rescue analgesia.

Methadone, 0.5 mg/kg, injected into the epidural space of experimental dogs significantly decreased the requirement for isoflurane by 30% when tested by electrical stimulation of the hind limb (Campagnol et al., 2012). This effect was present at 2.5 hours after administration but was waning at 5 hours. Analgesia in the forelimb appeared to persist for longer than in the hind limb. A lower dose of methadone, 0.3 mg/kg, was employed for epidural analgesia in clinical patients undergoing stifle surgery, however, no difference was detected in the duration of postoperative analgesia comparing epidural or IV methadone administration (Leibetseder et al., 2006). Fentanyl, 0.002–0.010 mg/kg, has been added to epidural injections of local anaesthetic. Almeida et al. (2007) investigated in dogs anaesthetized with propofol the quality of analgesia for ovariohysterectomy by epidural injections of bupivacaine, 1 mg/kg, alone or with fentanyl, 0.002 mg/kg, or sufentanil, 0.001 mg/kg. The epidural drugs were diluted to a total volume of 0.36 mL/kg to facilitate cranial migration into the thoracic dermatomes in order to provide analgesia of the ovaries. There were no differences in the three treatments during surgery with regard to HR, SAP, MAP, or propofol dose. The duration of sensory block for bupivacaine and fentanyl–bupivacaine was a mean of 3.4 hours, and for sufentanil–bupivacaine was 4 hours. None of the dogs required rescue analgesia, however, pain scores 6 hours after epidural injection were significantly lower in dogs that had received sufentanil–bupivacaine compared with bupivacaine alone.

Xylazine, medetomidine, and dexmedetomidine can also be administered by the epidural route. Significant decreases in the isoflurane concentration needed to prevent response to a noxious stimulus were measured in experimental dogs 2 hours after administration of 0.003 or 0.006 mg/kg dexmedetomidine, and the decrease was still significant 4.5 hours after administration of the higher

dose (Campagnol et al., 2007). Analgesia was restricted to the hind limbs.

Potential complications

Hypotension may develop acutely 5–20 minutes after epidural injection of a local anaesthetic in some dogs, presumably due to the onset of vasodilation in the dermatomes that are blocked. Results from one study indicated that hypotension was 8.1 times more likely to occur in dogs given bupivacaine, 1 mg/kg, and morphine compared with morphine alone (Kona-Boun et al., 2006). Hypotension was measured 5 minutes after epidural administration of 0.76% ropivacaine, 1.65 mg/kg (0.23 mL/kg), in isoflurane-anaesthetized Beagles, and lasted for 30 minutes (Bosmans et al., 2011). Infusion of 6% hetastarch 200/0.5, 7 mL/kg, over 30 minutes before epidural injection did not prevent hypotension. One dog did not regain consciousness after anaesthesia despite restoration of satisfactory blood pressure with dobutamine. Other factors may contribute to the severity of low pressure, such as pre-existing decreased circulating blood volume or low cardiac output, and use of larger volumes of local anaesthetic solution that result in more cranial spread in the epidural space increasing the extent and magnitude of sympathetic nerve block. Effective treatment of hypotension induced by epidural bupivacaine is not always straightforward and usually comprises a combination of decreased inhalant administration, balanced electrolyte 10 mL/kg bolus, dobutamine infusion with or without ephedrine, and hetastarch 5–10 mL/kg. Cardiac arrest is rare in dogs given epidural nerve block but has been reported after injection of lidocaine and lidocaine, bupivacaine and morphine (Savvas et al., 2006; Mosing et al., 2008). In each case, arrest occurred almost immediately after epidural injection. Spontaneous circulation was restored by cardiopulmonary resuscitation but soon asystole recurred and the dogs had to be resuscitated again. Cause of arrest may have been an acute decrease in venous return resulting in asystole since IV injection was ruled out. These cases are a reminder that cardiovascular function should be monitored closely after an epidural injection.

Agents other than local anaesthetics may be absorbed from the epidural space and cause significant systemic effects. The dose of epidural morphine is too low to produce significant systemic effect (Valverde et al., 1991). However, oxymorphone is systemically absorbed and causes dose-dependent sedation and significant decreases in HR and CO (Vesal et al., 1996; Torske et al., 1999). The addition of fentanyl, 0.01 mg/kg, to morphine for epidural injection resulted in significant decreases in MAP and vascular resistance, and increased $PaCO_2$ compared with morphine alone (Naganobu et al., 2004). Administration of glycopyrrolate IM/IV may improve HR and MAP in dogs with opioid-induced bradycardia. Medetomidine and dexmedetomidine are absorbed from the epidural space resulting in decreased HR and moderately increased

MAP (Vesal et al., 1996; Campagnol et al., 2007). In humans, respiratory depression has been reported to occur several hours after epidural morphine injection, but this does not appear to be a problem in dogs.

The incidence of other complications after epidural nerve block is low, but includes urine retention, pruritus, myoclonus, and persistent sensory or motor blockade (Troncy et al., 2002). Direct trauma of the spinal cord is a possible complication. Some agents may be neurotoxic, including lidocaine, and the addition of ketamine to lidocaine in an *in vitro* study increased cell toxicity in an additive manner (Werdehausen et al., 2011). However, no clinical or histological alterations in spinal tissue were found in dogs that had been given an intrathecal injection of ketamine, 1 mg/kg in 1 mL (Rojas et al., 2012). Postoperative urinary retention was reported in a dog following epidural analgesia with morphine and bupivacaine (Herperger, 1998).

A complication that may be regarded adversely by clients is inability of hair to grow back over the epidural site at the same rate as expected for other parts of the body and new hair may be darker than the original hair.

Infiltration; Soaker catheters

Infiltration of surgical sites with local anaesthetic solution is a common practice. Infiltration provides analgesia for the procedure in order to decrease the need for anaesthetic agents, for example, suturing of lacerations or midline infiltration of lidocaine before caesarian section. For incisional infiltration to be most effective for abdominal incisions, local anaesthetic must be injected subcutaneously and into the muscle down to the peritoneum. The effect of local infiltration on the patients' pain after surgery has been the focus of several investigations. Infiltration of 0.25% bupivacaine, 2 mg/kg, before the laparotomy incision or after closure of subcutaneous tissues was associated with decreased pain scores after anaesthesia (Savvas et al., 2008). Infiltration before skin incision was more effective than infiltration after surgery. Carpenter et al. (2004) found that bupivacaine, but not lidocaine, administered into the abdominal cavity or as a splash block on the closed linea alba after surgery decreased pain scores after surgery, although most dogs required rescue analgesia. Lidocaine, 8.8 mg/kg 2% with epinephrine 1 : 200 000, was diluted with an equal volume of isotonic saline and inserted into the peritoneal cavity just before close of the abdominal wall and a further injection of 2 mg/kg was administered as a splash block before closure of the incision (Wilson et al., 2004). Lidocaine was rapidly absorbed into the systemic circulation but plasma concentrations were only about half the reported concentrations achieved by IV infusions of lidocaine and were sustained for less than an hour. No signs of toxicity were observed in the dogs after anaesthesia.

Soaker catheters

Specific peripheral surgical sites or areas of trauma can be targeted for intermittent or continuous infusion of local anaesthetic solution. A soaker catheter is sealed at the end and has a series of pinpoint holes extending along the catheter for a distance that fits the size of the wound, typically ranging from 2.5 to 25 cm (1–10 inches) (Fig. 5.3). The sterile catheter is placed within the wound at the time of surgical closure with the free end exiting through the skin. Local anaesthetic solution, bupivacaine or lidocaine, can be injected as intermittent boluses or the catheter can be connected to a pressurized ball pump or continuous infusion pump. The anaesthetic solution slowly emerges from the holes in droplets to bathe the wound. The ON-Q® infusion system has been used in dogs with bupivacaine (Radlinsky et al., 2005) and with lidocaine (Wolfe et al., 2006). In another series of cases, either purchased or homemade sterile soaker catheters were used to deliver either 0.5% bupivacaine as boluses or 2% lidocaine as a continuous infusion of 2 mg/kg/h (Abelson et al., 2009). The concentration of the solutions was adjusted on an individual basis depending on the volume of solution needed to bathe the size of the wound. Extreme care must be taken to avoid bacterial contamination when administering anaesthetic solution or changing connections.

Intercostal nerve block

This block is commonly used to provide analgesia after lateral thoracotomy and can be performed before the start of surgery or by the surgeon during closure of the thoracic wall. The intercostal nerve should be blocked where it lies on the caudal surface of the rib. Injection of bupivacaine should be made as close to the head of the rib as possible before the nerve begins to send off branches. The nerve runs alongside a vein and artery, consequently, the syringe must be aspirated before injection to prevent intravascular injection. An acute and dramatic drop in blood pressure can follow accidental IV injection of bupivacaine. Generally, two nerves cranial to the thoracotomy and two caudal are blocked. The total maximum dose of 2.5 mg/kg of 0.5% bupivacaine is calculated and the volume divided between the sites and not to exceed administration of the total volume. Any bupivacaine remaining after perineural infiltration can be injected down the chest tube to minimize pain associated with pleural friction from the chest tube. A 75% success rate for analgesia for 12 hours after thoracotomy was reported in one investigation of this block (Pascoe & Dyson, 1993). Blockade of too many nerves will impair ventilation.

Interpleural block

Injection of bupivacaine, 1.5–2.5 mg/kg, into the interpleural space will provide analgesia after thoracotomy. The bupivacaine can be instilled into the pleural cavity at the end of surgery before starting wound closure or instilled down a chest tube, flushed in by a small amount of sterile saline. Analgesia develops most effectively when the dog is in dorsal recumbency so that the bupivacaine collects near the vertebral column, and blocks the nerves at that point. Injection with the dog in sternal position may only result in ventral analgesia.

Injection of 1.5 mg/kg after lateral thoracotomy was found to produce a significant improvement in PaO$_2$ and some measures of pulmonary function for several hours after anaesthesia when compared to systemic administration of morphine, 1 mg/kg (Stobie et al., 1995) or buprenorphine (Conzemius et al., 1994). Furthermore, analgesia was at least as good from interpleural bupivacaine as morphine (pain scores were lower after bupivacaine for 10 hours) and better than buprenorphine. A larger dose may be needed for analgesia after median sternotomy, however, it should be noted that a dose rate of 3 mg/kg 0.5% bupivacaine caused hypotension in some anaesthetized dogs (Kushner et al., 1995). This occurred 15 minutes after interpleural injection and was coincident with peak blood bupivacaine concentrations. A maximum total dose at one time of 2.5 mg/kg is recommended.

Supplemental injections of 1.5 mg/kg bupivacaine can be made down the chest tube as analgesia fades several hours later. Transient 30 second discomfort after injection may be observed in the conscious dog.

Intra-articular analgesia

Postoperative analgesia after arthrotomy may be provided by injection of 0.5% bupivacaine, 0.5 mg/kg, or preservative-free morphine, 0.1 mg/kg. A prospective blinded study comparing analgesic effects of these drugs after stifle surgery in dogs confirmed that less supplemental analgesia was needed in dogs receiving intra-articular bupivacaine or morphine compared with dogs receiving a placebo (Sammarco et al., 1996). Injections were made after the joint capsule and subcutaneous tissues were closed. Intra-articular bupivacaine provided the greatest analgesia for up to 24 hours and HR, MAP, RR, and pain scores were the lowest values postoperatively.

In humans, postoperative analgesia for shoulder, knee, and hip surgeries frequently includes infiltration of bupivacaine into the joint and periarticular tissues. This is followed by continued postoperative analgesia for 2–3 days using a catheter implanted at the time of surgery and continuous infusion of local anaesthetic solution from a ball pump. Recently, the toxicity effects of bupivacaine and lidocaine on articular cartilage were discussed in light of reports of chondrolysis after arthroscopy in humans. Analyses of reports indicate that the cases were associated with continuous infusion of the local anaesthetic into the joint postoperatively and the effect of a single injection has yet to be determined. Chondrolysis in humans has been associated with both bupivacaine and lidocaine, however, an in vitro comparison using equine articular chondrocytes revealed that although both agents caused cell death, bupivacaine was more toxic than lidocaine (Park et al., 2011).

Administration of morphine into the joint provides some analgesia though not as effective as bupivacaine. Non-inflamed canine joint tissue has been shown to contain minimal specific opioid binding sites but by 12 hours after initiation of inflammation there is approximately a 50-fold increase in the mean density of specific morphine binding sites in articular and periarticular tissues (Keates et al., 1999).

Intravenous regional analgesia (IVRA)

This method provides a safe and simple way of providing analgesia in a tractable or sedated or lightly anaesthetized dog of the distal part of the limb for suturing lacerations, excision of tissue masses, and surgery of the toes.

The dog should be restrained on its side and the appropriate limb held above heart level for 2–3 minutes partially to exsanguinate it prior to application of a tourniquet. Thin rubber tourniquets can be painful and a blood pressure cuff inflated to a pressure above systolic arterial pressure is least likely to cause the dog distress. On the forelimb, the tourniquet is placed either high on the forearm or above the elbow and on the hind limb above the hock. Lidocaine, 4 mg/kg, is injected with a 25 gauge needle into any vein distal to the occluding cuff, with the direction of injection being made towards the toes. The lidocaine should not include epinephrine which will cause vasoconstriction, impair diffusion of lidocaine and possibly result in tissue ischaemia. Onset of analgesia will be in about 15 minutes and this will persist as long as the tourniquet is in place. Failure of analgesia will occur if the tourniquet does not effectively occlude arterial or venous blood flow. Sensation will return to the limb within a few minutes of removal of the tourniquet.

Intravenous injection may be difficult in thick-skinned dogs and this problem can be circumvented by preplacement of a small indwelling catheter or Butterfly needle prior to application of the tourniquet.

The dog can be sedated with any drug combination appropriate for the dog. If the sedatives are to be reversed at the end of the procedure, it must be remembered that IVRA confers no lasting analgesia after the tourniquet is removed. Other agents have been investigated as additives to lidocaine for IVRA with limited success.

Mandibular and maxillary nerve blocks

Blockade of these nerves will achieve analgesia for a variety of procedures in the anaesthetized dog, including teeth extractions, tumour excisions and reconstructive surgery of the face rostral to the last molar, maxillary and mandibular fracture repairs, rhinotomy, and rhinoscopy. The nerves are commonly blocked where they enter or exit the skull

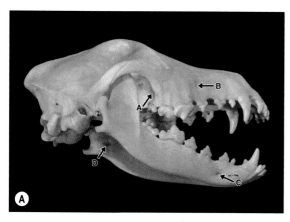
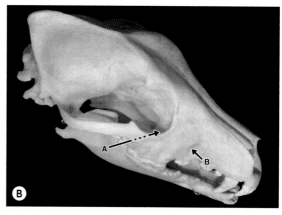

Figure 15.30 Nerve blocks of the rostral half of the head and the mandible. (A) Angle of the arrow indicates the direction of needle insertion through the mouth, alongside the caudal border of the maxilla adjacent to the last molar tooth to reach the sphenopalatine and posterior palatine foramina; B: infraorbital foramen; C: mental foramen adjacent to the second premolar tooth; D: mandibular foramen. The angle of the arrow indicates direction of insertion of the needle, perpendicular to the mandible just rostral to the angular process of the mandible and adjacent to the bone on the medial surface of the mandible. (B) A: Arrow is pointing to the sphenopalatine and posterior palatine foramina. The angle of the arrow indicates a lateral approach to the head with the direction of the needle inserted perpendicular to the skull beneath the anterior border of the zygomatic arch, and angled slightly dorsally and rostrally; B: arrow indicates direction of needle insertion to enter the infraorbital foramen.

(Fig. 15.30). Local anaesthetic solution deposited on the maxillary nerve as it enters the sphenopalatine and posterior palatine foramina will desensitize the hard and soft palate, upper teeth, gingivae and skin over the maxilla. There are two approaches employed, intraoral and percutaneous, and the choice may be dictated by the conformation of the dog. For the intraoral approach, with the dog on its side and the ventral surface of the neck next to the anaesthetist, the anaesthetist places a hand on the dog's forehead and straightens the head and neck to open the dog's mouth. The thumb is used to push up on the dog's lip to expose the last upper cheek tooth. The needle with syringe attached is introduced through the gum adjacent to the last molar tooth and is inserted along the caudal border of the maxilla as shown (Fig. 15.30A). A 25 gauge needle can be used for medium or small dogs and a 22 gauge needle for bigger dogs. For the percutaneous approach, the rostral end of the zygomatic arch is palpated where it joins the maxilla and the needle is inserted through the skin perpendicular to the skull and ventral to the end of the zygomatic arch (Fig. 15.30B). The needle is then directed slightly dorsally and rostrally. Contact may be made with the palatine bone and the needle withdrawn slightly. As always, the syringe must be aspirated before injecting local anaesthetic solution to ensure that the tip of the needle is not in an artery or vein.

The infraorbital nerve is a continuation of the maxillary nerve that emerges from the vertically oval infraorbital foramen positioned dorsal to the septum between the third and fourth cheek teeth. Just before the infraorbital nerve emerges from the infraorbital canal it gives off the rostral maxillary alveolar nerve that supplies the upper canine and incisor teeth. The infraorbital foramen can be approached through the mouth by lifting the upper lip or approached directly through the skin. The direction of the 25 gauge needle (or even smaller in tiny dogs) should be parallel to the infraorbital canal and the tip introduced gently for a short distance, remembering that the canal is short in brachycephalic dog breeds. The dog's nose is elevated, the infraorbital foramen occluded by finger pressure, the syringe aspirated to ensure the needle is not in a blood vessel, and local anaesthetic agent injected slowly to encourage caudal flow.

The mandibular alveolar nerve that is sensory to the lower teeth enters the mandible on the medial surface just rostral to the angular process (see Fig. 15.30A). To block this nerve before it enters the mandibular foramen, the needle is introduced through the skin perpendicular to the edge of the mandible at the caudal end of the concave edge of the body of the mandible. The needle must be inserted next to the bone and beneath the muscle to a distance that depends on the size of the dog. The needle can be inserted a little deeper than anticipated and, after aspiration of the syringe, local anaesthetic agent injected in a stream while partly withdrawing the needle. The mandibular foramen can also be approached through the mouth but locating the site and inserting the syringe may be a problem due to lack of space. The rostral, middle, and caudal mental nerves exit the mandible at the rostral end of the mandible. The middle mental foramen is largest and is located adjacent to the second premolar tooth. The lip is depressed, the foramen palpated and injection just inside the foramen will desensitize the canine and incisors.

The total volume to be injected for all sites should not exceed 4 mg/kg lidocaine or 2.5 mg/kg bupivacaine and, if combined, not more than 50% of the maximum dose of each. The plunger should always be withdrawn before injection to ensure that the needle is not in a blood vessel as IV injection of bupivacaine will cause serious cardiovascular depression. The volume injected at each site is usually about 0.5 mg/kg lidocaine or 0.25 mg/kg bupivacaine. Lidocaine has a rapid onset and duration of approximately 1.0–1.5 hours; bupivacaine has a slow onset and duration of 6–12 hours. Choice of agent therefore depends on the procedure to be performed. Lidocaine and bupivacaine can be combined in the same syringe. Chloroprocaine, 1 mL of 2% per site depending on the size of the dog, has been described for producing analgesia of the infraorbital and inferior alveolar nerves in anaesthetized dogs (Gross et al., 1997). Onset of analgesia occurred within 10 minutes and duration lasted less than 90 minutes in the majority of dogs but persisted in isolated teeth for up to 96 hours.

There is always concern that blockade of the maxillary and mandibular nerves may put the dog at risk for chewing its tongue during recovery from anaesthesia and for aspiration of fluid collecting in the pharynx. To date, these problems have not been reported. It has been suggested that a precautionary measure is to place the dogs in sternal recumbency with their tongues positioned within their mouths after extubation.

Ocular nerve blocks

Topical application of 0.5% proparacaine (proxymetacaine) hydrochloride will desensitize the cornea. The palpebral reflex can be abolished by an auriculopalpebral nerve block. Administration of an NMBA will cause paralysis of extraocular muscles, a centrally placed eye in the orbit, decreased IOP, and abolish the palpebral reflex but provide no analgesia.

Peribulbar and retrobulbar

A retrobulbar injection involves insertion of a needle into the orbit and advancing the tip behind the eyeball within the muscle cone and near the nerves. In contrast, peribulbar injection implies deposition of local anaesthetic solution less deep within the orbit and outside the muscle cone. Arguments against using either block for ocular surgery are that pressure on the eyeball in the presence of a corneal ulcer may induce eye rupture, that laceration of a blood vessel may cause haemorrhage that puts pressure on the eye and initiates an oculocardiac reflex or interferes with ocular blood flow, needle penetration of the globe may transfer bacteria, and insertion of the needle may introduce bacteria into the orbit. A life-threatening complication occurs when the needle penetrates the dural cuff near the optic nerve and local anaesthetic solution diffuses centrally to cause apnoea or cardiac arrest. The merits and disadvantages of retrobulbar and peribulbar blocks are argued in human ophthalmology. A 2008 Cochrane Database review found no differences in reported pain control and paralysis of the ocular muscles between the two techniques and a very small complication rate. Peribulbar and retrobulbar injections are commonly used for eye enucleations in veterinary medicine, but rarely for other procedures mainly owing to concern that should an increase in IOP occur it may have an adverse impact on the surgical outcome.

The surgical procedure of enucleation of the eye may elicit a response even from dogs apparently adequately anaesthetized. Analgesia may be provided by premedication with an opioid augmented by administration of IV lidocaine, 1–2 mg/kg, or a retrobulbar or peribulbar block of lidocaine and/or bupivacaine. Observation of dogs given a retrobulbar injection of preservative-free 0.5% bupivacaine approximately 20 minutes before the start of surgery identified a significant decrease in use of postoperative analgesics (Myrna et al., 2010). The dosage of bupivacaine in the trial never exceeded 2 mg/kg and the maximum volume injected did not exceed 3 mL in any patient. Doses were calculated using 0.5% bupivacaine: dogs weighing <5 kg were given bupivacaine, 0.05 mL/kg (0.25 mg/kg) diluted with an equal volume of saline, dogs 5–15 kg were given 2 mL of bupivacaine (0.7–2.0 mg/kg), and dogs >15 kg were injected with 3 mL bupivacaine (1 mg/kg for a 15 kg dog, decreased for heavier dogs). An experimental investigation of retrobulbar injection of latex and contrast agent followed by MRI in euthanized dogs and injection of 2 mL of 2% lidocaine in anaesthetized 10 kg dogs that were recovered from anaesthesia was not associated with complications (Accola et al., 2006). The duration of nerve block with this dose of lidocaine in this size dog was approximately 2 hours.

A technique for retrobulbar injection is as follows. The skin around the eye is cleaned as for a surgical procedure. The anaesthetist, wearing sterile gloves, takes a 22 gauge 3.8 cm (1.5 inch) spinal needle and bends it slightly in the middle to form a gentle crescent. The stilette is then removed. The tip of the needle is inserted at the edge of the orbital rim on the lower eyelid just lateral to the middle of the eyelid. The needle is advanced until a slight popping sensation is felt as the needle penetrates the orbital fascia and then the needle is advanced parallel to the curvature of the orbit to skirt the globe before being directed slightly dorsally and nasally. The syringe containing bupivacaine or lidocaine is attached to the needle and aspirated first to check that the tip of the needle is not in a blood vessel before injecting. Resistance to injection is a sign that the needle must be repositioned. The onset of nerve block is signified by the eye assuming a central position, complete pupillary dilation, and mild exophthalmia. Retrobulbar injection is contraindicated when infection is present in the eye or conjunctiva.

Technique for needle insertion for peribulbar injection is the same except that no attempt is made to redirect the needle within the muscle cone. Local anaesthetic solution is deposited between the ocular muscles and the orbit. A successful block is achieved by insertion of the needle dorsally as well as ventrally and dividing the total volume of anaesthetic solution to be injected between the two sites.

Intracameral lidocaine

The effects of intracameral injection of preservative-free 2% lidocaine, 0.3 mL, have been investigated in dogs anaesthetized for intraocular surgery including phaco-emulsification (Park et al., 2010). No increase in isoflurane was needed to maintain stable cardiovascular parameters during surgery in the dogs injected with lidocaine compared with balanced salt solution controls. The need for rescue analgesia after anaesthesia was significantly delayed by 3 hours. In this study, a 30 gauge needle on a 1 mL syringe was inserted into the anterior chamber slightly medial to the 12 o'clock position and 0.3 mL of fluid aspirated before injecting 0.3 mL of lidocaine 15 minutes before the start of surgery. A previous study (Gerding et al., 2004) had confirmed that injection of 0.1 mL of 1% or 2% preservative-free lidocaine produced no significant differences in IOP, central corneal thickness, endothelial cell density, cell area, or cell morphology in any eyes. An increase in the amount of aqueous flare was expected and was observed for 48 hours in injected eyes regardless of the use of lidocaine or salt solution.

Paravertebral nerve block (brachial plexus)

Paravertebral nerve blocks providing analgesia of the entire forelimb including the humerus involve injections of local anaesthetic solution on the nerves supplying the brachial plexus (sixth, seventh and eighth cervical nerves, first thoracic) as they leave the vertebral canal through intervertebral foramina between adjacent vertebrae (Fig. 15.31). Contributions from fifth cervical and second thoracic nerves to the brachial plexus are more often absent than present (Budras et al., 2007). The cranial nerves leave the vertebral canal cranial to the vertebra of the same name, except for the first and eighth cervical nerves. The phrenic nerve arises from the fifth to seventh cervical nerves and runs medial to the brachial plexus, and the axillary artery and vein lie ventromedial to the caudal portion of the brachial plexus. The transverse processes of the cervical vertebrae in this area are well developed and bifurcated and the transverse process of C6 has a large ventral expanded plate that can be used as a landmark. The cervical nerves to be blocked have been described ultrasonographically as lying beneath the scalenus muscles (Bagshaw et al., 2009). The sixth cervical nerve root passes obliquely across the cranial edge of the expanded plate of the transverse process of C6, the seventh cervical nerve lies between the transverse processes of C6 and C7, and the eighth cervical nerve lies immediately caudal to the transverse process of C7 (Fig. 15.31). The first thoracic nerve

root lies caudal to the head of the first rib. There are several recommendations for the angle of insertion of the needle to the appropriate sites and the procedure can be performed blindly or guided by use of a peripheral nerve stimulator or ultrasound (Lemke & Dawson, 2000; Hofmeister et al., 2007; Lemke & Creighton, 2008; Bagshaw et al., 2009; Rioja et al., 2012).

The dog is anaesthetized and the area to be injected must be clipped and the skin prepped as for a sterile procedure. An assistant can elevate the scapula away from the dog to facilitate palpation of the transverse process of C6 and the head of the first rib. These sites may be difficult to palpate in overweight or heavily muscled dogs. In one technique (Hofmeister et al., 2007), three separate needle insertions at the same angle are used to block the sixth to eighth cervical nerves. A 22 gauge, 3.75–7.5 cm (1.5–3 inch) spinal needle is inserted 2–3 cm from dorsal midline (for dogs 10–30 kg), in a sagittal plane parallel to the median and passing from craniodorsal to caudoventral at a 45° angle to the dorsal (horizontal) plane at the level of the nerve. Palpation of the head of the first rib is the landmark to guide the needle towards the eighth cervical nerve, at an angle as described for the first two nerves, to deposit local anaesthetic cranial to the head of the rib. If the head of the rib cannot be palpated, the site of needle insertion for the eighth cervical nerve is the distance between the first two skin punctures measured caudally from the second puncture. The T1–2 intervertebral space is identified by palpation of the head of the first rib or by palpating the first rib and extrapolating dorsally to the probable intersection of the rib and the spinal column. The needle to block the first thoracic nerve should be inserted at the same distance from dorsal midline but vertically and perpendicular to the dorsal (horizontal) plane. Keeping a finger on the head of the first rib identifies the maximum depth of the needle and may avoid penetration of the pleural space. The syringe should be always be aspirated before injection to minimize the risk of intravascular injection of local anaesthetic agent. The volume of 2% lidocaine or 0.5% bupivacaine to be injected at each site is not fully defined but the total volume for all nerves should not exceed 8 mg/kg of lidocaine or 2.5 mg/kg of bupivacaine. Onset of action of bupivacaine may be long, similar to its use for other nerve blocks, although a decrease in twitch strength induced by a peripheral nerve stimulator may be observed even during injection. Significant spread of anaesthetic solution will occur at an injection volume of 0.1 mL/kg, increasing the likelihood of phrenic nerve and epidural block (Bagshaw et al., 2009). Although volumes as low as 0.3 mL per site have been injected using ultrasonography with 100% accuracy in canine cadavers, the lowest volume that will produce analgesia is yet to be determined.

An alternative technique for this nerve block has been described (Lemke & Creighton, 2008; Rioja et al., 2012). After identifying the transverse process of C6 by palpation, a 22 gauge 3.8 cm (1.5 inch) or 20 gauge 7.6 cm (3 inch)

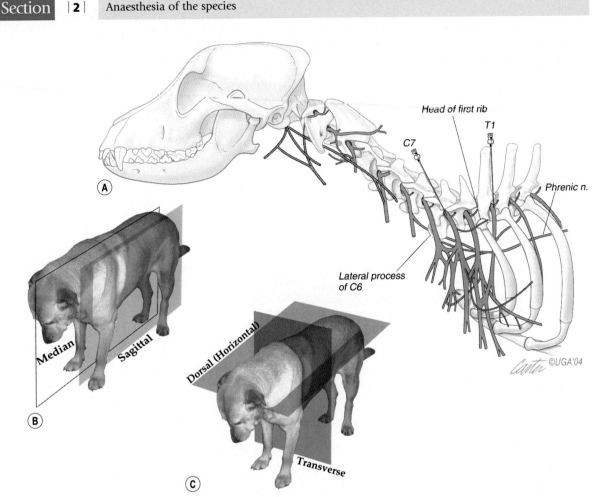

Figure 15.31 Anatomic landmarks for performing the paravertebral nerve block in the dog. Note the angle of insertion for the needle at the first three sites (45°) is different from the angle of insertion for the needle at the caudal site (90°) ©2000–2012 University of Georgia Research Foundation, Inc. Art by William 'Kip' Carter (University of Georgia), with permission from John Wiley & Sons Ltd (Hofmeister et al., 2007). Inserts: the median plane divides the body into equal right and left halves. A sagittal plane is parallel and lateral to the median plane and divides the body longitudinally but into unequal parts. The transverse plane is perpendicular to the median plane and cuts the body into cranial and caudal parts. The dorsal (horizontal) plane is perpendicular to both median and transverse planes and cuts the body into dorsal and ventral parts or the extremities into proximal and distal. Drawn from descriptions in Budras et al. (2007).

hypodermic needle is inserted 2–5 cm from dorsal midline, depending on the dog's bodyweight, dorsal to the cranial and caudal margins of the transverse process of C6 and directed ventrally and medially in the transverse plane but at a 30–45° angle to the sagittal plane, until the needle contacts the transverse process. The needle is then reoriented to become parallel to the sagittal plane and advanced cranially beyond the transverse process, where an injection is made to block the sixth cervical nerve. The tip of the needle is then reoriented caudally to the edge of the transverse process and a second injection is made to block the seventh cervical nerve. The eighth cervical and first thoracic nerves are blocked where they converge at a place dorsal to the axillary artery and costochondral junction along the

cranial margin of the first rib. The axillary artery and the first rib are palpated. The needle is inserted slightly dorsal to the spine of the scapula and is directed ventromedially at a 30° angle to the sagittal plane along the cranial edge of the rib. Local anaesthetic solution is injected when the tip of the needle is 1–2 cm dorsal to the chostrochondral junction and after aspiration to confirm that the tip is not in a blood vessel.

Blockade of some but not all nerves might decrease postsurgical analgesia requirement but is likely to result in an uneven plane of anaesthesia during the surgical procedure. The nerves may be more accurately located with the aid of electrical nerve stimulation or ultrasound. An experimental study involving injection of contrast agent and methylene blue under ultrasound guidance has identified ultrasonographic landmarks for cervical paravertebral injections and confirmed staining of all four nerves in every cadaver (Bagshaw et al., 2009). Injections of methylene blue made only by palpation of landmarks achieved staining of all four nerves in 33% (Hofmeister et al., 2007) or 17% of legs (Rioja et al., 2012). However, a comparison between techniques involving palpation only or with aid of peripheral nerve stimulation or ultrasound, determined that the palpation only technique was 2.37 and 2.25 times more likely to stain a greater number of nerves than the nerve stimulation or ultrasound techniques, respectively (Rioja et al., 2012). One explanation may be that a considerable degree of experience with ultrasound at this anatomical area is required for accuracy. Increased practice with ultrasound-guided needle insertion and a change to an axillary approach with the dog in dorsal recumbency appears to have increased performance accuracy of this block (Campoy L, presented at the 11th World Congress of Veterinary Anaesthesia, Cape Town, South Africa 2012).

The injected anaesthetic solution will spread to the spinal cord or phrenic nerve in a proportion of blocks and the degree of spread is decreased by use of smaller volumes of local anaesthetic (Lemke & Dawson, 2000; Lemke & Creighton, 2008; Bagshaw et al., 2009; Rioja et al., 2012). Paralysis of the cervical spinal cord or phrenic nerve may result in adverse cardiovascular or respiratory effects. Adverse effects of this block in clinical patients have not been reported in the veterinary literature. Experimental unilateral phrenic nerve blockade with interpleural bupivacaine in dogs resulted in partial or complete loss of diaphragmatic function on the side of the block (Kowalski et al., 1992). Phrenic nerve transection resulting in hemidiaphragmatic paralysis was documented to cause a direct detrimental effect on the expansion of both lungs (De Troyer et al., 2009). Pneumothorax is a potential complication when the needle penetrates the thorax. Staining of the visceral pleura indicating thoracic puncture was observed in 1/24 dogs injected using the palpation method, 1/21 dogs using electrical nerve stimulation location, and 3/23 dogs using the ultrasound-guided technique (Rioja et al., 2012).

Safety of the cervical paravertebral block requires a detailed knowledge of the anatomy of the area and close monitoring of respiratory function during blockade. Further investigation is needed to determine the lowest dose/site that will provide analgesia.

Pelvic limb blocks

Femoral and sciatic nerve blocks provide analgesia during surgery allowing the concentration of inhalation agent to be decreased, reduce spinal cord sensitization, and provide analgesia for some hours following anaesthesia. Epidural analgesia will provide the same benefits but causes greater vasodilation that significantly decreases arterial pressure, and may cause urinary retention in recovery that will necessitate manual compression of the bladder to express urine. The femoral and sciatic nerves can be blocked by injecting local anaesthetic solution as the nerves emerge from the spinal column (paralumbar plexus block and parasacral plexus block) resulting in complete sensory and motor blockade of the entire limb. Potential complications of paravertebral injections are the risk of spread into the epidural space, resulting in bilateral hind limb paralysis, and the risk of needle penetration of the abdominal cavity. An alternative to paravertebral injection is to target the nerves more distally in the limb. Potential disadvantages of this technique are that some proximal branches may be unblocked such that analgesia may not be complete, and that the femoral artery and vein are adjacent to the femoral nerve at the site of injection introducing risk of intravascular injection or haematoma formation. The landmarks to perform these blocks have been described following detailed dissections. Techniques involving ultrasound-guided placement of an electrical needle locator are evolving to facilitate accurate, safe, and effective nerve blocks. Direct nerve trauma during performance of nerve block is a possibility. If resistance to injection is felt, pressure on the syringe should cease immediately and the needle tip repositioned. However, no neurological deficits were recorded in 265 dogs that had received femoral and sciatic nerve blocks for stifle surgery (Vettorato et al., 2012). Sciatic nerve damage has been reported in dogs and cats as a consequence of pelvic, femoral, and stifle surgery, or intramuscular injections, that were not caused by regional nerve blocks (Forterre et al., 2007).

General principles applying to femoral and sciatic nerve blocks include clipping the hair over the injection sites, aseptic preparation of the skin, and aspiration before injection of local anaesthetic solution. The dog should be adequately sedated or anaesthetized and lying in lateral recumbency with the leg to be blocked uppermost. Nerve stimulating needles 21 or 22 gauge and 50 mm and 100 mm are used according to the size of the dog and the positive electrode can be clipped to the skin of the ventral abdomen.

Paralumbar plexus block

The femoral nerve is formed from branches of the fourth, fifth and sixth lumbar nerves. Lumbar nerves emerge caudal to their corresponding vertebrae. One published technique is to block all three nerves with separate injections (Portela et al., 2010). The nerve stimulator needle was inserted between L4 and L5, 1–2 cm lateral to midline and with the duration of electrical stimulus set at 0.1 milliseconds (ms), the frequency at 2 Hz, and the current at 2 mA, advanced within the sagittal plane. The electrical current was progressively decreased until contraction of the quadriceps or sartorius muscles was elicited with 0.5 mA. This procedure was repeated for the fifth lumbar nerve by insertion of the needle between L5 and L6 and observing contraction of the quadriceps muscle and extension of the knee joint. The needle was introduced between L6 and L7 to block the sixth lumbar nerve and injection was made after observation of contraction of the gluteal or biceps femoris muscles with extension of the hip. In this experimental study comparing three anaesthetic dose rates, the longest and most complete block was obtained following injection of 0.5% bupivacaine, 0.05 mL/kg/site (total 0.75 mg/kg). The duration of complete femoral nerve blockade was 6 ± 2 hours (Portela et al., 2010).

An alternative technique has been described where the dorsal spinous process of L5 was identified and the nerve stimulator needle inserted 1–2 cm lateral to midline and advanced parallel to the sagittal plane. When bone was contacted, needle was redirected into a slightly more caudal direction so as to pass over the transverse process until a contraction of the quadriceps muscle was observed at a current of 0.6 mA (Campoy et al., 2008). This was an experimental study that included injection of bupivacaine and methylene blue followed by euthanasia and dissection. No nerve staining was found in six dogs receiving either 0.1 or 0.2 mL/kg of injectate, epidural spread was found in two dogs and traces of dye were found in the abdominal cavity of two dogs. The results indicate that this approach did not produce consistent nerve blockade unless a higher dose of 0.4 mL/kg was used. These authors used a more distal blockade of the femoral nerve in a later clinical study. An investigation of 265 client-owned dogs administered pelvic limb blocks for surgery identified complete records for 115 dogs, 95 of which received paralumbar plexus and sciatic nerve blocks and 20 received femoral nerve and sciatic nerve blocks that were performed according to the techniques described by Campoy et al. in 2008 (Vettorato et al., 2012). The dose rates of 0.5% bupivacaine or 0.75% ropivacaine administered were for the paralumbar plexus, 1 ± 0.4 mg/kg, femoral nerve, 0.4 ± 0.2 mg/kg, and sciatic nerve 0.6 ± 0.3 mg/kg. The overall success rate for the nerve blocks was 77% with a slightly higher success rate in dogs receiving femoral nerve blocks compared with paralumbar plexus blocks. Postoperative analgesia was assessed every 2 hours by a 'blinded' observer. Interestingly, there was no difference in rescue doses of methadone given to dogs with successful or unsuccessful blocks. The authors proposed that although unsuccessful blocks may not provide sufficient analgesia to prevent responses to surgical manipulation, partial analgesia may have contributed to patient comfort in recovery.

Femoral nerve block

With the dog lying on its side, the limb to be blocked is abducted and elevated to an angle of 90° to the table and extended caudally. The femoral triangle is identified by palpating the pectineus muscle caudally, the sartorius muscle cranially, and the iliopsoas muscle proximally. A 50 mm stimulating needle with current set at 1 mA is advanced through the skin towards the iliopsoas muscle, medially to the femoral artery pulsation, while maintaining a 20–30° angle to the skin (Campoy et al., 2012a; Vettorato et al., 2012). Current is reduced towards 0.2 mA and contraction of the quadriceps muscle indicates proximity for injection of 0.5% bupivacaine, 0.1 mL/kg (Campoy et al., 2012a).

Sciatic nerve block

This nerve block can be performed with the anaesthetized dog lying in lateral recumbency with the leg to be blocked in a normal position. The site of needle insertion is described as one-third of the distance along a line from the greater trochanter of the femur to the ischiatic tuberosity (Campoy et al., 2008; Vettorato et al., 2012). The needle is inserted perpendicularly to the skin and advanced until a current >0.2–0.4 mA elicits contraction of the cranial tibial or gastrocnemius muscles (dorsiflexion or plantar extension of the foot). At this point bupivacaine, 0.1 mL/kg is injected.

A slightly different site for sciatic nerve block has been described using both nerve stimulator and ultrasound in 10 dogs sedated with infusions of propofol and dexmedetomidine for orthopaedic surgery (Campoy et al., 2012b). The needle was introduced through the skin immediately distal to the ischial tuberosity in the caudal aspect of the thigh. The sciatic nerve was located using a stimulating current of 0.4 mA. Bupivacaine 0.5% or 0.75% ropivacaine, mixed with an equal volume of dexmedetomidine, 0.5 µg/mL, was injected as a total volume of 0.1 mL/kg/nerve. Carprofen was administered at the end of surgery. Rescue analgesia with hydromorphone was not required until 9 hours after the nerves were blocked.

Parasacral plexus block

The parasacral plexus block has been performed in experimental dogs (Portela et al., 2010). An imaginary line drawn between the cranial dorsal iliac crest and the ischiatic tuberosity was divided into three equal parts. The site of the electrical stimulating needle insertion was at the junction of the cranial and middle thirds. The needle was inserted perpendicular to the skin and deep enough that electrical stimulation induced contraction of the gastrocnemius muscle or digital or tarsal flexion or extension. This site for injection is in the area where the seventh lumbar nerve joins the first and second sacral nerves. In the clinical study, results of injection of 0.05 mL/kg of 0.5% bupivacaine were inconsistent and the authors suggested that a higher dose rate might be more successful.

Peroneal and tibial nerve blocks

The peroneal and tibial nerves are easily blocked by infiltration of 2% lidocaine or 0.5% bupivacaine. The peroneal nerve is located along the craniolateral surface of the tibia just lateral to the tibial crest or more distally at the level of the hock. At the proximal site, local anaesthetic should be injected subcutaneously to block the superficial peroneal nerve and more deeply between the long and lateral digital extensor muscles to block the deep peroneal nerve. The tibial nerve is located on the medial aspect of the limb, just above the hock and cranial to the gastrocnemius tendon. A smaller bleb of local anaesthetic solution should be injected at a similar location on the lateral aspect of the limb to block a cutaneous branch. Aspiration of the syringe before injection to check for blood is essential to avoid injection into adjacent blood vessels.

RUMM blocks

The radial, ulnar, musculocutaneous, and median nerves (RUMM) can be blocked at mid-humerus level and a detailed description with diagrams has been published (Trumpatori et al., 2010). There is a case report of RUMM blocks in a conscious dog using an electrical nerve locator to identify nerves to be blocked (Bortolami & Love, 2012).

Transdermal lidocaine patch

Transdermal lidocaine patches available for use on human skin comprise of a matrix that binds the drug and controls its release. The amount of drug absorbed is proportional to the area of skin contact. Analgesia is primarily local as the amount of lidocaine absorbed is insufficient to cause

skin numbness in humans, and systemic analgesic effects are likely to be minimal because plasma lidocaine concentrations are low when the patch is properly applied. Consequently, transdermal lidocaine patches are used as part of a multimodal analgesia protocol. Measurements in experimental dogs have documented low and highly variable plasma lidocaine concentrations, peak concentrations at 24 hours after patch application, and steady state concentrations maintained for 48 hours (Ko et al., 2007) or 60 hours (Weiland et al., 2006). A depilatory agent was applied to the skin before application of the patch in one experiment and was associated with a significant increase in plasma lidocaine concentration within 5 hours (Weiland et al., 2006). Plasma lidocaine concentrations decreased over 3–6 hours after patch removal. One 700 mg lidocaine patch was used in dogs of mean weight 12 kg and two patches were used in dogs averaging 20 kg. The hair was clipped from the skin at the site of application (over the thorax or either side of midline) and the skin prepared with chlorhexidine as for a surgical procedure. An adhesive protective dressing was placed over the patch(es) to promote retention. Lidocaine patches are recommended for unbroken skin and the absorption may be different if placed over a surgical wound. The patches are clean but not sterile. Investigations of analgesic effects in clinical canine patients are needed to determine optimal use.

REFERENCES

Abelson, A.L., McCobb, E.C., Shaw, S., et al., 2009. Use of wound soaker catheters for the administration of local anesthetic for post-operative analgesia: 56 cases. Vet Anaesth Analg 36, 597–602.

Accola, P.J., Bentley, E., Smith, L.J., et al., 2006. Development of a retrobulbar injection technique for ocular surgery and analgesia in dogs. J Am Vet Med Assoc 229, 220–225.

Adams, V.J., Evans, K.M., Sampson, J., et al., 2010. Methods and mortality results of a health survey of purebred dogs in the UK. J Small Anim Pract 51, 512–524.

Aguado, D., Benito, J., Gómez de Segura, I.A., 2011. Reduction of the minimum alveolar concentration of isoflurane in dogs using a constant rate of infusion of lidocaine-ketamine in combination with either morphine or fentanyl. Vet J 189, 63–66.

Albert, S.G., Ariyan, S., Rather, A., 2011. The effect of etomidate on adrenal function in critical illness: a systematic review. Intensive Care Med 37, 901–910.

Alderson, B., Senior, M.J., Jones, R.S., et al., 2007. Use of rocuronium administered by continuous infusion in dogs. Vet Anaesth Analg 34, 251–256.

Allweiler, S., Brodbelt, D.C., Borer, K., et al., 2007. The isoflurane-sparing and clinical effects of a constant rate infusion of remifentanil in dogs. Vet Anaesth Analg 34, 388–393.

Almeida, D.E., Rezende, M.L., Nunes, N., et al., 2004. Evaluation of intraocular pressure in association with cardiovascular parameters in normocapnic dogs anesthetised with sevoflurane and desflurane. Vet Ophthalm 7, 265–269.

Almeida, T.F., Fantoni, D.T., Mastrocinque, S., et al., 2007. Epidural anesthesia with bupivacaine, bupivacaine and fentanyl, or bupivacaine and sufentanil during intravenous administration of propofol for ovariohysterectomy in dogs. J Am Vet Med Assoc 230, 45–51.

Ambros, B., Duke-Novakovski, T., Pasloske, K.S., 2008. Comparison of the anesthetic efficacy and

cardiopulmonary effects of continuous rate infusions of alfaxalone-2-hydroxypropyl-beta-cyclodextrin and propofol in dogs. Am J Vet Res 69, 1391–1398.

American Veterinary Dental Association, 2004. Companion animal dental scaling without anesthesia. www.AVDC.org

Andreoni, V., Hughes, J.M., 2009. Propofol and fentanyl infusions in dogs of various breeds undergoing surgery. Vet Anaesth Analg 36, 523–531.

Auer, U., 2007. Clinical observations on the use of the muscle relaxant rocuronium bromide in the dog. Vet J 173, 422–427.

Auer, U., Mosing, M., Moens, Y.P.S., 2007. The effect of low dose rocuronium on globe position, muscle relaxation and ventilation in dogs: a clinical study. Vet Ophthalm 10, 295–298.

Bagshaw, H., Larenza, P., Seiler, G., 2009. A technique for ultrasound-guided paravertebral brachial plexus injections in dogs. Vet Radiol Ultrasound 50, 649–654.

Baldwin, K., Bartges, J., Buffington, T., et al., 2010. AAHA nutritional assessment guidelines for dogs and cats. J Am Anim Hosp Assoc 46, 285–296.

Barletta, M., Austin, B.R., Ko, J.C., et al., 2011. Evaluation of dexmedetomidine and ketamine in combination with opioids as injectable anesthesia for castration in dogs. J Am Vet Med Assoc 238, 1159–1167.

Bartges, J., Boynton, B., Vogt, A.H., et al., 2012. AAHA Canine life stage guidelines. J Am Anim Hosp Assoc 48, 1–11.

Baum, V.C., Palmisano, B.W., 1997. The immature heart and anesthesia. Anesthesiology 87, 1529–1548.

Beck, J.J., Staatz, A.J., Pelsue, D.H., et al., 2006. Risk factors associated with short-term outcome and development of perioperative complications in dogs undergoing surgery because of gastric dilatation-volvulus: 166 cases (1992–2003). J Am Vet Med Assoc 229, 1934–1939.

Bednarski, R.M., Grimm, K.A., Harvey, R., et al., 2011. AAHA Anesthesia guidelines for dogs and cats. J Am Anim Hosp Assoc 47, 377–385.

Bellei, E., Roncada, P., Pisoni, L., et al., 2011. The use of fentanyl-patch in dogs undergoing spinal surgery: plasma concentration and analgesic efficacy. J Vet Pharmacol Ther 34, 437–441.

Belsõ, N., Kui, R., Szegesdi, I., et al., 2011. Propofol and fentanyl induced perioperative anaphylaxis. Br J Anaesth 106, 283–284.

Benchaoui, H.A., Cox, S.R., Schneider, R.P., et al., 2007. The pharmacokinetics of maropitant, a novel neurokinin type-1 receptor antagonist, in dogs. J Vet Pharmacol Ther 30, 336–344.

Berasategui, M.T.A., 2011. Potential hypersensitivity due to food or food additive content of medicinal products in Spain. J Investig Allergol Clin Immunol 21, 496–506.

Bersenas, A.M.E., Mathews, K.A., Allen, D.G., et al., 2005. Effects of ranitidine, famotidine, pantoprazole, and omeprazole on intragastric pH in dogs. Am J Vet Res 66, 425–431.

Bonath, K., Saleh, A., 1985. Long term treatment in the dog by peridural morphine. 2nd International Congress of Veterinary Anesthesia, Sacramento, California. p 161.

Bortolami, E., Love, E.J., 2012. Use of mid-humeral block of the radial, ulnar, musculocutaneous and median (RUMM block) nerves for extensor carpi radialis muscle biopsy in a conscious dog with generalized neuro-muscular disease. Vet Anaesth Analg 39, 446–447.

Boscan, P., Monnet, E., Mama, K., et al., 2011. Effect of maropitant, a neurokinin 1 receptor antagonist, on anesthetic requirements during noxious visceral stimulation of the ovary in dogs. Am J Vet Res 72, 1576–1579.

Bosmans, T., Schauvliege, S., Gasthuys, F., et al., 2011. Influence of a preload of hydroxyethylstarch 6% on the cardiovascular effects of epidural administration of ropivacaine 0.75% in anaesthetized dogs. Vet Anaesth Analg 38, 494–504.

Branson, K.R., Ko, J., Tranquilli, W., et al., 1993. Duration of analgesia induced by epidurally administered morphine and medetomidine in dogs. J Vet Pharmacol Ther 16, 369–372.

Branson, K.R., Quandt, J.E., Martinez, E.A., et al., 2001. A multisite case report on the clinical use of sevoflurane in dogs. J Am Anim Hosp Assoc 37, 420–432.

Brodbelt, D.C., Pfeiffer, D.U., Young, L.E., et al., 2008. Results of the confidential enquiry into perioperative small animal fatalities regarding risk factors for anesthetic-related death in dogs. J Am Vet Med Assoc 233, 1096–1104.

Brownlie, S.E., 1991. An electrocardiographic survey of cardiac rhythm in Irish wolfhounds. Vet Rec 129, 470–471.

Brull, S.J., Murphy, G.S., 2010. Residual neuromuscular block: Lessons unlearned. Part II: Methods to reduce the risk of residual weakness. Anesth Analg 111, 129–140.

Buber, T., Saragusty, J., Ranen, E., et al., 2007. Evaluation of lidocaine treatment and risk factors for death associated with gastric dilatation and volvulus in dogs: 112 cases (1997–2005). J Am Vet Med Assoc 230, 1334–1339.

Budras, K.-D., McCarthy, P.H., Horowitz, A., et al., 2007. Anatomy of the Dog. Schlütersche, Hannover.

Burkitt, J.M., Haskins, S.C., Nelson, R.W., et al., 2007. Relative adrenal insufficiency in dogs with sepsis. J Vet Intern Med 21, 226–231.

Burton, S.A., Lemke, K.A., Ihle, S.L., et al., 1997. Effects of medetomidine on serum insulin and plasma glucose concentrations in clinically normal dogs. Am J Vet Res 58, 1440–1442.

Campagnol, D., Teixeira Neto, F.J., Giordano, T., et al., 2007. Effects of epidural administration of dexmedetomidine on the minimum alveolar concentration of isoflurane in dogs. Am J Vet Res 68, 1308–1318.

Campagnol, D., Teixeira-Neto, F.J., Peccinini, R., et al., 2012. Comparison of the effects of epidural or intravenous methadone on the minimum alveolar concentration of isoflurane in dogs. Vet J 192, 311–315.

Campoy, L., Martin-Flores, M., Looney, A.L., et al., 2008. Distribution of a lidocaine-methylene blue solution staining in brachial plexus, lumbar plexus and sciatic nerve blocks in the dog. Vet Anaesth Analg 35, 348–354.

Campoy, L., Martin-Flores, M., Ludders, J.W., et al., 2012a. Comparison of bupivacaine femoral and sciatic nerve block *versus* bupivacaine and morphine epidural for stifle surgery in dogs. Vet Anaesth Analg 39, 91–98.

Campoy, L., Martin-Flores, M., Ludders, J.W., et al., 2012b. Procedural sedation combined with locoregional anesthesia for orthopedic surgery of the pelvic limb in 10 dogs: case series. Vet Anaesth Analg 39, 436–440.

Carpenter, R.E., Wilson, D.V., Evans, A.T., 2004. Evaluation of intraperitoneal and incisional lidocaine or bupivacaine for analgesia following ovariohysterectomy in the dog. Vet Anaesth Analg 31, 46–52.

Chandrasekharan, N.V., Dai, H., Roos, L.T., et al., 2002. COX-3, a cyclooxygenase-1 variant inhibited by acetaminophen and other analgesic/antipyretic drugs: Cloning, structure, and expression. Proc Natl Acad Sci USA 99, 13926–13931.

Chilvers, J., Geoghegan, J., Moore, P., et al., 2007. Internal jugular vein compression to assess the correct placement of an epidural catheter in postpartum women. Anaesthesia 62, 332–334.

Clarke, K., Hall, L.W., 1975. World Veterinary Congress, Thessaloniki, Greece. p. 1688.

Clutton, R.E., 1992. Combined bolus and infusion of vecuronium in dogs. J Vet Anaesth 19, 74–77.

Columbano, N., Secci, F., Careddu, G.M., et al., 2012. Effects of lidocaine constant rate infusion on sevoflurane requirement, autonomic responses, and postoperative analgesia in dogs undergoing ovariectomy under opioid-based balanced anesthesia. Vet J 193, 448–455.

Congdon, J.M., Marquez, M., Niyom, S., et al., 2011. Evaluation of the sedative and cardiovascular effects of intramuscular administration of dexmedetomidine with and without concurrent atropine administration in dogs. J Am Vet Med Assoc 239, 81–89.

Conzemius, M.G., Brockman, D.J., King, L.G., et al., 1994. Analgesia in dogs after intercostal thoracotomy: A clinical trial comparing intravenous buprenorphine and interpleural bupivacaine. Vet Surg 23, 291–298.

Conzemius, M.G., Hill, C.M., Sammarco, J.L., et al., 1997. Correlation between subjective and objective measures used to determine severity of postoperative pain in dogs. J Am Vet Med Assoc 210, 1619–1622.

Crawford, M.W., Pehora, C., Lopez, A.V., 2009. Drug-induced acute pancreatitis in children receiving chemotherapy for acute leukemia: Does propofol increase the risk? Anesth Analg 109, 379–381.

Credie, R.G., Teixeira Neto, F.J., Ferreira, T.H., et al., 2010. Effects of methadone on the minimum alveolar concentration of isoflurane in dogs. Vet Anaesthes Analges 37, 240–249.

Cremer, J., Sum, S.O., Braun, C., et al., 2013. Assessment of maxillary and infraorbital nerve blockade for rhinoscopy in sevoflurane anesthetized dogs. Vet Anaesth Analg In press.

Crowther, J., Hrazdil, J., Jolly, D.T., et al., 1996. Growth of microorganisms in propofol, thiopental, and a 1:1 mixture of propofol and thiopental. Anesth Analg 82, 475–478.

Cullen, L.K., Raffe, M.R., Randall, D.A., et al., 1999. Assessment of the respiratory actions of intramuscular morphine in conscious dogs. Res Vet Sci 67, 141–148.

Curtis, M.B., Bednarski, R.M., Majors, L., 1989. Cardiovascular effects of vasopressors in isoflurane-anesthetized dogs before and after hemorrhage. Am J Vet Res 50, 1866–1871.

Dalens, B., Bazin, J.-E., Haberer, J.-P., 1987. Epidural bubbles as a cause of incomplete analgesia during epidural anesthesia. Anesth Analg 66, 679–683.

De Kock, M.F., Lavand'homme, P.M., 2007. The clinical role of NMDA receptor antagonists for the treatment of postoperative pain. Best Pract Res Clin Anaesthesiol 21, 85–98.

de Medicis, E., Tetrault, J.-P., Martin, R., et al., 2005. A prospective comparative study of two indirect methods for confirming the localization of an epidural catheter for postoperative analgesia. Anesth Analg 101, 1830–1833.

De Troyer, A., Leduc, D., Cappello, M., 2009. Bilateral impact on the lung of hemidiaphragmatic paralysis in the dog. Respir Physiol Neurobiol 166, 68–72.

Dewachter, P., Mouton-Faivre, C., Castells, M.C., et al., 2011. Anesthesia in the patient with multiple drug allergies: are all allergies the same? Curr Opin Anaesthesiol 24, 320–325.

Dodam, J.R., Cohn, L.A., Durham, H.E., et al., 2004. Cardiopulmonary effects of medetomidine, oxymorphone, or butorphanol in selegiline-treated dogs. Vet Anaesth Analg 31, 129–137.

Dohoo, S.E., O'Connor, M.K., McDonell, W.N., et al., 1986. A clinical comparison of oxymorphone/acepromazine and fentanyl/droperidol sedation in dogs. J Am Anim Hosp Assoc 22, 313–317.

Donaldson, L.L., Leib, M.S., Boyd, C., et al., 1993. Effect of preanesthetic medication on ease of endoscopic intubation of the duodenum in anesthetized dogs. Am J Vet Res 54, 1489–1495.

Dugdale, A.H., Pinchbeck, G.L., Jones, R.S., et al., 2005. Comparison of two thiopental infusion rates for the induction of anaesthesia in dogs. Vet Anaesth Analg 32, 360–366.

Du Pen, S.L., Ramsey, D., Chin, S., 1987. Chronic epidural morphine and preservative-induced injury. Anesthesiology 67, 987–988.

Duke, T., Caulkett, N.A., Ball, S.D., et al., 2000. Comparative analgesic and cardiopulmonary effects of bupivacaine and ropivacaine in the epidural space of the conscious dog. Vet Anaesth Analg 27, 13–21.

Duke, T., Caulkett, N.A., Tataryn, J.M., 2006. The effect of nitrous oxide on halothane, isoflurane and sevoflurane requirements in ventilated dogs undergoing ovariohysterectomy. Vet Anaesth Analg 33, 343–350.

Dyson, D.H., Doherty, T., Anderson, G.I., et al., 1990. Reversal of oxymorphone sedation by naloxone, nalmefene, and butorphanol. Vet Surg 19, 398–403.

Dyson, D.H., Sinclair, M.D., 2006. Impact of dopamine or dobutamine infusions on cardiovascular variables after rapid blood loss and volume replacement during isoflurane-induced anesthesia in dogs. Am J Vet Res 67, 1121–1130.

Dyson, H.D., Maxie, M.G., Schnurr, D., 1998. Morbidity and mortality associated with anesthetic management in small animal veterinary practice in Ontario. J Am Anim Hosp Assoc 34, 325–335.

Edwin, S.B., Walker, P.L., 2010. Controversies surrounding the use of etomidate for rapid sequence intubation in patients with suspected sepsis. Ann Pharmacother 44, 1307–1313.

Eger, E.I. II, 2001. Age, minimum alveolar anesthetic concentration, and minimum alveolar anesthetic concentration-awake. Anesth Analg 93, 947–953.

Egger, C.M., Duke, T., Archer, J., et al., 1998. Comparison of plasma fentanyl concentrations by using three transdermal fentanyl patch sizes in dogs. Vet Surg 27, 159–166.

Ehrman, R., Wira, C., Lomax, A., et al., 2011. Etomidate use in severe sepsis and septic shock patients does not contribute to mortality. Intern Emerg Med 6, 253–257.

England, G.C.W., Hammond, R., 1997. Dose-sparing effects of romifidine premedication for thiopentone and halothane anaesthesia in the dog. J Small Anim Pract 38, 141–146.

England, G.C.W., Andrews, F., Hammond, R.A., 1996. Romifidine as a premedicant to propofol induction and infusion anaesthesia in the dog. J Small Anim Pract 37, 79–83.

Favarato, E.S., de Souza, M.V., dos Santos Costa, P.R., et al., 2012. Evaluation of metoclopramide and ranitidine on the prevention of gastroesophageal reflux episodes in anesthetized dogs. Res Vet Sci 93, 466–467.

Feldman, H.S., Arthur, G.R., Pitkanen, M., et al., 1991. Treatment of acute systemic toxicity after the rapid intravenous injection of ropivacaine and bupivacaine in the conscious dog. Anesth Analg 73, 373–384.

Firth, A., Haldane, S.L., 1999. Development of a score to evaluate postoperative pain in dogs. J Am Vet Med Assoc 214, 651–660.

Forterre, F., Tomek, A., Rytz, U., et al., 2007. Iatrogenic sciatic nerve injury in eighteen dogs and nine cats. Vet Surg 36, 464–471.

Fowler, D., Isakow, K., Caulkett, N., et al., 2003. An evaluation of the analgesic effects of meloxicam in addition to epidural morphine/mepivacaine in dogs undergoing cranial cruciate ligament repair. Can Vet J 44, 643–648.

Friese, K.J., Linton, D.D., Newbound, G.C., et al., 2012a. Population pharmacokinetics of transdermal fentanyl solution following a single dose administered prior to soft tissue and orthopedic surgery. J Vet Pharmacol Ther 35 (Suppl. 2), 65–72.

Friese, K.J., Newbound, G.C., Tudan, C., et al., 2012b. Pharmacokinetics and the effect of application site on a novel, long-acting transdermal fentanyl solution in healthy laboratory Beagles. J Vet Pharmacol Ther 35 (Suppl. 2), 27–33.

Frischmeyer, K.J., Miller, P.E., Bellay, Y., et al., 1993. Parenteral anticholinergics in dogs with normal and elevated intraocular pressure. Vet Surg 22, 230–234.

Galatos, A.D., Raptopoulos, D., 1995. Gastro-oesophageal reflux during anaesthesia in the dog: the effect of age, positioning and type of surgical procedure. Vet Rec 137, 513–516.

Galloway, D.S., Ko, J.C.H., Reaugh, H.F., et al., 2004. Anesthetic indices of sevoflurane and isoflurane in unpremedicated dogs. J Am Vet Med Assoc 225, 700–704.

Garcia-Pereira, F.L., Hauptman, J., Shih, A., et al., 2010. Evaluation of electric neurostimulation to confirm correct placement of lumbosacral epidural injections in dogs. Am J Vet Res 71, 157–160.

Gerding, P.A., Turner, T.L., Hamor, R.E., et al., 2004. Effects of intracameral injection of preservative-free lidocaine on the anterior segment of the eyes in dogs. Am J Vet Res 65, 1325–1330.

Gorgi, A.A., Hofmeister, E.H., Higginbotham, M.J., et al., 2006. Effect of body position on cranial migration of epidurally injected methylene blue in recumbent dogs. Am J Vet Res 67, 219–221.

Goyenechea Jaramillo, G., Murrell, J.C., Hellebrekers, L.J., 2006. Investigation of the interaction between buprenorphine and sufentanil during anaesthesia for ovariectomy in dogs. Vet Anaesth Analg 33, 399–407.

Gross, M.E., Pope, E.R., O'Brien, D., et al., 1997. Regional anesthesia of the infraorbital and inferior alveolar nerves during noninvasive tooth pulp stimulation in halothane-anesthetized dogs. J Am Vet Med Assoc 211, 1403–1405.

Gurney, M., Cripps, P., Mosing, M., 2009. Subcutaneous pre-anaesthetic medication with acepromazine-buprenorphine is effective as and less painful than the intramuscular route. J Small Anim Pract 50, 474–477.

Gwaltney-Brant, S.M., Albretsen, J.C., Khan, S.A., 2000. 5-Hydroxytryptophan toxicosis in dogs: 21 cases (1989–1999). J Am Vet Med Assoc 216, 1937–1940.

Hall, L.W., Nolan, A.M., Sear, J.W., 1997. Disposition of propofol after medetomidine premedication in beagle dogs. J Vet Anaesth 24, 23–30.

Hammond, R.A., Alibhai, H.I.K., Walsh, K.P., et al., 1994. Desflurane in the dog; Minimum alveolar concentration (MAC) alone and in combination with nitrous oxide. J Vet Anaesth 21, 21–23.

Hardie, E.M., Hansen, B.D., Carroll, G.S., 1997. Behavior after ovariohysterectomy in the dog: what's normal? Appl Anim Behav Sci 51, 111–128.

Hashim, M.A., Waterman, A.E., Pearson, H., 1995. A comparison of the effects of halothane and isoflurane in combination with nitrous oxide on lower oesophageal sphincter pressure and barrier pressure in anaesthetised dogs. Vet Rec 137, 658–661.

Haskins, S.C., Farver, T.B., Patz, J.D., 1985. Ketamine in dogs. Am J Vet Res 46, 1855–1985.

Haskins, S.C., Farver, T.B., Patz, J.D., 1986. Cardiovascular changes in dogs given diazepam and diazepam-ketamine. Am J Vet Res 47, 795–798.

Hayes, G., Mathews, K., Kruth, S., et al., 2010. Illness severity scores in veterinary medicine: What can we learn? J Vet Intern Med 24, 457–466.

Heath, R.B., Broadstone, R.V., Wright, M., et al., 1989. Using bupivacaine hydrochloride for lumbosacral epidural analgesia. Comp Cont Educ 11, 50–55.

Heldmann, E., Brown, D.C., Shofer, F., 1999. The association of propofol usage with postoperative wound infection rate in clean wounds: a retrospective study. Vet Surg 28, 256–259.

Hellebrekers, L.J., Sap, R., 1997. Medetomidine as a premedicant for ketamine, propofol or fentanyl anaesthesia in dogs. Vet Rec 140, 545–548.

Hellebrekers, L.J., vanHerpen, H., Hird, J.F.R., et al., 1998. Clinical efficacy and safety of propofol or ketamine anaesthesia in dogs premedicated with medetomidine. Vet Rec 142, 631–634.

Hellyer, P., Muir III, W.W., Hubbell, J.A.E., et al., 1989. Cardiorespiratory effects of the intravenous administration of tiletamine-zolazepam to dogs. Vet Surg 18, 160–165.

Hellyer, P.W., Mama, K.R., Shafford, H.L., et al., 2001. Effects of diazepam and flumazenil on minimum alveolar concentrations for dogs anesthetized with isoflurane or a combination of isoflurane and fentanyl. Am J Vet Res 62, 555–560.

Hendrix, P.K., Raffe, M.R., Robinson, E.P., et al., 1996. Epidural administration of bupivacaine, morphine, or their combination for postoperative analgesia in dogs. J Am Vet Med Assoc 209, 598–607.

Herperger, L., 1998. Postoperative urinary retention in a dog following morphine with bupivacaine epidural analgesia. Can Vet J 39, 650–652.

Hill, R.C., Scott, K.C., 2004. Energy requirements and body surface area of cats and dogs. J Am Vet Med Assoc 225, 689–694.

Hoffman, W.D., Banks, S.M., Alling, D.W., et al., 1991. Factors that determine the hemodynamic response to inhalation anesthetics. J Appl Physiol 70, 2155–2163.

Hofmeister, E.H., Egger, C.M., 2004. Transdermal fentanyl patches in small animals. J Am Anim Hosp Assoc 40, 468–478.

Hofmeister, E.H., Kent, M., Read, M.R., 2007. Paravertebral block for forelimb anesthesia in the dog-an anatomic study. Vet Anaesth Analg 34, 139–142.

Hofmeister, E.H., Mosunic, C.B., Torres, B.T., et al., 2006a. Effects of ketamine, diazepam, and their combination on intraocular pressures in clinically normal dogs. Am J Vet Res 67, 1136–1139.

Hofmeister, E.H., Williams, C.O., Braun, C., et al., 2006b. Influence of lidocaine and diazepam on peri-induction intraocular pressures in dogs anesthetized with propofol-atracurium. Can J Vet Res 70, 251–256.

Holton, L.L., Scott, E.M., Nolan, A.M., et al., 1998a. Relationship between physiological factors and clinical pain in dogs scored using a numerical rating scale. J Small Anim Pract 39, 469–474.

Holton, L.L., Scott, E.M., Nolan, A.M., et al., 1998b. Comparison of three methods used for assessment of pain in dogs. J Am Vet Med Assoc 212, 61–66.

Hoskins, J.D., 1995. The geriatric dog. Perspectives May/June, 39–46.

Hysing, E.S., Celly, J.E., Doursout, M.-F., et al., 1992. Comparative effects of halothane, enflurane, and isoflurane at equihypotensive doses on cardiac performance and coronary and renal blood flows in chronically instrumented dogs. Anesthesiology 76, 979–984.

Iff, I., Moens, Y.P.S., 2010. Evaluation of extradural pressure waves and the 'lack of resistance' test to confirm extradural needle placement in dogs. Vet J 185, 328–331.

Iff, I., Moens, Y., Schatzmann, U., 2007. Use of pressure waves to confirm the correct placement of epidural needles in dogs. Vet Rec 161, 22–25.

Ilkiw, J.E., Pascoe, P.J., Haskins, S.C., et al., 1992. Cardiovascular and respiratory effects of propofol administration in hypovolemic dogs. Am J Vet Res 53, 2323–2327.

Imagawa, V.H., Fantoni, D.T., Tatarunas, A.C., et al., 2011. The use of different doses of metamizole for post-operative analgesia in dogs. Vet Anaesth Analg 38, 385–393.

Ingvast-Larsson, C., Holgersson, A., Bondesson, U., et al., 2010. Clinical pharmacology of methadone. Vet Anaesth Analg 37, 48–56.

Iseri, T., Nishimura, R., Nagahama, S., et al., 2010. Epidural spread of iohexol following the use of air or saline in the 'loss of resistance' test. Vet Anaesth Analg 37, 526–530.

Itami, T., Tamaru, N., Kawase, K., et al., 2011. Cardiovascular effects of tramadol in dogs anesthetized with sevoflurane. J Vet Med Sci 73, 1603–1609.

Jackson, A.M., Tobias, K., Long, C., et al., 2004. Effects of various agents on laryngeal motion during laryngoscopy in normal dogs. Vet Surg 33, 102–106.

Jacobson, J.D., McGrath, C.J., Smith, E.P., 1994. Cardiorespiratory effects of four opioid-tranquilizer combinations in dogs. Vet Surg 23, 299–306.

Jones, R.S., Brearley, J.C., 1987. Atracurium infusion in the dog. J Small Anim Pract 28, 197–201.

Jones, R.S., Young, L.E., 1991. Vecuronium infusion in the dog. J Small Anim Pract 32, 509–512.

Joubert, K.E., 2009. Computer simulations of propofol infusions for total intravenous anaesthesia in dogs. J S Afr Vet Assoc 80, 2–9.

Joubert, K.E., Picard, J., Sethusa, M., 2005. Inhibition of bacterial growth by different mixtures of propofol and thiopentone. J S Afr Vet Assoc 76, 85–89.

Kastrup, M.R., Marsico, F.F., Ascoli, F.O., et al., 2005. Neuromuscular blocking properties of atracurium during sevoflurane or propofol anaesthesia in dogs. Vet Anaesth Analg 32, 222–227.

Katz, J., Clarke, H., Seltzer, Z., 2011. Preventive analgesia: quo vadimus? Anesth Analg 113, 1242–1253.

Keates, H.L., Cramond, T., Smith, M.T., 1999. Intraarticular and periarticular opioid binding in inflamed tissue in experimental canine arthritis. Anesth Analg 89, 409–415.

Ko, J.C.H., Weil, A.B., 2009. Effects of carprofen and morphine on the minimum alveolar concentration of isoflurane in dogs. J Am Anim Hosp Assoc 45, 19–23.

Ko, J., Weil, A., Maxwell, L., et al., 2007. Plasma concentrations of lidocaine in dogs following lidocaine patch application. J Am Anim Hosp Assoc 43, 280–283.

Ko, J.C., Golder, F.J., Mandsager, R.E., et al., 1999. Anesthetic and cardiorespiratory effects of a 1:1 mixture of propofol and thiopental sodium in dogs. J Am Vet Med Assoc 215, 1292–1296.

Ko, J.C.H., Fox, S.M., Mandsager, R.E., 2001a. Anesthetic effects of ketamine or isoflurane induction prior to isoflurane anesthesia in medetomidiine-premedicated dogs. J Am Anim Hosp Assoc 37, 411–419.

Ko, J.C.H., Fox, S.M., Mandsager, R.E., 2001b. Effects of preemptive atropine administration on incidence of medetomidine-induced bradycardia in dogs. J Am Vet Med Assoc 218, 52–58.

Kolata, R.J., Rawlings, C.A., 1982. Cardiopulmonary effects of intravenous xylazine, ketamine, and atropine in the dog. Am J Vet Res 43, 2196–2198.

Kona-Boun, J.-J., Cuvielliez, S., Troncy, E., 2006. Evaluation of epidural administration of morphine or morphine and bupivacaine for postoperative analgesia after premedication with an opioid analgesic and orthopedic surgery in dogs. J Am Vet Med Assoc 229, 1103–1112.

Kongara, K., Chamber, J.P., Johnson, C.B., 2012. Effects of tramadol, morphine or their combination in dogs undergoing ovariohysterectomy on peri-operative electroencephalographic responses and post-operative pain. N Z Vet J 60, 129–135.

Kopman, A.F., Eikermann, M., 2009. Antagonism of non-depolarising neuromuscular block: current practice. Anaesthesia 64 (Suppl 1), 22–30.

Kowalski, S.E., Bradley, B.D., Greengrass, R.A., et al., 1992. Effects of interpleural bupivacaine (0.5%) on canine diaphragmatic function. Anesth Analg 75, 400–404.

KuKanich, B., Bidgood, T., Knesl, O., 2012. Clinical pharmacology of nonsteroidal anti-inflammatory drugs in dogs. Vet Anesth Analg 39, 69–90.

Kulka, A.M., Otto, K.A., Bergfeld, C., et al., 2012. Effect of isoflurane anesthesia with and without dexmedetomidine or remifentanil on quantitative electroencephalographic variables before and after nociceptive stimulation in dogs. Am J Vet Res 73, 602–609.

Kuo, W.-C., Keegan, R.D., 2004. Comparative cardiovascular, analgesic, and sedative effects of medetomidine, medetomidine-hydromorphone, and medetomidine-butorphanol in dogs. Am J Vet Res 65, 931–937.

Kushner, L.I., Trim, C.M., Madhusudhan, S., et al., 1995. Evaluation of the hemodynamic effects of interpleural bupivacaine in dogs. Vet Surg 24, 180–187.

Kyles, A.E., Hardie, E.M., Hansen, B.D., et al., 1998. Comparison of transdermal fentanyl and intramuscular oxymorphone on post-operative behaviour after ovariohysterectomy in dogs. Res Vet Sci 65, 245–251.

Lantz, G.C., Badylak, S.F., Hiles, M.C., et al., 1992. Treatment of reperfusion injury in dogs with experimentally induced gastric dilatation-volvulus. Am J Vet Res 53, 1594–1598.

Lee, D.D., Mayer, R.E., Sullivan, T.C., et al., 1998. Respiratory depressant and skeletal muscle relaxant effects of low-dose pancuronium bromide in spontaneously breathing, isoflurane-anesthetized dogs. Vet Surg 27, 473–479.

Leibetseder, E.N., Mosing, M., Jones, R.S., 2006. A comparison of extradural and intravenous methadone on intraoperative isoflurane and postoperative analgesia requirements in dogs. Vet Anaesth Analg 33, 128–136.

Lemke, K.A., 2001. Electrocardiographic and cardiopulmonary effects of intramuscular administration of glycopyrrolate and romifidine in conscious beagle dogs. Vet Anaesth Analg 28, 75–86.

Lemke, K.A., Creighton, C.M., 2008. Paravertebral blockade of the brachial plexus in dogs. Vet Clin N Am Small Anim Pract 38, 1231–1241.

Lemke, K.A., Dawson, S.D., 2000. Local and regional anesthesia. Vet Clin N Am Small Anim Pract 30, 839–857.

Lemo, N., Vnuk, D., Radisic, B., et al., 2007. Determination of the toxic dose of lidocaine in dogs and its corresponding serum concentration. Vet Rec 160, 374–375.

Lennox, P.H., Umedaly, H.S., Grant, R.P., et al., 2006. A pulsatile pressure waveform is a sensitive marker for confirming the location of the thoracic epidural space. J Cardiothor Vasc Anesth 20, 659–663.

Lerche, P., Muir III, W.W., 2004. Effect of medetomidine on breathing and inspiratory neuromuscular drive in conscious dogs. Am J Vet Res 65, 720–724.

Lerche, P., Nolan, A.M., Reid, J., 2000. Comparative study of propofol or propofol and ketamine for the induction of anaesthesia in dogs. Vet Rec 146, 571–574.

Lin, G.-Y., Robben, J.H., Murrell, J.C., et al., 2008. Dexmedetomidine constant rate infusion for 24 hours during and after propofol or isoflurane anaesthesia in dogs. Vet Anaesth Analg 35, 141–153.

Linton, D.D., Wilson, M.G., Newbound, G.C., et al., 2012. The effectiveness of a long-acting transdermal fentanyl solution compared to buprenorphine for the control of postoperative pain in dogs in a randomized, multicentered clinical study. J Vet Pharmacol Ther 35 (Suppl. 2), 53–64.

Liu, Q., Kong, A., Chen, R., et al., 2011. Propofol and arrhythmias: two sides of the coin. Acta Pharmacol Sin 32, 817–823.

MacDougall, L.M., Hethey, J.A., Livingston, A., et al., 2009. Antinociceptive, cardiopulmonary, and sedative effects of five intravenous infusion rates of lidocaine in conscious dogs. Vet Anaesth Analg 36, 512–522.

Maddern, K., Adams, V.J., Hill, N.A.T., et al., 2010. Alfaxalone induction dose following administration of medetomidine and butorphanol in the dog. Vet Anaesth Analg 37, 7–13.

Magnusson, K.R., Scanga, C., Wagner, A.E., et al., 2000. Changes in anesthetic sensitivity and glutamate receptors in the aging canine brain. J Gerontol A Biol Sci Med Sci 55A, B448–B454.

Maney, J.K., Shepard, M.K., Braun, C., et al., 2013. A comparison of cardiopulmonary and anesthetic effects of an induction dose of alfaxalone or propofol in dogs. Vet Anaesth Analg, doi:10.1111/vaa.12006.

Mapleson, W.W., 1996. Effect of age on MAC in humans: a meta-analysis. Br J Anaesth 76, 179–185.

Margetts, L., Sawyer, R., 2007. Transdermal drug delivery: principles and opioid therapy. Cont Educ Anaesth, Crit Care & Pain 7, 171–176.

Marquez, M., Boscan, P., Weir, H., et al., 2011. The anesthetic sparing effect of maropitant as a pre-anesthetic agent during canine ovariohysterectomy. In: Proc Am Coll Vet Anesth Ann Mtg, Knoxville, TN, USA.

Martins, T.L., Kahvegian, M.A.P., Noel-Morgan, J., et al., 2010. Comparison of the effects of tramadol, codeine, and ketoprofen alone or in combination on postoperative pain and on concentrations of blood glucose, serum cortisol, and serum interleukin-6 in dogs undergoing maxillectomy or mandibulectomy. Am J Vet Res 71, 1019–1026.

Mathews, L., Reichl, L., Graham, L., et al., 2011. Comparison of the cardiovascular effects of acepromazine versus trazodone as pre-medication in dogs anesthetized for TPLO or TTA surgical procedures. In: Proc Am Coll Vet Anesth Ann Mtg, Nashville, TN, USA.

Matsubara, L.M., Oliva, V.N.L.S., Gabas, D.T., et al., 2009. Effect of lidocaine on the minimum alveolar concentration of sevoflurane in dogs. Vet Anaesth Analg 36, 407–413.

Mawbry, D.I., Bartges, J.W., d'Avignon, A., et al., 2004. Comparison of various methods for estimating body fat in dogs. J Am Anim Hosp Assoc 40, 109–114.

McMurphy, R.M., Davidson, H.J., Hodgson, D.S., 2004. Effects of atracurium on intraocular pressure, eye position, and blood pressure in eucapnic and hypocapnic isoflurane-anesthetized dogs. Am J Vet Res 65, 179–182.

Mehler, S.J., Mayhew, P.D., Drobatz, K.J., et al., 2004. Variables associated with outcome in dogs undergoing extrahepatic biliary surgery: 60 cases (1988–2002). Vet Surg 33, 644–649.

Michelsen, L.G., Salmenperä, M., Hug, C.H., et al., 1996. Anesthetic potency of remifentanil in dogs. Anesthesiology 84, 865–872.

Miller, C.J., McKiernan, B.C., Pace, J., et al., 2002. The effects of doxapram hydrochloride (dopram-V) on laryngeal function in healthy dogs. J Vet Intern Med 16, 524–528.

Mohammad-Zadeh, L.F., Moses, L., Gwaltney-Brant, S.M., 2008. Serotonin: a review. J Vet Pharmacol Ther 31, 187–199.

Monteiro, E.R., Teixeira Neto, F.J., Campagnol, D., et al., 2010a. Hemodynamic effects in dogs anesthetized with isoflurane and remifentanil-isoflurane. Am J Vet Res 71, 1133–1141.

Monteiro, E.R., Teixeira-Neto, F.J., Campagnol, D., et al., 2010b. Effects of remifentanil on the minimum alveolar concentration of isoflurane in dogs. Am J Vet Res 71, 150–156.

Morgaz, J., Granados, M.M., Domínguez, J.M., et al., 2009. Relationship of bispectral index to hemodynamic variables and alveolar concentration multiples of sevoflurane in puppies. Res Vet Sci 86, 508–513.

Mosing, M., Auer, U., West, E., et al., 2012. Reversal of profound rocuronium or vecuronium-induced neuromuscular block with sugammadex in isoflurane-anaesthetized dogs. Vet J 192, 467–471.

Mosing, M., Iff, I.K., Nemetz, W., 2008. Cardiopulmonary arrest and resuscitation following an extradural injection in a normovolemic dog. J Vet Emerg Crit Care 18, 532–536.

Muir, W.W. III, Wiese, A.J., March, P.A., 2003. Effects of morphine, lidocaine, ketamine, and morphine-lidocaine-ketamine drug combination on minimum alveolar concentration in dogs anesthetized with isoflurane. Am J Vet Res 64, 1155–1160.

Muir, W., Lerche, P., Wiese, A., et al., 2008. Cardiorespiratory and anesthetic effects of clinical and supraclinical doses of alfaxalone in dogs. Vet Anaesth Analg 35, 451–462.

Muir, W.W., Gadawski, J., 1998. Cardiorespiratory effects of low-flow and closed circuit inhalation anesthesia, using sevoflurane delivered with an in-circuit vaporizer and concentrations of compound A. Am J Vet Res 59, 603–608.

Murphy, A., Campbell, D.E., Baines, D., et al., 2011a. Allergic reactions to propofol in egg-allergic children. Anesth Analg 113, 140–144.

Murphy, G.S., Szokol, J.W., Avram, M.J., et al., 2011b. Intraoperative acceleromyography monitoring reduces symptoms of muscle weakness and improves quality of recovery in the early postoperative period. Anesthesiology 115, 946–954.

Mutoh, T., Nishimura, R., Kim, H.-Y., et al., 1997. Cardopulmonary effects of sevoflurane, compared with halothane, enflurane, and isoflurane, in dogs. Am J Vet Res 58, 885–890.

Mutoh, T., Nishimura, R., Sasaki, N., 2001. Effects of nitrous oxide on mask induction of anesthesia with sevoflurane or isoflurane in dogs. Am J Vet Res 62, 1727–1733.

Mutoh, T., Nishimura, R., Sasaki, N., 2002. Effects of medetomidine-midazolam, midazolam-butorphanol, or acepromazine-butorphanol as premedicants for mask induction of anesthesia with sevoflurane in dogs. Am J Vet Res 63, 1022–1028.

Myrna, K.E., Bentley, E., Smith, L.J., 2010. Effectiveness of injection of local anesthetic into the retrobulbar space for postoperative analgesia following eye enucleation in dogs. J Am Vet Med Assoc 237, 174–177.

Nagahama, S., Nishimura, R., Mochizuki, M., et al., 2006. The effects of propofol, isoflurane and sevoflurane on vecuronium infusion rates for surgical muscle relaxation in dogs. Vet Anaesth Analg 33, 169–174.

Naganobu, K., Maeda, N., Miyamoto, T., et al., 2004. Cardiorespiratory effects of epidural administration of morphine and fentanyl in dogs anesthetized with sevoflurane. J Am Vet Med Assoc 224, 67–70.

Nickalls, R.W.D., Mapleson, W.W., 2003. Age-related iso-MAC charts for isoflurane, sevoflurane and desflurane in man. Br J Anaesth 91, 170–174.

Nunes de Morales, A., Dyson, D.H., O'Grady, M.R., et al., 1998. Plasma concentrations and cardiovascular influence of lidocaine infusions during isoflurane anesthesia in healthy dogs and dogs with subaortic stenosis. Vet Surg 27, 486–497.

Ortega, M., Cruz, I., 2011. Evaluation of a constant rate infusion of lidocaine for balanced anesthesia in dogs undergoing surgery. Can Vet J 52, 856–860.

Pacharinsak, C., Greene, S.A., Keegan, R.D., et al., 2003. Postoperative analgesia in dogs receiving epidural morphine plus medetomidine. J Vet Pharmacol Ther 26, 71–77.

Panti, A., Bennett, R.C., Corletto, F., et al., 2009. The effect of omeprazole on oesophageal pH in dogs during anaesthesia. J Small Anim Pract 50, 540–544.

Park, J., Sutradhar, B.C., Hong, G., et al., 2011. Comparison of the cytotoxic effects of bupivacaine, lidocaine, and mepivacaine in equine articular chondrocytes. Vet Anaesth Analg 38, 127–133.

Park, S.A., Park, Y.W., Son, W.G., et al., 2010. Evaluation of the analgesic effect of intracameral lidocaine hydrochloride injection on intraoperative and postoperative pain in healthy dogs undergoing phacoemulsification. Am J Vet Res 71, 216–222.

Pascoe, P.J., Dyson, D.H., 1993. Analgesia after lateral thoracotomy in dogs. Epidural morphine vs. intercostal bupivacaine. Vet Surg 22, 141–147.

Pascoe, P.J., Raekallio, M., Kuusela, E., et al., 2006. Changes in the minimum alveolar concentration of isoflurane and some cardiopulmonary measurements during three continuous infusion rates of dexmedetomidine in dogs. Vet Anaesth Analg 33, 97–103.

Picker, O., Scheeren, T.W., Arndt, J.O., 2001. Inhalation anaesthetics increase heart rate by decreasing cardiac vagal activity in dogs. Br J Anaesth 87, 748–754.

Pieper, K., Schuster, T., Levionnois, O., et al., 2011. Antinociceptive efficacy and plasma concentrations of transdermal buprenorphine in dogs. Vet J 187, 335–341.

Poffenbarger, E.M., Ralston, S.L., Chandler, M.J., et al., 1990. Canine neonatology. Part I. Physiologic differences between puppies and adults. Comp Cont Educ 12, 1601–1609.

Popilskis, S., Kohn, D., Sanchez, J., et al., 1991. Epidural vs intramuscular oxymorphone analgesia after thoracotomy in dogs. Vet Surg 20, 462–467.

Portela, D.A., Otero, P.E., Tarragona, L., et al., 2010. Combined paravertebral plexus block and parasacral sciatic block in healthy dogs. Vet Anaesth Analg 37, 531–541.

Psatha, E., Alibhai, H.I., Jiminez-Lozano, A., et al., 2011. Clinical efficacy and cardiorespiratory effects of alfaxalone, or diazepam/fentanyl for induction of anaesthesia in dogs that are a poor anaesthetic risk. Vet Anaesth Analg 38, 24–36.

Pypendop, B.H., Ilkiw, J.E., 2006. Comparison of variability in cardiorespiratory measurements following desflurane anesthesia at a multiple of the minimum alveolar concentration for each dog versus a multiple of a single predetermined minimum alveolar concentration for all dogs in a group. Am J Vet Res 67, 1956–1961.

Pypendop, B.H., Verstegen, J.P., 1998. Hemodynamic effects of medetomidine in the dog: a dose titration study. Vet Surg 27, 612–622.

Pypendop, B.H., Verstegen, J.P., 2000. Effects of a medetomidine-midazolam-butorphanol combination on renal cortical, intestinal and muscle microvascular blood flow in isoflurane anaesthetized dogs: a laser Doppler study. Vet Anaesth Analg 27, 36–44.

Pypendop, B.H., Verstegen, J.P., 2001. Cardiovascular effects of romifidine in dogs. Am J Vet Res 62, 490–495.

Quandt, J.E., Robinson, E.P., Rivers, W.J., et al., 1998. Cardiorespiratory and anesthetic effects of propofol and thiopental in dogs. Am J Vet Res 59, 1137–1143.

Radlinsky, M.G., Mason, D.E., Hodgson, D., 2004. Transnasal laryngoscopy for the diagnosis of laryngeal paralysis in dogs. J Am Anim Hosp Assoc 40, 211–215.

Radlinsky, M.G., Mason, D.E., Roush, J.K., et al., 2005. Use of a continuous, local infusion of bupivacaine for postoperative analgesia in dogs undergoing total ear canal ablation. J Am Vet Med Assoc 227, 414–419.

Raptopoulos, D., Galatos, A.D., 1995. Post anaesthetic reflux esophagitis in dogs and cats. J Vet Anaesth 22, 6–8.

Raptopoulos, D., Galatos, A.D., 1997. Gastro-oesophageal reflux during anaesthesia induced with either thiopentone or propofol in the dog. J Vet Anaesth 24, 20–22.

Redondo, J.I., Gómez-Villamandos, R.J., Santisteban, J.M., et al., 1999. Romifidine, medetomidine or xylazine before propofol-halothane-N₂O anesthesia in dogs. Can J Vet Res 63, 31–36.

Reed, F., Burrow, R., Poels, K.L.C., et al., 2011. Evaluation of transdermal fentanyl patch attachment in dogs and analysis of residual fentanyl content following removal. Vet Anaesth Analg 38, 407–412.

Reid, J., Nolan, A.M., 1996. Pharmacokinetics of propofol as an induction agent in geriatric dogs. Res Vet Sci 61, 169–171.

Rioja, E., Sinclair, M., Chalmers, H., et al., 2012. Comparison of three techniques for paravertebral brachial plexus blockade in dogs. Vet Anaesth Analg 39, 190–200.

Robertson, S.M., 2009. Anesthesia for patients treated with behavioral medication. North Am Vet Conf, Orlando, FL, USA.

Robinson, T.M., Kruse-Elliott, K.T., Markel, M.D., et al., 1999. A comparison of transdermal fentanyl versus epidural morphine for analgesia in dogs undergoing major orthopedic surgery. J Am Anim Hosp Assoc 35, 95–100.

Rodríguez, J.M., Muñoz-Rascon, P., Navarrete-Calvo, R., et al., 2012. Comparison of the cardiopulmonary parameters after induction of anaesthesia with alphaxalone or etomidate in dogs. Vet Anaesth Analg 39, 357–365.

Rojas, A.C., Alves, J.G., Moreira e Lima, R., et al., 2012. The effects of subarachnoid administration of preservative-free S(+)-ketamine on spinal cord and meninges in dogs. Anesth Analg 114, 450–455.

Sammarco, J.L., Conzemius, M.G., Perkowski, S.Z., et al., 1996. Postoperative analgesia for stifle surgery: a comparison of intra-articular bupivacaine, morphine, or saline. Vet Surg 25, 59–69.

Sano, T., Nishimura, R., Kanazawa, H., et al., 2006. Pharmacokinetics of fentanyl after single intravenous injection and constant rate infusion in dogs. Vet Anaesth Analg 33, 266–273.

Savvas, I., Anagnostou, T., Papazoglou, L.G., et al., 2006. Successful resuscitation from cardiac arrest associated with extradural lidocaine in a dog. Vet Anaesth Analg 33, 175–178.

Savvas, I., Papazoglou, L.G., Kazakos, G.M., et al., 2008. Incisional block with bupivacaine for analgesia after celiotomy in dogs. J Am Anim Hosp Assoc 44, 60–66.

Savvas, I., Rallis, T., Raptopoulos, D., 2009. The effect of pre-anaesthetic fasting time and type of food on gastric content volume and acidity in dogs. Vet Anaesth Analg 36, 539–546.

Schertel, E.R., Allen, D.A., Muir, W.W., et al., 1997. Evaluation of a hypertonic saline-dextran solution for treatment of dogs with shock induced by gastric dilatation-volvulus. J Am Vet Med Assoc 210, 226–230.

Schmiedt, C.W., Bjorling, D.E., 2007. Accidental prehension and suspected transmucosal or oral absorption of fentanyl from a transdermal patch in a dog. Vet Anaesth Analg 34, 70–73.

Scroggin, R.D., Quandt, J., 2009. The use of vasopressin for treating vasodilatory shock and cardiopulmonary arrest. J Vet Emerg Crit Care 19, 145–157.

Seddighi, R., Egger, C.M., Rohrbach, B.W., et al., 2012. Effect of nitrous oxide on the minimum alveolar concentration for sevoflurane and the minimum alveolar concentration derivatives that prevent motor movement and autonomic responses in dogs. Am J Vet Res 73, 341–345.

Sedlacek, H.S., Ramsey, D.S., Boucher, J.F., et al., 2008. Comparative efficacy of maropitant and selected drugs in preventing emesis induced by centrally or peripherally acting emetogens in dogs. J Vet Pharmacol Ther 31, 533–537.

Self, I.A., Hughes, J.M., Kenny, D.A., et al., 2009. Effect of muscle injection site on preanaesthetic sedation in dogs. Vet Rec 164, 323–326.

Shaver, S.L., Jimenez, D.A., Brainard, B.M., et al., 2011. Evaluation of perioperative gastroesophageal reflux in dogs with brachycephalic syndrome. ACVS Conf, Chicago, IL, USA.

Smith, J.A., Gaynor, J.S., Bednarski, R.M., et al., 1993. Adverse effects of administration of propofol with various preanesthetic regimens in dogs. J Am Vet Med Assoc 202, 1111–1115.

Smith, L.J., Bentley, E., Shih, A., et al., 2004. Systemic lidocaine infusion as an analgesic for intraocular surgery in dogs: a pilot study. Vet Anaesth Analg 31, 53–63.

Smith, L.J., Yu, J.K.-A., 2001. A comparison of epidural buprenorphine with epidural morphine for postoperative analgesia following stifle surgery in dogs. Vet Anaesth Analg 28, 87–96.

Sneyd, J.R., Rigby-Jones, A.E., 2010. New drugs and technologies, intravenous anaesthesia is on the move (again). Br J Anaesth 105, 246–254.

Stephan, D.D., Vestre, W.A., Stiles, J., et al., 2003. Changes in intraocular pressure and pupil size following intramuscular administration of hydromorphone hydrochloride and acepromazine in clinically normal dogs. Vet Ophthalmol 6, 73–76.

Stobie, D., Caywood, D.D., Rozanski, E.A., et al., 1995. Evaluation of pulmonary function and analgesia in dogs after intercostal thoracotomy and use of morphine administered intramuscularly or intrapleurally and bupivacaine administered intrapleurally. Am J Vet Res 56, 1098–1109.

Stubhaug, A., Breivik, H., Eide, P.K., et al., 1997. Mapping of punctate hyperalgesia around a surgical incision demonstrates that ketamine is a powerful suppressor of central sensitization to pain following surgery. Acta Anaesth Scand 41, 1124–1132.

Tobias, K.M., Jackson, A.M., Harvey, R.C., 2004. Effects of doxapram HCl on laryngeal function of normal dogs and dogs with naturally occurring laryngeal paralysis. Vet Anaesth Analg 31, 258–263.

Tobias, K.M., Marioni-Henry, K., Wagner, R., 2006. A retrospective study on the use of acepromazine maleate in dogs with seizures. J Am Anim Hosp Assoc 42, 283–289.

Tolbert, K., Bissett, S., King, A., et al., 2011. Efficacy of oral famotidine and 2 omeprazole formulations for the control of intragastric pH in dogs. J Vet Intern Med 25, 47–54.

Torske, K.E., Dyson, D.H., Conlon, P.D., 1999. Cardiovascular effects of epidurally administered oxymorphone and an oxymorphone-bupivacaine combination in halothane-anesthetized dogs. Am J Vet Res 60, 194–200.

Torske, K.E., Dyson, D.H., Pettifer, G., 1998. End tidal halothane concentration and postoperative analgesia requirements in dogs: a comparison between intravenous oxymorphone and epidural bupivacaine alone and in combination with oxymorphone. Can Vet J 39, 361–368.

Troncy, E., Junot, S., Keroack, S., et al., 2002. Results of preemptive epidural administration of morphine with or without bupivacaine in dogs and cats undergoing surgery: 265 cases (1997–1999). J Am Vet Med Assoc 221, 666–672.

Trumpatori, B.J., Carter, J.E., Hash, J., et al., 2010. Evaluation of a midhumeral block of the radial, ulnar, musculocutaneous and median (RUMM block) nerves for analgesia of the distal aspect of the thoracic limb in dogs. Vet Surg 39, 1–12.

Tsuneyoshi, I., Akata, T., Boyle, W.A., 2004. Vascular reactivity. In: Evers,

A.S., Maze, M. (Eds). Anesthetic Pharmacology: Physiologic Principles and Clinical Practice. Churchill Livingstone, Philadelphia, pp. 297–321.

Tyner, C.L., Woody, B.J., Reid, J.S., et al., 1997. Multicenter clinical comparison of sedative and analgesic effects of medetomidine and xylazine in dogs. J Am Anim Hosp Assoc 211, 1413–1417.

Ueyama, Y., Lerche, P., Eppler, C.M., et al., 2009. Effects of intravenous administration of perzinfotel, fentanyl, and a combination of both drugs on the minimum alveolar concentration of isoflurane in dogs. Am J Vet Res 70, 1459–1464.

Ueyema, Y., Waselau, A.-C., Wiese, A.J., et al., 2008. Anesthetic and cardiopulmonary effects of intramuscular morphine, medetomidine, ketamine injection in dogs. Vet Anaesth Analg 35, 480–487.

Uilenreef, J.J., Murrell, J.C., McKusick, B.C., et al., 2008. Dexmedetomidine continuous rate infusion during isoflurane anaesthesia in canine surgical patients. Vet Anaesth Analg 35, 1–12.

Valverde, A., 2008. Epidural analgesia in dogs and cats. Vet Clin Small Anim 38, 1205–1230.

Valverde, A., Doherty, T.J., Hernández, J., et al., 2004. Effect of lidocaine on the minimum alveolar concentration of isoflurane in dogs. Vet Anaesth Analg 31, 264–271.

Valverde, A., Dyson, D., Cockshutt, J.R., et al., 1991. Comparison of the hemodynamic effects of halothane alone and halothane combined with epidurally administered morphine for anesthesia in ventilated dogs. Am J Vet Res 52, 505–509.

Valverde, A., Dyson, D.H., McDonell, W.N., 1989. Epidural morphine reduces halothane MAC in the dog. Can J Anaesth 36, 629–632.

van Oostrom, H., Doornenbal, A., Schot, A., et al., 2011. Neurophysiological assessment of the sedative and analgesic effects of a constant rate infusion of dexmedetomidine in the dog. Vet J 190, 338–344.

Vanio, O., 1991. Propofol infusion anaesthesia in dogs premedicated with medetomidine. J Vet Anaesth 18, 35–37.

Verbruggen, A.M., Akkerdaas, L.C., Hellebrekers, L.J., et al., 2000. The

effect of intravenous medetomidine on pupil size and intraocular pressure in normotensive dogs. Vet Quarterly 22, 179–180.

Vesal, N., Cribb, P.H., Frketic, M.M., 1996. Postoperative analgesic and cardiopulmonary effects in dogs of oxymorphone administered epidurally and intramuscularly, and medetomidine administered epidurally: A comparative clinical study. Vet Surg 25, 361–369.

Vettorato, E., Bradbrook, C., Gurney, M., et al., 2012. Peripheral nerve blocks of the pelvic limb in dogs: A retrospective clinical study. Vet Comp Orthop Traumatol 25, 314–320.

Vinclair, M., Broux, C., Faure, P., et al., 2008. Duration of adrenal inhibition following a single dose of etomidate in critically ill patients. Intensive Care Med 34, 714–719.

Waterman, A.E., Hashim, M.A., 1992. Effects of thiopentone and propofol on lower oesophageal sphincter and barrier pressure in the dog. J Small Anim Pract 33, 530–533.

Watkins, S., Hall, L., Clarke, K., 1987. Propofol as an intravenous anaesthetic agent for dogs. Vet Rec 120, 326–329.

Wehrenberg, A.P., Freeman, L.M., Ko, J.C., et al., 2009. Evaluation of topical epidural morphine for postoperative analgesia following hemilaminectomy in dogs. Vet Ther 10, E1–E12.

Weiland, L., Croubels, S., Baert, K., et al., 2006. Pharmacokinetics of a lidocaine patch 5% in dogs. J Vet Med A Physiol Pathol Clin Med 53, 34–39.

Werdehausen, R., Braun, S., Hermans, H., et al., 2011. The influence of adjuvants used in regional anesthesia on lidocaine-induced neurotoxicity in vitro. Regional Anesth Pain Med 36, 436–443.

Wiles, M.D., Nathanson, M.H., 2010. Local anaesthetics and adjuvants – future developments. Anaesthesia 65 (Suppl. 1), 22–37.

Wilson, D.V., Walshaw, R., 2004. Postanesthetic esophageal dysfunction in 13 dogs. J Am Anim Hosp Assoc 40, 455–460.

Wilson, D.V., Barnes, K.S., Hauptman, J.G., 2004. Pharmacokinetics of combined intraperitoneal and incisional lidocaine in the dog following ovariohysterectomy. J Vet Pharmacol Ther 27, 105–109.

Wilson, D.V., Boruta, D.T., Evans, A.T., 2006a. Influence of halothane, isoflurane, and sevoflurane on gastroesophageal reflux during anesthesia in dogs. Am J Vet Res 67, 1821–1825.

Wilson, D.V., Evans, A.T., Mauer, W.A., 2006b. Influence of metoclopramide on gastroesophageal reflux in anesthetized dogs. Am J Vet Res 67, 26–31.

Wilson, D.V., Pettifer, G.R., Hosgood, G., 2006c. Effect of transdermally administered fentanyl on minimum alveolar concentration of isoflurane in normothermic and hypothermic dogs. J Am Vet Med Assoc 228, 1042–1046.

Wilson, D.V., Evans, A.T., Mauer, W.A., 2007. Pre-anesthetic meperidine: associated vomiting and gastroesophageal reflux during the subsequent anesthetic in dogs. Vet Anaesth Analg 34, 15–22.

Wilson, D.V., Evans, A.T., Miller, R., 2005. Effects of preanesthetic administration of morphine on gastroesophageal reflux and regurgitation during anesthesia in dogs. Am J Vet Res 66, 386–390.

Wilson, J., Doherty, T.J., Egger, C.M., et al., 2008. Effects of intravenous lidocaine, ketamine, and the combination on the minimum alveolar concentration of sevoflurane in dogs. Vet Anaesth Analg 35, 289–296.

Wilson, M.J.A., 2007. Epidural endeavour and the pressure principle. Anaesthesia 62, 319–322.

Wolfe, T.M., Bateman, S.W., Cole, L.K., et al., 2006. Evaluation of a local anesthetic delivery system for the postoperative analgesic management of canine total ear canal ablation – a randomized, controlled, double-blinded study. Vet Anaesth Analg 33, 328–339.

Xenoulis, P.G., Steiner, J.M., 2010. Lipid metabolism and hyperlipidemia in dogs. Vet J 183, 12–21.

Yamashita, K., Yoshihiko, O., Yamashita, M., et al., 2008. Effects of carprofen and meloxicam with or without butorphanol on the minimum alveolar concentration of sevoflurane in dogs. J Vet Med Sci 70, 29–35.

Zhao, Y., Sun, L., 2008. Antidepressants modulate the in vitro inhibitory effects of propofol and ketamine on norepinephrine and serotonin transporter function. J Clin Neurosci 15, 1264–1269.

Chapter | **16** |

Anaesthesia of the cat

INTRODUCTION

General principles and recommendations for good anaesthetic practice that are discussed in the previous chapter are applicable to anaesthesia of cats. This chapter will focus on aspects of anaesthetic management that are influenced by feline behaviour, anatomy, physiology, pharmacology and disease. Other reading sources include the guidelines published by veterinary organizations with specific interest in the feline species, including the Association for Veterinary Anaesthesia (AVA), the American College of Veterinary Anesthesia and Analgesia (ACVAA), the International Society of Feline Medicine (ISFM) and the American Association of Feline Practitioners (AAFP).

The risk of death from anaesthesia or sedation has decreased. Recent data have led to approximate estimates of mortality of 0.1% in healthy cats and 1.4% in sick cats, with cats apparently at greater risk than dogs (Brodbelt et al., 2008a,b). Administration of anaesthesia in cats is not identical to that in dogs as the behavioural responses to and metabolism of some anaesthetic agents differ between cats and dogs. In a 2-year prospective survey of anaesthesia of 79 178 cats in the UK, physical status, age and weight increased the risk of death. Cats that were sicker, over 12 years of age, and weighing ≤2 kg or ≥6 kg were more likely to die during or after anaesthesia. Furthermore, cats weighing ≤2 kg were nearly 16 times more likely to die than cats weighing between 2 and 6 kg (Brodbelt et al., 2007). As with other species, illness and increasing age may exaggerate or diminish physiological responses to anaesthetic agents as well as decrease the dose rates required. Overweight cats are at increased risk for hypoventilation and hypoxaemia and the dose rates of anaesthetic agents must be decreased for these patients. Small cats are at risk for unintended drug overdose, especially if correct weights are not used. Accuracy of administration of small volumes is improved by use of 1 mL syringes with 24 gauge needles or insulin syringes. Larger needles may contain as much as 0.1–0.2 mL of drug that can increase the dose administered when injected into a small patient. Drugs should be diluted when the volume to be injected is too small to be accurately administered with available syringes/needles. Published factors associated with anaesthetic- and sedation-related deaths included the urgency and severity of the procedure, and use of endotracheal intubation and fluid therapy. Possible explanations are that preanaesthetic evaluation and preparation are curtailed with emergency and out-of-hours surgery. Less or inadequate time is spent restoring fluid and electrolyte balance, and fewer personnel may be available for optimum management. Endotracheal intubation is not quite as easy in cats due to the smaller size of the larynx and increased tendency for laryngospasm to interfere with insertion of the tube. Use of force or repeated attempts may cause trauma leading to laryngeal and tracheal mucosal swelling that obstructs airflow after extubation. Increased risk of death associated with fluid therapy may be a consequence of fluid overload. Not only is the blood volume of a cat smaller than that of a dog on a per kg basis such that a relatively smaller volume of fluid is required, but also accurate assessment of the fluid volume delivered may be difficult when using gravity flow from a 500 mL bag of balanced electrolyte solution, even with a paediatric (60 drops/mL) administration set. The anaesthetist must maintain close control of fluid administration and this can be facilitated by use of an infusion pump or syringe driver. A running tally of all fluid administered should be recorded, including any volumes administered with adjunct therapies such as dopamine or dobutamine and 5% dextrose in water (D5W).

PATIENT EVALUATION

Evaluation of the cat before sedation or anaesthesia should include assessment in each of the following areas.

History

The effects and elimination of anaesthetic agents may be altered by specific diseases and anaesthesia may result in a long-term adverse effect on organ function that was already compromised. Drugs administered to control fear or anxiety, such as amitriptyline, paroxetine, sertraline, fluoxetine, or selegiline may have interaction with anaesthetic agents. Although related complications are not documented in cats, there are potential problems with these agents and they have been discussed in the previous chapter. Concurrent administration of drugs to control hypertension may potentiate hypotension during anaesthesia. Frequent measurement of blood glucose perioperatively is important for cats with diabetes and some cats will require infusion of glucose-containing fluid. Knowledge of previous adverse responses to anaesthesia, such as excitement, hypotension, or difficult recovery, is useful so that the current protocol can be modified accordingly.

Physical examination

The physical characteristics of the patient may immediately suggest a potential problem, such as brachycephalic syndrome in Persian and Exotic shorthair cats. With severe brachycephalia, the upper canine teeth rotate from the normal nearly vertically aligned position to pronounced dorsorotation or nearly horizontal position. The greater the degree of brachycephalia and dorsorotation, the narrower the nasal cavity, nasal airways and nares (Schlueter et al., 2009). In the previous study, hypoplasia of the trachea was not present in the brachycephalic cats studied. Brachycephalic cats must not be left alone after premedication for fear of airway obstruction. Obese cats have impaired ventilation and are predisposed to hypoxaemia during sedation and anaesthesia. Dose rates of anaesthetic agents should be calculated on the ideal weights of these patients to avoid overdosage. Very thin cats are at increased risk for hypothermia and warming methods must be used throughout the anaesthetic episode, particularly during the time between induction of anaesthesia and start of surgery, and continued into recovery.

As in other species, age affects aspects of anaesthesia in feline patients. Although the demarcations between life stages are arbitrary, the AAFP and AAHA (American Animal Hospital Association) have determined feline life-stages as follows (Hoyumpa Vogt et al., 2010):

- Kitten Birth–6 months of age
- Junior 7 months–2 years
- Prime 3–6 years
- Mature 7–10 years
- Senior 11–14 years
- Geriatric >15 years.

Senior and geriatric cats will have decreased requirements for anaesthetic agents and are more likely than younger animals to develop hypoventilation, hypoxaemia, and hypotension during anaesthesia.

Auscultation of a heart murmur on routine physical examination should be further investigated. Cardiac pathology was identified using echocardiography in 53% of apparently healthy cats with a murmur (Nakamura et al., 2011). A heart murmur may be auscultated in animals without underlying structural heart disease, and in cats that are hypovolaemic, anaemic or febrile, or may be absent despite the presence of significant heart disease such as hypertrophic cardiomyopathy (HCM). Nevertheless, the presence of cardiac disease such as cardiomyopathy, mitral insufficiency, or a patent ductus arteriosus (PDA) requires modification of the anaesthetic protocol to avoid an adverse outcome. The lungs should be auscultated for abnormal or absent air sounds that suggest the presence of pulmonary disease or diaphragmatic rupture. Some breeds are associated with increased incidence of certain diseases, such as the Maine Coon and cardiac disease.

The range of normal values for physiological parameters is wide and the measurements obtained may be influenced by the surroundings and method of monitoring (Table 16.1). Respiratory rates (RR), heart rates (HR), and Doppler systolic arterial pressures (SAP) have been found to be slightly higher when obtained in the hospital compared with the home environment although, even at home, some cats struggle during measurements (Quimby et al., 2011). Cats ≥11 years of age were found to have significantly higher SAP, diastolic arterial pressures (DAP) and mean arterial pressures (MAP) than younger cats (Bodey & Sansom, 1998) and, in a later study, the increases in blood pressures were progressive with increasing age (Sansom et al., 2004). Increased systolic arterial pressures of 160–179 mmHg and DAP 100–119 mmHg carry

Table 16.1 Reference physiological values for awake unsedated cats

Parameter	Range of published means ± SD		
RR breaths/min	39 ± 13 to 52 ± 15		
ETCO$_2$ mmHg	29 ± 4		
PaO$_2$ mmHg	81 ± 7 to 103		
PaCO$_2$ mmHg	26 ± 3 to 32 ± 3		
pHa	7.30 ± 0.1 to 7.39 ± 0.04		
HCO$_3$ mmol/L	16 ± 3.1 to 18.6 ± 1.7		
BE mmol/L	−5 ± 1.8		
Temperature °C (°F)	37.0 ± 0.9 (98.6 ± 1.6) to 38.6 ± 0.6 (101.5 ± 1.1)		
Heart rate beats/min	118 ± 14 to 240 ± 21		
Systolic arterial pressure mmHg Invasive	174 ± 45 (aorta) 163 ± 12 (femoral artery)		
Diastolic arterial pressure mmHg Invasive	124 ± 27 (aorta) 111 ± 6 (femoral artery)		
Mean arterial pressure mmHg Invasive	146 ± 29 (aorta) 137 ± 8 (femoral artery)		
Systolic arterial pressure mmHg Oscillometric DINAMAP 1846SX, tail, 94 cats	Age (years) < 5 5–10 >10	Mean value 116 128 147	
Diastolic arterial pressure mmHg Oscillometric DINAMAP 1846SX, tail, 94 cats	Age (years) < 5 5–10 >10	Mean value 62 77 87	
Mean arterial pressure mmHg Oscillometric DINAMAP 1846SX, tail, 94 cats	Age (years) < 5 5–10 >10	Mean value 81 97 110	

Allen et al., 1986; Hikasa et al., 1996; Sansom et al., 2004; Souza et al., 2005; Wiese & Muir, 2007; Cleale et al., 2009; Muir et al., 2009; Taylor et al., 2012

a moderate risk for organ damage, and SAP ≥180 mmHg with DAP ≥120 mmHg as carrying a severe risk for organ damage (Brown et al., 2007). Cardiac abnormalities are frequent in cats with hypertension. Hypertension is present in 19–65% of cats with chronic kidney disease, although cats with extreme renal compromise may have lower pressures and cats with chronic kidney disease and hypertension may not have azotaemia (Bodey & Sansom, 1998; Brown et al., 2007). Cats with hyperthyroidism may or may not be hypertensive but hypertension has been measured in 50–100% of cats with primary hyperaldosteronism. Hypertension is considered pathological in cats when ocular pathology is also present. Hypokalaemia and muscle weakness are also features of primary hyperaldosteronism. Measurement of blood pressure is advisable in older cats as part of the preanaesthetic evaluation. The cat must be completely relaxed, preferably in its cage, and the final values recorded should be the average of several measurements.

Diagnostic tests

Further information may be desired based on the patient's history and physical examination. Requirement for preoperative laboratory data is based on the patient's age, preexisting disease, and the type and complexity of the planned procedure. Since organ malfunction increases with increasing age, haematological and biochemical measurements should be determined in mature and older animals and the results may provide warning of a problem that requires specific anaesthetic management. Laboratory tests should be performed on all cats with comorbidities. Preoperative test results from healthy or sick cats scheduled for complicated surgical procedures will provide baseline values for postoperative evaluation. Measurement of haematocrit, total protein, and blood urea nitrogen (BUN) is recommended in any dog or cat that has not had laboratory tests within 2–4 weeks of anaesthesia. The clinician has an obligation to determine clinical relevance of an abnormal result and need for further investigation (Epstein et al., 2005; Klein & Arrowsmith, 2010). Administration of sedation or anaesthesia before collection of blood will alter the results (Frankel & Hawkey, 1980; Dhumeaux et al., 2012; Reynolds et al., 2012). Even a small IV dose of ketamine, 2 mg/kg, with diazepam, 0.1 mg/kg, decreased red and white blood cell and platelet counts, albumin and triglycerides (Reynolds et al., 2012). Some laboratory reference values may be different for various breeds. An investigation of 525 Birman, Chartreux, Maine Coon, and Persian cats in France identified clinically relevant differences for creatinine, glucose, and total protein (Reynolds et al., 2010). The Birman cats were found to have higher creatinine concentrations than cats of the other breeds, and plasma glucose concentrations were higher in Chartreux and Maine Coon cats.

Impact of disease

The presence of abnormalities may indicate the need to adjust choice of agents and dose rates or anaesthetic management to improve safety. Cats with kidney disease or urethral obstruction have reduced urine flow and prolonged recovery from anaesthesia will result from use of agents that rely on renal excretion for elimination, specifically ketamine and tiletamine–zolazepam. Azotaemia decreases anaesthetic requirement, therefore, lower doses should be used and the drugs titrated to effect. Cats with chronic kidney disease should be administered balanced electrolyte solution IV during anaesthesia and even preoperatively and through the recovery period to encourage diuresis. The cats should be monitored after anaesthesia until confirmation of urine voiding.

Medications for cardiac disease should be continued on the morning of the day of surgery. Some medications used to treat hypertension increase the risk for hypotension during inhalation anaesthesia and preparations for treatment should be available. Increased HR may adversely impact cardiac function in cats with HCM. Atropine or glycopyrrolate should not be used for premedication in these patients but reserved for therapeutic use if necessary. Vasoconstriction will decrease cardiac output in the presence of mitral insufficiency. Medetomidine and dexmedetomidine or acepromazine should be used cautiously to avoid exacerbation of hypertension or hypotension, respectively. Fluid overloading should be avoided in cats with severe cardiac disease.

Consideration of the results from the physical examination and diagnostic tests should culminate in an overall assessment of the health status of the patient. Commonly, the patient is then assigned a category of 1–5, with 1 representing a healthy animal and 5 moribund, and with the suffix E in situations of emergency anaesthesia (Chapter 1; ASA categories). This is a useful exercise because categories 3–5 have been associated with increased incidence of complications. Potential complications of the proposed medical or surgical procedure are not included with ASA status, therefore, the assigned category does not represent the total risk of anaesthesia and surgery.

Vaccination

The effect of anaesthesia on serological responses to vaccination at the time of neutering has been of concern. One investigation of serological responses to vaccinations before, during or after neutering kittens at 7, 8, or 9 weeks of age measured antibody titres that were comparable to kittens that were not anaesthetized, suggesting that anaesthesia and surgery did not have a significant impact (Reese et al., 2008).

Handling

The ISFM and AAFP guidelines for handling cats encourages the veterinary team to 'think like a cat' (Rodan et al., 2011). Since cats often respond to confrontation by avoidance or hiding, allowing a cat to feel hidden using towels or carriers may facilitate handling. Cats should be handled gently (unless unavoidable) using slow steady movements, a quiet voice and avoiding direct eye contact. Spraying synthetic feline facial pheromone in advance into the cage and on towels used for handling may reduce anxiety and fear aggression. Use of pheromones was found to add an additional calming effect in cats given acepromazine and to a lesser extent when cats were not given acepromazine, but had no appreciable effect on the ease of IV catheter insertion (Kronen et al., 2006). When approaching a cat in a cage, the opening should not be completely blocked (which the cat perceives as a threat) and the cat should be allowed to approach the handler. If the cat is reluctant to approach, the top of some carriers can be removed to gain access to the cat. The ISFM/AAFP guidelines recommend that the carrier should not be tipped up and the cat shaken out but to reach in and support the caudal end of the cat and back legs to encourage it to move forward. Sliding a towel around or over the cat before laying on hands may sufficiently relax the cat to facilitate easy removal from the cage. Most cats prefer touch on their heads and neck than other parts of the body. Signs of anxiety or fear include ears that are lowered and swiveled out, head drawn into the body, back slightly hunched, tail moved in to cover the feet, and sweaty paws. Immobility ('freezing') may also indicate anxiety.

'Scruffing' is a term for a variety of holds on the skin of the cat's neck. Opinions vary about use of scruffing (Rodan et al., 2011). Some clinicians will never use scruffing, others use scruffing only if necessary to protect a cat or person from injury, while others believe that it is acceptable for short procedures or to prevent escape. A gentle hold is sufficient for most pets. Chemical restraint may be needed when an aggressive response is anticipated. Preanaesthetic medication reduces patient struggling during insertion of an IV catheter before general anaesthesia.

Nets of the clam-shell design with small holes are available commercially to capture cats reluctant to be handled (Fig. 16.1). Any part of the cat is then available for IM injection. Also available are clear plastic boxes with one side that can be moved to immobilize the cat for IM injection.

SEDATION AND ANALGESIA

The goal for sedation is a quiet tractable animal to facilitate procedures such as examination or IV injection. Sedation will modify sympathetic nervous system stimulation and minimize increases in cardiac output and blood pressure that would increase the dose rate of subsequent anaesthetic agents. High dose rates result in greater cardiopulmonary depression and a narrower margin of safety. Minimizing conflict between cat and handler also minimizes stress on the veterinary personnel and contributes

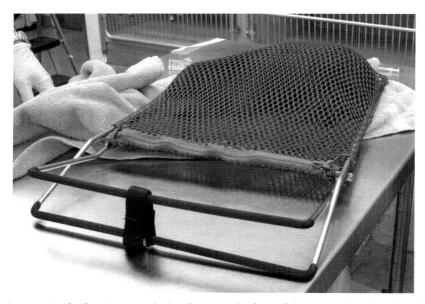

Figure 16.1 Net bag restraint for fractious cats. The handles are at the front of the picture, kept closed by Velcro. The hinge in the middle allows the far side to open like jaws to scoop up the cat. IM injection can be made through the holes in the netting.

to efficiency by allowing them to stay focused and complete the job in hand more quickly.

Agents

Acepromazine

Acepromazine may be given to cats at dose rates of 0.02–0.1 mg/kg IM, IV or SC (Table 16.2). Acepromazine given alone provides mild sedation that can be intensified by the addition of an opioid. It is used to provide a base for anaesthesia, to increase sedation from an opioid, to decrease signs of CNS stimulation seen with an opioid or

Table 16.2 Injectable drugs for sedation, analgesia, or premedication in cats

Drug	Dose (mg/kg)
Anticholinergic	
Atropine	0.04 IM, SC; 0.02 IV
Glycopyrrolate	0.01 IM; 0.005 IV
Phenothiazine	
Acepromazine	0.02–0.1 IM; 0.02–0.05 IV
Benzodiazepine	
Diazepam	0.2–0.5 IV
Midazolam	0.1–0.5 IM, 0.1–0.3 IV
α₂-Agonist sedative	
Xylazine	1–2 IM, 0.2–0.5 IV
Medetomidine*	0.005–0.08 IM
Dexmedetomidine*	0.002–0.04 IM
Opioid	
Butorphanol	0.1–0.4 IM, IV, SC
Buprenorphine	0.005–0.02 IM; 0.005–0.01 IV
Morphine	0.2–0.3 IM
Meperidine	2–5 IM, SC
Hydromorphone	0.05–0.1 IM, IV
Oxymorphone	0.05–0.1 IM, IV
Methadone	0.2–0.5 IM; 0.1–0.3 IV
Other	
Tramadol	2 SC

*0.005 mg/kg = 5 µg/kg, 0.08 mg/kg = 80 µg/kg

ketamine, and to provide a quieter recovery from anaesthesia.

α₂-Agonist sedatives

Experimental and clinical studies confirm that medetomidine and dexmedetomidine reliably produce sedation and analgesia in cats in 15–20 minutes after IM administration, although pre-injection excitement or aggression may result in sedation of less intensity. Dose rates based on body surface area are available in the product package, indicating that the µg/kg dose rate decreases as the animal's body weight increases. The duration of sedation is dose dependent. Equivalent sedative doses for dexmedetomidine are approximately one-half those for medetomidine. Analgesia produced by dexmedetomidine, 0.04 mg/kg (40 µg/kg), was reported to be equivalent to that provided by medetomidine, 0.08 mg/kg (80 µg/kg), IM (Slingsby & Taylor, 2008).

Dexmedetomidine given at doses varying from 0.015 to 0.04 mg/kg (15–40 µg/kg), IM induced lateral recumbency in cats in approximately 20–30 minutes (Monteiro et al., 2009; Slingsby et al., 2010). Maximum sedation without responsiveness lasted about 30 minutes from the highest dose and the sedative effects began to wane at 60 minutes after administration (Slingsby et al., 2010). Although times vary somewhat between reports, in general, the duration of maximum sedation was similar for all the doses but the total duration of sedation tended to be longer the higher the dose rate. Experimental tests of analgesia indicated that dexmedetomidine does not produce analgesia at low dose rates but that analgesia is present when the dose of dexmedetomidine is increased to 0.04 mg/kg, IM. Further, the intensity and duration of analgesia from dexmedetomidine, 0.04 mg/kg, was less than that provided by buprenorphine, 0.02 mg/kg (Slingsby et al., 2010). Dexmedetomidine, 0.04 mg/kg, administered by the buccal transmucosal (TM) route achieved the same effect as from IM administration (Slingsby & Taylor, 2009). Onset of sedation was on average 30–35 minutes and duration an average of 98 minutes from both IM and TM routes. Medetomidine, at a lower dose of 0.02 mg/kg (20 µg/kg), produced sedation lasting 30–60 minutes in experimental cats (Lamont et al., 2001).

The cardiovascular effects of medetomidine and dexmedetomidine are similar for all dose rates. After administration of medetomidine, 0.02 mg/kg, HR were decreased by 40% from the preadministration values and, although systemic vascular resistance (SVR) increased significantly at 15 minutes (vasoconstriction), MAP was unchanged. Cardiac output (CO) was decreased by 63% at 15 minutes, an effect due to a combination of decreased HR and decreased stroke index, the latter presumed due to the increase in afterload. No significant changes in blood gas values were noted. Similarly, HR decreased after administration of dexmedetomidine and SAP as measured by Doppler non-invasive blood pressure measurement (NIBP) was unchanged for 60 minutes (Monteiro et al., 2009). Prior administration of atropine, 0.05 mg/kg, IM significantly increased HR and SAP for 45 minutes, although not to the high levels recorded in dogs. Concurrent administration of atropine with these sedatives is not usually recommended.

The sedative effects following administration of xylazine, 1 mg/kg, or romifidine, 0.2 mg/kg, IM are similar although muscle relaxation and analgesia were less with romifidine and were not increased significantly by increasing dose rate (Selmi et al., 2004). Medetomidine and dexmedetomidine are generally chosen over romifidine for use in cats.

α_2-Agonist sedatives are commonly administered in combination with an opioid. The addition of butorphanol, 0.2 mg/kg, IM to a low dose of dexmedetomidine, 0.01 mg/kg, significantly increased sedation and muscle relaxation over administration of dexmedetomidine alone (Selmi et al., 2003). The combination of buprenorphine, 0.01 mg/kg, with dexmedetomidine, 0.02 mg/kg, IM produced a similar duration and degree of maximum sedation as dexmedetomidine, 0.04 mg/kg, and a greater duration of analgesia (Slingsby et al., 2010). A combination of midazolam, 0.4 mg/kg, butorphanol, 0.4 mg/kg, and dexmedetomidine, 0.005 mg/kg (5 µg/kg), IM produced deep and long-lasting sedation (Biermann et al., 2012). With this combination, HR decreased, CO decreased by approximately 50%, and blood pressure was unchanged.

The addition of ketamine to the combination of medetomidine or dexmedetomidine and butorphanol (popularly known as 'kitty magic') can produce sedation at low doses and anaesthesia at higher doses. The combination of 0.1 mL each of medetomidine (1 mg/mL) or dexmedetomidine (0.5 mg/mL), butorphanol (10 mg/mL), and ketamine (100 mg/mL) mixed in one syringe and administered IM will induce heavy sedation within 5 minutes (Ko et al., 2009). These volumes are calculated for cats weighing 4.5 kg and are equivalent to dexmedetomidine, 0.011 mg/kg, butorphanol, 0.22 mg/kg, and ketamine, 2.2 mg/kg. More or less of the total volume may be administered depending on the desired effect. The volume of each drug may be increased to 0.2 mL/4.5 kg or 0.13 mL/3 kg to induce general anaesthesia for castration and to 0.3 mL/4.5 kg or 0.2 mL/3 kg to produce 40 minutes of anaesthesia suitable for ovariohysterectomy. Administration of this drug combination IV is generally at half the IM dose. Substitution with buprenorphine for butorphanol is not as satisfactory for injectable anaesthesia because the onset time for buprenorphine is long, but is suitable for premedication to inhalation anaesthesia.

The sedative effects of medetomidine and dexmedetomidine may be antagonized by administration of atipamezole IM. The optimal recommended dose for atipamezole is 2.5× the dose of medetomidine, which equals half the volume of medetomidine previously administered, or up to 5× the dose of dexmedetomidine for deeply sedated cats. Allowance should be made for the time elapsed since administration of the α_2-sedative, as less atipamezole will be necessary over time. Overantagonism can lead to the cat becoming excessively alert. Antagonism of the sedative will remove analgesia and reveal excitatory effects of ketamine, when present. In an emergency, administration of atipamezole, 5–20 µg/kg has been recommended slowly IV (off label) over several minutes. Atipamezole is not FDA licensed for use in cats in the USA.

Vomiting has been recorded in cats after administration of xylazine, medetomidine, dexmedetomidine, and romifidine in most (Lamont et al., 2001; Selmi et al., 2004; Slingsby & Taylor, 2009; Slingsby et al., 2010; Biermann et al., 2012) but not all reports (Selmi et al., 2003). The cats are usually still standing at this point which decreases the risk of aspiration.

Concerns with use of α_2-agonists centre on their sedative and cardiovascular effects. When any of these agents is used for premedication, the dose of subsequently administered anaesthetic agent may be decreased by half or even more, especially when an opioid or a low dose of ketamine has been included. α_2-Sedatives profoundly decrease CO and this must be taken into consideration when selecting an anaesthetic protocol for old or sick cats and cats with cardiac disease. Use of medetomidine or dexmedetomidine is not recommended in very young kittens.

Benzodiazepines

Diazepam and midazolam are rarely used alone as they produce minimal sedative effects and may cause agitation or restlessness in healthy patients. Benzodiazepines are commonly administered as adjunct agents to opioids or anaesthetic agents to increase sedation or to block excitatory effects of ketamine. Midazolam, 0.1–0.5 mg/kg, may be administered IM or IV and diazepam, 0.1–0.5 mg/kg, may be administered IV. Oral forms of diazepam are not recommended because of the risk of hepatotoxicity.

Opioids

Factors to be considered when choosing an opioid are the preferred route of administration, speed of onset of effect, duration of effect, efficacy of analgesia in relation to the species and procedure to be performed, and adverse effects.

The speed of onset is of significance depending on the time available between administration and the start of anaesthesia or painful process, with IV and IM administration as the most reliable routes. Onset after IV administration is rapid for butorphanol, hydromorphone, oxymorphone, fentanyl, and methadone. Onset of analgesia following administration of buprenorphine,

0.02 mg/kg, was 15 minutes after IV administration in one study (Steagall et al., 2008a), 35 minutes for both IV and IM routes in another (Slingsby & Taylor, 2008), and 4 hours after IM administration in another (Robertson et al., 2003). Onset of effect after IM administration is relatively rapid with butorphanol and hydromorphone at 15–20 minutes (Lascelles & Robertson, 2004; Wells et al., 2008) and peak effect of hydromorphone, 0.1 mg/kg, was measured at 30 minutes (Robertson et al., 2009). Onset after IM injection of meperidine (pethidine) 5 mg/kg, was approximately 20 minutes with analgesia persisting for 60 minutes (Millette et al., 2008).

Methadone, 0.3 mg/kg, IV quickly causes sedation that lasts 30 minutes. Antinociception was detected 5 minutes after IV administration, was most intense for 60 minutes and a significant effect persisted for 4 hours (Ferreira et al., 2011). In a clinical investigation of cats undergoing ovariohysterectomy, premedication with methadone, 0.6 mg/kg, IM provided pain relief for 4 hours after surgery (Rohrer-Bley et al., 2004). The duration of analgesia from hydromorphone, 0.1 mg/kg, against experimental nociception was twice as long after IM than IV administration, 5.7 hours compared with 2.7 hours, respectively, and this dose rate produced significantly more analgesia than half that dose rate (Lascelles & Robertson, 2004; Wegner & Robertson, 2007). Thermal antinociception was recorded at 4–6 hours after IM injection of morphine, 0.2 mg/kg (Robertson et al., 2003). Morphine may not be as analgesic in cats as in other species because the glucuronidation pathway is less efficient in cats, preventing formation of a morphine active metabolite (Taylor et al., 2001). Evaluations of the duration of antinociception from butorphanol, 0.1–0.8 mg/kg, IM vary from 5 to 480 minutes (Robertson et al., 2003; Wells et al., 2008). A clinical perception is that the duration of analgesia from butorphanol is up to 2 hours and that while analgesia may be satisfactory for soft tissue surgery, butorphanol does not provide sufficient analgesia for orthopaedic procedures. No sedation should be expected after administration of buprenorphine alone. Duration of analgesia from buprenorphine, 0.02 mg/kg, was recorded as 7–8 hours (Slingsby & Taylor, 2008).

Care must be taken when mixing opioids in the same patient as μ agonists, buprenorphine, and butorphanol possess different receptor affinities that may result in diminished analgesia. Administration of hydromorphone and buprenorphine together resulted in minimal analgesia for the first 2 hours followed by onset of analgesia (Lascelles & Robertson, 2004) and, in another investigation, simultaneous administration of butorphanol and buprenorphine resulted in some cats without analgesia (Johnson et al., 2007).

Tramadol, 1 mg/kg, SC was an inefficient analgesic agent in an experimental investigation (Steagall et al., 2008b) whereas 2 mg/kg, administered SC 1 hour before ovariohysterectomy provided adequate analgesia postoperatively in 50% of cats (Brondani et al., 2009). Cats given both tramadol and a non-steroidal anti-inflammatory drug (NSAID) did not need rescue analgesia and did not develop hyperalgesia. A longer elimination half-life for tramadol was measured in cats than in dogs (Pypendop & Ilkiw, 2007).

Routes of administration other than IV and IM are not reliable for all opioids. Subcutaneous injection of hydromorphone has a slower onset of peak effect, a shorter duration of antinociception and is associated with more undesirable side effects (Robertson et al., 2009). Buprenorphine administered SC or by buccal transmucosal (TM) routes produced significantly less analgesia than from IV or IM injection (Slingsby & Taylor, 2008; Giordano et al., 2010), although one investigation using thermal nociception found the efficacy and duration of analgesia from buprenorphine similar after TM and IV administration (Robertson et al., 2005). TM administration is accomplished by squirting the drug from a 1 mL syringe inserted between the teeth and the cheek. Interestingly, administration was found to be significantly easier (without the cat turning its head away) using preservative-free buprenorphine than buprenorphine from a multidose bottle (Bortolami et al., 2012b). The authors proposed that the smell or taste of the chlorocresol preservative in the product intended for multiple injections could be responsible for the aversive behaviour and that the cat's response to the preservative might result in less precise administration or increased swallowing of buprenorphine. Plasma concentrations of butorphanol after TM administration remained below the concentrations anticipated for effective antinociception (Wells et al., 2008). Butorphanol is not as lipophilic as buprenorphine and the authors proposed that the cats' oral pH was not high enough to promote maximal absorption. TM administration of methadone resulted in a lower peak plasma concentration than after IV even though the TM dose was double the IV (Ferreira et al., 2011).

Naloxone is an opioid antagonist and will reverse opioid-induced sedation, analgesia and hyperthermia. Naloxone, 0.01–0.02 mg/kg, is administered IM or slowly IV.

Transdermal (TD) fentanyl

Most investigations have described the effects of a reservoir system fentanyl patch using one 25 µg/h patch per cat (see previous chapter for precautions for use and dangers for human toxicity). Despite considerable variability between cats, the increase in plasma concentration of fentanyl is quicker in cats than in dogs reaching a presumed analgesic threshold by 12–18 hours (Lee et al., 2000; Egger et al., 2003). Maximum plasma concentration was measured at 44 hours after application in one group of cats and mean values remained constant for 4 days (Lee et al., 2000). In contrast to dogs, plasma concentrations of fentanyl decreased more slowly in cats after the patches were removed, presumably due to a slow depletion of a cutaneous depot of fentanyl. Differences in skin structure may partly explain interspecies variability in serum or plasma fentanyl concentrations achieved following application or removal of a patch. Arbitrarily decreasing the surface area of the patch by removing part of the adhesive layer was not recommended for the reservoir type patch as that action would not correspond to a predictably linear decrease in fentanyl transfer (Lee et al., 2000). Nonetheless, comparison of full or partial exposure in cats weighing 1.3–4.3 kg anaesthetized for ovariohysterectomy revealed significantly higher plasma concentrations in cats with full exposure (Davidson et al., 2004). The authors proposed a 38% decrease in calculated delivery rate of fentanyl resulting from a 50% decrease in surface area. Dysphoria was observed in several cats that were fully exposed to the patch membrane. Application of a 25 µg/h patch to cats weighing 2.2–5 kg scheduled for anaesthesia and onychectomy resulted in a similar range of plasma fentanyl concentrations without adverse effects (Gellasch et al., 2002). In a study comparing serum cortisol concentrations in conscious cats and during anaesthesia with or without surgery, application of a TD fentanyl patch 12 hours before anaesthesia was associated with significantly decreased cortisol during and after surgery, supporting the authors' conclusion that the TD patch diminished pain or stress (Glerum et al., 2001). After application of a fentanyl patch, cats' behaviours should be observed for signs of overdosage, such as dysphoria, lethargy, inappetence. Cats should also be monitored for signs of pain. Adequate analgesia should not be assumed as plasma fentanyl concentrations may be low or undetectable in some cats after application of a patch (Lee et al., 2000).

TD fentanyl results in a small (18%) but significant decrease in isoflurane requirement in experimental cats (Yackey et al., 2004). A decrease in serum fentanyl concentrations after induction of anaesthesia has been measured in cats that developed hypothermia (35°C, 95°F), presumably due to decreased cutaneous blood flow from vasoconstriction (Pettifer & Hosgood, 2003). The mean fentanyl concentrations of all the cats were within values believed to be associated with analgesia so that the decrease may be of clinical relevance only in some cats. A further concern is that plasma fentanyl concentrations may increase when a cat is positioned with the fentanyl patch (and skin) in direct contact with a heating pad or heated cage floor.

Side effects of opioid administration

Side effects of opioids in cats are excessive salivation, vomiting, euphoria or dysphoria, and increased body temperature, with some variations between agents. Signs of euphoria (behaviour including more than usual meowing, purring, rubbing, rolling, and kneading with forepaws) was present for 2–6 hours after IV methadone and 6–12 hours after TM administration (Ferreira et al., 2011). Euphoria has been observed after administration of other opioids, lasting from 30 minutes with butorphanol to 24 hours with buprenorphine (Gellasch et al., 2002; Robertson et al., 2003; Steagall et al., 2008a; Bortolami et al., 2012a). Euphoria has also been observed after administration of tramadol (Pypendop & Ilkiw, 2007; Steagall et al., 2008b). Dysphoria (staring into space, wary of people, pacing, jumping at the cage walls) has been observed in some cats given oxymorphone, hydromorphone, fentanyl, or tramadol. Mydriasis is induced in cats by µ opioids, butorphanol, and buprenorphine, and dilated pupils may persist for 6–8 hours or even 2–3 days. Cats may vomit or excessively salivate after administration of morphine, hydromorphone, methadone, and tramadol. The addition of acepromazine may decrease the incidence of vomiting. Cats given butorphanol, buprenorphine, or fentanyl are not likely to vomit.

Increased body temperature frequently occurs when cats have been given an opioid. Cats with hyperthermia may pant or behave no differently from the expected effects of the drug(s) administered. Body temperature was monitored for 24 hours in experimental cats with a wireless thermistor implanted within the abdomen that were given different opioids and combinations (Posner et al., 2010). Moderate hyperthermia was defined as 40.1°C (104°F). Hydromorphone, morphine, buprenorphine and butorphanol produced mild to moderate increases in body temperature. Various doses of hydromorphone increased cats' temperatures to similar extents with a peak around 1.5–2 hours after administration and a return to baseline by about 5 hours. The maximum temperature recorded for any cat in this study was 40.7°C (105.3°F) but temperatures up to 42.5°C (108.5°F) have been reported (Niedfeldt & Robertson, 2006). Greater increases in temperature have been noted after opioid administration in conjunction with inhalation anaesthesia compared with opioid administration without general anaesthesia. It has also been noted that cats that were coldest during anaesthesia developed the highest peak temperatures during recovery (Posner et al., 2010). Increased body temperatures were also recorded for several hours after anaesthesia in cats with fentanyl patches applied for premedication (Lee et al., 2000; Glerum et al., 2001). Mild to moderate increases in temperature should resolve without treatment. Cooling measures should be instituted to treat severe hyperthermia and injection of naloxone may further decrease body temperature.

Non-steroidal anti-inflammatory agents

An NSAID will contribute to the comfort of a cat after a surgical procedure. Recommended dose rates for use in cats are given in Table 16.3, however, not all NSAIDs are licensed in all countries and the clinician should refer to local information and regulations (Sparkes et al., 2010). Single doses administered for treatment of acute pain may have a duration of 18–20 hours. Although the risk of acute

Table 16.3 NSAID dose rates in cats

NSAID	Formulation	Dose	Route	Frequency
Carprofen	Injectable 50 mg/mL	4 mg/kg	SC IV	Once only
Ketoprofen	Injectable 10 mg/mL	2 mg/kg	SC	Q24h up to 3 days
	Tablets 5 mg	1 mg/kg	PO	Q24 h up to 5 days
Meloxicam	Injectable 5 mg/mL	0.3 mg/kg	SC	Once only
	Injectable 2 mg/mL	0.2 mg/kg	SC	Once ± 0.05 mg/kg PO Q24h for 4 days
	Oral suspension 0.5 mg/mL	0.1 mg/kg (= 0.2 mL/kg day 1, then 0.05 mg/kg (0.1 mL/kg)	PO	Q24h indefinite
Robenacoxib	Injectable 20 mg/mL	2 mg/kg	SC	Once only
	Tablets 6 mg	1 mg/kg	PO	Q24h up to 6 days (longer in some countries)
Tolfenamic acid	Injectable 40 mg/mL	4 mg/kg	SC	Q24h for 2 days
	Tablets 6 mg	4 mg/kg	PO	Q24h for 3 days
Acetylsalicylic acid (aspirin)	Toxic to cats, except for very low dosage, 10–20 mg/kg, PO Q3-4 days (Grace 2011)			
Paracetamol (also known as acetaminophen) is extremely toxic to cats				

Sparkes et al., 2010. Note that not all drugs are licensed for cats in all countries.

renal failure is low in healthy cats, the ISFM and AAFP panel recommendations list increased risk of adverse renal effects associated with hypotension during anaesthesia, cats that are dehydrated or hypovolaemic, older cats, cats with concurrent cardiovascular, renal or hepatic disease, and concurrent administration of ACE inhibitors, diuretics, and beta-blocking drugs. NSAIDs should be used with extreme caution if at all in cats with severe liver dysfunction or hypoalbuminaemia.

CONTROVERSIAL ISSUES

This section addresses some areas where there are differences of opinion. One opinion may not be better or safer than another but they illustrate varying practices in different circumstances and the need for further evaluation.

Evaluation of pain

The presence and severity of pain in cats may be difficult to assess. Observation alone appears to be an inadequate assessment of pain and changes in HR or RR may be unrelated. Cats in pain tend to become quiet and less interactive and evaluation of their responses to stroking their fur or handling of the damaged or surgical site may be more

informative. Cats that hunch their backs, lower their ears, hiss, or are aggressive may be showing signs of anxiety, fearfulness, or pain. There are many pain scoring systems that may be employed (Chapter 5):

- The Visual Analogue Scale (VAS) is a line with a scale from 0 to 100 mm on which an observer marks a score based on observation of the cat. A VAS score can be assigned for evaluating pain or sedation or response to palpation of the incision. Generally 0 indicates no pain or no sedation and 100 mm represents the maximum possible score
- The Dynamic and Interactive Visual Analogue Scale (DIVAS) is a VAS that is a combined assessment of observation from a distance, the cat's behaviour when approached, and response to palpation of the surgical site
- The Numerical Rating Scale (NRS) includes observation of the cat from outside the cage and evaluation of the animal's behaviour after opening the cage door, stroking the cat, and finally palpation over or near the surgical incision. These behaviours are each graded by assigning a number from 0 to 3 or 0–4 based on the cat's responses. An exact description of the possible responses for 0, 1, 2, and 3 are predetermined. The total score represents the intensity of pain and the higher the score the greater the pain.

In many studies, these evaluations are performed before anaesthesia to provide a baseline value for comparison with postoperative values. The difficulty in designing a scale that is sufficiently sensitive to detect pain or a difference between two or more analgesic treatments lies in the interpretation of the cat's behaviour or response and in the relative ranking of the individual components of the scoring system. Healthy cats normally spend 40% of their day sleeping and 20% resting (Robertson & Lascelles, 2010). Thus, sternal recumbency may be normal or a result of agent-induced sedation, and lateral recumbency may be normal or the cat may be lying in this position because sternal position is uncomfortable or painful after a midline incision. A cat that is at the back of the cage, hunched over, tail wrapped around forepaws, eyes closed and ears down may be sedated or exhibiting the effects of residual anaesthetic agents or may be in pain. Cats will tear at bandages and exhibit abnormal behaviour whether they are in pain or not. Palpation of the surgical site followed by the cat moving away from the pressure may be the cat's normal aversion to being touched or may be a consequence of induced discomfort. Palpation of the wound during clinical evaluation and for experimental studies, use of a calibrated force testing instrument or device on or adjacent to the incision may be a more accurate measure of tenderness of the surgical area and existence of hyperalgesia (Benito-de-la-Víbora et al., 2008; Brondani et al., 2009; Bortolami et al., 2012a).

A further dilemma is the designated threshold of the scoring system at which rescue (interventional) analgesia is administered, that is, the point where there is recognition that the current analgesia protocol is providing insufficient analgesia for the individual cat. A frequently used threshold is a score that is 55–62% of the total points possible, a value that may be too high since, in many publications, the need for rescue analgesia does not fit an intuitive expectation of induced pain and authors have concluded that the assessment system was not sensitive enough to pick up the more subtle signs of pain. A threshold of 33% of the total possible score was utilized in one study for identifying need for rescue analgesia in cats undergoing ovariohysterectomy and this value appeared to demarcate clearly differences between cats that did or did not receive analgesic drugs (Brondani et al., 2009).

Experimental studies of the analgesic effects of drugs employ the application of a noxious stimulus, thermal, mechanical, or electrical, to a leg or the skin over the thorax in stepwise increments before and after administration of the drug to determine the threshold at which the cat responds. The stimulus ceases when the cat responds by turning towards the device or attempts to move away, and has an automatic cut-off to prevent tissue damage in the event the drug has prevented the cat from feeling the stimulus. The nature of these stimuli may not accurately mimic a naturally occurring painful process but allows comparison of drugs. The results have demonstrated that many drugs are associated with wide variations in responses within a cat population.

Pain induced by elective surgery of short duration generally lasts only a few days. Persistence of post-surgical pain occurs in a proportion of patients but, even in human medicine, this condition is under-diagnosed and under-recognized (Schug, 2012). Persistent pain was reported in 40%, 18% with moderate to severe pain, of over 2000 human patients that had surgery 3 months to 3 years previously (Johansen et al., 2012). The survey identified a strong association between persistent pain and the presence and intensity of the immediate post-surgical pain, and many of the patients were experiencing pain before surgery. Hyperaesthesia, indicating sensitization, occurred in most patients but hypoaesthesia, indicating nerve damage, was also often present. Cats clearly experience pain after surgery when not treated with analgesic agents. The incidence of persistent pain is unknown, however, experiences with human patients highlight the need to deal effectively with surgical pain. Preventive analgesia to minimize central sensitization of the spinal nociceptive neurons aims to block noxious stimuli pre-, intra-, and postoperatively and requires use of more than one ('multimodal') approach (Katz et al., 2011; Gurney, 2012). Acepromazine, thiopental, propofol, alfaxalone, and the volatile inhalation anaesthetics do not provide analgesia for painful procedures. Thus, the multimodal approach employs combinations of systemic opioid(s), NSAIDs, infiltration or regional nerve blocks with local anaesthetic or other drugs, and an NMDA-receptor antagonist. Effective analgesia is demonstrated by the reduction in pain and analgesic drug use beyond the duration of the drugs administered, defined as 5.5 half-lives (Katz et al., 2011). Long-term pain persisting for more than 2–3 weeks in cats may be associated with signs of decreased mobility, decreased interaction with humans and other animals, poor appetite, and aggression. Long-term pain from non-surgical causes, such as degenerative joint disease, cystitis, neoplasia, and dental disease requires consideration of agents that may 'reset' the CNS and agents that are considered to be safe for continued administration in cats, such as tramadol, NSAIDs, and 'off label' use of other drugs (Robertson & Lascelles, 2010).

Ovariohysterectomy, castration

Pain scoring has identified that cats exhibit signs attributable to pain after ovariohysterectomy and castration, and pain has been present in some cats for at least 24 hours (Balmer et al., 1998; Slingsby & Waterman-Pearson, 1998, 2002; Glerum et al., 2001; Al-Gizawiy & Rudé, 2004; Rohrer-Bley et al., 2004; Gassel et al., 2005; Grint et al., 2006; Tobias et al., 2006; Benito-de-la-Víbora et al., 2008; Brondani et al., 2009; Steagall et al., 2009b; Giordano et al., 2010; Murison & Martinez Taboada, 2010). A comparison of the flank and midline surgical approaches confirmed that wound tenderness was greater following a flank incision (Grint et al., 2006), as might be expected from muscle involvement in the flank incision. An inexperienced surgeon may cause more tissue trauma than an experienced surgeon, however, a study evaluating postoperative behaviours after ovariohysterectomy in dogs found no significant association with experience of the surgeon or duration of surgery (Wagner et al., 2008).

Frequently, in clinical practice, a sedative such as acepromazine, medetomidine or dexmedetomidine, an opioid and an NSAID are administered in conjunction with anaesthetic agent(s) in order to achieve both intra- and postoperative analgesia (Bortolami et al., 2012a; Mathis et al., 2012). Anaesthesia for ovariohysterectomy may be maintained with an inhalant agent preceded by premedication and induction of anaesthesia with ketamine, ketamine with diazepam or midazolam, tiletamine–zolazepam, thiopental, propofol, or alfaxalone. Anaesthetic protocols using only injectable agents are commonly used when surgery time is likely to be less than 30 minutes (Table 16.4). Published investigations involving cats

presented for ovariohysterectomy or castration should be evaluated cautiously because the anaesthetic protocols may have been limited combinations to facilitate study of a single analgesic drug. It is important when selecting analgesic drugs to consider their onset times to avoid start of surgery before onset of analgesia. For example, administration of buprenorphine or an NSAID at induction of anaesthesia does not provide sufficient time for onset of analgesia before the surgical procedure and, in some cases, recovery from anaesthesia. The durations of analgesia of the agents chosen must also be known for scheduling of the redosing interval. Butorphanol and pethidine (meperidine) have short durations of action of about 2 hours and a single administration of these drugs for premedication will be insufficient for postoperative analgesia (Balmer et al., 1998; Slingsby & Waterman-Pearson, 1998). Methadone, hydromorphone, oxymorphone, and buprenorphine may provide analgesia for 4–6 hours. Published research indicates that administration of only an NSAID for analgesia does not provide sufficient analgesia after ovariohysterectomy (Brondani et al., 2009; Murison &

Table 16.4 Examples of anaesthetic agent combinations for general anaesthesia in domestic cats

Premedication*	Induction of anaesthesia†	Maintenance of anaesthesia
Acepromazine 0.05 mg/kg Butorphanol 0.3 mg/kg IM or Buprenorphine 0.01–0.02 mg/kg IM Atropine 0.04 mg/kg IM	Ketamine 5 mg/kg mixed with diazepam 0.25 mg/kg or ketamine 5–10 mg/kg IV	10 min anaesthesia
Medetomidine 0.08 mg/kg Ketamine 5–7.5 mg/kg IM	—	50 min anaesthesia
Dexmedetomidine 0.03 mg/kg Butorphanol 0.4 mg/kg Ketamine 7 mg/kg IM	—	40 min anaesthesia
Tiletamine–zolazepam 4 mg/kg IM Butorphanol 0.2 mg/kg IM	Ketamine 2–4 mg/kg IV if needed for intubation	Isoflurane or sevoflurane starting with no/low vaporizer setting
Acepromazine 0.05 mg/kg IM Buprenorphine 0.02 mg/kg IM or other opioid‡	Propofol 4 mg/kg or alfaxalone 2–5 mg/kg or ketamine 5 mg/kg mixed with diazepam 0.25 mg/kg IV	Isoflurane or sevoflurane
Medetomidine 0.01–0.02 mg/kg or dexmedetomidine 0.005–0.01 mg/kg IM Opioid IM	Propofol 2 mg/kg or alfaxalone 2 mg/kg or ketamine 2 mg/kg IV	Isoflurane or sevoflurane
Acepromazine 0.05 mg/kg IM Opioid IM	Propofol 4 mg/kg or alfaxalone 2–5 mg/kg IV	Propofol 6–18 mg/kg/h or alfaxalone 11 mg/kg/h, respectively
Ill or cardiac patients: Butorphanol 0.2–0.3 mg/kg IM or Buprenorphine 0.01 mg/kg IM	Diazepam 0.25 mg/kg or midazolam IV before Etomidate 1.5 mg/kg IV	Isoflurane or sevoflurane

*Onset time depends on drugs chosen; † Approximate dose rates, drugs should be given 'to effect'; ‡ Or substitute with IM injection of butorphanol 0.3 mg/kg IM, or oxymorphone 0.1 mg/kg, or hydromorphone 0.1 mg/kg, or methadone 0.3 mg/kg, or morphine 0.3 mg/kg
Verstegen et al., 1990; Ko et al., 2009; O'Hagan et al., 2012.

Martinez Taboada, 2010) although, in some studies, cats receiving an NSAID had better total pain scores than those receiving an opioid only (Slingsby & Waterman-Pearson, 1998; Gassel et al., 2005). Inclusion of an NSAID was found to decrease incisional hyperalgesia (Al-Gizawiy & Rudé, 2004; Benito-de-la-Víbora et al., 2008) and decrease pain scores when administered in combination with an opioid (Brondani et al., 2009; Steagall et al., 2009b).

Rescue (interventional) analgesia is usually in the form of an opioid at the same or reduced dose that is used for premedication, and is commonly administered IM for rapid onset of analgesia. An NSAID (SC administration) may be included if one has not already been administered. Examples of drugs used for rescue analgesia in cats after ovariohysterectomy are:

- Morphine 0.2–0.3 mg/kg IM
- Pethidine (meperidine) 4 mg/kg IM
- Buprenorphine 0.01–0.02 mg/kg IM
- Butorphanol 0.2–0.4 mg/kg IM
- Hydromorphone or oxymorphone 0.05 mg/kg IM
- Methadone 0.2–0.3 mg/kg IM
- Tramadol 2 mg/kg SC.

Management of anaesthesia in high volume practices and animal shelter programmes may of necessity be more regimented than tailored to the individual patient, and preanaesthetic evaluation of feral cats may not be possible. Guidelines for spay-neuter programmes published by the Association of Shelter Veterinarians are detailed and contain many suggestions for good patient care (Looney et al., 2008). The guidelines stress that a standard volume dose rate of anaesthetic agents for all cats should be avoided and suggest that doses either be calculated on a per kg basis or calculated for cats in several weight ranges, for example <1 kg, 1–2 kg, and 2–4 kg, and the volume of each drug be written out in a chart for easy reference. Anaesthetic protocols should provide analgesia. Reversible drugs are useful, especially in feral cats, but recognizing that reversal of medetomidine or dexmedetomidine removes some of the analgesia. In the context of shelter medicine, an animal with a mild infection or non-infectious medical condition may be anaesthetized because of the likelihood that the animal will not be available for neutering at a later date (Looney et al., 2008). The presence of disease may be responsible for deaths during or following anaesthesia (Gerdin et al., 2011).

Feral cats

Feral cats are defined as free-roaming cats without owners. A feral cat is caught in a special trap that can be adjusted to immobilize the cat for IM injection. The anaesthetic agent combination must reliably induce anaesthesia in unsocialized cats without causing overdosage. A small number of cats may need supplementation with additional anaesthetic agent to provide a sufficient depth of anaesthesia for ovariohysterectomy or castration. In one series of 101 feral cats (Harrison et al., 2011), the weight of each cat was determined by subtracting the known weight of the trap from the combined total weight. Medetomidine, 0.1 mg/kg (100 µg/kg), ketamine, 10 mg/kg, and buprenorphine, 0.01 mg/kg, were administered into the paralumbar muscles. If the cat was still responsive after the first injection, additional medetomidine, 0.02 mg/kg, was administered IM. Ketamine, 2.5 mg/kg, was injected IM if anaesthesia was still insufficient. Atipamezole, 0.125 mg/kg, SC was administered at the completion of surgery and the cats were released the next day. Eleven cats required additional medetomidine ± ketamine and 11 cats required supplemental isoflurane, half of which were after 45 minutes of satisfactory anaesthesia. The initial injection induced recumbency in 5 ± 5 minutes and the median time from injection to start of surgery was 23 minutes. Monitoring the cats immediately after induction and during anaesthesia is important and support treatment must be available. In the previous investigation, significant decreases in SpO$_2$ were observed in cats in the first few minutes of anaesthesia, one cat was apnoeic after induction of anaesthesia, one cat was cyanotic and responded sluggishly to O$_2$ supplementation, one cat had bradycardia (<60 beats/min), and three cats were hypotensive (Doppler SAP <90 mmHg).

An older review of 7501 feral cats anaesthetized for ovariohysterectomy (59%) or castration (41%) utilized a combination of tiletamine–zolazepam, ketamine, and xylazine (TKX) (Williams et al., 2002). A vial of 500 mg of lyophilized tiletamine–zolazepam was reconstituted with 4 mL of ketamine (100 mg/mL) and 1 mL of 10% xylazine (100 mg/mL) so that each mL of solution contained 50 mg tiletamine, 50 mg zolazepam, 80 mg ketamine, and 20 mg xylazine. The average dose per cat was 0.25 mL of the combination injected IM. Using the average weight of 3 kg from 194 cats, the dose rates can be calculated as tiletamine–zolazepam, 8.3 mg/kg, ketamine, 7 mg/kg, and xylazine 1.7 mg/kg. The standard dose of 0.25 mL was adjusted according to the estimated size of the cat and additional small doses were administered when the first dose was insufficient. A single dose provided adequate anaesthesia for 79.5% of cats. Yohimbine, 0.5 mg for adults and 0.3 mg for kittens, was injected at the end of surgery to reverse the xylazine. Twenty-six cats (0.35%) died before hospital discharge, of which 17 were considered to be anaesthetic deaths. In another report, the same anaesthetic drug combination (0.25 mL IM) was administered to 22 male and 67 female feral cats, and a single injection provided sufficient anaesthesia in 92% of all cats (Cistola et al., 2004). The mean time to start of ovariohysterectomy was 28 minutes and surgery time was 11 minutes. All cats survived to discharge but hypoxaemia, detected by pulse oximetry, was prevalent and some cats became hypotensive. These abnormalities are potential causes of anaesthetic death but all the cats in this study survived without treatment. The authors stressed the difficulty of routinely supplying supplemental O_2 in a high volume Trap-Neuter-Return programme when, for example, 12 cats are anaesthetized simultaneously. The authors also noted that MAP increased at the start of surgery and questioned the adequacy of the combination for providing postoperative analgesia.

When dealing with a small number of feral cats in a practice environment, addition of pulse oximetry and Doppler or oscillometric arterial pressure monitoring, and supplementation with O_2 when needed, is feasible and advisable.

Regional nerve blocks

Nerve blocks can be a valuable part of an anaesthetic protocol by blocking central sensitization and extending analgesia postoperatively. The brachial plexus block provides analgesia below the elbow for radius/ulna and metacarpal orthopaedic surgery. Epidural analgesia can be included for pelvis and hind limb surgery and an epidural opioid provides some analgesia for thoracotomy. Epidural analgesia has been used for many years in cats with urethral obstruction but, more recently, a sacrococcygeal nerve block has been recommended for pain relief in cats with this disease (O'Hearn & Wright, 2011). Peroneal and tibial nerve blocks are easily performed and bupivacaine may provide at least 6 hours of analgesia for metatarsal surgery. Digital nerve blocks can provide effective analgesia after onychectomy, 'declawing', where performed, and anecdotally have been associated with a decrease in owners' concerns after the cat's return home. Dental nerve blocks are commonly employed for tooth extractions and major oral surgery. Soaker catheters can provide substantial pain relief in cats with major superficial wounds.

Euthanasia

This section is not a discussion of the ethical concerns of euthanasia, a topic that has been addressed elsewhere (Yeates, 2010). The new 2013 American Veterinary Medical Association (AVMA) Guidelines for the Euthanasia of Animals is an extensive document that includes discussions of ethical concerns and techniques of euthanasia in all species and scenarios (www.avma.org). Injectable euthanasia agents provide the most rapid and reliable method of performing euthanasia. Intraperitoneal injection of a non-irritating euthanasia agent that does *not* contain a neuromuscular blocking agent (not T61) may be acceptable when IV administration is considered impracticable or impossible. Absorption of the drug by this route may be slow and signs of Stage 2 anaesthesia may be manifested before the cat progresses to anaesthesia and overdose. Intrahepatic injection by trained personnel of a combination of pentobarbital and lidocaine may have

limited application in cats. Intracardiac injection in awake cats is not considered acceptable. Intracardiac injection is acceptable only when the cat is unconscious or anaesthetized. Use of a supersaturated solution of potassium chloride in unanaesthetized animals is also unacceptable. Euthanasia should be performed in accordance with applicable federal, state, and local laws governing handling of drugs and methods used for euthanasia.

Euthanasia of pregnant animals must take into consideration euthanasia of the fetuses. Studies in other species have documented that after euthanasia with pentobarbital solution, cardiac function continues in the fetuses for 25 minutes (Peisker et al., 2010). The 2013 AVMA Guidelines recommend that after euthanasia of a pregnant cat by barbiturate injection, the fetuses should be left undisturbed in the uterus for 20 minutes after the queen has been confirmed dead. During ovariohysterectomy of a pregnant queen, the uterine blood vessels should be ligated and the uterus should not be opened for an hour after removal from the abdomen. IP injection of pentobarbital is recommended for late-term pregnancy fetuses that have been removed from the uterus.

A quiet and painless death should be the aim for euthanasia. This may be easier said than done given the tendency of some cats to resist even minimal restraint during routine physical examination and collection of blood for laboratory tests. The presence of a grieving owner may impact on the cat's behaviour and impose unrealistic expectations for an uncomplicated procedure. Induction of sedation or general anaesthesia before injection of a euthanasia drug may be less stressful for the patient and client and avoid terminal gasping, however, administration of an α_2-sedative may induce vomiting that is upsetting for the client to observe. Ketamine is absorbed through mucous membranes and sedation can be achieved by squirting ketamine into the mouth of a hissing cat and leaving it undisturbed for 30 minutes before attempting IV injection. A large dose of acepromazine IM or SC may induce sufficient sedation in 10–15 minutes for IV injection.

GENERAL ANAESTHESIA

Preanaesthetic preparation

Fasting before anaesthesia is recommended to minimize the likelihood of solid food in the stomach at the time of anaesthesia. This may reduce the risk of pulmonary aspiration should the cat vomit during induction or recovery from anaesthesia or if regurgitation occurs during anaesthesia. Overnight fasting is recommended for animals >16 weeks of age and scheduled for anaesthesia in the morning (Bednarski et al., 2011). Fasting is limited to <4 hours for young kittens. Water must be removed at the time of premedication.

Premedication

Administration of sedatives and opioids before induction of anaesthesia increases the safety of the patient by reducing anxiety, providing analgesia, decreasing the dose rates of anaesthetic agents, and preventing adverse effects of other drugs. The sedative and cardiopulmonary effects and duration of action will depend on the combination of drugs chosen. There are several anaesthetic protocols that can be used safely in young healthy cats scheduled for elective procedures and choice of protocol is influenced by personal preference (see Table 16.4). Anaesthetic agents must be selected more carefully for old or sick cats with regard for potential impact of the disease on agent effects, and vice versa.

Sedatives and analgesics

Acepromazine, 0.05 mg/kg, is commonly used in combination with any of the opioids for premedication to general anaesthesia. Sedation is not usually profound but is generally sufficient to allow IV injection of anaesthetic agent or placement of an IV catheter prior to induction of anaesthesia. The degree of sedation from an acepromazine–opioid combination varies according to the opioid chosen, for example, minimal with buprenorphine to appreciable with methadone. Similarly, the reduction in dose rate for anaesthetic agents depends on the opioid used, for example, less reduction with butorphanol and greater with hydromorphone. The duration of preanaesthetic drug effects is generally longer after IM injection than IV, and effects of some drugs are unpredictable after SC administration. A benzodiazepine may contribute significantly to sedation when paired with an opioid or administered immediately before or with injection of an anaesthetic agent. An α_2-agonist sedative may be used alone or with an opioid for premedication and the sedative effect is dose and drug dependent. Ketamine can be added to any IM combination to induce profound sedation or anaesthesia.

Anticholinergic agents

Use of an anticholinergic agent, atropine or glycopyrrolate, is not routine. This author generally administers an anticholinergic in cats (atropine 0.04 mg/kg IM or, more frequently, glycopyrrolate 0.01 mg/kg IM) to minimize oral secretions especially with drugs that increase salivation such as ketamine and tiletamine, and to counter bradycardia with pure μ opioids such as oxymorphone, hydromorphone, or fentanyl. An anticholinergic is not commonly used in cats given medetomidine or dexmedetomidine because the increased heart rate may cause hypertension in an animal with an already high pressure. Anticholinergics are not used routinely in cats with myocardial disease, tachyarrhythmias, traumatic myocarditis, pathological tachycardia, hyperthyroidism, pneumonia, or disease-induced hyperthermia.

Intravenous injection

Whenever possible, restraint for IV injection should be minimal. Cats may respond strongly to forced restraint resulting in sympathetic stimulation that increases the dose rate for anaesthetic agents to achieve anaesthesia. Intravenous injections are commonly made into the cephalic vein on the dorsal surface of the forelimb between elbow and carpus or the saphenous vein on the medial surface of the hind limb. For injection into the cephalic vein, the cat is placed in a sitting position on a table of convenient height and for injection into the right cephalic vein the assistant stands to the cat's left side, raising and supporting its head between the thumb and fingers of the left hand (Fig. 16.2). The assistant's right hand is placed so the middle, third and fourth fingers are behind the olecranon, and the thumb is around the front of the cat's right forelimb. The limb is extended by pushing on the olecranon and the vein is raised by applying gentle pressure with the thumb. If the limb is held in a vice-like grip, the cat is likely to respond adversely. Clipping the hair over the vein should be accomplished quickly using quiet electric clippers. When more restraint is needed, the assistant

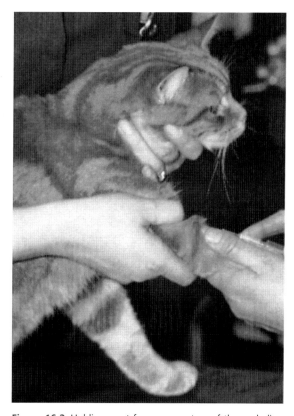

Figure 16.2 Holding a cat for venepuncture of the cephalic vein.

should hold the cat between his or her body and right arm while preventing movement from the hind limbs by pressing the cat gently on to the table surface. An effective restraint technique is to wrap the cat in a towel leaving exposed a leg for injection; the head may be covered or uncovered. Nylon feline restraint bags are available commercially that have a zipper over the back of the cat and front leg openings through which one limb can be exposed for catheterization. Ultimately, it may be necessary for the assistant to control the cat's head by a firm grip with the left hand on the scruff at the back of the head. Sometimes injection into the saphenous vein is less stressful than using the cephalic vein. There is always the option of administering additional agents IM for sedation and waiting an appropriate time for sedation to deepen before again attempting IV injection.

A 25 gauge or 22 gauge needle is commonly used for percutaneous venepuncture. Greater venous access security is achieved by use of a Butterfly needle or a 22 gauge or 20 gauge indwelling catheter. A surgical scrub should be applied to the skin before catheter placement. If desired, the skin can be desensitized by application of local analgesic cream (e.g. EMLA), wrapped with an occlusive dressing and left for 30–45 minutes. The dressing is removed and the skin cleansed before venepuncture. The cephalic vein is located on the dorsal surface of the forearm. The needle or catheter should be inserted gently, without jabbing. Once blood is observed in the hub of the needle, both the needle and catheter must be advanced a small distance (3 mm) to be sure that the catheter is also within the vein, and then, without moving the needle, the catheter should be advanced as far as possible. The needle is removed and the catheter cap or T-port attached. White tape is wrapped around the catheter and then around the leg. A second piece of tape is inserted first under the catheter hub, sticky side next to the skin, and then wrapped around the leg and back around the catheter. If the cap or T-port is not a luer lock, then additional tape should be wrapped around the junction to prevent accidental disconnection. Every attempt should be made to accomplish IV catheterization as smoothly and quietly as possible leaving the cat calm for induction of anaesthesia (Fig. 16.3).

The medial saphenous vein is located medial to the tibia (Fig 16.4). The hair should be clipped down to the hock and up to the stifle to prevent contamination of the catheter during placement. After preparation of the skin, a catheter is inserted and secured in the same manner as just described. This vein is frequently used for cats with point colours as clipping over the cephalic vein, or other parts of the body, may be followed by regrowth of hair in the point colour (Fig. 16.5). The lateral saphenous vein, located on the caudolateral surface of the hind limb above the hock, is a much smaller vein and difficult to catheterize. Longer catheters may be inserted in the jugular vein, generally during general anaesthesia.

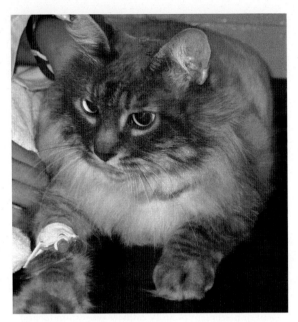

Figure 16.3 Catheter in the cephalic vein capped with a T-port. The fluid administration set is attached to the tube extension so that the cap on the catheter is available for drug administration. Mydriasis is obvious after opioid premedication.

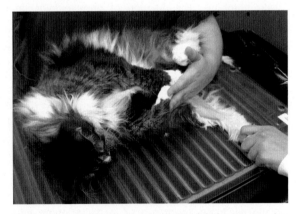

Figure 16.4 Fractious cat heavily sedated with acepromazine and ketamine in preparation for insertion of a 20 gauge catheter into the medial saphenous vein on the medial aspect of the right hind limb. The cat is lying on a hot water circulating acrylic pad.

Endotracheal intubation

Intubation may be unnecessary for short periods of general anaesthesia. A mask can be applied to provide oxygen or for short-term administration of an inhalation anaesthetic agent (see Fig. 10.26). Induction and maintenance of

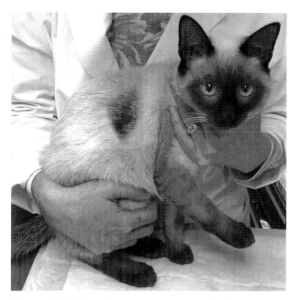

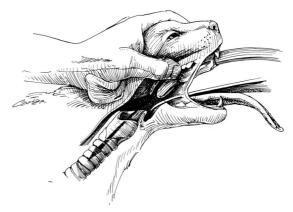

Figure 16.6 The cat's head must be extended to align the pharynx with the trachea for intubation. The laryngoscope blade has been introduced over the tongue until the tip is ventral to the epiglottis.

© *2000–2012 University of Georgia Research Foundation, Inc. Art by William 'Kip' Carter (University of Georgia).*

Figure 16.5 Hair on Siamese cats may grow back as point colour after clipping. This cat had a square of hair clipped over its chest for application of a fentanyl patch.

anaesthesia with inhalation agent by facemask is not recommended as a routine procedure as room pollution with waste gases is unacceptable, wastage occurs because of dilution with room air, and inadequate ventilation cannot be assisted for long due to stomach inflation. Further, proficiency in endotracheal intubation in cats should be achieved using healthy patients so that in an emergency or during difficult situations there is no delay to intubation. Should a cat develop cyanosis during induction of anaesthesia or during the process of intubation, oxygen should be supplied using a well-fitting cat mask. Artificial ventilation, two or three breaths, can be given by squeezing the reservoir bag before attempting intubation. When gastric regurgitation has occurred, the pharynx should rapidly be scooped clean first to provide a clear airway.

Tracheal intubation can be performed with the cat in any position but it is commonly done with the cat in sternal position. The assistant places his/her palm on the top of the cat's head and grasps it with the thumb on one side and fingers on the other. The thumb and fingers can either use the zygomatic arch on each side for leverage or the thumb and forefinger can be placed further forward on the maxilla just caudal to the upper canine teeth. The cat's head and neck must be lifted and stretched into a straight line for optimal position for intubation (Fig. 16.6). The assistant's other hand is used to depress the mandible. The assistant or anaesthetist will pull the tongue gently rostrally to expose the laryngeal entrance. Vision is further assisted by placement of a laryngoscope blade on the tongue with the tip of the blade ventral to

the epiglottis. The cat has a sensitive larynx and touch is likely to induce laryngospasm. Topical application of lidocaine, either as a spray or by dripping from a syringe, will promote easy intubation and avoid the need for undue pressure of the tube on the arytenoids, minimizing trauma. The dose of lidocaine used for topical analgesia must not exceed 2 mg/kg because lidocaine is rapidly absorbed from the tracheal mucosa and may produce a blood concentration that causes cardiovascular depression or arrest. Lidocaine for injection, without epinephrine, 0.1 mL drawn into a 1 mL syringe and dripped into the larynx delivers 2 mg that is an effective and safe dose for most cats and one squirt of Intubeaze™ spray (20 mg/mL) will deliver 0.1–0.2 mL or 2–4 mg. Xylocaine spray marketed for intubation in humans should not be used as it has a variety of additives that cause laryngeal and tracheal mucosal swelling in cats resulting in potentially lethal airway obstruction (Taylor, 1992; Fisher, 2010). Laryngospasm may temporarily occur after application of lidocaine and it is advisable to wait for 20–30 seconds before intubating. The tip of the endotracheal tube should be placed ventrally at the entrance to the larynx (with the cat in sternal position) (Fig. 16.7) with the bevel of the tube vertically. The tube should be rotated 90° anticlockwise (to spread the arytenoids) while being advanced into the larynx. If difficulty in entering the larynx is encountered, an option is to wait for the cat to inhale before advancing the tube. When a stilette is used, for example for a guarded (metal spiral) endotracheal tube, care must be taken to ensure that the stilette tip does not extend past the tip of the endotracheal tube as it may cause tracheal laceration. Care should be taken to limit the force used to push the endotracheal tube into the larynx as the tube may rupture

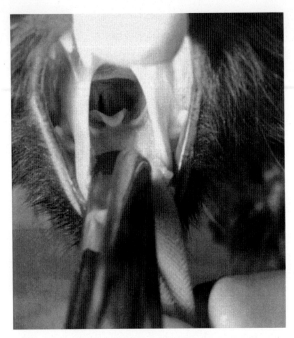

Figure 16.7 View of the epiglottis and arytenoids before intubation in a cat in sternal recumbency.

Table 16.5 Range of dose rates for injectable anaesthetic agents*

Anaesthetic agent	Dose rates mg/kg and route
Alfaxalone	0.5–5 IV
Etomidate	1–3 IV
Ketamine	2–10 IV, 2–33 IM
Propofol	2–10 IV
Thiopental	2–20 IV
Tiletamine–zolazepam	1–2 IV, 2–15 IM

*Dose rate depends on premedicant and concurrent drugs. In general, the heavier the preanaesthetic sedation the lower the dose rate.

the larynx or be diverted into subcutaneous tissues (Hofmeister et al., 2007). There is often a temptation to use a tube that is too small because it is easier to introduce, but this should be resisted because a small tube constitutes a partial airway obstruction. Endotracheal tubes with thin walls and thin-walled soft cuffs are optimal and for most junior and adult cats tubes of 4.0–4.5 mm internal diameter (ID) are suitable. The tip of the tube should be inserted to the approximate level of the thoracic inlet, 12–14 cm for most cats. Large cats and large breeds, such as the Maine Coon, will accommodate larger (5.0 and 5.5 mm ID) and longer tubes. The position of the tip of the tube can be verified by palpation of the tip of the tube in the trachea at the base of the cat's neck, whereupon the tube is advanced a further 1 cm distance. Alternatively, the length of the endotracheal tube can be approximated before intubation but measuring the tube alongside the cat, from incisors to thoracic inlet. Once placed, the position of the tube at the incisors should be memorized by observation of the centimetre distance on the tube, or adjacent lettering, so that any movement of the tube can be recognized early before accidental extubation occurs. The tube should be secured in place using gauze, tape, or plastic tubing tied tightly around the tube and then behind the cat's head or around the bottom jaw and before the cuff is inflated. The position of the tube at the incisors should be rechecked to ensure that the tube has not been inserted more deeply during the process. The cuff should

be inflated by injection of small increments of air until no air leak can be heard when the cat's lungs are artificially inflated to 15–20 cm H_2O. A variety of types of small endotracheal tubes are available for use in small cats, including uncuffed and Cole tubes (see Fig. 10.30). The pharynx is usually packed with moistened gauze when an uncuffed tube is used to avoid tracheal aspiration of fluid and anaesthetic pollution of the room, and to facilitate artificial ventilation. An excess of tube between the mouth and anaesthetic breathing system adds significantly to the apparatus dead space and CO_2 rebreathing. In most cases, the endotracheal tubes can be cut short to different lengths without interfering with the inflation tube supplying the cuff.

Endotracheal intubation through the pharyngostomy site to facilitate exposure for oral surgery has been described in the previous chapter.

Injectable anaesthetic agents

There are several injectable anaesthetic agents that are used to provide anaesthesia in cats (Table 16.5). Some agents, such as thiopental, propofol, and etomidate must be administered IV whereas the dissociative agents ketamine and tiletamine can be administered IV or IM. Alfaxalone is currently licensed for IV use in many countries. Investigations of IM doses of the new formulation of alfaxalone were not published at the time of writing.

Thiopental

Thiopental may only be administered IV and in cats it should be used as a 1, 2 or 2.5% solution. Induction doses are up to 12 mg/kg depending on the degree of preanaesthetic sedation and very small doses (2 mg/kg) will be needed after heavy premedication. The agent is titrated to jaw relaxation and rostroventral rotation of the eye with a weak palpebral reflex. Laryngeal reflexes are retained to some extent with thiopental and use of lidocaine for intubation is advisable. Swallowing during attempted intubation is an indication for additional thiopental administration. Withdrawal of a limb after a toe pinch is an indication of a light plane of anaesthesia. Use of thiopental without preanaesthetic sedation may require incremental doses up to a maximum of 20 mg/kg. This protocol is not advisable because higher doses of thiopental induce excessive respiratory and cardiovascular depression, and prolonged recovery from anaesthesia. Furthermore, thiopental is not analgesic and other agents should be included to supply analgesia. Thiopental is a satisfactory agent for induction of anaesthesia in healthy premedicated cats prior to maintenance of anaesthesia with an inhalation agent but adequacy of ventilation and blood pressure should be closely monitored. Cats are likely to be lethargic the day following thiopental administration.

Methohexital

Methohexital has been used in the past as a 0.5 or 1.0% solution at 6 mg/kg IV for induction of anaesthesia in premedicated cats. The agent is administered in a similar fashion to thiopental, that is, injection of one-third the anticipated dose over 5 seconds and additional increments over 60 seconds to achieve the desired depth of anaesthesia. Recovery from anaesthesia from methohexital without sufficient sedation is accompanied by hyperreflexia, exaggerated muscle response to a stimulus such as nose contact to the side of the cage, or body jerks. The duration of effect of methohexital is extremely short-lived necessitating efficient transfer to an inhalation agent. Agents other than methohexital are currently used for anaesthesia in cats.

Pentobarbital

Pentobarbital is not used for anaesthesia in clinical patients but may be used in experimental protocols. Pentobarbital must be given by IV injection up to 25 mg/kg in unpremedicated animals. Onset of anaesthesia is slow, therefore, administration involves injection of half the anticipated dose to speed transition through the early stages of anaesthesia and then injection of small increments to achieve the desired depth of anaesthesia. The interval between increments must be much longer than with thiopental otherwise overdosage will occur. Total administration time is about 5 minutes. Signs used to titrate the anaesthetic dose include presence or absence of limb withdrawal in response to a toe pinch and twitching of the whiskers in response to pinching the ear pinna. Administration should cease when these reflexes are weak or gone because anaesthesia will continue to deepen for several minutes after the last administration. Duration of surgical anaesthesia may be as long as 2 hours. Recovery

from anaesthesia is largely due to metabolism of pentobarbital and consequently recovery from anaesthesia is prolonged for hours, and will be even longer if the cat becomes cold.

Propofol

Propofol is injected IV at 2–6 mg/kg, depending on the degree of preanaesthetic sedation, and up to 10 mg/kg in the absence of premedication. Approximately one-third of the anticipated dose is administered over 10 seconds and then propofol is titrated in small increments. Injection of the total dose of propofol should be over 1 minute, slower than thiopental, to decrease the incidence and severity of apnoea. The signs and stages observed during induction of anaesthesia with propofol are very similar to those of thiopental except that jaw relaxation occurs earlier and laryngeal spasm is less. Oral mucous membranes may develop a deep red-blue colour that is due to a combination of low oxygenation and low blood pressure. A few artificial breaths with O_2 may be necessary to restore quickly a normal pink mucous membrane colour. Femoral artery pulse strength or blood pressure should be immediately assessed. Apnoea may occur immediately after induction of anaesthesia. Cyanosis or apnoea may occur more frequently when larger doses of propofol are administered or when propofol is administered rapidly (Hall et al., 1999; Matthews et al., 2004). The duration of anaesthesia from an initial anaesthetic dose of propofol is 6–8 minutes. Anaesthesia may be prolonged by additional administration of propofol, 0.1–0.3 mg/kg/min, or an inhalation agent. The significantly longer time for recovery from an infusion of propofol for 150 minutes compared with administration for induction or for 30 minutes has been attributed to the inefficiency of the hepatic metabolic pathway for propofol in cats (Pascoe et al., 2006a). Recovery from propofol is more complete than from thiopental and without the hyperreflexia of ketamine. The cat may exhibit disorientation for a short time and can be loosely wrapped in a towel under supervision until full awareness returns.

The drugs used for premedication will influence the cardiovascular effects of propofol administration. Propofol alone decreases arterial blood pressure and some cats will develop hypotension (Pascoe et al., 2006a; Cleale et al. 2009). SpO_2 ≤90% develops in some cats, indicating the need for O_2 supplementation (Matthews et al., 2004; Selmi et al., 2005; Cleale et al., 2009; Taylor et al., 2012). Mild to moderate hypoventilation develops during a light plane of anaesthesia.

Mild to moderate increases in Heinz bodies have been detected after propofol anaesthesia on consecutive or alternate days reflecting the susceptibility of feline red blood cells to oxidative injury (Andress et al., 1995; Matthews et al., 2004; Bley et al., 2007; Taylor et al., 2012). The numbers of Heinz bodies varied between cats

517

and were considered not to be clinically significant in the majority of studies. However, after anaesthesia on 4 successive days in one study (Andress et al., 1995), five out of six cats exhibited general malaise, anorexia, and diarrhoea. Routine haematological monitoring is recommended as a precaution in cats receiving multiple propofol anaesthesias for radiotherapy (Bley et al., 2007). A concern has been expressed that propofol may be associated with postanaesthetic deterioration in cats with hepatic lipidosis. A retrospective survey of 44 cats with hepatic lipidosis requiring anaesthesia for feeding tube placement, of which 27 received propofol, found no significant association between use of propofol and morbidity or mortality (Posner et al., 2008).

Currently, propofol is marketed as a 1 % and 2% emulsion containing soybean oil and egg phospholipid. This product supports bacterial growth and once a vial or bottle has been opened (it should be marked with the date and time of first use), the remaining propofol should be discarded after 8 hours. Propofol emulsion containing benzyl alcohol as a preservative is also available (PropoFlo™ 28 and PropoFlo™ Plus). The benzyl alcohol is of concern as cats are deficient in glucuronidating metabolic pathways involved in benzyl alcohol metabolism. Evaluation of this product in cats with multiple anaesthetic episodes at 48-hour intervals confirmed no significant differences in haematological and biochemical laboratory test results between propofol without preservative and propofol with benzyl alcohol (Taylor et al., 2012). More details on formulation are given in Chapter 6.

Alfaxalone

Alfaxalone was first used in cats in combination with alphadolone solubilized in Cremophor-EL (Saffan®), but is no longer available. Despite well-documented problems due to Cremophor-EL-induced histamine release, it still proved to be a useful anaesthetic agent in cats and had a wide therapeutic index. A large survey of anaesthetic deaths in general practice showed that cats anaesthetized with Saffan® were three times less likely to die than those anaesthetized by any other method available at that time (Clarke & Hall, 1990).

Alfaxalone (alphaxalone), 10 mg/mL, is now available in a cyclodextrin formulation that should avoid the problem of histamine release. The recommended dose for cats is up to 5 mg/kg IV to be administered over 1 minute. In one study of young cats premedicated with acepromazine, 0.03 mg/kg, and butorphanol, 0.3 mg/kg, SC, induction of anaesthesia with alfaxalone injected over 60–90 seconds was achieved with a mean dose of 2.7 mg/kg compared with 4.3 mg/kg in unpremedicated cats (Zaki et al., 2009). The dose rate for induction of anaesthesia was significantly decreased by dilution of the alfaxalone to 5 mg/mL with sterile water before injection. This modification may have been effective by facilitating

control over the volume injected or by slowing administration. In another clinical study of cats premedicated with acepromazine, 0.05 mg/kg, IM, alfaxalone administered at a rate of 5 mg/kg/min required a mean dose of 4.7 mg/kg to achieve intubation (Martinez Taboada & Murison, 2010). The duration from a single administration of alfaxalone, 5 mg/kg, has been reported as 7 ± 3 and 15 ± 4 minutes (Whittem et al., 2008; Muir et al., 2009). The quality of induction is described as fair to excellent. Recovery may be good or accompanied by paddling, and may be improved by the addition of premedication and a quiet environment.

Administration of alfaxalone, 5 mg/kg, IV to eight unpremedicated instrumented experimental cats caused no significant change in HR, CO, and SVR and a slow progressive decrease in MAP that reached statistical significance at 102 ± 26 mmHg (aortic pressure) by 15 minutes (Muir et al., 2009). Apnoea occurred in one cat and PaO_2 was <60 mmHg in five cats. RR decreased but $PaCO_2$ was unchanged, leading the authors to attribute the immediate decrease in PaO_2 to altered pulmonary perfusion. Administration of an excessive dose (15 mg/kg) caused vasodilation and negative inotropic effects. The addition of isoflurane is likely to induce hypotension (Zaki et al., 2009).

Etomidate

Etomidate is most commonly used for induction of anaesthesia in cats with cardiac disease because etomidate does not cause alterations in the cardiovascular haemodynamics as do the other agents. Premedication is essential to provide analgesia and for a smooth induction with etomidate, and may consist of butorphanol, buprenorphine, or another opioid, with or without midazolam IM. Diazepam, 0.2 mg/kg, may be injected IV immediately before etomidate. Etomidate is administered IV at a dose of 1.5 mg/kg, although occasionally up to 50% less may be needed in cats with poor cardiovascular function, or additional etomidate up to a total of 3 mg/kg, may be needed in some healthy cats. Etomidate has a short duration of action, consequently, administration should be a bit faster than with propofol or alfaxalone. Approximately half of the anticipated dose is injected over 5–10 seconds and additional increments injected after 15 seconds. Jaw relaxation, rostroventral rotation of the eye, and a weak palpebral reflex are goals for tracheal intubation. Anaesthesia must be maintained with an inhalation agent because increasing dose administration of etomidate increases its depressant effect on adrenal function. The carrier for etomidate includes ethylene glycol, which is toxic to red cells. No adverse effect of the small dose described has been observed but some clinicians prefer to administer etomidate into a catheter through which balanced electrolyte solution is flowing in order to produce rapid dilution. Lack of adequate preinduction sedation or delay in intubation and delivery of the inhalant anaesthetic will contribute to need of a higher dose of etomidate.

Ketamine

Ketamine is available as the water-soluble racemic mixture of two isomers and the standard for veterinary use is a solution containing 100 mg/mL ketamine hydrochloride with a preservative. Ketamine is subject to abuse and must be kept under locked storage and, in some countries, ketamine is a controlled substance requiring records of individual patient administration. Ketamine is a commonly used anaesthetic agent in cats and can be administered IM, IV, or SC and is absorbed through oral membranes. Accidental introduction into the eyes during oral administration does not cause corneal damage despite the low pH of ketamine (Macy & Siwe, 1977). Intramuscular injection appears to be painful and the cat must be restrained to avoid sudden movement that might result in needle breakage or only partial injection of the calculated dose. Onset of sedation or anaesthesia after IM injection of ketamine is rapid. When the cat is left in its cage during onset of anaesthesia, the water bowl and litter box must be removed to prevent accidental airway obstruction or inhalation of water or litter particles.

Ketamine induces catalepsy so that cats receiving ketamine alone have high muscle tone, rigid limbs, and spontaneous movement. Consequently, ketamine is usually administered in combination with sedatives and opioids. Ketamine has a wide variety of uses, such as providing mild sedation, immobilization, anaesthesia with injectable agents only, induction of anaesthesia for tracheal intubation before using inhalation anaesthesia, or as a continuous low dose infusion as an adjunct to inhalation anaesthesia or postoperatively. Many combinations have been described using low (2–4 mg/kg IM or IV), medium (5–10 mg/kg IM or IV) or high dosage (25–33 mg/kg IM) based on the degree of CNS depression desired, the route of administration, and the pharmacological effects of the combination drugs (see Table 16.4). The ketamine dose rate is generally low to medium when ketamine is combined with medetomidine or dexmedetomidine, or when used IV for induction of anaesthesia to be maintained with an inhalation agent. High dosage in combination with acepromazine and butorphanol or buprenorphine has been used for anaesthesia for ovariohysterectomy in healthy cats. Recovery may be prolonged after high dose rates when fluid therapy is not included because urine formation is necessary for elimination of ketamine in cats (Heavner & Bloedow, 1979). Since no antagonist is available for ketamine, some have recommended inclusion of medetomidine or dexmedetomidine in the combination in order to decrease the ketamine dose rate, for example, medetomidine, 0.08 mg/kg (80 µg/kg) with ketamine 5 or 7.5 mg/kg, IM for ovariectomy (Verstegen et al., 1990). Shorter recovery time can be facilitated, if necessary, by administration of an α_2-antagonist (see earlier for dose rates).

Low to medium dose rates of ketamine can be used in combination with other drugs for premedication and induction of anaesthesia prior to inhalation anaesthesia. For example, acepromazine, 0.05 mg/kg, with or without an opioid, plus ketamine, 4–5 mg/kg, IM for premedication. This is followed in 15–30 minutes by induction of anaesthesia with ketamine, 5 mg/kg, IV with or without diazepam, titrated to accomplish intubation and transfer to an inhalation agent.

Ketamine is often mixed with diazepam in the same syringe for IV administration. A commonly used calculated dose rate is ketamine, 5 mg/kg, and diazepam, 0.25 mg/kg; a 1:1 ratio when using ketamine 100 mg/mL and diazepam 5 mg/mL. One-half to two-thirds of the calculated dose, depending on the premedication, is administered rapidly IV to healthy animals and the remainder titrated in two to three increments to the desired effect. Onset of action is slow at 40–50 seconds and is slower than the other anaesthetic agents. The anaesthetist must be patient and allow time for full effect before intubation, at which point jaw tone will be moderate, the eye in a central position in the orbit, and the palpebral reflex will be brisk. Swallowing is a common occurrence during intubation and is 'normal' for this anaesthetic agent. Despite the appearance of swallowing, pharyngeal and laryngeal reflexes will be depressed and cats are still at risk for pulmonary aspiration of fluid during ketamine anaesthesia in the absence of endotracheal intubation.

A combination of xylazine, 1 mg/kg, with ketamine, 10 mg/kg, administered together IM has been in use for many years to provide 30 minutes of anaesthesia for ovariohysterectomy. Occasionally, apnoea and cyanosis ensue requiring administration of O_2 and artificial ventilation. A study monitoring cardiopulmonary function after administration of this combination measured significant decreases in cardiac output, HR and MAP at 5 minutes after xylazine and ketamine administration that continued throughout the 150-minute monitoring period, but no changes in arterial pH and blood gases (Allen et al., 1986).

Fatal pulmonary oedema has been associated with ketamine anaesthesia (Trim CM, recipient of personal communications, Van der Linde-Sipman et al., 1992). The presence of fluid or froth in the endotracheal tube during anaesthesia or laboured breathing with crackles during thoracic auscultation developing hours after anaesthesia are common signs. Aggressive treatment with O_2 and furosemide are usually necessary to avoid a fatal outcome.

Tiletamine

The combination of tiletamine with zolazepam (Telazol® or Zoletil®) is frequently used to produce heavy sedation or anaesthesia in cats. Administration of tiletamine–zolazepam, 4.0–4.4 mg/kg, IM with an opioid will induce a light plane of anaesthesia sufficient for intubation in most cats. Onset of anaesthesia is rapid. Because the duration of anaesthetic effect is extended, in contrast to induction of anaesthesia with thiopental or propofol, initially the vaporizer is not turned on or set at a very low % to avoid overdose. As the effect of tiletamine wanes and signs of a lightening plane of anaesthesia are observed, administration of the inhalation agent can be started or increased. Hypotension is an indication to decrease the vaporizer setting.

Hyperthermia develops in cats after opioid administration but also may occur after tiletamine–zolazepam-inhalation anaesthesia, with rectal temperatures up to 41 °C (106 °F). The cats exhibit typical dissociative recovery activity with restless jerky movements about the cage and head bobbing. Treatment to decrease their body temperatures may include administration of a sedative, such as acepromazine, 0.05 mg/kg, IM where appropriate and application of a draft of cold air from a fan, ice packs, or a pad for the cat to lie on that circulates iced water.

Higher dose rates for tiletamine–zolazepam are licensed in the cat, up to 10 mg/kg IM for minor procedures and 15 mg/kg IM for surgical procedures. Tiletamine-zolazepam may be incorporated into an injectable anaesthetic protocol with ketamine and xylazine (TKX) that has been described earlier in the section on feral cats. Tiletamine-zolazepam is contraindicated for use in animals with pancreatitis. Recovery from anaesthesia will be excessively prolonged when tiletamine–zolazepam is administered to cats with renal disease or urethral obstruction. Postanaesthetic pulmonary oedema has been reported.

Total intravenous anaesthesia (TIVA)

Ketamine and tiletamine–zolazepam anaesthetic combinations with a sedative and/or opioid administered as a single injection may provide anaesthesia that is of satisfactory duration for short procedures. Additional small doses of ketamine may be administered to prolong anaesthesia, but will also prolong recovery time.

Currently, preservative-free propofol is the agent most commonly used for TIVA. Premedication with a sedative and an opioid is advisable, induction of anaesthesia with propofol, and either top-up doses at appropriate intervals depending on the opioid or a continuous infusion of opioid should be administered during anaesthesia to maintain analgesia. Propofol is continuously infused at a rate of 0.1–0.3 mg/kg/min (6–18 mg/kg/h) using a syringe driver. Endotracheal intubation and administration of oxygen are necessary as hypoventilation may be moderate to severe. The cats may appear to be lightly anaesthetized and absence of movement or autonomic stimulation in response to surgery should be used to assess depth of anaesthesia. Cats do not metabolize propofol as rapidly

as dogs, and recovery will be progressively prolonged with increased hours of anaesthesia.

Concurrent continuous infusions of fentanyl and propofol, with or without midazolam, have been used to maintain anaesthesia for cats with neurological disease and those undergoing craniotomy for tumour excision. The technique is similar to that already described in Chapter 15 for dogs. Others have reported using infusions of sufentanil, alfentanil, or low loses of ketamine with propofol for TIVA.

Investigations of alfaxalone administered for maintenance of anaesthesia are only just appearing in the literature. Short surgical procedures can be performed in cats premedicated with acepromazine and an opioid and anaesthesia induced with alfaxalone, 5 mg/kg, IV. Intermittent administration or a continuous infusion of alfaxalone at a rate of 0.18 mg/kg/min (11 mg/kg/h) have been used to prolong anaesthesia for ovariectomy ± hysterectomy. Cats were premedicated with acepromazine, 0.03 mg/kg, morphine, 0.3 mg/kg, and atropine, 0.04 mg/kg, SC, followed by induction of anaesthesia with alfaxalone, mean dose 4.7 mg/kg (O'Hagan et al., 2012) or premedicated with medetomidine, 0.02 mg/kg, and morphine, 0.3–0.5 mg/kg, IM and anaesthesia induced with alfaxalone, mean dose 1.8 mg/kg, IV (Beths et al., 2009). The cats were administered oxygen in both studies.

Inhalation anaesthesia

The minimum alveolar concentration (MAC) value or potency for isoflurane in cats was initially measured at 1.6% (Steffey & Howland, 1977; Drummond et al., 1983) but, since that time, mean MAC values have been measured from 1.3% to 2.2% (Ilkiw et al., 1997; Yackey et al., 2004; Pypendop & Ilkiw, 2005b). Published mean MAC values for sevoflurane in cats are 2.4% (Ko et al., 2008a), 2.6% (Doi et al., 1988), and 3.2–3.4% (Lamont et al., 2004; Pypendop & Ilkiw, 2004; Ferreira et al., 2011). The MAC value for desflurane in cats was reported to be a mean of 9.8% (range 8.6–10.6%) (McMurphy & Hodgson, 1995) and 10.3 ± 1.1% (Barter et al., 2004). The cats in these publications were anaesthetized with the inhalation agent only. Differences in mean MAC value may be due to different experimental conditions, such as cats with different genetic origins and degree of socialization, the time of the day, and slight differences in methods of application of the noxious stimulus. Halothane is more potent than isoflurane, sevoflurane or desflurane, with a MAC value in cats of 1.1–1.2% (Steffey et al., 1974; Drummond et al., 1983). Nitrous oxide (N_2O) is not sufficiently potent to provide unconsciousness in cats when administered alone, and the MAC value has been calculated as 255% at normal barometric pressure, higher than the MAC in dogs. Addition of 50–70% N_2O to inspired gases provides some analgesia and decreases the requirement for the primary inhalation agent. The requirements for isoflurane and sevoflurane in cats were decreased by a mean of 26% or 23%, respectively, by the addition of 66% N_2O (Hikasa et al., 1996). Although N_2O causes myocardial depression, it also causes some sympathetic stimulation so that the addition of 50% or 70% N_2O to isoflurane does not further decrease cardiac output, and arterial pressure increases due to peripheral vasoconstriction (Pypendop et al., 2003).

The speed of induction of anaesthesia with an inhalant agent depends on the technique used, with administration through a facemask potentially faster than induction of anaesthesia with the cat in a chamber before transferring to a facemask, and faster with a non-rebreathing circuit than a circle rebreathing circuit. The vaporizer setting and O_2 flow rate also influence the speed of induction using rebreathing circuits by controlling the rate of increase in inspired anaesthetic concentration. Induction times in cats sedated with acepromazine, 0.05 mg/kg, IM using a facemask and non-rebreathing circuit were 5 ± 1 minutes with isoflurane and 4 ± 1 minutes with sevoflurane (Lerche et al., 2002). Use of a chamber slows the time to intubation. Using an O_2 flow of 6 L/min and a desflurane vaporizer setting of 1.5× MAC or higher, cats in a chamber lost their righting reflexes on average in 2.3 minutes. The cats were removed from the chamber and desflurane administered using a facemask, O_2 flow appropriate for the circuit used, and the vaporizer set at 1.5× MAC until intubation was accomplished, a total time of 6.3 ± 1 minutes (McMurphy & Hodgson, 1995; Barter et al., 2004). A significant disadvantage to induction of anaesthesia with an inhalation agent compared with an IV injectable agent is the relatively long time that the pharyngeal reflexes are depressed before tracheal intubation, increasing the risk of pulmonary aspiration in the event that the cat vomits. Vomition during induction of anaesthesia with an inhalant is not common but can occur (Barter et al., 2004). Atmospheric pollution with the anaesthetic agent can be a problem with chamber inductions.

Anaesthetic gas analysers measure the end-tidal (end-expiration, alveolar) agent concentration and this value most closely approximates brain concentration. The inspiratory concentration will generally be 0.2–0.3% higher. Without concurrent administration of sedatives, analgesics, or other anaesthetic agents, an end-tidal value of 1.3–1.5× MAC is considered to be a light to moderate plane of anaesthesia whereas deep anaesthesia is a concentration equivalent to 2× MAC. Concentrations in excess of MAC, in the absence of other drugs, are necessary because inhalation agents block the motor response to a noxious stimulus at a lower concentration than will block autonomic and CNS responses. All the inhalation agents induce a dose-dependent decrease in MAP and, in most investigations, this was accompanied by a decrease in CO during deep anaesthesia. The mode of ventilation, spontaneous versus controlled, did not influence the cardiovascular effects except during deep anaesthesia when controlled ventilation significantly decreased CO during isoflurane (Hodgson et al., 1998) and MAP during desflurane anaesthesia (McMurphy & Hodgson, 1996). Heart rates were significantly decreased with increasing concentrations of isoflurane from 1× MAC to 2× MAC but not by sevoflurane or desflurane in the majority of studies (Steffey & Howland, 1977; Poterack et al., 1991; McMurphy & Hodgson, 1996; Hikasa et al., 1997; Hodgson et al., 1998; Lamont et al., 2004; Pypendop & Ilkiw, 2004; Souza et al., 2005). Increasing concentrations of isoflurane induced vasodilation (decreased systemic vascular resistance, SVR) (Hodgson et al., 1998) but no changes in SVR were measured during sevoflurane or desflurane anaesthesia (McMurphy & Hodgson, 1996; Pypendop & Ilkiw, 2004). A study comparing isoflurane and sevoflurane determined that MAP was significantly higher during deep sevoflurane anaesthesia than isoflurane when the cats were breathing spontaneously (Hikasa et al., 1997). One effect of halothane that is significantly different from the other agents is the increased incidence of cardiac dysrhythmias, primarily premature ventricular complexes (PVCs), caused by sensitization of the myocardium in situations such as myocardial ischaemia, increased sympathetic nervous system activity during light anaesthesia, hypercarbia, increased endogenous or exogenous catecholamine concentrations, or increased HR or blood pressure (Hubbell et al., 1984).

Increasing depth of anaesthesia with all agents results in moderate to severe hypoventilation and increased $PaCO_2$, generally with no decrease in RR (Hodgson et al., 1998; Souza et al., 2005). Consequently, although monitoring RR during anaesthesia is necessary to detect apnoea, RR will not be a warning of hypoventilation.

Administration of inhalation agents

Two factors that may increase $PaCO_2$ are resistance to breathing and large apparatus dead space that cause decreased tidal volume and increased rebreathing of CO_2. A circle rebreathing circuit is frequently used for cats weighing more than 2.5 kg as the O_2 inflow is low and the circuit is convenient to use with a mechanical ventilator. When using a low O_2 inflow, the cats' respiratory movements are responsible for flow of the gases around the circle and through the CO_2 absorbent. The absorbent granules offer resistance to air flow as does turbulence created in wide bore tubing and the presence of valves. The impact of these factors on small cats can be minimized by increasing O_2 flow rate to 1 L/min and using paediatric hoses that have a small (12 mm) internal diameter. The total volume of the circle is high in relation to the fresh gas inflow so that the anaesthetic concentration is slow to change. Overswing in anaesthetic concentration may occur during a dynamic change that may result in overdosage.

Non-rebreathing circuits have no CO_2 absorbent and may not have valves to offer resistance to airflow. The inspired anaesthetic concentration is the same as the vaporizer setting thus, changing the vaporizer % results in an immediate change in inspired concentration and facilitates rapid changes in depth of anaesthesia. Since the total flow of gas is fixed by the design of the circuit, N_2O can be added without changing total gas inflow.

Apparatus dead space begins at the endotracheal tube level with the incisors and extends into the anaesthetic delivery circuit to the point at which CO_2-free gases are available to the cat. The apparatus dead space gas contains CO_2 that will be inhaled at the beginning of the next inspiration. A large volume of apparatus dead space in relation to the cat's tidal volume significantly increases the inspired CO_2 concentration and thus the $PaCO_2$. Some Y-pieces on circle circuits have median dividers that cut down on dead space and non-rebreathing circuits may be designed to deliver fresh gases at the level of the endotracheal tube. Any addition between the endotracheal tube and circuit, such as a T-piece for a gas analyser or a humidity and moisture exchanger, increases dead space. Adapters are available for 2 or 3 mm ID endotracheal tubes that have lumens the same ID as the endotracheal tube and a side port for the gas analyser (see Fig. 10.30A), and both features decrease dead space.

Adjunct agents

Balanced anaesthesia employs administration of several drugs to achieve unconsciousness, analgesia, and muscle relaxation and by doing so allows use of smaller dose rates of each drug. In dogs, opioids are frequently administered not only for analgesia but also to decrease the concentration of inhalation agent, thereby diminishing the impact on MAP. Opioid administration in cats does not decrease the concentration of inhalant required to the same extent as in dogs. Continuous infusions of fentanyl, 5 µg/kg/h, or morphine, 0.1 mg/kg/h, have been used to maintain analgesia during inhalation anaesthesia. Ketamine continuous infusion, 0.1–0.5 mg/kg/h, is also used to provide some sedation and in the hope that it attenuates central sensitization induced by surgery.

Continuous infusion of lidocaine is often used in dogs to decrease inhalant concentration and provide analgesia. Increasing plasma lidocaine concentrations in cats produces a dose-dependent decrease in MAC of isoflurane (Pypendop & Ilkiw, 2005b). However, significant decreases in cardiac index and increased SVR have been measured during lidocaine administration such that cardiovascular function was no better by inclusion of lidocaine and decreasing the isoflurane concentration than maintaining anaesthesia at an equipotent concentration of isoflurane alone (Pypendop & Ilkiw, 2005a). Many clinicians avoid the use of lidocaine infusion in cats because of the adverse cardiovascular effects.

Neuromuscular blockade

Paralysis with a non-depolarizing neuromuscular blocking agent (NMBA) during anaesthesia is commonly used for ocular surgical procedures such as cataract extraction, corneal transplant, or conjunctival flap attachment for a corneal ulcer or laceration. This author currently uses atracurium but pancuronium, vecuronium, and rocuronium are also used. The pharmacological effects of NMBAs are given in Chapter 8 and the clinical use of these agents in cats is similar to that described for dogs in Chapter 15.

When the cat is paralysed, even with low doses of NMBA for ocular surgery, breathing is abolished or inadequate and artificial ventilation is required. If paralysis is not required until the start of surgery then the cat can be taken to an adequate depth for surgery before administration of the NMBA. Once paralysed, eye position, palpebral reflex, and breathing are lost monitoring aids. It is important to achieve in the patient an adequate depth of anaesthesia and analgesia without excessive anaesthetic administration. Administration of an NMBA without the monitoring capability for measuring blood pressure is not recommended. Intraoperative fluid therapy is advisable to contribute to maintaining adequate circulation and redistribution of the NMBA.

Evaluation of neuromuscular transmission using a peripheral nerve stimulator is used to guide administration of additional NMBA to maintain paralysis without excessive dosage, and to determine at what point it is safe to allow the animal to begin spontaneous breathing. The need for a reversal agent depends on the NMBA used, dose rates used, the duration of drug administration, time elapsed since the last administration, and information provided by peripheral nerve stimulation. The cat should not be allowed to breathe spontaneously until four twitches of equal strength are obtained with the train-of-four (TOF). Atracurium does not require hepatic or renal function for elimination and is short lived when used in small doses for ocular surgery. Use of a reversal agent is not always necessary but, if needed, edrophonium is the cholinesterase inhibitor of choice.

MONITORING AND MANAGEMENT

Continuous observation of cat behaviour and vital signs after premedication and during induction, maintenance and recovery from anaesthesia is important to enable recognition of normal and abnormal responses to anaesthetic agents. Attached monitors and alarms serve as alerts for potential or actual problems. Anaesthetic agents may induce cardiopulmonary abnormalities in any animal whether the duration of anaesthesia is 10 minutes or 2 hours, consequently, application of monitoring equipment is advisable from the start of anaesthesia whatever the intended duration or the patient's health status. Even just changing the body position of an anaesthetized cat can result in life-threatening hypotension. A record of drug administrations and monitored parameters should be maintained and is a legal requirement in some states or countries. An anaesthetic record identifies gradual trends that require action, provides information for retrospective evaluation of patient care and for future anaesthetics in the same patient. The record is a framework for legal defence in the event of a serious complication.

Signs to be observed during induction of anaesthesia for assessment of depth of anaesthesia include assumption of recumbency and loss of righting reflex, diminished pedal withdrawal reflex, eye position, palpebral reflex, and relaxation of jaw muscles just sufficient to open the mouth. Observation of RR and character of breathing, mucous membrane colour, and palpation of the femoral artery for pulse rate, rhythm, and strength should be included to evaluate the cat's physiological status. Apnoea, cyanosis (remembering that a cat's tongue may remain pinkish during hypoxia), bradycardia, or a weak or absent pulse are indicators that anaesthetic drug administration should be stopped and O_2 administered. If need be, cats can be effectively artificially ventilated using a tight-fitting mask.

The eye signs vary according to the anaesthetic agents administered. Ketamine and tiletamine are associated with the presence of a brisk palpebral reflex whereas this sign reflects a light plane of anaesthesia during inhalation anaesthesia. The eye is centrally placed in the orbit during ketamine anaesthesia but rolls rostroventrally during other injectable and inhalation anaesthesia, returning to a central position as anaesthesia deepens. The presence of limb withdrawal after a toe pinch can be a useful sign of inadequacy of anaesthesia, however, the absence of withdrawal does not necessarily reflect adequacy of analgesia for intensely nociceptive procedures. Monitoring RR, HR, and blood pressure for changes in response to surgical stimulus may be a more reliable guide.

Ventilation

Magnitude of ventilation can be difficult to assess by observation of chest excursion. Ketamine induces a characteristic pattern of breathing, 'apneustic breathing', whereby the cat inhales and holds inspiration for several seconds before exhaling. The duration of inspiration can be so long that the cat appears apnoeic, except that eventually it exhales (a pattern that is opposite to apnoea). RR within the normal range is characteristic of inhalation anaesthetic agents during light or deep anaesthesia. The volume of each breath progressively decreases as anaesthesia deepens so that the cat may be breathing 30 breaths/min but severely hypoventilating. Adequacy of ventilation can be measured indirectly using capnography (Figs 16.8 & 16.9, see Fig. 2.28) and invasively using blood gas analysis. Significant hypoventilation is present in a cat when the

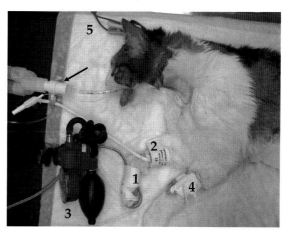

Figure 16.8 The endotracheal tube is connected to an adapter for a side-stream gas analyser (arrow) that in turn is connected to paediatric circle hoses. A Doppler probe has been placed distal to the carpal pad and taped to the leg (1). The probe wire was passed between the toes and taped to the leg for added security. A cuff (2) is placed proximal to the probe and connected to a manometer (3) for systolic blood pressure measurement. A 20 gauge catheter has been inserted in the cephalic vein on the opposite leg and taped in place (4). A T-port has been connected and the IV administration set tubing connected to the side arm. A pulse oximeter probe (5) is attached to a pinna.

end-tidal carbon dioxide ($ETCO_2$) value exceeds 6 kPa (45 mmHg). Further increase should be prevented by either decreasing anaesthetic administration or providing assisted or controlled ventilation. A low $ETCO_2$ value (<30 mmHg; 4 kPa) may represent adequate/increased ventilation or may be an error when using a side-stream capnograph. Dilution of exhaled gas with fresh gas results in a low $ETCO_2$ measurement that is not representative of $PaCO_2$. This will occur in cats with a small tidal volume, slow RR, and when the cat is connected to a non-rebreathing circuit. The pulse oximeter probe can be clipped on the tongue, ear, lip, or toe web (Fig. 16.8). The pulse oximeter provides a pulse rate and indicates haemoglobin O_2 saturation but is not a measure of adequacy of ventilation. Use of a pulse oximeter has been associated with decreased risk of death during anaesthesia (Brodbelt et al., 2008b).

Hypoventilation may be caused by anaesthetic depression of cerebral respiratory neurons or due to mechanical impairment of ventilation from obesity, a large uterus or abdominal mass, or from certain body positioning such as a head-down prone position for perineal surgery. Hypoventilation may result in inadequate uptake of inhalation anaesthetic and an uneven depth of anaesthesia, in which case, assisted or controlled ventilation may stabilize the depth. Hypercarbia causes sympathetic stimulation in some animals and increased SVR that elevates MAP.

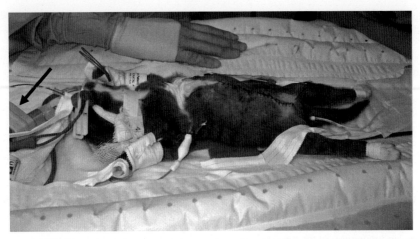

Figure 16.9 It is the end of surgery for this 0.5 kg 5-week old kitten lying within a hot air blanket to preserve body temperature. Monitoring included an ECG, Doppler systolic blood pressure, pulse oximeter with the probe on the tongue, main stream capnography (arrow), and a rectal probe for temperature. A 24 gauge catheter was inserted in a cephalic vein for fluid and drug administration. A red rubber feeding tube had been inserted (through an uncuffed endotracheal tube) into the stomach for decompression.

However, hypercarbia also causes vasodilation and increased intracranial and spinal pressure. Controlled ventilation is essential for cats with head trauma, or for craniotomy, dorsal laminectomy, or fractured vertebra stabilization, cats undergoing diaphragmatic rupture repair, thoracotomy or thoracoscopy, and cats that are paralysed with an NMBA.

A respiratory rate of 12–15 breaths/min and tidal volume approximately 12–15 mL/kg will usually maintain normocarbia. Inflation time should be just over 1 second and 15 cm H_2O (11.4 mmHg) inspiratory pressure is sufficient to achieve a suitable tidal volume in many cats. For most patients, the airway pressure must decrease to zero between breaths to allow adequate venous return to the heart. When controlled ventilation is used to treat hypoventilation, the vaporizer setting should be decreased to avoid increased depth of anaesthesia caused by delivery of anaesthetic to more pulmonary capillaries. A mechanical ventilator with a small bellows (capacity 100 mL or 300 mL) is ideal for adjusting to the small tidal volume of a cat. Manual ventilation may be the best option when the ventilator cannot be adjusted to deliver a small enough tidal volume. The Hallowell Workstation (see Fig. 10.17) is an example of an anaesthesia machine/ventilator designed specifically for very small animals.

Cardiovascular system

Minimal cardiovascular monitoring includes HR, CRT, mucous membrane colour, and palpation of a femoral pulse. Heart rate and rhythm can be obtained from an ECG, oesophageal stethoscope, pulse oximeter, or a Doppler probe over a peripheral artery. In general, a decrease in intensity of Doppler sound occurs with a decrease in blood pressure (the opposite effect is not necessarily true – that a loud sound heard when the Doppler probe is initially attached represents adequate blood pressure). Hypotension is frequently associated with use of propofol, tiletamine–zolazepam, and inhalation anaesthesia. The values obtained from oscillometric and Doppler ultrasound methods may or may not be accurate for individual cats and the recording from the Doppler method may be closer to MAP than SAP (see Chapter 2). Differences in recorded measurements are influenced by the site of cuff application, cuff diameter, and the relationship between cuff position and heart level as well as the technique and model employed (Cannon & Brett, 2012). Nonetheless, NIBP monitors are easy to use and provide warning of a severely decreased blood pressure or a change in pressure (see Fig. 16.8). Actions initiated by a low blood pressure measurement may prevent progression to cardiac arrest (Fig. 16.10). Invasive blood pressure monitoring provides valuable information in cats with significant cardiac disease, very ill cats, and during complicated surgical procedures. A 22 or 24 gauge catheter is inserted in the dorsal pedal or coccygeal artery after the skin at the site has had a presurgical preparation. The coccygeal artery midline on the ventral surface of the tail may be easier to catheterize but skin preparation and protection of cleanliness of the catheter must be high quality because of the potential contamination of the site. A 22 gauge catheter is less likely to require frequent flushing. Attaching a continuous flush device (see Fig. 2.20) to the catheter is useful for maintaining patency for long-term pressure monitoring. The pressure transducer should be placed level with the thoracic inlet. Central venous pressure can be

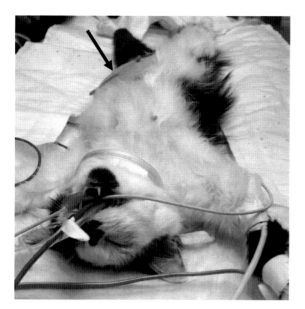

Figure 16.10 This pregnant cat is anaesthetized for ovariohysterectomy. Systolic arterial pressure decreased to 40 mmHg (aortocaval compression) when the cat was placed in dorsal recumbency but rebounded after the cat was turned onto its side. Blood pressure was minimally improved by administration of dopamine. The left lateral tilt of the abdomen illustrated in the picture by the arrow pointed at midline was the closest position to dorsal recumbency that allowed adequate blood pressure. Removal of the uterus was immediately followed by a dramatic increase in blood pressure.

measured in cats with a long jugular catheter in place. An ECG is essential for the diagnosis of irregular rhythms.

Maintenance fluid therapy during anaesthesia is usually balanced electrolyte solution, 5–10 mL/kg/h for the first 1–2 hours followed by 5 mL/kg/h for subsequent hours. The circulating blood volume of cats is approximately 56 mL/kg body weight. Accidental delivery of 100–300 mL of fluid may constitute overload, depending on the size of the cat, and a bolus of 60 mL/kg of fluid is likely to cause pulmonary oedema. Administration of furosemide is indicated when an excessive volume of fluid has been administered.

Hypotension, MAP <60–65 mmHg or SAP ≤80 mmHg, should be treated according to the cause. Hypotension induced by inhalation anaesthetic agents should be managed initially by decreasing the vaporizer setting. Expansion of blood volume can be accomplished by one fluid bolus of 5–10 mL/kg and infusion of hydroxethyl starch (hetastarch) 5 mL/kg over 10 minutes with one repeat dose. Hypotension may also be reversed by infusion of a vasoactive agent, such as dopamine, 7 μg/kg/min. The cardiovascular effects of dopamine, dobutamine, epinephrine, and phenylephrine have been evaluated in healthy

experimental cats made hypotensive with isoflurane (Pascoe et al., 2006b). An infusion of dopamine, 5 μg/kg/min, IV resulted in a significant increase in HR and cardiac index (CI) and an infusion of 10 μg/kg/min increased MAP >70 mmHg in all cats. SVR was unchanged at these infusion rates. HR and CI were increased significantly by dobutamine infusion ≥5 μg/kg/min but MAP increased only in 3/6 cats, and overall increases in MAP were not significant at infusion rates of 5 or 10 μg/kg/min. SVR was decreased from baseline at all infusion rates. Infusion of epinephrine, 0.5 μg/kg/min, significantly increased HR, CI and MAP without significant changes in SVR. Infusions of phenylephrine, 1 and 2 μg/kg/min, increased MAP and SVR with no significant change in HR. CI was significantly increased by infusion of the higher dose rate. In this investigation, dopamine was the most useful drug to increase MAP and perfusion, and phenylephrine could be used to increase MAP by vasoconstriction. MAP decreased rapidly after stopping infusions of dopamine and epinephrine, so these infusions should be decreased in step-wise fashion.

A concentration of 100 μg/mL dopamine or dobutamine is commonly used as it can be reasonably regulated and avoids excessive infusion of saline (see Box 15.9). The rate of infusion must be closely controlled using a paediatric 60 drop/mL administration set or, even better, a syringe driver where the rate of infusion is not influenced by other solutions entering the same catheter. It is important in cats (and small dogs) to insert the needle as close to the IV catheter as possible so that any change in infusion rate can occur quickly, which is not the case if the vasoactive line is inserted into a fluid extension distant from the catheter. Dopamine is started at a rate of 7 μg/kg/min. The rate of infusion may be decreased once the blood pressure has increased. In refractory situations, dopamine dose rate may be increased to 10 μg/kg/min, or dobutamine added, or a change made to phenylephrine.

The volume of blood lost during a surgical or medical procedure must be assessed closely. Hidden losses must also be included, such as blood on the drapes, between the drapes and the table, or on the floor. The pharynx should be packed with gauze during nasal or oral surgery to prevent blood passing down the oesophagus into the stomach where it cannot be quantitated. One fully soaked 4″×4″ (10 cm square) gauze can hold 8–15 mL blood, depending on the type of gauze. A loss of 30–40 mL blood in a 3.5 kg cat (15–20% of circulating blood volume) will have a significant adverse effect on cardiac output. Initial replacement of blood loss in a previously healthy cat can be with crystalloid solution at 2 times the volume lost, however, administration of a colloid is indicated if the blood pressure remains low, if the TP decreases below 4 g/dL, or by 15% blood loss. A blood transfusion may be necessary at 20% loss of circulating blood volume, or earlier in patients starting with lower than normal Hct, or when Hct decreases to 20%. When major haemorrhage is anticipated based on the type of surgical procedure, e.g. rhinotomy, it is advisable to blood type the cat and have a donor with the same blood type available. Feline packed red blood cells and plasma are also commercially available. Cats scheduled for potentially haemorrhagic surgical procedures, such as exploratory laparotomy or pelvic limb fracture repair, that have a preoperative Hct <24% should receive a blood transfusion before or from the beginning of anaesthesia.

Temperature

An anaesthetized cat can quickly lose body heat when placed on a metal table, in a cold environment, skin prepared with cold solutions and alcohol, and connected to a non-rebreathing circuit. In one report, anaesthetic agents did not contribute to heat loss (Haskins, 1981).

The definition of hypothermia is not universally recognized, however, low body temperature developing during anaesthesia is accompanied by decreased metabolism, decreased end-tidal CO_2, cardiovascular instability, and slows recovery time, increases postanaesthetic catabolism, and decreases resistance to infection. Hypothermia <35.5°C (<96°F) is of concern and temperatures <33.3°C (<92°F) should be considered as serious as they are associated with a significant decrease in anaesthetic requirement and decreased cardiovascular function. Temperature can be measured rectally or with a long probe inserted through the mouth into the oesophagus with the tip just caudal to the thoracic inlet. It is important to prevent the initial heat loss that occurs between induction of anaesthesia and start of surgery. A foam pad and a hot water circulating pad (rigid plastic to prevent puncture from cat claws) between the cat and the table will help (see Fig. 16.4). Overhead radiant heaters are particularly effective for use during the initial preparation and recovery times. Warm IV fluids and towels covering the cat should be utilized wherever possible but are not very effective. Warm air blankets or tubes (e.g. Bair Hugger) placed over or around the cat can be used to slow heat loss or to warm up a cat (see Fig. 16.9). Wrapping the legs in plastic or bubble wrap may help to retain heat. Using low flow systems of administration for inhalation agents, such as a paediatric circle circuit may assist to retain heat by maintaining moisture laden inspired gases. Circle circuit hoses with embedded heating elements are now available (www.darvallvet.com). It is a clinical impression that a heat and moisture exchanger (HME) inserted between the endotracheal tube and anaesthetic circuit helps to maintain body heat but at least one investigation found no improvement in body temperature with the use of an HME in dogs (Hofmeister et al., 2011).

Hyperthermia is rare during anaesthesia in cats although a few cases of malignant hyperthermia syndrome have been reported. Hyperthermia not infrequently develops in cats during recovery from anaesthesia, partly due to the increased activity associated with dissociative agents and

partly due to the effects of opioid administration (see earlier).

Recovery from anaesthesia

The cat's urinary bladder should be expressed by gentle compression of the abdomen at the end of anaesthesia before the anaesthetic depth lightens to provide evidence that urine was formed during anaesthesia and to prevent soiling during recovery; exceptions are following a laparotomy or urinary tract surgery. At the end of inhalation anaesthesia, O_2 should be continued for a period of time (10 min) after the vaporizer has been turned off to allow waste gases to be scavenged, and to allow ventilation and blood pressure to increase before inspired O_2 is replaced by air. The cat should not be flipped from side to side for stimulation as this action will result in a significant decrease in blood pressure in some individuals.

During recovery from routine anaesthesia, the endotracheal tube cuff is deflated and the tie around the back of the head loosened or undone. A hand should always remain on the cat for control in case the cat abruptly moves. Signs of recovery may include an increase in RR, pupillary dilation, tongue curling, and shivering. Extubation should be performed when the anaesthetic plane is light, jaw muscle tone is moderate, and swallowing is observed when the tube is moved. Extubation should be performed with the head and neck extended to minimize closing strength of the lower jaw and the tube should be removed rostrally between the incisors to reduce the likelihood of the endotracheal tube being accidentally bitten in half. The cat should be monitored for adequate ventilation after extubation, particularly in the presence of a head and neck bandage, thoracic or abdominal bandage, or an Elizabethan collar. Chest movement does not guarantee adequate airflow. Observation should be supported by listening for the sound of air movement, observation of movement of a few cat hairs held near the nostrils, auscultation of the trachea or thorax with a stethoscope, or sustained SpO_2 >93% from a pulse oximeter probe. Hypoxaemia accompanied by some air movement is characteristic of a thoracic or abdominal bandage that is too tight. Releasing some of the pressure by splitting the bandage is followed by a satisfactory increase in SpO_2. Cats that are overweight or brachycephalic should be monitored with a pulse oximeter after extubation. Oxygenation may be improved by placing the cat in prone position with the head supported in a normal position by a small towel.

Laryngospasm may occur during induction or recovery from anaesthesia. Laryngospasm is characterized by a harsh 'crowing' noise on inspiration (partial airway obstruction) and retraction of the chin to the cat's chest. Initial treatment involves overextending the cat's head and neck (prevent neck flexure) and grasping the tongue to pull it forward out of the mouth in order to move the epiglottis rostrally. In most cases, the repositioning is sufficient to allow satisfactory airflow and the laryngospasm dissipates. If the cat's mouth can be opened, dripping lidocaine, approximately 0.5 mg/kg, into the larynx may abort the laryngospasm. The cat must be intubated in those rare cases in which the laryngospasm persists as complete airway obstruction and cyanosis develops.

Partially anaesthetized cats should not be carried or cradled because of increased stimulation and possibility of airway obstruction; rather they should be stretched out on a flat surface. All water bowls and litter trays must be removed from cages in which cats are recovering from anaesthesia to avoid accidental pulmonary aspiration of water or dust or airway obstruction due to a kinked neck. Cages with a heated floor are a justified investment in facilities where hypothermia is a common occurrence. Postoperative management of feral cats is curtailed because of limited access, however, for domesticated cats, rectal temperature should be measured at 30–60-minute intervals to detect either a decrease or an increase in the recovery period. Hyperthermia is a common occurrence after administration of opioids or with increased muscle activity following anaesthesia with ketamine or tiletamine. Excessively high temperatures should be treated as previously described.

The need for analgesic agents will depend largely on agents used in the anaesthetic protocol and on the anticipated pain induced by the surgery. Cats that have received morphine, meperidine, hydromorphone, oxymorphone or methadone during anaesthesia may be given supplemental doses at appropriate time intervals for the drugs. Butorphanol may require supplementation by 2 hours after initial administration whereas analgesia from buprenorphine may persist for 6 hours. Immediately switching from a μ opioid for anaesthesia to buprenorphine in recovery is unwise in painful cats as this will result in a gap in analgesia. A smoother transition will be obtained if μ opioid analgesia is continued for a few hours after anaesthesia. A fentanyl patch applied the day before anaesthesia may not supply sufficient analgesia for the immediate recovery period and should be supplemented by administration of another μ opioid. An NSAID provides synergistic analgesic effect with an opioid by modulating the inflammatory response to surgery. An option for continuous analgesia in the ICU for postoperative major surgery is a continuous infusion of fentanyl, with or without ketamine. Analgesia for the client to administer may include, but not limited to, buccal TM buprenorphine or tramadol tablets.

Specific postanaesthetic intensive care for individual patients might involve administration of O_2 with the cat in an O_2 cage, turning the cat hourly, lubrication of the eyes, and measurement of blood pressure, RR, SpO_2, and temperature at specified intervals. Continued IV fluid administration, care of feeding tubes, chest tubes, urinary catheters and collection bags, will be accompanied by recording of volumes in and volumes out, and daily weighing.

LOCAL ANALGESIA

Local nerve blocks can be included with general anaesthesia to allow a decreased administration of general anaesthetic agents and continued analgesia into recovery. The major precaution for use of local anaesthetic solutions in cats is to calculate accurately dose rates for small cats to avoid toxicity. When two local anaesthetics are used together, the dose rates of each should be proportionately reduced. Secondly, the syringe must always be aspirated before injection because inadvertent intravascular injection of local anaesthetic solution will be followed by an acute decrease in blood pressure, even cardiac arrest.

Brachial plexus nerve block

Brachial plexus nerve block is a useful block for orthopaedic surgery performed distal to the elbow. The landmarks and procedure are the same as for the dog and have been described in detail in Chapter 15. Bupivacaine is the drug of choice and is administered at 2 mg/kg (slightly less than for the dog).

Dental nerve blocks

Landmarks for location of the dental nerves for nerve blocks with local anaesthetic solution are essentially the same as for the dog with a few exceptions. The infraorbital canal is short and the tip of the 24 or 26 gauge needle should only be inserted a few millimetres into the infraorbital foramen. The ventral border of the mandible is straight but the mandibular foramen is located approximately 20% of the distance from the angular process to the ramus of the mandible (Boyd & Paterson, 2001). The mental foramen is on the lateral aspect of the mandible just rostral to the premolar teeth.

Digital nerve blocks

Local anaesthetic solution must be infiltrated SC on the dorsal and palmar aspects of the forelimb just proximal to the radiocarpal joint (Fig. 16.11). Total lidocaine, 2 mg/kg, or bupivacaine, 2 mg/kg, is divided between all sites. Bupivacaine is preferred because of the much longer duration of anaesthesia but it has a longer onset time. If lidocaine and bupivacaine are combined, half of each maximum dose is used to avoid toxicity. The syringe must be aspirated before each injection to avoid inadvertent vascular injection.

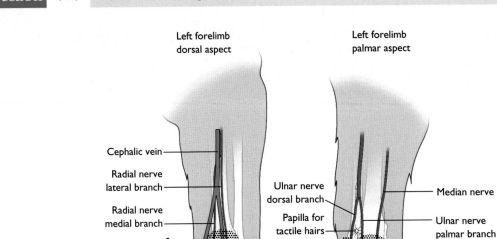

Figure 16.11 Sites for nerve blocks for onychectomy in the forelimb are illustrated by the stippled areas. (A) On the dorsal aspect, local anaesthetic solution is infiltrated on either side of the accessory cephalic vein at the level of the distal radius. The combination of the distal radius and ulna are easily palpated as the widest osseous structure just proximal to the carpus. (B) On the palmar aspect, local anaesthetic solution is injected just proximal to the carpal pad and accessory carpal bone on either side of the superficial flexor tendon and extending the width of the limb. In the stippled zone lateral to the accessory carpal bone, the needle should be inserted into the subcutaneous space as the dorsal branch of the ulnar nerve is very superficial. In the stippled zone beginning dorsal to the accessory carpal bone and extending medially, the needle should be inserted through the skin and antebrachial fascia because the palmar branch of the ulnar nerve and the median nerve pass through the carpal canal adjacent and deep to the superficial digital flexor tendon and flexor retinaculum. Based on anatomical dissection by Dr CJ Roberts.

Epidural analgesia

Epidural injection is easily accomplished at the lumbosacral space in cats. The cat may be restrained squarely in a crouching position or on its side with the hind limbs pulled cranially. The area for injection is located by palpation of the cranial dorsal iliac spines and the spinous processes of the last lumbar and first sacral vertebrae. The lumbosacral space and site of needle insertion in the cat is immediately cranial to the sacrum in contrast to its position in the dog of halfway between L7 and S1 (König & Liebich, 2009). In addition, in the cat, the vertebral body length of L7 is shorter than that of L6 and L5 which must be taken into account if using inter-vertebral distances to locate the lumbosacral space. Aseptic technique is essential and the skin must be clipped and prepared as for a surgical procedure. A 22, 23, or 25 gauge, 2.5 or 3.75 cm (1 or 1.5 inch), spinal needle is inserted midline through the skin perpendicular to the cat's back to a depth of about 1 cm. The resistance to penetration of the ligamentum flavum is characteristic of needle placement in dogs but may not be obvious in cats. A 'hanging drop' technique can be used to assess insertion of the needle tip into the epidural space in cats in sternal position. The spinal cord ends in most cats between L7 and S3 vertebrae, and the dural sac continues through the sacrum. The hub of the needle must be inspected for cerebrospinal fluid (CSF) or blood after removing the stilette. In either case, the needle should be removed and replaced with a new one. Injection of local anaesthetic solution into the epidural space after penetration of the dura is likely to increase the intensity and duration of block due to increased uptake into CSF. An epidural needle should be inserted with care, without excessive force, and the needle hub held firmly to prevent the tip from moving around in the epidural space. Complications are rare, however, they may occur. Neurological dysfunction of micturition and defaecation persisting for more than a year in a cat has been attributed to probable traumatic injury during epidural needle placement (Song et al., 2011).

After the stilette is removed, a 3 mL syringe containing 0.25 mL of saline or air, or a syringe specifically manufactured for 'loss of resistance' test, should be firmly attached to the needle (by holding the needle hub firmly with one hand and screwing, not pushing, the syringe on with the other). Aspiration of the plunger first is essential to identify a negative aspiration of blood or CSF. Compression of the plunger should be easy – hence the term 'loss of resistance'. Only a small volume of air must be injected because the bubbles that form interfere with uniform neural blockade. The bevel of the needle should be directed cranially and the local anaesthetic solution injected over 30–60 seconds.

The volume for injection into the epidural space is commonly 0.2 mL/kg and frequently drugs are diluted with sterile saline to achieve this volume. Lidocaine, 4 mg/kg, has a rapid onset of analgesia up to 10 minutes with a reported mean duration of 40–90 minutes (Klide & Soma, 1968; DeRossi et al., 2009; Lawal & Adetunji, 2009). Bupivacaine, 1 mg/kg, has a reported similar rapid onset of action with variable duration measured at 79 ± 6 minutes (Lawal & Adetunji, 2009) or 2–6 hours (Lamont, 2002). Morphine and buprenorphine are probably the most common opioids administered in the epidural space in clinical feline practice. Our clinical impression is that combinations of bupivacaine, 0.5 mg/kg, with morphine, 0.1 mg/kg, or buprenorphine, 0.005–0.01 mg/kg, provide postoperative analgesia in cats after orthopaedic pelvic limb surgery. The effects of administering opioids or sedatives have been investigated in experimental cats using tests of analgesia such as needle pricks or skin pinches with a haemostat forceps, thermal or mechanical antinociception measuring devices. Experimental tests of analgesia from epidural morphine, 0.1 mg/kg, revealed significant analgesia for at least 12 hours (Castro et al., 2009). Tests of analgesia from epidural morphine in cats anesthetized with isoflurane were equivocal, providing a reduction in isoflurane requirement in one study (Golder, 1998) but none in another (Pypendop et al., 2006). Epidural injection of buprenorphine, 0.02 mg/kg, induced thermal antinociception for up to 24 hours, but only 8 hours from half that dose combined with medetomidine (Steagall et al., 2009a). Sufficient buprenorphine was absorbed systemically to induce euphoria in the cats starting 2 hours after injection and lasting 24 hours in some cats. Medetomidine is quickly absorbed from the epidural space into the systemic circulation and induces sedation, vomiting, and decreased RR, HR, and MAP. Epidural injection of medetomidine, 0.01 mg/kg, produced significant analgesia in the forelimb for 2 hours and in the hind limbs for 4 hours in experimental cats tested by electrical stimulation (Duke et al., 1994). Medetomidine provided hind limb analgesia for 4–6 hours in another study that used thermal and mechanical testing (Steagall et al., 2009a). There is considerable variability between cats and it is unclear whether analgesia is due to epidural or systemic effects. The addition of S(+)-ketamine, 2.5 mg/kg, to lidocaine, 4 mg/kg, diluted to a total volume of 0.33 mL/kg and injected into the epidural space doubled the duration of analgesia from lidocaine alone to a mean of 140 minutes as determined by skin pinches over the hind limbs, abdominal wall, and perineum (DeRossi et al., 2009). S(+)-ketamine is available as a preservative-free product. Racemic ketamine such as is used to induce anaesthesia by IM or IV route should not be used for epidural injection because cell toxicity has been observed. No response to clamping of the skin over the tail was obtained for 6 hours after epidural administration of tramadol, 1 mg/kg (Castro et al., 2009).

Peroneal and tibial nerve block

These nerve blocks are easy to perform using a 25 gauge hypodermic needle for infiltration of lidocaine or bupivacaine. The common peroneal (fibular) nerve crosses the lateral surface of the gastrocnemius muscle obliquely from caudal to cranial at the level of the stifle and divides into superficial and deep branches just distal to the stifle joint. The bellies of the relevant muscles can be separated by thumb pressure to identify the location for needle insertion. The superficial branch can be blocked by infiltration of local anaesthetic solution between the long digital flexor muscle caudally and the long peroneal muscle cranially. The needle should then be advanced a few millimetres in depth in a slightly cranial direction to infiltrate around the deep peroneal nerve where it runs between the long digital extensor muscle caudally and the long peroneal muscle cranially. The nerves can also be located with the aid of a peripheral nerve stimulator that is used for monitoring blockade with an NMBA or a specific needle locator. The tibial nerve can be blocked just above the hock by SC infiltration on the medial aspect immediately caudal to the tibia and cranial to the gastrocnemius tendon. A small branch of the tibial nerve, caudal cutaneous sural nerve, is blocked at the same level on the lateral aspect of the limb. Bupivacaine 0.5%, total maximum dose for all nerves of 2 mg/kg, will provide several hours of analgesia for metatarsal surgery.

Sciatic nerve block

Location of nerves with use of electrical stimulation or ultrasound is becoming popular for more accurate placement of local anaesthetic around nerves in dogs. A recent publication described anatomical dissections and use of ultrasound to locate the sciatic nerve in cats (Haro et al., 2012). The cats were positioned in lateral recumbency with the limb to be blocked uppermost and hair clipped from the lateral and caudal aspects of the limb. After surgical preparation of the skin, a stab incision was made through the skin on the caudal aspect at approximately mid-femur level to facilitate insertion of an atraumatic peripheral nerve block needle (Stimuplex® by B. Braun is an insulated echogenic peripheral nerve block needle with a short 30° bevel to decrease the risk of nerve injury). Ultrasound was used to identify the sciatic nerve and allowed precise positioning of the needle next to the nerve and observation of the spread of anaesthetic solution during injection. Paralysis of the limb was achieved by injecting lidocaine, 2 mg/kg diluted in saline to a 1 mL volume, in multiple small volume injections around the nerve to achieve the ultrasound 'doughnut' sign that is indicative of perineural infiltration. Onset time and duration of analgesia were not given.

Topical or transdermal

A mixture of lidocaine and prilocaine (EMLA) is available as a cream or patch that is used to provide dermal anaesthesia and prevent or minimize pain associated with intravenous insertion of a needle or catheter. The site is prepared for venepuncture and a 2–3 mm layer of cream spread on the skin and covered with an occlusive dressing for approximately 45 minutes (Flecknell, 1994). Jugular catheters were successfully inserted in a higher percentage of awake sick cats that were pretreated with 1 mL of EMLA cream over a 2×5 cm area of skin than were not, although the difference was not statistically significant (Wagner et al., 2006). Methaemoglobin blood concentrations measured in five cats were within normal range and plasma lidocaine/prilocaine concentrations were undetectable. No adverse effects attributable to toxic effects of the local anaesthetic agents were observed.

In humans, lidocaine patches are used for controlling postsurgical incisional pain. Lidocaine patches are of a matrix system construction whereby lidocaine is within the adhesive layer and diffuses across the skin from high to low concentration. A study investigating the effects of a 700 mg lidocaine patch applied to skin over the thorax of experimental cats determined that plasma lidocaine concentrations increased for about 12 hours after patch application and remained constant for 72 hours (Ko et al., 2008b). The plasma concentrations remained 25-fold less than concentrations achieved by a bolus IV injection of lidocaine, 2 mg/kg. Concentration of lidocaine in the skin under the patch was much higher than plasma concentration. Further investigation is necessary to determine a role for this form of analgesia in clinical feline practice.

REFERENCES

Al-Gizawiy, M.M., Rudé, E.P., 2004. Comparison of preoperative carprofen and postoperative butorphanol as postsurgical analgesics in cats undergoing ovariohysterectomy. Vet Anaesth Analg 31, 164–174.

Allen, D.G., Dyson, D.H., Pascoe, P.J., et al., 1986. Evaluation of a xylazine-ketamine hydrochloride combination in the cat. Can J Vet Res 50, 23–26.

Andress, J.L., Day, T.K., Day, D., 1995. The effects of consecutive day propofol anesthesia on feline red blood cells. Vet Surg 24, 277–282.

Balmer, T.V., Irvine, D., Jones, R.S., et al., 1998. Comparison of carprofen and pethidine as postoperative analgesics in the cat. J Small Anim Pract 39, 158–164.

Barter, L.S., Ilkiw, J.E., Pypendop, B.H., et al., 2004. Evaluation of the induction and recovery characteristics of anesthesia with desflurane in cats. Am J Vet Res 65, 748–751.

Bednarski, R.M., Grimm, K.A., Harvey, R., et al., 2011. AAHA Anesthesia guidelines for dogs and cats. J Am Anim Hosp Assoc 47, 377–385.

Benito-de-la-Víbora, J., Lascelles, B.D.X., García-Fernández, P., et al., 2008. Efficacy of tolfenamic acid and meloxicam in the control of postoperative pain following ovariohysterectomy in the cat. Vet Anaesth Analg 35, 501–510.

Beths, T., Touzot-Jourde, G., Musk, G., et al., 2009. Total intravenous anesthesia (TIVA) in cats: Evaluation of Alfaxan® to induce and maintain anesthesia in feral and domestic cats undergoing neutering procedures. 10th World Veterinary Anaesthesia Congress, Glasgow, Scotland.

Biermann, K., Hungerbühler, S., Mischke, R., et al., 2012. Sedative, cardiovascular, haematologic and biochemical effects of four different drug combinations administered intramuscularly in cats. Vet Anaesth Analg 39, 137–150.

Bley, C.R., Roos, M., Price, J., et al., 2007. Clinical assessment of repeated propofol-associated anesthesia in cats. J Am Vet Med Assoc 231, 1347–1353.

Bodey, A.R., Sansom, J., 1998. Epidemiological study of blood pressure in domestic cats. J Small Anim Pract 39, 567–573.

Bortolami, E., Murrell, J.C., Slingsby, L.S., 2012a. Methadone in combination with acepromazine as premedication prior to neutering in the cat. Vet Anaesth Analg 40, 181–193.

Bortolami, E., Slingsby, L., Love, E.J., 2012b. Comparison of two formulations of buprenorphine in cats administered by the oral transmucosal route. J Feline Med Surg 14, 534–539.

Boyd, J.S., Paterson, C., 2001. Clinical Anatomy of the Dog and Cat. Mosby International Limited, London.

Brodbelt, D.C., Pfeifer, D.U., Young, L., et al., 2007. Risk factors for anaesthetic-related death in cats:

results from the confidential enquiry into perioperative small animal fatalities (CEPSAF). Br J Anaesth 99, 617–623.

Brodbelt, D.C., Blissett, K.J., Hammond, R.A., et al., 2008a. The risk of death: the confidential enquiry into perioperative small animal fatalities. Vet Anaesth Analg 35, 365–373.

Brodbelt, D.C., Pfeiffer, D.U., Young, L.E., et al., 2008b. Results of the confidential enquiry into perioperative small animal fatalities regarding risk factors for anesthetic-related death in dogs. J Am Vet Med Assoc 233, 1096–1104.

Brondani, J.T., Luna, S.P.L., Beier, S.L., et al., 2009. Analgesic efficacy of perioperative use of vedaprofen, tramadol or their combination in cats undergoing ovariohysterectomy. J Feline Med Surg 11, 420–429.

Brown, S.A., Atkins, C., Bagley, R., et al., 2007. Guidelines for the identification, evaluation and management of systemic hypertension in dogs and cats. J Vet Intern Med 21, 542–558

Cannon, M.J., Brett, J., 2012. Comparison of how well conscious cats tolerate blood pressure measurement from the radial and coccygeal arteries. J Feline Med Surg 14, 906–909.

Castro, D.S., Silva, M.F.A., Shih, A.C., et al., 2009. Comparison between the analgesic effects of morphine and tramadol delivered epidurally in cats receiving a standardized noxious stimulation. J Feline Med Surg 11, 948–953.

Cistola, A.M., Golder, F.J., Centonze, L.A., et al., 2004. Anesthetic and physiologic effects of tiletamine, zolazepam, ketamine, and xylazine combination (TKX) in feral cats undergoing surgical sterilization. J Feline Med Surg 6, 297–303.

Clarke, K.W., Hall, L.W., 1990. A survey of anaesthetic practice in small animals. J Assoc Vet Anaesth 17, 4–10.

Cleale, R.M., Muir, W.W., Waselau, A.-C., et al., 2009. Pharmacokinetic and pharmacodynamic evaluation of propofol administered to cats in a novel, aqueous, nano-droplet formulation or as an oil-in-water macroemulsion. J Vet Pharmacol Ther 32, 436–445.

Davidson, C.D., Pettifer, G.R., Henry, J.D. Jr, 2004. Plasma fentanyl concentrations and analgesic effects during full or partial exposure to transdermal fentanyl patches in cats. J Am Vet Med Assoc 224, 700–705.

DeRossi, R., Benites, A.P., Ferreira, J.Z., et al., 2009. Effects of lumbosacral epidural and lidocaine in xylazine-sedated cats. J S Afr Vet Assoc 80, 79–83.

Dhumeaux, M.P., Snead, E.C.R., Epp, T.Y., et al., 2012. Effects of a standardized anesthetic protocol on hematologic variables in healthy cats. J Feline Med Surg 14, 701–705.

Doi, M., Yunoki, H., Ikeda, K., 1988. The minimum alveolar concentration of sevoflurane in cats. J Anesth 2, 113–114.

Drummond, J.C., Todd, M.M., Shapiro, H.M., 1983. Minimal alveolar concentrations for halothane, enflurane, and isoflurane in the cat. J Am Vet Med Assoc 182, 1099–1101.

Duke, T., Komulainen Cox, A.-M., Remedios, A.M., et al., 1994. The analgesic effects of administering fentanyl or medetomidine in the lumbosacral epidural space of cats. Vet Surg 23, 143–148.

Egger, C.M., Glerum, L.E., Allen, S.W., et al., 2003. Plasma fentanyl concentrations in awake cats and cats undergoing anesthesia and ovariohysterectomy using transdermal administration. Vet Anaesth Analg 30, 229–236.

Epstein, M., Kuehn, N.F., Landsberg, G., et al., 2005. AAHA senior care guidelines for dogs and cats. J Am Anim Hosp Assoc 41, 81–91.

Ferreira, T.H., Rezende, M.L., Mama, K.R., et al., 2011. Plasma concentrations and behavioral, antinociceptive, and physiologic effects of methadone after intravenous and oral transmucosal administration in cats. Am J Vet Res 72, 764–771.

Fisher, J., 2010. Use of Xylocaine spray in cats. Vet Rec 167, 500.

Flecknell, P.A., 1994. Injectable anaesthetics. In: Hall, L.W., Taylor, P.M. (Eds), Anaesthesia of the Cat. Baillière Tindall, London, pp. 129–156.

Frankel, T., Hawkey, C.M., 1980. Haematological changes during sedation in cats. Vet Rec 107, 512–513.

Gassel, A.D., Tobias, K.M., Egger, C.M., et al., 2005. Comparison of oral and subcutaneous administration of buprenorphine and meloxicam for preemptive analgesia in cats

undergoing ovariohysterectomy. J Am Vet Med Assoc 227, 1937–1944.

Gellasch, K.L., Kruse-Elliot, K.T., Osmond, C.S., et al., 2002. Comparison of transdermal administration of fentanyl versus intramuscular administration of butorphanol for analgesia after onychectomy in cats. J Am Vet Med Assoc 220, 1020–1024.

Gerdin, J.A., Slater, M.R., Makolinski, K., et al., 2011. Post-mortem findings in 54 cases of anesthetic associated death in cats from two spay-neuter programs in New York State. J Feline Med Surg 13, 959–966.

Giordano, T., Steagall, P.V.M., Ferreira, T.H., et al., 2010. Postoperative analgesic effects of intravenous, intramuscular, subcutaneous or oral transmucosal buprenorphine administered to cats undergoing ovariohysterectomy. Vet Anaesth Analg 37, 357–366.

Glerum, L.E., Egger, C.M., Allen, S.W., et al., 2001. Analgesic effect of the transdermal fentanyl patch during and after feline ovariohysterectomy. Vet Surg 30, 351–358.

Golder, F.J., Pascoe, P.J., Bailey, C.S., et al., 1998. The effect of epidural morphine on the minimum alveolar concentration of isoflurane in cats. J Vet Anaesth 25, 52–56.

Grace, S.F., 2011. Aspirin toxicosis. In: Norsworthy, G.D. (Ed.), The Feline Patient, 4 ed. Wiley-Blackwell, Ames, p 32.

Grint, N.J., Murison, P.J., Coe, R.J., et al., 2006. Assessment of the influence of surgical technique on postoperative pain and wound tenderness in cats following ovariohysterectomy. J Feline Med Surg 8, 15–21.

Gurney, M.A., 2012. Pharmacological options for intra-operative and early postoperative analgesia: an update. J Small Anim Pract 53, 377–386.

Hall, T.L., Duke, T., Townsend, H.G.C., et al., 1999. The effect of opioid and acepromazine premedication on the anesthetic induction dose of propofol in cats. Can Vet J 40, 867–870.

Haro, P., Laredo, F.G., Belda, E., et al., 2012. Ultrasound-guided block of the feline sciatic nerve. J Feline Med Surg 14, 545–552.

Harrison, K.A., Robertson, S.A., Levy, J.K., et al., 2011. Evaluation of medetomidine, ketamine and buprenorphine for neutering feral cats. J Feline Med Surg 13, 896–902.

Haskins, S.C., 1981. Hypothermia and its prevention during general anesthesia in cats. Am J Vet Res 42, 856–861.

Heavner, J.E., Bloedow, D.C., 1979. Ketamine pharmacokinetics in domestic cats. Vet Anesth 6, 16–19.

Hikasa, Y., Kawanabe, H., Takase, K., et al., 1996. Comparisons of sevoflurane, isoflurane, and halothane anesthesia in spontaneously breathing cats. Vet Surg 25, 234–243.

Hikasa, Y., Ohe, N., Takase, S., et al., 1997. Cardiopulmonary effects of sevoflurane in cats: comparison with isoflurane, halothane, and enflurane. Res Vet Sci 63, 205–210.

Hodgson, D.S., Dunlop, C.I., Chapman, P.L., et al., 1998. Cardiopulmonary effects of anesthesia induced and maintained with isoflurane in cats. Am J Vet Res 59, 182–185.

Hofmeister, E.H., Brainard, B.M., Braun, C., et al., 2011. Effect of a heat-moisture exchanger on heat loss in isoflurane-anesthetized dogs undergoing single-limb orthopedic procedures. J Am Vet Med Assoc 239, 1561–1565.

Hofmeister, E.H., Trim, C.M., Kley, S., et al., 2007. Traumatic intubation in a cat. Vet Anaesth Analg 34, 213–216.

Hoyumpa Vogt, A., Rodan, I., Brown, M., et al., 2010. AAFP-AAHA Feline life stage guidelines. J Feline Med Surg 12, 43–54.

Hubbell, J.A.E., Muir III, W.W., Bednarski, R.M., et al., 1984. Change of inhalation anesthetic agents for management of ventricular premature depolarizations in anesthetized cats and dogs. J Am Vet Med Assoc 185, 643–646.

Ilkiw, J.E., Pascoe, P.J., Fisher, L.D., 1997. Effect of alfentanil on the minimum alveolar concentration of isoflurane in cats. Am J Vet Res 58, 1274–1279.

Johansen, A., Romundstad, L., Nielsen, C.S., et al., 2012. Persistent postsurgical pain in a general population: prevalence and predictors in the Tromsø study. Pain 153, 1390–1396.

Johnson, J.A., Robertson, S.A., Pypendop, B.H., 2007. Antinociceptive effects of butorphanol, buprenorphine, or both administered intramuscularly in cats. Am J Vet Res 68, 699–703.

Katz, J., Clarke, H., Seltzer, Z., 2011. Preventive analgesia: quo vadimus? Anesth Analg 113, 1242–1253.

Klein, A.A., Arrowsmith, J.E., 2010. Should routine pre-operative testing be abandoned? Anaesthesia 65, 974–976.

Klide, A.M., Soma, L.R., 1968. Epidural analgesia in the dog and cat. J Am Vet Med Assoc 153, 165–172.

Ko, J.C., Knesl, O., Weil, A.B., et al., 2009. Analgesia, sedation, and anesthesia – Making the switch from medetomidine to dexmedetomidine. Compend Contin Educ Vets 31 (suppl 1A), 1–24.

Ko, J.C.H., Abbo, L.A., Weil, A.B., et al., 2008a. Effect of orally administered tramadol alone or with an intravenously administered opioid on minimum alveolar concentration of sevoflurane in cats. J Am Vet Med Assoc 232, 1834–1840.

Ko, J.C.H., Maxwell, L.K., Abbo, L.A., et al., 2008b. Pharmacokinetics of lidocaine following the application of 5% lidocaine patches to cats. J Vet Pharmacol Ther 31, 359–367.

König, H.E., Liebich, H.-G., 2009. Veterinary Anatomy of Domestic Mammals. Schattauer, Stuttgart.

Kronen, P.W., Ludders, J.W., Erb, H.N., et al., 2006. A synthetic fraction of feline facial pheromones calms but does not reduce struggling in cats before venous catheterization. Vet Anaesth Analg 33, 258–265.

Lamont, L.A., 2002. Feline perioperative pain management. Vet Clin N Am Small Anim Pract 32, 747–763.

Lamont, L.A., Bulmer, B.J., Grimm, K.A., et al., 2001. Cardiopulmonary evaluation of the use of medetomidine hydrochloride in cats. Am J Vet Res 62, 1745–1762.

Lamont, L.A., Greene, S.A., Grimm, K.A., et al., 2004. Relationship of bispectral index to minimum alveolar concentration multiples of sevoflurane in cats. Am J Vet Res 65, 93–98.

Lascelles, B.D., Robertson, S.A., 2004. Antinociceptive effects of hydromorphone, butorphanol, or the combination in cats. J Vet Intern Med 18, 190–195.

Lawal, F.M., Adetunji, A., 2009. A comparison of epidural anaesthesia with lignocaine, bupivacaine and lignocaine-bupivacaine mixture in cats. J S Afr Vet Assoc 80, 243–246.

Lee, D.D., Papich, M.G., Hardie, E.M., 2000. Comparison of

pharmacokinetics of fentanyl after intravenous and transdermal administration in cats. Am J Vet Res 61, 672–677.

Lerche, P., Muir, W.W., Grubb, T.L., 2002. Mask induction of anaesthesia with isoflurane or sevoflurane in premedicated cats. J Small Anim Pract 43, 12–15.

Looney, A.L., Bohling, M.W., Bushby, P.A., et al., 2008. The Association of Shelter Veterinarians veterinary medical care guidelines for spay-neuter programs. J Am Vet Med Assoc 233, 74–86.

Macy, D.W., Siwe, S.T., 1977. The use of ketamine as an oral anesthetic in cats. Feline Pract 7, 44–66.

Martinez Taboada, F., Murison, P.J., 2010. Induction of anaesthesia with alfaxalone or propofol before isoflurane maintenance in cats. Vet Rec 167, 85–89.

Mathis, A., Pinelas, R., Brodbelt, D.C., et al., 2012. Comparison of quality of recovery from anaesthesia in cats induced with propofol or alfaxalone. Vet Anaesth Analg 39, 282–290.

Matthews, N.S., Brown, R.M., Barling, K.S., et al., 2004. Repetitive propofol administration in dogs and cats. J Am Anim Hosp Assoc 40, 255–260.

McMurphy, R.M., Hodgson, D.S., 1995. The minimum alveolar concentration of desflurane in cats. Vet Surg 24, 453–455.

McMurphy, R.M., Hodgson, D.S., 1996. Cardiopulmonary effects of desflurane in cats. Am J Vet Res 57, 367–370.

Millette, V.M., Steagall, P.V.M., Duke-Novakovski, T., et al., 2008. Effects of meperidine or saline on thermal, mechanical and electrical nociceptive thresholds in cats. Vet Anaesth Analg 35, 543–547.

Monteiro, E.R., Campagnol, D., Parrilha, L.R., et al., 2009. Evaluation of cardiorespiratory effects of combinations of dexmedetomidine and atropine in cats. J Feline Med Surg 11, 783–792.

Muir, W., Lerche, P., Wiese, A., et al., 2009. The cardiorespiratory and anesthetic effects of clinical and supraclinical doses of alfaxalone in cats. Vet Anaesth Analg 36, 42–54.

Murison, P.J., Martinez Taboada, F., 2010. Effect of propofol and alfaxalone on pain after ovariohysterectomy in cats. Vet Rec 166, 334–335.

Nakamura, R.K., Rishniw, M., King, M.K., et al., 2011. Prevalence of echocardiographic evidence of cardiac disease in apparently healthy cats with murmurs. J Feline Med Surg 13, 266–271.

Niedfeldt, R.L., Robertson, S.A., 2006. Postanesthetic hyperthermia in cats: a retrospective comparison between hydromorphone and buprenorphine. Vet Anaesth Analg 33, 381–389.

O'Hagan, B.J., Pasloske, K., McKinnon, C., et al., 2012. Clinical evaluation of alfaxalone as an anaesthetic induction agent in cats less than 12 weeks of age. Aust Vet J 90, 395–401.

O'Hearn, A.K., Wright, B.D., 2011. Coccygeal epidural with local anesthetic for catheterization and pain management in the treatment of feline urethral obstruction. J Vet Emerg Crit Care 21, 50–52.

Pascoe, P.J., Ilkiw, J.E., Frischmeyer, K.J., 2006a. The effect of the duration of propofol administration on recovery from anaesthesia in cats. Vet Anaesth Analg 33, 2–7.

Pascoe, P.J., Ilkiw, J.E., Pypendop, B.H., 2006b. Effects of increasing infusion rates of dopamine, dobutamine, epinephrine, and phenylephrine in healthy anesthetized cats. Am J Vet Res 67, 1491–1499.

Peisker, N., Preissel, A.K., Reichenbach, H.D., et al., 2010. Foetal stress response to euthanasia of pregnant sheep. Berl Munch Tierarztl Wochenschr 123, 2–10.

Pettifer, G.R., Hosgood, G., 2003. The effect of rectal temperature on perianesthetic serum concentrations of transdermally administered fentanyl in cats anesthetized with isoflurane. Am J Vet Res 64, 1557–1561.

Posner, L.P., Asakawa, M., Erb, H.N., 2008. Use of propofol for anesthesia in cats with primary hepatic lipidosis: 44 cases (1995–2004). J Am Vet Med Assoc 232, 1841–1843.

Posner, L.P., Pavuk, A.A., Rokshar, J.L., et al., 2010. Effects of opioids and anesthetic drugs on body temperature in cats. Vet Anaesth Analg 37, 35–43

Poterack, K.A., Kampine, J.P., Schmeling, W.T., 1991. Effects of isoflurane, midazolam, and etomidate on cardiovascular responses to stimulation of central nervous system pressor sites in

chronically instrumented cats. Anesth Analg 73, 64–75.

Pypendop, B.H., Ilkiw, J.E., 2004. Hemodynamic effects of sevoflurane in cats. Am J Vet Res 65, 20–25.

Pypendop, B.H., Ilkiw, J.E., 2005a. Assessment of the hemodynamic effects of lidocaine administered IV in isoflurane-anesthetized cats. Am J Vet Res 66, 661–668.

Pypendop, B.H., Ilkiw, J.E., 2005b. The effects of intravenous lidocaine administration on the minimum alveolar concentration of isoflurane in cats. Anesth Analg 100, 97–101.

Pypendop, B.H., Ilkiw, J.E., 2007. Pharmacokinetics of tramadol, and its metabolite O-desmethyl-tramadol, in cats. J Vet Pharmacol Ther 31, 52–59.

Pypendop, B.H., Ilkiw, J.E., Bolich, J.A., 2003. Hemodynamic effects of nitrous oxide in isoflurane-anesthetized cats. Am J Vet Res 64, 273–278.

Pypendop, B.H., Pascoe, P.J., Ilkiw, J.E., 2006. Effects of epidural administration of morphine and buprenorphine on the minimum alveolar concentration of isoflurane in cats. Am J Vet Res 67, 1471–1475.

Quimby, J.M., Smith, M.L., Lunn, K.F., 2011. Evaluation of the effects of hospital visit stress on physiologic parameters in the cat. J Feline Med Surg 13, 733–737.

Reese, M.J., Patterson, E.V., Tucker, S.J., et al., 2008. Effects of anesthesia and surgery on serologic responses to vaccination in kittens. J Am Vet Med Assoc 233, 116–121.

Reynolds, B.S., Concordet, D., Germain, C.A., et al., 2010. Breed dependency of reference intervals for plasma biochemical values in cats. J Vet Intern Med 24, 809–818.

Reynolds, B.S., Geffré, A., Bourgès-Abella, N.H., et al., 2012. Effects of intravenous, low-dose ketamine-diazepam sedation on the results of hematologic, plasma biochemical, and coagulation analyses in cats. J Am Vet Med Assoc 240, 287–293.

Robertson, S.A., Lascelles, B.D.X., 2010. Long term pain in cats How much do we know about this important welfare issue? J Feline Med Surg 12, 188–199.

Robertson, S.A., Lascelles, B.D., Taylor, P.M., et al., 2005. PK-PD modeling of buprenorphine in cats: intravenous and oral transmucosal administration. J Vet Pharmacol Ther 5, 453–460.

Robertson, S.A., Taylor, P.M., Lascelles, B.D.X., et al., 2003. Changes in thermal threshold response in eight cats after administration of buprenorphine, butorphanol and morphine. Vet Rec 153, 462–465.

Robertson, S.A., Wegner, K., Lascelles, B.D.X., 2009. Antinociceptive and side-effects of hydromorphone after subcutaneous administration in cats. J Feline Med Surg 11, 76–81.

Rodan, I., Sundahl, E., Carney, H., et al., 2011. AAFP and ISFM feline-friendly handling guidelines. J Feline Med Surg 13, 364–375.

Rohrer-Bley, C., Neiger-Aeschbacher, G., Busato, A., et al., 2004. Comparison of perioperative racemic methadone, levo-methadone and dextromoramide in cats using indicators of post-operative pain. Vet Anaesth Analg 31, 175–182.

Sansom, J., Rogers, K., Wood, J.L.N., 2004. Blood pressure assessment in healthy cats and cats with hypertensive retinopathy. Am J Vet Res 65, 245–252.

Schlueter, C., Budras, K.D., Ludewig, E., et al., 2009. Brachycephalic feline noses CT and anatomical study of the relationship between head conformation and the nasolacrimal drainage system. J Feline Med Surg 11, 891–900.

Schug, S.A., 2012. Persistent post-surgical pain: A view from the other side of the fence. Pain 153, 1344–1345.

Selmi, A.L., Barbudo-Selmi, G.R., Mendes, G.M., et al., 2004. Sedative, analgesic and cardiorespiratory effects of romifidine in cats. Vet Anaesth Analg 31, 195–206.

Selmi, A.L., Mendes, G.M., Lins, B.T., et al., 2003. Evaluation of the sedative and cardiorespiratory effects of dexmedetomidine, dexmedetomidine-butorphanol, and dexmedetomidine-ketamine in cats. J Am Vet Med Assoc 222, 37–41.

Selmi, A.L., Mendes, G.M., Lins, B.T., et al., 2005. Comparison of xylazine and medetomidine as premedicants for cats being anaesthetised with propofol-sevoflurane. Vet Rec 157, 139–143.

Slingsby, L.S., Taylor, P.M., 2008. Thermal antinociception after dexmedetomidine administration in cats: a dose-finding study. J Vet Pharmacol Ther 31, 135–142.

Slingsby, L.S., Taylor, P.M., 2009. Thermal antinociception after dexmedetomidine administration in cats: a comparison between intramuscular and oral transmucosal administration. J Feline Med Surg 11, 829–834.

Slingsby, L.S., Waterman-Pearson, A.E., 1998. Comparison of pethidine, buprenorphine and ketoprofen for postoperative analgesia after ovariohysterectomy in the cat. Vet Rec 143, 185–189.

Slingsby, L.S., Waterman-Pearson, A.E., 2002. Comparison between meloxicam and carprofen for postoperative analgesia after feline ovariohysterectomy. J Small Anim Pract 43, 286–289.

Slingsby, L.S., Murrell, J.C., Taylor, P.M., 2010. Combination of dexmedetomidine with buprenorphine enhances the antinociceptive effect to a thermal stimulus in the cat compared with either agent alone. Vet Anaesth Analg 37, 162–170.

Song, R.B., Cross, J.R., Golder, F.J., et al., 2011. Suspected epidural morphine analgesia induced chronic urinary and bowel dysfunction in a cat. J Feline Med Surg 13, 602–605.

Souza, A.P., Guerrero, P.N.H., Nishimori, C.T., et al., 2005. Cardiopulmonary and acid-base effects of desflurane and sevoflurane in spontaneously breathing cats. J Feline Med Surg 7, 95–100.

Sparkes, A.H., Heiene, R., Lascelles, B.D.X., et al., 2010. ISFM and AAFP consensus guidelines Long-term use of NSAIDs in cats. J Feline Med Surg 12, 521–538.

Steagall, P.V.M., Mantovani, F.B., Taylor, P.M., et al., 2008a. Dose-related antinociceptive effects of intravenous buprenorphine in cats. Vet J 182, 203–209.

Steagall, P.V.M., Taylor, P.M., Brondani, J.T., et al., 2008b. Antinociceptive effects of tramadol and acepromazine in cats. J Feline Med Surg 10, 24–31.

Steagall, P.V.M., Millette, V., Mantovani, F.B., et al., 2009a. Antinociceptive effects of epidural buprenorphine or medetomidine, or the combination, in conscious cats. J Vet Pharmacol Ther 32, 477–484.

Steagall, P.V.M., Taylor, P.M., Rodrigues, L.C.C., et al., 2009b. Analgesia for cats after ovariohysterectomy with either buprenorphine or carprofen alone or in combination. Vet Rec 164, 359–363.

Steffey, E.P., Howland, D. Jr, 1977. Isoflurane potency in the dog and cat. Am J Vet Res 38, 1833–1836.

Steffey, E.P., Gillespie, J.R., Berry, J.D., et al., 1974. Anesthetic potency (MAC) of nitrous oxide in the dog, cat, and stump-tail monkey. J Appl Physiol 36, 530–532.

Taylor, P.M., 1992. Use of Xylocaine pump spray for intubation in cats. Vet Rec 130, 583.

Taylor, P.M., Chengelis, C.P., Miller, W.R., et al., 2012. Evaluation of propofol containing 2% benzyl alcohol preservative in cats. J Feline Med Surg 14, 516–526.

Taylor, P.M., Robertson, S.A., Dixon, M.J., et al., 2001. Morphine, pethidine and buprenorphine disposition in the cat. J Vet Pharmacol Ther 24, 391–398.

Tobias, K.M., Harvey, R.C., Byarley, J.M., 2006. A comparison of four methods of analgesia in cats following ovariohysterectomy. Vet Anaesth Analg 33, 390–398.

Van der Linde-Sipman, J.S., Hellebrekers, L.J., Lagerwey, E., 1992. Myocardial damage in cats that died after anaesthesia. Vet Quarterly 15, 91–94.

Verstegen, J., Fargetton, X., Donnay, I., et al., 1990. Comparison of the clinical utility of medetomidine/ketamine and xylazine/ketamine combinations for the ovariectomy of cats. Vet Rec 127, 424–426.

Wagner, A.E., Worland, G.A., Glawe, J.C., et al., 2008. Multicenter, randomized controlled trial of pain-related behaviors following routine neutering in dogs. J Am Vet Med Assoc 232, 109–115.

Wagner, K.A., Gibbon, K.J., Strom, T.L., et al., 2006. Adverse effects of EMLA (lidocaine/prilocaine) cream and efficacy for the placement of jugular catheters in hospitalized cats. J Feline Med Surg 8, 141–144.

Wegner, K., Robertson, S.A., 2007. Dose-related thermal antinociceptive effects of intravenous hydromorphone in cats. Vet Anaesth Analg 34, 132–138.

Wells, S.M., Glerum, L.E., Papich, M.G., 2008. Pharmacokinetics of butorphanol in cats after intramuscular and buccal transmucosal administration. Am J Vet Res 69, 1548–1554.

Whittem, T., Pasloske, K.S., Heit, M.C., et al., 2008. The pharmacokinetics and pharmacodynamics of alfaxalone in cats after single and multiple intravenous administration of Alfaxan® at clinical and supraclinical doses. J Vet Pharmacol Ther 31, 571–579.

Wiese, A.J., Muir, W.W., 2007. Anaesthetic and cardiopulmonary effects of intramuscular morphine, medetomidine and ketamine administered to telemetered cats. J Feline Med Surg 9, 150–156.

Williams, L.S., Levy, J.K., Robertson, S.A., et al., 2002. Use of the anesthetic combination of tiletamine, zolazepam, ketamine, and xylazine for neutering feral cats. J Am Vet Med Assoc 220, 1491–1495.

Yackey, M., Ilkiw, J.E., Pascoe, P.J., et al., 2004. Effect of transdermally administered fentanyl on the minimum alveolar concentration of isoflurane in cats. Vet Anaesth Analg 31, 183–189.

Yeates, J., 2010. Ethical aspects of euthanasia of owned animals. In Practice 32, 70–73.

Zaki, S., Ticehurst, K.E., Miyaki, Y., 2009. Clinical evaluation of Alfaxan-CD® as an intravenous anaesthetic in young cats. Aust Vet J 87, 82–87.

Chapter | **17** |

Anaesthesia of zoological species (exotic pets, zoo, aquatic, and wild animals)

Stephen J. Divers

INTRODUCTION

The problems involved in anaesthetizing such diverse taxa as birds, reptiles, fish, and exotic mammals present unique and varied challenges. Dangerous animals (e.g. venomous snakes, large carnivores, etc.) are often impossible to evaluate and examine thoroughly prior to induction for reasons of human safety. Laboratory animals (e.g. rabbits and rodents) are often healthy and, when anaesthetized for experimental purposes, it is particularly important that methodologies have little or no influence on the result of the study. Conversely, pet rabbits and rodents are often unhealthy and considerably older. The techniques to be described in this chapter are those which the author has found to be satisfactory in general practice for most clinical purposes in the various species of animal presented. In some cases, specialized drugs and equipment not commonly found in general practice are required, which only adds to the importance of advanced planning. Readers are directed to specialized texts for more in-depth descriptions as only brief overviews can be provided here (Brown, 1993; Heard, 2004; Edling, 2006; Schumacher & Yelen, 2006; West et al., 2007).

SMALL MAMMALS

With over 10 million pet rabbits (*Oryctolagus cuniculus*), ferrets (*Mustela putorius furo*), and rodents (order Rodentia) in the USA, these small mammals represent the third largest group of companion mammals, after dogs and cats (AVMA, 2007). Although similar demographic data have not been located for Europe, this group nevertheless represents an expanding component of small animal practice, with many clients expecting the same level of medicine for them as for more traditional pet species. Many diagnostic and surgical procedures warrant anaesthesia, therefore, acquiring skills for competent anaesthesia is an indispensable skill for the exotic animal practitioner. Short anaesthetic procedures are commonplace for completing tasks such as thorough examination, phlebotomy, radiography, or other short diagnostic/therapeutic procedures. In addition, many small mammal clinical problems necessitate surgery. Readers are directed to detailed reviews that are available on the subject, as personal preferences will largely be presented here (Heard, 2004, 2007a,b; Carpenter, 2005). Practitioners are also finding that sedation, especially when combined with local anaesthesia, is often a viable option to general anaesthesia for such procedures as sample collection and catheterization.

Although rodents and other small mammals are anaesthetized in large numbers for laboratory procedures with apparently few serious problems, when similar species are anaesthetized for clinical purposes, the mortality is higher. The cause of the higher clinical mortality probably results from unfamiliarity with the species and the generally poor health of many companion animals. Therefore, success can be improved by:

1. Preparing the veterinary team by reviewing the species-specific anatomy/physiology of the patient, the procedure(s) to be performed, anticipating potential problems, and having back-up plans
2. Calculate emergency drugs, or consider a dedicated emergency drug chart (Table 17.1). For critical cases, prepare individual emergency drug doses before induction
3. Preparing all equipment and supplies ahead of time (anaesthetic drugs, catheters, fluids, fluid additives, non-rebreathing anaesthetic circuits with appropriately sized bags and masks, surgical equipment, etc.)
4. Ensuring the patient has been stabilized as much as possible prior to sedation or anaesthesia (e.g. patient is normothermic, rehydrated, previous good plane of nutrition, fasted if needed, no metabolic derangements).

Table 17.1 Emergency drug calculator chart for a rabbit

Patient Name:		Roger			
Patient Number:		319902			
Patient weight (kg):		1.230			
Drug	**Concentration**	**Dose**	**Route**	**Bolus**	**Units**
Glycopyrrolate	0.2 mg/mL	0.02 mg/kg	IV/IO/IT	0.12	mL
Epinepherine (1:1000)	1 mg/mL	0.2 mg/kg	IV/IO/IT	0.25	mL
Diazepam	5 mg/mL	2 mg/kg	IV/IO	0.49	mL
Furosemide	50 mg/mL	2 mg/kg	IV/IO	0.05	mL
Shock fluids		90 mL/kg/h	IV/IO	111	mL/h
Maintenance fluids		70 mL/kg/day	IV/IO	4	mL/h
Naloxone	0.4 mg/mL	0.01 mg/kg	IV/IO	0.03	mL

Table 17.2 Common problems, complications, and possible solutions associated with small mammal anaesthesia

Problem	Potential complication	Possible solution
Small size	Mechanical obstruction of airway due to positioning; compression of thoracic cavity during handling/surgery	Be careful to keep head/neck extended; do not place heavy drapes, equipment or rest hands/arms on the animal during anaesthesia and surgery
High metabolic rate	Hypoglycaemia, especially if prolonged fasting prior to procedure; rapid drug metabolism; higher fluid requirements; unexpected drug effects of interactions (e.g. atropine and tiletamine in rabbits)	Plan to be able to deliver higher fluid requirements and administer fluids pre-, intra- and postoperatively; consider dextrose in IV fluids if hypoglycaemic; minimize fasting time; utilize drug dosages based on species-specific pharmacokinetic studies; know the species idiosyncrasies, avoid drug contraindications, be prepared to reverse drugs if undesirable effects are appreciated, be prepared to provide respiratory support
High surface area : volume ratio	Hypothermia (small animals lose heat more readily) especially during abdominal/thoracic surgery; hypothermia can lead to decreased anaesthetic requirements, prolonged recovery, bradycardia, and terminal ventricular fibrillation	Provide warmth from the point of induction; monitor body temperature carefully and frequently; plan for different types of supplemental heat during anaesthetic episode and use them simultaneously (radiant source, heating pad, warm fluids, warm air); administer heat prior to animal becoming hypothermic and continue until the animal can thermoregulate
Catecholamine-driven prey animals	Stressed prey species release endogenous catecholamines that sensitize the myocardium (among other effects); this effect is much more pronounced in certain species (especially rabbits)	Minimize handling of untamed animals preoperatively; plan for hospital environment to be stress-free (shelter boxes, quiet wards away from predators); premedicate patient with anxiolytics prior to induction; utilize strategies such as rapid induction agents and induction chambers (instead of facemask) to minimize handling
Present with underlying cardiovascular disease	Small thorax, limited tidal volume, little respiratory or cardiovascular reserve	Perform a preanaesthetic evaluation; minimize anaesthetic time through efficiency (not rushing); carefully monitor patient ($ETCO_2$, SpO_2, blood pressure, blood gases); be able to ventilate animal; have crystalloids, colloids, dopamine/dobutamine, and emergency drugs available
Difficult to intubate	No control over ventilation; potential for hypoxaemia and hypercapnia	Study anatomy of the animal prior to scheduling procedure and research intubation methods; practice on cadavers; many small mammals can be safely intubated with practice and proper equipment; if unable to intubate, realize limitations of lack of control of airway, keep procedure short; utilize well-fitting mask and appropriate lab animal anaesthetic circuit (*not* a traditional non-rebreather or T-piece circuit)
Difficult to gain vascular access	Unable to administer maintenance fluids during anaesthetic procedure to maintain proper blood pressure and blood flow to vital organs; unable to administer emergency agents if needed	Study anatomy of the animal prior to scheduling procedure and research catheterization methods; many small mammals can be catheterized, either IV or IO with practice and proper equipment; if unable, administer maintenance fluid requirements SC before the procedure (or at induction), and repeat just prior to recovery

There are some basic principles that apply when using general anaesthesia in small mammalian patients in addition to the sound, basic principles of domestic animal anaesthesiology. These additional comments are based on the fact that exotic mammals are often small in size, have high metabolic rates, have high body surface area : volume ratios and are prone to hypothermia, are often catecholamine-driven prey animals that 'stress' easily, are typically presented in advanced stages of disease (often respiratory) with little respiratory or cardiovascular reserve, and have anatomy that challenges endotracheal intubation and intravenous access. However, there are solutions that can help address these problems (Table 17.2). It should be kept in mind that patients under sedation alone must still be carefully monitored.

Many small mammals become distressed by handling, increasing the risk of physical damage and of adrenaline release leading to problems under subsequent anaesthesia. Respiratory rate should be recorded before the animal is disturbed and removed from the cage. The risk of physical damage is considerably reduced by proper handling. Many rabbits and rodents can be secured using the dorsal scruff,

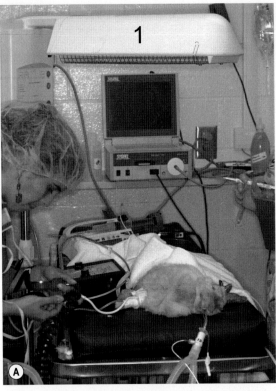 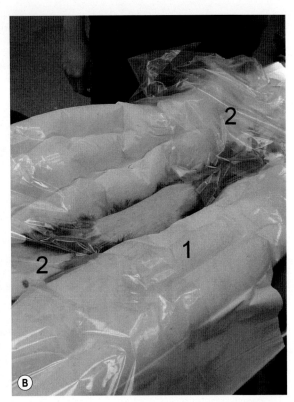

Figure 17.1 Warming devices. (A) Radiant heating element (1) positioned above an anaesthetized rabbit; (B) ferret positioned on top of a warm forced air blanket (1), with additional clear drapes (2) to maintain temperature following aseptic preparation of the abdomen. Note blood pressure measurement on the rabbit is Doppler ultrasound technique.
Courtesy of Dr Stephen Divers, University of Georgia.

while a towel over the eyes can further reduce stress and struggling. Small mammals can be placed into a small bag or box and accurately weighed. Adequate preanaesthetic examination is often difficult but many have respiratory disease so oxygen should be available even if only injectable agents are to be used. The high metabolic rate of these small mammals means that they require an almost constant supply of food, so preanaesthetic fasting should not exceed 2 hours. In general, the cardiac sphincter of most rabbits and rodents prevents regurgitation, while the majority of the gastrointestinal ingesta are located in the hind-gut such that prolonged fasting would be required to reduce volume, and likely lead to hepatic lipidosis. The main purpose of short-term fasting is, therefore, to reduce food material within the oral cavity. There is no need to curtail the water supply up to the time of induction of anaesthesia; however, fasting typically requires not only the removal of all food but also all bedding materials that may be chewed. During anaesthesia, small mammals are particularly prone to hypothermia (<37.8°C, <100°F) and precautions to avoid this should be taken from the time of induction. Removal of hair and wetting (particularly

with alcohol-based preparations) should be kept to a minimum; the use of overhead radiant heat sources, warmed-water and warmed-air blankets should be employed at induction, as well as during maintenance and recovery periods to maintain core temperatures (Fig. 17.1). Heat loss can be considerably reduced by wrapping the animal in foil or bubble wrap during non-surgical procedures, while the application of clear plastic surgical drapes helps maintain temperature during surgery. When inhalation agents are used, carrier gases also contribute to cooling effects, thus gas flows should be adequate but not excessive. In-line gas warmers can be used as long as increased circuit resistance is overcome. Intravenous or intraosseous catheterization should also be considered routinely and, in cases where this is likely to prove difficult, subcutaneous fluid therapy should be instituted prior to induction and repeated during anaesthesia (Fig. 17.2). Maintenance of hydration status and circulation, ventilation and temperature appear to be key. Adequate monitoring of the animal's condition, including cardiac and respiratory function is essential until recovery is complete.

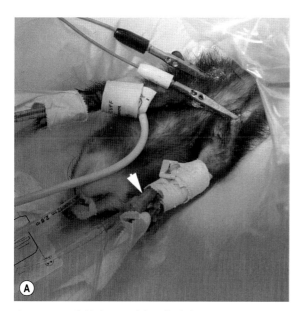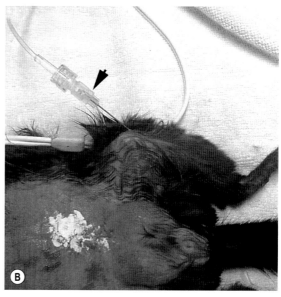

Figure 17.2 Fluid therapy. (A) IV fluid therapy via a cephalic catheter (arrow) in a ferret; (B) IO fluid therapy via a spinal needle placed into the tibia (arrow) in a guinea pig.
Courtesy of Dr Stephen Divers, University of Georgia.

The commonest cause of death is respiratory failure. Ideally, O_2 and the ability to administer artificial ventilation of the lungs should always be available. However, intubation of rabbits and rodents requires practice as the narrow mouth makes viewing the larynx difficult. Suitable antagonists should be at hand and there may be a place for analeptic agents, such as doxapram, in circumstances where intubation is difficult. The other common cause of mortality is surgical blood loss so that care must be taken to minimize this and, whenever possible, to replace that which does occur, with crystalloid boluses (such as Normosol-R), volume expanders (colloids), or blood transfusion products.

The use of anticholinergic premedication is controversial as in other species, but as small airways can be easily blocked by saliva or mucus, their use may be desirable. Glycopyrrolate is preferred for rabbits as they possess increased atropinase activity that reduces the efficacy and duration of atropine. The author prefers an opioid and benzodiazepine combination for premedication, and these drugs can be given by intramuscular or, in smaller animals, by subcutaneous injection (Table 17.3). General anaesthesia is preferred for most purposes and may be induced and maintained with volatile agents, induced with injectable drugs and maintained with volatile agents, or maintained with injectable drugs alone. There are many different protocols available and only those routinely used and preferred by the author are presented here (Table 17.3). A more complete listing can be found in the references (Brown, 1993; Carpenter, 2005; AVMA, 2007; Chinnadurai et al., 2010).

Preanaesthetic sedation and analgesia

Midazolam is commonly used in human and traditional pet medicine for purposes of preanaesthesia and sedation. It has a wide margin of safety in many species. When combined with an opioid, effects are synergistic, allowing a reduction of the amount of either drug (see Table 17.3). Effects in exotic species are promising, and this author has not observed severe adverse effects in any species in which it has been utilized (avian, exotic mammals including rabbits, ferrets, rodents, primates, carnivores, and others). Effects are variable, from slight decrease in activity to lateral recumbency. Effects appear to be more pronounced in the rabbit and ferret and in compromised patients, and less pronounced in rats and mice unless higher dose rates are used. These effects are likely related to species variability in response and the varying dose rates suggested for different species/groups. However, with the availability of inexpensive flumazenil, the sedative effects can, if deemed necessary, be reversed postoperatively. In all cases, patients still react somewhat to handling and noxious stimuli. When midazolam is combined with an opioid, greater sedation and analgesia result. Depending on overall patient condition and goal of the sedation procedure, additional sedation can be provided with subanaesthetic dosages of ketamine (see Table 17.3). If additional immobilization is essential, low concentrations of inhalant gas can be considered. This combination of drugs for sedation allows overall reduction of required inhalant gases, decreasing risk associated with the use of general anaesthesia.

Table 17.3 Sedative, premedication, induction and maintenance drugs preferred for small mammals

Species	Premedication/sedation (mg/kg)	Induction typically 5–15 mins after premedication (mg/kg)	Maintenance	Additional analgesics (mg/kg)
Ferret	Butorphanol (0.1–0.3) SC/IM *or* Buprenorphine (0.01–0.03) SC/IM/IV *or* Oxymorphone (0.05–0.2) SC/IM plus (if necessary) Midazolam (0.1–0.3) SC/IM	Isoflurane or Sevoflurane by mask Ketamine (5–10) IV *or* (10–15) IM Propofol (3–6) IV	Isoflurane 1–2.5% Sevoflurane 2–4%	Meloxicam (0.2) SC/IM/PO q 12–24 h Buprenorphine (0.01–0.03) SC/IM/IV q 6–12 h Oxymorphone (0.05–0.2) SC/IM q 8–12 h
Rabbit	Butorphanol (0.2–0.4) SC/IM *or* Buprenorphine (0.01–0.05) SC/IM/IV *or* Oxymorphone (0.05–0.2) SC/IM plus Midazolam (0.5) SC/IM	Ketamine (5–10) plus additional Midazolam (0.25–0.50) IV *or*, if IV inaccessible Ketamine (25–30) IM *or* induction using Sevoflurane	Isoflurane 1.5–2.5% Sevoflurane 2–4%	Meloxicam (0.5) SC/IM/PO q 12 h Buprenorphine (0.01–0.05) SC/IM/IV q 6–12 h Oxymorphone (0.05–0.2) SC/IM q 8–12 h
Rat Mouse Gerbil Hamster Guinea pig Chinchilla	Butorphanol (2–4) SC/IM/IP *or* Buprenorphine (0.05–0.1) SC/IM/IP *or* Oxymorphone (0.2–0.5) SC/IM/IP plus Midazolam (1–2) SC/IM/IP	Ketamine (25–50) IM/IP if intubating. Sevoflurane (8%) with induction chamber if to be maintained by mask	Isoflurane 1.5–3% Sevoflurane 2–5%	Meloxicam (1–2) SC/PO q 12 h Buprenorphine (0.05–0.1) SC q 6–12 h Oxymorphone (0.2–0.5) SC q 8–12 h

α_2-Agonists (medetomidine, dexmedetomidine, xylazine) can also be used alone or in combination with opiates for sedation. However, given the profound cardio-respiratory effects of the modern potent drugs, the author prefers not to use these agents and restrict their use to young healthy animals.

Regional anaesthesia and local blocks

It should be kept in mind that use of sedation and manual restraint alone is inappropriate in clinical practice for any procedure expected to produce discomfort. An exception may be in a calm patient with judicious and efficient use of local anaesthesia in the form of a local or regional block. In addition, when used in combination with general anaesthesia, the use of local blocks can help reduce general anaesthetic requirements. For example, epidural blocks for pelvic orthopaedic surgery, and dental blocks for tooth extractions appear to be particularly worthwhile. Local anaesthetic drugs should be carefully calculated and diluted if necessary to avoid overdose. The most commonly utilized agents for local block are 1 mg/kg lidocaine and 1 mg/kg bupivacaine. The onset of action of lidocaine is rapid but short lived, while bupivacaine is slower to act but, in some species, may provide analgesia for up to 6–8 hours. Lidocaine is painful when injected and should therefore be buffered with bicarbonate unless the animal is unconscious.

Inhalation anaesthetic agents

The most popular agents for use in these species are isoflurane and sevoflurane. Halothane is still available in some countries and can certainly be used, albeit with a reduced margin of safety. Mask induction can lead to handling stress, particularly when using agents other than sevoflurane, and the use of an induction chamber, although preferable, in some individuals does lead to greater volatile drug use, and often greater environmental contamination unless active scavenging is available. Several such chambers are commercially available but they are relatively easy to improvise and there is no reason why they should not be available in most general veterinary practices. Induction of anaesthesia with inhalants provides very little time for intubation, unless the operator is highly skilled, and therefore, once induced, anaesthesia is generally maintained by administering the volatile agent in oxygen through a T-piece or similar low-resistance breathing system and a facemask. Rodents and other mammals <1 kg benefit from a dedicated rodent circuit (Fig. 17.3). Unlike the T-piece or similar circuits used for cats and dogs that rely on active inspiration for taking in gas, a dedicated rodent circuit forces gas into the oral cavity and this

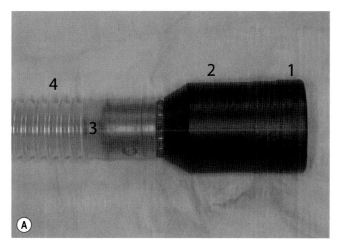
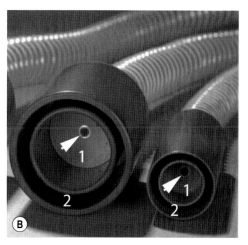

Figure 17.3 Dedicated rodent masks and circuits. (A) The rubber skirt (1) ensures that the mask (2) is secure around the rodent's head, a small diameter tube (3) delivers gas as a jet into the oral cavity while the large diameter outer tube (4) provides a low resistance path for expired gases. (B) Close-up view of rodent masks demonstrating the small diameter gas delivery (arrow) to the breathing chamber (1), and the outer tube (2) that carries away expired gases.
Courtesy of Dr Stephen Divers, University of Georgia.

positive pressure improves ventilation. These circuits including suitable facemasks are commercially available, or can be made from plastic syringe barrels and rubber gloves. Facemasks should incorporate a close-fitting rubber skirt to reduce leaks that cause atmospheric pollution. Some form of passive or active scavenging of gases should be used.

Injectable anaesthetic agents

Theoretically, any injectable anaesthetic can be used in small mammals and usually the necessary doses for healthy animals are well known from the original developmental work in laboratory animals carried out by the company that marketed the drug. However, practical limitations are set by the possible methods of administration. In some animals with easily accessible veins (e.g. in rabbits), drugs such as propofol or rapidly-acting barbiturates can be used as in cats and dogs (although the duration of effect is generally much shorter). Where IV injection is more difficult, drugs can be given by IM, IP, or SC routes. The most popular combinations of drugs are the neuroleptanalgesics or mixtures incorporating ketamine. There are marked differences between species responses and, even within one species of animal, many drug actions may be unreliable, such that a given drug producing deep anaesthesia in one animal may only provide some sedation in another of the same species.

Ketamine

Ketamine has the advantage that it is effective no matter what the route of administration. Doses required and

efficacy vary greatly between the various species. Lower doses may be used for sedation and immobilization for non-surgical procedures. As in other species of animal, ketamine is used in combination with drugs such as the benzodiazepines (diazepam or midazolam) and/or α_2-adrenoceptor agonists (xylazine or medetomidine) in order to reduce the dose of ketamine, improve muscle relaxation and to increase the effectiveness of the dissociative agent as an anaesthetic. Many of the animals seen in clinical practice are ill and/or aged, and therefore potent α_2-adrenoceptor agonists like medetomidine and dexmedetomidine are usually avoided. The author prefers to induce anaesthesia using intravenous ketamine, often in combination with additional benzodiazepine, as this induction provides more time for endotracheal intubation, compared to inhalant induction.

Neuroleptanalgesia

Although most commercially available neuroleptanalgesic combinations can be used, the mixture of fentanyl and fluanisone (Hypnorm®) has proved to be the most popular in the UK, and it can be administered by any route. The dose of fentanyl in Hypnorm® is high, resulting in a prolonged length of action and, occasionally, in respiratory arrest. Combinations of Hypnorm® with diazepam or midazolam give better muscle relaxation and allow a reduction of some 50% in the dose of Hypnorm®. If anaesthesia becomes too deep, the fentanyl component may be antagonized with naloxone (0.01 mg/kg). Buprenorphine can be used to antagonize the fentanyl in the drug combination. The technique is termed sequential analgesia and relates to the selective displacement of a

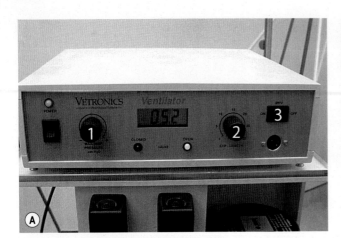
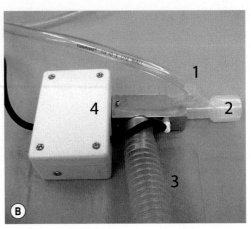

Figure 17.4 Pressure-cycled ventilator. (A) Main control unit featuring maximum inspired pressure control (1), expiration length (2), and passive/ventilator switch (3); (B) patient delivery system with gas inlet (1), endotracheal tube connector (2), waste gas removal (3) and solenoid switch (4).
Courtesy of Dr Stephen Divers, University of Georgia.

pure agonist with a partial agonist/antagonist in the hope of reducing respiratory depression and sedation while maintaining analgesia.

Other agents

A mixture that is often used, although unlicensed, is known as the 'Hellabrunn Mixture'. It was developed primarily for administration to zoo animals and is prepared by adding 4 mL of ketamine (100 mg/mL) to a vial of dry xylazine (500 mg). This yields a stable injectable solution containing xylazine 125 mg/mL together with ketamine 100 mg/mL. Its stability means that it is immediately available and it is relatively safe for the administrator. Ketamine and medetomidine/dexmedetomidine combinations are also very effective, but their use is best restricted to young healthy animals.

Propofol has been recommended for intravenous use in rabbits, rats, mice and hamsters, however, its short duration of action combined with apnoea necessitates rapid intubation. Alfaxalone has proven useful in some species when given IV. Pentobarbital and thiopental may be used but given their prolonged sedation and respiratory depression, they cannot be recommended for clinical use. The shorter acting methohexital appears safer and has been used in various small mammals (Smith, 1993).

Ventilation

This author prefers to connect all intubated small mammals <8 kg to a pressure-cycled ventilator (e.g. Small Animal Ventilator VT-5000, BASi Vetronics, USA, or SAV03 Vetronics, UK). The ventilator is routinely set to the non-rebreathing passive circuit, with active ventilation selected if required (Fig. 17.4). This has the advantage of being able to select the mode of ventilation by flicking a switch and without changing circuits. Ventilation is used whenever end-tidal CO_2 ($ETCO_2$) rises above 45 mmHg or SpO_2 falls below 95%. Ventilation is used routinely for laparoscopy involving abdominal insufflation with CO_2. This inexpensive pressure-cycled ventilator is simple to use and has a proven track record in exotic mammal practice. Depth and frequency of ventilation are initially set to mimic preanaesthetic respiration, but are modified to maintain $ETCO_2$ readings of between 35 and 45 mmHg.

Monitoring

The primary goal of anaesthetic monitoring should be to minimize morbidity by preventing, identifying, and correcting hypotension, bradycardia, arrhythmias, hypoxaemia, hypercapnia, and metabolic disturbances. Although the size and anatomy of some small mammal patients often preclude some anaesthetic monitoring techniques, this should not discourage the practitioner from including the following steps:

1. Perform a basic preanaesthetic examination to record heart and respiratory rates and character, and if possible collect baseline clinicopathological data. Complete blood counts and full biochemistry profiles are not always possible (and, indeed, anaesthesia is often used to facilitate blood collection), however, haematocrit, total protein, urea, and glucose can be run as a minimum using small samples. Alternatively, blood samples may be collected and run immediately following induction using point-of-care analysers (e.g. Abaxis biochemistry machine, I-Stat analyser).

Table 17.4 Normal physiological values for selected small mammals

Species	Body weight (g) Male/female	Life span (years)	Temperature °C (°F)	Heart rate	Respiratory rate
Chinchilla	450–600/550–800	8–10	36.1–37.8 (97.0–100.0)	40–100	40–80
Gerbil	65–100/55–85	3–4	37.0–38.5 (98.6–101.3)	360	90
Guinea pig	900–1200/700–900	4–5	37.2–39.5 (99.0–103.1)	230–380	40–100
Hamster	85–130/95–150	1.5–2	37.0–38.0 (98.6–100.4)	250–500	35–135
Mouse	20–40/25–40	1.5–3	35.4–39.1 (95.7–102.3)	325–780	60–220
Rat	450–520/250–300	2.5–3.5	35.9–37.5 (96.6–99.5)	250–450	115
Prairie dog	1000–2200/500–1500	6–10	35.4–39.1 (95.7–102.3)	83–318	40–60
Rabbit	2000–5000/2000–6000	5–15	38.5–40.0 (101.3–104.0)	130–325	30–60
Ferret	1000–2000/500–1000	5–8 (US) 6–12 (UK)	37.8–40.0 (100.0–104.0)	200–400	33–36

Modified from Carpenter 2005.

2. Record the precise time of premedication/induction. This step is often overlooked but it is important to know how long an animal has been anaesthetized, and to maximize efforts in expediting procedures.
3. Gauge the depth of anaesthesia by observation of mentation and reflexes.
4. Utilize simple monitoring techniques rather than elaborate systems that are prone to failure. First, take a heart rate and note cardiac rhythm with a simple stethoscope and note the depth and frequency of ventilation, and judging the information based upon preanaesthetic values (Table 17.4).
5. Utilize equipment that will give you the most information with least problems, for example, ultrasound Doppler probe for heart rate and rhythm, end-tidal capnography, and ECG are easy to use. Pulse oximetry can be temperamental but still useful when a reliable pulse wave is obtained (irregular or poor pulse wave leads to untrustworthy readings that must not be relied upon). Pulse oximetry readings (SpO$_2$) <90% is taken to correlate with hypoxaemia PaO$_2$ ≤60 mmHg. Indirect blood pressure readings taken from the radial artery of the forelimb using a sphygmomanometer and ultrasound Doppler have been shown to be accurate and reliable compared to direct arterial blood pressures in rabbits

(Ypsilantis et al., 2005). A 22 or 24 gauge catheter inserted in an ear artery is used for invasive blood pressure monitoring in rabbits.
6. Do not rely totally on the monitoring equipment – always rely on human evaluation of the patient which means that there must be an anaesthetist dedicated to the case at all times. No anaesthetic monitoring equipment can ever replace an attentive, experienced veterinary anaesthetist.
7. Maintain a contemporaneous record throughout the anaesthetic period. Record quantitative readings and qualitative evaluations every 5 minutes on a dedicated anaesthesia sheet that should form part of the medical record.

Recovery and postoperative care

Recovery and the immediate postoperative period can be just as critical as the maintenance period in ensuring that your small mammal patient recovers completely. Indeed, the point of initial recovery and extubation can often be the most critical stage of the anaesthetic procedure, because critical support mechanisms have been withdrawn. In general, the following steps should be taken for patient support:

1. When discontinuing inhalation anaesthesia, consider administration of applicable reversal drugs (e.g. flumazenil for benzodiazepines).
2. Maintain oxygen administration after extubation until fully conscious.
3. Recovery areas should be quiet, warm and in a place where the animal can be placed in sternal recumbency, and readily monitored. Hypothermic animals should be placed into an incubator until normothermic. Do not add water/food bowls or cage furniture/substrate until the animal is ambulatory.
4. Monitor the animal frequently and administer additional fluids or antagonists as and when needed.

Postoperative analgesia is important and must not be neglected. It should be a continuation/modification of the pre-emptive analgesic protocol employed for premedication. Some opioid drugs are suitable and other methods utilizing local analgesics should be considered. It is regrettable that the rat, which has probably contributed more than most animals to advances in medical and veterinary sciences, still is ignored in many laboratories in circumstances where postoperative analgesia would be regarded as essential for other animals. Meloxicam is a preferential COX-2 inhibitor that has been tried and tested in laboratory rodents and, although multidose pharmacokinetics have yet to be determined, the author uses this analgesic routinely with good effects.

Monitor temperature regularly and remove from incubators once normothermic. Some mustelids, especially otters, appear prone to anaesthesia-induced hyperthermia that can be fatal if uncontrolled.

LAGOMORPHS – RABBITS (*ORYCTOLAGUS CUNICULUS*) AND HARES (*LEPUS EUROPAEUS*)

Rabbits and hares need to be handled carefully as they tend to panic if placed on slippery surfaces. These animals are best held for injection wrapped in a towel in the arms of an assistant or placed in a restraining box. A rabbit or hare struggling against forcible restraint may fracture a vertebra, so any restraint technique used should only entail the minimum of force. The animal should be caught by grasping the scruff of the neck firmly and pressing down on a flat surface until it relaxes, then it may be lifted by supplementing the neck grip with support for the hindquarters. Rabbits, especially when kept as pets, can be calmed by scratching behind the ears and stroking the back. Respiratory problems, usually due to various bacteria including but not limited to *Pasteurella*, are common in rabbits that may appear to be healthy. Auscultation of the lungs for diagnosis is not easy and many authorities advise conscious thoracic radiography prior to general anaesthesia so that owners may be warned of the anaesthetic risks associated with the presence of lung disease.

Intramuscular injections are made into the quadriceps or triceps, epaxial or lumbar muscles. Intravenous injections can be most easily given into the marginal ear, cephalic, and lateral saphenous veins. Intravenous injection is greatly facilitated by the use of a restraining box that leaves the ears accessible, or good quality restraint following sedation. Rabbits produce atropinase, which rapidly inactivates atropine, so to be effective doses of this agent must be high (1–2 mg/kg) and repeated every 15–20 minutes. Alternatively, glycopyrrolate (0.01–0.02 mg/kg) is preferred as an anticholinergic.

Although IV anaesthetic agents can be used to induce anaesthesia in rabbits they are not good for maintaining anaesthesia for even very small incremental doses may cause death through respiratory arrest. Induction of anaesthesia is satisfactory with methohexital (5–10 mg/kg), alfaxalone (2–8 mg/kg), propofol (3–6 mg/kg), or ketamine (10–15 mg/kg) and midazolam (0.5–1.0 mg/kg) given IV to effect. These agents can be given IV through a 21 gauge or 23 gauge catheter placed into an ear, cephalic, or lateral saphenous vein. The ketamine/midazolam combination is preferred by the author as it provides a longer duration of action for placing an endotracheal tube. Diazepam injected into an ear vein may cause tissue necrosis.

Induction of anaesthesia is usually quiet with sevoflurane administered in O_2 1–2 L/min through a facemask from a non-rebreathing system. Induction with isoflurane is facilitated when the animal is first heavily sedated and the concentration of isoflurane increased in small step increments up to 3 or 4%. Alternatively, the rabbit can be placed in an induction chamber or plastic box with a charcoal canister on the outlet for scavenging and isoflurane in O_2 introduced into the box until the animal is unconscious. Inhalation agents are eliminated rapidly after the mask is removed and leave little time for the process of endotracheal intubation.

Endotracheal intubation is relatively difficult because of the long, narrow oropharynx and long incisor teeth limiting access through the mouth. The tongue is thick, fleshy, friable, and easily torn. The soft palate is long and the epiglottis is large. In all cases, it is essential to have an adequately anaesthetized patient that is completely relaxed – attempts to intubate a semiconscious small mammal are likely to cause damage and fail. Endotracheal intubation is accomplished by either (1) direct view of the larynx using a straight, premature human infant blade (Wisconsin 00) or endoscope, or (2) blindly. A semi-rigid stylet can be used as a guide to aid in the passage of the endotracheal tube. Tubes of 2.0–4.0 mm internal diameter are suitable for use in most rabbits. Direct view of the larynx is considered the gold standard in human and veterinary medicine, and typically enables a larger endotracheal tube to be placed compared to blind techniques (Fig. 17.5).

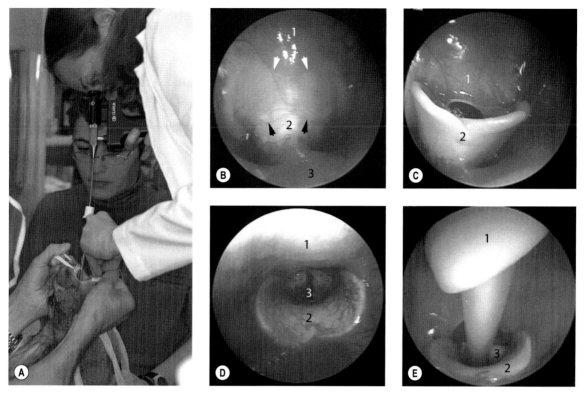

Figure 17.5 (A) Endotracheal intubation in a rabbit using a fibreoptic laryngoscope; (B) first reveals the caudal edge of the soft palate (black arrows) buttoned below the epiglottis (2) at the base of the fleshy tongue (3). The cranial margin of the epiglottis can be seen through the caudal soft palate (white arrows); (C) gentle dorsal deflection of the soft palate (1) enables the epiglottis to fall ventrad (2); (D) with the soft palate (1) now disengaged from the epiglottis (2), the glottis (3) can be seen; (E) endotracheal tube (1) containing a stylet is being passed over the epiglottis (2) and through the glottis (3) into the trachea. *Courtesy of Dr Stephen Divers, University of Georgia.*

Placement of the largest possible tube becomes especially critical in smaller animals where significant decreases in airway resistance and gas flow can be obtained (see Table 17.4). The chances of successful intubation in small rabbits and rodents can be maximized by:

1. Ensuring adequate anaesthesia (see Table 17.3). Ketamine and midazolam anaesthesia will provide 5+ minutes of good restraint and relaxation for intubation (compared to 20–40 seconds following inhalant induction).
2. Maintaining the animal on oxygen by holding a small facemask over the nose during induction. A pulse oximeter probe attached to a foot will provide warning of low oxygenation during intubation.

There are two main techniques for endotracheal intubation of rabbits and rodents:

1. Laryngoscope or endoscope-guided intubation. With the rabbit in sternal (or dorsal) recumbency, use gauze to open the mouth fully and hyperextend the head and neck. Insert the laryngoscope (Wisconsin 00, long blade) or endoscope to view the epiglottis and ensure that it is not engaged above the soft palate (rabbits and many rodents are obligate nasal breathers) (see Fig. 17.5A,B). Applying mild dorsal pressure on the soft palate will cause the epiglottis to fall ventrally and expose the glottis (see Fig. 17.5C,D). Apply (<2 mg/kg) lidocaine to the glottis, and wait for 30–60 seconds while administering nasal oxygen. The endotracheal tube can be advanced alongside the laryngoscope, or slid off the endoscope, and advanced through the glottis and into the trachea (see Fig. 17.5E). Many experienced lab animal vets are able to perform a blind intubation technique in rabbits; however, given the smaller size of most pet rabbits compared to the 3–5 kg laboratory New Zealand white, varied breed/conformation and disease status, direct viewing is preferred for clinical practice.
2. Blind intubation. The rabbit is positioned in sternal or dorsal recumbency with the head and neck overextended. Introduce the endotracheal tube into the oral cavity and over the tongue while listening

Table 17.5 Cross-sectional area, changes in gas flow and resistance associated with different endotracheal tube diameters

Endotracheal tube size, internal diameter (mm)	Cross-sectional area, πr^2 (mm²)	Relative resistance for tubes of the same length at the same flow rate*
1.0	0.79	410
1.5	1.77	81
2.0	3.14	26
2.5	4.91	10
3.0	7.07	5
3.5	9.62	3
4.0	12.57	2
4.5	15.90	1

*Hagen–Poiseuille equation for airway resistance is $R = 8ln/\pi r^4$. In this case as 8ln represents a constant, and so the values have been made relative to a 4.5 mm tube with R = 1.

for the sound of air movement as the tube advances. The tube is positioned over the glottis when the sound of air movement is the loudest. Alternatively, watch for the presence of condensation in the tube. The tube is gently rotated while moving forward and back until the tube slides into the trachea. At no time must any pressure be used to insert the tube. Blind techniques are more acceptable for larger animals because the size of the endotracheal tube that can be easily inserted is generally smaller compared to a direct view technique. Such reductions in tube size become increasingly critical as tube diameter decreases (Table 17.5).

In addition to endotracheal intubation, nasal intubation has also been used effectively in various small mammals, particularly rabbits and rodents undergoing dental evaluations where the presence of an endotracheal tube can be a hindrance. Following induction, lidocaine (<2 mg/kg total) is instilled into one or both nostrils before the insertion of fine-diameter tubes. Nasal tubes should be inserted carefully to avoid trauma and haemorrhage to nasal turbinates and, if placed deeply, will often simply enter the trachea of obligate nasal breathers like the rabbit. The airway resistance of nasal tubes is typically high and therefore they must be connected directly to the anaesthesia machine and (low flow) oxygen supply, and not via a T-piece or other low-resistance circuit. It is generally impossible to ventilate an animal using an intranasal tube and waste gases will contaminate the environment

unless active scavenging is placed near the animal's mouth and nose. Therefore, the author primarily uses this technique to provide supplemental oxygen to animals under injectable anaesthesia.

If two attempts at intubation are unsuccessful, the animal should be placed on a tight-fitting facemask. Pharyngeal oedema and dyspnoea associated with repeated intubation attempts are not uncommon. Anti-inflammatory drugs may be necessary and can be administered by the IV or intratracheal routes (e.g. NSAIDs or, less favourably unless severe, steroids). Anaesthesia is usually maintained with vaporizer settings of 1.5–3% isoflurane, or 2–4% when administered by facemask. Oxygen administration is essential since anaesthetized rabbits rapidly develop hypoxaemia. In many circumstances, controlled ventilation is important to maintain adequate ventilation. Recently, the use of laryngeal cuffs (supraglottic devices) have gained some popularity. They can be more easily placed than endotracheal tubes and in many cases can be used to provide ventilation.

The MAC values for isoflurane and sevoflurane in New Zealand white rabbits are 2.05% and 3.7%, respectively (Drummond, 1985; Scheller et al., 1988). The depth of anaesthesia is assessed by tickling the inside of the ear pinnae. Eye rotation occurs at 0.8 MAC while toe-pinch withdrawal and pain reflexes are abolished >1 MAC. Palpebral and corneal reflexes are lost at ≥2 MAC, and indicate dangerously deep anaesthesia. Postoperative analgesia may be provided by opioids such as buprenorphine and NSAIDs, for example, meloxicam. Postoperatively, hypothermic rabbits should be kept warm (e.g. in an incubator) until normothermic, remembering that a normothermic rabbit kept in an ambient temperature above 30°C (86°F) can quickly result in heat stress.

RODENTS – RATS (*RATTUS NORVEGICUS*), MICE (*MUS MUSCULUS*), GUINEA PIGS (*CAVIA PORCELLUS*), HAMSTERS AND GERBILS (*MESOCRICETUS AURATUS* AND *GERBILLIDAE*)

Rats that are not tame can be very difficult to handle because they cannot be restrained by the tail for any long time for they will turn and climb up their own tails to bite the restraining hand. They can be restrained in a towel that is folded over the rat and rolled, making sure that the legs are secure. Experienced handlers often grasp the rat with the palm of the hand over the animal's back and restrain the forelegs by folding them across each other under the chin so that the chin cannot be depressed enough to bite. Mice should be lifted by holding the base of the tail between the thumb and forefinger and immediately transferred to a horizontal cloth surface (e.g. the coat of the handler). As it attempts to escape, it is grasped by the loose scruff of the neck and the tail is gripped. Guinea pigs lack a true scruff and are best restrained by grasping around their pectoral and pelvic structures. It should be remembered that hamsters are nocturnal and often greatly resent being disturbed during daytime, making them liable to bite. The hamster's scruff is quite loose so restraint by grasping the scruff needs to be quite vigorous. Chinchillas are prone to 'hair slip' where they expel large tufts of hair in response to being grasped.

Pre-existing chronic respiratory disease due to variety of viral or bacterial agents is common in non-laboratory rodents. There are very many ways of anaesthetizing rodents but simple gaseous anaesthesia is satisfactory for most clinical purposes. Intravenous injections into the dorsal metatarsal or tail vein of conscious rats are possible, but difficult to impossible in most other small rodents. Subcutaneous (and intraperitoneal) injections are more frequently used, and appear to be as effective as the IM route for induction.

Induction of anaesthesia with injectable agents is useful in larger rodents prior to tracheal intubation. Accurate bodyweights to the nearest gram (or 0.1 grams for rodents <30 g) are critical for the precise calculation of drug doses. Ketamine is generally unsatisfactory as a sole agent, and must be combined with either a benzodiazepine or α_2-agonist (see Table 17.3). There are species, age and sex differences in responses of rodents to ketamine. Duration of effect decreases as young rats mature from 1 to 3 weeks of age, whereas after 3 weeks of age females sleep longer than males.

In inexperienced hands, inhalation anaesthesia is safer for most rodents, and anaesthesia is best induced in a chamber or by facemask. Isoflurane or sevoflurane in O_2 1–2 L/min is administered, starting with a minimal concentration and gradually increasing it until the animal loses consciousness. Scavenging of anaesthetic gases from the chamber or facemask is important and should not be overlooked. Unconsciousness is equated with loss of the righting reflex when the box is tilted. Anaesthesia is usually produced in about 2–3 minutes and can be maintained with concentrations of isoflurane (2–3%) or sevoflurane (2–4%) through a facemask from a dedicated rodent circuit (see Fig. 17.3). A useful alternative that has proven effective for maintaining anaesthesia during intra-oral dentistry is the use of a nose cone or nasal catheter. Following induction and the instillation of 1–2 drops of lidocaine (diluted if necessary to keep the total dose <2 mg/kg) into the nares, a fine diameter catheter is placed into one or both nares (Fig. 17.6). The tube is then connected directly to the anaesthesia machine without the use of any form of circuit. Oxygen 0.5 L/min is then forced into the nares and nasopharynx to maintain anaesthesia if carrying an anaesthetic agent or to provide O_2 if using injectable agents. Excess gases escape through the mouth or around the nasal catheter(s) and must be actively scavenged using a negative pressure hose to avoid room contamination.

Maintenance of a clear airway is not always easy in the absence of endotracheal intubation since nasal and oropharyngeal secretions tend to become viscid during anaesthesia and are liable to give rise to obstruction. The

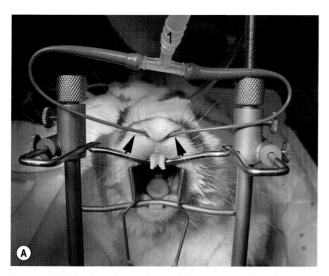
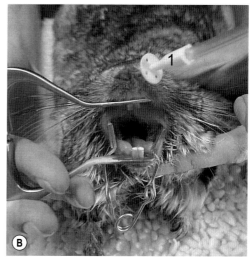

Figure 17.6 Nasal intubation in a rabbit using 5 Fr red rubber tubes (A) and guinea pig using a 3 Fr urinary catheter (B) to provide oxygen during oral surgery performed under injectable anaesthesia. This system can be used to provide inhalant agents but scavenging near the oral cavity is required.
Courtesy of Dr Stephen Divers, University of Georgia.

risk may be countered by frequent aspiration of the mouth and oropharynx using a fine rubber catheter attached to a 60 mL syringe. Endotracheal intubation is possible and the author prefers the use of a 1 mm diameter endoscope with appropriately small endotracheal tubes (1–2 mm). Intubation using a small otoscope to insert a stylet as a guide for a 14 gauge IV catheter cut short and with the end blunted in a flame has also been advocated for rats (Trim, personal communication). As with all small mammals, conservation of body heat is critically important and a warm environment must always be provided from the point of induction to recovery. Intraoperative fluids may be administered by IV catheters (larger rodents only) or the IO (femur or humerus) route. Where only maintenance fluids are required (e.g. elective castration), a fluid bolus can be given SC following induction, and will be absorbed during anaesthesia. Rodents regain consciousness quickly within a few minutes of discontinuing inhalants, and full recovery takes less than 10–30 minutes.

MUSTELIDS – FERRETS (*MUSTELA PUTORIUS FURO*), MINK (*MUSTELA LUTREAOLA*), EUROPEAN OTTER (*LUTRA LUTRA*), STOAT OR SHORT-TAILED WEASEL (*MUSTELA ERMINE*), POLECAT (*MUSTELA PUTORIUS*), BADGER (*MELES MELES*)

Domesticated, neutered ferrets are generally tame, and can be handled in a similar way to cats and small dogs. They readily vomit when anaesthetized so they should be fasted for 6–8 hours before induction of anaesthesia. Ferrets can be anaesthetized with isoflurane or sevoflurane passed into an induction box or by facemask until they are unconscious (see Table 17.3). Alternatively, propofol IV can be used with tractable individuals, while IM ketamine combinations can be used in those that are unable to be handled (Table 17.6).

Mink, stoats, weasels, and otters are not domestic animals – they are nervous, fast and can be vicious. They are best handled by persuading them to enter a clear-sided induction box or squeeze cage. Most mustelids dislike a human blowing into their face and will retreat from such an onslaught. Moreover, they are very inquisitive and will investigate the source of gentle scratching noises such as can be made on the side of a box. Once in the box, they can be anaesthetized with a volatile anaesthetic such as isoflurane or sevoflurane. If necessary, the box may be covered with transparent plastic sheeting to make it more gas-tight and, until the animal is unconscious, it should not be removed from the box. Experienced handlers can net individual animals and inject by hand an anaesthetic combination of ketamine, α_2-sedative or benzodiazepine (see Table 17.6).

Badgers resist handling by biting and scratching. The safest procedure for handling them is to immobilize them with a squeeze cage and an IM ketamine combination, followed by intubation and maintenance of anaesthesia with conventional inhalation techniques (see Table 17.6).

Like other carnivores, endotracheal intubation is generally straightforward, and maintenance using a T-piece or other non-rebreathing system is recommended for animals <6–8 kg. Temperature monitoring is critical as hypothermia and life-threatening hyperthermia (especially in otters) are not uncommon.

Table 17.6 Injectable anaesthetic regimens recommended for European mustelids

Species, adult weight range (kg)	Agents and doses (mg/kg)	Reversal agent (mg/kg)	Comments
European mink (*Mustela lutreaola*), 0.4–1 kg	Ketamine (10) Medetomidine (0.20)	Atipamezole (1)	Beware of hypothermia
European otter (*Lutra lutra*), 3–14 kg	Ketamine (15–18) + diazepam (0.4–0.5) Ketamine (5) + medetomidine (0.05)	Atipamezole (0.25)	Respiratory depression Bradycardia, apnoea, hypothermia
Stoat or short-tailed weasel (*Mustela ermine*), 0.05–0.36 kg	Ketamine (5) + medetomidine (0.1)	Atipamezole (0.5)	
European polecat (*Mustela putorius*), 0.7–1.7 kg	Ketamine (10) + medetomidine (0.20)	Atipamezole (1)	Beware hypothermia
European badger (*Meles meles*), 5.5–12.5 kg	Ketamine (10–15) + midazolam (0.4–1) Ketamine (5–10) + medetomidine (0.05–0.10)	Atipamezole (0.25–0.50)	Preferred combination

INSECTIVORES – EUROPEAN HEDGEHOGS (*ERINACEUS EUROPAEUS*), AFRICAN PYGMY HEDGEHOGS (*ATELERIX ALBIVENTRIS*)

Hedgehogs are insectivores with rapid metabolism and, as such, should not be fasted for more than 1 hour. Efforts must be made to maintain temperature, especially in the smaller pygmy species. Inhalational anaesthesia using chamber induction is preferred as even a tightly rolled-up hedgehog will succumb. Intubation can be challenging and is most readily accomplished using endoscopic guidance of small diameter endotracheal tubes (Fig. 17.7). Alternatively, facemask maintenance is often acceptable for short procedures. Parenteral drugs may be indicated for fieldwork but details are scant.

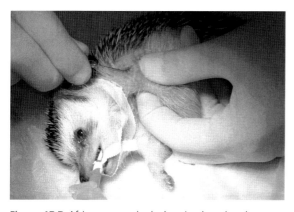

Figure 17.7 African pygmy hedgehog intubated and maintained on isoflurane/O$_2$ while a needle is placed into the humerus for IO access.
Courtesy of Dr Stephen Divers, University of Georgia.

REPTILES

The Class Reptilia consists of over 8000 species, but only a few dozen species are likely to be encountered with any regularity in general practice. All the crocodylia, front-fanged poisonous snakes (but not all backed-fanged poisonous species) and both species of poisonous lizard (*Heloderma* spp.) are considered to be dangerous animals and are usually covered by national and/or state legislation. The following description will concentrate on companion reptiles that are frequently presented to practitioners.

Class Reptilia
  Order Crocodyla (crocodiles, alligators, gharials)
  Order Testudines, suborders
  a) Pleurodira (side-necked turtles, snake-neck turtles)
  b) Cryptodira (tortoises, terrapins, soft-shelled turtles)
  Order Squamata, suborders
  a) Sauria (lizards)
  b) Serpentes (snakes)
  c) Amphisbaenia (worm lizards)
  Order Rhynchocephalia (tuataras)

Reptiles are vertebrates with similar organ systems to mammals. However, they are ectothermic and rely on environmental temperature and behaviour to control their core body temperature. They possess both renal and hepatic portal circulations, and predominantly excrete ammonia, urea, or uric acid depending upon their evolutionary adaptations. They possess nucleated red blood cells and their metabolic rates are typically only around 15% those of mammals.

The diversity of evolutionary adaptations within the Reptilia necessitates generalities. Reptiles possess a common cloaca that receives the lower gastrointestinal, reproductive, and urinary tracts. In addition, lungs are simpler and composed of vascular pockets, more like a cavitated sponge than alveoli. Lizards are quadrupeds and have a similar organ distribution. Of particular note is the lack of a diaphragm such that all organs are contained within a single coelomic cavity. Some lizards (e.g. tegus and monitors) possess post-pulmonary and/or post-hepatic membranes that are thin but divide the coelom into compartments. Snakes have their organs distributed in a longitudinal arrangement. While the general location of organs is similar between species, variations do occur. However, the heart is typically located 22–35% from snout-to-vent, while the respiratory surface areas of the lungs are situated between 25 and 50% snout-to-vent (the caudal air sac may extend far further caudad). Boas and pythons are primitive snakes and having more recently evolved from quadripedal reptiles still possess both left and right lungs; however, more evolved members of the Serpentes lack a developed left lung. Snakes and lizards have incomplete tracheal rings. The chelonians (Testudines) are characterized by their shell, which comprises of a dorsal carapace and ventral plastron. The shell may be leathery or rigid. The internal organs are not dissimilar in distribution between different chelonian species. The cranioventral heart is located within a pericardial membrane, while the lungs are dorsad and separated from the remaining viscera by a post-pulmonary membrane (or septum horizontale). Chelonians have complete tracheal rings, and males possess a single copulatory phallus. Crocodilians have a four-chambered heart, and a functional diaphragm that utilizes the ventral body wall skeletal

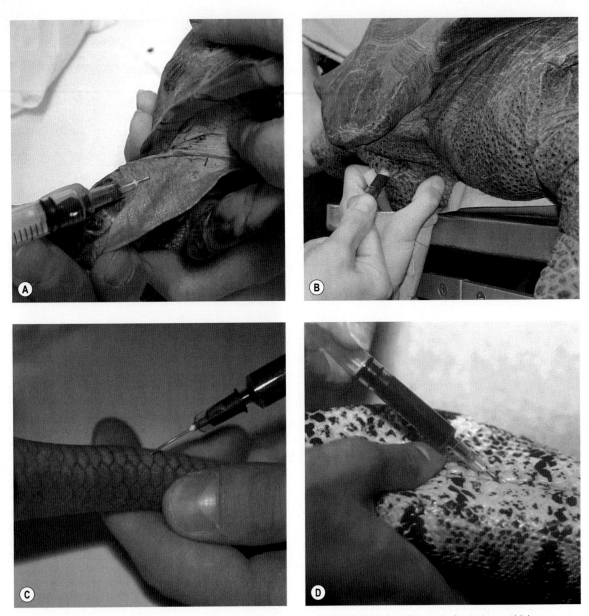

Figure 17.8 Reptile venipuncture sites: (A) left jugular vein in a Greek tortoise; (B) dorsal coccygeal vein in an Aldabra tortoise; (C) caudal (ventral tail) vein in a monkey-tailed skink; (D) cardiocentesis in a sedated boa constrictor.
Courtesy of Dr Stephen Divers, University of Georgia.

musculature and liver to create a 'diaphragmatic pump'. The gular flap must first be displaced ventrad to expose the glottis for tracheal intubation. The trachea is composed of complete tracheal rings. All reptiles have both pulmonary and systemic circulations (similar to mammals). In non-crocodilian reptiles, functional separation of venous and arterial blood is largely maintained by a muscular ridge within the ventricle. The total blood volume of reptiles is approximately 4–8% of body weight and of this, up to 10% may be withdrawn safely in healthy animals. A range of IV routes are available for blood collection and the administration of anaesthetics and other agents (Fig. 17.8):

Tortoises, turtles and terrapins – Jugular vein, subcarapacial sinus, post-occipital sinus, dorsal coccygeal vein

Table 17.7 Important husbandry requirements for some popular reptiles

Species	Habitat/vivarium type	POTZ °C	Humidity %*	Lighting	Hibernation	Diet
Corn/rat snake	Terrestrial, scrubland	25–30	30–70	NS	Yes	C
Boa constrictor	Terrestrial, rainforest (semi-arboreal/aquatic)	28–31	70–95	NS	No	C
Ball python	Terrestrial, scrubland	25–30	50–80	NS	No	C
Leopard gecko	Terrestrial, arid scrub	25–30	20–30	NS	No	I, c
Green iguana	Arboreal, rainforest	29–33	60–85	BS	No	H
Bearded dragon	Terrestrial, desert	20–32	20–30	BS	No	I, c, h
Water dragon	Arboreal, rainforest	24–30	80–90	BS	No	I, c, h
Savannah monitor	Terrestrial, arid scrub	25–32	20–40	BS	No	C, i
Greek tortoise	Terrestrial, temperate to subtropical	20–26	30–50	BS	Yes	H, c
Box tortoise	Terrestrial, temperate to subtropical	22–28	50–80	BS	Yes	H, I, c
Leopard tortoise	Terrestrial, tropical	25–30	30–50	BS	No	H, c
Red-footed tortoise	Terrestrial, tropical	25–30	50–90	BS	No	H, c
Red-eared terrapin	Temperate to subtropical, semi-aquatic, water depth 30 cm min, land area ⅓ of tank	24–28	aquatic	BS	Yes	H, I, c

*Humidity requirements will be significantly greater during ecdysis. Temperature requirements shown are air temperature gradients. In general, basking temperatures should be 5°C greater, while at night these temperatures should fall by 5°C. BS: broad spectrum lighting (UVB 290–320 nm) essential; NS: no special lighting requirements known or able to utilize dietary Vit D3; Ii: insectivorous, Hh: herbivorous, Cc: carnivorous. Upper case indicates major food items, lower case minor food items.

Lizards – Caudal (ventral tail) vein, caudal to cloaca
Snakes – Caudal (ventral tail) vein, caudal to cloaca; cardiocentesis
Crocodilians – Caudal (ventral tail) vein (small animals), supravertebral sinus (just caudal to the skull in the dorsal midline).

Reptiles rely on environmental temperature and behaviour to maintain their body temperature within their preferred optimum temperature zone (POTZ) (Table 17.7). Maintenance of species-specific POTZ before, during, and after anaesthesia is important to ensure proper drug metabolism and complete recovery. For some minor procedures, for example blood sampling, simple restraint may be all that is required. This can be enhanced by temporary immobilization techniques, for example dorsal recumbency, reduced light intensity, or by gentle ocular pressure (vaso-vagal response). However, for more invasive and painful procedures sedation or anaesthesia is required.

Preanaesthetic stabilization, sedation and analgesia

A full clinical examination should be performed, and the animal accurately weighed. The fluid status of all reptiles should be assessed, especially if debilitated or presented post-hibernation. Reduced skin elasticity is an unreliable sign of dehydration, but together with enophthalmos and reduced body weight compared to previous records, evidence of dry mucous membranes and lethargy may be suggestive. However, determination of packed cell volume and total solids by blood sampling provides a more quantitative measure of dehydration. Normal haematocrit values vary between species, but tend to be approximately 20–35%. Lithium-heparin tubes should be used for biochemical profiles, while EDTA is preferred for haematology (unless it is known to cause haemolysis in which case heparin is used, e.g. for some species of chelonians).

For elective procedures (e.g. neutering), underweight, dehydrated or debilitated animals should be nursed for days, weeks or months until their condition improves. For non-elective cases, attempts to correct dehydration should be started prior to anaesthesia. Even the most moribund reptile will usually benefit from stabilization for 24–48 hours before embarking on general anaesthesia. In the author's experience, reptiles that fail to stabilize prior to surgery tend to succumb intra- or postoperatively. While oral fluids are non-invasive to administer and provide the most physiologically normal method of rehydration, they are sufficient only for mildly dehydrated tractable animals

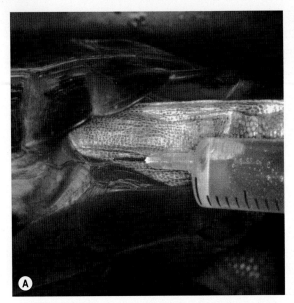
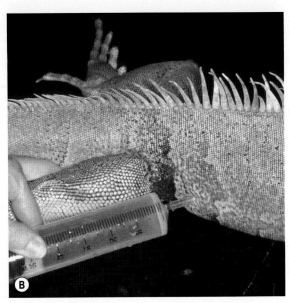

Figure 17.9 Intracoelomic fluid therapy administration (A) in a tortoise via the ventrocranial aspect of the prefemoral fossa, cranial to the left hind limb; (B) in a green iguana cranial to the right hind limb. Care is required to avoid the often voluminous bladder of chelonians and some lizards.
Courtesy of Dr Stephen Divers, University of Georgia.

and are contraindicated immediately prior to surgery due to the risks associated with regurgitation. Intracoelomic fluids are more suitable but uptake can take many hours and their use is obviously problematic if coeliotomy or coelioscopy is scheduled (Fig. 17.9). Thus, for dehydrated surgical candidates, IV or IO fluid therapy should be considered.

The osmolarity of reptile plasma is generally lower than that of mammals, although desert species are certainly capable of profound physiological haemoconcentration that would be fatal to mammals. In addition, reptiles possess a larger intracellular fluid compartment than mammals. Consequently, for both IV and IO fluid therapy, isotonic (hypotonic compared to mammals) electrolyte fluids (260–290 mOsm/L) are favoured to encourage the intracellular diffusion of water. Fluids are administered at 20–35 mL/kg/day (rates of up to 5 mL/kg/h may be initially used for the first 3 hours, although maintenance rates of 3 mL/kg/h are typically used during anaesthesia). Use of an infusion pump or syringe driver achieves accurate dosing but multiple bolus injections are a practical alternative. The catheter site should be prepared aseptically. For lizards and snakes, ventral tail vein catheters, size dependent upon animal size, can be placed and maintained during anaesthesia (Fig. 17.10A,B). In addition, IO tibial or femoral catheters are well tolerated in lizards (Fig. 17.10C). Jugular catheterization can be used in chelonians and snakes, while cephalic catheters can also be practical in larger lizards. Most IV catheterizations require a surgical cut-down procedure. (Fig. 17.10D).

All reptiles should be hospitalized and maintained at their POTZ at all times to minimize physiological disturbance, facilitate recovery, and ensure immunocompetence (see Table 17.7). It should be noted that although hypothermia will reduce movement, it does not provide analgesia, and is therefore unacceptable as a means of anaesthesia. It can also dramatically affect the pharmacokinetics of any drugs administered and greatly prolong recovery. Fasting should be carried out before all elective procedures in order to avoid the compression of lung(s) associated with large meals and potential regurgitation. Fasting time depends on the feeding regimen of the reptile but, in general, one feeding cycle should be omitted prior to surgery.

Phenothiazines and parasympatholytics are rarely employed, however, benzodiazepines have been used. The presurgical administration of analgesics should be routine, although taxa-specific effects have been documented (Table 17.8). Morphine (but not butorphanol) has been shown to be analgesic in bearded dragons and red-eared terrapins, whereas high doses of butorphanol (but not morphine) is effective in snakes (Sladky et al., 2007, 2008).

Regional anaesthesia and local block

Inadequate knowledge of precise nerve positions is probably responsible for the current lack of regional nerve blocks in reptiles, however, nerve locators may help

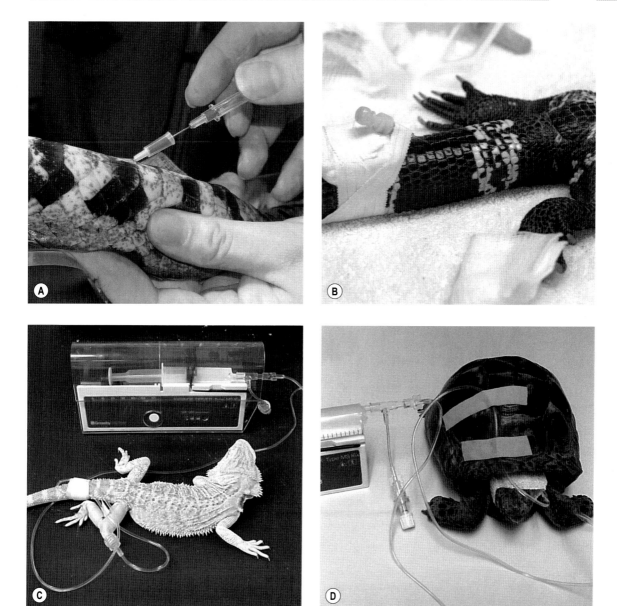

Figure 17.10 (A) Intravenous catheterization of the caudal (ventral tail) vein in an anaconda; (B) caudal (ventral tail) vein catheter taped in position in an anaesthetized beaded lizard in dorsal recumbency; (C) intraosseous fluid therapy via a tibial needle in a conscious bearded dragon; (D) intravenous fluid therapy via a left jugular catheter in a Greek tortoise. *Courtesy of Dr Stephen Divers, University of Georgia.*

alleviate this problem (Wellehan et al., 2006). Certainly, local anaesthetics have been used at coeliotomy sites, and although inadequate for major surgery, they may be useful for decreasing general anaesthetic requirements (Hernandez-Divers et al., 2009). Recently, a local anaesthetic technique was used for surgical phallectomy of hybrid Galapagos tortoises (Rivera et al., 2011). The

authors used 2% lidocaine, 1 mL/25 kg or 0.8 mg/kg, injected intrathecally by insertion of a needle from the dorsal aspect of the tail into the intercoccygeal vertebral space located by digital palpation. Complete analgesia and relaxation of the cloaca and phallus developed in 4 ± 3 minutes. Mild hind limb paresis was noted in some animals but resolved within 2–3 hours.

Table 17.8 Analgesics, sedatives, and anaesthetics used in reptiles

Drug	Dose (mg/kg)	Comments
Morphine	1.5 IM,SC 10 IM, SC	Chelonia Lizards Not analgesic for snakes. May cause respiratory depression
Hydromorphone	0.5 IM, SC	Chelonia (causes less respiratory depression than morphine)
Butorphanol	20 IM	Corn snakes Not analgesic for bearded dragons or red-eared sliders. May cause respiratory depression
Meloxicam	0.2 IV, IM, SC	Pharmacokinetic data in iguanas
Ketamine	10–40 IM 40–60 IM Ketamine (10), combined with medetomidine (0.1) *or* dexmedetomidine (0.05), and morphine (1.5) IM (or 50% dose IV)	Sedation, prolonged hangover effects Deeper sedation but not sufficient for painful procedures and care in debilitated individuals Deep sedation/anaesthesia in many chelonia. More pronounced effects in aquatic species. Can be reversed using atipamezole (0.5 mg/kg IM) and naloxone (0.2 mg/kg IM)
Midazolam	2 IM or IV	Given with ketamine to increase sedative effects or promote similar effects at lower ketamine doses. Little effect by itself
Tiletamine/zolazepam	3–12 IM	Tortoises, lizards, snakes
Propofol	3–10 IV, IO	Low dose rate for larger reptiles Subanaesthetic doses produce variable short-term sedation
Alfaxalone	5–10 IV 10–20 IM	Low dose rate for larger reptiles Has the advantage of being effective IV or IM
Isoflurane	1–5%	Routine gaseous agent, subanaesthetic levels provide short-term sedation. Mask down or conscious (sedated) intubation possible in some species
Sevoflurane	2–7%	Very similar effects to isoflurane but recoveries appear to be faster Preferred agent for critical or giant reptiles

Injectable anaesthetic agents

Propofol, 3–10 mg/kg, IV or IO or alphaxolone, 5–10 mg/kg, IV provide a rapid, controlled mode of induction (Fig. 17.11; see Table 17.8). These agents are relatively non-toxic and there is minimal risk of thrombophlebitis if injected perivascularly, a particular concern since IV access may be relatively difficult especially in active animals undergoing elective procedures. Alfaxalone also has the added advantage of being effective when administered IM at 10–20 mg/kg.

If IV access is impractical or dangerous to attempt, IM agents can be used to induce sufficient chemical restraint for intubation. For IM injections in lizards and chelonia, the forelimb musculature is preferable, while for snakes, the epaxial muscles are used. Recently, an IM combination of ketamine, 10–20 mg/kg, medetomidine, 0.1–0.2 mg/kg, or dexmedetomidine, 0.05–0.1 mg/kg, and morphine, 1.0–1.5 mg/kg, has proven effective for a variety of chelonians, and anaesthesia can be readily reversed using atipamezole, 0.5–1.0 mg/kg, and naloxone, 0.2–0.4 mg/kg.

Inhalation anaesthetic agents

Isoflurane, desflurane, or sevoflurane are the agents of choice for maintenance of anaesthesia. These volatile agents have faster modes of action, are more controllable, and facilitate faster recoveries than most alternatives. Furthermore, their lack of reliance on hepatic metabolism or renal excretion further reduces the anaesthetic risk to debilitated reptiles or those with questionable renal or hepatic function. Some reptiles can be induced by inhalation agents in an induction chamber or by mask. A small lizard or snake can be placed into a Ziplock bag which is then flushed with 5% isoflurane or 8% sevoflurane (Fig. 17.12). Induction typically takes 10–20 minutes. Prolonged breath-holding is common with chelonians and crocodilians, and anaesthetic induction with inhalation agents is seldom, if ever, possible. Intubation of conscious patients has been suggested following local lidocaine spray, but cannot be recommended given the stress and risks of trauma to reptile and staff.

Intubation is relatively straightforward in snakes and lizards as the glottis is positioned craniad, but more

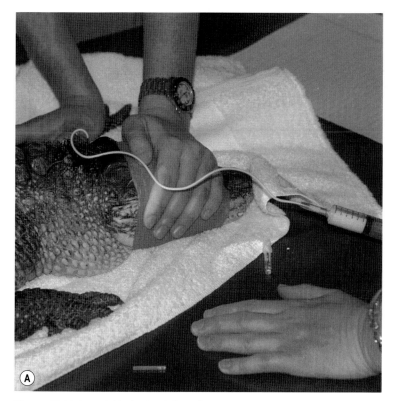

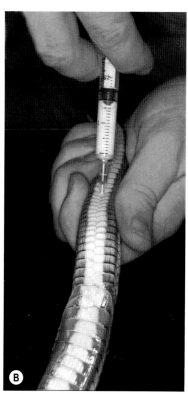

Figure 17.11 Propofol induction (A) via the supravertebral sinus in an American alligator; (B) via the caudal (ventral tail) vein in a colubrid snake.
Courtesy of Dr Stephen Divers, University of Georgia.

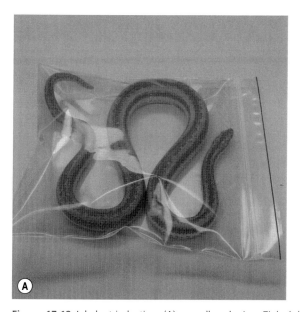

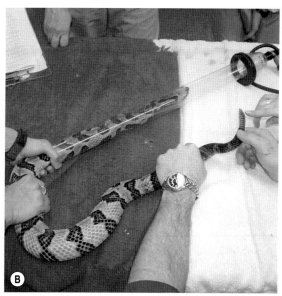

Figure 17.12 Inhalant induction: (A) a small snake in a Ziplock bag flushed with 8% sevoflurane; (B) a rattlesnake having been coerced and restrained within the plastic tube receiving 5% isoflurane from a non-rebreathing mask circuit.
Courtesy of Dr Stephen Divers, University of Georgia.

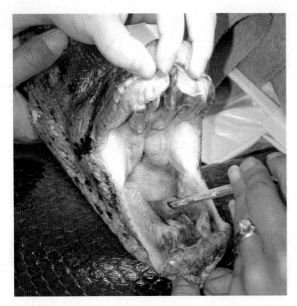

Figure 17.13 Intubation of a large snake. Even though this is a non-venomous constrictor, care is still required to avoid the needle-sharp teeth. The reptile glottis remains closed and only opens during active inspiration.
Courtesy of Dr Stephen Divers, University of Georgia.

difficult in chelonia and crocodylia (Figs 17.13, 17.14). Many chelonians, lizards and crocodilians have a powerful bite and a strong mouth gag is required for protection during intubation and throughout anaesthesia (Fig. 17.15). In addition, crocodilians possess a gular flap that must be deflected ventrad to expose the glottis. When dealing with venomous snakes, it is important to keep well clear of the fangs and use a head guard on the anaesthetized snake to prevent accidental envenomation. For most pet reptiles, small diameter endotracheal tubes or catheters are inserted through the glottis immediately caudal to the tongue, and this may be aided by forcing the tongue up and forward by pressing a finger into the intermandibular space from under the jaw. The reptilian glottis is actively dilated, and therefore its movement will often be abolished once anaesthetized. A guiding stylet can be useful in facilitating endotracheal tube placement. The bifurcation of the trachea may be sited far craniad in some chelonia, and gaseous exchange has also been reported within the tracheal lung of some snakes. Care should therefore be taken to use a short endotracheal tube that is securely taped into position.

Ventilation

Apart from crocodilians, reptiles lack a functional diaphragm, instead relying on skeletal intercostal muscles (lizards and snakes) or limb movements (chelonia). The action of these muscles is abolished at surgical anaesthetic planes, and intermittent positive pressure ventilation is essential for all reptiles that are anaesthetized for prolonged periods. Ventilation rates should initially mirror preanaesthesia evaluations, and then be adjusted to maintain end-tidal capnography readings of above 10 mmHg and, ideally, 15–25 mmHg. The use of electrical ventilators enables precise and consistent ventilation rates and pressures thus preventing some of the variables associated with manual ventilation and unstable anaesthetic depths. Large reptiles are prone to ventilation–perfusion mismatch if placed into lateral or dorsal position, and therefore it is wise to achieve a surgical plane of anaesthesia before positioning for surgery.

Monitoring

Monitoring anaesthesia in reptiles can be different compared to that of mammals. Palpebral and corneal reflexes are reliable in those species in which they can be elicited (snakes and some lizards have spectacles, fused transparent palpebrae). Corneal reflexes are abolished at excessive depth, while pupillary diameter may bear little relation to the depth of anaesthesia (unless fixed and dilated which indicates excessive anaesthetic depth or brain anoxia and death). Jaw tone (not recommended in venomous species) and withdrawal reflexes (tongue, limb or tail) are useful, becoming abolished only at a surgical plane. This also correlates with full loss of righting reflex, loss of spontaneous movement, and complete muscle relaxation. Cloacal tone is lost at excessively deep levels. Temperature should be monitored as metabolism of drugs is directly related to core temperature with decreased temperature commonly associated with protracted recoveries. Pulse oximetry, using either an oesophageal or cloacal reflectance probe is useful for monitoring pulse rate. In addition, although the SpO_2 readings are often low and have not been conclusively validated for reptiles, monitoring the trend in SpO_2 is often helpful. Doppler ultrasound is often more reliable for detection of a heart beat than pulse oximetry when the probe is placed and taped over the heart of lizards and snakes or positioned over the carotid artery or placed at the caudolateral aspect of the neck of chelonia and directed towards the heart. End-tidal capnography has proven useful to assess adequacy of ventilation (Fig. 17.16). Excessive ventilation and low $ETCO_2$ readings tend to correlate with a delayed return to spontaneous respiration and slower recoveries.

Arterial catheters are difficult to place in reptiles and require a surgical cut-down procedure to the carotid or femoral arteries. Average MAP in conscious green iguanas was 79 mmHg and decreased to 47 mmHg when anaesthetized with 1.5% isoflurane (Chinnadurai et al., 2010). A poor correlation between oscillometric and direct blood pressure measurements was obtained in a recent study

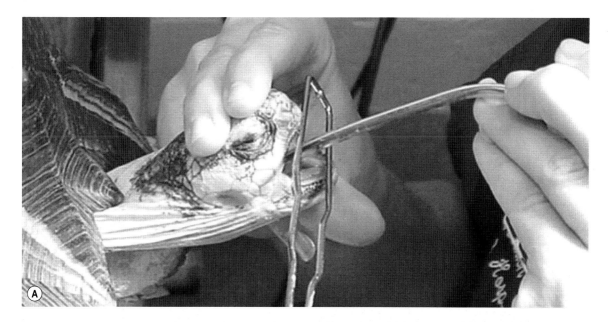

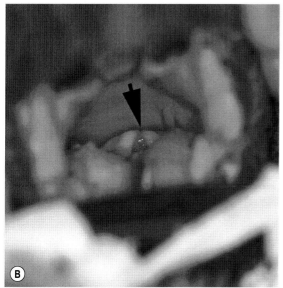
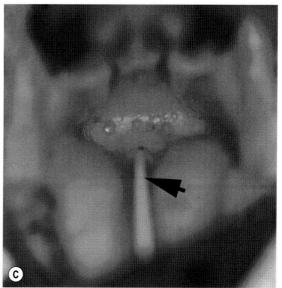

Figure 17.14 (A) Endotracheal intubation in red-foot tortoise induced with propofol. Note the use of the metal gag to protect the anaesthesiologist and endotracheal tube from being bitten. (B) View of the glottis (arrow) as it opens during inspiration and (C) following intubation (arrow indicates endotracheal tube).
Courtesy of Dr Stephen Divers, University of Georgia.

of green iguanas (Chinnadurai et al., 2010). The same researchers also discovered that only norepinephrine, 0.3–0.5 µg/kg/min, resulted in a significant increase in blood pressure when used in hypotensive iguanas (unpublished data). Blood gas measurements are often affected by intracardiac or pulmonary shunts, especially in aquatic species.

Recovery and postoperative care

Towards the end of surgery, the anaesthetic gas should be discontinued while maintaining ventilation for a further 5–10 minutes to facilitate inhalation agent excretion. At this point, oxygen should be discontinued in favour of decreased ventilation (once every 1–3 minutes) using room air delivered by an ambulance bag as this will help reduce PaO_2 and increase CO_2 levels which stimulate spontaneous respiration (Fig. 17.17A). Once breathing spontaneously, the reptile can be extubated, and returned to an incubator to recover fully. Continued monitoring remains essential until righting reflexes return and the animal is ambulatory. It is not unusual for a recovering reptile to revert back to unconsciousness and apnoea (Fig. 17.17B). Additional analgesia and fluid support should be provided as indicated.

BIRDS

There are over 10 000 species of birds that vary tremendously in their anatomical, physiological, and ecological adaptations. It would be impossible to cover all species and therefore this review has been purposefully restricted to those likely to be encountered in companion animal practice, namely the psittacines (parrots), passerines (song birds), raptors (birds of prey), waterfowl (ducks and geese), and backyard chicken. Readers are directed to the dedicated literature on avian medicine and anaesthesia for further details, as only a brief overview can be provided here (Forbes & Harcourt-Brown, 1996; Harcourt-Brown & Chitty, 2005; Harrison & Lightfoot 2006).

Birds possess a unique and highly efficient cardiorespiratory system that has evolved to cope with the high metabolic demands of flight. Several of these anatomical and physiological adaptations have a significant impact on anaesthesia. The glottis is positioned at the base of the tongue, while the trachea is long and wide and extends from the oral cavity to the syrinx. While the avian trachea shows dramatic taxonomic variation

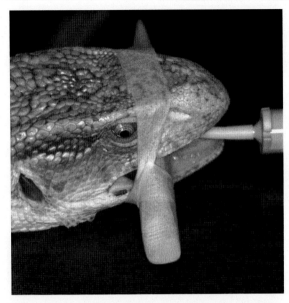

Figure 17.15 Monitor lizards have powerful bites and the use of a mouth gag helps protect the endotracheal tube.
Courtesy of Dr Stephen Divers, University of Georgia.

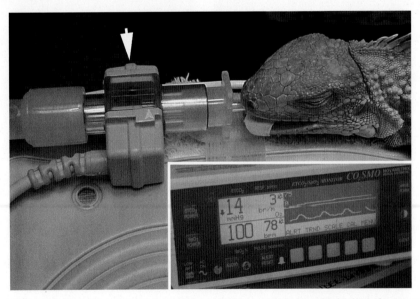

Figure 17.16 End-tidal capnography in a green iguana using a paediatric mainstream adapter (arrow) connected between endotracheal tube and the circuit. Insert: capnography readout indicates an $ETCO_2$ of 14 mmHg and a ventilation rate of 3 per minute. The pulse oximeter probe (not shown) is reading 100% saturation and a pulse of 78 per minute.
Courtesy of Dr Stephen Divers, University of Georgia.

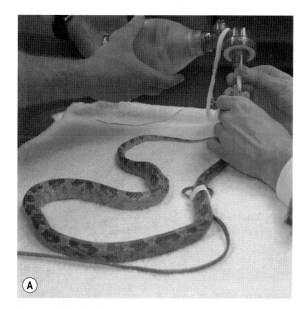
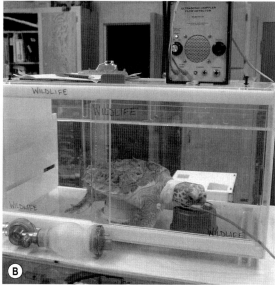

Figure 17.17 (A) Use of an ambulance bag to deliver air to a corn snake recovering from general anaesthesia; (B) recovering reptiles, like this sea turtle, should be closely monitored, even after extubation, and until ambulatory. *Courtesy of Dr Stephen Divers, University of Georgia.*

(e.g. complete septum and division in penguins, mallards and petrels; inflatable sac-like diverticulum in emus and ducks; complex tracheal loops within the keel of cranes), the most common concern is the considerable increase in dead space compared to mammals. The two primary bronchi are divided into extrapulmonary (from syrinx to lung parenchyma) and intrapulmonary (throughout length of lung to abdominal air sacs). Further bronchial division gives rise to the secondary bronchi, one group of which, the ventrobronchi, communicates with the cranial air sacs (cervical, interclavicular, and cranial thoracic). The dorsal and lateral secondary bronchi terminate in the caudal air sacs (abdominal and caudal thoracic air sacs). The dorsal and ventral bronchi are joined by narrow tubes, the parabronchi, which form the analogue to mammalian lungs and are where gaseous exchange takes place between the air and the blood. In birds, inspiration and expiration are active processes requiring muscular activity, and the air sacs act as bellows, delivering air in a unidirectional manner through the non-expansible lungs.

Air passing through the parabronchi moves in one direction only during both inspiration and expiration: blood flows across the direction of gas flow in a cross-current design. Thus, the gas composition must change from the inspiratory to expiratory ends of the parabronchi so that capillary blood must equilibrate with parabronchial gas at widely different PO_2 and $PaCO_2$. The arrangement is such that gas exchange takes place during both inspiration and expiration and its efficiency is dependent on an uninterrupted flow of air through the lungs. Tidal exchange is generated through the air sacs.

The respiratory volume per unit body mass of the avian respiratory system is two to four times that of the dog; however, the volume of gas in the lungs is only 10% of total volume (compared to 96% in mammals). Therefore, birds have a much smaller functional reserve capacity and even short periods of apnoea are serious and will produce marked hypoxia. The cross-current relationship between the respiratory and vascular structures enables improved efficiency regarding gas exchange, including anaesthetic gas exchange. Consequently, anaesthetic depth can change quickly, necessitating a focused and attentive anaesthetist at all times.

Preanaesthetic stabilization, sedation and analgesia

Many birds will hide clinical signs of disease until advanced and so seemingly healthy individuals may actually be seriously compromised. Anorectic, depressed or 'fluffed' birds carry a high anaesthetic risk (Fig. 17.18). Prior to anaesthesia, every bird should be physically restrained as described below (especially for assessment of body condition, and cardiorespiratory function), and accurately weighed. High-risk patients are often subjected to a cursory physical examination and weight determination, before being stabilized for 1–2 hours prior to a more detailed examination. Maintenance in a heated incubator at 28–30°C (82–88°F), SC fluid therapy, and oxygen

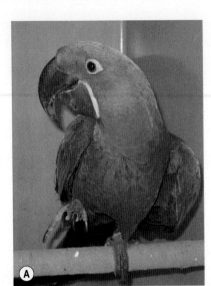
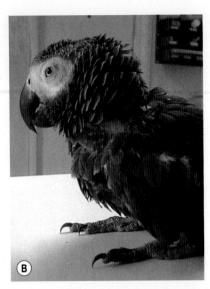

Figure 17.18 (A) A healthy bird, like this hyacinth macaw is bright, alert and responsive, especially when in strange surroundings and confronted by a veterinarian. (B) A sick bird, like this African grey parrot is fluffed-up, depressed, and lethargic, and should be considered a high anaesthetic risk.
Courtesy of Dr Stephen Divers, University of Georgia.

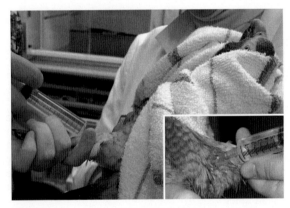

Figure 17.19 Subcutaneous fluid administration into the medial inguinal skin fold of a conscious parrot.
Courtesy of Dr Stephen Divers, University of Georgia.

provision are commonly used during triage (Fig. 17.19). Nutritional support is also critical for many birds, especially for smaller passerines that require a near-constant food supply.

Physical restraint should be kept to a minimum because small birds, such as budgerigars and canaries, are prone to become very distressed and large birds may struggle violently. Poultry should be grasped so that the wings are held back along the body to quieten them. Small passerines and psittacines should be cradled in the palm of the hand with the neck between the index and middle fingers, taking care not to apply pressure to the neck or the coelom

(Fig. 17.20A). For larger birds, it helps to use a towel to keep the wings under control (Fig. 17.20B). Raptors can be examined after being caste onto a table in either dorsal or ventral recumbency, and wrapped in a towel, while some hawks and falcons can be hooded. As birds do not have a functional diaphragm, any disease process, or space-occupying lesion anywhere within the coelom can have adverse effects on cardiorespiratory function.

Birds tend to have fast gastrointestinal transit times and preanaesthetic fasting times are generally reduced with the objective of emptying the crop (if present) and stomach (proventriculus and ventriculus) prior to induction. Small birds (e.g. budgerigars and cockatiels) are often fasted for 1–2 hours, medium-sized parrots (e.g. African greys, Amazons) for 2–3 hours, and large parrots (e.g. cockatoos and macaws) for 4–6 hours. These times can be extended or reduced following palpable evaluation of the crop. Large raptors that feed once daily can be fasted for 8–12 hours.

Avian analgesia has received little attention, but butorphanol appears to be more efficacious as an analgesic than buprenorphine in some parrots (Paul-Murphy et al., 1999; Sladky et al., 2006).

Regional anaesthesia and local block

While local anaesthesia can be useful to reduce the need for volatile agents, they are seldom sufficient by themselves as general restraint is required. Overdosage is likely in small species such as budgerigars but, in larger

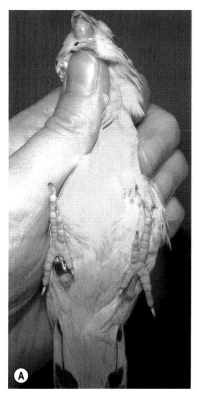 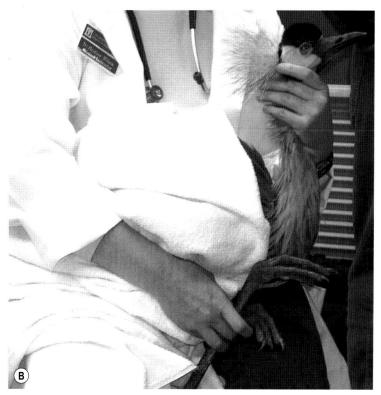

Figure 17.20 (A) Small birds like this budgerigar can be held using one hand to control the head, but care is required not to compress the coelom and compromise breathing. (B) Large birds like this African crowned crane require two-handed restraint and the use of a towel can help control the wings.
Courtesy of Dr Stephen Divers, University of Georgia.

birds, local analgesia can be used quite safely as long as the total dose is calculated and maintained under 4 mg/kg lidocaine.

Injectable anaesthetic agents

Intramuscular injection is made into the pectoral muscles on either side of the cariniform sternum or into the thigh muscles. Intravenous injections are made into the ulnar or basilic vein (e.g. parrots, raptors), right jugular vein (more difficult in pigeons), or medial metatarsal vein (e.g. waterfowl, chickens, large parrots). Although many injectable agents have been used in birds of all kinds, the proven effectiveness and improved safety of modern inhalation agents has largely relegated injectable agents to situations where gas is not practical, possible, or is cost prohibitive. Currently, most injectable anaesthetic agents are restricted to instructional or free-ranging field applications. It would be difficult for a practitioner to defend the use of an injectable agent for induction or maintenance in companion avian practice.

Ketamine has been used alone and in combination with medetomidine, midazolam, and butorphanol in pigeons,

chickens, guinea fowl, hawks, and ostriches (Gandini et al., 1986; Teare, 1987; Degernes et al., 1988; Langan et al., 2000; Lumeij & Deenik, 2003; Mohammad et al., 2007). The response to some of these drugs (especially α_2-agonists) is inconsistent but may be of value in specific situations (Table 17.9). The bird should be confined in a warm, darkened box as soon as the injection has been made and the depth of anaesthesia produced is assessed by noting response to withdrawal reflexes and, although the eyelids often close, the corneal reflex should persist throughout. Increments can be given to produce the desired degree of unconsciousness. Propofol has also been used in pigeons, as well as larger species including ostriches and waterfowl (Fitzgerald & Cooper, 1990; Langan et al., 2000); however, concerns exist regarding narrow safety margins.

Inhalation anaesthetic agents

Whenever possible, it is desirable following premedication, to induce and maintain anaesthesia with an inhalation agent, namely isoflurane or sevoflurane. Most birds may be restrained so that anaesthesia can be induced using

Table 17.9 Injectable analgesic, sedative, and anaesthetic agents used in birds

Drug	Dose (mg/kg) and route	Indications	Comments
Diazepam	0.2–2.0 IV	Most species, premedicant, sedative, anticonvulsant	May cause ataxia, remove perches. IM may cause muscle irritation Reversed with flumazenil
Midazolam	0.2–2.0 IM, IV, intranasal	Most species, premedicant, sedative	May cause regurgitation, and ataxia at higher doses
Ketamine Medetomidine	20–50 IM 0.1–0.35 IM	Most species, often inadequate for major surgery	High doses generally required for surgery. Reduced safety margin compared to inhalants
Ketamine Xylazine	20–50 IM 1–10 IM	Most species, often inadequate for major surgery	High doses generally required for surgery. Reduced safety margin compared to inhalants
Meloxicam	0.25–1.0 IM, PO	NSAID	Care if used repeatedly
Butorphanol	2–4 IM q 2–6 h	Analgesia	Proven efficacy in parrots
Buprenorphine	0.01–0.05 IM q 8–12 h	Analgesia	Ineffective in parrots

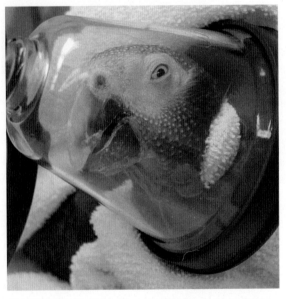

Figure 17.21 Mask induction using isoflurane in oxygen in an African grey parrot.
Courtesy of Dr Stephen Divers, University of Georgia.

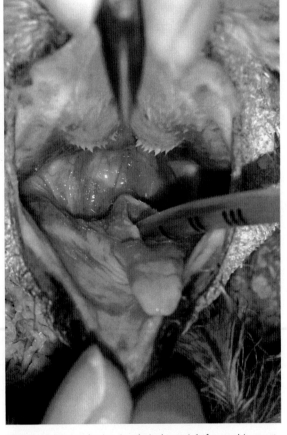

Figure 17.22 Intubation is relatively straightforward in most birds. The glottis of an owl after intubation.
Courtesy of Dr Stephen Divers, University of Georgia.

a facemask or they can be confined in a box made of transparent plastic material while anaesthetic gases are introduced into the box (Fig. 17.21). When working with trained raptors, the use of a hood can reduce stress and struggling during induction. Endotracheal intubation is not difficult in most birds but uncuffed tubes are preferred as the avian trachea is composed of complete rings (Fig. 17.22). Endotracheal tubes should be lubricated and placed gently to avoid trauma. Airway secretions may block the flow of gas in both intubated and non-intubated birds so it is always wise to have suction available for their removal by aspiration. Adequate suction can be provided from a 60 mL syringe fitted with a short length of fine catheter.

Most birds can be induced with 4–5% isoflurane or 6–8% sevoflurane, and maintained on 1.0–2.0% isoflurane or 2.0–4.0% sevoflurane in O_2 delivered by mask or endotracheal tube. While non-rebreathing circuits (e.g. T-piece system) are often adequate for larger birds, the air sacs should be flushed at about 1–5-minute intervals by occlusion of the open arm of the T-piece system, their over distension being prevented by escape of gas around the endotracheal tube or by partial lifting of the facemask away from the face. The author prefers to use a ventilator (Small Animal Ventilator, Vetronics) that can be used as a passive non-rebreather circuit or as an active ventilator, simply by pushing a button (Fig. 17.23). Total gas flow rates should be about two to three times the estimated minute volume of respiration of the bird (respiratory rate/ min × tidal volume 15–30 ml/kg). Inhalation anaesthetics may also be administered through a cannula inserted into the caudal thoracic air sac, but not the clavicular air sac (Jaensch et al., 2001). This is particularly useful when performing surgery in the oral cavity or the trachea, and when dealing with an upper respiratory obstruction. The air sac cannula can be placed through the lateral body wall (either in front of or behind the left pelvic limb),

behind the last rib, and just ventral to the flexor cruris medialis muscle.

Unlike injectable agents, modern inhalants provide reliable induction, consistent dose-dependent cardiorespiratory effects across a wide taxonomic range of birds, wide safety margin, and rapid recovery with minimal hangover effects. The greatest challenges when using gas appear to be maintaining ventilation and core body temperature. These can be largely overcome by the careful use of patient warming blankets (warm water blankets and forced air heaters), and mechanical ventilation (see Fig. 17.23).

Ventilation

Large birds placed on their backs may not ventilate adequately due to the weight of their keel and pectoral muscles. Even smaller birds may suffer from a gradual deterioration in ventilation. Consequently, all birds generally benefit from continuous or intermittent ventilation; however, accurate monitoring of both $ETCO_2$ and SpO_2 is required (see monitoring below) (see Fig. 17.23). The author prefers a pressure-cycled ventilator that can overcome a small leak associated with an uncuffed endotracheal tube. In general, $ETCO_2$ concentration should be maintained between 35 and 45 mmHg, and SpO_2 above 95%. Overventilation results in decreased $ETCO_2$, respiratory alkalosis and delayed return to spontaneous respiration necessitating a gradual weaning off the ventilator. When controlled ventilation is employed, in-line

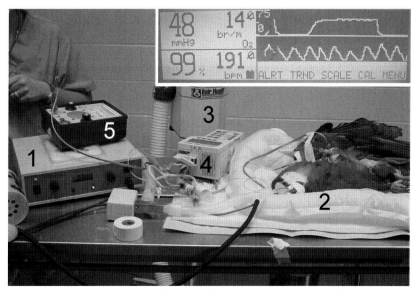

Figure 17.23 An anaesthetized macaw receiving isoflurane/O_2 from a dedicated ventilator (1) positioned on a warm air blanket (2) supplied by a forced air heater (3). Fluids are being delivered IV from a syringe driver (4) into the ulnar vein and a Doppler probe is being used to monitor the ulnar pulse (5). Inset shows measurements and waveforms for respiratory rate, $ETCO_2$, heart rate and SpO_2.
Courtesy of Dr Stephen Divers, University of Georgia.

humidifiers and warmers can be used to reduce the cooling effects of inhaled O_2.

Monitoring

Respiratory rate can be monitored visually or by using a respiratory monitor or capnography, or can be set by the ventilator. Pulse rates can most easily be monitored using a Doppler probe over the ulnar artery as it courses medially, close to the elbow. Thermometers with a remote probe are most useful with the probe inserted into the cloaca or oesophagus. Maintenance of core temperatures around 39.4–40.6°C (103–105°F) are ideal but can be difficult to maintain in small birds. $ETCO_2$ can be reliably measured using a mainstream capnography unit with a paediatric adaptor – side stream units often have too high a sampling volume to be accurate for small birds. Pulse oximetry can be unreliable but intermittent readings may be obtained from the tongue, oral commissure, cloaca, or oesophagus. SaO_2 and SpO_2 are not well correlated but observed trends may be useful (Schmitt et al., 1998).

Intraosseous (ulnar, tibiotarsus) or IV (jugular, ulnar/basilic, medial metatarsal) catheterization is recommended for the provision of crystalloid fluids at 10 mL/kg/h, or emergency medications (Fig. 17.24). Arterial catheterization for direct blood pressure and arterial blood gas measurements is certainly possible in birds over 400 g but can take practice to perfect (Touzot-Jourde et al., 2004) (Fig. 17.25).

Recovery and postoperative care

Recovery is often the most critical time when support measures are withdrawn. If adequately ventilated, hydrated and normothermic, healthy birds recover quickly from inhalant anaesthesia and can be perching within minutes. More compromised patients should be wrapped in a towel to maintain warmth, held upright, and directly observed. Following extubation, critical birds should be maintained on O_2 using a mask (without the rubber skirt), and once struggling, placed back into an oxygenated incubator (Fig. 17.26). Continued fluid therapy and analgesia are important for a quick return to normal behaviour and feeding. Assisted feeding (crop tubing) should be instituted within a few hours if the bird is anorectic.

FISH

Fish are usually anaesthetized by allowing them to swim in a solution of the anaesthetic agent that has been made up in some of the water in which they are normally maintained (*not* in tap water which is often heavily chlorinated) and the temperature and pH matched to their tank water.

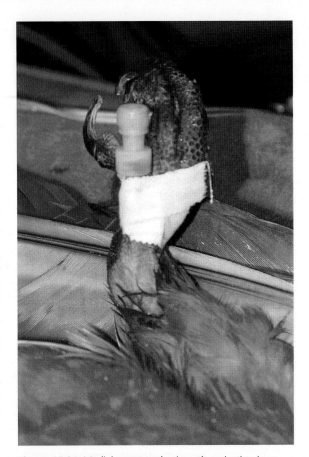

Figure 17.24 Medial metatarsal vein catheterization in a parrot.
Courtesy of Dr Stephen Divers, University of Georgia.

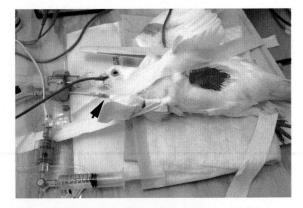

Figure 17.25 Arterial catheterization of the cranial tibial artery (arrow) for invasive blood pressure monitoring in a pigeon. A mainstream capnograph is attached to the endotracheal tube, a Doppler probe held over the radial artery by a clamp fashioned from two tongue depressors, and an oesophageal probe is inserted to measure temperature.
Courtesy of Dr Stephen Divers, University of Georgia.

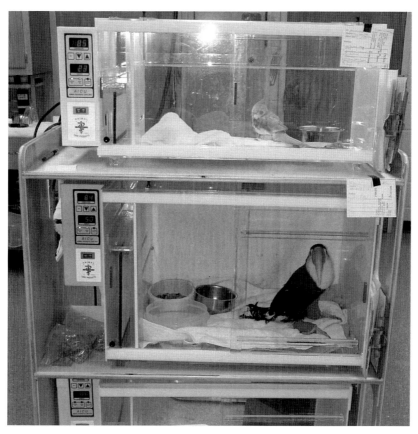

Figure 17.26 Heated incubators capable of temperature control and oxygen support are useful for critical birds, and those recovering from anaesthesia.
Courtesy of Dr Stephen Divers, University of Georgia.

Furthermore, additional clean, aerated tank water is required for recovery. Various drugs have been used for fish anaesthesia including carbon dioxide, ketamine, medetomidine, metomidate, alphaxalone/alphadolone, diethylether, propoxate hydrochloride, tiletamine–zolazepam, benzocaine, (iso)eugenol (clove oil) and tricaine methanesulphonate (MS222) (Neiffer, 2007). Of these, eugenol and tricaine methanesulphonate are probably the most common agents in use, although carcinogenic concerns have been raised.

Preanaesthetic stabilization, sedation and analgesia

It can be challenging to stabilize a fish prior to anaesthesia and generally anaesthesia is required for detailed examination. Nevertheless, visual evaluation can be useful, and regular observations by trained personnel are invaluable

at identifying potential problems before they become advanced. While subanaesthetic doses of MS222 and eugenol may be used to sedate fish, most situations require general anaesthesia. It is preferable to fast fish by one feeding cycle in order to reduce ammonia contamination in the anaesthetic solution.

Fish analgesia is still an area of contention because some argue that fish lack the cerebral centres required for cognitive assessment of pain and suffering. Nevertheless, there is increasing evidence to support the notion that fish should receive analgesics. In koi carp, butorphanol (0.4 mg/kg IM) has been has been shown to decrease the negative effects of anaesthesia and surgery (Harms et al., 2005), while the analgesic effects of morphine in goldfish can be blocked by opiate antagonists like naloxone (Ehrensing et al., 1982). Of the non-steroidal anti-inflammatory drugs, ketoprofen has been evaluated in koi carp but shown to be ineffective compared to controls (Harms et al., 2005).

Anaesthesia, monitoring and recovery

MS222, a widely licensed fish anaesthetic, is a white powder that dissolves in both fresh and seawater. It is highly acidic and must be buffered close to that of the original fish tank water using sodium bicarbonate. For general freshwater applications, two parts sodium bicarbonate to one part MS222 is often acceptable, while 1:1 is adequate in salt water due to the intrinsic buffering capacity of the marine environment. Induction results vary with species and temperature but 100–200 mg/L MS222 often induces stage 3 anaesthesia within 5 minutes (Fig. 17.27).

Isoeugenol is licensed for use in fish in some countries, but is frequently employed by the ornamental fish industry by using the non-pharmaceutical grade product known as clove oil. A recent study in koi carp has demonstrated a wide margin of safety with doses of 40–80 mg/L inducing stage 3 anaesthesia within 4–11 minutes (Gladden et al., 2010).

Following placement in the aerated induction solution, fish often exhibit a brief period of excitement, before losing their righting reflex, becoming inactive, and sinking to the bottom of the container (see Fig. 17.27B). Stage 3 anaesthesia is characterized by slowed opercular movements and an absence of withdrawal reflexes. Fish should be removed at this point to prevent excessively deep anaesthesia and medullary collapse. Fish can be kept out of water for 5 minutes which is often sufficient time for minor procedures. For longer procedures, fish are removed from the induction tank and placed on a water recirculating machine (Fig. 17.28). A water reservoir containing maintenance anaesthetic solution (generally 50% of induction dose) is positioned under a perforated surgery platform. The fish is positioned on foam or in a V-slot on the surgery platform, and receives water from a small submersible pump in the reservoir. The rubber tube is positioned inside the buccal cavity to facilitate water flow over both sets of gills. Water flows out of the opercula and drips back into the aquarium and for recirculation. Such anaesthesia machines have enabled fish to be anaesthetized for prolonged periods of time for lengthy procedures including major surgery.

Anaesthetic monitoring is limited but should minimally include visual appraisal of spontaneous movement and tail/mouth pinch withdrawal reflexes. Heart rate can be monitored using an ultrasonic Doppler flow detector, or a pulse oximeter placed across the commissure of the mouth (Fig. 17.29). For recovery, fish are placed in non-medicated tank water that is strongly aerated. Return of righting reflexes and swimming behaviours typically return in 5–15 minutes. Ram ventilators (i.e. fish that must be actively swimming to ventilate), like some sharks, require a constant stream of aerated water over the gills until they can actively swim.

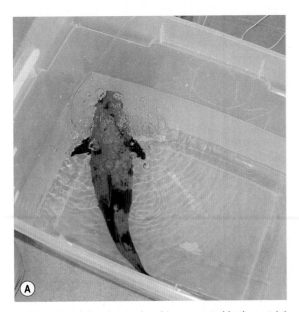
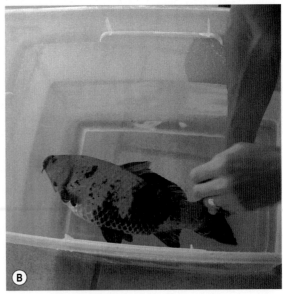

Figure 17.27 (A) Koi carp placed in an aerated bath containing the anaesthetic agent MS222 is initially in a normal position in the water column. (B) The same fish following induction of anaesthesia has rolled into lateral recumbency and is non-responsive to a tail pinch.
Courtesy of Dr Stephen Divers, University of Georgia.

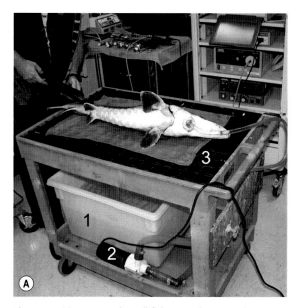
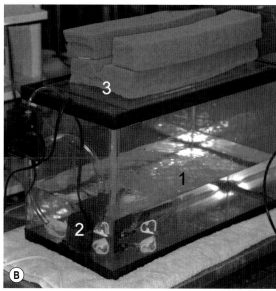

Figure 17.28 Large and small fish anaesthesia machines possess the same essential elements including a reservoir (1) containing maintenance anaesthetic solution, a pump (2) to deliver the water to the surgery platform (3), which is fenestrated to allow drainage back into the reservoir. Water temperature and pH must be matched to the original tank water. *Courtesy of Dr Stephen Divers, University of Georgia.*

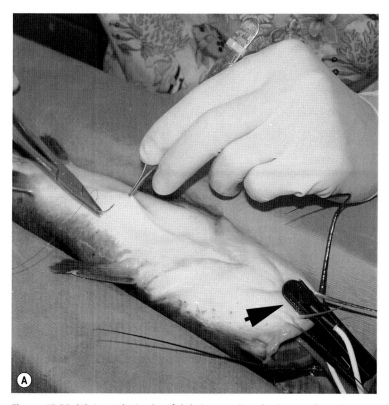
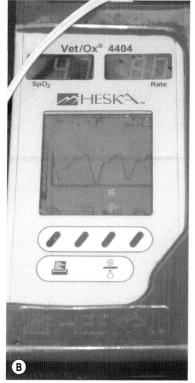

Figure 17.29 (A) Anaesthetized catfish being monitored using a pulse oximeter and tongue clip placed over the mandible. (B) Pulse oximetry display from the same fish indicates a pulse rate of 80 and SpO_2 of 47%. It is important to note that the heartbeat of fish is biphasic due to the extended contraction of the sinus arteriosus and sinus venosus. Consequently, many commercial monitors record the piscine heartbeat as two separate events and indicate a heart rate that is double the actual rate. In this case, the true heart rate is 40. In addition, the SpO_2 values recorded by machines calibrated for mammals are not accurate in fish. *Courtesy of Dr Stephen Divers, University of Georgia.*

REFERENCES

AVMA, 2007. US Pet Ownership & Demographics Sourcebook. American Veterinary Medical Association. Accessed online, http://www.avma.org/reference/marketstats/ownership.asp

Brown, L., 1993. Anesthesia and restraint. In: Stoskopf, M.K. (Ed.), Fish Medicine. W.B. Saunders, Philadelphia, pp. 79–90.

Carpenter, J.W., 2005. Exotic Animal Formulary, third ed. W.B. Saunders Co, St Louis.

Chinnadurai, S.K., DeVoe, R., Koenig, A., et al., 2010. Comparison of an implantable telemetry device and an oscillometric monitor for measurement of blood pressure in anaesthetized and unrestrained green iguanas (Iguana iguana). Vet Anaesth Analg 37, 434–439.

Degernes, L.A., Kreeger, T.J., Mandsager, R., et al., 1988. Ketamine-xylazine anesthesia in red-tailed hawks with antagonism by yohimbine. J Wildlife Dis 24, 322–326.

Drummond, J.C., 1985. MAC for halothane, enflurane, and isoflurane in the New Zealand white rabbit: and a test for the validity of MAC determinations. Anesthesiology 62, 336–338.

Edling, T.M., 2006. Updates in anesthesia and monitoring. In: Harrison, G.J., Lightfoot, T.L. (Eds.), Clinical Avian Medicine, vol. 2. Spix Publishing, Palm Beach, pp. 747–760.

Ehrensing, R.H., Michell, G.F., Kastin, A.J., 1982. Similar antagonism of morphine analgesia by MIF-1 and naloxone in Carassius auratus. Pharmacol Biochem Behav 17, 757–761.

Fitzgerald, G., Cooper, J.E., 1990. Preliminary studies on the use of propofol in the domestic pigeon (Columba livia). Res Vet Sci 49, 334–338.

Forbes, N.A., Harcourt-Brown, N.H., 1996. BSAVA Manual of Raptors, Pigeons and Waterfowl, second ed. British Small Animal Veterinary Association, Cheltenham.

Gandini, G.C., Keffen, R.H., Burroughs, R.E., et al., 1986. An anaesthetic combination of ketamine, xylazine and alphaxalone-alphadolone in ostriches (Struthio camelus). Vet Rec 118, 729–730.

Cladden, J.N., Brainard, B.M., Shelton, J.L., et al., 2010. Evaluation of isoeugenol for anesthesia of koi carp (Cyprinus carpio). Am J Vet Res 71, 859–866.

Harcourt-Brown, N.H., Chitty, J., 2005. BSAVA Manual of Psittacine Birds, second ed. British Small Animal Veterinary Association, Cheltenham.

Harms, C.A., Lewbart, G.A., Swanson, C.R., et al., 2005. Behavioral and clinical pathology changes in koi carp (Cyprinus carpio) subjected to anesthesia and surgery with and without intra-operative analgesics. Comp Med 55, 221–226.

Harrison, G.J., Lightfoot, T.L., 2006. Clinical Avian Medicine. Spix Publishing, Palm Beach.

Heard, D.J., 2004. Anesthesia, analgesia, and sedation of small mammals. In: Quesenberry, K.E., Carpenter, J.W. (Eds.), Ferrets, Rabbits, and Rodents: Clinical Medicine and Surgery, second ed. W.B. Saunders Co, Philadelphia, pp. 356–369.

Heard, D.J., 2007a. Lagomorphs (rabbits, hares and pikas). In: West, G., Heard, D., Caulkett, N. (Eds.), Zoo Animal & Wildlife Immobilization and Anesthesia. Blackwell Publishing, Ames, pp. 647–653.

Heard, D.J., 2007b. Rodents. In: West, G., Heard, D., Caulkett, N. (Eds.), Zoo Animal & Wildlife Immobilization and Anesthesia. Blackwell Publishing, Ames, pp. 655–663.

Hernandez-Divers, S.J., Stahl, S.J., Farrell, R., 2009. Endoscopic gender identification of hatchling Chinese box turtles (Cuora flavomarginata) under local and general anesthesia. J Am Vet Med Assoc 234, 800–804.

Jaensch, S.M., Cullen, L., Raidal, S.R., 2001. Comparison of endotracheal, caudal thoracic air sac, and clavicular air sac administration of isoflurane in sulphur-crested cockatoos (Cacatua galerita). J Avian Med Surg 15, 170–177.

Langan, J.N., Ramsay, E.C., Blackford, J.T., et al., 2000. Cardiopulmonary and sedative effects of intramuscular medetomidine-ketamine and intravenous propofol in ostriches (Struthio camelus). J Avian Med Surg 14, 2–7.

Lumeij, J.T., Deenik, J.W., 2003. Medetomidine-ketamine and diazepam-ketamine anesthesia in racing pigeons (Columba livia domestica) – A comparative study. J Avian Med Surg 17, 191–196.

Mohammad, F.K., Al-Zubaidy, M.H., Alias, A.S., 2007. Sedative and hypnotic effects of combined administration of metoclopramide and ketamine in chickens. Lab Anim (NY) 36, 35–39.

Neiffer, D.L., 2007. Boney fish (lungfish, sturgeon and teleosts). In: West, G., Heard, D., Caulkett, N. (Eds.), Zoo Animal & Wildlife Immobilization and Anesthesia. Blackwell Publishing, Ames, pp. 159–196.

Paul-Murphy, J.R., Brunson, D.B., Miletic, V., 1999. Analgesic effects of butorphanol and buprenorphine in conscious African grey parrots (Psittacus erithacus erithacus and Psittacus erithacus timneh). Am J Vet Res 60, 1218–1221.

Rivera, S., Divers, S.J., Knafo, S.E., et al., 2011. Sterilisation of hybrid Galapagos tortoises (Geochelone nigra) for island restoration. Part 2: male phallectomy under intrathecal anaesthesia. Vet Rec 168, 78–81.

Scheller, M.S., Saidman, L.J., Partridge, B.L., 1988. MAC of sevoflurane in humans and the New Zealand white rabbit. Can J Anaesth 35, 153–156.

Schmitt, P.M., Göbel, T., Trautvetter, E., 1998. Evaluation of pulse oximetry as a monitoring method in avian anesthesia. J Avian Med Surg 12, 91–99.

Schumacher, J., Yelen, T., 2006. Anesthesia and analgesia. In: Mader, D.R. (Ed.), Reptile Medicine and Surgery, second ed. Elsevier, St Louis, pp. 442–452.

Sladky, K.K., Kinney, M.E., Johnson, S.M., 2008. Analgesic efficacy of butorphanol and morphine in bearded dragons and corn snakes. J Am Vet Med Assoc 233, 267–273.

Sladky, K.K., Krugner-Higby, L., Meek-Walker, E., et al., 2006. Serum concentrations and analgesic effects of liposome-encapsulated and standard butorphanol tartrate in parrots. Am J Vet Res 67, 775–781.

Sladky, K.K., Miletic, V., Paul-Murphy, J., et al., 2007. Analgesic efficacy and respiratory effects of butorphanol and morphine in turtles. J Am Vet Med Assoc 230, 1356–1362.

Smith, W., 1993. Responses of laboratory animals to some injectable anaesthetics. Lab Anim 27, 30–39.

Teare, J.A., 1987. Antagonism of xylazine hydrochloride-ketamine

hydrochloride immobilization in guineafowl (Numida meleagris) by yohimbine hydrochloride. J Wildlife Dis 23, 301–305.

Touzot-Jourde, G., Hernandez-Divers, S.J., Trim, C.M., 2004. Cardiopulmonary effects of controlled versus spontaneous ventilation in pigeons anesthetized for coelioscopy. J Am Vet Med Assoc 227, 1424–1428.

Wellehan, J.F., Gunkel, C.I., Kledzik, D., et al., 2006. Use of a nerve locator to facilitate administration of

mandibular nerve blocks in crocodilians. J Zoo Wildlife Med 37, 405–408.

West, G., Heard, D., Caulkett, N., 2007. Zoo Animal & Wildlife Immobilization and Anesthesia. Blackwell Publishing, Ames.

Ypsilantis, P., Didilis, V.N., Politou, M., et al., 2005. A comparative study of invasive and oscillometric methods of arterial blood pressure measurement in the anesthetized rabbit. Res Vet Sci 78, 269–275.

Chapter | 18 |

Chemical immobilization of wild animals

Sonia M. Hernandez

INTRODUCTION AND GENERAL CONCEPTS

The nature of wild animals dictates that any manipulation that requires handling will necessitate chemical immobilization. Anaesthetizing wild animals is typically done to mark an animal, to apply a radio transmitter, administer individual animal treatment, or for the purpose of research. Anaesthesia of wildlife can be challenging and requires that veterinarians adjust the general principles of anaesthesia to the unique anatomy and physiology of wildlife species and challenging field conditions. Specific anatomical and physiological details are not always available, although the reader is directed to excellent resources for specifics (Fowler & Cubas, 2001; Fowler & Miller, 2003). In most cases, anaesthetic protocols have been adjusted from doses in domestic species and rarely are detailed pharmacokinetic studies available. Unlike working with small animal patients, veterinarians planning to anaesthetize wildlife are not often afforded the opportunity to physically examine patients, or acquire biological samples to assess their physical status prior to anaesthesia, and that sometimes translates to choosing anaesthetic cocktails with a wider safety margin while sacrificing other parameters such as recovery time. Additionally, capture and chemical immobilization of wildlife can pose some significant human safety considerations. Lastly, morbidity and mortality of patients undergoing field anaesthetic procedures is not uncommon. For example, high ambient temperature can lead to hyperthermia.

This review will focus on the general principles of wildlife anaesthesia, with an emphasis on free-ranging North American species; however, for more in-depth information, particularly species-specific details, the reader is directed to more detailed references (Kreeger & Arnemo, 2002; Carpenter, 2005; West et al., 2007). Other texts such as *Research and Management Techniques For Wildlife and Habitats* are also very helpful for capture, identification and handling of wildlife species (Brookhout, 1996). Veterinarians working with wildlife will benefit from collaboration with wildlife biologists and ecologists who can help design capture techniques that minimize stress and provide invaluable knowledge about the animal's behaviour. When anaesthetizing a species for the first time, it is very useful to contact zoo and wildlife veterinarians who routinely work with these species for their expertise. Important modification to protocols often take time to be published, yet experienced practitioners have a wealth of knowledge.

PRIOR TO CAPTURE AND ANAESTHESIA

As much as possible, veterinarians working in wildlife capture teams should become familiar with the anatomy, physiology and population dynamics of the species at hand. In some cases, humane and effective methods of physical capture of wildlife species have been described often negating, or at least facilitating, chemical immobilization (Schemnitz, 1999). The team responsible for the anaesthetic event should meet several times in advance to plan and organize the logistical, equipment and personnel needs for the procedures. It is important to assign each person a specific duty, so that at the time of the anaesthetic procedure everyone's responsibilities are clear. When working with dangerous animals, a specific person trained and equipped with firearms may be needed. In addition, a visit to the site of capture prior to the procedure is paramount to determine environmental factors, such as landscape characteristics that may pose a threat to the personnel or the animals. Field sites can be rocky, muddy, traversed by creeks that pose a drowning hazard, or cliffs. It may be possible to estimate the time of the day that the animal in question may have had the least amount of food, or remove available food resources. Finally, the team should discuss the realistic potential for morbidity and mortality and should agree on what may be considered an 'acceptable rate'. For example, when working with common and abundant species, it may be acceptable to expect a 10% loss, while when working with endangered species, even the loss of one individual might not be acceptable. These decisions may translate to utilizing more expensive anaesthetic protocols, or designing back-up plans that require more personnel and equipment.

Anaesthetic procedures should be planned at a time of year and time of day when they pose the least hazard to the species. For example, if working with bears, it is important to take into consideration the metabolic changes associated with hibernation and avoid anaesthesia during this period. Ungulates are best anaesthetized in the early spring or fall and during the coolest period of the day to avoid hyperthermia. On the other hand, in temperate zones, hypothermia during winter months is also a major concern. In addition, vehicles required for the anaesthetic procedure (e.g. helicopters, trucks) may not be efficient during rainy, ice or snowy conditions. Some landscape characteristics can pose real dangers. For example, steep, rocky terrain, or nearby water sources may require additional personnel to corral or herd animals away from danger and working in such conditions requires protocols that produce the shortest induction time. The social

hierarchy of some animals may be important if individuals are going to be separated from a group, or if, for example, a herd may become 'protective' or aggressive towards an animal showing drug effects, or towards the capture team. Predation can occur, particularly during induction and recovery, before or after the anaesthetic team can protect the animals.

Unfortunately, the body weight of the animal often needs to be estimated. This may prove difficult in larger species that cannot be examined up close prior to darting. However, there are several resources which publish the range of body weight expected for common species (Kreeger & Arnemo, 2002; Fowler & Miller, 2003). The gender, life stage and reproductive status are also important details. For example, xylazine is a common ingredient in anaesthetic cocktails utilized to immobilize free-ranging bison, yet it may cause abortion. All of this information should be carefully recorded. Record sheets should be designed ahead of time to collect important data that can facilitate future anaesthetic periods.

Premedication is rarely possible in wildlife species. However, it may be useful to contain animals in large enclosures and remotely administer neuroleptics, particularly to those species prone to anxiety or stress and particularly if transport is planned. Azaperone has been used to facilitate translocations and zuclopenthixol acetate provides up to 4 days of tranquilization in cervids (Read et al., 2000; Woodbury et al., 2001; Read and McCorkell, 2002).

CAPTURE TECHNIQUES AND REMOTE DRUG DELIVERY

Physical restraint, whenever possible, will facilitate administration of anaesthesia and reduce stress for the animal. This is particularly useful for small mesopredators (e.g. raccoons, coyotes, otters) in which leghold traps, cage traps or squeeze cages allow the anaesthetist to hand inject, or use a pole syringe (Figs 18.1, 18.2). Small rodents can also be trapped in cage traps, transferred to mesh bags and hand-injected (Fig. 18.3). Other animals may be baited to food sources, or attracted to areas with pheromones, allowing the anaesthetist to see and dart them more easily. If physical restraint is not possible, animals may need to be located and chased with the use of hunting dogs, helicopters or trucks (Fig. 18.4).

HUMAN SAFETY

Chemical immobilization of wildlife is inherently a dangerous job, particularly for those that lack experience

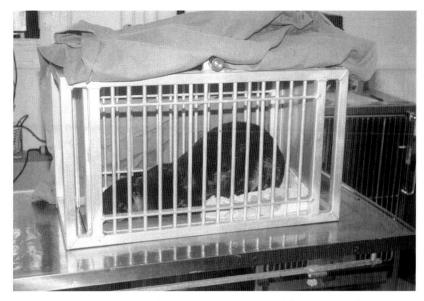

Figure 18.1 A river otter was transferred directly from its transport cage to a laboratory animal-type squeeze cage where it can easily be hand-injected.

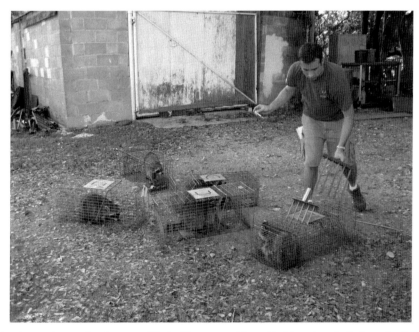

Figure 18.2 A Havahart style cage has been modified with a removable welded-bar piece that allows for the biologist to hand inject a raccoon.
Photo courtesy of M. J. Yabsley.

(Caulkett & Shury, 2007). It is wise for at least two people in the team to be trained in safety, first aid and CPR. It is also useful, particularly when working with anaesthetics in the field, that a relationship has been established with a nearby hospital or physician who is familiar with field chemical immobilization procedures. Human safety should be paramount in any chemical immobilization procedure and the team leader should not be afraid to cancel or postpone a procedure if human safety is at risk of being compromised. There are a variety of hazards that

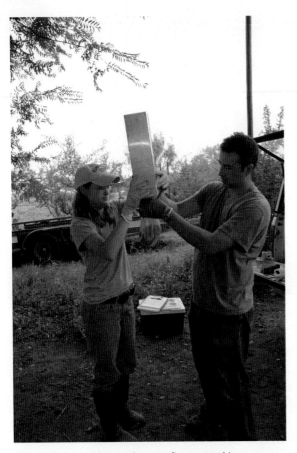

Figure 18.3 A pocket gopher was first trapped in a modified cage trap, then transferred to a zippered mesh bag for hand injection of anaesthetic agents.

can be encountered and easily overlooked. As mentioned before, the capture team should become intimately familiar with the terrain, weather conditions and equipment available at the field site well in advance to any procedure to identify potential hazards. Procedures can take longer than expected and the team should be prepared for a variety of situations, including incoming inclement weather.

The team should be composed of someone who is very familiar with the behaviour of the animal to be immobilized. Most animal species have some inherent defence system, particularly when chased, trapped or cornered. Hill et al. (1998) reported on the increase of animal-related injuries to veterinarians working with wildlife. If an animal is cornered, formulating an escape route for the capture team should be discussed in advance. Although the danger associated with some species like carnivores is obvious, ungulates can be just as lethal, especially aggressive males during rut. Even when anaesthetized, premature arousal or stimulation can cause an animal to bite or kick. Large ungulates should be hobbled and other forms of physical restraint, such as a dedicated person holding the head of a carnivore, are wise. Members of a herd can become curious or aggressive towards the capture team (Fig. 18.5).

Darts and dart delivery equipment should be treated like firearms. Anyone handling the equipment should be adequately trained. Shooting should not take place in areas where a person may inadvertently become the target. Drug exposure or other types of injury (e.g. inadvertent needle sticks, explosions) usually occur when darts are being loaded. Ideally, a dart should be loaded in a quiet place where the loader is not distracted by the activities of the capture, but where at least another person can

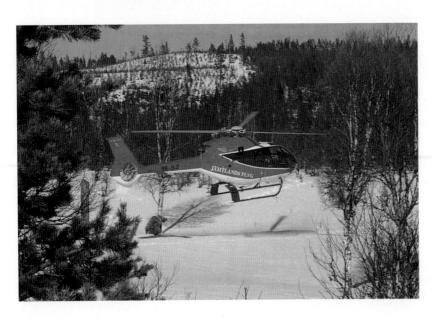

Figure 18.4 A brown bear is darted from a helicopter.
Photo courtesy of Åsa Fahlman.

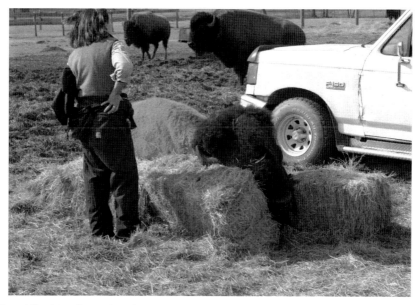

Figure 18.5 An immobilized North American bison in sternal recumbency is surrounded by trucks and personnel to protect the capture team from the rest of the curious herd.

watch the loader in the event of injury. The loader should wear minimum standard personal protective equipment, including gloves, long sleeve attire and a face shield. Damaged darts sometimes cannot be identified until they are pressurized and thus the same equipment should be donned when a dart is pressurized. Not uncommonly, in two-chambered gas darts, the needle is not secured properly and can shoot forward when the dart is initially pressurized. The author always uses a large empty syringe case slipped over the dart while it is being pressurized. When working with large dangerous species, a dedicated, trained security person with a backup firearm is essential. This person should be adequately trained and familiar with the firepower necessary to incapacitate the species at hand.

Most anaesthetics pose some safety hazard for people. The 'super narcotics' (etorphine and carfentanil) can cause rapid, severe and profound sedation, respiratory depression, hypotension and cardiac arrest. For perspective, carfentanil is 10 000 times as potent as morphine. Therefore, any exposure has to be taken seriously. Inadvertent intoxication can occur through small skin cuts, needle sticks or ocular and nasal exposure. Symptoms of exposure include nausea, dizziness, respiratory depression, miosis and quick progression to loss of consciousness, seizures or coma. Anyone working with anaesthetics, particularly in the field, should have a written emergency protocol clearly to identify and determine the steps that should be taken in the event of an exposure. This protocol should be discussed with all participating personnel.

Handling and treatment of accidental exposure to carfentanil or etorphine

Whenever carfentanil or etorphine are used, multiple vials of naloxone should be readily available and kept in date. The exposure kit should also contain: naloxone: 1 mg/mL, 10 mL multidose vials (total 10); five additional vials should be stored in the emergency box. Other items that are essential include: normal saline intravenous fluids, IV administration set, various gauge IV Butterfly catheters, various sized IV catheters and needles, various size syringes (including large sizes for fluid administration), various size gauge needles, tourniquet (used to help establish IV access), alcohol swabs, gauze pads, tape, disposable gloves, pocket mask with one way valve, non-rebreathing mask, SPU resuscitator (AMBU) with reservoir attachment and tubing, carfentanil/etorphine emergency protocol, and drug package inserts. Lastly, a portable oxygen tank should be available whenever potent narcotics are being used.

The protocol for treatment of human narcotic exposure includes:

1. Do not leave the patient unattended!
2. Call for help. One person should be designated to radio or call emergency services. This person should clearly state that someone has been exposed to a potent narcotic and immediate emergency assistance is needed. That person should also be responsible for providing emergency personnel exact directions to the site

3. Flush the exposed areas with copious amounts of water or saline. Avoid contamination of additional personnel while doing this
4. Bring the Human Narcotic Exposure Emergency Kit and oxygen to the patient
5. Draw up 30 mL of naloxone (3 bottles, 30 mg total) into a 35 mL syringe
6. Draw up 10 mL of naloxone (1 bottle, 10 mg) into a 12 mL syringe
7. Monitor the patient's pulse and respiration rate
8. Place the patient on his/her side to prevent aspiration and obstruction of airway by the tongue, elevate the legs, maintain body temperature and do not give anything by mouth
9. If the patient is awake and talking continue to monitor
10. If the patient is losing consciousness or becomes symptomatic proceed to establishing IV access. If the patient is unconscious, and IV access cannot be quickly established, proceed immediately to administering 10 mL naloxone IM into a large muscle mass. Continue to repeat naloxone doses (10–30 mL) until the patient wakes up and is able to talk. Multiple doses may be required. If IV access is still inaccessible, repeat the 10 mL naloxone IM until help arrives. Initiate respiratory and cardiac resuscitation as needed. If the patient is conscious but symptomatic, administer 8–10 L of oxygen using the non-rebreathing facemask. If the patient is unconscious, and in respiratory arrest, begin CPR. All treatments and actions should be clearly recorded. Ideally, one person will be dedicated to noting all actions and becomes responsible for transferring the information to the emergency personnel when they arrive. The capture team, along with a physician, should determine, in advance, how far they should proceed with treatment.

It is important to remember that many other anaesthetic agents aside from the potent narcotics pose serious hazards. For example, α_2-agonists can cause bradycardia, hypotension and respiratory depression, while ketamine and related compounds can cause confusion, tachycardia, hypertension and respiratory depression. Personal protective equipment should be used any time these drugs are handled during wildlife immobilization.

EQUIPMENT

Field equipment needed for anaesthetic procedures should be packed into well-organized and easy to carry tackleboxes or backpacks. Tackleboxes should be labelled or coloured for the different jobs, for example, 'physical exam', such that they are easily recognized. Field conditions are unpredictable and packing for several scenarios is wise. An emergency tacklebox should contain standard emergency drugs (e.g. epinephrine, lidocaine, atropine), additional anaesthetic and reversal drugs and items to support ventilation such as a laryngoscope, endotracheal tubes, and nasal insufflation lines. Oxygen cylinders of the appropriate size are paramount, although not always practical. Additionally, equipment to support blood pressure, such as IV catheters and fluids, is important. It is important to foresee and plan for equipment to deal with other emergency conditions, such as hyperthermia (water or alcohol) or blankets or tarps to combat hypothermia. Finally, traumatic injuries are common, and an emergency laceration surgical pack, or at minimum, antiseptics and suture packs should be available. Other field equipment I often find useful includes binoculars, multipurpose tools, duct tape, and thick permanent markers.

Remote delivery systems

Chemical immobilization of wildlife typically requires remote drug delivery. In the case of small animals that are trapped, inhalation agents can be delivered in makeshift anaesthetic chambers. Otherwise, delivery of injectable anaesthetics can be accomplished via hand-injection, pole syringes, blowguns or other power projection systems via darts. Darts can cause significant impact trauma. They should be delivered at the lowest velocity that still provides accuracy at the distance needed. Dart-associated problems include: (1) improper dart placement into body cavities, joints or other vital structures; (2) dart-impact trauma from high velocity; (3) drug-delivery trauma from darts that contain an internal explosive charge; (4) infection of dart wounds. Most dart-associated trauma results from inappropriately planned pre-capture periods, inappropriate use of equipment, or inexperienced personnel. Only personnel that have been trained on the use of power projection systems and have practised should be responsible for darting. Pole syringes are typically used on animals already under some form of physical restraint but are not efficient when the animal can easily move away, as pole syringes require some resistance for accurate delivery. These systems are basically modified syringes 'on a pole' measuring 3–4 m and allow some distance between an animal and the anaesthetist. The pole syringes typically require large gauge needles for fast delivery of drugs. Blowguns are hollow barrels through which a dart is propelled by the anaesthetist blowing in one, firm exhalation. The forced exhalation requires practice and blowguns are only useful in relatively short distances (up to 10 m) with lightweight darts (3 mL). Internal explosive darts typically cannot be delivered fast enough to discharge with a blowgun.

Power projection systems include pistols or rifles that use two systems to propel darts: (1) powder charges; or

(2) carbon dioxide or compressed air. There are basically three types of rifles and pistols: (1) blowgun-like projectors that utilize compressed gas or CO_2; (2) compressed gas rifles and pistols with permanent barrels; and (3) power load powered rifles. Blowgun-like projectors use either compressed air or carbon dioxide to propel darts. Their basic components are a source of compressed gas, some way to control the gas pressure through a pressure gauge and valve system, a trigger mechanism, and a detachable barrel. Rifles for long-distance work can be fitted with telescopic sights. A common compressed air projector is the Dan-Inject projector (Fig. 18.6). Both Palmer Cap-Chur and Pneu-Dart manufacture rifle and pistol systems that use compressed gas or air with a permanently mounted barrel. These types of projectors are not very accurate at long distances, lack accurate pressure gauges and valve systems but rather have two to three preset steps for selecting power levels. They are useful for moderate distances. Power load powered rifles look like typical rifles with permanently mounted barrels, and utilize .22 caliber blanks in several charge strengths with different amounts of powder. These rifles are only for long distance work and have the longest accuracy range. In all cases, training is paramount. As with any firearm, appropriate cleaning and maintenance is essential to ensure appropriate dart delivery.

Darts

There are several types of dart and the type dictates the method by which drug is delivered into the animal. The two types currently available commercially in the USA include: (1) two-chambered compressed gas darts; and (2) powder explosive powered darts. Two-chambered compressed gas darts are lightweight, typically made of plastic and reusable (Fig. 18.7). The anterior chamber contains the drug to be delivered and is separated from the posterior chamber by a movable, rubber syringe plunger. The anterior chamber is attached to a hollow needle that is sealed at the end and has a small side-hole. The posterior chamber is where the compressed gas is injected and contains a plunger valve that acts as a one-way valve, allowing air to be forcefully introduced to build up pressure. The posterior chamber ends in a syringe hub that is fitted with a tailpiece that acts like a rudder. The dart is charged by filling the anterior drug chamber,

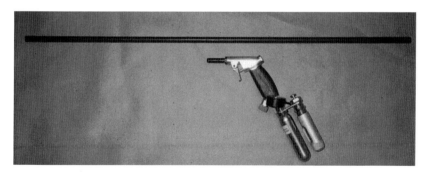

Figure 18.6 The Dan-Inject compressed gas pistol/rifle system is a very versatile system for short distance darting. The barrels (available in two sizes) are removable for ease of transport.

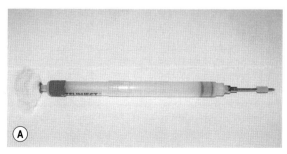

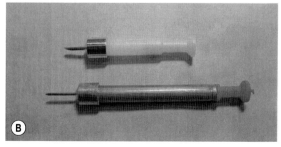

Figure 18.7 (A) An example of a two-chambered gas dart is the Tel-Inject dart. The needles for two-chambered gas darts are sealed on the end but have two holes that open on the shaft of the needle. These holes are covered by a silicone collar while the dart is pressurized. This collar will slide down when the dart enters the animal, allowing drugs to escape through the holes. (B) Two sizes of internally charged darts (Pneu-Dart).

placing the needle in front, securing a silicone collar over the needle hole (Fig. 18.7A) and then charging the posterior chamber with air (or liquid butane) with a syringe. As the dart hits the animal, the silicone collar is pushed down the needle, the pressurized gas in the posterior chamber forces the plunger forward, pushing the drug in the anterior chamber out through the needle hole. These darts can be gas sterilized and the needles autoclaved. Blowguns necessitate the use of blow darts, which are lighter versions of the two-chambered compressed gas dart. Powder explosive powered darts contain an explosive cap that, when discharged, forces the drug into the animal (Fig. 18.7B). They are composed of an anterior drug chamber, a plunger, a posterior chamber that holds the explosive cap, a weighted firing pin and a spring that keeps the firing pin away from the cap. When the dart hits the animal, the impact causes the metal firing capsule to shift forward, overcoming the force of the spring and allowing the firing pin to impact the cap, causing it to explode. The expanding gas forces the plunger forward, pushing the drug through the needle. These darts deliver drug at a speed that can cause tissue trauma. The success of delivery depends on the dart hitting the animal with enough force to trigger the explosion. There are both reusable (Palmer Cap-Chur) and disposable (Pneu-Darts) powered explosive darts. Disadvantages of these darts include explosive cap failure and cost. In addition, these darts are either aluminium or opaque plastic, which does not allow the anaesthetist to see if the plunger has moved forward indicating drug delivery. The advantage of the prefabricated darts (Pneu-Dart) is that they are simple and do not have to be handled for cleaning, which is important when human safety is a concern. Some general rules of thumb apply to darts and dart delivery. The size of the dart chosen should be as close as possible to the volume of the anaesthetic drug cocktail volume. If there is space leftover, the aerodynamic properties of the dart will be improved if the chamber is topped off with a sterile solution that is compatible with the anaesthetics used, for example, 0.9% NaCl. All dart components should be checked the day of the procedure. For example, the plunger should be forced to slide back and forth to be certain it is sliding smoothly, and the dart should be pressurized with sterile water or saline in the anterior chamber to observe for leakages or cracks. Finally, several back-up darts should be available, as dart failure is not uncommon.

Ideal dart sites are large muscle masses that will allow accurate intramuscular delivery. In most animals, the muscles of the upper hind legs are best; however, in some species, particularly those that have substantial subcutaneous fat over the hindquarters, the base of the neck or the triceps muscle are preferred. Needle lengths for darts are chosen based on the thickness of the skin and the depth of the muscle mass targeted. Darts are typically loaded with anaesthetic agents prior to locating an animal, but they should only be pressurized at the last minute to avoid leaking of pressure and accidental discharge.

Anaesthetic agents

The ideal anaesthetic drug protocol has a wide safety margin, low mortality rate, rapid and smooth onset of action after intramuscular administration, causes minimal excitement phase, allows the retention of some reflexes that allow monitoring, and produce relaxation that facilitates ease of handling of the animal. Additionally, ideal anaesthetics are water soluble, stable, have a long shelf life, are non-irritating, do not cause hypersensitivity, cause minimal cardiovascular or respiratory depression, are rapidly metabolized, are analgesic at subanaesthetic doses, and produce rapid and smooth recovery with minimal side effects. As most experienced anaesthetists know, there is no such drug! Therefore, all drug and drug combinations will require compromising some of the properties and the anaesthetist will have to determine which compromises are most appropriate.

INDUCTION OF ANAESTHESIA

Once the animal has been darted or injected, the capture team should remain quiet for several minutes, to allow the anaesthetics to take effect without further stimulating the animal. The induction time is dependent upon the properties of the drugs delivered, the level of anxiety or stress under which the animal was darted, the animal's physiological and physical status, its innate sensitivity to the drugs delivered, and the placement of the dart (e.g. if drug is inadvertently delivered subcutaneously, induction time will be longer and unpredictable). One should expect that animals can cover large distances walking or running prior to becoming ataxic. The capture team should have explored the terrain ahead of time and anticipated where an animal may travel, or potential dangers in the way. In some cases, vehicles can be used to herd animals away from dangerous areas. It is best to remain within visual distance, although monitoring could be done, for example, with binoculars to avoid stressing the animal further. Once the animal becomes recumbent, the anaesthetist should ensure there is no voluntary movement prior to approaching. When an α_2-agonist has been included in the anaesthetic protocol, head lifting or limb movement indicate that the level of anaesthesia is very light. Premature arousal at this time can be dangerous, particularly with large animals. One person should carefully approach the animal. Clapping can be used to determine if the animal is capable of responding (e.g. observe to see if the ears twitch). If there is no response, a long pole can be used to stimulate the animal from a safe distance. If the animal fails to respond, the airway should

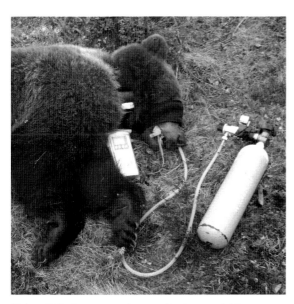

Figure 18.8 Oxygen supplementation is essential for free-ranging wild animal anaesthesia. A blindfold and gauze in the ears decrease external stimuli that might promote premature arousal, particularly when using protocols that contain α_2-agonists. A pulse oximeter clip on the tongue monitors oxygenation and heart rate.
Photo courtesy of Åsa Fahlman.

be checked. If the animal becomes recumbent in an awkward position, such as the head is facing downhill so that the abdominal viscera place excessive pressure on the thoracic cavity, its position should be adjusted. In all cases, ruminants should be propped in sternal recumbency to prevent pressure on the rumen and bloating and the head should be supported in an anatomic position. The head and neck should be extended to open the airway as much as possible. At this time, a blindfold should be placed over the eyes and cotton inserted in the ears to decrease visual and auditory stimuli (Fig. 18.8). Once a first set of vital signs measurements are obtained, the eyes should be lubricated. Additional physical restraint, such as tying the legs with ropes, may be considered if there is a concern over premature arousal. The dart should be recovered and safely discarded to avoid human exposure. The dart site should be identified and inspected for trauma that might require wound treatment. The fur of the animal at the dart site can be soaked with anaesthetic agent and thus exam gloves should be used to examine the site. If needed, the site can be flushed with copious amounts of water to rinse off the anaesthetic and prevent human exposure.

At least one person should be assigned to monitoring the animal, paying particular attention to ventilation, cardiac function, body temperature, and depth of anaesthesia. That person should be in charge of informing the teams if any problems arise that necessitate shortening the procedure. If the animal is determined to be stable, it can be manipulated to obtain a body weight, perform a physical exam, and obtain morphometric measurements or biological samples. The anaesthetist should be allowed access to the animal for monitoring at least every 5–10 minutes. Whenever possible, equipment that allows continuous monitoring, such as pulse oximetry, should be employed (see Fig. 18.8).

STRESS AND CAPTURE MYOPATHY

Animals undergoing capture and chemical immobilization are likely to be under some degree of stress. Anxiety, fear, excessive exercise, trauma, exposure to inclement weather, pain and anaesthetic drugs are all potential triggers of stress. As much as possible, capture and anaesthetic protocols should be designed to reduce stress. Stress prevention is largely aimed at avoiding prolonged pursuit or restraint and minimizing adverse effects of the environment and anaesthetics on the animal. Because pain can be a significant stress trigger, analgesics should be incorporated into the anaesthetic protocol whenever painful procedures such as tooth extractions, biopsies or surgery are to be performed.

It is important to understand how stress affects the physiology of animals to anticipate, monitor and treat such effects. Stress is a cumulative and adaptive response that allows an animal to interact with its environment through receptors. Stress responses are directed at coping with changes and include a change in behaviour, and significant physiological changes led by the autonomic nervous system and the neuroendocrine system. These changes result in an increase in muscle activity, body temperature, and overall oxygen demand. The autonomic nervous system provides the rapid response to stress commonly known as the fight-or-flight response, engaging the sympathetic nervous system and withdrawing the parasympathetic nervous system, thereby enacting cardiovascular, respiratory, gastrointestinal, renal, and endocrine changes. The hypothalamic–pituitary–adrenal axis (HPA), a major part of the neuroendocrine system involving the interactions of the hypothalamus, the pituitary gland, and the adrenal glands, is also activated by release of corticotropin-releasing hormone (CRH) and arginine–vasopressin (AVP). This causes release of adrenocorticotropic hormone (ACTH) from the pituitary into the circulation, resulting in secretion of cortisol and other glucocorticoids from the adrenal cortex. Catecholamine secretion by the adrenal medulla, controlled by the sympathetic nervous system, induces changes such as increased heart rate, blood pressure, and cardiac output. Blood flow is increased to the muscles and decreased to non-essential

Table 18.1 Capture myopathy can be classified into four categories that are helpful in determining the outcome of the case

Syndrome classification	Characteristics	Clinical signs	Pathology
Hyperacute or capture shock syndrome	Occurs within a short period after capture and immobilization	Depression, tachypnoea, tachycardia, hyperthermia, hypotension and death	Small areas of necrosis of skeletal muscle, brain, liver, heart and other organs
Ataxic myoglobinuric syndrome	Becomes evident hours to days after capture	Ataxia, torticollis, myoglobinuria. Animals with severe clinical signs are likely to die	Swollen and dark kidneys, bladder contains dark urine, appendicular skeletal muscle groups contain multifocal, pale, soft, dry areas. Renal lesions include dilation of tubules, tubular necrosis, myoglobin casts
Ruptured muscle syndrome	Manifests 24–48 h after capture	Dropped hindquarter, hyperflexion of hock due to uni- or bilateral rupture of the gastrocnemius	Subcutaneous haemorrhage, multifocal small–large, pale lesions of the limbs. Muscle necrosis can be diffuse
Delayed-peracute syndrome	Manifest after restraint for 24 h	Animals can look normal, but when disturbed may try to run and then suddenly die due to ventricular fibrillation	There are typically no lesions or few small, pale foci of the skeletal muscle

organs. Splenic contraction can acutely increase packed cell volume. Blood glucose levels increase due both to increased liver and muscle glycogenolysis, and conversion of lactic acid into glucose in the liver. Ventilation increases, bronchodilation occurs, mental activity and alertness become more acute. All of these physiological changes are appropriate to provide an animal the tools needed for an effective escape.

Capture myopathy

Capture myopathy (CM) is a generic name given to a syndrome clinically characterized by pain, muscular stiffness, incoordination, ataxia, oliguria, paresis, paralysis, metabolic acidosis, depression, and potentially death. The condition is associated with the stress of capture, exertion, trauma, handling, long periods of restraint, and transportation. This condition was originally described in free-ranging herbivores, but has since been reported in a variety of mammalian and avian species, including primates, pinnipeds, marsupials, canids, mustelids, tayassuids, ratites and anatids. Some factors appear to predispose animals to the development of CM. These include high environmental temperatures and relative humidity during capture, handling and transportation, deficiencies in vitamin E/selenium, fear, perception of danger, and a complex interaction between the sympathetic nervous system, the endocrine system and muscular activity. Some anaesthetics, such as opioids, that can promote excitement, muscle rigidity, hypoventilation, catecholamine release and hyperthermia may also contribute to CM.

Dehydration and underlying disease can also be important contributors.

The pathophysiology of CM is complex and has been thoroughly reviewed elsewhere (Spraker, 1993). Generally, CM is a result of altered blood flow to tissues, exhaustion of aerobic energy, decreased delivery of oxygen and nutrients, increased circulating lactic acid and inadequate removal of cellular waste from tissues. Increased levels of circulating myoglobin resulting from rupture of cells can lead to tubular necrosis of the kidneys and renal failure. Capture myopathy is a form of rhabdomyolysis that consists of breakdown of skeletal muscle and leakage of the intracellular contents into the blood. Depending on the predominating mechanism, CM has been classified into four temporal syndromes: hyperacute, acute, subacute and chronic; however, a descriptive classification system is preferred (Table 18.1). Although classifications of CM are artificial and the pathogenesis of CM is a continuum, they are useful for predicting the outcome.

Treatment of CM is difficult and logistically difficult in wild animals. In the early stages, treatments such as fluid administration, analgesics, muscle relaxants (e.g. methocarbamol), benzodiazepines (e.g. diazepam), dantrolene (used to treat malignant hyperthermia syndrome), vitamins (e.g. vitamins B, E), oxygen therapy, and sodium bicarbonate (to combat acidaemia) have all been recommended and achieve various degrees of efficacy. Because treatment is unreliable and not always effective, the focus should be on prevention. Restraint and handling should be minimized and transportation should be as short as possible. The anaesthetic protocol should be designed to produce a rapid induction and recovery and provide as much physiological stability as possible. Adverse effects, such as depressed ventilation, should be addressed quickly and oxygen supplementation is recommended in all cases.

MONITORING

Once induction of anaesthesia is successful, the animal should be carefully monitored. Excellent reviews have been written to address the peculiarities of monitoring non-domestic animals (Heard, 2007). Among all the excitement, the anaesthetist might have trouble remembering the simplest of details. A written protocol and data sheet are useful to implement an adequate monitoring plan and will become vital when reviewing the anaesthetic protocols in the future. Appropriate monitoring relies on detailed knowledge of the baseline vital values of the species at hand and those should be researched prior to any procedure. Vital signs should be recorded at least every 5–10 minutes. If manipulation is necessary, such as to place the animal on a scale, it should be done early in the procedure. There is ample evidence to suggest that hypoxaemia is very common during anaesthesia in free-ranging animals (Caulkett & Arnemo, 2007; Fahlman et al., 2010). Oxygenation should be monitored by a pulse oximeter, the observation of mucous membrane colour, or measurement of blood gases using portable blood gas analysers, and hypoxaemia prevented or treated with supplemental oxygen. Oxygen "E" tanks have wide applicability as they are relatively easy to get to the field and can provide 10 L/min for approximately 1 hour. Smaller tanks are also useful for shorter periods (see Fig. 18.8). Oxygen can be administered via nasal insufflation, by mask, or following endotracheal intubation.

Anaesthetic depth should be monitored carefully as the safety of the entire capture team depends on the animal remaining anaesthetized. The team should become familiar with the signs associated with premature arousal (ear or facial twitching, chewing, blinking, etc.) for the particular species and anaesthetic protocol in use. Supplemental doses of drugs, such as ketamine, should be calculated and drawn up in advance. If the procedure is likely to take more than 30 minutes, an IV catheter can be placed to administer supplemental drugs and fluids. Specific drug combinations, such as those that include α_2-agonists are notorious for being associated with premature arousal in certain species, particularly carnivores. Loud noises and physical manipulation are stimulatory and should be avoided or kept to a minimum when utilizing those protocols.

Heart rate and pulse quality should be carefully monitored. Peripheral pulses, such as the auricular or pedal, should be strong and regular. Portable equipment to

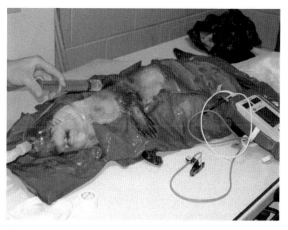

Figure 18.9 Otters can easily become hyperthermic during anaesthetic periods due to their extremely dense and insulating pelts. Ice packs are useful for cooling down such species.

measure blood pressure directly or indirectly has become commonplace.

Body temperature monitoring is essential. Small animals with a large surface to body ratio, young and old animals, and those with underlying diseases, are particularly susceptible to hypothermia. Tarpaulins, blankets and other insulation are needed for capture events during wintertime. Hypothermia should be treated using warm packs, friction, etc., otherwise recovery will be prolonged. Hyperthermia is common after chasing animals, during warm seasons or in animals with particularly dense coats. Hyperthermia can also induce increased respiratory rates and fast, weak or irregular heart beats. Hyperthermia can exacerbate hypoxaemia and is directly associated with increased mortality. The capture team should be ready to cool the animal with water, alcohol or ice packs (Fig. 18.9). If the body temperature of an animal continues to rise despite attempts to cool it, the immediate administration of reversal agents to antagonize the effects of anaesthesia is recommended.

RECOVERY

Recovery quality and duration will depend on the capture and field situation, the anaesthetic protocol, and the species of animal. Most modern anaesthetic protocols for wildlife include agents that have antagonists that will either completely or partially reverse the effects of the anaesthetic. Ketamine cannot be antagonized, consequently, when using ketamine in combination with an α_2-agonist, enough time should be allowed prior to reversal of the sedative to allow for ketamine redistribution, otherwise the animal will be ataxic upon reversal which can lead to injury. All equipment should be removed and carried away to a safe distance. In the case of dangerous animals, all but essential personnel should retreat. One person is assigned to remain with the animal until signs of recovery appear to be progressing as expected (Fig. 18.10). If possible, animals should be observed from a safe distance until they have fully recovered.

ANAESTHETIC AGENTS FOR SELECTED COMMON WILDLIFE SPECIES

Protocols for capturing and anaesthetizing common species wildlife species in North America are summarized on Table 18.2.

Table 18.2 Anaesthetic protocols for capturing wildlife

Species	Preferred IM anaesthetic combination	Comments	References
White-tailed deer (*Odocoileus virginianus*)	4.4 mg/kg of tiletamine–zolazepam with 2.2 mg/kg xylazine Antagonists: 0.125 mg/kg yohimbine Alternative protocol: 7.5 mg/kg ketamine with 1.5 mg/kg xylazine, antagonized as above	White-tailed deer are fairly easy to immobilize as long as they are calm. They can become hyperthermic if chased, and develop hypoxaemia and capture myopathy easily	Kreeger & Arnemo, 2002; Caulkett & Arnemo, 2007
American Black bear (*Ursus americanus*)	4–7 mg/kg tiletamine–zolazepam Antagonist: None Alternative protocols: (1) 4.4 mg/kg ketamine with 2 mg/kg xylazine, antagonized with 0.15 mg/kg yohimbine 2) 0.05 mg/kg medetomidine and 2 mg/kg tiletamine–zolazepam antagonized with atipamezole at 4 × the medetomidine dose	Physical capture in snares or culvert traps facilitates immobilizations. Tiletamine–zolazepam produces long inductions and recoveries. Premature arousal is possible with xylazine–ketamine combinations	Kreeger & Arnemo, 2002; Caulkett, 2007
Bobcat (*Lynx rufus*)	0.8–2 mg/kg ketamine with 0.0037–0.0057 mg/kg medetomidine and 0.15–0.2 mg/kg butorphanol and antagonized with atipamezole. Alternative protocols: 10 mg/kg tiletamine–zolazepam	Physical capture with leghold trap is preferred. Tiletamine–zolazepam can produce long recoveries	Kreeger & Arnemo, 2002; Gunkel & Lafortune, 2007
Coyote (*Canis latrans*)	10 mg/kg ketamine with 2 mg/kg xylazine Antagonist: 0.15 mg/kg yohimbine Alternative protocol: 10 mg/kg tiletamine–zolazepam	Physical capture with leghold trap is preferred	Kreeger & Arnemo, 2002
North American river otter (*Lontra canadensis*)	15 mg/kg ketamine with 0.5 mg/kg diazepam or 0.4 mg/kg midazolam Alternative protocol: 2.5 mg/kg ketamine with 0.025 mg/kg medetomidine antagonized with 0.1 mg/kg atipamezole	Physical capture with leghold trap is preferred. Hyperthermia is common in this species, particularly if muscle relaxation is not complete or premature arousal occurs	Hernandez-Divers et al., 2001; Kreeger & Arnemo, 2002
Raccoon (*Procyon lotor*)	20 mg/kg ketamine with 4 mg/kg xylazine Antagonist: 0.15 mg/kg yohimbine	Physical capture in Havahart-style traps is preferred	Kollias & Abou-Madi, 2007
Virginia Opossum (*Didelphis virginiana*)	10 mg/kg ketamine with 2 mg/kg xylazine Alternative protocol: 0.1 mg/kg medetomidine with 10 mg/kg ketamine	Opossums can be easily physically restrained by hand and respond well to inhalant anaesthesia in small induction chambers. Given the slow metabolic rate of marsupials, recoveries may be prolonged and careful body temperature monitoring is recommended	Holz, 2007

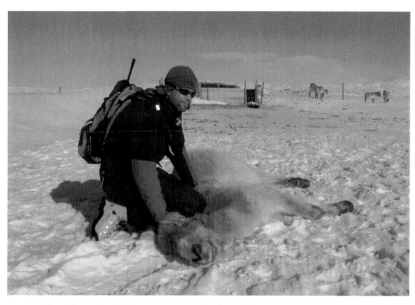

Figure 18.10 One person should remain with a recovering animal until the animal shows signs of progressing towards recovery normally and while it is still safe for personnel to remain close. In this case, the anaesthetist is preventing a Przewalski horse from raising its head until it is fully recovered.
Photo courtesy of Christian Walzer.

REFERENCES

Brookhout, T.A., 1996. Research and Management Techniques for Wildlife and Habitats, fifth ed. The Wildlife Society, Bethesda.

Carpenter, J.W., 2005. Exotic Animal Formulary. Elsevier Saunders, St Louis.

Caulkett, N., 2007. Bears. In: West, G., Heard, D., Caulkett, N. (Eds.), Zoo Animal and Wildlife Immobilization and Anesthesia. Blackwell Publishing, Ames, pp. 409–415.

Caulkett, N., Arnemo, J., 2007. Chemical immobilization of free-ranging terrestrial mammals. In: Tranquilli, W.J., Thurmon, J.C., Grimm, K.A. (Eds.), Lumb and Jones' Veterinary Anesthesia and Analgesia, fourth ed. Blackwell Publishing, Ames, pp. 807–831.

Caulkett, N., Shury, T., 2007. Human safety during wildlife capture. In: West, G., Heard, D., Caulkett, N. (Eds.), Zoo Animal and Wildlife Immobilization and Anesthesia. Blackwell Publishing, Ames, pp. 147–158.

Fahlman, Å., Pringle, J., Arnemo, J., et al., 2010. Treatment of hypoxemia during anesthesia of brown bears (Ursus arctos). J Zoo Wild Med 41, 160–163.

Fowler, M.E., Cubas, Z.S., 2001. Biology, Medicine and Surgery of South American Wild Animals. Iowa State University Press, Ames.

Fowler, M.E., Miller, R.E., 2003. Zoo and Wild Animal Medicine. W.B. Saunders Co, Philadelphia.

Gunkel, C., Lafortune, M., 2007. Felids. In: West, G., Heard, D., Caulkett, N. (Eds.), Zoo Animal and Wildlife Immobilization and Anesthesia. Blackwell Publishing, Ames, pp. 443–457.

Heard, D., 2007. Monitoring. In: West, G., Heard, D., Caulkett, N. (Eds.), Zoo Animal and Wildlife Immobilization and Anesthesia. Blackwell Publishing, Ames, pp. 83–91.

Hernandez-Divers, S.M., Kollias, G.V., Abou-Madi, N., et al., 2001. Surgical technique for intra-abdominal

radiotransmitter placement in North American river otters (Lontra canadensis). J Zoo Wildl Med 32, 202–205.

Hill, D.J., Langley, R.L., Morrow, W.M., 1998. Occupational injuries and illnesses reported by zoo veterinarians in the United States. J Zoo Wildl Med 29, 371–385.

Holz, P., 2007. Marsupials. In: West, G., Heard, D., Caulkett, N. (Eds.), Zoo Animal and Wildlife Immobilization and Anesthesia. Blackwell Publishing, Ames, pp. 341–346.

Kollias, G.V., Abou-Madi, N., 2007. Procyonids and Mustelids. In: West, G., Heard, D., Caulkett, N. (Eds.), Zoo Animal and Wildlife Immobilization and Anesthesia. Blackwell Publishing, Ames, pp. 417–427.

Kreeger, T.J., Arnemo, J.M., 2002. Handbook of Wildlife Chemical Immobilization. Sunquest, Laramie.

Read, M., Caulkett, N., McCallister, M., 2000. Evaluation of zuclopenthixol acetate to decrease handling stress in wapiti. J Wildl Dis 36, 450–459.

Read, M.R., McCorkell, R.B., 2002. Use of azaperone and zuclopenthixol acetate to facilitate translocation of white-tailed deer (Odocoileus virginianus). J Zoo Wildl Med 33, 163–165.

Schemnitz, S.D., 1999. Capturing and handling wild animals. In:

Brookhout, T.A. (Ed.), Research and Management Techniques For Wildlife and Habitats, fifth ed. The Wildlife Society, Bethesda, pp. 106–124.

Spraker, T.R., 1993. Stress and capture myopathy in Artiodactylid. In: Fowler, M.E. (Ed.), Zoo and Wildlife Animal Medicine Current Therapy 3. W.B. Saunders Company, Philadelphia, pp. 481–488.

West, G., Heard, D., Caulkett, N., 2007. Zoo Animal and Wildlife Immobilization and Anesthesia. Blackwell Publishing, Ames.

Woodbury, M.R., Caulkett, N.A., Baumann, D., et al., 2001. Comparison of analgesic techniques for antler removal in wapiti. Can Vet J 42, 929–935.

Section | 3 |

Special anaesthesia

Anaesthesia for obstetrics

INTRODUCTION

There is no one anaesthetic agent or technique that is ideal for all parturient animals. In veterinary practice, the choice of anaesthetic methods and drugs is often influenced by whether the fetus(es) are alive and wanted, unwanted, or dead due to obstetrical problems. In any case, the choice must be such as to ensure the safety of the mother and any living fetus(es), comfort of the mother during parturition or hysterotomy and convenience of the obstetrician/surgeon. To make a rational choice, the anaesthetist must be familiar with physiological alterations induced by pregnancy and labour, the pharmacology of the agents used, and significance of obstetric complications necessitating assisted delivery of the newborn. Most studies have been carried out in ewes, but physiological alterations are broadly comparable in other species of animal even if their magnitude differs. The following brief account of changes in physiology and in actions of drugs administered during pregnancy and parturition is a summary of many published papers and accounts in standard textbooks and should apply to all species of domestic animals. A referenced review of this topic has been published by Pascoe and Moon (2001).

THE STATE OF PREGNANCY

Physiological and anatomical alterations occur in many organ systems during pregnancy and delivery of the fetuses. Early in pregnancy changes are due, at least in part, to metabolic demands of the fetus(es), placenta and uterus, due largely to increasing levels of progesterone and oestrogen. Later changes starting around mid-pregnancy are anatomical in nature and are caused by mechanical pressure from the enlarging uterus.

Table 19.1 Physiological changes with pregnancy and impact on anaesthesia

Physiological changes	Significance for anaesthesia
Central nervous system	
Decreased requirement for anaesthetic agents	Risk of deep anaesthesia
Respiratory system	
Increased volume of ventilation Increased oxygen consumption and decreased functional residual capacity	Uptake of inhalation agents more rapid PaO_2 decreases more rapidly during decreased ventilation; onset of hypoxia more rapid during apnoea
Cardiovascular system	
Blood volume increases to accommodate uterus and fetus(es) Heart rate increases but blood pressure remains unchanged Cardiac output increases	Factors decreasing blood volume and cardiac output decrease blood pressure; maternal hypotension decreases uterine blood flow and causes fetal metabolic acidosis
Gastrointestinal tract	
Gastric emptying slowed	Retention of gastric contents increases risk for aspiration pneumonia in dogs and cats
Reproductive tract	
Enlarged uterus	Uterus compresses diaphragm and decreases ventilation during anaesthesia; uterus may compress caudal vena cava during dorsal recumbency and cause hypotension

Circulatory changes

Circulatory changes develop primarily to meet increased metabolic demands of the mother and fetus(es) (Table 19.1). Blood volume increases progressively, most of the added volume being accommodated in the increased capacity of vessels in the uterus, mammary glands, renal, striated muscle and cutaneous tissues so that there is no evidence of circulatory overload in healthy pregnant animals. Increase in plasma volume is relatively greater than that of red cells, resulting in haemodilution with decreased haemoglobin content and haematocrit. The purpose of this increase in blood volume is usually assumed to be twofold. First, it increases placental exchanges of respiratory gases, nutrients and waste metabolites. Secondly, it acts as a reserve if there is any abnormal maternal blood loss at parturition so that increased autotransfusion of blood can occur from the involuting uterus. Cardiac output increases in pregnancy to a similar degree as blood volume and there is an additional increase in cardiac output during all stages of labour. In 3rd stage labour it probably results from blood being expelled from the involuting uterus into the general circulation. Peripheral vascular resistance usually decreases during pregnancy so that mean arterial pressure (MAP) does not change. A serious decrease in venous return due to compression of the vena cava and aorta by the enlarged uterus and its contents can occur if the animal is restrained or positioned in dorsal recumbency. This decrease in venous return will, of course, cause a fall in cardiac output for the heart cannot pump more blood than is being returned to it. Cardiac work is increased during pregnancy so that at parturition cardiac reserve is reduced and pulmonary congestion and heart failure may occur in animals that had previously well compensated cardiac disease.

Respiratory system changes

During pregnancy, the sensitivity of the respiratory centre to carbon dioxide is increased, presumably due to changes in hormone levels, so that $PaCO_2$ and serum bicarbonate decrease, although arterial pH is maintained due to long-term renal compensation. Oxygen consumption is increased by the demands of the developing fetus(es), placenta, uterine muscle and mammary glands. During labour, ventilation may be further increased by apprehension or anxiety. Airway conductance is increased and total pulmonary resistance is decreased, apparently from hormone-induced relaxation of bronchial smooth muscle. Cranial displacement of the diaphragm results from increasing volume of the gravid uterus leading to a decrease in functional residual capacity (FRC), so that it is possible for airway closure to occur at end-expiration. Reduction in oxygen storage capacity from reduced FRC leads to an unusually rapid decline in PaO_2 during apnoea. Some compensation for the tendency of the FRC to decrease is achieved by increases in the transverse and craniocaudal diameters of the chest cavity and flaring of the ribs.

Other systems

Liver function is generally well maintained during pregnancy. Plasma protein concentration is decreased but total plasma protein is increased due to increase in blood volume.

Renal plasma flow (RPF) and glomerular filtration rate (GFR) increase progressively, paralleling the increases in blood volume and cardiac output. Due to increases in renal clearances blood urea and creatinine levels are lower than in non-pregnant animals.

Uterine blood flow is directly proportional to perfusion pressure and inversely proportional to uterine vascular resistance, so that it can be compromised from vasoconstriction due to catecholamine release from fright or anxiety.

PHARMACOLOGY OF DRUGS ADMINISTERED DURING PREGNANCY

The effects of pregnancy on drug disposition, biotransformation and excretion are largely unknown in domestic animals. The minimum alveolar concentration (MAC) of inhalation agents is decreased due to inconclusive mechanisms. The increase in RPF and GFR favours renal excretion of drugs. Any drug administered to the mother is liable to cross the placenta to the fetus(es) and induce effects similar to those observed in the mother.

Placental transfer of drugs is governed by the physiochemical properties of the drug and anatomical features of the placenta. Transfer of drugs can occur by simple diffusion, facilitated diffusion via transport systems, active transport and pinocytosis. Of these, simple diffusion is by far the most important and this will be affected by the surface area and thickness of the placenta. The larger farm animals have thick epitheliochorial placentae with relatively small areas for diffusion due to their cotyledonary or patchy diffuse distribution, whereas dogs and cats have thinner endotheliochorial placentae with larger zonular areas of implantation. Thus, the placental diffusion barrier is greatest in ruminants, pigs and horses and least in dogs and cats. However, the diffusion barrier does not appear to be of great clinical significance in the transfer of drugs from mother to fetus(es) in any species of animal.

More important is the diffusion constant which is unique to each drug and determined by molecular weight, degree of protein binding in maternal blood, lipid solubility and degree of ionization in the plasma. Most drugs

used in anaesthesia have large diffusion constants – low molecular weights, high lipid solubility and poor ionization – and diffuse rapidly across the placenta. The exceptions are the neuromuscular blocking drugs, which are highly ionized and of low lipid solubility.

Maternal blood concentrations of drug depend on total dose administered, site or route of administration, rate of distribution and uptake of it by maternal tissues and maternal detoxification and excretion. Thus drugs with rapidly declining plasma concentration after administration of a fixed dose (e.g. thiopental) result in a short exposure of the placenta, and hence fetus(es), to high maternal concentrations. Drugs administered continuously (e.g. inhalation anaesthetics, infused agents during TIVA) are associated with a continuous placental transfer to the fetus(es).

The concentration of drug in the umbilical vein of a fetus is not that to which the fetal target organs such as the heart and brain are exposed, for most of the umbilical blood passes initially through the liver, where the drug may be metabolized or sequestered. The remainder of the umbilical blood passes through the ductus venosus to the vena cava where it is diluted by drug-free blood from the hind end of the fetus. Thus, the fetal circulation protects vital tissues and organs from exposure to sudden high drug concentrations.

Clinical significance of changes during pregnancy and parturition

Circulatory changes of pregnancy and parturition can put a mother suffering from even normally well compensated heart disease at risk unless care is taken to ensure a minimum cardiac depression from anaesthetic drugs. Ecbolics used early on in labour can have an adverse effect on cardiovascular function. Oxytocin will induce vasodilation and hypotension that will have an adverse effect on both mother and fetus(es) due to decreased tissue and placental perfusion. Venous engorgement of the epidural space decreases the volume of solutions needed to produce block to any given level.

Reduction in FRC means that any respiratory depression caused by drugs is more significant in pregnant than in non-pregnant animals and hypoventilation will lead to hypercapnia and hypoxaemia; the hypoxaemia is particularly undesirable during labour when oxygen consumption is increased. In small animals, induction of anaesthesia with inhalational agents will be more rapid than in non-pregnant animals due to the decrease in FRC and increased alveolar ventilation as well as the decrease in MAC, but in recumbent large animals shunting of pulmonary blood may make the maintenance of inhalation anaesthesia more difficult.

In monogastric animals, there is an increased risk of both vomiting and silent aspiration of gastric contents in parturient animals for the time of last feeding is frequently unknown, and intragastric pressure is increased in the stomach displaced by the gravid uterus. Risk of regurgitation of ruminal contents when general anaesthesia is induced seems to be great in cattle, but perhaps not in sheep and goats which normally have less fluid rumen contents.

Drug actions

Opioids

Opioids rapidly cross the placenta from mother to fetus(es) and can cause marked respiratory and central nervous depression in neonate(s) with sleepiness and reluctance to feed. Some clinicians use a short-acting opioid for premedication in small animals, others wait until the puppies or kittens are delivered before administering an opioid to the dam. An opioid antagonist such as naloxone can be given to the neonate(s). Because the action of naloxone is shorter than that of some opioids, depression may return when naloxone is metabolized and careful observation is indicated to allow this to be detected and treated by the injection of more naloxone.

α_2-Agonists; ketamine

All α_2-adrenoceptor agonists rapidly cross the placenta and can cause respiratory and cardiovascular depression in both mother and babies, although the magnitude differs between species and can be counteracted by antagonists. Unless used in small dosage, xylazine causes significant newborn depression when administered to cows and small ruminants. Xylazine–ketamine combinations are not recommended for caesarean section (CS) in dogs due to excessive newborn depression. Xylazine–ketamine appears to be a satisfactory combination for induction of anaesthesia in mares and sows with satisfactory activity in foals and piglets after vaginal delivery or CS. Information about the fetal depressant effects of medetomidine or dexmedetomidine in small animals is confusing. Some clinicians avoid using this agent while others have used it to their satisfaction as premedication in dogs prior to mask induction with an inhalant. Atipamezole is the reversal agent for medetomidine and, if injected into the newborn, may be sufficiently absorbed to reverse the sedative effects caused by placental transmission.

Intravenous anaesthetics; neuromuscular blockers

Low doses of thiopental, methohexital, propofol and alfaxalone produce varying degrees of respiratory and central nervous depression in neonates. Thiopental has been used in low dose for induction of anaesthesia prior to maintenance with an inhalation agent for CS in humans and other species of animals. Newborns exhibit a degree of depression after maternal administration of thiopental and clinical studies have shown that newborns are more vigorous when IV agents other than thiopental are used for induction of anaesthesia (Copland, 1977; Elovsson et al., 1996; Luna et al., 2004). A study comparing thiopental and alphaxalone/alphadalone for induction of anaesthesia prior to maintenance with halothane for CS in ewes confirmed that a low dose of the steroid anaesthetic was associated with less neonatal depression than thiopental (Copland, 1977). Measurements of cardiovascular parameters in late-term pregnant ewes were used to compare anaesthesia induced and maintained with isoflurane 1.3% with anaesthesia induced with propofol, 2.5 mg/kg, IV followed by an infusion of 0.3 mg/kg/min, tracheal intubation and ventilation with oxygen (Gaynor et al., 1998). Maternal mean heart rate (HR), MAP, and cardiac output were higher during propofol than isoflurane anaesthesia (depths of anaesthesia may not have been equivalent) but uterine arterial and umbilical venous flows were not different between the agents. In a study using higher dose rates, anaesthesia induced with propofol, 6 mg/kg, IV and maintained with an infusion of 0.4 mg/kg/min in pregnant ewes induced significant maternal and fetal respiratory acidosis and a significant decrease in maternal MAP at 5–15 minutes (Andaluz et al., 2005). The pharmacokinetic parameters of an injection of propofol, 6 mg/kg, IV with or without a continuous infusion have been determined in instrumented pregnant ewes (Andaluz et al., 2003). Although propofol rapidly crossed the placenta, fetal blood concentrations were low compared with maternal concentrations. In dogs, administration of one small supplemental bolus of propofol before puppy removal has been advocated as causing minimal fetal depression but maintenance of anaesthesia with an infusion of propofol has yet to be evaluated regarding the degree of puppy depression. Neuromuscular blocking agents may cross the placenta in small amounts but are seldom needed in obstetrical anaesthesia.

Inhalation anaesthetics

Inhalation anaesthetics readily cross the placental barrier with rapid equilibration between the mother and fetus(es). The degree of depression they cause in the neonate is directly proportional to the depth of anaesthesia induced in the mother. While light (1 MAC) anaesthesia with isoflurane induced no significant effect on uterine blood flow or fetal metabolic status, it has been found that deep (2 MAC) anaesthesia induces significant decreases in uterine blood flow and fetal metabolic acidosis within 15 minutes of start of administration (Palahniuk & Shnider, 1974a). At 2 MAC isoflurane or sevoflurane, maternal and fetal MAP and fetal HR were significantly decreased from awake and 1 MAC values (Okutomi et al., 2009). Values were not different between isoflurane and sevoflurane. There is a reduction in requirement for anaesthetic drugs and a decrease in MAC of inhalation agents at term pregnancy. When measured in ewes, MAC is 21–40% lower in gravid as compared with non-pregnant animals (Palahniuk et al., 1974; Okutomi et al., 2009). Use of the less soluble agents isoflurane, sevoflurane and desflurane will lead to more rapid recovery of the newly delivered animals than when more soluble agents such as halothane are employed. Nitrous oxide will often enable concentration of more potent soluble anaesthetic agent to be reduced and its use does not add to depression of the newborn, however, oxygen must be administered for a few minutes after delivery to prevent diffusion hypoxia.

Fetal haemoglobin can carry more O_2 for a given PO_2 due to the low concentration of 2,3-diphosphoglycerate (2,3-DPG) in fetal red cells. This ensures a higher level of haemoglobin saturation at the normally low PO_2 of umbilical venous blood. Administration of O_2 to the mother results in a significant increase in fetal oxygenation and maternal inspired O_2 concentrations of over 50% during general anaesthesia are associated with delivery of more vigorous newborn.

Local analgesics

Local analgesics are not as harmless as sometimes supposed. Amide derivatives (e.g. lidocaine, mepivacaine, bupivacaine) are broken down by hepatic microsomal enzymes. After absorption from the site of injection, significant concentrations may be reached in the fetus(es) causing depression in the neonate. Sufficiently high concentrations seldom occur after epidural or paravertebral administration, but may occur after local infiltration of large volumes of local analgesic solutions. Epidural block may produce hypotension and this may be treated by infusing fluid to fill the dilated vascular bed, or better, by injection of ephedrine. Ephedrine increases venous tone and thus cardiac preload; it has minimal vasoconstrictor effect on the arterial system. In the past few years, there have been a number of published investigations comparing ephedrine and phenylephrine for the treatment of epidural-induced hypotension in humans during CS. These indicate that blood pressure support is better during infusion of phenylephrine and that ephedrine administration results in more fetal acidosis. In contrast, administration of ephedrine to pregnant sheep with epidural-induced hypotension increased maternal arterial pressure and uterine blood flow with no change in fetal acid-base status (Strümper et al., 2005).

Anticholinergics

Because glycopyrrolate does not readily cross the placental barrier, it is probably the anticholinergic of choice if anticholinergics are to be used to minimize the effects of traction on the uterus and broad ligaments by the surgeon. In contrast, atropine crosses the placenta and elevates fetal heart rate.

ANAESTHESIA FOR DYSTOCIA AND CAESAREAN SECTION

Horses

The ideal anaesthesia for vaginal delivery of a live foal from a healthy mare with dystocia is sedation and epidural (see Chapter 11 for suitable combinations and doses). Where short duration general anaesthesia becomes necessary, for example for vaginal delivery in a mare with a ruptured prepubic tendon, administration of xylazine, 1.1 mg, followed by ketamine, 2.2 mg/kg, IV with the dose rates calculated on the mare's estimated non-pregnant weight induce recumbency without depression of the foal. Total intravenous anaesthesia (TIVA) or inhalation anaesthesia will be required when extensive manipulation and repositioning of a dead foal is anticipated. Different approaches to delivery of the foal may alter the choice of anaesthetic agents. When the mare is to be hoisted by the hind limbs so that the mare's head, neck and shoulders are on the ground and the hindquarters are elevated into the air, a combination of xylazine or romifidine, guaifenesin, and ketamine with oxygen supplied to the mare has been used without maternal mortality. The protocol involves premedication of the mare with decreased doses of xylazine or romifidine with butorphanol, 0.02 mg/kg, followed by induction of anaesthesia with ketamine or diazepam–ketamine. Maintenance of anaesthesia is 'to effect' with guaifenesin–ketamine–xylazine (GKX) drip (e.g. 1 L 5% guaifenesin to which has been added 1300 mg ketamine and 650 mg xylazine that is administered IV at a rate that is less than the usual 2 mL/kg/h). Endotracheal intubation facilitates an increase in the inspired oxygen % by insufflation into the tube with oxygen, 15 L/min for a full-sized horse or, preferably, artificial ventilation with oxygen using a demand valve. Monitoring may be limited to counting heart rate, respiratory rate, and palpation of the facial artery pulse. After the foal is removed, the floor must be totally dried to avoid the mare slipping when trying to stand. Xylazine-induced ataxia may be reversed after the mare is standing by IV injection of tolazoline at approximately 25% of the manufacturer's dose rate. In one retrospective survey of mares in which dystocia was managed by fetotomy, mares were initially sedated with xylazine or detomidine and butorphanol IV, with or without an epidural nerve block (Nimmo et al., 2007). General anaesthesia was subsequently induced with xylazine–ketamine–guaifenesin and maintained with halothane.

Anaesthesia for caesarean section

Caesarian section (CS) can be accomplished under TIVA with added local analgesia, but general anaesthesia maintained by an inhalation agent is most common. Induction of anaesthesia with xylazine or romifidine and ketamine, with or without guaifenesin, should provide a satisfactory outcome when the foal is alive. Guaifenesin has been documented to cross the placenta in cattle and slow activity of calves *in utero*. Clinical impression is that foals may be similarly affected after delivery but that breathing is satisfactory and the delay before standing is short. Any technique compatible with anaesthesia of a sick horse can be used when the foal is known to be dead. Since the mare has a distended abdomen and will be in dorsal recumbency for a midline incision, controlled ventilation should be instituted and blood pressure monitored to identify hypotension. Hypotension may result from pre-existing hypovolaemia (dehydration), exaggerated adverse effects of anaesthetic agents due to exhaustion or toxaemia, or from aortocaval compression from the uterus and foal. Blood loss during the procedure may be significant and should be replaced with balanced electrolyte solution IV. Hypertonic saline solution, 4 mL/kg, may be required for blood volume expansion. Administration of dobutamine and ephedrine may be used to support arterial blood pressure. Recovery from anaesthesia should be managed in a similar fashion as for horses after colic surgery.

Care of the newborn foal

Foals should start regular breathing of 10–20 breaths/minute within 30 seconds of birth and normal heart rates are approximately 70 beats/minute (Corley & Axon, 2005). Resuscitation is indicated for foals with no breathing or heart beat, with a delay to breathing or have obvious abnormal breathing patterns, or have heart rates <50 beats/min. Oxygen supplementation can be achieved with an O_2 flow rate of 5 L/min delivered through a loose fitting mask or through a rubber tube inserted into the ventral nasal meatus. Nasotracheal intubation (see Chapter 11) is the best option for assisted ventilation, with the tracheal tube connected to an anaesthesia machine circle circuit or a resuscitator (Ambu) bag that allows artificial ventilation with air or oxygen (see Fig. 22.1). The reservoir bag should be compressed and the chest wall observed to expand. An adequate tidal volume should be achieved with a peak inspiratory pressure of 15–20 cmH_2O. A less optimal situation is use of a tight fitting mask and ventilation with the resuscitator bag. The foals should be rubbed down and dried with a towel and placed in a warm environment. Foals delivered by CS may not have received umbilical cord blood and will benefit from IV bolus of crystalloid fluid (10 mL/kg lactated or acetated Ringer's solution) or colloid (2 mL/kg hetastarch). Management of cardiac arrest is covered in Chapter 22 and elsewhere (Palmer, 2007).

Cattle

In cattle, caudal epidural nerve block with lidocaine, procaine, or xylazine is often administered prior to attempting vaginal delivery or CS to decrease abdominal straining. Recommended dose rates used for the caudal epidural are lidocaine, 5 mL of 2%, 2 mL (80 mg) procaine 4% with epinephrine (Kolkman et al., 2007), xylazine, 0.05–0.07 mg/kg diluted with saline to 5–7.5 mL (Newman, 2008) or xylazine, 0.01–0.016 mg/kg (Kolkman et al., 2007). When the cow is weak, a lidocaine or procaine epidural may be avoided as these agents may induce ataxia and increase the risk for recumbency. Clenbuterol, 0.15 mg injected into a tail vein, has also been recommended before CS to relax the uterus (Kolkman et al., 2007, 2010b). Clenbuterol is prohibited for use in food producing species in some countries.

There are eight available approaches to coeliotomy for CS in cattle that are left or right paralumbar in standing or recumbent cows, left oblique in standing cows, and paramedian, ventrolateral, or midline in recumbent cows (Schultz et al., 2008). Sedation with xylazine is often avoided because it may increase contractions of the uterus (Newman, 2008; Schultz et al., 2008), although this effect can be counteracted by administration of clenbuterol where permitted. Administration of xylazine, 0.04 mg/kg, IV to pregnant cows resulted in a 56% reduction in uterine artery blood flow after 5 minutes accompanied by an increase in uterine artery vascular resistance and a substantial decrease in maternal PaO_2 (Hodgson et al., 2002). These changes significantly decreased oxygen delivery to the calf and may be clinically important for the viability of the calf. Except for a 5% decrease in PaO_2 at 5 minutes, these changes did not occur after administration of acepromazine, 0.02 mg/kg. Recumbent cows sedated with xylazine may also be at increased risk for pulmonary aspiration after regurgitation. Nevertheless, xylazine sedation has been used in cows for CS for many years with satisfactory outcomes. Detomidine, 0.01–0.02 mg/kg, IV or 0.02–0.04 mg/kg, IM is an alternative sedative for this purpose. The cow is more likely to remain standing and the ecbolic effects are less. Other drug combinations that have been recommended for standing restraint are 7.5 mg of acepromazine with 10 mg butorphanol IV in standing healthy dairy heifers or xylazine, 0.02 mg/kg, butorphanol, 0.01 mg/kg, and ketamine, 0.04 mg/kg, all injected IM for anxious cows (Newman, 2008). Choice of sedative may be limited by the milk-withdrawal times dictated by country specific legislation.

A preferred technique for CS is the left paralumbar approach in standing cows. Ideally, the farm has a covered area with fixed restraints that can be used but some clinics have a portable chute and other facilities, such as an overhead winch and resuscitation equipment, that can be transported to the site. A halter is placed on the cow and tied to the left. A blindfold on the cow may decrease kicking by preventing observation of the surgeon's movements. Forcible elevation of the tail is a distracting technique that can be used to immobilize cattle during injection of local anaesthetic solution unless a caudal epidural has been administered. Options for analgesic techniques for surgery are proximal or distal paravertebral nerve blocks or local infiltration. The latter is administered subcutaneously and into the abdominal muscle as an inverted-L block or as a line block at the incision site. Choice of technique may be clinician preference. Less local anaesthetic solution is used in the paravertebral block and analgesia may be more complete when compared with infiltration. Cows that will be recumbent for surgery are cast with ropes and the head and legs tied to prevent movement. A paramedian incision is usually blocked by infiltration of local anaesthetic solution in an L-shape across the cranial end of the incision and 2–5 cm lateral to the proposed incision with injections extending the depth of the abdominal wall. A midline incision is blocked by line infiltration. Cows that are sick as a result of toxaemia from a dead fetus or uterine torsion should receive balanced electrolyte fluid IV to restore blood volume and, if recumbent, intranasal administration of oxygen, 15 L/min.

Care of the newborn calf

One study has evaluated the effect of body position of calves after delivery by caesarean section and rupture of the umbilical cord (Uystepruyst et al., 2002). Lateral recumbency, manual positioning in sternal recumbency, and suspension of the calves by the hind limbs for up to 90 seconds (until the calf resisted) were compared by blood gas analysis and pulmonary function tests at intervals up to 24 hours. PaO_2 tensions were significantly higher in the sternal and suspended calves, and tidal volumes were greater in the first hour after birth in the suspended calves. A significant enhancement of passive transfer of colostral immunoglobulins was documented in the suspended calves compared with calves that were not suspended. All calves had low PaO_2 tensions immediately after birth that progressively increased over the subsequent 24 hours, and $PaCO_2$ tensions were high (>8 kPa, >60 mmHg) initially and decreased to 5.3 kPa (40 mmHg) at 12 hours. All groups had a mean base deficit at birth that converted to base excess by 12 hours.

Postoperative behaviour

Postoperative analgesia is often neglected in cows undergoing caesarean section. Questionnaires investigating current use of non-steroidal anti-inflammatory drugs (NSAIDs) have not had a high response rate but the information obtained indicates administration may be to 50% or less of cows (Hewson et al., 2007). Administration of an NSAID is recommended within the restrictions of the

country's licensing, and appropriate meat and milk withdrawals need to be followed.

Behaviour of cows with no postoperative analgesic drugs after caesarian section were compared and evaluated with cows that had natural vaginal delivery using behaviour analysis software (Noldus Observer®). The analysis included activities such as general activity and body positions, limb movement, licking, eating, rumination, vocalization, and interaction with neighbours (Kolkman et al., 2010a). On the day after surgery, the cows had significantly less limb movement and more positional transitions, and spent less time eating and ruminating, than the cows that had vaginal delivery. The cows' behaviour was not different from the control cows on the third day but they continued to respond to pressure on the flank incision when tested on the first, third, and fourteenth day after surgery. The degree of pain experienced by cows after caesarian section is not known but it is inconceivable that none is present. The results of this study indicate that in the absence of NSAID administration there is general malaise for at least 24 hours and local surgical site discomfort for 2 weeks.

Sheep and goats

Caudal epidural nerve block can be used to reduce straining and provide analgesia for vaginal delivery of lambs. Analgesia for CS through a left flank incision can be supplied by epidural nerve block with lidocaine injected at the lumbosacral space, paravertebral nerve block of the 13th thoracic, first, second and third lumbar nerves, or local infiltration using an inverted L block or line block. A disadvantage of an epidural nerve block is that there will be a delay before the ewe or doe is able to stand by herself to nurse the lambs or kids. It must be remembered that the dose rate for local anaesthetic solution for a lumbosacral epidural should be calculated on the estimated nonpregnant weight.

Dehydration and hypovolaemia should be corrected by IV administration of electrolyte fluids. Animals with multiple fetuses may have difficulty breathing when restrained in lateral recumbency and flow-by administration of 5 L/min oxygen using a mask will maintain oxygenation of the dam and fetuses, and probably minimize struggling initiated by hypoxaemia.

General anaesthesia is an option in a clinic setting but the lambs or kids will likely be more depressed than when only local analgesia is used. Sufficient numbers of personnel must be available for one-to-one resuscitation of the newborns. Low doses of midazolam–ketamine or propofol can be used for induction of anaesthesia followed by maintenance with sevoflurane or isoflurane. Publications describing use of alfaxalone for CS are yet to appear but based on experiences with its predecessor, alfaxalone is likely to be a satisfactory induction agent for this purpose.

When administered, IV oxytocin must be injected slowly as it may acutely induce hypotension. Postoperative analgesia may be supplied by administration of an NSAID. Opioids such as buprenorphine, 0.01 mg/kg, IM may also be administered at intervals of 6 hours (see Chapter 13).

Camelids

Dystocia is relatively uncommon in llamas and alpacas but may be indicated for fetal malpositioning or uterine torsion (Anderson, 2009). In contrast to cattle practice, elective caesarean section is not recommended because mortality of crias is high. Rather, the viability of the fetus is monitored by observation of dam behaviour, ultrasonography, and Doppler ultrasound determination of the fetal heart rate. Oxygen therapy may be indicated for a severely distressed pregnant female. A jugular catheter should be inserted and a dehydrated animal should be resuscitated with IV electrolyte solution. Surgery is performed with the female haltered and tied in recumbency and local infiltration with lidocaine as a line block at the proposed incision site. A maximum total dose of 4 mg/kg lidocaine is recommended for these species (Anderson, 2009). The dam may be sedated with butorphanol, 0.03–0.1 mg/kg. Xylazine may not be a good choice because the decrease in cardiac output and peripheral vasoconstriction will result in a decrease in uterine blood flow, maternal oxygenation is decreased unless oxygen is supplied by tube or mask and, at least in other ruminants, xylazine increases myometrial activity. If used, only low doses, 0.1–0.2 mg/kg, IM should be administered. Induction of anaesthesia with propofol and maintenance with isoflurane or sevoflurane may be satisfactory when general anaesthesia is required (Tibary et al., 2008). Antibiotics and an NSAID should also be administered (Anderson, 2009).

Care of the newborn

Normal alpaca crias should weigh at least 5.5 kg and llama crias 7 kg, and preferably more (Whitehead, 2009). Normal body temperatures are 37.8–38.9°C (100–102°F), heart rates 70–100 beats/minute and respiratory rates 20–30 breaths/minute. Crias must be kept warm and adequate colostrum intake in the first 24 hours must be ensured. Assessment of the newborn should include a full physical examination. Crias born earlier than 315 (Tibary et al., 2008) or 335 (Whitehead, 2009) days of pregnancy are termed premature. Premature or compromised crias should also receive oxygen, IV fluid therapy and dextrose-containing fluids, and possibly plasma. Administration of aminophylline, 2 mg/kg SC, for 3 days initially at 4-hour intervals and finishing at 8-hour intervals has been recommended for premature crias based on clinical experience (Whitehead, 2009).

Pigs

The general principles of anaesthesia for CS in sows are similar to those in all other species of animal – it is necessary to provide adequate surgical conditions to prevent the sow from experiencing pain and to use a method that produces minimal depression of the piglets. Ideally, both the sow and piglets should recover from the effects of the anaesthetic in the minimum of time.

Caesarean section may be carried out under conditions which vary from those encountered on the farm to those provided in an operating theatre. Elective CS is carried out more commonly for the production of minimal disease herds of pigs, or gnotobiotic animals for research purposes, than in farm sows, and is more likely to be performed in a well-equipped operating room.

On the farm, CS is probably best carried out under local or regional analgesia. The sow may be restrained in lateral recumbency with ropes and the site of incision infiltrated with local anaesthetic solution. An epidural nerve block may also be used. The sow may be toxic and depressed and supplementation with oxygen through a mask appears to decrease mortality in the sows and piglets.

Sows that are relatively healthy can be restrained by IV injection of xylazine, 1 mg/kg, and ketamine, 2 mg/kg and rope ties on the limbs, and analgesia supplied by a local anaesthetic line block. Alternatively, azaperone, where available, can be used to provide sedation prior to local analgesia, although the drug does cross the placental barrier and the piglets are sleepy when delivered. However, respiratory depression in the offspring seems minimal and if kept warm they usually survive. The sedative effects of azaperone on the sow are rather prolonged and she may not be able to suckle the piglets for some hours; if left unattended with the neonatal piglets she may suffocate some by lying on them.

Under conditions encountered in hospitals, techniques are not usually limited by availability and a wide variety of techniques can be employed. The piglets are not always returned to the dam and, in these circumstances, speed of recovery of the sow is less important than under farm conditions.

Viable piglets are obtained when anaesthesia is induced via facemask and maintained with an inhalation anaesthetic and a high concentration of inspired oxygen. In the majority of sows, anaesthesia is rapidly attained with agents such as halothane, isoflurane or sevoflurane, especially if a mild sedative is administered first. If the sow is very large or difficult to handle, administration of a sedative or a minimal dose of thiopental or propofol can be employed.

Involution of the uterus after delivery of the piglets may, if the animal is not hypoxic or hypercapnic, be helped by IV 2–10 IU oxytocin.

Dogs and cats

Many anaesthetic agent combinations have been employed to provide operating conditions in dogs and cats for CS. Epidural analgesia with lidocaine, with or without an opioid, has been used for many years in dogs and results in vigorous puppies. Disadvantages of epidural analgesia for this purpose include failure of satisfactory analgesia at the cranial end of the midline incision, movement of the bitch in response to intra-abdominal manipulation and mesenteric traction or ovariectomy, and hypotension. The addition of a sedative or opioid may facilitate restraint but does not adequately prevent the complications. In early years, fentanyl–droperidol or barbiturate were the only injectable induction agents used, and while fentanyl remains a useful option, thiopental is better substituted with propofol or alfaxalone for more vigorous newborns. It was quickly discovered that the combination of xylazine and ketamine was not suitable for anaesthesia for CS in dogs (Navarro & Friedman, 1975). In an extensive survey of 109 veterinary practices in Canada and the USA, involving 807 CS producing 3908 puppies, survival rate was 87% at 2 hours after delivery and 80% at 7 days (Moon et al., 2000). Of these, 58% were emergency CS. A wide variety of anaesthetic protocols were used (1994–1997) with one-third being propofol–isoflurane and one-third mask induction, intubation, and maintenance with isoflurane. Protocols that included the use of xylazine, ketamine, or methoxyflurane were associated with increased risk of puppy deaths. Survival was greater when surgery was not an emergency, the dam was not brachycephalic, there were ≤4 puppies per litter, and that there were no naturally delivered or deformed puppies in the litter.

In one comparison of anaesthetic combinations for CS in 24 pregnant bitches following premedication with chlorpromazine, puppies were most depressed after delivery from midazolam–ketamine–enflurane and thiopental–enflurane, whereas puppies were less depressed when the dam was anaesthetized with propofol–enflurane and most vigorous when delivered during a lidocaine–bupivacaine epidural block (Luna et al., 2004). In another study, no difference in puppy mortality (86% overall survival) was recorded between 62 puppies born by CS during propofol–isoflurane and bupivacaine line block for anaesthesia and 127 puppies born by natural or assisted vaginal birth (Veronesi et al., 2009). Similar results were obtained in a study of 141 bitches and 412 puppies born by CS where survival rate of puppies born by propofol–isoflurane anaesthesia was the same as delivered by epidural analgesia, but the survival rate of puppies from thiopental–isoflurane anaesthesia was lower (Funkquist et al., 1997). Diazepam has been associated with muscle weakness and decreased ability to nurse or maintain body heat in human babies for hours after delivery. Clinical impression is that diazepam administration to the dam has the same effect in puppies and, therefore, should be avoided.

Combination of epidural with general anaesthesia has also been recommended (Brock, 1996; Traas, 2008). An example of a sequence of events would be an opioid epidural performed in the conscious animal followed by administration of hydromorphone or fentanyl and atropine before propofol for induction of anaesthesia, tracheal intubation and administration of oxygen. Inhalation anaesthesia is administered once the puppies are delivered and a line block at the incision site is performed with bupivacaine, 2.5 mg/kg, at the end of surgery (Traas, 2008).

Mask induction of anaesthesia with an inhalation agent after preanaesthetic sedation is a technique for CS that that results in vigorous kittens. It is important to note that, in contrast to experience with anaesthesia in dogs, the inclusion of propofol in the CS anaesthetic protocol for cats has been found to result in unacceptable kitten depression. In a retrospective evaluation of CS in 159 cats over 13 years, it was discovered that epidural analgesia had the best kitten survival rate (Elovsson et al., 1996). The percentage of kittens born dead increased five to six times when anaesthesia was provided with xylazine or medetomidine–ketamine and was seven times greater when anaesthesia was propofol–isoflurane. The percentage of drowsy kittens of those born alive was dramatically higher when anaesthesia was thiopental–halothane or propofol–isoflurane. Infiltration of the incision site after the abdomen is closed with bupivacaine, 2 mg/kg, will provide several hours of analgesia. If TIVA has to be used for CS in cats, alfaxalone may turn out to be the best. Although alfaxalone crosses the placental barrier and will affect the kittens, no noticeable respiratory depression was observed when the earlier product 'Saffan' was used. Information about use of alfaxalone in CS is yet to be published.

When the bitch or queen is depressed or toxic and it is known that the fetuses are dead, the anaesthetic protocol chosen should be appropriate for management of a patient with a reduced anaesthetic requirement at high risk for circulatory failure.

Anaesthetic management

Preparation before anaesthesia should include placement of an IV catheter for administration of anaesthetic agents and balanced electrolyte solution during surgery (Box 19.1). Crystalloid fluid should be administered before anaesthesia to animals judged to be dehydrated or toxaemic. Hair should be clipped from the abdomen. All equipment for newborn resuscitation should be assembled. As just described, anaesthesia provided by epidural nerve block, or sedation and mask induction and maintenance with an inhalation agent, or induction with propofol (dogs only) and maintenance with an inhalation agent are protocols that preserve newborn vigour. Drugs to be administered IV should be calculated on the dams estimated non-pregnant weight. A low dose of an opioid may be administered for premedication. Heavy or long-acting sedation is avoided because it may depress the dam in the postoperative period, interfering with her tending the neonates. Administration of oxygen by facemask for 3 minutes before induction of general anaesthesia (preoxygenation) is advisable for brachycephalic breeds and animals that are toxic, if not for all CS patients. The patient owners may know the time of last feeding or contents of the stomach may be observed on a radiograph. Induction of anaesthesia using an inhalant delivered by facemask is not advisable in animals that are known to have food or fetal membranes in their stomachs because the time taken increases the risk for regurgitation and pulmonary aspiration. Animals with gastric contents should be induced rather quickly in a sternal or upright position and not allowed to lie down until endotracheal intubation and inflation of the cuff has been accomplished.

Local infiltration of the midline with lidocaine, 2 mg/kg, in dogs is useful adjunct analgesia and minimizes response of the dam to the incision. Depression of the newborns by inhalation anaesthetic is related to the concentration and duration of administration. Thus, use of the lowest effective vaporizer setting and a short time between induction and delivery are optimal. Depending on the anaesthetic protocol chosen, once the neonates have been delivered, additional anaesthetic agent can be administered for closure of the uterus and abdomen, for example, start or increase inhalant administration or injection of an opioid such as butorphanol if none has already been given (Box 19.2).

Experimental studies failed to demonstrate aortocaval compression and hypotension in pregnant anaesthetized bitches positioned in dorsal recumbency (Probst & Webb, 1983). Nevertheless, this may occur in some animals and blood pressure should be checked shortly after the animal is turned onto its back. Rotation into a left lateral oblique position may be sufficient to correct hypotension from this cause. Controlled or assisted ventilation may be necessary until the abdominal pressure is relieved by removal of the fetuses. *En bloc* excision of the uterus and puppies or kittens is not advisable when the puppies and kittens are wanted alive because the extra time taken for ligation will result in hypoxia of the fetuses. Blood loss during this surgical procedure can be significant and rate of administration of IV fluids should be increased in compensation. Administration of oxytocin may be indicated to aid uterine involution but should be administered very slowly to avoid abrupt hypotension. Local infiltration of the incision site with bupivacaine, ≤2 mg/kg, at the end of surgery may help to provide pain relief postoperatively.

Care of the newborns

Upon delivery, fluid should be suctioned carefully, a few seconds at a time, from the puppies' or kittens' noses using a blue bulb syringe or nasal aspirator sold for use in human babies. A few minutes of oxygen should be supplied when the dam has been breathing nitrous oxide. The newborns should be rubbed with a towel and dried and stimulated. Breathing spontaneously and vocalizing within one minute of delivery are indicators of puppy vigour and of increased survival (Moon et al., 2000). Normal newborn puppy respiratory rates are 10–18 breaths/minute. Hypoxia and irregular breathing patterns have been observed in puppies born after normal vaginal delivery or CS (Silva et al., 2009). Cardiac massage should be applied if the heart beat is slow (<170 beats/minute). When the newborn puppies and kittens are not vigorous and an opioid has been administered to the dam before delivery, naloxone can be injected to antagonize its effects.

Other reversal agents are flumazenil for diazepam and atipamezole for medetomidine. Doxapram is a respiratory stimulant that may also induce arousal due to release of norepinephrine and has been advocated for use in newborn animals but may be ineffective. Lawler (2008) has described neonatal care in detail, including environmental temperature guidelines, nutritional support, normal haematological and chemical values, from birth to weaning.

LIMITATIONS OF OUR KNOWLEDGE

Intrathecal or epidural analgesia is frequently employed for elective or emergency caesarean delivery in humans, with conversion to general anaesthesia in cases of analgesia failure or for maternal safety. Post-spinal hypotension requiring treatment with a vasopressor occurs in approximately 60% of elective caesarean deliveries (Mhyre, 2011). Administration of colloid solution before or during surgery did not maintain an acceptable maternal blood pressure in several clinical studies. There are many scientific publications documenting that, in this specific situation, phenylephrine infusion is more effective in increasing blood pressure than the traditionally recommended ephedrine. These findings may be relevant to obstetrical management of sheep, goats, dogs and cats where epidural analgesia with local anaesthetic solution is used for caesarian section. However, phenylephrine infusion decreases cardiac output and causes peripheral vasoconstriction, and these changes may decrease uterine blood flow.

Specialized abdominal wall nerve blocks, the transversus abdominal plane or TAP blocks, have been evaluated in parturient women for their value in postoperative pain management. The technique of TAP blocks in dogs and their potential value for analgesia are currently being investigated.

Published scientific literature documenting outcomes from different anaesthetic techniques for obstetrical procedures in different species of animals is sparse. Much more information needs to be available before reliable consensus statements can be constructed for anaesthetic management of the domestic species for surgical delivery of newborns in optimum condition.

REFERENCES

Andaluz, A., Trasserras, O., Garcia, F., 2005. Maternal and fetal effects of propofol anaesthesia in the pregnant ewe. Vet J 170, 77–83.

Andaluz, A., Tusell, J., Trasserras, O., et al., 2003. Transplacental transfer of propofol in pregnant ewes. Vet J 166, 198–204.

Anderson, D.E., 2009. Uterine torsion and cesarean section in llamas and alpacas. Vet Clin Food Anim 25, 523–538.

Brock, N., 1996. Anesthesia for canine cesarian section. Can Vet J 37, 117–118.

Copland, M.D., 1977. The effects of CT1341, thiopentone and induction-delivery time on the blood gas and acid-base status of lambs delivered by caesarean operation and on the onset of respiration. Aust Vet J 53, 436–439.

Corley, K.T.T., Axon, J.E., 2005. Resuscitation and emergency management for neonatal foals. Vet Clin Equine 21, 431–455.

Elovsson, L., Funkquist, P., Nyman, G., 1996. Retrospective evaluation of anaesthetic techniques for Caesarian section in the cat. J Vet Anaesth 23, 80.

Funkquist, P.M., Nyman, G.C., Löfgren, A.J., et al., 1997. Use of propofol-isoflurane as an anesthetic regimen for cesarean section in dogs. J Am Vet Med Assoc 211, 313–317.

Gaynor, J.S., Wertz, E.M., Alvis, M., et al., 1998. A comparison of the haemodynamic effects of propofol and isoflurane in pregnant ewes. J Vet Pharmacol Ther 21, 69–73.

Hewson, C.J., Dohoo, I.R., Lemke, K.A., et al., 2007. Canadian veterinarians' use of analgesics in cattle, pigs, and horses in 2004 and 2005. Can Vet J 48, 155–164.

Hodgson, D.S., Dunlop, C.I., Chapman, P.L., et al., 2002. Cardiopulmonary effects of xylazine and acepromazine in pregnant cows in late gestation. Am J Vet Res 63, 1695–1699.

Kolkman, I., Aerts, S., Vervaecke, H., et al., 2010a. Assessment of differences in some indicators of pain in double muscled Belgian Blue cows following naturally calving vs caesarean section. Reprod Dom Anim 45, 160–167.

Kolkman, I., Opsomer, G., Lips, D., et al., 2010b. Pre-operative and operative difficulties during bovine caesarean section in Belgium and associated risk factors. Reprod Dom Anim 45, 1020–1027.

Kolkman, I., De Vliegher, S., Hoflack, G., et al., 2007. Protocol of the caesarean section as performed in daily bovine practice in Belgium. Reprod Dom Anim 42, 583–589.

Lawler, D.F., 2008. Neonatal and pediatric care of the puppy and kitten. Theriogenology 70, 384–392.

Luna, S.P.L., Cassu, R.N., Castro, G.B., et al., 2004. Effects of four anaesthetic protocols on the neurological and cardiorespiratory variables of puppies born by caesarean section. Vet Rec 154, 387–389.

Mhyre, J.M., 2011. What's new in obstetric anesthesia? Int J Obstet Anesth 20, 149–159.

Moon, P.F., Erb, H.N., Ludders, J.W., et al., 2000. Perioperative risk factors for puppies delivered by cesarean section in the United States and Canada. J Am Anim Hosp Assoc 36, 359–368.

Navarro, J.A., Friedman, J.R., 1975. A clinical evaluation of xylazine and ketamine HCL for cesarean section in the dog. Vet Med Small Anim Clin 70, 1075–1079.

Newman, K.D., 2008. Bovine cesarian section in the field. Vet Clin Food Anim 24, 273–293.

Nimmo, M.R., Slone, D.E., Hughes, F.E., et al., 2007. Fertility and complications after fetotomy in 20 brood mares (2001–2006). Vet Surg 36, 771–774.

Okutomi, T., Whittington, R.A., Stein, D.J., et al., 2009. Comparison of the effects of sevoflurane and isoflurane anesthesia on the maternal-fetal unit in sheep. J Anesth 23, 392–398.

Palahniuk, R.J., Shnider, S.M., 1974a. Maternal and fetal cardiovascular and acid-base changes during halothane and isoflurane anesthesia in the pregnant ewe. Anesthesiology 41, 462–472.

Palahniuk, R.J., Shnider, S.M., Eger, E.I., 1974b. Pregnancy decreases the requirements for inhaled anesthetic gases. Anesthesiology 41, 82–83.

Palmer, J.E., 2007. Neonatal foal resuscitation. Vet Clin Equine 23, 159–182.

Pascoe, P.J., Moon, P.F., 2001. Periparturient and neonatal anesthesia. Vet Clin N Am Small Anim Pract 31, 315–341.

Probst, C.W., Webb, A.I., 1983. Postural influence on systemic blood pressure, gas exchange, and acid/base status in the term-pregnant bitch during general anesthesia. Am J Vet Res 44, 1963–1965.

Schultz, L.G., Tyler, J.W., Moll, H.D., et al., 2008. Surgical approaches for cesarian section in cattle. Can Vet J 49, 565–568.

Silva, L.C.G., Lúcio, C.F., Veiga, G.A.L., et al., 2009. Neonatal clinical evaluation, blood gas and radiographic assessment after normal birth, vaginal dystocia or caesarean section in dogs. Reprod Dom Anim s44, 160–163.

Strümper, D., Gogarten, W., Durieux, M.E., et al., 2005. Effects of cafedrine/theodrenaline, etilefrine and ephedrine on uterine blood flow during epidural-induced hypotension in pregnant sheep. Fetal Diagn Ther 20, 377–382.

Tibary, A., Rodriguez, J., Sandoval, S., 2008. Reproductive emergencies in camelids. Theriogenology 70, 515–534.

Traas, A.M., 2008. Surgical management of canine and feline dystocia. Theriogenology 70, 337–342.

Uystepruyst, C., Coghe, J., Dorts, T., et al., 2002. Sternal recumbency or suspension by the hind legs immediately after delivery improves respiratory and metabolic adaptation to extra uterine life in newborn calves delivered by caesarian section. Vet Res 33, 709–724.

Veronesi, M.C., Panzani, S., Faustini, M., et al., 2009. An Apgar scoring system for routine assessment of newborn puppy viability and short-term survival prognosis. Theriogenology 72, 401–407.

Whitehead, C.E., 2009. Management of neonatal llamas and alpacas. Vet Clin Food Anim 25, 353–366.

Anaesthesia for intrathoracic procedures

The primary concern for anaesthesia of intrathoracic procedures is management of the pneumothorax that is necessary for surgical access created by opening the chest wall and/or the diaphragm. Ventilation must therefore be controlled and monitored closely by the anaesthetist or an individual on the anaesthesia team to maintain appropriate oxygenation and gas exchange (see Chapter 9). Manual ventilation can be satisfactory but the use of a mechanical ventilator ensures accurate delivery of minute ventilation, a rhythmic cycle of breathing that the surgeon can anticipate during the procedure, and more time for the anaesthetist to devote to patient monitoring. Clinical intrathoracic procedures are most commonly performed in dogs and cats; specific management details are included in latter sections of this chapter. Some surgical or medical procedures may inadvertently penetrate the pleural cavity and create a pneumothorax, for example, ventral cervical surgery near the thoracic inlet (tracheal ring repair, ventral cervical decompression, or mass excision), oesophageal endoscopy, cranial abdominal surgery resulting in a crural tear, mass excisions over the thorax, and trauma disrupting the integrity of the thoracic wall (fractured ribs, pulmonary bullae, or penetrating wound). Experimental thoracotomy is frequently performed in pigs and sheep. The general principles for anaesthetic management are the same for all species.

GENERAL PRINCIPLES

Preanaesthetic evaluation and preparation

The incidence of postoperative pulmonary complications is high in human patients after thoracic and upper abdominal surgery (Duggan & Kavanagh, 2010). Factors associated with such complications are a history of smoking, increasing age, degree of preoperative dyspnoea, increasing ASA score, extent of an intrathoracic tumour, presence of cardiac disease, and duration of surgery exceeding 3 hours. Low serum albumin has also been found to be an important predictor of postoperative pulmonary complications and 30-day mortality (Duggan & Kavanagh, 2010). Thus, the physical status of the veterinary patient

Table 20.1 Impact of presenting problem on anaesthetic management, in addition to considerations specific to thoracotomy or thoracoscopy

Inability adequately to oxygenate or ventilate

Aspiration pneumonia	Persistent right aortic arch (PRAA)
Pulmonary contusions	Vehicular trauma, diaphragmatic rupture, big dog-little dog/cat trauma
Restricted lung inflation	Chylothorax, pyothorax, pneumothorax, flail chest, diaphragmatic rupture, lung mass (abscess, neoplasia, lobe torsion), thoracic mass, gastro-oesophageal intussusception

Potential for hypotension or cardiovascular collapse

Cardiac disease, congenital defects, cardiac surgery	Requires pacemaker, neoplasia, pericardial effusion, heartworms, peritoneal-pericardial hernia, patent ductus arteriosus
Generalized trauma with haemorrhage	
Sepsis	

Decreased anaesthetic requirement

Pre-existing CNS depression	Sepsis, oesophageal rupture, pyothorax
Cardiac disease	Requires pacemaker, heartworm removal, neoplasia, myocardial contusions

scheduled for thoracic procedures should be evaluated with a thorough physical examination. Some patients may be relatively healthy, others will have specific abnormalities that must be considered in the anaesthetic management (Table 20.1). These might include pneumonia, diffuse pulmonary neoplasia, a space-occupying mass(es), pulmonary or myocardial contusions, restricted lung inflation from pulmonary or external causes, cardiac disease, pre-existing central nervous system (CNS) depression, or sepsis.

Lung function should be evaluated when respiratory disease is present by assessing the degree of exercise intolerance (ability to walk without dyspnoea), the pattern of breathing, auscultation of the lungs for abnormal sounds, arterial blood gas analysis ($PaCO_2$ and PaO_2), and thoracic radiography (Miller, 2007). An electrocardiogram (ECG) should be obtained to identify any dysrhythmias. Lung function may be evaluated in dogs and horses with spirometry. Flow-volume loops are obtained with a pneumotachometer and a tightly fitting mask over the patient's muzzle. Further information may be obtained from computerized tomography (CT) in some patients. Whenever

possible, medical treatment should be instituted before anaesthesia to improve the patients' physical status, for example, removal of air or drainage of pleural fluid.

The surgical approach varies depending on the specific lesion and location, and the surgical techniques utilized – abdominal, left or right thoracotomy, and median sternotomy are most common; thoracoscopy may be performed instead of or in addition to thoracotomy. Requirements for management of the various approaches may differ, for example, analgesic techniques for a lateral thoracotomy will be different from a thoracoscopy.

Preanaesthetic preparation of both patient and equipment is key to avoid or prevent complications. Basic needs include one or more often two venous catheters sufficient for rapid fluid therapy, warming devices as heat loss can be severe, and a thermometer, a pulse oximeter, and blood pressure monitor. Controlled ventilation, either manual or by mechanical ventilator, is necessary. Blood for transfusion should be available for some procedures and blood typing or cross-matching before anaesthesia may also be advisable for procedures where blood loss is common. Suction equipment should be available for procedures involving surgery of pulmonary tissue so that blood and fluid can be removed from the airway as needed. Suction technique of the trachea should be intermittent rather than continuous to avoid collapsing the lung from excessive suction.

Ideally, facilities should be available for intensive monitoring that include capnography, blood gas analysis, and invasive pressure measurements, however, management of an acute diaphragmatic rupture in a dog or cat is likely to be much less complex than a thoracotomy for pericardectomy or experimental cardiac surgery. Many procedures in dogs, such as lobectomy, pericardectomy, thoracic duct ligation, and exploratory, can be performed by thoracoscopy when the equipment is available. Although this technique has the benefit of decreased postoperative pain for the patient, it presents some difficulties for the anaesthetist particularly involving provision of adequate ventilation and oxygenation. One-lung ventilation (OLV) requires additional equipment preparation and lengthens the time from induction to start of the surgical procedure.

The species of the patient will have a significant impact on choice of anaesthetic agents and anaesthetic management. Anaesthesia of a sheep for experimental thoracotomy must include plans for management of bloat and prevention of aspiration in the event of regurgitation. Maintenance of adequate $PaCO_2$ and PaO_2 is often difficult in a horse with a diaphragmatic rupture, and management of recovery is more difficult than in a dog.

Ventilation and oxygenation

The effects of artificial ventilation and of opening the chest on cardiopulmonary function have been discussed in Chapter 9. Controlled ventilation (IPPV) with cyclical stretching of the lungs may cause lung damage that results in complications postoperatively. Toll-like receptors are thought to play a key role by activating a series of complex signalling pathways that initiate inflammation (Curley et al., 2009). The impact of IPPV strategy on healthy lungs may be minimal since several studies comparing ventilation at tidal volumes of 12–15 mL/kg with 6 mL/kg for relatively short times (5 hours) have not identified differences between ventilation protocols when measuring plasma tumour necrosis factor α (TNFα) and interleukin concentrations (Curley et al., 2009; Beck-Schimmer & Schimmer, 2010). It has been suggested that a two-hit process may be required for ventilator-induced injury. Also recommended is further research into the effect of anaesthetic agents on the mechanisms of lung injury as downregulation of these processes offering a degree of protection has been documented with some anaesthetic agents (Curley et al., 2009).

Use of low tidal volumes of 6 mL/kg of ideal body weight is recommended for ventilation of human patients with acute lung injury and acute respiratory distress syndrome (ARDS) of various aetiologies (Bigatello & Pesenti, 2009). Injury in the lung is not homogeneous but occurs in small areas. Delivery of a fixed volume breath to the lung results in areas of pressures within the lung that are different to the measured tracheal pressure. Alveoli that are closed with fluid-filled terminal airways will not be ventilated and air is then directed at a higher pressure into alveoli that are already ventilated (compliant alveoli) resulting in their overventilation. A disadvantage of restriction of tidal volume to avoid barotrauma is that, despite an increase in respiratory rate, it may result in an inability effectively to maintain $PaCO_2$ within normal limits. In this instance, an option is to allow 'permissive hypercapnia' where a higher than normal $PaCO_2$ (<55 mmHg) is purposely allowed to avoid high airway pressure or tidal volume. The body of information on ventilator-induced lung trauma has largely been acquired from investigations involving humans and mice, and research involving the varied domestic species is needed for accurate veterinary relevance.

It is usual to modify the parameters used for ventilation of healthy lungs for ventilation of animals with damaged lungs, such as pulmonary contusions, pneumonia, and collapsed lung lobes, by limiting the peak inspiratory pressure to ≤15 cmH_2O whenever possible. The decrease in tidal volume achieved by this low pressure is compensated for by an increase in respiratory rate. Similarly, tidal volume must be decreased after lung lobectomy and at the change from two-lung ventilation (2LV) to OLV to avoid over distension of the one lung being ventilated, barotrauma, and pneumothorax.

Lung collapse will occur even in healthy patients without thoracic disease during anaesthesia. Three areas for potential collapse are: (1) the alveoli (atelectasis, loss of aeration of a whole acinus) caused by resorption of oxygen, inadequate distending pressure, or physical compression in the dependent lung; (2) bronchiolar collapse (airway closure) in areas of lung with low ventilation; and (3) capillary collapse for a number of reasons including absolute or relative hypovolaemia (Tusman & Böhm, 2010). Administration of 100% oxygen will potentiate atelectasis because of the absence of nitrogen to keep the alveoli open after O_2 is absorbed. However, reducing the inspired oxygen % increases the risk of hypoxaemia in patients with acute lung injury; 100% oxygen may be needed for OLV, in the event of cardiovascular collapse, and during colonic surgery.

Lung recruitment manoeuvre

A lung recruitment manoeuvre is a ventilator strategy designed to reverse lung collapse, restore more uniform expansion of the lungs, and improve arterial oxygenation (see Chapter 9). It is a brief and controlled increment in airway pressure to open alveoli and bronchioles and is generally followed by the application of positive endexpiratory pressure (PEEP) to maintain the improvement in oxygenation (Tusman & Böhm, 2010). The optimal PEEP varies with the individual patient and does not always increase PaO_2. Natural recruitment manoeuvres in awake subjects include coughing, sighing, sneezing, and postural changes, and they may play a part in quick reversal of lung collapse in healthy patients after anaesthesia. The recommended technique for recruitment in human patients involves increasing PEEP at 5 cmH_2O increments every 5 breaths up to 20 cmH_2O and then increasing the airway pressure to 40 cmH_2O to deliver a larger tidal volume for 10 breaths before a stepwise decrease of PEEP in increments of 2 cmH_2O (Tusman & Böhm, 2010). PEEP may have a significant adverse effect on cardiovascular function, usually starting at 10 cmH_2O PEEP, that can be recognized by decreases in heart rate (HR) or mean arterial pressure (MAP) or decreased MAP to below 55 mmHg. The procedure is then halted and PEEP decreased. Blood volume is expanded by infusion of crystalloid or colloid solution before the next attempt at recruitment.

A gradual progressive decrease in SpO_2 to below 90% in dogs with diseased lungs could have one of several origins, such as progressive lung collapse, decreased cardiovascular function, or developing pneumothorax. Recruitment may be indicated when cardiovascular failure and pneumothorax have been ruled out and lung collapse is suspected. A simple recruitment technique is to increase the peak inspiratory pressure over several breaths to 30–40 cmH_2O, holding inspiration for 7–15 seconds. The lung inflation should be performed gently.

One-lung ventilation

Bilateral lung ventilation (2LV) is most frequently used for thoracic surgery or thoracoscopy in veterinary patients and is satisfactory for most procedures (Leasure et al., 2011). However, OLV may be advantageous in some cases. The main indications for OLV are: (1) to isolate diseased lung to prevent contamination of the healthy lung during extirpation of an abscess or when excessive haemorrhage is anticipated; and (2) to control distribution of ventilation to a selected lung. This situation is desirable when lung collapse would improve surgical exposure, to prevent ventilation of a lung with a major bronchial or alveolar tear, or to improve visibility or surgical access during thoracoscopy. Lung separation can be accomplished by using a bronchial blocker or a double lumen endotracheal tube (Brodsky, 2009). Occlusion of the bronchus to the right cranial lobe may be difficult to achieve (Caccamo et al., 2007).

Bronchial blocker

A bronchial blocker (BB) is a narrow-diameter tube with a cuff or balloon at the end that is inserted into the bronchus of the lung to be collapsed (Fig. 20.1). Inflation of the BB balloon after exhalation allows the lung distal to the inflated balloon to remain collapsed. The BB can be inserted through the lumen of a standard endotracheal tube or the BB may be an integral moving part in the wall of a special endotracheal tube. Several BBs with different designs are manufactured for use in humans (Narayanaswamy et al., 2009). The Arndt endobronchial blocker (Cooke Critical Care) is a balloon-tipped catheter with an inner lumen that contains a flexible wire. The wire exits the end of the catheter as a flexible wire loop that can be guided into a selected bronchus by the tip of a flexible endoscope. Once the blocker is positioned, the wire loop

is withdrawn from the catheter and the balloon is inflated. The endoscope is then used to observe the accuracy of balloon inflation. The lumen of the BB can be used to insufflate O_2 into the collapsed lung. One problem is that a BB may slide around within the bronchus during surgical manipulation and is at risk of being displaced into the trachea when the patient is moved or during surgery. Some catheters intended for other uses have been used as BB but complications have been seen, such as damage to the bronchial mucosa from a very high pressure created by the balloon (Brodsky, 2009).

Double lumen tube

A double lumen endotracheal tube (Carlens and Robertshaw/Roberts-Shaw) is designed to allow selective ventilation of the left and right lungs in human patients. The main body of the endotracheal tube has a cuff that resides within the trachea. One lumen extends beyond the tip of the other and can be inserted into one main bronchus and the cuff of that extension can be inflated to isolate the lung. Double lumen endotracheal tubes are available as right or left sided depending on which main bronchus is to be isolated. The tubes can be effectively positioned in large dogs but not so easily in smaller patients. The position of the tube can be checked using a flexible endoscope. One lung can then be ventilated as usual and the other either deflated or insufflated with oxygen to achieve continuous positive airway pressure (CPAP) (see Chapter 9). Problems associated with use of double lumen tubes include difficulty in placement, difficulty in occluding the bronchus to the right cranial lung lobe, and the need to change (ideally) to a single lumen

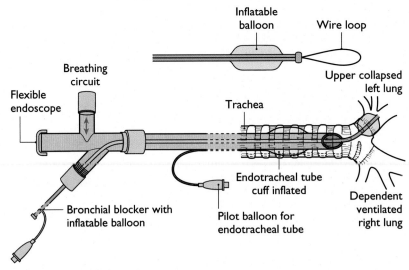

Figure 20.1 Schematic diagram of lung separation using a bronchial blocker (BB) introduced through an endotracheal tube in a dog. The tip of the Arndt BB (shown expanded) has a wire loop that a flexible endoscope can push into the desired bronchus.

tube for recovery to allow total lung inflation. A recent report described the use of a 37 Fr right double lumen endobronchial tube (Portex Ltd) in a 30 kg Pointer anaesthetized in left lateral recumbency for right middle lung lobectomy (Jiménez Peláez & Jolliffe, 2012). During surgery, the left lung and right cranial lung lobe were ventilated. Intraoperative PaO_2 was not reported.

Pulmonary effects of OLV

The effects of change from 2LV to OLV have been studied in experimental dogs and pigs. OLV results in a significant decrease in PaO_2 due to the increase in venous admixture from the collapsed lung. In one study in healthy experimental dogs, shunt fraction increased from 17% to 30% during OLV, although cardiac output, MAP, and O_2 delivery were unchanged (Kudnig et al., 2003).

When ventilation ceases in one lung, the alveoli progressively collapse. OLV with a decreased inspired FIO_2 may result in desaturation (SpO_2<90%). Mechanisms to manage this include intermittent insufflation of the non-dependent (collapsed) lung with oxygen, maintaining CPAP by slow continuous insufflation of oxygen in the non-dependent (collapsed) lung, and instituting PEEP in the dependent (ventilated) lung. PEEP may expand collapsed alveoli and improve expansion of poorly ventilated alveoli, however, the increase in intrathoracic pressure when the chest is closed will decrease cardiac output. In one study using large healthy dogs and OLV, thoracoscopy was simulated by placement of three ports (pleural cavity open to the air), and the cardiovascular effects of IPPV with 2.5 and 5.0 cmH$_2$O PEEP were compared with zero PEEP (Kudnig et al., 2006). Under these conditions, cardiac index and MAP were not affected by 5 cmH$_2$O. PaO_2 and arterial oxygen content were significantly increased, although since these dogs were healthy the change was not great.

Re-expansion pulmonary oedema

It is believed that the first report of re-expansion pulmonary oedema (REPE) was in 1853 (Sohara, 2008). In more recent years, there have been case reports of REPE in human patients and a few reports in the veterinary literature. REPE is a rare complication that occurs following rapid expansion of a chronically collapsed lung, for example, after removal of a large amount of air or fluid from the pleural space (Fossum et al., 1992; Soderstrom et al., 1995; Tarver et al., 1996) or when forceful ventilations are used during anaesthesia rapidly to expand lung that has been collapsed for days or weeks due to an intrathoracic mass or a diaphragmatic hernia (Stampley & Waldron, 1993). Experimental studies in a variety of species have indicated re-expansion of lungs that have been collapsed for 24 hours or more results in leakage of plasma albumin from the pulmonary microvessels. REPE may be a permeability pulmonary oedema associated with

Box 20.1 **Anaesthetic management for thoracotomy**

- Analgesia, unconsciousness, relaxation
- Artificial ventilation, manual or mechanical
- Minimum monitoring is ECG, pulse oximeter, NIBP, thermometer

injury of pulmonary microvessels (Sohara, 2008). Strategies to prevent the occurrence of REPE in clinical patients include avoiding strong negative pressure in the thorax when aspirating air or fluid, and during surgery making no specific effort to re-expand lung that has been collapsed for 12 hours or more; the lung should be allowed to re-expand progressively with time. Treatment of REPE is symptomatic.

Choice of anaesthetic agents

Anaesthetic agents must be chosen to provide analgesia and, in most cases, unconsciousness and muscle relaxation (Box 20.1). An exception would be a unilateral thoracotomy performed on standing horses, using only sedation and nerve blocks. This is possible because the intact mediastinum allows a horse to continue breathing when one pleural cavity is penetrated. For the majority of procedures, general anaesthesia is necessary, most frequently inhalation anaesthesia, and the choice of agents is influenced by the anaesthetist's preferences. Some anaesthetic agents have beneficial effects on the respiratory system. For example, the inhalation agents that decrease airway reactivity, ketamine induces bronchodilation, lidocaine IV prevents surgically-induced reflex bronchospasm, and atropine can block cholinergic bronchospasm. Except for some analgesic techniques, the selection of anaesthetic protocols is not specific for intrathoracic procedures but is governed by many factors including the patient's age and physical health status and the reason for performing the procedure. These have been discussed in the species chapters.

Analgesia

Thoracic surgery is described as being extremely painful. Choice of analgesia for thoracic surgery is influenced by the species of patient and the surgical approach. Analgesia for lateral thoracotomy, for example, can be provided by bolus, continuous infusion, or transdermal administration of an opioid, nerve blocks that include paravertebral or intercostal nerve blocks with bupivacaine, epidural morphine, interpleural bupivacaine, and a non-steroidal anti-inflammatory drug. Local infiltration with bupivacaine around the thoracoscopy ports appears to minimize discomfort in recovery.

An advantage of epidural opioid administration is the long duration of analgesia and lack of respiratory depression obtained compared with systemic administration of an opioid. Epidural administration of morphine, 0.1 mg/kg, or oxymorphone, 0.1 mg/kg, provided analgesia after thoracotomy in dogs for up to 24 hours, and at least for 10 hours, respectively (Popilskis et al., 1991; Pascoe & Dyson, 1993). Not all dogs in these studies were analgesic and some required rescue analgesia. Intercostal nerve blocks performed with bupivacaine for a lateral thoracotomy were found to provide analgesia similar to that obtained from epidural morphine (Pascoe & Dyson, 1993). A comparison of analgesic techniques in dogs after left thoracotomy revealed significant decreases in PaO_2 in dogs for the first 2 hours after subcutaneous administration of morphine compared with intercostal or interpleural injection of bupivacaine (Thompson & Johnson, 1991). Interpleural instillation of bupivacaine with repeat doses also provides equivalent and longer lasting analgesia for thoracotomy with less adverse impact on PaO_2 (Thompson & Johnson, 1991; Conzemius et al., 1994). In experimental dogs, lidocaine, 1.5 mg/kg, and bupivacaine, 1.5 mg/kg, were injected into the pericardial space to mimic interpleural administration in patients with a pericardial window (Bernard et al., 2006). Stroke volume was significantly decreased but the effect was not different between interpleural administration with or without access to the myocardium. None of these techniques provide analgesia for all animals, consequently, more than one method of analgesia should be included in the anaesthetic protocol.

Neuromuscular blockade

Respiratory movements do not cease in some dogs and cats despite ventilation to a low $PaCO_2$. In these patients, administration of a neuromuscular blocking agent (NMBA) may be necessary to facilitate the surgical procedure. Neuromuscular blockade is commonly used to provide complete muscle relaxation and controlled conditions for experimental intrathoracic surgery. Provision of adequate analgesia and unconsciousness is essential whenever an NMBA is used. Residual neuromuscular blockade during recovery from anaesthesia may contribute to hypoventilation and postoperative complications.

Monitoring

Monitoring of animals during anaesthesia has been discussed in detail in previous chapters. Essential monitoring will vary between patients and should be planned on an individual basis. Some patients that are healthy and without special intraoperative conditions may be adequately managed with a pulse oximeter, ECG, non-invasive blood pressure (NIBP) monitoring, and temperature. Other patients may have significant systemic disease or be relatively healthy but require specific management relevant

to the surgical procedure, and will be better managed with the inclusion of capnography, invasive pressure monitoring, and pH and blood gas analysis. Adequate arterial oxygenation will largely depend on whether the lungs are healthy or diseased and the mode of ventilation employed. Animals with preanaesthetic pulmonary contusions, pneumonia, or pulmonary collapse are at greater risk for hypoxaemia when anaesthetized and during thoracotomy. Medical treatment, such as pleurocentesis of fluid or air, or systemic antibiotics, can improve pulmonary function in these patients and should be done before anaesthesia. Monitoring of oxygen saturation using pulse oximetry in the pre-, intra-, and postoperative periods is essential and blood gas analysis should be performed for confirmation of accuracy, if available. Some pulse oximeters consistently provide values that are lower than that obtained from measurement of saturation by blood gas analysis. Controlled ventilation is necessary during thoracic surgery. End-tidal CO_2 ($ETCO_2$) monitoring is useful except when there is significant lung collapse during the surgical procedure, especially thoroscopy or thoracotomy. $ETCO_2$ is no longer representative of $PaCO_2$ when there is a severe ventilation–perfusion mismatch such that $ETCO_2$ may be in the normal range when the $PaCO_2$ is as high as 90 mmHg. Arterial blood gas analysis can be used to determine the accuracy of $ETCO_2$ measurement in the individual case. Alternatively, during a pause in the surgical procedure the tidal volume can be increased to see if there is a corresponding increase in $ETCO_2$, indicating that hypercarbia is present.

Surgery within the chest may obstruct blood flow in the aorta and vena cava or change the position of the heart and interfere with blood flow. The sound from a Doppler ultrasound probe over a peripheral artery may diminish or change character as blood flow is affected. Observation of a direct arterial pressure waveform may also warn of an acute decrease in blood pressure or cardiac output. Measurement of arterial blood pressure, either indirectly or invasively, is advisable. Monitoring of cardiac rhythm with an ECG is necessary to interpret dysrhythmias that may originate from preanaesthetic traumatic damage or cardiac disease, or from surgical manipulation.

Closure of the thorax

There may be a substantial amount of air remaining in the pleural cavity at the end of surgery, which will limit normal expansion of the lungs. Therefore, it is common practice to insert a chest tube to facilitate evacuation of this air at the end of surgery and during the recovery period. It is important to note, however, that the diameter of the chest tube is insufficient to allow movement of a normal tidal volume during inhalation and exhalation, and that hypoxemia may develop if the chest tube remains open during closure of subcutaneous tissues. Aspiration of the air from the chest and occlusion of the chest tube should improve oxygenation.

Recovery from anaesthesia

Specific attention must be paid to the adequacy of ventilation (CO_2 elimination), oxygenation, and the control of pain in patients recovering from anaesthesia for thoracic surgery. Animals with thoracic pain breathe shallowly, potentiating lung collapse and exacerbating inadequate gas exchange. Thoracic excursion, respiratory rate and pattern of breathing are used to assess ventilation with more information provided by measurement of $ETCO_2$ and blood gas analysis. A pulse oximeter should be used to track oxygenation before and after disconnection from the anaesthesia machine circuit. Supplementation with oxygen is usual after thoracotomy at least for a few hours. When SpO_2 is low, placing the patient in sternal position may serve to decrease ventilation–perfusion mismatch and improve oxygenation. Measurement of functional residual capacity (FRC) by helium dilution in lightly sedated healthy experimental dogs confirmed that FRC was significantly improved when the dogs were in sternal compared with lateral recumbency (Rozanski et al., 2010). Application of a circumferential thoracic bandage, such as is often applied after thoracotomy, resulted in a further significant decrease in FRC. Oxygenation should be measured after bandaging; tight bandages should be loosened to correct iatrogenic hypoxaemia.

ANAESTHESIA FOR SPECIFIC PROCEDURES

Diaphragmatic rupture in dogs and cats

Although the majority of diaphragmatic ruptures are repaired through an abdominal incision, the pleural cavity is open to the air and the procedure qualifies as a thoracotomy. The damage frequently occurs as a result of trauma and other injuries may have been incurred (Box 20.2). Most commonly in dogs and cats, the diaphragm is repaired first with any other abdominal trauma, such as abdominal wall lacerations, ruptured urinary bladder, or caesarian section. The patient is reanaesthetized at a later date for orthopaedic repair of fractured bones. The urgency of the surgery for diaphragm repair depends on the degree of respiratory compromise. Anaesthesia may be induced within a short time of admission to the hospital when breathing is laboured and oxgenation is tenuous. Ideally, anaesthesia can be postponed for up to 24 hours if oxygenation can be maintained to allow restoration of fluid balance and adequate evaluation of other organ functions. Management of anaesthesia is smoother when several hours have elapsed from the incident. Chronic diaphragmatic rupture, when the trauma occurred several months previously, may be associated

> **Box 20.2 Anaesthetic management of dogs and cats for diaphragmatic rupture repair**
>
> - Evaluate patient for severity of respiratory compromise and other organ trauma
> - Choose anaesthetic agents appropriate to individual patient
> - Preoxygenate before induction of anaesthesia
> - Premedicate with an opioid ± diazepam or midazolam, induction with ketamine, propofol, or alfaxalone
> - Intubate and maintain anaesthesia with an inhalation anaesthetic
> - Check SpO_2 immediately after induction and correct abnormal value with IPPV and/or change in body position
> - Be prepared for hypotension when organs are extracted from pleural cavity; treat with infusion of dobutamine or dopamine
> - Do not try to re-inflate collapsed lung
> - Continue to supply O_2 into recovery and monitor SpO_2
> - Options for analgesia include systemic opioid and epidural opioid ± incisional infiltration with bupivacaine

with significant cardiac dysrhythmias during surgical breakdown of adhesions. Anaesthetic requirement is often markedly reduced in these patients.

Choice of anaesthetic agents

The choice of anaesthetic agents must be made after listing the specific problems of the individual patient, including age, presence of brachycephalia, ASA physical status, and other damage that may have incurred such as traumatic myocarditis or haemorrhage. Anticholinergic agents would most likely be omitted in patients with pulmonary and myocardial contusions to avoid increased heart rates and potentiation of ventricular dysrhythmias. It should be remembered that while myocardial damage is likely present, indicators of damage such as premature ventricular complexes (PVCs) do not appear until approximately 36 hours after the initial trauma.

Premedication should not be heavy due to respiratory depression, unless incorporated into the anaesthesia induction sequence. For cats, buprenorphine, 0.01–0.02 mg/kg, or butorphanol, 0.2–0.4 mg/kg, IM or IV can be used, followed by induction of anaesthesia with the combination of ketamine, 5 mg/kg, and diazepam or midazolam, 0.25 mg/kg, given IV in increments 'to effect', and maintenance of anaesthesia with isoflurane or sevoflurane. Hydromorphone and oxymorphone, 0.05–0.1 mg/kg, IM or IV or methadone can be used where greater analgesia is required, however, these agents cause respiratory depression and the cats may vomit, causing greater respiratory distress in patients with already compromised breathing. Medetomidine and dexmedetomidine are not suitable choices as vomiting may be induced and cardiac output severely decreased. Anaesthesia may be induced with propofol or alfaxalone, although propofol is associated with hypotension in cats. The duration of butorphanol may be longer in cats (2.5 hours) than in dogs, but will require supplementation.

Dogs with acute diaphragmatic rupture should not be premedicated with opioids that induce vomiting. Vomiting should not occur after administration of butorphanol, buprenorphine, methadone, or fentanyl. Hydromorphone, oxymorphone, or morphine can be administered after the patient is anaesthetized, for example following premedication with fentanyl and midazolam. Induction of anaesthesia should be with an IV injectable agent such as ketamine, alfaxalone or propofol, with or without midazolam or diazepam, 0.2 mg/kg. Thiopental and propofol may potentiate ventricular dysrhythmias during anaesthesia. Lidocaine, 1–2 mg/kg, IV can be incorporated into the induction protocol and then continued as an infusion during anaesthesia, 0.025–0.05 mg/kg/min (1.5–3.0 mg/kg/h) IV where it will decrease the concentration of inhalation agent needed for anaesthesia. Anaesthesia is generally maintained by an inhalation agent. Nitrous oxide should not be administered until the abdomen is open and only used when oxygenation is adequate. N_2O must be turned off before the diaphragm is closed to avoid expansion of air remaining in the pleural cavity.

Epidural opioid administration may be indicated for prolonged postoperative analgesia in some patients.

Anaesthetic management

Sedation may adversely affect the animal's ability to breathe adequately and result in hypoxaemia. Therefore, premedication and induction of anaesthesia are generally administered within a few minutes of each other and the patient is kept under direct observation after administration of any sedative, analgesic, or anaesthetic agents. If possible, the abdomen is clipped before anaesthesia while the animal is being held in a standing upright position. When a full stomach is suspected, the animal is also held upright during the induction phase until the endotracheal tube is placed and the cuff inflated.

There are five specific areas of concern during anaesthesia for repair of ruptured diaphragm:

1. *Artificial ventilation is essential.* The depth of breathing may severely decrease immediately after induction of anaesthesia and artificial ventilation should be initiated. Inspiratory pressure should initially be limited to less than 20 cmH$_2$O in an attempt to avoid barotrauma. Depth of breathing should be altered to accommodate stiff and compressed lungs by using a fast rate and small breaths, i.e. 15–20

breaths/min and 11 mL/kg. The anaesthetist who is providing manual ventilation should be focused on monitoring the patient and providing consistent and appropriate ventilation. Use of a mechanical ventilator will allow the anaesthetist to focus more on the patient but the breathing circuit pressure gauge must be observed frequently to ensure that an increase in airway pressure is recognized immediately.

2. *Oxygenation may be influenced by body position.* The patient may become hypoxaemic immediately after induction of anaesthesia and the pulse oximeter should be attached as early as possible. Oxygenation may be improved by the start of IPPV. Sometimes lung collapse is greater in one body position, for example, the dog is hypoxaemic in left lateral recumbency but not in right lateral or dorsal oblique recumbency and in these cases a change in body position may improve oxygenation.

3. *Hypotension occurring when abdominal organs are removed from the chest.* Hypotension can develop any time after induction of anaesthesia but specifically may occur during surgery when the abdominal organs are retrieved from the thoracic cavity. The probable mechanism is vasodilation in the abdominal organs resulting in sequestration of blood. Treatment with a large bolus of crystalloid fluid is not advisable as return of vascular tone later creates hypervolaemia that may induce pulmonary oedema. Management of low blood pressure in this situation is best with an IV infusion of vasoactive agent such as dobutamine or dopamine, 5–7 µg/kg/min.

4. *Do not re-inflate collapsed lung.* Lung that has been collapsed for several hours by compression from the intestines and liver will have the appearance of a light-coloured liver. The lung should be allowed to re-expand at a slow rate determined by normal breathing and not by delivery of artificially high volume breaths. Re-expansion of the lung in this clinical condition may result in barotrauma and subsequent development of life-threatening generalized pulmonary oedema.

5. *Dysrhythmias during surgery.* The occurrence of PVCs during this surgery is common in dogs. Lidocaine is the treatment of choice when the frequency of PVCs is judged adversely to affect blood pressure. Lidocaine can be injected as a bolus of 1–2 mg/kg IV that will last 10–15 minutes or the bolus can be followed by a continuous infusion for the duration of anaesthesia. Lidocaine infusion is not generally recommended in cats, but a bolus of lidocaine, 1 mg/kg, IV can be administered provided that the volume injected is precisely controlled.

Recovery from anaesthesia

After surgery, oxygen should be supplied into recovery and oxygenation checked with a pulse oximeter when the patient is switched to air breathing. Nasal or cage oxygen supplementation, or 'flow-by' oxygen with a mask, oxygen cylinder and regulator, may be needed. Analgesia is continued by means generally recommended for ovariohysterectomy, unless other surgical repairs have been performed and then analgesia must be matched to those procedures.

Patent ductus arteriosus (PDA)

This abnormality is frequently detected in young animals by auscultation of a characteristic machinery murmur. Echocardiography will determine the direction of blood flow through the defect, the size of the defect, and the extent of myocardial abnormality. Repair may involve either sedation or anaesthesia without thoracotomy for insertion of a catheter into a vein or artery to introduce a device that will occlude the PDA, or a thoracotomy for direct surgical ligation or to facilitate occlusion. Anaesthesia will be the same for the two techniques but thoracotomy includes specific management of ventilation and oxygenation and increased attention to provision of analgesia. Anaesthesia should be relatively straightforward in the younger animals but may require greater attention to treatment of hypotension in dogs with cardiac abnormalities. Both occlusion achieved by catheter introduction and surgical ligation can be associated with significant haemorrhage from a tear at the PDA or further down the vascular tree.

A PDA is associated with low diastolic and mean arterial pressures that contribute to hypotension during the first part of anaesthesia (Box 20.3). Mean arterial pressure increases after ligation or occlusion and, therefore, hypotension should be managed by use of dobutamine or dopamine which can be discontinued at that time. Infusion of IV fluids to treat hypotension will result in fluid

overload after ligation and pulmonary oedema in some patients. Animals less than 3 months of age or lean body type may be at risk for hypoglycaemia during and after anaesthesia and should receive an infusion of 5% dextrose in water (D5W) at 3 mL/kg/h with an acetated or lactated Ringer's solution infusion rate of 3 mL/kg/h. Blood glucose should be measured at the start and end of anaesthesia. Dogs and cats with a PDA may be extremely small such that monitoring may be more difficult than usual and requires intense concentration on the part of the anaesthetist. Older dogs may have left atrial and left ventricular enlargement, pulmonary hypertension and oedema and dictate that the anaesthetic management be adjusted to the inadequacies of cardiovascular function.

Choice of anaesthetic agents

Several anaesthetic drug protocols have been used satisfactorily and all include opioid administration for premedication. Induction of anaesthesia with etomidate or alfaxalone will be less likely to potentiate hypotension. In dogs, premedication with fentanyl and midazolam IV can be used to decrease significantly the dose of propofol required for tracheal intubation. Thiopental is least popular in these patients as it may further decrease blood pressure and sensitize the myocardium to dysrhythmias during surgical manipulation. Anaesthesia is usually maintained with an inhalation agent and, for these patients, sevoflurane or isoflurane are superior to halothane. Lidocaine infusion in dogs will further decrease the inhalant concentration and protect against surgically-induced dysrhythmias. A continuous infusion of fentanyl, 5–8 µg/kg/h, IV in dogs is another option for continuous analgesia and reduction in inhalant anaesthetic concentration.

Analgesia for lateral thoracotomy should include intercostal nerve blocks using bupivacaine, 1 mg/kg, with the balance of the total dose of bupivacaine instilled into the thorax at the end of the surgical procedure for interpleural analgesia. Epidural administration of morphine or oxymorphone will provide additional long-term analgesia.

Anaesthetic management

Infusion of balanced electrolyte solution IV during anaesthesia should be restricted to 6 mL/kg/h to avoid fluid overload after ligation. The fluid rate should be reduced proportionately when D5W, 3 mL/kg/h, is infused for paediatric patients. Methods to control and measure accurately fluid infusion in the little animals should be in place (syringes, syringe driver, burette). Ligation of the PDA is accompanied by a significant increase in diastolic and mean arterial pressures, sometimes accompanied by bradycardia. The ECG should be observed for PVCs but they rarely require treatment. Infusion of dobutamine or

---

Box 20.3 Anaesthetic management of PDA

- Anticipate hypotension; treat with dobutamine or dopamine, and not by fluid challenge
- Limit total IV fluid administration to ≤6 mL/kg/h
- Monitor and control blood glucose in patients <3 months of age
- Thoracotomy requires IPPV and increased use of techniques for analgesia
- Monitor SpO₂ in recovery; supplemental O₂ and blood gas analysis if needed/available
- Thoracic bandage may limit breathing

dopamine is usually discontinued at this time. Management for recovery from anaesthesia is the same as for any thoracotomy.

Persistent right aortic arch (PRAA)

The main concern for anaesthesia of dogs with PRAA is the presence of pneumonia and its impact on oxygenation. Preoxygenation is recommended. Anaesthesia should be induced with the animal in upright position, as for any patient at risk for regurgitation, and the trachea intubated and cuff inflated before the patient is allowed to assume lateral recumbency. There are no specific anaesthetic agents recommended for this procedure. Anaesthetic management follows the principles of management of a thoracotomy.

Thoracoscopy

Thoracoscopy has been used in dogs and cats for lung and mediastinal mass biopsy, pericardectomy, lung lobectomy, ligation of the thoracic duct, ligation of a persistent right aortic arch, lavage for pyothorax, and investigation of spontaneous pneumothorax (Radlinsky, 2009). Dogs may be positioned in lateral, dorsal or sternal recumbency depending on the area to be viewed. The most common complications are inadequate oxygenation, hypercarbia, haemorrhage, and trauma to tissues outside the area of view. Thoracic insufflation is rarely required and should be discouraged. Incremental positive insufflation of the pleural cavity in anaesthetized experimental dogs was found to decrease cardiac output significantly by 21% at an interpleural pressure of 3 mmHg and by 39.4% at a pressure of 6 mmHg (Daly et al., 2002). Monitoring the patient by usual means may be misleading as to the extent of cardiac depression since, in this study, animals' SpO_2 did not reach 90% until an interpleural pressure of 10 mmHg, at which point cardiac output was decreased by 51.5% from baseline.

Bilateral lung inflation may obscure the surgeon's view and this is partly offset by decreasing the tidal volume and increasing the respiratory rate. The surgeon's view may be expanded by use of OLV, as previously described. Spontaneous thoracic movement can be controlled by administration of an NMBA and the relaxation will facilitate the surgical procedure. Management of neuromuscular blockade is described in several previous chapters.

Conversion from thoroscopy to thoracotomy should always be anticipated when preparing for a thoroscopy procedure. Reasons for the conversion include an inability to ventilate the patient with the amount of lung collapse required for surgical view, adhesions or large lesions that are not conducive to thoracoscopic treatment, a procedure that is taking too long, or because of difficulties relating to surgeon inexperience.

Analgesia can be provided by administration of a systemic opioid. Epidural opioid analgesia can be provided if the surgical procedure is assessed as painful. Postoperative pain after thoracoscopy has been ascribed to pressure of the ports on intercostal nerves. Infiltration with 0.5% bupivacaine, up to 2.5 mg/kg for dogs or 2 mg/kg for cats, around the port sites appears to prevent local pain in the recovery. Any bupivacaine remaining from the local infiltration can be instilled into the pleural cavity. Excision of pericardium is thought not to be a specific contraindication to interpleural bupivacaine.

REFERENCES

Beck-Schimmer, B., Schimmer, R.C., 2010. Perioperative tidal volume and intraoperative open lung strategy in healthy lungs: where are we going? Best Prac Res Clin Anaesthesiol 24, 199–210.

Bernard, F., Kudnig, S.T., Monnet, E., 2006. Hemodynamic effects of interpleural lidocaine and bupivacaine combination in anesthetized dogs with and without an open pericardium. Vet Surg 35, 252–258.

Bigatello, L.M., Pesenti, A., 2009. Ventilator-induced lung injury (Editorial). Anesthesiology 111, 699–700.

Brodsky, J.B., 2009. Lung separation and the difficult airway. Br J Anaesth 103 (Suppl), i66–i75.

Caccamo, R., Twedt, D.C., Buracco, P., et al., 2007. Endoscopic bronchial anatomy in the cat. J Feline Med Surg 9, 140–149.

Conzemius, M.G., Brockman, D.J., King, L.G., et al., 1994. Analgesia in dogs after intercostal thoracotomy: A clinical trial comparing intravenous buprenorphine and interpleural bupivacaine. Vet Surg 23, 291–298.

Curley, G.F., Kevin, L.G., Laffey, J.G., 2009. Mechanical ventilation: Taking its toll on the lung. Anesthesiology 111, 701–703.

Daly, C.M., Swalec-Tobias, K., Tobias, A.H., et al., 2002. Cardiopulmonary effects of intrathoracic insufflation in dogs. J Am Anim Hosp Assoc 38, 515–520.

Duggan, M., Kavanagh, B.P., 2010. Perioperative modifications of respiratory function. Best Prac Res Clin Anaesthesiol 24, 145–155.

Fossum, T.W., Evering, W.N., Miller, M.W., et al., 1992. Severe bilateral fibrosing pleuritis associated with chronic chylothorax in five cats and two dogs. J Am Vet Med Assoc 201, 317–324.

Jiménez Peláez, M., Jolliffe, C., 2012. Thoracoscopic foreign body removal and right middle lung lobectomy to treat pyothorax in a dog. J Small Anim Pract 53, 240–244.

Kudnig, S.T., Monnet, E., Riquelme, M., et al., 2006. Effect of positive end-expiratory pressure on oxygen delivery during 1-lung ventilation in thoracoscopy in normal dogs. Vet Surg 35, 534–542.

Kudnig, S.T., Monnet, E., Riquelme, R., et al., 2003. Effect of one-lung ventilation on oxygen delivery in anesthetized dogs with an open thoracic cavity. Am J Vet Res 64, 443–448.

Leasure, C.S., Ellisone, G.W., Roberts, J.F., et al., 2011. Occlusion of the thoracic duct using ultrasonically activated shears in six dogs. Vet Surg 40, 802–810.

Miller, C.J., 2007. Approach to the respiratory patient. Vet Clin Small Anim 37, 861–878.

Narayanaswamy, M., McRae, K., Slinger, P., et al., 2009. Choosing a lung isolation device for thoracic surgery: A randomized trial of three bronchial blockers versus double-lumen tubes. Anesth Analg 108, 1097–1101.

Pascoe, P.J., Dyson, D.H., 1993. Analgesia after lateral thoracotomy

in dogs epidural morphine vs. intercostal bupivacaine. Vet Surg 22, 141–147.

Popilskis, S., Kohn, D., Sanchez, J.A., et al., 1991. Epidural vs. intramuscular oxymorphone analgesia after thoracotomy in dogs. Vet Surg 20, 462–467.

Radlinsky, M.G., 2009. Need for conversion from thoracoscopy to thoracotomy in small animals. Vet Clin Small Anim 39, 977–984.

Rozanski, E.A., Bedenice, D., Lofgren, J., et al., 2010. The effect of body position, sedation, and thoracic bandaging on functional residual capacity in healthy deep-chested dogs. Can J Vet Res 74, 34–39.

Soderstrom, M.J., Gilson, S.D., Gulbas, N., 1995. Fatal reexpansion pulmonary edema in a kitten following surgical correction of pectus excavatum. J Am Anim Hosp Assoc 31, 133–136.

Sohara, Y., 2008. Reexpansion pulmonary edema. Ann Thorac Cardiovasc Surg 14, 205–209.

Stampley, A.R., Waldron, D.R., 1993. Reexpansion pulmonary edema after surgery to repair a diaphragmatic hernia in a cat. J Am Vet Med Assoc 203, 1699–1701.

Tarver, R.D., Broderick, L.S., Conces, D.J. Jr, 1996. Reexpansion pulmonary edema. J Thorac Imaging 11, 198–209.

Thompson, S.E., Johnson, J.M., 1991. Analgesia in dogs after intercostal thoracotomy A comparison of morphine, selective intercostal nerve block, and interpleural regional analgesia with bupivacaine. Vet Surg 20, 73–77.

Tusman, G., Böhm, S.H., 2010. Prevention and reversal of lung collapse during the intra-operative period. Best Prac Res Clin Anaesthesiol 24, 183–197.

Chapter |21|

Complications

INTRODUCTION

The layout of this chapter is based on identification of an abnormal behaviour or measurement in the perianaesthetic period, such as an arrhythmia, cyanosis, hypotension, or laboured breathing. Sometimes the cause of the abnormality is immediately obvious, such as hypotension following injection of an anaesthetic agent or change in patient body position, other times it is necessary to work through a checklist to identify the origin of the abnormality. Potential causes are listed for abnormal signs and have been classified according to categories to aid differential diagnosis. The following eight categories comprise a good checklist when troubleshooting a patient's problem: Drugs, Equipment, Mechanical, Other patient problems (than cardiac or respiratory) and procedure, Cardiac, Respiratory, Allergic, and Toxic. The first letter of each category forms the acronym DEMOCRAT, which is helpful to ensure a thorough and systematic evaluation of the patient is performed. Suggestions for management of each cause are included and further explanations are presented in the following boxes and text. Details of events leading up to cardiac arrest and the current approach to cardiopulmonary cerebral resuscitation (CPCR) are given in the next chapter. Hypothermia and hyperthermia are covered in Chapter 2. Regurgitation is discussed in Chapter 15 and the ruminant chapters. Myopathy and neuropathy that may occur after anaesthesia in horses is discussed in Chapter 11.

ABNORMAL BREATHING

An animal's breathing pattern during anaesthesia is not the same as in the conscious state, varies between species, and may be influenced by the specific anaesthetic agent administered. The breathing pattern may also be changed by the patient's current health status, acid–base status, depth of anaesthesia, or other conditions that may develop during anaesthesia.

Abnormal or laboured breathing

Breathing that is gasping, jerky, shallow, or has excessively large thoracic excursions, flexion of head and neck, and/or tracheal airflow that is zero, reduced, or increased, is usually associated with abnormalities that may have serious consequences for the patient (Table 21.1, Boxes 21.1-3).

Bronchodilation

Albuterol (USA name) is the same as salbutamol (International name) and is administered by inhalation for its direct β_2-adrenergic agonist effect on bronchial smooth muscle as rescue medicine for bronchoconstriction in humans. The stated time of onset is 5–20 minutes. There are several products commercially available and Ventolin® is the only product that does not contain ethanol as a co-solvent. Albuterol/salbutamol has been used to treat horses with recurrent airway obstruction (RAO, 'heaves') that have increased airway resistance and decreased lung compliance from bronchoconstriction, airway wall oedema and mucus accumulation in small airways (Derksen et al., 1999; Bertin et al., 2011). Measurements of pulmonary function determined that 360 µg of aerosolized albuterol/salbutamol in conscious horses with RAO caused significant bronchodilation and that increasing the dose to 720 µg did not significantly enhance bronchodilation or increase the duration of action (Derksen et al., 1999). Onset of bronchodilation was rapid within 5 minutes and the effect lasted 0.5–3 hours. Another experimental study (Bertin et al., 2011) administered albuterol (Ventolin) by metered-dose inhaler that delivered 90 µg albuterol/actuation (puff) in 10 conscious horses with RAO. Measured changes in transpulmonary pressures and lung compliance confirmed that the average dose of albuterol/salbutamol required for maximal bronchodilation in the horses studied was 6 actuations (540 µg) but that there was a large variation between horses, with maximum bronchodilation achieved between 2 (180 µg) and 10 (900 µg) actuations.

Administration of albuterol/salbutamol may be an effective treatment of hypoxaemia in anaesthetized horses. In a clinical study, horses anaesthetized for surgery for colic were administered albuterol into the Y-piece of the circle breathing circuit during inhalation at a dose rate of 2 µg/kg (Robertson & Bailey, 2002). Arterial blood collected 20 minutes later revealed a significant increase in average PaO_2 from 8.25 kPa (62 mmHg) to 15.8 kPa (119 mmHg). The bronchodilation may have improved ventilation in underventilated parts of the lungs and thereby increased O_2 uptake. No significant changes in

heart rate (HR) or blood pressures were recorded. A dose rate of 2 µg/kg (equivalent to 10 actuations for a 450 kg horse) is higher than the requirement for bronchodilation measured in conscious horses, and it may be that less albuterol/salbutamol will produce satisfactory results in some anaesthetized horses.

Bronchoconstriction is also a component of an allergic or anaphylactic reaction. Albuterol was administered as part of treatment to one horse that developed respiratory failure in response to injection of contrast media during imaging (Gunkel et al., 2004). The response to albuterol was minimal, although subsequent injection of atropine, also a bronchodilator, produced a slight positive effect. The clinicians involved with this horse were persistent with their heroic efforts despite an extremely low PaO_2 of 4.26–5.2 kPa (32–39 mmHg) that increased to 5.6 kPa (42 mmHg) after the horse was standing. Treatment included albuterol/salbutamol, atropine, furosemide, and O_2, and the horse survived to be reanaesthetized without complications one month later.

Albuterol/salbutamol has been studied in healthy cats with drug-induced bronchoconstriction using measurements of lung function by whole body plethysmography (Leemans et al., 2009). One puff from a metered-dose inhaler (Ventolin®) induced a significant antispasmodic effect lasting for 4 hours. In an emergency situation in cats with asthma, further doses may be given, such as an additional dose every 30 minutes for up to 4 hours (Padrid, 2006).

Tachypnoea or panting

Tachypnoea or panting may result in hyperventilation or hypoventilation depending on the adequacy of alveolar ventilation. Panting is a common side effect of opioid administration in dogs, most frequently seen with morphine, oxymorphone and hydromorphone and less frequently with butorphanol and buprenorphine. Rapid respiratory rates may be seen, especially in small dogs, during inhalation anaesthesia. Small ruminants have a relatively fast respiratory rate that generally decreases with increasing depth of anaesthesia. α_2-Agonist sedative administration to healthy or febrile horses occasionally causes short-lived increases in respiratory rates to 40–100 breaths/min, with minimal decreases in $PaCO_2$. No specific treatment is recommended for the tachypnoea.

Differential diagnoses of a faster than normal respiratory rate include:

- Light plane of anaesthesia
- Hypoxaemia
- High inspired CO_2 from an incorrectly connected circuit, exhausted CO_2 absorbent, or a malfunctioning one-way valve in a rebreathing circuit
- Hyperthermia from excessive application of external heat, anaesthetic-induced impairment of

Table 21.1 Abnormal or laboured breathing: causes and management

Species	Causes	Management
Drugs		
All species	Excessive depth of anaesthesia, immediately preceding (or sometimes following) cardiac arrest	Check pulse exists Discontinue anaesthetic administration, flush circuit with O_2, may need dobutamine or antagonists
	Anaesthesia too light can result in jerky breathing, may be accompanied by body tremors, brisk palpebral reflex	Increase anaesthetic administration
	Fentanyl-induced chest splinting	Discontinue fentanyl, spontaneous ventilation if oxygenation adequate, ± naloxone
Dogs, cats	Residual curarization after NMBA administration	Check response to peripheral nerve stimulation and eye position, ± IPPV, administer edrophonium or neostigmine
Equipment		
All species	Airway obstruction from kinked ETT, endobronchial intubation, oesophagal intubation, ETT too small, mucus plug in ETT, by pharyngeal or tracheal foreign body after extubation	Assess endotracheal tube placement and size, pharyngeal packing removed?
	Bain disconnect at ETT connector resulting in hypercarbia, non-rebreathing circuit broken or incorrectly connected	Check assembly and integrity of circuit
	Rebreathing from one-way valve malfunction, exhausted CO_2 absorbent in circle circuit, rebreathing diagnosed by capnography waveform (see Fig. 2.33A)	No movement of one-way valve (open or shut) with breathing – dislodge and clean, absent valve flap – replace it, check absorbent indicator colour – change it if 75% used or when capnography indicates rebreathing
Mechanical		
Dogs, cats	External chest compression	Remove compression
	Airway obstruction when not intubated, e.g. brachycephalic breeds, nasal polyp, retropharyngeal abscess, neoplasia, collapsing trachea, laryngeal paralysis, swelling after oral surgery	Endotracheal intubation, breathing may be easier with sedation for collapsing trachea or laryngeal paralysis, for postsurgical swelling obstruction – dexamethasone, 0.5 mg/kg, IV and reanaesthetize and reintubate with head elevated for an hour, ± tracheotomy (see Box 21.1)
	Laryngospasm, occurs in cats most frequently and resolves with repositioning	Extend head and neck, open mouth, pull tongue rostrally, ± topical lidocaine on larynx, ± tracheal intubation
Horses	Laryngeal hemiplegia	Endo- or nasotracheal intubation
	Nasal mucosa congestion limits air flow after extubation	Assess swelling before extubation, oral or nasal ETT until horse stands, ± phenylephrine spray into nasal meatus
	Tracheal obstruction by blood clot from sinus, pharyngeal, dental surgery	Head elevated/nose down during surgery, leave orotracheal tube until standing and extubate with head down, if tracheotomy during anaesthesia – be prepared to extract large clot
	Laryngospasm, or total laryngeal paralysis, most commonly seen when trying to stand during recovery from anaesthesia, usually complete obstruction in horses until unconscious or dead	Nasotracheal or orotracheal intubation when horse goes unconscious + O_2 by demand valve, ± emergency tracheotomy (see Box 21.1)
	Abdominal distension (colic) causing hypoxia	Nasogastric tube, ± caecal trocharization, immediate induction of anaesthesia (if in clinic) with IPPV rapid RR with O_2 before transport to OR

Table 21.1 Continued

Species	Causes	Management
Llamas	Obligate nasal breathers, nasal mucosal congestion causes airway obstruction	Elevate head during anaesthesia to avoid congestion, sternal position as soon as surgery ends, ± nasotracheal intubation until animal sternal enough time for congestion to resolve
Pigs	Laryngospasm, or pharyngeal obstruction from flexed head/neck	Topical lidocaine on larynx, O_2, dexamethasone IV, put head and neck in normal position

Other patient problems & procedure

Species	Causes	Management
All species	Hypoxaemia from blood loss Pain/inadequate analgesia thoracic or upper abdominal surgery	Restore blood volume, blood transfusion Increase analgesia medication
Dogs, cats	Cervical/thoracic spinal cord damage (big dog-little dog-cat-piglet trauma)	Measure SpO_2, supply O_2, IPPV when anaesthetized

Cardiac

Species	Causes	Management
All species	Cerebral hypoxia from hypotension, severe hypercarbia, or cardiac failure	Monitor circulation, cardiovascular support, ± IPPV, define specific cause

Respiratory

Species	Causes	Management
All species	Pulmonary oedema: excessive negative intrathoracic pressure in response to hypoxia, laryngospasm, airway obstruction (see Box 21.2)	Relieve airway obstruction, measure PaO_2, furosemide IV, supply O_2 by nasal tube
Dogs, cats	Hypoxaemia, hypercarbia from limited lung expansion: flail chest, pneumothorax, pleural effusion, pulmonary oedema	Supply O_2, treat individual cause

Allergic

Species	Causes	Management
Dogs, cats	Bronchoconstriction: feline asthma Anaphylactic shock: thiopental, radiological contrast agents	Albuterol/salbutamol inhaled (1 or 2 actuations), see text CPCR or circulatory and respiratory support (see Box 21.3)
Horses	Bronchoconstriction: recurrent airway obstruction (heaves), contrast agent, blood transfusion	Atropine, albuterol/salbutamol inhaled (6–10 actuations/adult horse), see text, antihistamine, ACVC if hypotensive
Ruminants	Bronchoconstriction: aspiration of ruminal fluid	Head down, O_2, avoid IPPV, postpone surgery, antibiotic, monitor PaO_2

Toxic

Species	Causes	Management
All species	Acute release of vasoactive substances from manipulation of ischaemic tissues	Decrease anaesthetic administration, treat hypotension and low cardiac output

NMBA: Neuromuscular blocking agent; ETT: endotracheal tube; OR: operating room/theatre, CPCR: cardiopulmonary cerebral resuscitation (see Chapter 22).

Box 21.1 **Tracheotomy**

An emergency tracheotomy should be a rare occurrence. Preferably, airway obstruction should be anticipated and either avoided by modification of anaesthetic management or by performing a tracheotomy aseptically under local or general anaesthesia before induction or before recovery from anaesthesia.

Technique in dogs and cats

The animal should be positioned on its back with a sandbag or roll of towels placed under its neck, and the forelimbs pulled caudally. The skin should be incised midline over the first to the eighth tracheal rings and the trachea exposed by separation of the sternohyoideus muscles. The trachea may be incised between the third and fourth or fourth and fifth tracheal rings to approximately 40% of the circumference. A suture placed around the distal tracheal ring, or around the proximal and distal rings, will be helpful in manipulating the trachea during insertion of the tracheotomy tube (Fig. 21.1). The diameter of the tube should be only slightly smaller than the size normally used for orotracheal intubation. The tube should be inserted gently and secured so that it cannot be moved. The incision should remain open to avoid subcutaneous emphysema, although a few sutures may be placed at either end if the incision is exceptionally long. Sterile gauze should be placed between the incision and the external part of the tracheotomy tube, and the tube secured by

non-adhesive tapes tied around the neck. Postoperative nursing care will be easier if a tracheotomy tube with an inner cannula is used. The external end of most tracheotomy tubes will connect directly to an anaesthesia circuit. Care should be taken to prevent the weight of the breathing circuit from rotating the tracheotomy tube (cuffed or uncuffed), which will abrade the tracheal mucosa.

Technique in horses

An emergency tracheotomy is performed with the horse standing or recumbent. The best site for incision is midcervical ventral midline, where the sternocephalic muscles diverge and the omohyoid muscles converge (Honnas, 1999). If there is time, the hair is clipped and cleaned for a surgical procedure. Local anaesthetic solution is infiltrated subcutaneously for an elective tracheotomy. A 4–6 cm (1.5–2.5 inch) incision is made midline through the skin and subcutis and the paired sternothyrohyoideus muscles are separated by dissection to expose the trachea. An annular ligament between two tracheal rings is incised transversely to separate the tracheal rings enough to allow insertion of a tracheotomy tube. The tracheal rings should not be incised longitudinally because healing may result in a tracheal stricture. Further details about types of tubes and care of the tracheotomy site should be obtained from an equine medicine and surgery textbook.

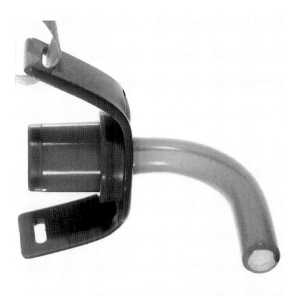

Figure 21.1 A tracheotomy tube is a short tube with a right-angled bend. Tracheotomy tubes may be plain or with a cuff similar to an endotracheal tube, and may have an inside sleeve that can easily be removed for cleaning. Some tracheotomy tubes may have a central solid obturator to provide stiffness and a rounded end for initial insertion. Tracheotomy tubes for horses may be constructed of metal, and of a different design whereby the tube is in two halves with flanges that insert both rostrally and caudally within the trachea to ensure retention.

Box 21.2 **Pulmonary oedema**

Cats

There are both published and many anecdotal reports of fatal pulmonary oedema associated with ketamine anaesthesia in cats (Van der Linde-Sipman et al., 1992). Pulmonary oedema has developed during anaesthesia, observed during recovery from anaesthesia or developed several hours after anaesthesia. The anaesthetic protocol xylazine–ketamine was initially under suspicion but protocols including a variety of preanaesthetic drugs with ketamine have been involved. The occurrence is unpredictable as one clinician may see an isolated case and then not another for 10 years whereas another clinician may see several in one week. The cause of the pulmonary oedema is not clear but immediate development after induction of anaesthesia may be a consequence of pulmonary hypertension while the delayed response may follow myocardial ischaemia. Pre-existing cardiac disease as a contributing cause cannot be ruled out. In a survey of 120 cats with hypertrophic cardiomyopathy, 15 developed congestive heart failure in association with anaesthesia, of which nine cats received ketamine and one cat received tiletamine–zolazepam (Rush et al., 2002). Cardiac auscultation before anaesthesia to identify a murmur is recommended, even in young apparently healthy cats. The need for treatment is urgent and includes O_2 and diuretic therapy.

Dogs

There is little reported on pulmonary oedema associated with anaesthesia in dogs. Pulmonary oedema developed in one dog following induction of anaesthesia with diazepam–ketamine (Boutureira et al., 2007). Treatment included postponing surgery, administration of O_2 by nasal insufflation and furosemide, 2 mg/kg, IV. Abnormality of

cardiac rhythm (PVCs) was recorded the following day and for 24 hours. Anaesthesia with different agents 4 days later for resection of rectal masses was without complication.

Horses

There are anecdotal cases of frothy fluid appearing in the endotracheal tube soon after induction of anaesthesia with xylazine–ketamine. Most reports of pulmonary oedema in horses cite first observation during recovery from anaesthesia (Kollias-Baker et al., 1993; Ball & Trim, 1996; Borer, 2005; Holbrook et al., 2007). In these situations, the cause is usually strong negative intrathoracic pressures as the result of laboured breathing during hypoxia from lung collapse or air embolism, or airway obstruction after extubation from laryngospasm, excessive nasal mucosal congestion or oedema, or abnormal body position such as a kinked head and neck or nostril occlusion while in a head pressing stance. Hypoxaemia increases capillary permeability further contributing to oedema formation. Fluid will pour from the nostrils when the horse is standing. Treatment includes administration of O_2 15 L/min by insufflation through a nasal tube, and furosemide, 1 mg/kg, IV. Blood gas analysis will determine the duration of O_2 therapy, which may be required for up to 48 hours. Other pharmacological agents will be necessary, such as an antibiotic and NSAID, especially when the horse has developed neurological deficits.

Ruminants

Pulmonary oedema in sheep has been reported following administration of xylazine and other α_2-agonists. Hypoxaemia and pulmonary oedema with subsequent death occurred in a sheep following anaesthesia with xylazine–ketamine (Stegmann, 2000).

---

thermoregulation, bacteraemia, or malignant hyperthermia.

Opioid-induced panting is usually controllable by intermittent positive pressure ventilation (IPPV). Depth of anaesthesia should be assessed using the known amount of anaesthetic agent administered and observation of eye signs and reflexes. The anaesthesia machine and circuit should be checked for faults and corrected. Hyperthermia should be treated by removal of external heating devices and application of ice packs if considered necessary. Malignant hyperthermia is usually differentiated from other forms of hyperthermia by the production of excessive amounts of CO_2 seen as a rapid increase in indicator colour and temperature of the CO_2 absorbent, tachycardia, hypertension, and a pH and blood gas analysis confirming respiratory and metabolic acidoses (see Chapter 2).

Irregular breathing patterns

Some irregular breathing patterns observed during anaesthesia indicate respiratory centre depression but may be characteristic of a particular anaesthetic agent, such as ketamine. Some breathing patterns occur frequently and are considered to be a 'normal' abnormality. Irregular breathing is an indication that respiratory control is impaired and that fluctuations in PaO_2 and $PaCO_2$ are probably occurring.

- Cheyne–Stokes: The depth of breathing is at first shallow but becomes progressively deeper. Breathing then gradually decreases in volume and may cease before the pattern begins again. This crescendo–decrescendo pattern of breathing is commonly observed in horses anaesthetized with xylazine and ketamine.

Box 21.3 **Anaphylaxis and allergic reactions**

Anaphylaxis can be caused by either an anaphylactic or anaphylactoid reaction, they have the same clinical appearance and are treated identically (Waddell, 2010). Onset of circulatory collapse may be within 1 minute or may be delayed 30 minutes after exposure to the initiating substance. In dogs, the shock organ is the liver resulting in portal hypertension, and in cats and horses the lung is the shock organ and bronchoconstriction contributes to respiratory distress. Clinical signs include respiratory distress, bradycardia and extreme hypotension, and dogs and cats that are conscious will vomit and defaecate. In mild allergic reactions, dogs and cats may exhibit swollen eyelids and lips, bright red colour on the inside of the ears and between the toes, and flushed pink abdominal skin, all of which generally respond to administration of diphenhydramine, 2 mg/kg, IM.

Causes

Anaesthetic drugs: morphine, meperidine/pethidine, thiopental, atracurium, rocuronium, procaine HCl
Antibiotics: procaine penicillin
Blood products or substitutes: blood, plasma, hetastarch, dextran
Radiographic contrast agent injected IV, intraarterial, or intrathecal for angiography, pyelography, myelography, computed tomography (CT), and MRI

Management

CPCR if cardiac arrest or severe hypotension, including epinephrine, 0.015 mg/kg, and O_2. Hypotension is treated with rapid infusion of crystalloid fluid 20–30 mL/kg in dogs and 10–20 mL/kg in cats and horses, hetastarch 5 mL/kg, and dopamine, 7–10 µg/kg/min. Blood pressure and CRT response are reassessed and further fluid administered as indicated.

Other drugs that may be needed are diphenhydramine, 1–2 mg/kg, IV for dogs and cats, and options for treatment of bronchoconstriction are aminophylline for dogs and cats, 5–10 mg/kg, IV respectively, atropine, 0.02–0.04 mg/kg, IV for dogs and cats, or 0.01–0.02 mg/kg for horses, and inhaled albuterol/salbutamol (for dose rates see text under abnormal breathing).

Continue to monitor following resuscitation for evidence of prolonged clotting time and disseminated intravascular coagulation (DIC) and treat appropriately. Antibiotic therapy and intestinal protectants are advisable if there is blood in faeces or vomitus indicating mucosal damage.

Significance for future anaesthesia

A recent editorial describes the problems with differentiation between types and mechanisms of anaphylaxis (Armitage-Chan, 2010). The article cites the limited number of published cases of anaphylaxis in animals, despite the much higher number of cases seen clinically (confirmed by this author's experience of a relatively large number of allergic/anaphylactic cases). The link between documented existing allergies in a patient and potential adverse reaction to anaesthetic or associated drugs has not been elucidated. In event of a severe reaction in a previous anaesthesia, the cause of the reaction may not be determined and a subsequent anaesthesia protocol would have to avoid all injectable anaesthetic agents previously used. Pretreatment with an antihistamine may not prevent a severe anaphylactic response (Armitage-Chan, 2010). Emergency drugs and equipment should always be in close proximity to the location of any anaesthetized animal, and that may be particularly important for patients anaesthetized for CT scans and myelography.

- Apneustic: This pattern has prolonged end-inspiratory pauses of several seconds duration where the lungs remain inflated longer than usual. This pattern is commonly associated with ketamine anaesthesia and can be observed in cats and horses anaesthetized with ketamine.
- Cluster breathing: This pattern is defined as a disorderly breathing pattern with grouped series of breaths interrupted by non-regular pauses.
- Biot's breathing: This is an alternating pattern with two to several breaths and apnoea. This pattern may be observed in horses during early return of spontaneous breathing while recovering from inhalation anaesthesia.
- Ataxic breathing: Both rhythm and depth of breathing are irregular.
- Kussmaul's breathing: This is a pattern of regular deep laboured breaths without pauses commonly associated with severe metabolic acidosis.

- Hiccups: Occasionally hiccups are observed in anaesthetized dogs as jerky inspirations resembling hiccups in humans. Management involves squeezing the reservoir bag on the anaesthesia machine to hold the lungs inflated for 5 seconds. This manoeuvre may have to be repeated several times and arterial pressure should be allowed to stabilize between inflations.

ARRHYTHMIAS

Causes and management

This section covers some of the most common arrhythmias detected during the perianaesthetic period (Table 21.2). Second degree AV block is a common finding on preanaesthetic evaluation of conscious horses and often

617

Table 21.2 Some electrocardiographic abnormalities occurring during anaesthesia; causes and management

Arrhythmia*	Recognition	Causes	Management

Sinus arrhythmia

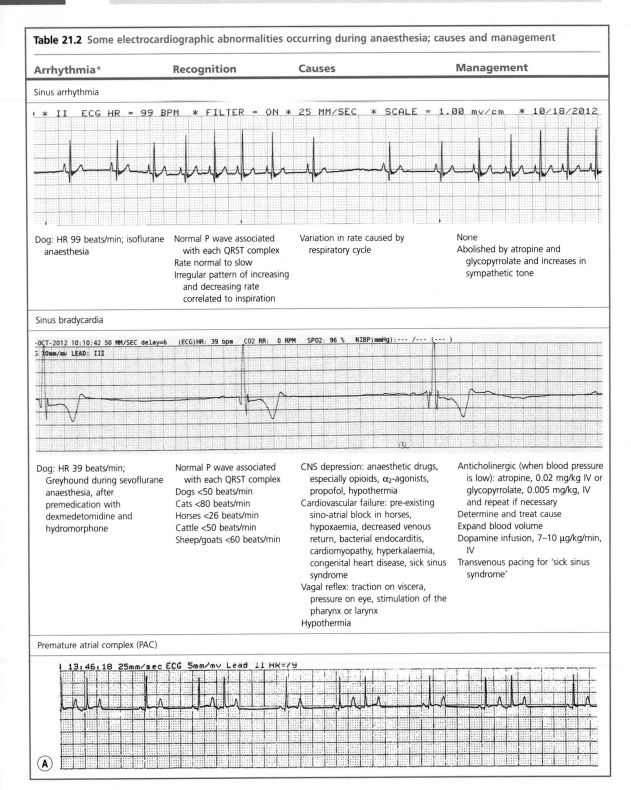

Dog: HR 99 beats/min; isoflurane anaesthesia	Normal P wave associated with each QRST complex Rate normal to slow Irregular pattern of increasing and decreasing rate correlated to inspiration	Variation in rate caused by respiratory cycle	None Abolished by atropine and glycopyrrolate and increases in sympathetic tone

Sinus bradycardia

Dog: HR 39 beats/min; Greyhound during sevoflurane anaesthesia, after premedication with dexmedetomidine and hydromorphone	Normal P wave associated with each QRST complex Dogs <50 beats/min Cats <80 beats/min Horses <26 beats/min Cattle <50 beats/min Sheep/goats <60 beats/min	CNS depression: anaesthetic drugs, especially opioids, α_2-agonists, propofol, hypothermia Cardiovascular failure: pre-existing sino-atrial block in horses, hypoxaemia, decreased venous return, bacterial endocarditis, cardiomyopathy, hyperkalaemia, congenital heart disease, sick sinus syndrome Vagal reflex: traction on viscera, pressure on eye, stimulation of the pharynx or larynx Hypothermia	Anticholinergic (when blood pressure is low): atropine, 0.02 mg/kg IV or glycopyrrolate, 0.005 mg/kg, IV and repeat if necessary Determine and treat cause Expand blood volume Dopamine infusion, 7–10 µg/kg/min, IV Transvenous pacing for 'sick sinus syndrome'

Premature atrial complex (PAC)

Table 21.2 Continued

Arrhythmia*	Recognition	Causes	Management

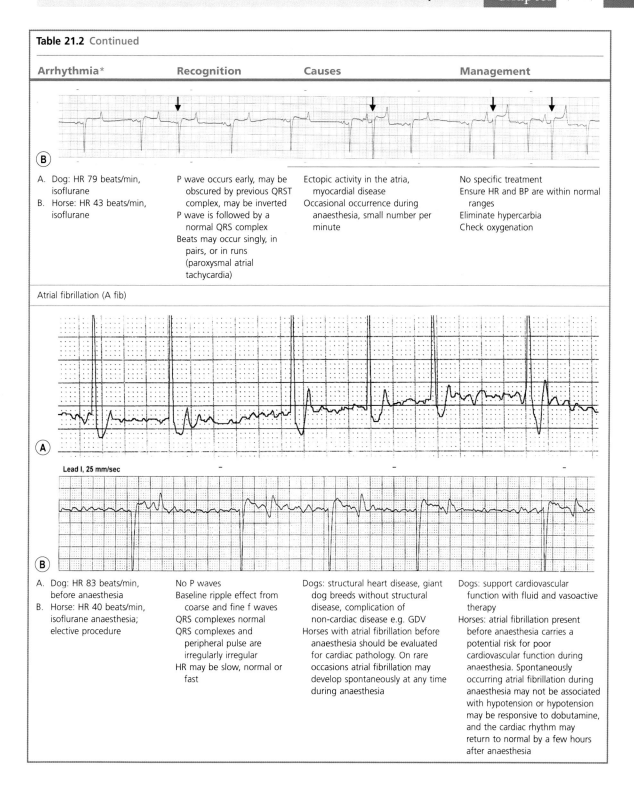

A. Dog: HR 79 beats/min, isoflurane
B. Horse: HR 43 beats/min, isoflurane

P wave occurs early, may be obscured by previous QRST complex, may be inverted
P wave is followed by a normal QRS complex
Beats may occur singly, in pairs, or in runs (paroxysmal atrial tachycardia)

Ectopic activity in the atria, myocardial disease
Occasional occurrence during anaesthesia, small number per minute

No specific treatment
Ensure HR and BP are within normal ranges
Eliminate hypercarbia
Check oxygenation

Atrial fibrillation (A fib)

Lead I, 25 mm/sec

A. Dog: HR 83 beats/min, before anaesthesia
B. Horse: HR 40 beats/min, isoflurane anaesthesia; elective procedure

No P waves
Baseline ripple effect from coarse and fine f waves
QRS complexes normal
QRS complexes and peripheral pulse are irregularly irregular
HR may be slow, normal or fast

Dogs: structural heart disease, giant dog breeds without structural disease, complication of non-cardiac disease e.g. GDV
Horses with atrial fibrillation before anaesthesia should be evaluated for cardiac pathology. On rare occasions atrial fibrillation may develop spontaneously at any time during anaesthesia

Dogs: support cardiovascular function with fluid and vasoactive therapy
Horses: atrial fibrillation present before anaesthesia carries a potential risk for poor cardiovascular function during anaesthesia. Spontaneously occurring atrial fibrillation during anaesthesia may not be associated with hypotension or hypotension may be responsive to dobutamine, and the cardiac rhythm may return to normal by a few hours after anaesthesia

Table 21.2 Continued

Arrhythmia*	Recognition	Causes	Management

Second degree atrioventricular block

(OX)HR=93 SPO2=97%

Hg *UNPLUGGED

Arrhythmia*	Recognition	Causes	Management
A. Horse: Preanaesthetic ECG, 2nd degree AV block Mobitz Type 1 B. Dog: During isoflurane anaesthesia, HR 93 beats/min, advanced 2nd degree AV block, ECG shows 2 P waves without QRS complexes with normal complexes on either side	Impaired conduction of electrical impulse through the AV node, bundle of His, or bundle branches 1st degree AV block is prolongation of PR interval 2nd degree AV block is when some P waves are not followed by a QRS complex (no peripheral pulse) Mobitz Type I (Wenkebach) is progressive prolongation of PR interval before a non-conducted P wave occurs Mobitz Type II has uniform PR intervals preceding blocked impulses Advanced 2nd degree AV block when more than one P wave in a row is blocked	Mobitz Type I AV block common in awake horses due to increased vagal tone α_2-Agonist sedatives May occur transiently after administration of atropine or glycopyrrolate	Usually benign, not usually present during anaesthesia except after α_2-agonist No treatment if infrequent and when blood pressure is adequate Anticholinergic if frequency increases or when blood pressure is low

Third degree atrioventricular block

Table 21.2 Continued

Arrhythmia*	Recognition	Causes	Management

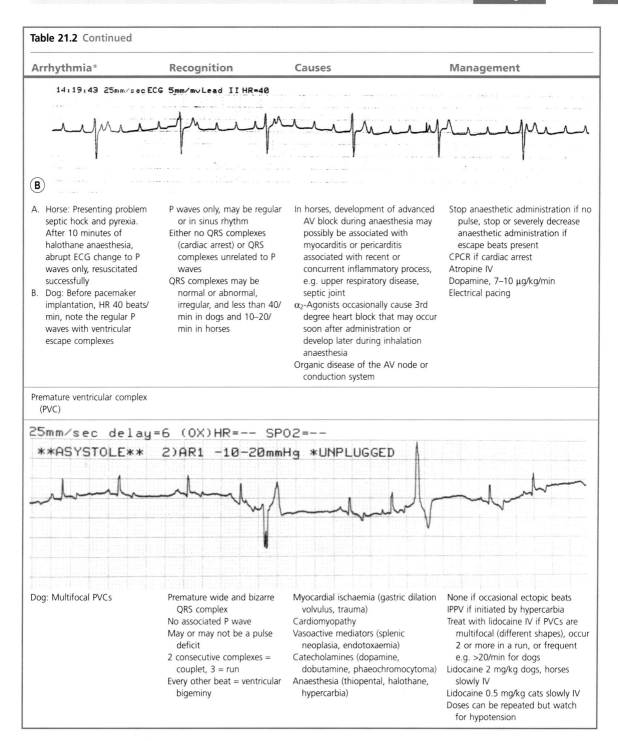

14:19:43 25mm/sec ECG 5mm/mv Lead II HR=40

Ⓑ

A. Horse: Presenting problem septic hock and pyrexia. After 10 minutes of halothane anaesthesia, abrupt ECG change to P waves only, resuscitated successfully

B. Dog: Before pacemaker implantation, HR 40 beats/min, note the regular P waves with ventricular escape complexes

P waves only, may be regular or in sinus rhythm Either no QRS complexes (cardiac arrest) or QRS complexes unrelated to P waves QRS complexes may be normal or abnormal, irregular, and less than 40/min in dogs and 10–20/min in horses	In horses, development of advanced AV block during anaesthesia may possibly be associated with myocarditis or pericarditis associated with recent or concurrent inflammatory process, e.g. upper respiratory disease, septic joint α_2-Agonists occasionally cause 3rd degree heart block that may occur soon after administration or develop later during inhalation anaesthesia Organic disease of the AV node or conduction system	Stop anaesthetic administration if no pulse, stop or severely decrease anaesthetic administration if escape beats present CPCR if cardiac arrest Atropine IV Dopamine, 7–10 μg/kg/min Electrical pacing

Premature ventricular complex (PVC)

25mm/sec delay=6 (OX)HR=-- SPO2=--

ASYSTOLE 2)AR1 -10-20mmHg *UNPLUGGED

| Dog: Multifocal PVCs | Premature wide and bizarre QRS complex
No associated P wave
May or may not be a pulse deficit
2 consecutive complexes = couplet, 3 = run
Every other beat = ventricular bigeminy | Myocardial ischaemia (gastric dilation volvulus, trauma)
Cardiomyopathy
Vasoactive mediators (splenic neoplasia, endotoxaemia)
Catecholamines (dopamine, dobutamine, phaeochromocytoma)
Anaesthesia (thiopental, halothane, hypercarbia) | None if occasional ectopic beats
IPPV if initiated by hypercarbia
Treat with lidocaine IV if PVCs are multifocal (different shapes), occur 2 or more in a run, or frequent e.g. >20/min for dogs
Lidocaine 2 mg/kg dogs, horses slowly IV
Lidocaine 0.5 mg/kg cats slowly IV
Doses can be repeated but watch for hypotension |

Table 21.2 Continued

Arrhythmia*	Recognition	Causes	Management

Ventricular tachycardia (V tach)

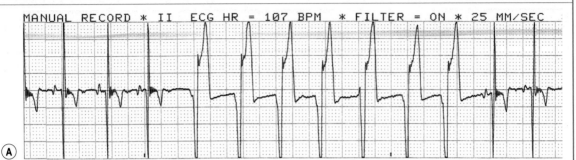

Dog: Weimeraner after splenectomy
A. HR 107 beats/min; slow accelerated idioventricular rhythm
B. HR 170 beats/min; fast ventricular tachycardia (rate >160 beats/min)

Wide abnormal QRS complexes
At least 3 PVCs in a row
Ventricular rate > 100 beats/min in dogs, >150 beats/min in cats
Rhythm may be regular
Independent or retrograde P waves
May be interspersed with normal complexes and fusion beats (simultaneous normal and premature beats)

Myocardial ischaemia (gastric dilatation volvulus, trauma)
Cardiomyopathy
Vasoactive mediators (splenic neoplasia, endotoxaemia)
Phaeochromocytoma

Lidocaine in dogs and horses
Cardiac output may be significantly impaired
CPCR if no accompanying pulses

ECG artifact

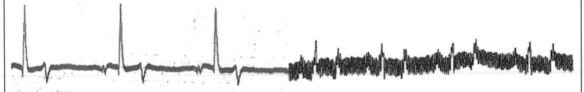

60 cycle interference seen as a thickened baseline, horse ECG on the left and dog ECG on the right

QRS rhythm regular
Extra waves of equal size, upright form, or
60 cycle electrical interference, or
Wandering baseline due to movement of electrodes (see Fig. 2.10B)

Electrical interference from other monitoring equipment, electrical heating pad, thermocautery
ECG leads over the chest and respiratory movements cause wandering baseline

Adjust electrodes, improve skin contact, check wires for breaks
Minimize electrical interference by running ECG leads together, try turning off cautery or hot water circulating pad
No ECG lead lying over the thorax

*Configuration of the ECG will depend on the Lead that is recorded. Commonly, during anaesthesia standard Lead II is used for cats, dogs, pigs, and small ruminants, and a base-apex Lead I for horses. Equine atrial premature complex, equine atrial fibrillation, and canine third degree AV block ECGs courtesy of Dr Jennifer Adams.

develops in all species after administration of α_2-agonists. Premature ventricular complexes (PVC) are a common consequence of myocardial ischaemia in dogs with gastric dilation-volvulus, splenic neoplasia, and thoracic contusions acquired during a road traffic accident. PVCs occur commonly in dogs for several minutes after induction of anaesthesia with thiopental, often as a bigeminal rhythm. PVCs may occur during halothane anaesthesia in dogs and cats with hypercarbia from hypoventilation. They are not a common occurrence during anaesthesia in other species.

Tachycardia

Tachycardia denotes a rapid heart rate, with the rate exceeding 180 beats/min in dogs, 240 beats/min in cats, and 50 beats/min in horses (Physick-Sheard, 1999; Carr et al., 2001). Sinus tachycardia is regular and continuous. When the rhythm originates outside the sinoatrial node (atrial tachycardia), the P waves may be a different shape from normal but the QRS complexes are normal. Tachycardia may also be paroxysmal.

Ketamine, atropine, or glycopyrrolate injected IV frequently cause a fast heart rate in dogs and cats that is close to but does not usually achieve the strict definition of tachycardia. Hypoxaemia, and sometimes hypercarbia, cause increased heart rates. Excessively increased heart rate does not usually accompany hypotension induced by deep anaesthesia or inhalant agents. Heart rate may not change during blood loss in the anaesthetized animal until blood volume is moderately to severely depleted, but will generally occur in response to an abrupt severe decrease in blood pressure caused by anaphylactic reactions. Heart rates may increase when analgesia is inadequate during surgery. A heart rate increased above that normally expected for the anaesthetic protocol can be caused by ruminal distension (bloat) in ruminants, gastric distension in horses, or urinary bladder distension in dogs. Tachycardia due to endotoxaemia during anaesthesia of horses with colic has been associated with increased mortality. Endogenous (phaeochromocytoma) and exogenous catecholamines (administration of dopamine, dobutamine or ephedrine) can cause tachycardia or fast heart rates.

Clearly, management varies depending upon the cause of the fast heart rate. The effects of ketamine and anticholinergics generally wane within 20 minutes. Hypoxaemia and hypercarbia should be corrected. Blood pressure should be measured and treated if low. Tachycardia may occur in response to haemorrhage and low blood pressure following recovery from anaesthesia when the baroreceptor reflex is no longer depressed by the anaesthetic agents. Intra-abdominal haemorrhage after castration or laparotomy is an example where tachycardia is present but bleeding is not apparent. Observation of mucous membrane colour, CRT, and pulse pressure, and ultrasound or percutaneous needle aspiration of the abdominal cavity are required for the diagnosis of haemorrhage.

Pain should be managed appropriately. If feasible, a stomach tube should be passed in a small ruminant to decompress the rumen and the patency of a stomach tube in a horse should be checked. The presence of urinary retention can be assessed by palpation, ultrasound, or a walk outside for a dog after recovery from anaesthesia. Tachycardia and hypertension caused by release of catecholamines from a phaeochromocytoma should be managed by infusion of nitroprusside. For dogs, 25 mg of nitroprusside added to 500 mL saline produces a concentration of 50 μg/mL (a smaller volume or more dilute solution can be made up for small dogs). The dose to calculate for this clinical problem is 1 μg/kg/min, however, half that rate may be sufficient to treat hypertension and the infusion should be stopped or reduced before reaching the target mean arterial pressure (MAP) otherwise an overcorrection will occur. Catecholamines may be released from a phaeochromocytoma in surges resulting in rapid swings in blood pressure, therefore, the infusion rate must be tightly controlled and blood pressure must be continually monitored to facilitate immediate changes in nitroprusside infusion rate in response to changes in blood pressure.

CYANOSIS AND HYPOXAEMIA

Cyanosis is the bluish colour of skin or mucous membranes caused by the presence of more than 5 g desaturated haemoglobin per 100 mL of blood. The blue mucous membrane colour may be difficult to detect in an anaemic patient. The colour of mucous membranes may not accurately reflect haemoglobin O_2 saturation in the presence of excessive vasodilation or vasoconstriction.

- Oral mucous membranes observed to be blue or white. Assessment of mucous membrane colour may be inaccurate in poor lighting or with reflection from blue drapes or when a light is in close proximity. Vasoconstriction induced by α_2-agonists, pain, activated sympathetic system, or catecholamine release may cause oral membranes to look white even when hypoxaemia is not present. In dogs with good peripheral perfusion, mucous membranes may be a dull pink not bluish in the presence of hypoxaemia.
- Respiratory movements may be normal or rapid or appear laboured.
- The cardiovascular system is initially stimulated, resulting in tachycardia and hypertension. Prolonged hypoxaemia results in bradycardia and hypotension. ECG changes include reversed polarity of T wave with ST segment depression and slur.

Causes and management

Management involves administration of O_2 and correction of the initiating cause (Table 21.3, Box 21.4). Consequences

Table 21.3 Cyanosis or SpO_2 <90% (hypoxaemia): causes and management

Species	Causes	Management
Drugs		
Dogs, cats	Sedation plus partial airway obstruction (brachycephalics) at premedication	Monitor SpO_2, supply O_2 by mask
	Rapid IV administration at induction decreasing ventilation and/or cardiac output, propofol	Inject anaesthetic agents in increments, preoxygenation*
	Residual respiratory depression in recovery	Anticipate low PaO_2 in recovery, mask or insufflate O_2
Ruminants	α_2-agonists	Use low dose, supply O_2
Horses	Increased V/Q inequality during recumbency from anaesthesia even in healthy horses	Withhold food before anaesthesia, lateral preferable to dorsal recumbency, supply O_2
Equipment		
All species	O_2 supply failure: cylinder empty or not turned on, O_2 flow meter off or too low	Restore O_2 supply
	Delivery circuit failure: assembled incorrectly, disconnected, high circuit pressure because relief valve closed, rebreathing bag empty	Check circuit connections and circuit pressure
	Endotracheal tube malfunction: oesophageal intubation, tube is kinked, compressed, obstructed, in one bronchus	Check placement of endotracheal tube, air flow in tube, manually inflate lungs to assess flow and resistance
	N_2O: accumulation in rebreathing circuit, flow rate too high, 'diffusion hypoxia'	Check O_2 and N_2O flow meters, supply O_2 for >5 min after N_2O discontinued
	Measurement error: pulse oximeter low signal or poor contact	Observe signal strength on pulse oximeter, oximeter pulse rate should be the same as obtained by another method
Mechanical		
Dogs, cats	Surgeon leaning on the chest	Check personnel positions
	Thoracic or abdominal bandages limiting thoracic or diaphragm movements	Assess bandages for flexibility, longitudinal cut through bandage
	Head and neck bandages causing pharyngeal compression after extubation	Loosen or cut bandage
Horses, ruminants	Inadequate diaphragm movement and lung collapse: dorsal recumbency, abdominal distension (colic, bloat), table tilted head-down	IPPV, ± PEEP, for colic horses add albuterol/salbutamol during inhalation (6–10 actuations/adult horse) (see text), CPAP, recruitment manoeuvre (see Chapter 9)
Other patient problems & procedure		
All species	Obesity or abdominal distension limiting thoracic or diaphragm movements	Monitor SpO_2 and ventilation, IPPV, drain fluid/air if possible
	Inadequate lung expansion during thoracoscopy under general anaesthesia	Increase tidal volume, periodically expand lungs, change to one lung ventilation
	Postoperative pain resulting in reluctance to expand thorax	Analgesia

Table 21.3 Continued

Species	Causes	Management
Cardiac		
All species	Low cardiac output or blood pressure: anaesthetic drug depression	Assess adequacy of circulation, improve by appropriate treatment
Respiratory		
All species	Apnoea or severe respiratory depression when breathing air	IPPV from anaesthesia machine, intubate trachea if not intubated and ventilate from anaesthesia machine or demand valve, AMBU bag if <80 kg, if no endotracheal tube (large animals) consider doxapram IV (see Box 21.4) or relevant antagonists and external compression of thoracic cage
	Pathology or disease: traumatic injury to ribs, diaphragm or lungs, pneumothorax, pneumonia, pleural effusion, intrathoracic masses	Supply O_2, aspirate pleural air or fluid, IPPV with low inspiratory pressure <20 cmH$_2$O
Allergic		
	See Table 21.1 for causes	Table 21.1, Box 21.3, see text
Toxic		
All species	Endotoxaemia	NSAID, ACVC

*Preoxygenation: administration of O_2 by mask for a few minutes before and during induction of anaesthesia; V/Q: ventilation/perfusion inequality within the lungs; PEEP: positive end-expiratory pressure (see Chapter 9); CPAP: continuous positive airway pressure (see Chapter 9); CPR/CPCR: cardiopulmonary cerebral resuscitation (see Chapter 22); ACVC: circulatory support (see Box 21.5).

of hypoxaemia depend on the timing and effectiveness of intervention and may range from death during anaesthesia to blindness after anaesthesia.

α₂-Antagonists

Administration of an antagonist may be life saving for an animal in a life-threatening situation. However, the consequences of sedative (or opioid) reversal must be considered. α₂-Agonist sedatives provide profound sedation and drug and dose-dependent analgesia and may play a large part in maintaining anaesthesia. Abrupt reversal can result in the patient becoming suddenly awake and trying to stand up, unmask ketamine resulting in CNS excitement, or cardiac arrest as the patient suddenly experiences pain and a surge of catecholamines is released. If there is time,

administration of an antagonist should be incremental over a period of minutes, allowing progressive assessment and control of the animal.

Yohimbine is a competitive α₂-receptor antagonist. It is licensed as an antagonist to xylazine in dogs and has been used in horses but may cause a serious adverse reaction, including death, in this species.

- Dogs and cats: Yohimbine, 0.1 mg/kg IV slowly, SC or IM 0.25–0.5 mg/kg.
- Horses: Yohimbine, 0.075 mg/kg, IV slowly (Hsu, 2008a).

Tolazoline is a competitive α₁- and α₂-receptor antagonist. In some countries, it is marketed for reversal of xylazine sedation in horses and is an effective reversal agent for xylazine in cattle. Measurement of the decline in blood concentration has led to the recommendation of a cattle slaughter withdrawal time of 8 days and withholding of

---

Box 21.4 Doxapram

What is it?

Doxapram is a respiratory stimulant and an analeptic (CNS stimulant) that is used to treat drug-induced ventilatory depression and apnoea in newborn animals and humans. At low doses, doxapram increases ventilation primarily through action on the carotid bodies and higher doses may increase ventilation through direct stimulation of respiratory neurons in the CNS. The tandem pore (K_{2P}) potassium channel family mediates background 'leak' K^+ current regulating excitability in neurons and is expressed in carotid bodies and the brainstem. Doxapram increases carotid body discharge by inhibition of K^+ current through pH sensitive K^+ TASK-1 and TASK-3 channels (Duprat et al., 1997; Cotten et al., 2006; Mulkey et al., 2007; Wilkinson et al., 2010). Doxapram induces noticeable arousal effects in animals given xylazine or thiopental.

The increase in breathing may speed elimination of inhalation agents.

Dose rates

- Dogs and cats: Doxapram, 0.5–2.0 mg/kg, during inhalation anaesthesia; 5–10 mg/kg for emergency treatment of barbiturate overdose
- Horses: Doxapram, 0.2–0.5 mg/kg, IV
- Small ruminants: Doxapram, 1–2 mg/kg, IM, IV
- Calves, newborn: Doxapram, 2 mg/kg, IM, IV

The effect is short-lived and doxapram may have to be repeated in 15–20 minutes.

Adverse effects

Doxapram induces arousal through central stimulation and release of catecholamines results in increased blood pressure (Lumb & Jones, 1984). Doxapram may also induce PVCs in animals with hearts sensitized to catecholamines, for example, during halothane anaesthesia. Doxapram has a wide margin of safety between the convulsive dose and respiratory stimulant dose.

---

milk for 48 hours (Hsu, 2008b). Adverse side effects of tolazoline administration are tachycardia and hypotension, thus it is advisable to administer tolazoline slowly over several minutes to avoid cardiovascular collapse. When tolazoline is used to decrease ataxia attributed to xylazine after total IV anaesthesia in horses, as opposed to an emergency situation, a low dose of 0.8–1.0 mg/kg IV provides a satisfactory effect.

- Horses and cattle: Tolazoline, 1–4 mg/kg, IV slowly over several minutes.

Tolazoline has also been evaluated for effectiveness of antagonism in horses sedated with detomidine, 0.02 mg/kg, IV (Hubbell & Muir, 2006). Although tolazoline did not produce complete reversal, time to recovery was shortened, ease of walking was improved, and ataxia minimized. The horses appeared to be nervous for 15 minutes after reversal. Administration of tolazoline, 4 mg/kg, IV 20 minutes after horses were sedated with detomidine, 0.04 mg/kg, IV decreased sedation, head position returned to normal, and cutaneous analgesia was lost (Carroll et al., 1997). No effect of tolazoline on HR, MAP, respiration rate (RR), or temperature was recorded. Use of tolazoline and atipamezole in cattle has been described in Chapter 12.

Atipamezole is licensed as an antagonist to medetomidine and dexmedetomidine sedation in dogs to be dosed IM as an equal volume as the volume of sedative administered, equivalent to a dose of atipamezole five times that of medetomidine or dexmedetomidine (see product package information sheet). Various dose rates of atipamezole antagonize detomidine sedation in horses (see Chapter 11). Sedation provided by a continuous infusion of detomidine in standing horses for laparoscopy was reversed within 10 minutes of injection of atipamezole given at a dose equal to the cumulative dose of detomidine for each horse (van Dijk et al., 2003). No relapse into sedation was noted. A case report has described the use of atipamezole to treat detomidine overdose. A pony received a 10-fold overdose of detomidine (total 0.3 mg/kg) with ketamine, a mistake that was recognized when the pony failed to recover at the expected time (Di Concetto et al., 2007). Increments of atipamezole injected over 30 minutes reached a dose (1.1 mg/kg) that was 3.6 times the dose of detomidine and decreased sedation enough for the pony to stand. In experimental investigations of horses sedated with detomidine, 0.01 or 0.02 mg/kg, IV, atipamezole, 0.1 mg/kg, IV produced incomplete antagonism but significant improvement in locomotion (Buchner et al., 1999; Hubbell & Muir, 2006). The degree of antagonism was less than obtained after tolazoline administration (Hubbell & Muir, 2006).

HYPOTENSION

Extreme changes in clinical signs, such as white mucous membranes (hypotension or hypertension), slow heart rate, or lack of peripheral arterial pulse, clearly warn about the need for intense, aggressive treatment. Of concern is the fact that these parameters may be within the normal ranges and yet the cardiovascular system may need support. For example, heart rate may be normal but the arterial blood pressure too low, or mucous membranes may be pink but the blood pressure too low. Except for the extreme values, evaluation of several parameters is necessary to assess accurately cardiovascular status of anaesthetized patients.

Mean arterial pressure in awake, healthy adult dogs and cats is 90–100 mm Hg (systolic pressure 135–160 mm Hg, diastolic pressure 65–80 mm Hg), MAP in conscious horses is 95–115 mmHg, and in sheep 90–110 mmHg. Hypotension is MAP ≤60–65 mm Hg or systolic pressure ≤80 mmHg. Other clinical signs are:

- Prolonged CRT, blood oozing at the operative site rather than free flowing
- Weak pulse on palpation. Note that a weak pulse may not be indicative of hypotension when an α_2-agonist has been recently administered because of vasoconstriction; conversely, the pulse can feel strong during hypotension if the artery is dilated
- Bradycardia may or may not be present. Tachycardia occurring in response to hypotension in the conscious animal is often absent during anaesthesia due to baroreceptor receptor reflex suppression
- ST segment slur on the ECG indicating myocardial hypoxia
- Dysrhythmias may cause hypotension
- During laparotomy, intestines may be pale pink or white.

Significance of hypotension

- MAP <55 mm Hg is life threatening.
- Hypotension of only 15 minutes may contribute to organ malfunction or result in blindness after anaesthesia.

Causes and management

Treatment of hypotension should be directed at the cause (Table 21.4, Boxes 21.5-8).

Injection of water-soluble sodium or potassium penicillin IV to horses occasionally results in hypotension attributed to myocardial depression (Hubbell et al., 1987) or anaphylaxis (Olsén et al., 2007). Injection of procaine penicillin IM in horses can cause collapse and death or various CNS signs, including ataxia, muscle tremors, anxiety and nystagmus. Mechanisms proposed are anaphylaxis causing collapse and procaine toxicity following inadvertent IV injection during IM injection (Olsén et al., 2007). It is advisable to administer antibiotics at least 30 minutes before induction of anaesthesia so that abnormal behaviour can be recognized immediately. When IV administration during anaesthesia is unavoidable, the antibiotic must be injected in small increments and the blood pressure closely monitored for any adverse effect.

Crystalloids and colloids

Abbreviations:

- HES = hetastarch
- HSS = hypertonic saline solution
- HHES = hypertonic saline in hetastarch

Selection of fluid type and infusion rate for administration to healthy patients during anaesthesia is highly debated. Other requirements may be superimposed on intraoperative maintenance fluid choice, such as the need to treat hypotension or specific pre-existing component abnormalities, or management of blood loss, and choices may be limited by cost and availability. Searching for answers among the publications of experimental and clinical studies is not easy because experimental designs and patient populations differ and because the end-points for fluid therapy are variable and often not clearly defined.

Isotonic crystalloid fluid, such as 0.9% NaCl, lactated (lactated Ringer's solution [LRS], Hartmann's), or acetated (Normosol®-R, Plasma-Lyte A) balanced electrolyte solution is the usual choice for maintenance fluid during anaesthesia and is given to compensate for lack of oral water intake before and after anaesthesia, losses from the lungs, urinary and gastrointestinal tracts, evaporation from exposed viscera during laparotomy or thoracotomy, and losses created by surgical trauma. For the most part, balanced electrolyte solution is preferred to saline, even though saline produces a larger intravascular volume and more sustained expansion than LRS (Reid et al., 2011). Saline alone in large quantities induces a metabolic acidosis. Saline may be the fluid of choice for vomiting patients and those with adrenocortical insufficiency or diabetic ketoacidosis.

Under normal circumstances, fluid is filtered from the blood into the interstitial space under a pressure gradient created by the balance between hydrostatic and oncotic pressure gradients. Absorption into venous capillaries does not occur and most of the filtered fluid returns to the circulation as lymph (Woodcock & Woodcock, 2012). The endothelial glycocalyx layer (EGL) is a web of glycoproteins and proteoglycans on the luminal side of the endothelial cells of blood vessels. The subglycocalyx space separates plasma from the capillary wall and the colloid osmotic pressure (COP) of this space determines the transcapillary flow of fluid. Plasma albumin is the major determinant of plasma COP in health, but other proteins become important in acquired hypoalbuminaemia. During inflammation, the extravascular proportion of albumin will increase. Normal transcapillary escape rate of albumin (TCERA), an index of vascular permeability, in humans is about 5% of the plasma albumin per hour (Woodcock & Woodcock, 2012). This rate can double during surgery and may be increased 20% or more in septic shock, and evidence points to a compromised EGL in these patients. Plasma substitutes, such as HES, dextran 70, or gelatins, increase the circulating COP thus limiting

Table 21.4 Hypotension: causes and management

Species	Causes	Management
	Drugs	
All species	Injectable or inhalation anaesthesia Epidural bupivacaine or other local anaesthetic Accidental IV bupivacaine, local anaesthetic overdose Antibiotics causing myocardial depression	Check depth of anaesthesia, ACVC Crystalloid, colloid, dopamine or ephedrine ACVC, lipid rescue (ILE) (see text) ACVC, IV antibiotics over several minutes, IV antibiotics to horses minimum 30 min before induction
Dogs, cats	Acepromazine, ACE inhibitor Opioid IV during anaesthesia	ACVC ACVC, anticholinergic for bradycardia
Horses	Acepromazine IV on rare occasions induces acute hypotension, recumbency, sweating, ± signs of colic	May resolve in 20 min without treatment, IV fluid bolus
	Equipment	
All species	NIBP measurement error: either incorrect application or inherent monitor variation Direct blood pressure error: transducer position incorrect, catheter lumen obstructed (kink, accumulated red cells) Increased circuit pressure from closed or malfunctioning APL valve	Follow guidelines for correct NIBP measurement (see Chapter 2) Check transducer is level with manubrium, flush catheter, observe waveform for damping Check circuit pressure, release valve, decrease vaporizer, monitor pulse strength continuously, start CPR
	Mechanical	
All species	Change in body position (see Fig. 2.11) IPPV with decreased blood volume Laparoscopy Aortocaval compression (see Box 21.6)	Consider turning back to original position, try turning slowly, may need dobutamine infusion Check for systolic pressure variation, infuse balanced electrolyte solution Maintain low abdominal pressure, dobutamine or dopamine IV Tilt animal to one side, if possible, infuse vasoactive drug
Ruminants	Ruminal distension (bloat)	Pass stomach tube, rarely need to trocharize, monitor ventilation, sternal position as soon as possible
	Other patient problems & procedure	
All species	Pre-existing hypovolaemia Pre-existing azotaemia, CNS depression Sepsis and vasodilation Hypoproteinaemia Blood loss Air embolism (see Box 21.7)	Balanced electrolyte solution IV Decreased anaesthetic agent dose rates Fluids and vasoactive drugs Colloid or plasma IV Options: balanced electrolyte at 2× volume lost, colloid 1:1, hypertonic saline, blood transfusion (see Box 21.5, text) Stop air leak, flood operative site with saline, discontinue N$_2$O, vasopressors or CPCR, treat neurological deficits
Dogs, cats	Surgical compression of caudal vena cava	Release liver lobe or adjust surgical manipulation

Table 21.4 Continued

Species	Causes	Management
	Cardiac	
All species	Bradycardia, tachycardia Arrhythmia Decreased contractility Valvular disease	Search for further cause See Table 21.2 Dobutamine IV Avoid bradycardia/tachycardia, maintain cardiac contractility and blood volume
Dogs, cats	Congenital: PDA, PSS Cardiomyopathy Pericardial effusion	Dobutamine IV (see Chapters 15, 20) Appropriate selection of anaesthetic protocol to minimize cardiac depression, IV dobutamine, avoid volume overload Drain fluid before or at the beginning of anaesthesia
	Respiratory	
All species	Hypercarbia (may cause sympathetic stimulation or hypotension) Decreased venous return from incorrect IPPV: prolonged inspiratory time, PEEP, large lung inflations Tension pneumothorax: ruptured alveolus or oesophagus, thoracic inlet, intercostal penetration Pleural effusion Diaphragmatic rupture repair after removal of organs from thoracic cavity	IPPV Follow guidelines for correct application Aspirate air from pleural cavity, seek origin of leak (see Box 21.8) Remove fluid Dobutamine IV (no fluid bolus)
	Allergic	
Dogs, cats	Morphine, meperidine/pethidine, atracurium Thiopental Contrast agents Manipulation of mast cell tumour	Occasionally produce hypotension, most often after rapid IV Rarely, causes anaphylactic shock Frequently decrease MAP, occasionally cause acute cardiovascular collapse requiring CPCR High risk of cardiovascular collapse, diphenhydramine for preanaesthetic medication in dogs and cats
Horses	Meperidine/pethidine, procaine penicillin, contrast agent	Rare cases of cardiovascular collapse, CPCR
	Toxic	
All species	Release of vasoactive mediators: endotoxin, pancreatitis, pancreatic abscess, catecholamine-secreting tumours (Carcinoid syndrome)	Circulatory support

ACVC: circulatory support (see Box 21.5); ACE: angiotensin converting enzyme; NIBP: non-invasive blood pressure; APL valve: adjustable pressure limiting (pop-off) valve; PDA: patent ductus arteriosus; PSS: portosystemic shunt.

Box 21.5 ACVC: treatment of hypotension

Standard treatment of hypotension involves (A) decreasing anaesthetic agent administration, (C) IV infusion of crystalloid fluid, (V) stimulation of the cardiovascular system with one or more vasoactive drugs, and (C) IV infusion of colloid.

A. Anaesthetic administration

Since most anaesthetic agents decrease cardiovascular function, decreasing administration should result in improved blood pressure and/or increased cardiac output. Inhalation agents significantly decrease blood pressure at higher concentrations. Supplementation with other agents that induce less vasodilation while decreasing the concentration of inhalant may reverse hypotension.

C. Crystalloid fluids

Balanced electrolyte solutions, such as lactated or acetated Ringer's are commonly infused to maintain normovolaemia. The infusion rate during anaesthesia is initially 5–10 mL/kg/h followed by 3–5 mL/kg/h for maintenance. Rapid IV infusion of 10–20 mL/kg significantly increases cardiac output and MAP in conscious dogs but the increases are less dramatic in dogs anaesthetized with inhalation agents. An initial bolus of 10 mL/kg may be indicated when there is suspicion of a relative or absolute hypovolaemia (e.g. drug-induced vasodilation or no oral intake for several hours before anaesthesia). If there is no improvement in MAP, then treatment should include administration of a vasoactive agent ± colloid solution.

Hypertonic (7.5%) saline (HSS) may be infused IV over 10 minutes at 4 mL/kg when an immediate increase in blood pressure is desired and other efforts, such as decreasing anaesthetic administration and infusing a bolus of balanced electrolyte solution have failed. HSS is primarily used in situations of blood loss and the need for rapid blood volume expansion. The duration of effect is short-lived (30 minutes to 2 hours). Infusion of balanced electrolyte solution should be continued. Despite the short duration of effect, HSS may improve haemodynamic function sufficiently to allow time for institution of further appropriate treatment and for surgery to be completed. At the end of anaesthesia, elimination of anaesthetic agents should be followed by improved cardiovascular function and return of normal physiological compensatory mechanisms.

V. Vasoactive drugs

Infusion of dobutamine, 0.5–10 µg/kg/min, or dopamine, 3–10 µg/kg/min, may be sufficient to improve MAP and CRT in healthy animals. Dobutamine, 0.5–1.0 µg/kg/min may increase MAP in horses whereas a higher dose rate of 5 µg/kg/min should be started in dogs, cats, and small ruminants. Dobutamine occasionally induces bradycardia, such that the blood pressure remains low, and management can include decreasing the infusion rate, administration of atropine of glycopyrrolate in dogs and cats, or adding ephedrine, 0.06 mg/kg, IV. Dopamine should be started at 5–7 µg/kg/min in dogs, cats, and small ruminants, and the infusion rate decreased as the blood pressure increases. In horses, dopamine initially induces vasodilation and the MAP will decrease for 7–10 minutes before increasing, consequently dopamine is less effective than dobutamine in increasing blood pressure. Exceptions would be treatment of third degree heart block and cardiac arrest where dopamine, 7–10 µg/kg/min, is most appropriate.

Ephedrine, 0.06–0.1 mg/kg, is most effective when low blood pressure is the result of vasodilation. Ephedrine is given as a bolus injection that has up to a 5-minute onset of action and duration up to 40 minutes. The dose of ephedrine may be repeated. Transient tachycardia is a common side effect.

Phenylephrine and vasopressin may be administered to increase blood pressure by vasoconstriction in animals in septic shock. Discussion of use and adverse effects of these agents is addressed in the species-specific chapters. Use of vasoactive agents in management of cardiac arrest is described in Chapter 22.

C. Colloids

Hetastarch increases intravascular volume by an amount at least equal to the volume infused and increases the colloid oncotic pressure. During anaesthesia, an infusion of HES, 5–10 mL/kg, IV over 10–15 minutes may be sufficient to increase MAP. During haemorrhage, one regimen involves replacement of half the blood volume lost with HES and the remainder with LRS at twice the lost volume; an alternative is to continue crystalloid at maintenance rate and replace blood loss with colloid at a 1 : 1 ratio. When blood loss approaches 17–20% of blood volume a blood or packed red cell transfusion may be indicated. A discussion about the effects of HES is in the text.

---

fluid loss into the interstitial space and promote vascular expansion for a longer time than crystalloid solutions. Infused macromolecules do not easily penetrate the intact EGL but can escape through sinusoidal capillaries in the bone marrow, liver and spleen and return to the venous system via the lymphatics. Increasing intravascular COP

does not result in absorption of interstitial fluid; consequently, colloid therapy does not prevent or improve tissue oedema (Woodcock & Woodcock, 2012). Anaesthesia with inhalation agents alters the balance of fluid movement and movement of fluid from the intravascular compartment may be faster or slower than in a conscious

---

Box 21.6 **Aortocaval compression (AOC)**

What is it?

Compression of the aorta or caudal vena cava (AOC) may occur from pressure of an abdominal mass when an animal is placed in dorsal recumbency. Venous return may be limited, cardiac output decreases and hypotension develops. Pressure is immediately restored when the animal is moved back into lateral position. Decreased venous return may also be caused by a high intra-abdominal pressure.

Common scenarios

In cats, the weight of a gravid uterus may cause caval compression (see Fig. 16.12). In dogs, hypotension may develop in dorsal recumbency due to weight from an abdominal or splenic mass. It might be expected that the larger the size of the mass the greater likelihood of AOC but that is not necessarily the case. A small mass in a dog suffering from weight loss may cause hypotension whereas an enormous mass may or may not cause aortocaval compression. In horses with colic, impaction of the transverse colon will cause AOC and can be relieved by elevation of the intestine by the surgeon. Unfortunately, it is hard to keep the colon off the caudal vena cava during

enterotomy and infusion of a vasopressor just increases heart rate without increasing blood pressure. Occasionally, healthy horses placed in dorsal recumbency develop hypotension that can be immediately reversed by turning the horse into lateral recumbency.

Differential diagnoses

This is not the same as a decrease in blood pressure due to a change in body position. The exact cause of the latter effect is not clear but may be due to decreased venous return from a change in focus of gravity and slow mobilization of blood from previously congested areas. Other causes of hypotension should be investigated (see Table 21.4), however, AOC should always be suspected if the animal has an abdominal mass or large abdomen.

Management

Turn dog or cat into an oblique position to reposition the mass. Turning a horse into lateral position may result in an immediate increase in blood pressure. In the case of a horse with colon impaction, sometimes the only course is to rely on rapid surgical technique of colon evacuation.

---

subject depending on the composition of the fluid load. Induction of vasodilation with anaesthetic agents or epidural analgesia decreases MAP resulting in slowed transcapillary filtration and an increase in blood volume that in turn decreases COP. In one study of healthy client-owned horses anaesthetized with sevoflurane, COP decreased after 30 minutes of anaesthesia but increased back to the preanaesthesia value by 2 hours after anaesthesia (Wendt-Hornickle et al., 2011). Not only did the COP decrease below 15 mmHg (suggested as the level that intestinal oedema becomes significant) but COP was <15 mmHg before anaesthesia in some horses. Half of the horses received LRS at 7.5 mL/kg/h and the others LRS at same rate plus HES 2.5 mL/kg. Administration of HES at the rate studied failed to attenuate the decrease in COP. Dogs premedicated with acepromazine and morphine developed a significant decrease in COP (Wright & Hopkins, 2008). Further decreases were measured during 45 minutes of halothane or isoflurane anaesthesia for ovariohysterectomy, to a significantly lower value in dogs given LRS, 10 mL/kg/h, compared with dogs given no fluids. By 45 minutes after anaesthesia, COP had increased in all dogs and had returned to the baseline value in the no fluid group.

The goal of fluid therapy during anaesthesia is to restore and maintain normovolaemia. Overtransfusion has been associated with adverse effects, including tissue oedema

that may impair surgical site healing and dilution of clotting factors. Conversely, hypovolaemia results in decreased cardiovascular function and inadequate tissue perfusion. Attempts to define an intraoperative volume infusion rate ideal for all patients have revolved around discussions of 'liberal' or 'high' versus 'restrictive' or 'low' administration strategies (Chappell et al., 2008; Bundgaard-Nielsen et al., 2009). Unfortunately, there is frequent overlap in the definitions of liberal and restricted fluid volumes (Chappell et al., 2008). Furthermore, outcomes are not just influenced by intraoperative but also postoperative fluid infusion rates. A review of 187 articles relating to fluid therapy in adult humans identified only seven sufficiently similar to compare (Bundgaard-Nielsen et al., 2009). Of these, three reported improved outcomes after major abdominal surgery using restrictive fluid administration whereas two studies reported no differences in wound infection, gastrointestinal recovery, and length of hospital stay. One study involving colonic surgery identified improved pulmonary function, postoperative oxygenation, and reduced vasoactive hormonal concentrations on a liberal regimen. Another meta-analysis evaluated studies comparing perioperative fluid rates in human patients, separating them according to fluid rates consistent with supplying average daily fluid and sodium requirements ('balanced') with regimens that were 'unbalanced' (over or under administration) (Varadhan & Lobo, 2010). The number of

Box 21.7 **Air embolism**

Consequences of air embolism

Air embolism of the systemic arterial system usually occurs during cardiopulmonary bypass procedures or thoracic trauma. Embolism in the coronary circulation may be fatal and embolism in the cerebral circulation may cause neurological deficits. Air embolism of the venous circulation (VAE) is more common. Air travels to the right ventricle and some bubbles leaving the heart become trapped in the lungs and obstruct pulmonary arterioles. The lung is a filter of bubbles but when it becomes overwhelmed it releases bubbles and they may reach the cerebral circulation. One theory is that air bubbles collect in the ventricle and obstruct flow into the pulmonary artery, decreasing cardiac output. Another that cause of death is due to early development of myocardial ischaemia resulting from severe hypotension (Geissler et al., 1997). Injury to pulmonary capillaries can lead to pulmonary oedema and microbubbles from turbulence precipitate platelet aggregation, leading to a systemic inflammatory response (Mirski et al., 2007). The heart continues to beat and can be felt through the chest but when auscultated with a stethoscope, the heart sounds like a washing machine. In severe cases of VAE, the peripheral pulse disappears, NIBP Doppler sound ceases, and $ETCO_2$ decreases to 0–16 mmHg, signifying a cardiac arrest. The ECG complexes will be normal for several minutes after loss of peripheral pulse. Usually, small amounts of air have no clinical significance but that cannot be guaranteed as small bubbles in an IV line were reported to induce cardiac arrest in a small dog (Walsh et al., 2005) and this author has personal experience that rapid IV injection of 3 mL of air into a cephalic vein caused cardiac arrest in an anaesthetized 15 kg (research) dog.

Clinical scenarios

When a large vein is lacerated, for example, in dogs and cats during dorsal spinal surgery, ventral cervical decompression, forelimb amputation, intra-abdominal surgery, or mastectomy, air may be entrained when intrathoracic pressure decreases during inspiration (Trim, unpublished observations). Directing pressurized air into an empty tooth socket during dentistry has caused subcutaneous emphysema, hypotension, and fatalities in dogs, cat, and humans (Gunew et al., 2008). Accidental penetration of a vessel may occur during insufflation for laparoscopy and result in massive CO_2 embolism (Staffieri et al., 2007). Injection of air bubbles from a syringe or fluid IV administration set or disconnection of a fluid line are all causes of air embolism. In conscious horses during placement of a jugular catheter with the tip towards the heart, air entrainment can be heard when the stilette is removed unless jugular vein compression is maintained

further down the neck. If the cap on the jugular catheter is dislodged or removed to change the cap for a syringe or tubing, air may be entrained. Fatalities and non-fatal neurological deficits have been described as consequences of catheter cap failure in horses during the perianaesthetic period (Holbrook et al., 2007). Loss of a catheter cap when a horse is in its stall depends on whether the horse lowers its head, when blood flows from the catheter, or lifts its head, when air is entrained. If discovered quickly and stopped, the horse may develop signs referable to hypotension, such as appearance of sedation and mild colic. Severe haemorrhage and fatalities have been associated with cases of displaced catheter caps in horses.

Monitoring and prevention

A Doppler NIBP probe placed over the chest in the area of the right atrium can detect small amounts of air in small animals. Sudden acute decreases in $ETCO_2$ observed on the capnograph waveform indicate a significant decrease in cardiac output. Altered Doppler sounds from a peripheral artery without significant $ETCO_2$ changes probably indicate insignificant amounts of air. Controlled ventilation abolishes negative intrathoracic pressure and may prevent air entrainment in the event of an accidental vein transection.

Treatment

An open IV line should be immediately closed. If the air was entrained from a surgical site, the area should first be flooded with saline and then packed off. If an acute decrease in $ETCO_2$ occurs during insufflation for laparoscopy, the needle should be removed immediately and the abdominal pressure released. When a standing horse collapsed following VAE from a catheter, immediate cardiac compressions apparently contributed to a successful outcome. Changing body position in experimental dogs resulted in relocation of air within the heart but had detrimental effects on cardiac output (Geissler et al., 1997). O_2 should be supplied, if not already. N_2O should be discontinued, if being used. In event of cardiac arrest or hypotension, CPCR with use of vasopressors should be started. Air can be aspirated from the heart in dogs and cats using a jugular catheter with the tip in or close to the right atrium (central venous pressure catheter) but, unless the catheter is already in place, this may have a low success rate. Cardiac puncture is a high risk because it may initiate ventricular fibrillation, pericardial tamponade from myocardial bleeding, and laceration of a coronary vessel. Neurological deficits in survivors should be treated appropriately. Clinical experience and published reports indicate that air embolisms during anaesthesia in dogs and cats are often fatal whereas more horses survive to receive intensive care and recover. Early diagnosis of air embolism may decrease mortality.

NIBP: non-invasive blood pressure; $ETCO_2$: end-tidal CO_2 (capnography).

Box 21.8 **Tension pneumothorax**

A pneumothorax develops when air enters the thorax, a) through ruptured lung (e.g rupture of pulmonary contusions or pleural bleb (Fig. 21.2), pneumonia, high airway pressure), b) lacerated oesophagus (e.g. during extraction of a swallowed bone or bougienage or placement of a feeding tube), c) tracheal tear, d) penetration of the chest wall (e.g. dog fight, fractured ribs, invasive subcutaneous tumour excision), e) neck surgery near the thoracic inlet (e.g. cervical fenestration, repair of collapsing trachea, tumour excision), or f) through the diaphragm and its attachments to the body wall when the abdomen is open (e.g. congenital defect of the diaphragm or concussive trauma or surgery in the cranial abdomen or closure of a diaphragmatic rupture). A tension pneumothorax develops when the site of air entry into the thorax acts as a one-way valve. Air enters the pleural cavity or mediastinum on inspiration, but is trapped and does not leave during expiration. The volume of air in the thorax increases with each breath, progressively restricting lung inflation. Hypercapnia and, ultimately, hypoxia, decreased cardiac output and hypotension develop. Immediate treatment of severe or tension pneumothorax is to insert a Butterfly needle or catheter, with three-way stopcock and syringe attached, into the pleural space to aspirate air and decrease the intrathoracic pressure. O_2 should be supplied and controlled ventilation may be necessary if air aspiration does not correct the hypoxaemia. A chest tube must be inserted if the leak continues and surgical closure may be appropriate for some leaks. Pawloski & Broaddus (2010) have provided a detailed review of pneumothorax in dogs, including practical details of chest tube placement and drainage.

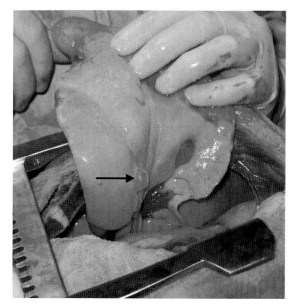

Figure 21.2 Pulmonary bleb in a dog. This dog was anaesthetized for lobectomy for treatment of persistent spontaneous pneumothorax.

patients with complications and length of hospital stay were significantly lower in the 'balanced' fluid administration compared with the 'unbalanced' protocols, although there was no apparent difference in outcomes.

In an attempt to limit the volume of isotonic crystalloid fluid needed to maintain a satisfactory MAP, one strategy has been to use a low infusion rate of crystalloid and to bump intravascular volume by periodic boluses or continuous infusion of colloid solutions. Hetastarch is a hydroxyethylstarch (HES) solution with a high *in vitro* molecular weight 450–600 kDal manufactured by hydroxyethylation of glucose molecules in the branched natural polymer, amylopectin. The molecular weight and degree of hydroxyl substitution influence the duration of effect. The duration of intravascular volume expansion for hetastarch is 12–48 h in humans but normal dogs have an increased concentration of serum amylase, the enzyme responsible for degradation of HES. Published durations

of HES or dextran 70, 20 mL/kg, in dogs are blood volume expansion maintained for at least 4 hours (Silverstein et al., 2005). After HES administration COP and blood volume had returned to preinfusion levels at 12 hours (Moore & Garvey, 1996) and at 24 hours (Chohan et al., 2011). Gelatins are modifications of bovine collagen with relatively low molecular weights of 30–35 kDal. The immediate plasma expansion is almost equal to the volume infused and the duration of effect is short (Niemi et al., 2010).

Hypertonic 7.5% saline solution (HSS) is used for rapid expansion of blood volume in treatment of severe blood loss because the much smaller volume, 4–5 mL/kg, can be infused quickly. The high osmolality decreases fluid filtration to the interstitial space, which subsequently becomes more osmolar and pulls out intracellular fluid. The duration of blood volume expansion by HSS is 1–2 hours and diuresis occurs. Crystalloid fluid must be given after HSS otherwise the patient will remain hypovolaemic (Barros et al., 2011). The cardiovascular response to resuscitation with HSS differs in conscious and anaesthetized animals. Infusion of HSS, 2 mL/kg, over 5 minutes to standing conscious instrumented sheep that were bled 20 mL/kg over 20 minutes resulted in blood volume expansion, an increase in MAP to above 70 mmHg within 3 minutes, increased cardiac output, and tachycardia (Frithiof et al., 2011). This experiment determined that HSS increased cardiac output beyond the effect of improved preload produced by volume expansion and that HES induced chronotropic and inotropic actions that depended on activation of the cardiac β-receptors. Hypertonic resuscitation causes peripheral vasodilation mainly due to the hyperosmolality-induced vascular smooth muscle relaxation. Consequently, in the presence of cardiovascular depression from anaesthetic agents, rapid IV administration of HSS may transiently augment hypotension in the anaesthetized animal (Kien et al., 1991; Frithiof et al., 2011).

Monitoring fluid infusion

The wide variation in fluid infusion rates, use of different animal species and patient populations, and the many alternative research protocols has interfered with the formation of a common agreement relating to intraoperative fluid administration. One unresolved issue is the best method for monitoring fluid administration to identify when a human or animal has received sufficient fluid (normovolaemia). Some studies were directed toward comparison of fluid types using infusions of fixed volumes and evaluation that included measurement of intravascular volume expansion by changes in haematocrit (Hct) or dilution of an injected dye (Evan's blue, indocyanine green) and measurement of haemodynamic parameters. Others have worked from the premise that administration of a fixed volume of fluid is unlikely to be ideal in every patient and measurements of MAP and HR can be within acceptable ranges in the presence of hypovolaemia. Therefore, goal-directed measurements are needed to aid in optimization of fluid load in individual patients, particularly patients that are sick or undergoing major surgery. Pulse pressure variation and systolic pressure variation can be used for goal-directed fluid therapy in patients with direct arterial pressure measurement, controlled ventilation with tidal volumes >7 mL/kg, and in the absence of arrhythmias (Kehlet & Bundgaard-Nielsen, 2009). Mixed venous oxygen saturation ($S_{mv}O_2$) >60% has been used as a target for goal-directed fluid therapy (Kimberger et al., 2009). Guiding fluid management using stroke volume and central venous pressure produced fewer episodes of hypotension and lower lactate concentrations at the end of surgery (Lansdorp et al., 2012). Recommendations for monitoring changes in stroke volume (using pulse contour or oesophageal Doppler methods) in response to fluid therapy in high-risk patients are being adopted by several societies associated with anaesthesia in humans (Michard & Biais, 2012). Some studies are attempting to define fluid protocols that go beyond normalization of systemic haemodynamics and investigate regimens that optimize tissue perfusion and oxygenation with minimal adverse effect. One such study involved pigs that were anaesthetized for laparotomy and intestinal anastomosis to compare intraoperative infusions of LRS or HES using $S_{mv}O_2$ >60% as a goal-directed fluid therapy target (Kimberger et al., 2009). Anaesthesia was maintained with infusions of injectable agents and ventilation was controlled using 30% O_2. The pigs were infused with LRS, 3 mL/

kg/h, or the same volume of LRS with periodic 250 mL boluses of LRS or HES (130/0.4) to achieve the target. Baseline measurements were made after instrumentation, colon anastomosis and closure of the abdomen. The mean $S_{mv}O_2$ of all groups was initially <60%. The MAP and cardiac index were improved in the goal-directed groups and the goal of $S_{mv}O_2$ >60% was achieved in the colloid group. Four hours later, the perianastomotic colon tissue O_2 tension was significantly increased to 147% or 245% above baseline in the goal-directed LRS and colloid groups, respectively. The microcirculatory blood flow in the healthy colon mucosa was highest in the colloid group but the anastomosis mucosal perfusion was unchanged. Total fluids infused included LRS, 3 mL/kg/h, average 928 mL for each pig for the duration of the experiment, plus an average of 831 mL HES in the colloid group or additional average 1794 mL LRS in the LRS goal-directed group. No differences were measured in gut wall glucose (an early marker of impaired intestinal perfusion) or lactate/pyruvate ratio between groups. There was no difference in the wet/dry weight ratios of lung tissue or healthy or anastomotic colon tissue between the two goal-directed groups. Infusion of HES improved systemic haemodynamic measurements and colon O_2 tension but not colon mucosa microcirculation. There are other options available in clinical anaesthesia to manipulate the patients' physiological parameters. In a similar experiment from the same laboratory comparing high and low crystalloid therapy, improvement in perianastomotic O_2 tension was only achieved by increasing the inspired O_2 to 100% (Kimberger et al., 2007).

Expansion capabilities of different colloids

Administration of a large volume of crystalloid solution may expand blood volume but fail adequately to treat hypotension. Healthy, normovolaemic experimental Beagles were made hypotensive by inducing deep isoflurane anaesthesia (Aarnes et al., 2009). Infusion of LRS, 80 mL/kg, over 1 hour increased blood volume and improved cardiac output but increased vasodilation prevented a change in systolic and MAP. In contrast, infusion of 6% HES reversed hypotension in four out of six dogs. The volume of HES required to achieve this effect was 4.3–40 mL/kg and the effect occurred within 5–46 minutes. Signs of fluid overload, fluid dripping from the nostrils, chemosis, and vomiting, were noted after anaesthesia in the dogs that received LRS. Infusion of such a large volume of LRS to animals with normovolaemia is not advisable and a smaller volume coupled with HES and decreasing isoflurane concentration will produce a better effect. Anaesthetized Beagles were made hypotensive by withdrawal of 14 mL/kg of blood (Muir, 2004). Administration of 6% HES (550/0.7) approximately equal to the volume of blood loss and given over 13 minutes rapidly reversed hypotension and increased cardiac output. In comparison, lactated Ringer's solution approximately 4.4 times the volume of blood loss was needed to correct hypotension. The haemodynamic parameters remained above baseline for the 2-hour monitoring period.

HSS in combination with colloids has been evaluated for expansion of blood volume in the absence of haemorrhage. Conscious instrumented sheep received, on separate occasions, LRS, 25 mL/kg, or 7.5% NaCl 6% dextran 70 (HSDex), 4 ml/kg IV, over 30 minutes (Tølløfsrud et al., 2001). The sheep may have been mildly dehydrated because water was withheld for 12 hours before the experiment. Using the Evans blue dilution technique to measure blood volume expansion, it was found that both fluids induced the same peak intravascular fluid expansion; decreasing rapidly by 30 minutes after LRS whereas HSDex maintained expansion for a further 30 minutes before decreasing slowly. Infusion of LRS resulted in increased extravascular volume. In contrast, HSDex resulted in a diuresis of several times its fluid volume and decreased extravascular volume, supporting the recommendation that HSS should be accompanied by infusion of crystalloid solution.

Conscious healthy normovolaemic dogs were given on separate occasions HHES as 7.5% NaCl in 6% HES (200/0.5), 4 mL/kg, or 20% mannitol, 4 mL/kg (1 g/kg), IV over 15 minutes and monitored for 2 hours (Robinson et al., 2011). Both agents produced a significant increase in blood volume, as calculated using the changes in Hct, lasting for the duration of the experiment. HHES induced significant hypernatraemia at 60 minutes. HHES and mannitol induced similar diuresis and the average amount of urine was approximately four times the volume infused. The authors concluded that HHES administration should not be repeated within 1–2 hours.

Management of septic shock generally requires administration of a vasoactive agent in addition to fluid therapy to treat hypotension. Administration of a sublethal dose of *E. coli* endotoxin to halothane-anaesthetized horses produced a wide variation in cardiopulmonary and biochemical responses consistent with previously published results (Pantaleon et al., 2006). In this experiment, resuscitation with crystalloid (Normosol®-R) at rates of 15 or 60 mL/kg, was compared with HSS 7.2% NaCl, 5 mL/kg, followed by HES (600/0.75), 10 mL/kg. Fluid infusions were started at the end of the 30-min endotoxin infusion and the horses were monitored for 3 hours. Mean pulmonary artery pressure was significantly increased and periorbital oedema was noticed more frequently in horses given the higher dose of crystalloid. No treatment had a beneficial effect on the changes induced by endotoxin as hypotension persisted and lactate increased in each group.

Adverse effects of colloid administration

Hetastarch can impair hemostasis by dilution of clotting factors and direct effect on coagulation factors and platelet function. The impact on coagulation was investigated in dogs anaesthetized with isoflurane and morphine epidurals for stifle arthroscopy (Chohan et al., 2011). Half of the dogs were infused with LRS, 10 mL/kg, IV over 20 minutes and the remainder with 6% HES (600/0.75), 10 mL/kg, over 20 minutes with all dogs then infused with LRS, 10 mL/kg/h. In both groups, buccal mucosa bleeding time (BMBT), considered to be the best test of platelet plug formation, and prothrombin time (PT) were significantly longer at 1 hour compared with before premedication. No significant changes were found in activated partial thromboplastin time (APTT), von Willebrand's factor antigen concentration (vWF:Ag) or factor VIII coagulant activity (FVIII:C). The surgeons, who were blinded to the fluid treatment, reported no indication of increased bleeding at the operative site. The COP was significantly higher in the HES group (14% below baseline compared with 24%) at 1 hour of anaesthesia but no difference was measured at 24 hours. The degree of impaired coagulation may not be significant for healthy patients but may have an impact on animals with abnormal coagulation profiles.

Anaphylaxis is a potential adverse effect of HES administration that is rarely reported. Package information for an HES (130/0.4) product in the veterinary market includes the recommendation for an initial slow infusion of a small volume of HES to allow time for observation of the signs of anaphylactic shock; also that HES is contraindicated in patients with pulmonary oedema, congestive heart failure, renal failure not related to hypovolaemia, and with intracranial bleeding.

The effect of HES administration in suppression of hepatic albumin synthesis may be a reason to minimize use of HES in animals with hypoproteinaemia.

Points to remember

Administration of a fixed volume of fluids as the main strategy is unlikely to prevent hypovolaemia or fluid excess in all patients; consequently fluid therapy must be based on knowledge of the individual's specific needs and continual assessment of peripheral perfusion during anaesthesia. Nonetheless, morbidity rather than mortality is primarily affected by the type of fluid and how it is administered (Rafie et al., 2004; Vallet, 2011). Fluid administration will depend on whether the patient is hypovolaemic or normovolaemic before induction of anaesthesia, and other factors, such as use of vasoactive agents or decreasing the inhalant anaesthetic concentration can be used to improve haemodynamic performance. When assessing response to colloid administration, it should be remembered that measurement of total protein using a refractometer will not reflect the contribution by the colloid.

Blood loss

Assessment of blood loss during anaesthesia is made from the following information:

- Estimation of the volume on the drapes, in a suction bottle, on the floor, or in a bucket placed under the surgical site. Sometimes visualizing the volume of fluid in a 50 mL drug bottle or 500/1000 mL fluid bag can be used for a reference point. Buckets used in large animal surgery can be premarked in litre volumes.
- When blood loss is anticipated, the Hct and TP should be measured after induction of anaesthesia and before the start of surgery. The Hct will change little during haemorrhage when fluid therapy is minimal, but will provide an idea of the impact of blood loss when measured during infusion of crystalloid at a 2–3 : 1 ratio. The Hct will progressively increase with time as the crystalloid fluid leaves the vascular space and increase further during recovery from anaesthesia due to splenic contraction.
- Blood loss can be measured during surgery on small animals by weighing the blood-soaked gauzes and subtracting the weight of dry gauzes. Using a gram scale, 1 dry gauze and a plastic bag are weighed separately. A known number of used gauzes are placed in the bag and weighed. Assuming that 1 gram weight = (approximately) 1 mL blood, then mL blood lost = weight of used gauzes in the plastic bag – (weight of one dry gauze × number of gauzes plus weight of the plastic bag).
- Blood pressure will decrease, cardiac output will decrease earlier and to a greater extent than blood pressure, and HR may not reliably change. Blood pressure may remain constant until severe blood loss has occurred when crystalloid or colloid fluid therapy is provided.
- Calculation of the % of blood loss to normal blood volume. Blood volume differs between species, for example, values published for conscious healthy animals are:
  - Thoroughbreds, 100 mL/kg
  - Pony and draft horses, 72 mL/kg
  - Dogs, 86 mL/kg
  - Sheep, 60 mL/kg
  - Cats, 56 mL/kg.

In experimental studies, the cardiovascular effects of blood loss are modified by the conscious state versus anaesthesia, the anaesthetic agents and the species, and influenced by the volume lost, the speed of loss, and whether the end-point was a predetermined volume or the volume determined by a target blood pressure. For example, when blood was removed from isoflurane-anaesthetized dogs until hypotension developed, mean blood loss was 14 mL/kg (approximately 17% of blood volume) withdrawn over 15 minutes (Muir, 2004). Cardiac output had decreased by >40%. In another study of dogs anaesthetized with halothane, isoflurane, or sevoflurane, removal of 32 mL/kg (37–40% of blood volume) over 30 minutes resulted in decreased MAP to about 40 mmHg in dogs anaesthetized with halothane or sevoflurane but only to 65 mmHg during isoflurane anaesthesia (Teixeira Neto et al., 2007). Cardiac outputs were decreased by 46.5–49.5% during all three anaesthetic agents and HRs were unchanged during halothane and sevoflurane but increased during isoflurane anaesthesia. There is little detailed information about effects of graded haemorrhage on cardiovascular parameters in horses. In one study of horses weighing an average 486 kg, anaesthetized with halothane (8) or isoflurane (1), and receiving lactated Ringer's solution, 10 mL/kg/h, an approximate blood loss of 10 L over 15 minutes caused hypotension and prolonged CRT (Wilson et al., 2003). That heart rates, Hct and base excess values were unchanged is of significance to monitoring of clinical patients.

It is important to realize that anaesthetized animals cannot tolerate the same blood loss as conscious animals because cardiovascular reflexes are depressed. Overall, significant haemodynamic changes occur in healthy anaesthetized animals after blood loss equivalent to 15–20% of the patient's blood volume. Circulatory shock may be produced in old, debilitated, or anaemic animals with a smaller blood loss.

Fluid resuscitation

When hypotension is caused by haemorrhage, the decrease in hydrostatic pressure reduces fluid loss from the intravascular space resulting in augmentation of blood volume 'autotransfusion'. This effect is short lived but is a significant physiological protective mechanism.

For many years, blood loss has been replaced by infusion of balanced electrolyte solution at a rate of 2.5–3 times the volume of shed blood. Frequently, this is an effective method to maintain arterial blood pressure, particularly when accompanied by a decrease in anaesthetic administration. The previous section has described the adverse effects of infusion of large volumes of crystalloid solution; therefore, addition of plasma substitute becomes necessary at some point during haemorrhage and, ultimately, the administration of an O_2-carrying solution.

There is evidence that when treating haemorrhagic hypotension, MAP 65 mmHg may be a suboptimal target. Conscious, instrumented sheep were subjected to blood loss of 35 mL/kg over 1 hour (Rafie et al., 2004). Haemorrhage resulted in a 65% decrease in cardiac output, MAP <45 mmHg, and HR increase to an average of 150 beats/min. The sheep were resuscitated using LRS or 6% HES (670/0.75) in LRS, beginning 30 minutes after the start of haemorrhage. The infusion rates were initially fast and then slowed as MAP of either 65 or 90 mmHg was approached, and the sheep were monitored for 3 hours. The total volumes of infused fluid to achieve MAP 65 mmHg were LRS, 18 mL/kg, or HES, 12 mL/kg, but cardiac outputs remained 15–20% below prehaemorrhage values. Infusion of LRS at an average of 61 mL/kg restored cardiac output and MAP increased to just short of 90 mmHg. Plasma volumes for all three treatments were similar for the first 90 minutes. Since half of the sheep resuscitated to MAP 65 mmHg developed a metabolic acidosis and two sheep died, the authors concluded that MAP 65 mmHg was too low for optimal outcome.

Small volume HES in hypertonic saline resuscitation may effectively restore cardiovascular parameters but not tissue perfusion. Isoflurane-anaesthetized dogs were bled 20 mL/kg and MAP and cardiac output were effectively resuscitated using saline 40 mL/kg (2:1 saline:blood loss) or HHES, 4 mL/kg, for the 60 minutes monitoring period (Udelsmann et al., 2009). In another study of dogs anaesthetized with isoflurane, splenectomized, and haemorrhaged approximately 30 mL/kg over 60 minutes to maintain MAP 40–50 mmHg, infusion of either LRS 3:1 volume of shed blood, HES (130/0.4) in a 1:1 volume of shed blood, or HHES (7.5% saline in 6% HES (130/0.4)), 4.4 mL/kg, reversed the hypotension and increased cardiac output to or above baseline measurements (Barros et al., 2011). However, blood volume expansion by HHES was significantly less than produced by HES, and beneficial effects were decreasing at 90 minutes. Gastric mucosal blood flow was restored by infusion of LRS and HES but measurements indicated hypoperfusion persisting in dogs given HHES.

Fluid therapy in pregnant animals is complicated as changes in the fetus may be significantly different from those in the mother. Haemorrhage of 20 mL/kg over 10 minutes in anaesthetized and instrumented pregnant sheep caused maternal hypotension, heart rate decreases from on average 119 beats/min to 88 (range 40–167) beats/min, and decreased blood O_2 content, uterine blood flow, and uterine O_2 delivery (Moon et al., 2001). Acute fetal hypoxaemia and acidaemia were induced, and one fetus died during haemorrhage. The ewes were successfully resuscitated by either an autologous blood transfusion (reinfusion of lost blood), with 6% HES at 20 mL/kg, or with oxyglobin at 20 mL/kg, however, HES did not restore O_2 delivery to the fetus. This investigation confirms the ability of HES to restore adequate circulatory function but, at some point, administration of crystalloid and/or colloid is insufficient and an O_2-carrying product must be included.

Blood product transfusion triggers

- Assessed blood loss at 20–25% of the anaesthetized patient's circulating blood volume.
- Hct ≤20% during anaesthesia or Hct ≤25% before anaesthesia for surgery (these values may vary according to whether anaemia is acute or chronic, and the planned procedure).
- Failure to restore haemodynamic parameters to acceptable values using a combination of crystalloid

and colloid fluid therapy, decreased anaesthetic agent, and vasoactive agent.
- Need to maintain O_2 delivery to fetus.
- Need for labile coagulation factors in fresh whole blood for patients with thrombocytopaenia, haemophilia, hepatic disease, disseminated intravascular coagulation.

Intravenous lipid emulsion (ILE)

Intravenous administration of lipid to counter CNS depression from barbiturate was first published in 1962, but interest in using the lipid effect against drug overdosage did not increase until the late 1990s. To date, there are many papers addressing 'lipid rescue™' (www.lipidrescue.org) of human patients and experimental animals after toxic effects of local anaesthetics and other lipophilic agents have caused cardiovascular collapse or cardiac arrest (Candela et al., 2010; Cave et al., 2011; Fernandez et al., 2011; Mauch et al., 2011; Weinberg & Warren, 2012). Reports of ILE in human patients and animals have involved the toxic effects of the local anaesthetic agents lidocaine, mepivacaine, bupivacaine and ropivacaine, and other drugs including tricyclic antidepressants, lipophilic β-blockers, and calcium channel blockers.

There are few published reports of use of ILE in the treatment of toxicities in clinical veterinary patients (Fernandez et al., 2011). One puppy with suspected moxidectin toxicosis from ingestion exhibited seizures, slow heart rate, severe respiratory acidosis, and high lactate concentration (Crandell & Weinberg, 2009). Treatment consisted of oral activated charcoal, IPPV with O_2, atropine, and IV fluids. Approximately 10 hours after toxic exposure, 20% soybean emulsion, 2 mL/kg, was injected IV as a bolus followed by 3.75 mL/kg/h for 4 hours. After 2 hours of ILE therapy, controlled ventilation was discontinued but the puppy remained unconscious. It received further intensive care until 25 hours after suspected toxic exposure when another infusion of lipid emulsion, 15 mL/kg given over 30 minutes was quickly followed by return to ambulation and improved behaviour.

A domestic shorthair cat that was recumbent and unresponsive, exhibiting respiratory distress and cardiovascular collapse was suspected of lidocaine toxicity after receiving local infiltration of lidocaine, 20 mg/kg (O'Brien et al., 2010). The cat was given O_2 to breathe but initial attempts at placing an IV catheter failed. Thirty minutes after admission (one hour after lidocaine injection), the cat was less lethargic, able to assume sternal position but unable to hold its head up. A 20% 50:50 emulsion of soybean and safflower oil, 1.5 mL/kg, was infused over 30 minutes and by the end of the infusion the cat was able to hold its head up, appeared aware of its surroundings and began grooming behaviour. The maximum suggested dose of lidocaine in cats for local analgesia is about 4 mg/kg. When three times that dose is infiltrated during general anaesthesia, the first indication may be death during the recovery period. The cat in the previous report received a massive overdose and was fortunate to survive transportation to a referral hospital. The half-life of lidocaine is quite short and supportive therapy may be sufficient to allow detoxification and patient survival.

An inadvertent IV injection of bupivacaine during local infiltration may result in an abrupt decrease in blood pressure that is responsive to discontinuing anaesthetic administration and IV infusion of dobutamine or dopamine. However, ILE seems to be a logical treatment for local anaesthetic overdose if conventional measures of resuscitation, such as O_2, IPPV, IV fluids, and vasoactive drugs, do not produce improvement. The optimal dose rate of lipid emulsion for this purpose in domestic animals has not been determined and may differ between species. Weinberg et al. (2003), in early experiments with isoflurane-anaesthetized dogs, induced circulatory collapse and cardiac arrest or bradycardia <10 beats/min by IV injection of bupivacaine, 10 mg/kg. Isoflurane was discontinued and cardiac massage instituted for 10 minutes before infusion of lipid emulsion (20% soybean oil), 4 mL/kg bolus followed by a continuous infusion of 0.5 mL/kg/min for 10 minutes, or saline. Normal sinus rhythm was established in 6/6 dogs within 5 minutes of starting the lipid infusion and cardiovascular parameters progressed to baseline values by 30 minutes. In contrast, no dogs given saline recovered adequate circulation (Weinberg et al., 2003). ILE has had positive results in animal experiments involving rats and rabbits but not in pigs.

The use of ILE has been included in practice advisories of the Association of Anaesthetists of Great Britain and Ireland, the American Society of Regional Anesthesia and Pain Medicine, endorsed by the American Heart Association Advanced Cardiac Life Support recommendations, and the Australian and New Zealand College of Anaesthetists (Cave et al., 2011; Weinberg & Warren, 2012). ILE is recommended after primary intensive care support, including O_2, IPPV, IV fluids, and specific antagonists, has failed to achieve improved responsiveness. It is important to establish good oxygenation in the patient as ILE administration may have deleterious effects, including cardiac arrhythmias, in the hypoxic subject. Interaction of ILE with concurrent administration of CPCR drugs is being investigated, with varying results. Some studies indicate a beneficial effect of a low (1 μg/kg) dose of epinephrine. Recommended dose rates for ILE in humans for toxic syndromes are 1.5 mL/kg IV over 1 minute followed by an infusion of 0.25 mL/kg/min IV over 30–60 minutes, and the bolus could be repeated 1–2 times for persistent asystole (www.lipidrescue.org). These dose rates are flexible depending on the circumstances. These instructions come with a recommendation that an emergency box containing the items needed for ILE be immediately available where

local anaesthesia is performed. Fernandez et al. (2011), in a review directed at the veterinary profession, suggested lipid dose rates for dogs and cats in the range 1.5–4 mL/kg (0.3–0.8 g/kg) followed by 0.25 mL/kg/min (0.05 g/kg/min) IV over 30–60 minutes. They noted that additional IV increments may be needed in animals that remain unresponsive such as 1.5 mL/kg every 4–6 h or an infusion of 0.5 mL/kg/h, given up to a maximum of 24 hours. Emulsions of long chain triglycerides (LCT) and mixtures of LCT and medium chain triglycerides have been used in clinical cases and experimental investigations. Further studies are needed to confirm whether one product is more effective than the other. Fernandez et al. (2011) included detailed descriptions of the different formulations of lipid emulsions in their review. Adverse effects following administration of lipid emulsion for resuscitation have not been reported but anaphylactoid and allergic reactions have been reported during use for parenteral nutrition.

There are currently three proposed mechanisms for the effect of lipid emulsion on lipophilic toxins: the 'lipid sink' theory; the carnitine metabolism theory; and the calcium agonist theory (Litonius et al., 2012). The 'lipid sink' theory proposes that the lipid infusion creates a large lipid fraction in the plasma that traps lipophilic toxins. An *in vitro* model adding lipid emulsion to water containing two lipophilic dyes with log P values comparable to lidocaine and bupivacaine and comparing the resultant colour changes seemed to support the concept of a 'lipid sink' effect (Papadopoulou et al., 2012). However, ILE administered to human volunteers given a non-toxic dose of bupivacaine IV moderately decreased the total plasma concentrations of bupivacaine but had no effect on the plasma non-lipid bound or free (non-protein bound) concentrations of bupivacaine (Litonius et al., 2012). The pharmacokinetic results of this study suggested that bupivacaine was redistributed into tissues at a faster rate during lipid emulsion infusion but the authors noted that there might be difference between a non-cardiotoxic dose and an overdose of bupivacaine. Carnitine acylcarnitine translocase is an enzyme that contributes to passage of free fatty acids bound to acetyl coA across mitochondrial membranes (Picard & Meek, 2006; Fernandez et al., 2011). Inhibition of this enzyme by local anaesthetics results in depleted energy supply for the myocardium. One suggestion is that a lipid infusion overcomes the enzyme inhibition thus restoring the myocardial energy supply.

INADEQUATE ANAESTHESIA

Signs of light anaesthesia differ between injectable and inhalant anaesthesia and between species. Signs associated with light or inadequate anaesthesia include any or all of the following: presence of a strong palpebral reflex;

nystagmus in horses; eyeball rolled rostroventrally in any animal or sometimes dorsocaudally (star-gazing) in horses and pigs; autonomic responses such as increased heart rate or blood pressure; increased respiratory rate; and muscle movements associated with an aspect of surgery or the procedure; or muscle tremors. Some of these signs can be caused by other conditions such as hypoxaemia, hypercarbia, and hyperthermia, and these must be ruled out. In horses, ketamine anaesthesia can be associated with spontaneous blinking and nystagmus and should not be assumed to be due to light anaesthesia. Horses susceptible to developing hyperkalaemic periodic paralysis may start twitching during anaesthesia if the syndrome is triggered. Management will depend on the cause (Table 21.5) and on the clinical scenario, for example, a dog wakening during inhalation anaesthesia in the operating room will be managed differently from a horse anaesthetized with injectable agents for castration or eye enucleation in the field. The reader is referred to anaesthetic management in the species-specific chapters. It is important to remember that during inhalation anaesthesia when the effects of premedicant and induction drugs begin to wane then the vaporizer setting must be increased to abolish response to surgery. The increased inspired inhalation agent is accompanied by a progressive decrease in blood pressure. Administration of a sedative or analgesic drug usually allows a decrease in the inhaled anaesthetic concentration that may result in an improvement in blood pressure.

MUSCLE MOVEMENTS

Twitching or jerks of the muzzle, ears, and legs occur occasionally in dogs and cats following administration of propofol or etomidate for induction of anaesthesia. No specific treatment is indicated as the twitches will disappear after about 10 minutes. Increasing anaesthetic administration is not the correct treatment for this abnormality.

Shivering or tremors may be observed in some animals during lightening of anaesthesia or recovery from inhalation anaesthesia or after epidural analgesia. Shivering is not always associated with hypothermia, although warming should be applied if the patient is cold.

INJURY ASSOCIATED WITH ANAESTHESIA

Contrast agents

Cardiovascular collapse and death occasionally occur after injection of contrast agents used for imaging. Management is listed in Tables 21.1, 21.3 and Box 21.3. Seizures may occur following myelography, particularly in large dogs with cervical lesions and cervical injections (da Costa et al., 2011). The risk for seizures in all species after myelography should be minimized by facilitating caudal movement of dye in the spinal cord after radiography by elevating the head by 45° to the spine and by promoting elimination of iohexol by diuresis with IV fluids, 10 mL/kg/h. Elimination of iohexol in horses is facilitated by premedication with an α_2-agonist such as xylazine through its diuretic effect. It is our practice to maintain anaesthesia in dogs and cats for 45 minutes after injection of iohexol as an arbitrary time for elimination before allowing the patient to recover slowly from anaesthesia (unless proceeding to surgery). Horses are not kept anaesthetized but moved to a quiet room for recovery, positioned with the head elevated, given xylazine 0.2 mg/kg IV if anaesthetized with an inhalation agent and O_2 by nasal insufflation. Some horses are more ataxic in recovery than before anaesthesia and may need assistance to stand. An NSAID should be administered some hours before anaesthesia.

Postoperative infection

Surgical site infections can be influenced by many factors, such as obesity that decreases wound O_2 tensions and predisposes towards more difficult hygienic practices, the site of the incision and its proximity to contamination, and the animal's licking or rubbing the surgical site. Anaesthetic management also influences postoperative infection. Regional analgesia has been documented in humans to decrease surgical site infection compared with general anaesthesia, possibly relating to vasodilation and increased wound blood flow facilitating migration of neutrophils. A long duration of anaesthesia is also associated with increased incidence of infection because anaesthetic agents decrease the immune response and decreased cardiovascular function decreases wound perfusion. Both hypovolaemia and overadministration of crystalloid fluid can affect the incidence of surgical site infection, and hypothermia in the patient has been associated with increased infection. There are studies comparing the effects of 30% with 80% inspired O_2 on surgical site infection and results of meta-analyses have been interpreted with varying results. One recent meta-analysis determined that hyperoxia did not have an impact on surgical site infection over a range of surgical procedures but that a subgroup analysis of trials in which human patients underwent only colorectal surgery there was a significant benefit of hyperoxia in decreasing surgical site infection (Togioka et al., 2012). These results might have relevance for horses undergoing colon surgery. Direct application of O_2 within the lumen of ischaemic intestine in anaesthetized experimental ponies was found to decrease the severity of intestinal mucosa damage (Moore et al., 1980).

Table 21.5 Inadequate anaesthesia: causes and management (Note that it is difficult to provide management for every situation and this table is intended only to provide a guide)

Species	Causes	Management
Drugs		
All species	Insufficient anaesthetic administration or inadequate analgesia, premedication and induction agent effects waning	Increase vaporizer setting and/or administer analgesic agent
	Hypoventilation	IPPV
Equipment		
All species	Circuit incorrectly assembled or disconnected	Check anaesthesia machine and circuit for faults
	Vaporizer: filler port open, insufficient liquid, room too cold	Check vaporizer, fluid level, output
	Inspired anaesthetic concentration lower than estimated: rebreathing circuit VOC, large patient with low O_2 flow	Transiently increase O_2 flow or increase vaporizer setting, compress rebreathing bag to empty and fill with fresh gas
	Endotracheal tube too small (resistance to airflow), cuff not airtight (inspired gas diluted with air), tube out or in oesophagus	Check endotracheal tube for placement, check for air leak by inflating lungs and listening or feeling neck for vibration (large animals)
	Syringe/infusion pump for adjunct agents not turned on or inaccurate delivery	Check infusion pump and check liquid flow from the extension tubing, check volume delivered : calculated
Other patient problems & procedure		
All species	Increased surgical or procedural stimulus intensity	Increase anaesthesia or analgesia
	Excited patient before anaesthesia resulting in decreased blood volume	Fluid bolus and vasoconstriction: dopamine for dogs and cats, ephedrine for horses
	Malignant hyperthermia may mimic light anaesthesia (signs in Chapter 2)	Discontinue inhalation anaesthesia, dantrolene, ice (see Chapter 2)
Cardiac		
All species	Intraventricular shunting of injectable drugs through ventricular septal defect = less effect from standard induction drug dose rate	Convert to inhalation anaesthesia, auscultation for murmur or ultrasound
Respiratory		
All species	Hypoxaemia may mimic light anaesthesia although many animals that are hypoxaemic show no signs	Check membrane colour and SpO_2 as part of troubleshooting
	Hypoventilation decreases delivery of inhalant agent: panting in dogs (brachycephalic breeds, opioids), V/Q inequality in large animals	IPPV usually results in an adequate and stable plane of anaesthesia

VOC: vaporizer-outside-circle.

Myopathy and nerve damage

Ischaemia of tissues due to compression or hypotension during anaesthesia is most often observed in horses and details of safe positioning during anaesthesia and differential diagnoses are discussed in Chapter 11. Injury can occur with horses in dorsal or lateral positions, and with flexed or frog-legged limbs. Damage varies from oedematous plaques present on the dependent side of the animal, over the masseter muscle and over the thorax, flank, or thigh, to neuropathy or myopathy of the forelimb or hind limb, facial nerve paralysis, and swelling of a masseter muscle or one or both gluteal muscles. An NSAID and analgesia are first line treatment. Sedation (acepromazine) may be needed for anxious or active horses, and ice may be necessary when hyperactivity or struggling has resulted in hyperthermia. When standing is difficult due to radial nerve or peroneal or femoral nerve paralysis, the opposite limb may need external bandage support. Some horses may need to be supported in a sling. Horses that remain recumbent will need intensive care that may include, in addition to just mentioned treatment, dimethylsulphoxide (DMSO), catheterization of the urinary bladder for drainage, frequent turning, O_2 by insufflation, and periodic laboratory tests to identify abnormalities. Myopathy may progress to renal failure due to release of massive amounts of myoglobin, and early aggressive IV fluid therapy is recommended in an attempt to prevent irreversible renal damage.

Radial nerve paralysis may develop in adult cattle and has been discussed in Chapter 12. Radial nerve damage is a rare complication after anaesthesia in large dogs (legs hanging off the table) but should be prevented by care with positioning and padding during anaesthesia. There are anecdotal reports of tongue paralysis in dogs, presumably due to excessive traction during intubation or positioning that causes occlusion of the lingual artery and ischaemia for a period of time.

Visual loss

Loss of vision after anaesthesia is rare but occurs in humans and animals. In human patients, the most common causes of perioperative visual loss (POVL) are retinal artery occlusion (RAO) and ischaemic optic neuropathy (ION) associated with a wide variety of procedures but commonly cardiothoracic surgery, spine, head and neck surgery where the patient is lying in prone position (Roth, 2009). Retinal ischaemia may result from occlusion of the central retinal artery due to external compression of the eye from improper patient positioning, including use of a horseshoe headrest where the head is moved during surgery and the eye becomes compressed. This results in unilateral partial or complete loss of vision. Occlusion of a branch of the central retinal artery has been associated with emboli created during cardiopulmonary

bypass. Many potential contributing causes have been listed for ION, including eye compression, hypotension, abnormalities in blood supply to the optic nerve, long duration surgery, large amounts of IV fluids during anaesthesia, and a possible impact of operating table position (head down) (Roth, 2009). The impact of blood loss and haemodilution on optic nerve O_2 delivery has been investigated as a possible cause of POVL. Studies in pigs and cats determined that isovolaemic haemodilution did not have a significant effect on O_2 delivery to the optic nerve. However, simultaneously decreasing the haematocrit and inducing hypotension significantly decreased O_2 delivery.

One might expect horses in dorsal recumbency to be at risk for external eye compression resulting in blindness, especially when the head is rotated into an oblique position, however, that does not seem to be the case. Twenty-five years ago, blindness in horses after halothane anaesthesia was an occasional occurrence and was attributed to cortical ischaemia from hypotension although unconfirmed because in those cases blood pressure was not measured. Similarly, there have been anecdotal reports over the years of POVL in dogs and cats after anaesthesia for elective procedures. Many years ago, two patients under my care had cardiac arrests during anaesthesia, a cat anaesthetized with methoxyflurane for ovariohysterectomy and a dog anaesthetized with halothane undergoing thoracotomy for ligation of a patent ductus arteriosus. After resuscitation, the cat was blind for 3 days and the dog for 2–3 months. In these cases involving cardiac arrest, it was assumed that the visual loss was due to cerebral cortical ischaemia as a result of hypotension.

Recently, the medical records of 20 cats with POVL were reviewed (Stiles et al., 2012). Three cats had suffered cardiac arrests and the blindness was presumed due to cerebral hypoxia. Eight cats were examined by an ophthalmologist who characterized the blindness as cortical in origin, based on normal size pupils, normal direct and indirect pupillary light reflexes, positive dazzle reflex, negative menace response, and lack of ocular lesions. Many of the cats had received acepromazine and an opioid, buprenorphine, butorphanol, oxymorphone, or hydromorphone, for premedication, anaesthesia was induced with propofol in 14 cats and, except for two cats that suffered cardiac arrest immediately, anaesthesia was maintained with isoflurane/O_2. The earliest recovery of vision was 1 day and the longest 6 weeks (average 4.5 days) in 11 cats that were monitored regularly, but vision improved over several months in all cats. Seventeen cats had additional neurological abnormalities after recovery from anaesthesia and 59% of 17 cats with follow-up records recovered fully; one cat was euthanized because of neurological abnormalities. Excluding the cats with cardiac arrest, 13 cats were undergoing dentistry and four were anaesthetized for endoscopy, and of these, a spring-held mouth gag was inserted in all but one cat. The authors were unable to prove by dissection of cadavers that the open-mouth position limited blood flow in the maxillary artery and to the brain, but postulated that the spring-held mouth gag may be a risk factor for POVL. A recent scientific presentation described imaging techniques identifying decreased maxillary artery blood flow in approximately 50% of a group of anaesthetized cats when the mouth was maximally opened using a spring-loaded mouth gag (Barton-Lamb et al., 2012). All the cats recovered uneventfully from anaesthesia. The anaesthetic combination of propofol and isoflurane frequently causes hypotension in cats. In Stiles et al. (2012), hypotension was measured in seven cats and no blood pressure monitoring was performed on a further seven cats. Consequently, hypotension cannot be ruled out as a cause of cerebral hypoxia, especially if the cats were also hypercarbic. Blood pressure monitoring and appropriate response to abnormal measurements should be an integral part of patient management during inhalation anaesthesia.

REFERENCES

Aarnes, T.K., Bednarski, R.M., Lerche, P., et al., 2009. Effect of intravenous administration of lactated Ringer's solution or hetastarch for the treatment of isoflurane-induced hypotension in dogs. Am J Vet Res 70, 1345–1353.

Armitage-Chan, E., 2010. Anaphylaxis and anaesthesia. Vet Anaesth Analg 37, 306–310.

Ball, M.A., Trim, C.M., 1996. Post anaesthetic pulmonary oedema in two horses. Equine Vet Educ 8, 13–16.

Barros, J.M.P., de Nascimento, P., Marinello, J.L.P., et al., 2011. The effects of 6% hydroxyethyl starch-hypertonic saline in resuscitation of dogs with hemorrhagic shock. Anesth Analg 112, 395–404.

Barton-Lamb, A., Martin-Flores, M., Ludders, J., et al., 2012. Evaluation of maxillary arterial flow in cats with and without use of a spring loaded dental mouth gag. In Proceedings of 18th IVEECS Symposium, San Antonio, TX, USA, p. 721.

Bertin, F.R., Ivester, K.M., Couëtil, L.L., 2011. Comparative efficacy of inhaled albuterol between two hand-held delivery devices in horses with recurrent airway obstruction. Equine Vet J 43, 393–398.

Borer, K.E., 2005. Pulmonary oedema associated with anaesthesia for colic surgery in a horse. Vet Anaesth Analg 32, 228–232.

Boutureira, J., Trim, C.M., Cornell, K.K., 2007. Acute pulmonary edema after diazepam-ketamine in a dog. Vet Anaesth Analg 34, 371–376.

Buchner, H.H.F., Kübber, P., Zohmann, E., et al., 1999. Sedation and antisedation as tools in equine lameness examination. Equine Vet J Suppl 30, 227–230.

Bundgaard-Nielsen, M., Secher, N.H., Kehlet, H., 2009. 'Liberal' vs. 'restrictive' perioperative fluid therapy – a critical assessment of the evidence. Acta Anaesthesiol Scand 53, 843–851.

Candela, D., Louart, G., Bousquet, J.-P., et al., 2010. Reversal of bupivacaine-induced cardiac electrophysiologic changes by two lipid emulsions in anesthetized and mechanically ventilated piglets. Anesth Analg 110, 1473–1479.

Carr, A.P., Tilley, L.P., Miller, M.S., 2001. Treatment of cardiac arrhythmias and conduction disturbances. In: Tilley, L.P., Goodwin, J.-K. (Eds.), Manual of Canine and Feline Cardiology. W.B. Saunders, Co, Philadelphia, pp. 371–405.

Carroll, G.L., Matthews, N.S., Hartsfield, S.M., et al., 1997. The effect of detomidine and its antagonism with tolazoline on stress-related hormones, metabolites, physiologic responses, and behavior in awake ponies. Vet Surg 26, 69–77.

Cave, G., Harvey, M., Graundins, A., 2011. Review article: Intravenous lipid emulsion as an antidote: A summary of published human experience. Emerg Med Austral 23, 123–141.

Chappell, D., Jacob, M., Hoffmann-Kiefer, K., et al., 2008. A rational approach to perioperative fluid management. Anesthesiology 109, 723–740.

Chohan, A.S., Greene, S.A., Grubb, T.L., et al., 2011. Effects of 6% hetastarch (600/0.75) or lactated Ringer's solution on hemostatic variables and clinical bleeding in healthy dogs anesthetized for orthopedic surgery. Vet Anaesth Analg 38, 94–105.

Cotten, J.F., Keshavaprasad, B., Laster, M.J., et al., 2006. The ventilatory stimulant doxapram inhibits TASK tandem pore (K2P) potassium channel function but does not affect minimum alveolar anesthetic concentration. Anesth Analg 102, 779–785.

Crandell, D.E., Weinberg, G.L., 2009. Moxidectin toxicosis in a puppy successfully treated with intravenous lipids. J Vet Emerg Crit Care 19, 181–186.

da Costa, R.C., Parent, J.M., Dobson, H., 2011. Incidence of and risk factors for seizures after myelography performed with iohexol in dogs: 503 cases (2002–2004). J Am Vet Med Assoc 238, 1296–1300.

Derksen, F.J., Olszewski, M.A., Robinson, N.E., et al., 1999. Aerosolized albuterol sulfate used as a bronchodilator in horses with recurrent airway obstruction. Am J Vet Res 60, 689–693.

Di Concetto, S., Archer, R.M., Sigurdsson, S.F., et al., 2007. Atipamezole in the management of detomidine overdose in a pony. Vet Anaesth Analg 34, 67–69.

Duprat, F., Lesage, F., Fink, M.P., et al., 1997. TASK, a human background K+ channel to sense external pH variations near physiological pH. EMBO J 16, 5464–5471.

Fernandez, A.L., Lee, J.A., Rahilly, L., et al., 2011. The use of intravenous lipid emulsion as an antidote in veterinary toxicology. J Vet Emerg Crit Care 21, 309–320.

Frithiof, R., Ramchandra, R., Hood, S.G., et al., 2011. Hypertonic sodium resuscitation after hemorrhage improves hemodynamic function by stimulating cardiac, but not renal, sympathetic nerve activity. Am J Physiol Heart Circ Physiol 300, H685–H692.

Geissler, H.J., Allen, S.J., Mehihorn, U., et al., 1997. Effect of body repositioning after venous air embolism. Anesthesiology 86, 710–717.

Gunew, M., Marshall, R., Lui, M., et al., 2008. Fatal venous air embolism in a cat undergoing dental extractions. J Small Anim Pract 49, 601–604.

Gunkel, C.I., Valverde, A., Robertson, S.A., et al., 2004. Treatment for a severe reaction to intravenous administration of diatrizoate in an anesthetized horse. J Am Vet Med Assoc 224, 1143–1146.

Holbrook, T.C., Dechant, J.E., Crowson, C.L., 2007. Suspected air embolism asssociated with post-anesthetic pulmonary edema and neurologic sequelae in a horse. Vet Anaesth Analg 34, 217–222.

Honnas, C.M., 1999. Principles of emergency respiratory therapy. In: Colahan, P.T., Mayhew, I.G., Merritt, A.M., Moore, J.N. (Eds.), Equine Medicine and Surgery, *Vol I*. Mosby, Inc, St Louis, pp. 458–460.

Hsu, W.H., 2008a. Appendix 2. In: Hsu, W.H. (Ed.), Handbook of Veterinary Pharmacology. Wiley-Blackwell, Ames, pp. 489–536.

Hsu, W.H., 2008b. Chapter 2. In: Hsu, W.H. (Ed.), Handbook of Veterinary Pharmacology. Wiley-Blackwell, Ames, pp. 29–58.

Hubbell, J.A.E., Muir, W.W., 2006. Antagonism of detomidine sedation in the horse using intravenous tolazoline or atipamezole. Equine Vet J 38, 238–241.

Hubbell, J.A.E., Muir, W.W., Robertson, J.T., et al., 1987. Cardiovascular effects of intravenous sodium penicillin, sodium cefazolin, and sodium citrate in awake and anesthetized horses. Vet Surg 16, 245–250.

Kehlet, H., Bundgaard-Nielsen, M., 2009. Goal-directed perioperative fluid management. Anesthesiology 110, 453–455.

Kien, N.D., Kramer, G.C., White, D.A., 1991. Acute hypotension caused by rapid hypertonic saline infusion in anesthetized dogs. Anesth Analg 73, 597–602.

Kimberger, O., Arnberger, M., Brandt, S., et al., 2009. Microcirculation of healthy and perianastomotic colon. Anesthesiology 110, 496–504.

Kimberger, O., Fleischmann, E., Brandt, S., et al., 2007. Supplemental oxygen, but not supplemental crystalloid fluid, increases tissue oxygen tension in healthy and anastomotic colon in pigs. Anesth Analg 105, 773–779.

Kollias-Baker, C.A., Pipers, F.S., Heard, D.J., et al., 1993. Pulmonary edema associated with transient airway obstruction in three horses. J Am Vet Med Assoc 202, 1116–1118.

Lansdorp, B., Lemson, J., van Putten, M.J.A.M., et al., 2012. Dynamic indices do not predict volume responsiveness in routine clinical practice. Br J Anaesth 108, 395–401.

Leemans, J., Kirschvink, N., Bernaerts, F., et al., 2009. A pilot study comparing the antispasmodic effects of inhaled salmeterol, salbutamol and ipratropium bromide using different aerosol devices on muscarinic bronchoconstriction in healthy cats. Vet J 180, 236–245.

Litonius, E., Tarkkila, P., Neuvonen, P.J., et al., 2012. Effect of intravenous lipid emulsion on bupivacaine plasma concentration in humans. Anaesthesia 67, 600–605.

Lumb, W.V., Jones, E.W., 1984. Veterinary Anesthesia. Lea & Febiger, Philadelphia.

Mauch, J., Jurado, O.M., Spielmann, N., et al., 2011. Comparison of epinephrine vs lipid rescue to treat severe local anesthetic toxicity – an experimental study in piglets. Ped Anesth 21, 1103–1108.

Michard, F., Biais, M., 2012. Rational fluid management: dissecting facts from fiction. Br J Anaesth 108, 369–371.

Mirski, M.A., Lele, A.V., Fitzsimmons, L., et al., 2007. Diagnosis and treatment of vascular air embolism. Anesthesiology 106, 164–177.

Moon, P.F., Bliss, S.P., Posner, L.P., et al., 2001. Fetal oxygen content is restored after maternal hemorrhage and fluid replacement, but not with hetastarch, in pregnant sheep. Anesth Analg 93, 142–150.

Moore, J.N., White, N.A., Trim, C.M., et al., 1980. Effect of intraluminal oxygen in intestinal strangulation obstruction in ponies. Am J Vet Res 41, 1615–1620.

Moore, L.E., Garvey, M.S., 1996. The effect of hetastarch on serum colloid oncotic pressure in hypoalbuminemic dogs. J Vet Intern Med 10, 300–303.

Muir, W.W. III, 2004. Comparison of lactated Ringer's solution and a physiologically balanced 6% hetastarch plasma expander for the treatment of hypotension induced

via blood withdrawal in isoflurane-anesthetized dogs. Am J Vet Res 65, 1189–1194.

Mulkey, D.K., Talley, E.M., Stornetta, R.L., et al., 2007. TASK channels determine pH sensitivity in select respiratory neurons but do not contribute to central respiratory chemosensitivity. J Neurosci 27, 14049–14058.

Niemi, T.T., Miyashita, R., Yamakage, M., 2010. Colloid solutions: a clinical update. J Anesth 24, 913–925.

O'Brien, T.Q., Clark-Price, S.C., Evans, E.E., et al., 2010. Infusion of a lipid emulsion to treat lidocaine intoxication in a cat. J Am Vet Med Assoc 237, 1455–1458.

Olsén, L., Ingvast-Larsson, C., Broström, H., et al., 2007. Clinical signs and etiology of adverse reactions to procaine benzylpenicillin and sodium/potassium benzylpenicillin in horses. J Vet Pharmacol Ther 30, 201–207.

Padrid, P., 2006. Use of inhaled medications to treat respiratory diseases in dogs and cats. J Am Anim Hosp Assoc 42, 165–169.

Pantaleon, L.G., Furr, M.O., McKenzie II, H.C., et al., 2006. Cardiovascular and pulmonary effects of hetastarch plus hypertonic saline solutions during experimental endotoxemia in anesthetized horses. J Vet Intern Med 20, 1422–1428.

Papadopoulou, A., Willers, J.W., Samuels, T.L., et al., 2012. The use of dye surrogates to illustrate local anesthetic drug sequestration by lipid emulsion: a visual demonstration of the lipid sink effect. Reg Anesth Pain Med 37, 183–187.

Pawloski, D.R., Broaddus, K.D., 2010. Pneumothorax: A review. J Am Anim Hosp Assoc 46, 385–397.

Physick-Sheard, P.W., 1999. Cardiovascular system: Pathophysiology and principles of therapy. In: Colahan, P.T., Mayhew, I.G., Merritt, A.M., Moore, J.N. (Eds.), Equine Medicine and Surgery, *Vol. 1*. Mosby, St Louis, pp. 337–380.

Picard, J., Meek, T., 2006. Lipid emulsion to treat overdose of local anaesthetic: the gift of the glob. Anaesthesia 61, 107–109.

Rafie, A.D., Rath, P.A., Michell, M.W., et al., 2004. Hypotensive resuscitation of multiple hemorrhages using crystalloid and colloids. Shock 22, 262–269.

Reid, F., Lobo, D.N., Williams, R.N., et al., 2011. (Ab)normal saline and physiological Hartmann's solution: a randomized double-blind crossover study. Clin Sci 104, 17–24.

Robertson, S.A., Bailey, J.E., 2002. Aerosolized salbutamol (albuterol) improves PaO$_2$ in hypoxaemic anaesthetized horses – a prospective clinical trial in 81 horses. Vet Anaesth Analg 29, 212–218.

Robinson, R., Schwendenwein, I., Wacek, S., et al., 2011. Plasma volume and electrolyte changes following intravenous infusion of hypertonic hydroxyethyl starch versus mannitol in healthy dogs. Vet J 190, 268–272.

Roth, S., 2009. Perioperative visual loss: what do we know, what can we do? Br J Anaesth 103 (Suppl 1), i31–i40.

Rush, J.E., Freeman, L.M., Fenollosa, N.K., et al., 2002. Population and survival characteristics of cats with hypertrophic cardiomyopathy: 260 cases (1990–1999). J Am Vet Med Assoc 220, 202–207.

Silverstein, D.C., Aldrich, J., Haskins, S.C., et al., 2005. Assessment of changes in blood volume in response to resuscitative fluid administration in dogs. J Vet Emerg Crit Care 15, 185–192.

Staffieri, F., Lacitignola, L., De Siena, R., et al., 2007. A case of spontaneous venous embolism with carbon dioxide during laparoscopic surgery in a pig. Vet Anaesth Analg 34, 63–66.

Stegmann, F.G., 2000. Hypoxaemia and suspected pulmonary oedema in a Dorper ewe after diazepam-ketamine induction of anaesthesia. J S Afr Vet Assoc 71, 64–65.

Stiles, J., Weil, A.B., Packer, R.A., et al., 2012. Post-anesthetic cortical blindness in cats: Twenty cases. Vet J 193, 367–373.

Teixeira Neto, F.J., Luna, S.P., Cruz, M.A., et al., 2007. A study of the effect of hemorrhage on the cardiorespiratory actions of halothane, isoflurane and sevoflurane in the dog. Vet Anaesth Analg 34, 107–116.

Togioka, B., Galvagno, S., Sumida, S., et al., 2012. The role of perioperative high inspired oxygen therapy in reducing surgical site infection: A meta-analysis. Anesth Analg 114, 334–342.

Tølløfsrud, S., Elgjo, G.I., Prough, D.S., et al., 2001. The dynamics of vascular volume and fluid shifts of lactated Ringer's solution and hypertonic-saline-dextran solutions infused in normovolemic sheep. Anesth Analg 93, 823–831.

Udelsmann, A., Bonfim, M.R., Silva, W.A., et al., 2009. Hemodynamic effect of volume replacement with saline solution and hypertonic hydroxylethyl starch in dogs. Acta Cirúrg Brasil 24, 87–92.

Vallet, B., 2011. Intravascular volume expansion: Which surrogate markers could help the clinician to assess improved tissue perfusion? Anesth Analg 112, 258–259.

Van der Linde-Sipman, J.S., Hellebrekers, L.J., Lagerwey, E., 1992. Myocardial damage in cats that died after anaesthesia. Vet Quart 15, 91–94.

van Dijk, P., Lankveld, D.P.K., Rijkenhuizen, A.B.M., et al., 2003. Hormonal, metabolic and physiological effects of laparoscopic surgery using a detomidine-buprenorphine combination in standing horses. Vet Anaesth Analg 30, 72–80.

Varadhan, K.K., Lobo, D.N., 2010. A meta-analysis of randomised controlled trials of intravenous fluid therapy in major elective open abdominal surgery: getting the balance right. Proc Nutr Soc 69, 488–498.

Waddell, L.S., 2010. Systemic anaphylaxis. In: Ettinger, S.J. & Feldman, E.C. (Eds.), Textbook of Veterinary Internal Medicine, Vol. 1. Saunders Elsevier, St Louis, pp. 531–537.

Walsh, V.P., Machon, R.G., Munday, J.S., et al., 2005. Suspected fatal air embolism during anaesthesia in a Pomeranian dog with pulmonary calcification. N Z Vet J 53, 359–362.

Weinberg, G., Warren, L., 2012. Lipid resuscitation: Listening to our patients and learning from our models. Anesth Analg 114, 710–712.

Weinberg, G., Ripper, R., Feinstein, D.L., et al., 2003. Lipid emulsion infusion rescues dogs from bupivacaine-induced cardiac toxicity. Reg Anesth Pain Med 28, 198–202.

Wendt-Hornickle, E.L., Snyder, L.B.C., Tang, R., et al., 2011. The effects of lactated Ringer's solution (LRS) or LRS and 6% hetastarch on the colloid osmotic pressure, total protein and osmolality in healthy horses under general anesthesia. Vet Anaesth Analg 38, 336–343.

Wilkinson, K.A., Huey, K., Dinger, B., et al., 2010. Chronic hypoxia increases the gain of the hypoxic ventilatory response by a mechanism in the central nervous system. J Appl Physiol 109, 424–430.

Wilson, D.V., Rondenay, Y., Shance, P.U., 2003. The cardiopulmonary effects of severe blood loss in anesthetized horses. Vet Anaesth Analg 30, 81–87.

Woodcock, T.E., Woodcock, T.M., 2012. Revised Starling equation and the glycocalyx model of transvascular fluid exchange: an improved paradigm for prescribing intravenous fluid therapy. Br J Anaesth 108, 384–394.

Wright, B.D., Hopkins, A., 2008. Changes in colloid osmotic pressure as a function of anesthesia and surgery in the presence and absence of isotonic fluid administration in dogs. Vet Anaesth Analg 35, 282–288.

Chapter | **22** |

Cardiopulmonary cerebral resuscitation (CPCR)

Jennifer G. Adams

HISTORY AND INTRODUCTION

Organized efforts to promote resuscitation began centuries ago. The Dutch Humane Society and the Royal Humane Society were both founded in the 1700s in Amsterdam and London, respectively, after realizing that drowned or otherwise injured individuals could be revived (Sternbach et al., 2005; Cooper et al., 2006). These groups sought to enlighten the public as to this phenomenon and to teach the techniques necessary for resuscitation. By the 1950s, concerted efforts to educate the lay public in cardiopulmonary resuscitation (CPR) techniques were underway. Currently, CPR classes are offered by numerous local and national agencies or institutions and many, many lay people have been trained in resuscitation techniques of humans. With the development of the automated external defibrillator (AED), 'bystander CPR' has become a significant factor in saving the lives of humans in cardiac arrest. In fact, AEDs are readily available in many public places, for example, the Hartsfield-Jackson International Airport in Atlanta, Georgia has more than 200 portable AEDs positioned throughout the facility (www.atlantaairport.com). CPR techniques for animals are published and available to pet owners in print form and on the Internet at numerous websites sponsored by pet rescue groups, pet care organizations, and veterinarians. Classes in 'pet CPR' are also available from many sources.

A report by Beecher and Todd published in 1954 reported an anaesthetic mortality of 1:2680 in humans following examination of the anaesthetic records of almost 600 000 cases at 10 institutions over a 5-year period. Mortality associated with anaesthesia has since greatly decreased in humans; one report states that death is expected to occur no more often than 1 in 200 200 cases (0.0005%) involving healthy patients (Eichhorn, 1989); another reports 1:13 000 (0.008%) when all cases are considered (Lagasse, 2002). Veterinary anaesthetic mortality rates have also improved since the 1950s, but are still much higher than humans. Rates of 1:555 (0.18%) in healthy dogs, 1:385 (0.26 %) in healthy cats (Brodbelt et al., 2008), and 1:111 (0.9%) (Johnston et al., 2002) to 1:1250 (0.08%) (Bidwell et al., 2007) in horses (excluding colic surgery) are reported most recently. In spite of advances in techniques and treatments and widespread training in cardiopulmonary cerebral resuscitation (CPCR), the overall success rate following CPCR attempts is still poor in both humans and animals; 17.6% of inpatients and 6.4% of outpatients survived cardiac arrest when the results of three human studies were combined (Cooper et al., 2006). A recent study of survival following CPCR at a veterinary teaching hospital reported that no patients requiring CPCR at admission survived. It also found that only 6% (12/204) of all dogs and cats experiencing in-hospital cardiopulmonary arrest (CPA) survived to discharge (Hofmeister et al., 2009). This is similar to an earlier review of CPA in hospitalized patients where only 4.1% of dogs and 9.6% of cats survived to discharge (Wingfield & Van Pelt, 1992). When patients experience cardiac arrest under anaesthesia, the % return of spontaneous circulation (ROSC) and survival to discharge from hospital is usually much higher. In Hofmeister et al. (2009), nine of the 12 (75%) animals that survived were anaesthetized at the time CPA occurred; the only survivors of CPA (4/135) in a 4-year period at another veterinary teaching hospital had been under anaesthesia when arrest occurred (Kass & Haskins, 1992). Even though the outcome of anaesthesia-related CPA may be better, successful CPCR is certainly not always likely; thus prevention of CPA is the best course.

CEREBRAL RESUSCITATION

Outcome measures in CPR studies originally focused on the return of spontaneous circulation and hospital discharge of patients. However, the number of patients with ROSC is much greater than those that actually survive to be discharged with normal or minimal neurological dysfunction. Hence, more emphasis is now placed on neurological outcome, long-term survival, and quality of life post cardiac arrest. The acronym was changed to CPCR to reflect this emphasis. Return of effective cerebral circulation begins with re-establishment of cardiopulmonary function

via the basic elements of CPR, such as timely recognition of arrest, immediate institution of effective CPR resulting in ROSC, and prevention of systemic complications in the post-arrest period. Attention to specific techniques such as using continuous cardiac compressions and avoiding pauses may allow improved neurological outcome. Optimal post-resuscitation therapy is important to minimize the damage that occurs following reperfusion of the ischaemic brain. Homeostatic parameters such as blood pressure, acid–base status, electrolytes, blood gases, glucose, should be maintained in the normal range. Treatment to decrease neuronal death and improve cerebral function such as therapeutic hypothermia has already been adopted; others are now being examined, including neuronal cell growth promotion, inhibition of reperfusion injury and neuronal apoptosis. Clinical signs, electrophysiological testing, diagnostic imaging, and measurement of neuron-specific proteins in serum are used to evaluate cerebral function and estimate a prognosis following resuscitation (Schneider et al., 2009).

The science behind CPCR techniques has been periodically evaluated by The International Liaison Committee on Resuscitation (ILCOR). This group was formed in 1992 to represent a consortium of scientists working in the resuscitation and critical care fields. It presently includes groups from the six major continents. The purpose of ILCOR is to identify information relevant to resuscitation, emergency and critical care medicine, perform an evidence-based review of this information, and develop a consensus of guidelines based on the strength of the scientific evidence. In cooperation with the American Heart Association, ILCOR produced the first International CPR Guidelines in 2000 and an International Consensus on CPR and Emergency and Critical Care (ECC) Science with Treatment Recommendations in 2005, published in the journals *Circulation* and *Resuscitation*. The group currently meets biannually and plans to publish updates every 5 years. The most recent reviews were published in October and November 2010, and can be obtained at the ILCOR website, www.ilcor.org/en/home/. Although the purpose of ILCOR is to define best practices for humans, much of the research is performed in anaesthetized animals, especially dogs and swine, and is potentially applicable to veterinary medicine. Since animals used in research are generally healthy, some differences will emerge when study findings are used in clinical populations. Plunkett and McMichael (2008) published a very thorough update of CPCR in small animals based on the 2005 ILCOR guidelines.

Most recently, an extensive review of the literature as it specifically pertains to resuscitation of small animal veterinary patients was conducted by a group of 101 veterinarians, specialists in internal medicine, anaesthesia, and critical care. The investigation was conducted very similarly to the protocol used by the ILCOR group. They developed topics pertinent to the performance of CPCR in animals and explored the literature for evidence. From their efforts, called the Reassessment Campaign on Veterinary Resuscitation (RECOVER) initiative, a set of consensus guidelines for CPCR in dogs and cats was published in a supplement to the *Journal of Veterinary Emergency and Critical Care* (2012) (see suggested reading) and is available at www.veccs.org or www.onlinelibrary.wiley.com.

PRIOR TO ANAESTHESIA

The prevention of anaesthetic complications including cardiac arrest begins prior to the anaesthetic episode. A thorough preanaesthetic evaluation including physical examination, laboratory evaluation, and diagnostics appropriate to the patient and problems present is vital to identify pertinent risk factors. A discussion of the anaesthetic plan and potential complications for each case should take place preoperatively between all members of the anaesthesia staff. All equipment, drugs, and supplies required for treatment of anaesthetic complications should be conveniently within reach of the anaesthetized patient at all times. Those specific to CPCR should be immediately available; standard doses of epinephrine and atropine should be calculated and even drawn up prior to induction for specific cases or patients (i.e. birds, small mammals, very small dogs and cats, severely ill patients). Reference charts with the CPCR protocol and emergency drug dosages should be posted in anaesthesia and surgery areas. All staff potentially involved in performance of CPCR should have formal training. Since cardiac arrest is not a common event, practice sessions of CPCR techniques should be performed on a regular basis. Review of the team's performance following resuscitation events can identify deficiencies and improve outcome of subsequent cases. Finally, phone numbers for immediate contact with owners should be available and resuscitation status should be determined from discussions with the owner at admission. This should be documented in the patient record, and posted on the patient's cage/stall. Suggested categories are: (1) do not attempt resuscitation (DNAR); (2) resuscitation efforts limited to external compressions and medical therapy; and (3) unlimited efforts including internal cardiac compressions (Rieser, 2000).

CAUSES OF CARDIAC ARREST/RISK FACTORS FOR ANAESTHETIC MORTALITY

The immediate cause of cardiac arrest under anaesthesia is always associated with respiratory and/or cardiac insufficiency, as lack of oxygen rapidly results in dysfunction of brain and myocardial cells. Hypoxaemia, hypoventilation,

Table 22.1 Causes of respiratory or cardiac dysfunction that may lead to arrest

Respiratory	Cardiac
Hypoxaemia	Hypoxaemia
Hypocarbia/hypercarbia	Hypercarbia
Non-respiratory acidosis	Non-respiratory acidosis
Hypothermia	Hypothermia
Hypoglycaemia	Hypoglycaemia
Electrolyte abnormalities	Electrolyte abnormalities
Airway problems	Hypotension
Endotracheal tube obstructed	Hypovolaemia
Endotracheal tube	Vasodilation
malpositioned	Decreased cardiac output
Anatomical airway obstruction	Poor cardiac contractility
Anaesthesia machine problems	Cardiac arrhythmias
Breathing hoses obstructed	Decreased venous return
No oxygen or wrong gas	Anaphylaxis
Medication errors	Medication errors
Overdose, incorrect dose	Overdose, incorrect dose
Wrong drug or vial	Wrong drug or vial
Drug interaction	Drug interaction
Surgical error/event	Surgical error/event

hypotension, hypovolaemia, cardiac arrhythmia, hypothermia, anaesthesia machine or equipment malfunction, drug interactions or overdose, and anaphylaxis are the most common precipitating causes (Table 22.1). These can be associated with or directly the result of the patient's condition, anaesthesia, or surgery. Occasionally, events occur that are not preventable. The classic clinical signs of cardiac arrest are loss of a palpable pulse, lack of heart sounds with auscultation, cyanotic mucous membranes (except in sudden arrest where mucous membranes remain pink for a few minutes), apnoea, pupillary dilation, and lack of bleeding from surgical incisions. Other signs include very slow capillary refill time, and loss of the palpebral reflex. Although it often seems to happen quite suddenly, some cases of arrest involve more than one problem, developing over the course of the anaesthetic episode.

Sudden changes in vital signs may not always occur prior to an arrest. Clinical signs that should prompt the anaesthetist to be suspicious of an impending arrest include gradually decreasing or increasing heart rate, continuing change in the mucous membrane colour, capillary refill time, pupil size, or ocular responses, frequent premature contractions, frequent atrioventricular heart block, decreasing end-tidal CO_2 levels, decreasing or increasing temperature, slower respiratory rates, and very irregular or gasping respiratory patterns.

Hypoventilation and the resulting hypercarbia produce clinical signs that may mimic a 'light' depth of anaesthesia as rapid deep breaths may occur (Kussmaul respiratory pattern); limb motion, muscular twitching, tachycardia, and hypertension may also be seen. This may mislead the anaesthetist into giving more drugs, further exacerbating respiratory insufficiency. Unusual respiratory patterns seen with some anaesthetic agents (Biot's, apneustic with ketamine) may also be confusing as deep or rapid ventilations may occur. Short periods of apnoea are not unusual especially following induction of anaesthesia. Overdose of anaesthetics results in prolonged periods of apnoea and a Cheyne–Stokes type of abnormal respiratory pattern in which breaths gradually increase and then decrease in depth. This pattern is seen when cerebral blood flow (CBF) is decreased and the respiratory centre becomes ischaemic (Muir & Hubbell, 2009). Cardiac arrest may be associated with specific types of patients or procedures, and at specific times during a procedure. Induction, intubation, extubation, during repositioning or movement onto or off transport carts/surgery tables, and during transport to other areas of hospital are times when conditions that could quickly lead to arrest are perhaps more likely to occur and be unnoticed. Repositioning under anaesthesia, especially from lateral to dorsal or to the opposite lateral can result in sudden severe hypotension in large animals, large dogs, and heavily pregnant females of any species, and patients with distension of the gastrointestinal tract or abdominal masses. However, small patients are not immune to problems during repositioning and even a cat may arrest immediately following a change from lateral to sternal recumbency. Dislodgement or kinking of the endotracheal tube, especially in small size patients, may also develop during repositioning. Risk of an unnoticed complication is increased when monitoring of anaesthetic depth is discontinued or decreased during the process of repositioning.

Some procedures may unexpectedly lead to arrest. Dental procedures and endoscopy of the upper airway or oesophagus have inadvertently resulted in pneumothorax, pneumomediastinum, and venous air embolism (Mitchell et al., 2000; Gunew et al., 2008; Ober et al., 2006). Laceration of a vein during limb amputation in patients breathing spontaneously and loss of the injection cap from a jugular catheter in horses can also result in venous air embolism. Insertion of central venous catheters and intraventricular pacemaker leads can stimulate cardiac arrhythmias, cause haemothorax or pneumothorax, and rarely, cardiac tamponade (Domino et al., 2004; Wess et al., 2006). Injection of contrast media or local anaesthetic intravenously or into the epidural or subarachnoid space can result in bradycardia, hypotension, and respiratory and/or cardiac arrest (Iff & Moens, 2008; Mosing et al., 2008). Ophthalmic and gastrointestinal (GI) procedures involving stimulation of parasympathetic nerves via the oculo-cardiac reflex or from tension on abdominal organs respectively, can cause bradycardia and arrest. GI procedures may also cause hypotension when diseased or large organs or masses are manipulated or exteriorized. Thoracic surgery may stimulate arrhythmias and cause haemorrhage. Manipulation of adrenal, thyroid, or pancreatic masses may also result in hypotension, hypertension, or arrhythmia (Gross & Giuliano, 2007; Greene & Marks, 2007; Harvey & Schaer, 2007).

Although cardiac arrest or situations that could lead to arrest may be anticipated more often in more critical patients, healthy patients may suffer as well when attention to monitoring is less vigilant. Anaesthetic errors persistently identified that have resulted in perioperative death include lack of monitoring, inattention to monitoring, lack of experience or knowledge, failure to treat complications such as hypotension or hypoventilation correctly, inadequate supervision, lack of communication, medication errors, and fatigue (Arbous et al., 2001, 2005; Johnston et al., 2002; Brodbelt, 2009). Medication errors such as overdose, incorrect choice of drug, improper route of administration, selection of the wrong syringe or vial, and incorrect labelling have resulted in mortality and severe morbidity (Abeysekera et al., 2005).

Risk of mortality associated with anaesthetic monitoring has been evaluated in many studies (Table 22.2). The presence of a technician to monitor the patient, the presence of experienced staff, and the use of full time staff have been associated with decreased risk of anaesthetic mortality in veterinary and human medicine. Use of documented equipment checklists, monitoring the pulse, and the use of pulse oximetry have also been associated with decreased risk of anaesthetic death. Lack of appropriate monitoring of patients during maintenance and recovery has been associated with increased anaesthetic mortality in humans. Veterinary studies have recently identified the recovery period as a factor with the deaths of 50% of dogs, and >60% of cats and rabbits, occurring postanaesthesia, especially in the first 3 hours postoperatively. These findings differ from earlier studies, suggesting that while intraoperative monitoring has improved, it should be continued into the postoperative period (Arbous et al., 2001, 2005; Brodbelt et al., 2008; Brodbelt 2009).

Older patients, sicker patients, emergency procedures, procedures of long duration, more complex procedures, and timing of procedures after hours and on weekends have also been consistently found to be associated with greater perioperative mortality in small animals, horses, and humans (Tiret et al., 1986; Gaynor et al., 1999; Johnston et al., 2002; Arbous et al., 2005; Lienhart et al., 2006; Brodbelt, 2009).

Consistent and thorough monitoring in *all* patients and anticipation of potential problems in patients and situations with higher risk throughout the anaesthetic episode and recovery period will minimize the incidence of CPA and potentially improve outcome if an arrest occurs.

CARDIOPULMONARY CEREBRAL RESUSCITATION PROTOCOL

Once the heart has stopped, it cannot be actively restarted. Since the cardiac pacemaker has inherent automaticity, resuscitation efforts focus on therapies to improve

Table 22.2 Risk factors for perioperative mortality in horses, small animals, and humans

Risk factor	Increased risk	Risk factor	Decreased risk
Patient characteristics	Older[a] Sicker[a] Very young[a] Very small[a] Larger[a] Some breeds brachycephalic, terriers, draft horses	Anaesthetic technique	Injectable only[e] Use of acepromazine[sa] Isoflurane (vs) halothane[e] Pain management postop[h] Reversal of NMB[h]
Procedure	Inadequate preoperative prep[a] Emergencies[a] Complicated procedures[a] Longer duration[a] After hours or on weekends[a]	Anaesthetic management	Pulse monitoring[sa] Pulse oximetry[sa,h] Technician present[sa] Experienced staff[h] Full time staff[h]
Anaesthetic management	Lack of monitoring[a] IV fluids given[c] Inhalant only used[d,f] Endotracheal tube used[c] Use of xylazine[sa] Use of romifidine[e]	Other	Checklists[h] Documentation of checklist[h]

[a]all species; [c]cats; [d]dogs; [e]equine; [f]foals; [h]human; [sa]small animals.
Arbous et al., 2001, 2005; Johnston et al., 2002; Brodbelt, 2009.

coronary perfusion and eliminate any specific causes of arrest so that the cardiac pacemaker can restart on its own. Successful outcome is dependent on the prior status of the myocardium, the amount of damage that has occurred to both the heart and the brain during the arrest, and the quality of resuscitation efforts. Cerebral resuscitation is now specifically considered in the protocol as neurological status is considered to be a more important outcome parameter than return of spontaneous or sustained circulation (ROSC).

Resuscitation protocols for all patients follow the universal 'A-B-C-D' algorithm that represents the major components of CPCR – the airway, breathing, circulation, and drugs. Guidelines also divide the components of this algorithm into two major categories – Basic Cardiac Life Support (BCLS) and Advanced Cardiac Life Support (ACLS), even though components of both may be used simultaneously. BCLS includes the initial steps of resuscitation, the 'A-B-C' portion of the algorithm, where the airway, breathing, and circulation are addressed. The patient is identified as in respiratory and/or cardiac arrest, mouth to mouth or nose ventilation may be given, and cardiac compressions are initiated. ILCOR currently emphasizes the circulation portion of the algorithm more heavily because of the high incidence of sudden cardiac arrest from coronary artery disease in humans, and is now using 'C-A-B' to describe initial resuscitation events. Cardiac compressions and defibrillation are considered more important to outcome than medical therapy (ICCOR, 2010). ACLS includes invasive airway control, cardiac rhythm identification, medical therapy, and electrical defibrillation or conversion. Medications used for ACLS include those for treatment of a primary cause, those which improve myocardial perfusion to enable the heart to restart, and those for treatment of intra- and post-resuscitation events or conditions. The CAB algorithm may not be as applicable to veterinary anaesthesia since coronary artery disease is not seen. Distinction between BCLS and ACLS may be primarily theoretical for veterinary medicine since most resuscitation events occur in hospital where access to medical therapy and defibrillation is available. However, pet owners are becoming increasingly educated in all aspects of their pets' health. Anecdotal reports of owner administered BCLS exist and are only likely to become more common.

Once an emergency situation has been identified, intervention must be swift, as the duration of arrest prior to both chest compressions and defibrillation is inversely related to the success of the return of spontaneous and/or sustained circulation (ROSC) and survival (Fecho et al., 2009). Although CPCR is performed by available personnel, an ideal team includes experienced individuals responsible for the following duties:

1. A leader to direct resuscitation efforts and evaluate response
2. Cardiac compressions – more than one individual to take turns
3. Ventilation of the patient, including placement of an endotracheal tube
4. Draw up and administer drugs
5. Monitors – electrocardiograph, Doppler on limb and/or cornea, capnography, oximetry

6. Vascular access – venous and arterial catheters
7. Recorder – events, medications, and time
8. Communication with owner (not the same as 1).

For both ethical and economic reasons, the decision to perform resuscitation should be based on the patient's overall prognosis in regard to the primary disease present, the suspected cause of the arrest, and the wishes of the owner. The financial and emotional costs of resuscitation and post-arrest care can be extreme. Healthy anaesthetized patients that develop a treatable arrhythmia might be easily resuscitated, whereas a dog with severe damage from a gastric volvulus, or a septic foal with uroperitoneum may not be as good a candidate for resuscitation. Cases where arrest is witnessed are also more likely to be successfully resuscitated.

Basic cardiac life support 'A-B-C'

Once an arrest or near arrest situation has been identified in an anaesthetized patient, the inhalant anaesthetic vaporizer should be turned off and sedatives or opioids should be reversed as soon as possible. A search for potentially reversible causes such as hypoxaemia, hypercarbia, hypovolaemia, hypothermia, and metabolic or electrolyte disturbances, should also be instituted as soon as possible. This can be performed while the CPCR team assembles, someone begins compressions, and others are gathering supplies and drawing up emergency drugs.

'A & B' – airway and breathing

Patients under general anaesthesia are often already intubated and, in these cases, correct placement, size, and patency of the endotracheal tube should be verified and corrected if necessary. Patients who have arrested at induction, in recovery, or elsewhere should be intubated as quickly as possible. Use of a laryngoscope is recommended, when appropriate for the species, to accomplish intubation quickly and allow immediate confirmation of correct placement. Other airway devices such as a laryngeal mask airway may be used only if the operator is proficient in their use. Orotracheal intubation in many veterinary species is usually not difficult. Proper placement of the endotracheal tube should be confirmed using auscultation of lung sounds, viewing the tube entering the larynx, and capnography. Capnography is a very reliable measure as CO_2 elimination is dependent on blood flow through the lungs. In patients with cardiac arrest, very low levels of end-tidal CO_2 ($ETCO_2$) are usually encountered. Negligible $ETCO_2$ will be detected when the oesophagus has been intubated. In rare instances, no waveform may register on the capnogram even though the endotracheal tube is correctly placed, such as severe bronchospasm, severe pulmonary embolism, obstruction of the endotracheal tube, and the presence of a large leak around the endotracheal tube (Sanehi & Calder, 1999). Patients with upper airway

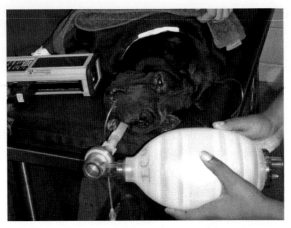

Figure 22.1 An Ambu bag being used in an anaesthetized dog. This is a manual resuscitation device originally developed by the Ambu company in Denmark over 50 years ago. It consists of a self-re-inflating bag and a non-rebreathing valve that can be used with a facemask or directly connected to an endotracheal tube. Room air is most commonly used but a line can be attached for oxygen supplementation.

obstruction may require intubation via a tracheostomy. A few breaths and attention to the precipitating cause (such as decreasing anaesthetic administration) may be all that is needed if the patient has suffered a primary respiratory arrest that was witnessed or very quickly identified. An AMBU bag (Fig. 22.1), demand valve (Fig. 22.2), or anaesthesia machine can be used to provide ventilation. Room air may suffice in some cases, but 100% oxygen is recommended if full cardiac arrest is present or resuscitation takes longer than a few minutes. Research and clinical investigations have shown that artificial ventilation may not be necessary for the first few minutes in some cases, the rate can be decreased from previous guidelines, and that excessive ventilation can be harmful (Aufderheide et al., 2004; Nagao, 2009). However, when arrest is associated with asphyxia, as seen with trauma, drowning, or any cause of primary respiratory arrest, especially when arrest is not witnessed and hypoxic conditions may have been present for several minutes, ventilation should be provided immediately. Cardiac compression : ventilation ratios of 15 : 1 or 30 : 2 both provided adequate oxygenation and haemodynamic profiles with minimal interruption of compressions in a dog CPR study, and are recommended when enough people are present (Hwang et al., 2008). Cardiac massage should **not stop** when breaths are given or intubation is performed, and compressions and ventilations should be performed simultaneously. Once intubated, ventilations should be performed in a consistent fashion at a regular rate. Hyperventilation and high peak inspiratory pressure must be avoided to avoid compromise of venous return; 10–12 breaths per minute is suggested for adult small animals, and 4–8 per minute for adult large animal species. Respiratory rate can be increased up to 20 per minute in neonates and very young animals. Inspirations should be as consistent as possible in duration and depth; approximately 1 second is recommended for most patients. Peak inspiratory

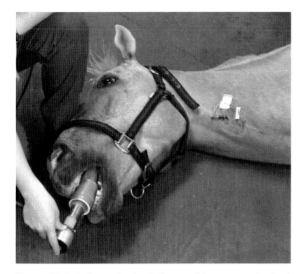

Figure 22.2 A demand valve being used in an anaesthetized horse. This is a manual resuscitation device that can be used in small or large animals to control or assist ventilation. It has a one-way valve connected via a pressure hose directly to an oxygen source. Flow of 100% oxygen is triggered by the negative pressure created by inspiration or when a button on the device is pushed. Flow stops when the button is released or the patient pauses for expiration and the negative pressure disappears. Expired gas is passively routed to the environment.

pressure should be ≤20 cmH$_2$O in small animals, and 20–30 cm H$_2$O in adult large animals (Table 22.3) (Plunkett & McMichael, 2008; Muir & Hubbell, 2009).

Doxapram increases ventilation by direct stimulation of the carotid chemoreceptors augmented by non-selective stimulation of central nervous system (CNS) neurons. It has been used to stimulate respiration and hasten recovery in sedated and anaesthetized small animals and horses. It may be useful if other methods to achieve breathing are not available, however, its effect is temporary. If the primary cause of respiratory arrest has not been corrected, apnoea or respiratory insufficiency will reoccur. Side effects of this drug can be significant and include cardiac arrhythmias, muscle fasciculation, seizures, increased oxygen requirement, and decreased CBF caused by the non-selective stimulation of the brain which results in increased sympathetic outflow. It is not recommended when intubation is possible and ventilation can be controlled.

Use of stimulation at the Jen Chung acupuncture point VG 26, at the nasal philtrum, is reported to stimulate respiration (Janssens et al., 1979). Although this is a simple and quick therapy, several minutes of stimulation may be required to see results, the technique has not been documented by experimental studies, and cardiac arrest occurred in two cats following nasal stimulation (K. Clarke, personal communication). Use of this technique should not preclude efforts to identify the primary cause of respiratory arrest and initiate CPCR. It is not recommended by this author.

'C' – circulation – cardiac compressions

In anaesthetized patients, treatment of a precipitating cause should be immediately instituted. Compressions

---

Table 22.3 Guidelines for ventilation during CPCR

Cardiac compression : ventilation ratios – 15 : 1 or 30 : 2

If not intubated, use tight mask with room air or 100% O$_2$; or mouth to nose.
Place ET tube and ventilate with room air or 100% O$_2$ with AMBU bag, demand valve, anaesthesia machine.
Use 100% oxygen for prolonged arrest (> few min)

	Small animal	Large animal	Neonates, very young, or very small
Respiratory rate	5–10/min	5–8/min	Up to 20/min
Inspiratory pressure	Max 20 cmH$_2$O	Up to 30 cmH$_2$O	Max 20 cmH$_2$O
Duration	1 second	1–1.5 second	1 second

Confirm patent airway – view larynx, auscultation of lungs, CO$_2$ monitoring.
Note: End-tidal CO$_2$ is proportional to PBF when ventilation is consistent. No CO$_2$ may be present in expired gas if asystole is present.

Do not stop compressions for intubation or ventilation.

PBF: pulmonary blood flow; ET: endotracheal tube. Plunkett & McMichael, 2008; Muir & Hubbell, 2009.

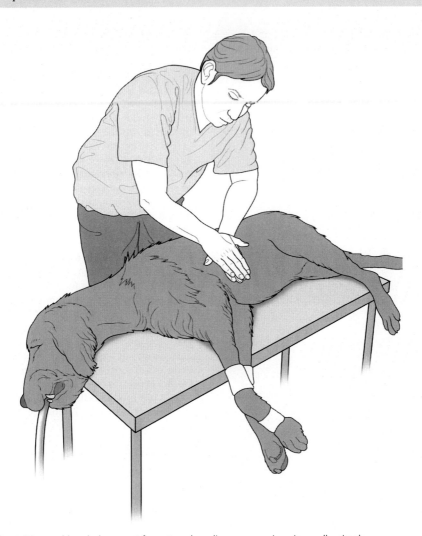

Figure 22.3 Body position and hand placement for external cardiac compressions in small animals.

should not be delayed or interrupted to await the outcome of any treatment. The quality of cardiac compressions has been shown to be associated with improved survival, so careful and consistent technique is important (Yu et al., 2002; Ristagno et al., 2007).

The arrested patient should be placed in right lateral recumbency on a *firm* surface. The individual performing compressions should be positioned above the patient to optimize compression and recoil distance. In animals 10–150 kg, the person's hands should be placed one on top of the other at the widest part of the chest (Fig. 22.3). Compressions should be performed as consistently as possible and should depress the chest diameter at least 30–40%. The duration of the components of each compression cycle should be approximately equal in duration, i.e. 50:50 active compression:passive recoil. Complete

recoil of the chest should be allowed between compressions to allow for maximal cardiac filling. In dogs and cats, rate of compressions should be 100–120 per minute. Compressions should continue with absolutely as few interruptions as possible. When unavoidable, interruptions should last <10 seconds. Compressions should continue following electrical shock or medical therapy for at least 2 minutes as continued perfusion of the coronary circulation is necessary for therapy to be effective. Even good compression technique produces only 20–25% of normal cardiac output in dogs. Coronary perfusion drops dramatically with cessation of compressions, and it then takes a few minutes for maximum coronary perfusion to return when compressions are resumed. Performance of external compressions is tiring and multiple rescuers should take turns at approximately 2-minute intervals (Box 22.1).

- Place patient on firm surface in right lateral recumbency
- Compressor should be positioned above patient; change compressor every 2 minutes
  80–100 compressions/minute for dogs; 100+ for cats
  40–80 for large animals; land on chest with knees in adults
- Compress chest 30% of chest diameter
- *Allow complete recoil* of chest between compressions
- Perform compressions *continuously*
- Avoid pauses; limit these to <10s
- Continue for 2 min following medical therapy *before* checking ECG

Hand placement for external cardiac compressions in small animals

Medium/large dogs – One at widest part of chest, second on top and parallel; use palms
7–10 kg – both hands over the apex of heart, 4th to 6th intercostal space, or slightly dorsal to the costochondral junction
>10 kg – place hands slightly more dorsal
<7 kg – fingers only one side, thumb of same hand or fist of second hand on opposite side; avoid compressing with tips of fingers

The use of interposed abdominal compressions was not supported by the ILCOR 2005 guidelines. However, since then, some animal studies have shown improved outcomes with the use of abdominal compressions without chest compressions. Using only rhythmic abdominal compressions provided effective circulation and ventilation in swine, and sustained abdominal compression has recently been shown to be advantageous as well, improving coronary blood flow to the same degree as the use of vasopressors (Lottes et al., 2007; Pargett et al., 2008). The 2010 guidelines now include a recommendation for interposed abdominal compressions with thoracic compressions in adult humans when enough well-trained rescuers are available. Use of this technique requires training and practice, and it has not been validated in veterinary patients.

Devices are available to enhance venous return or replace the human compressor. These provide consistent effects and avoid operator fatigue, and are used often in research models of CPR to standardize conditions. Since the quality of the compressions performed generally outweighs the use of particular devices or techniques, it is best to utilize techniques at which one is most skilled. Practice with any new technique is recommended before it is added to the CPCR protocol.

To accomplish effective compressions in adult horses and cows, the resuscitator must stand next to the ventral aspect of the left chest and fall onto one or both knees on the chest of the patient. The rate necessary to achieve ROSC in horses is uncertain. Only one study has measured cardiac output in adult horses following cardiac arrest. Three minutes of external compressions at 40, 60, or 80 times per minute were shown to generate average cardiac outputs of 5.65, 6.33, and 8.28 L/min (18–36 % of normal) respectively, enough to maintain temporarily coronary blood flow (Hubbell et al., 1993). The major emphasis of this study was to show that forward blood flow is possible with CPCR in adult horses. The faster heart rates are quite difficult to achieve with large horses and lower compression rates have been sufficient to result in return of ROSC and survival of clinical patients. Further studies are needed to determine optimal cardiac compression rates for horses in cardiac arrest. The technique of external compressions for adult horses is physically demanding and will be most effective if several individuals are available to assist. Compressions in foals and calves and smaller large animal patients are performed similarly to large dogs at rates of 60–80 times per minute.

The cardiac pump and thoracic pump theories are explanations proposed for the mechanisms of blood flow created by chest compressions. The cardiac pump theory suggests that chest compressions compress the ventricles against the chest wall, increasing ventricular pressure, which closes the atrioventricular valves and produces outflow from the heart. The thoracic pump theory maintains that the increase in intrathoracic pressure forces blood out of the chest. Backward flow of blood into the chest through the venous system is prevented by valves, however, the atrioventricular valves do not participate in this mechanism and remain open. In both mechanisms, recoil between compressions allows flow of blood back into the heart. The cardiac pump theory is likely possible only in cats and small dogs. Since the thoracic pump mechanism is most likely in larger animals, compression of a significant portion of the chest diameter (30–40%) and complete recoil between compressions is important to optimize both venous return and cardiac output (Cooper et al., 2006).

Internal cardiac compressions

Internal cardiac compressions should be instituted as soon as possible in resuscitation category 3 patients (unlimited efforts requested by owner) when external compressions are not successful. This is best initiated within 5 minutes of arrest. For patients with haemoperitoneum, cardiac tamponade, extreme obesity, or disease of the thorax such that appropriate pressure cannot be generated (e.g. rib fracture, pleural effusion, haemothorax, pneumothorax), only the internal technique will work. It should also be used in patients with an open abdomen as access via an incision through the diaphragm is readily available. For the thoracic approach (Haskins, 1992), the hair is clipped over the fifth intercostal space, the skin is disinfected with one swipe of antiseptic solution, an incision is made down to the parietal pleura with a scalpel, the thorax is opened with a haemostat, and retractors may be placed if needed. The pericardium may have to be opened to provide the best cardiac compressions. Depending on heart size, compressions may be performed with a finger and thumb, between fingers and the chest wall, or using one or two hands. Extra care should be taken with handling of the heart and vessels, especially in small patients. The operator must avoid rotation or displacement of the heart and avoid using the fingertips that could penetrate vessels or cardiac chambers. The distal aorta may be completely or partially occluded using digital pressure to improve blood flow to the heart and brain, but for not more than 10 minutes. Aortic occlusion can be maintained throughout CPCR and then gradually released over 15–20 minutes when stable ROSC occurs. The chest cavity and the incision should be thoroughly lavaged and then closed according to usual surgical guidelines. Placement of a chest tube is advisable. Antibiotics and pain management should be provided; local blocks and systemic therapy are described elsewhere as for a thoracotomy. Infection is not commonly reported in small animal patients, but has been a limiting factor in resuscitated horses (Muir & Hubbell, 2009).

'D' – advanced cardiac life support

Animals in cardiac arrest that do not respond to cardiac compressions and ventilation require medical therapy to improve coronary perfusion, and electrical therapy in appropriate cases. The cardiac rhythm present should be identified and appropriate treatment instituted. The following paragraphs, Figure 22.4 and Table 22.4 summarize ACLS treatment.

Cardiac arrest rhythms and electrical shock

Asystole, pulseless electrical activity (PEA, formerly known as electromechanical dissociation) (Fig. 22.5), ventricular fibrillation (VF) (Fig. 22.6) and pulseless ventricular tachycardia (PVT) are the rhythms most often associated with cardiac arrest. Asystole is most common in arrested veterinary patients. PEA includes any electrical activity that is not associated with a palpable pulse. Severe bradycardia as a cause of PEA is not uncommon especially in anaesthetized patients due to vagal stimulation. Hypothermia, increased intracranial pressure, electrolyte abnormalities, and medications can cause also cause bradycardia. Idioventricular tachycardia and ventricular escape rhythms are examples of PEA. Some ECG complexes appear quite

abnormal with wide QRS-T waves but others may look normal or only somewhat abnormal with changes in the ST segment (Figure 22.5). Only ventricular fibrillation and ventricular tachycardia are shockable rhythms. Since very fine ventricular fibrillation can be confused with asystole, different leads should be examined to determine the exact rhythm. Cardiac compressions should be used rather than defibrillation in cases with fine VF as this rhythm does not respond well to electrical shock. The presence of fine VF is thought to indicate a longer duration of arrest and poorer coronary perfusion. If fine VF rhythm changes to coarse VF during CPCR, electrical defibrillation can then be used (Rush & Wingfield, 1992).

Timing of electrical shocks has been the subject of much research and debate. Previous guidelines suggested that improvement of perfusion with cardiac compressions may be needed prior to defibrillation. This is no longer considered necessary when a shockable rhythm (VF or PVT) is present at the onset of CPCR. However, compressions should not be delayed while a defibrillator is located and prepared for use (ICCOR, 2010). Earlier guidelines also included up to 3 shocks in succession if needed, however, *one* electrical shock at a time is now recommended (ILCOR, 2005; ICCOR, 2010). Outcome is greatly affected when compressions are paused, due to the loss of coronary perfusion in the interim. Compressions should therefore continue immediately following each single shock. After 2 minutes, compressions are paused briefly to check the rhythm. For asystole and PEA, medical therapy and compressions are the only recourse. Applying current to a heart in asystole can result in myocardial damage and is contraindicated. If fibrillation develops during CPCR for asystole or PEA, electrical shock can then be used.

The CPCR algorithm

When cardiac arrest occurs during anaesthesia, the inhalation anaesthetic agent should be discontinued and antagonists for reversible agents administered (see Fig. 22.4). When the patient is intubated, it should be artificially ventilated twice, 1 s each, and cardiac compressions started. If not intubated, the patient's nose can be covered with a tight fitting facemask, the head and neck extended, and two manual breaths given with a rebreathing or resuscitator bag. This manoeuvre may reverse primary respiratory arrest and can improve oxygenation enough to facilitate the efficacy of cardiac compressions. Intubation can then be performed at the same time as compressions are started. Ideally, compressions and ventilation begin simultaneously when enough rescuers are present. When a shockable rhythm (VF or PVT) is present at the onset of arrest, defibrillation can be performed immediately, but compressions should be performed while the defibrillator is prepared for use. When a shockable rhythm is not present at onset (asystole or PEA), compressions should be performed for 2 minutes. If ROSC does not occur within 2 minutes,

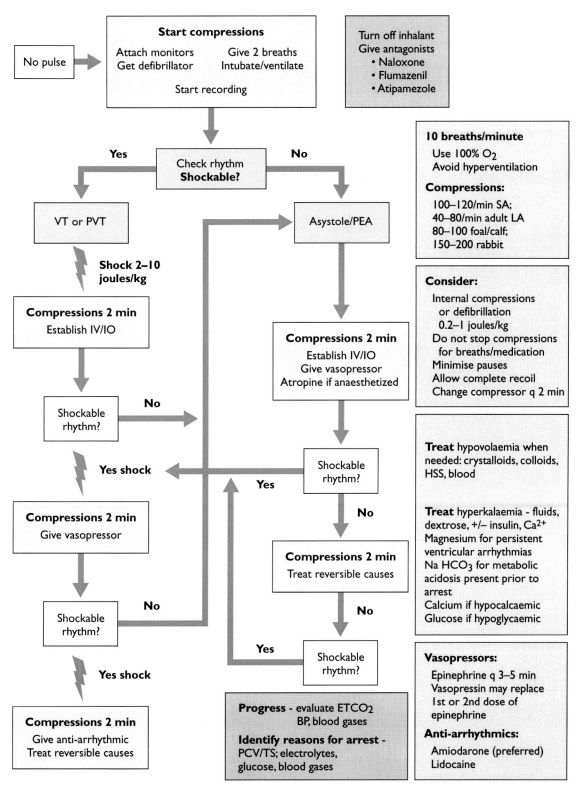

Figure 22.4 Algorithm for performance of CPCR (Source: American Heart Association, Inc., format). HSS: Hypertonic saline solution.

Table 22.4 Drug dosages for advanced life support

Treatment	Dose mg/kg IV	Indication and comments
Epinephrine	0.01	Cardiac arrest
1 mg/mL or 1:1000	1–5 µg/kg (LA)	
Dilute to 1:10000	0.05–5 µg/kg/min	Hypotension due to vasodilation
Vasopressin (20 U/mL)	0.1–0.8 U/kg 0.01–0.04 U/kg/min	Cardiac arrest Hypotension due to vasodilation
Atropine (0.54 mg/mL)	0.04 0.02–0.04 (LA)	Bradycardia; 3rd degree AV block; bronchoconstriction
Naloxone (0.4 mg/mL)	0.04	Opioid reversal
Flumazenil (0.1 mg/mL)	0.009–0.2	Benzodiazepine reversal
Atipamezole (5 mg/mL) Tolazoline (100 mg/mL) Yohimbine (25 mg/ml)	0.001-0.020 (SA) 0.02–0.20 (horse) 0.5–1.5 (horse or camelid) 0.5–2 (ruminants) 0.1 (SA) 0.075 (horse)	α_2-Agonist reversal; to avoid excitement, dilute and give **very** slowly IV; use lowest dose possible; decrease dose with time lapsed since administration; sudden death has been reported with use in awake horses and camelids
Amiodarone* (50 mg/ml)	5	Refractory ventricular tachycardia
Lidocaine 2%	1–2 (dog, horse) ± 0.02–.08 mg/kg/min 0.5–1 (cat)	Ventricular tachycardia when amiodarone not available
Dobutamine* (12.5 mg/mL diluted to 100 or 200 µg/mL)	1–15 µg/kg/min	Hypotension due to poor cardiac contractility
Dopamine* (40 mg/mL diluted to 100 or 200 µg/mL)	1–10 µg/kg/min to increase contractility; >10 = vasopressor activity	Hypotension due to poor cardiac contractility or vasodilation; AV conduction block
Ephedrine (50 mg/mL, or diluted)	0.06–0.2	Mild hypotension
Norepinephrine* (1 mg/mL)	0.05–0.3 µg/kg/min for vasoconstriction	Hypotension due to vasodilation
Phenylephrine 1%*	0.005–0.01	Hypotension due to vasodilation
Calcium chloride 10%	50 (SA)	Hypocalcaemia, hyperkalaemia, Ca channel blocker toxicity; give slowly, monitor for arrhythmias
Calcium gluconate 23%	0.5–1.5 mL/kg (SA) 0.2–0.4 mL/kg (LA)	Hypocalcaemia, hyperkalaemia, Ca channel blocker toxicity; give slowly, monitor for arrhythmias
Dextrose 25% Dextrose 50% Dextrose 5%	0.7–1 g/kg of 25% dextrose over 3–5 min 1 mL/kg dilute 1:4; give over 5 min (SA) 4.4–6.6 mL/kg of 5% (adult horse) 4–8 mL/kg/min (neonatal foals)	Hypoglycaemia or hyperkalaemia
Magnesium sulphate 50 %	0.2 mEq/kg (SA) 25-50; 2 mg/kg/min (horse)	Hypomagnesaemia, hypocalcaemia, torsades des pointes, persistent ventricular tachycardia
Na Bicarbonate 5 or 8.4%	mEq = BW (kg) × 0.3** × deficit (**0.5 for neonates) give ½ deficit initially and re-evaluate	Metabolic acidosis Prolonged CPR (>10 min)
Fluids Crystalloids	Normovolaemic patients 20 mL/kg dog, horse 10 mL/kg cat	Hypovolaemic patients should be treated as needed with crystalloids, colloids, blood, etc. Avoid hypervolaemia

Table 22.4 Continued

Treatment	Dose mg/kg IV	Indication and comments
Colloids Hypertonic saline 7.5%	5–10 mL/kg dog; 2–3 mL/kg cat 2–4 mL/kg	Avoid hypervolaemia
HSS/Hetastarch	2 mL/kg HSS and 5 mL/kg hetastarch (dog, horse) or 2–4 mL/kg of combination over 10 min	
Defibrillation	External 2–10 joules/kg Internal 0.2–1 joules/kg	Ventricular fibrillation; Pulseless ventricular tachycardia

LA: large animals; SA: small animals; HSS: hypertonic saline; * must be diluted prior to use.
Burns, 2008; Plunkett & McMichael, 2008; Cole, 2009; Muir & Hubbell, 2009; Riordan & Schaer, 2009; Scofield, et al, 2010.

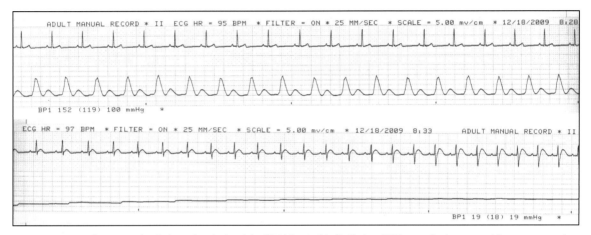

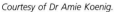

Figure 22.5 Development of pulseless electrical activity (PEA) in a critically ill dog (ECG trace is above arterial pressure trace). Note the only change at first is a small change in the size of the ST segment, at which time the patient had already been pulseless for over a minute.
Courtesy of Dr Amie Koenig.

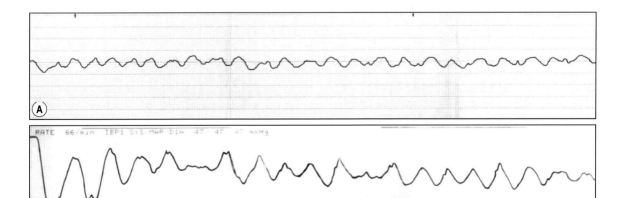

Figure 22.6 (A) Fine and (B) coarse ventricular fibrillation.

compressions can be paused *briefly* for a rhythm check. If a shockable rhythm is present, administer a vasopressor IV or IO, apply one shock, and continue compressions with minimal delay. After another 2 minutes, repeat the check, vasopressor, and shock when applicable, and then immediately continue compressions. The basic routine is repeated sequences of compressions 2 min, vasopressor IV or IO ± a shock, compressions 2 min, with the vasopressor IV or IO ± shock administered every 3-5 minutes. The individuals applying shocks and giving medications should be ready *before* compressions have stopped to minimize the duration of pauses. Since it takes time for drug levels to increase, medication is given during the same pause with the shock and followed by compressions so that drugs will be better circulated to the tissues in hopes of facilitating ROSC before the next pause. Compressions should not be stopped for administration of drugs, for intubation, or for ventilation. If PEA or asystole is present, the above routine is followed without the use of electrical shocks.

Anti-arrhythmic therapy should be administered when VF/PVT is not converted following three cycles of compressions/vasopressor therapy. Potentially reversible causes of arrest should be pursued throughout the resuscitation effort,, such as hypovolaemia, hypoxaemia, hypothermia, electrolyte abnormalities, and hypoglycaemia.

Defibrillation

Both monophasic and biphasic waveform defibrillators are available (Fig. 22.7). Biphasic units utilize current in two directions, using lower energy settings to achieve defibrillation. Monophasic machines generate greater current in one direction. Some authors feel the occurrence of myocardial damage secondary to electrical shock is less with biphasic machines, however, other studies using monophasic waveforms have not seen such damage. If a defibrillator

is available, familiarity with appropriate technique and settings is most important. Ideally, hair should be clipped from the chest. Both paddles and pads are now available with many defibrillators. The pads come in small sizes that work well for smaller patients. Conductive paste should be applied to defibrillator paddles; alcohol should not be used on the paddles or ECG leads as it may ignite during defibrillation. Paddles can be placed on the same side of the chest or on opposite sides (Fig. 22.8). The operator should ensure that good contact between the patient and the electrodes is present and that no one is touching the patient, the table, or anything attached to the patient before applying a shock. The defibrillator must be allowed to charge to the selected setting before the shock is applied to the chest. If unsuccessful, the energy setting should be increased for subsequent shocks. Recommended defibrillator settings are listed in Table 22.3, however, guidelines vary with different types of machines. Manufacturers' recommendations should be reviewed as they have usually validated the settings for their particular model. Great care should be taken with the use of defibrillators as injury to the patient and the resuscitation team including burns or electric shock can occur.

LARGE ANIMAL RESUSCITATION

Since anaesthetic recovery in adult large animals requires the attainment of a standing position, a prolonged course of CPCR may be a problem since hypotension (MAP <70 mmHg) for more than 20–30 minutes can result in myopathy even in patients that have not arrested. Recovery is often accompanied by excitement and further injury to the patient, especially if significant brain injury has also occurred. The anaesthetist must be mindful of human

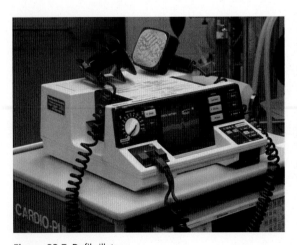

Figure 22.7 Defibrillator.

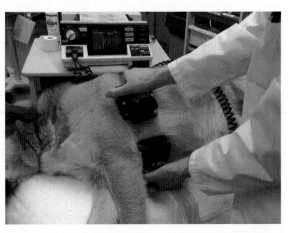

Figure 22.8 Defibrillator paddles are placed over the base of the heart and over the sternum at the apex of the heart.

safety as well as patient safety in these circumstances. In spite of these issues, successful resuscitation has been reported in ponies and adult horses (Frauenfelder et al., 1981; Kellagher & Watney, 1986; McGoldrick et al., 1998), and one cow (Raptopoulos & Karatzias, 1981) using both external and internal cardiac compression techniques. The eventual outcome following use of internal compressions was unfortunately most often euthanasia due to infection in the pleural cavity (Muir & Hubbell, 2009). The basic guidelines for BCLS in foals, calves, ponies, and small horses are the same as for small animals. Dosages of some drugs may differ (see Table 22.4). The major difference is in the technique for external cardiac compression in adults, as described earlier. Defibrillation is also similar in calves and foals and the smaller large animal species such as sheep, goats, and swine. Direct defibrillation of the heart is technically not a problem in large patients, but access through the thoracic wall may be inadequate without a rib resection, takes time, and the incidence of complications is high. Transthoracic defibrillation in patients >100 kg is reported to be difficult even in humans. The greater the body size, the more impedance of the flow of current and the less effective is the shock. Reports of successful electrical defibrillation performed in adult horses required several shocks in succession at high energy settings. The equipment was specifically designed for this purpose, including the defibrillator, the electrodes were implanted under the skin to decrease impedance, and a team of individuals was trained to perform external compressions (Tacker et al., 1973; Geddes et al., 1974).

MONITORING DURING CPCR

Some clinical signs and monitoring aids commonly used during anaesthesia are not useful during CPCR. Mucous membrane colour is unreliable due to poor peripheral perfusion and the use of vasopressors. Palpation of pulses is difficult, wastes time, and can be unreliable due to backflow into veins during compressions. Measurement of arterial blood gases taken before ROSC will be misleading. Poor perfusion of tissues should result in metabolic acidosis and hypercarbia, however, with oxygen supplementation, the respiratory alkalosis caused by controlled ventilation and the lack of adequate venous return, a normal or increased PaO_2 can be measured. $PaCO_2$ levels do not reflect tissue metabolism, but rather pulmonary blood flow and ventilation. Pulse oximetry may also be misleading initially as it can take several minutes for haemoglobin desaturation to develop after cardiac arrest when the patient was breathing 100% oxygen.

An indirect blood pressure monitor using Doppler ultrasound offers some information as the disappearance and reappearance of peripheral pulses is audible. If available, an extra probe can also be placed on the cornea under the third eyelid to identify arterial pulsation more readily than when placed on an extremity. Direct blood pressure monitoring provides real-time assessment of blood pressure. The presence of a waveform indicates a cardiac contraction or a compression strong enough to produce peripheral flow. Waveform changes may reveal the quality of cardiac contractility and the presence of vasodilation or vasoconstriction. Pupil size is a reliable indirect indicator of CBF. Dilation occurs when CBF is inadequate; therefore, a decrease in pupil size indicates improvement. Mixed venous oxygen saturation reflects overall tissue perfusion and oxygen extraction and is a more accurate measure of efficacy of blood flow to the body. However, a central venous catheter must be in place to obtain mixed venous samples. Jugular venous oxygen saturation can reflect cerebral oxygenation and extraction. Electrocardiography may reveal myocardial changes via waveform abnormalities but it is most important for identification and treatment of arrest rhythms. The best indirect monitor of cardiac output and pulmonary blood flow is $ETCO_2$ from capnography. When ventilation is consistent, $ETCO_2$ is proportional to blood flow through the lungs. As flow improves with effective CPCR, $ETCO_2$ increases and vice versa. In fact, decreasing $ETCO_2$ is one of the best indicators of impending cardiac arrest, while sudden or persistent increase is one of the best indicators of ROSC (ICCOR, 2010).

Goals of effective CPCR are: $ETCO_2$ ≥30–40 mmHg; mean arterial pressure ≥50 mmHg; normal K^+, Ca^{2+}, and glucose, normal acid base status, and normoxia (Box 22.2). Autoregulation of CBF is impaired following cardiac arrest and cerebral blood flow is greatly affected by oxygen, carbon dioxide concentration, and mean arterial blood pressure. Hypocarbia ($PaCO_2$ <30 mmHg) decreases CBF; hypercarbia ($PaCO_2$ ≥60 mmHg) causes vasodilation and increased CBF and increased ICP. Arterial oxygen levels should be maintained within the normal range (80–100 mmHg) to avoid further tissue damage. Poorer outcomes have been documented post resuscitation when hyperoxia persists (Pilchera et al, 2012; Kilgannon et al, 2010). Since reperfusion of ischaemic tissues results in the production of oxygen radicals and other deleterious substances when more oxygen is present, greater concentrations of these substances will be produced, and more tissue damage occurs.

Box 22.2 **Goals for performance of effective CPCR**

- ETCO2 30–40 mmHg
- MAP >50 mmHg
- Normal acid–base status via central or jugular venous blood gases
- Normal electrolytes and glucose

MEDICAL THERAPIES FOR CARDIAC ARREST (see Table 22.4)

Routes of administration

Intravenous (IV), intraosseous (IO), intratracheal (IT), or via an ET tube are all possible routes of administration of medications (Plunkett & McMichael, 2008). Venous access should be acquired as soon as possible without interfering with resuscitation. Patency of existing venous catheters should be verified to ensure appropriate drug delivery. Use of a central venous catheter is ideal. Medications administered through a peripheral catheter should be followed by larger than normal volumes of flush solution to facilitate their transfer into the systemic circulation. Medications administered by the IO route enter the circulation almost as quickly as when injected IV. An IO needle is relatively easy to install quickly when peripheral perfusion is poor. Intratracheal administration is now recommended only when IV or IO are not readily available. Larger doses are necessary for IT administration, up to 3–10× greater for epinephrine. Sterile water should be used for dilution of drugs rather than saline as absorption of the drug is greater. Drugs administered via the trachea or endotracheal tube should be instilled with a long catheter to reach the bronchi or flushed to transport them to the bronchi where absorption is faster. Calcium and sodium bicarbonate should not be administered IT. Intracardiac injection is not recommended due to damage to cardiac muscle. Cardiac compressions must be continued during and following administration of all medications to promote movement of the drugs into the coronary circulation.

Vasopressors

Both adrenergic and non-adrenergic drugs have been used in resuscitation of the arrested patient. Although no studies exist that document a better outcome when vasopressors are used versus a placebo, adrenergic therapy has been the mainstay of ACLS since the use of epinephrine was introduced in the early 1900s (Cooper et al., 2006). Intense vasoconstriction of peripheral vessels is thought to increase venous return to the heart and improve coronary perfusion. In some species, it may preferentially increase flow to the brain with greater constriction of the external versus the internal carotid arteries. Historically, epinephrine has been the primary medical therapy for cardiac arrest. A sympathomimetic catecholamine, epinephrine acts on both α- and β-receptors in the heart and periphery. It produces profound vasoconstriction via α_1-receptor activity on peripheral vasculature. Its cardiac β-effects increase heart rate and contractility. Negative effects of epinephrine include a tendency for increased cardiac metabolic oxygen requirements, decreased coronary blood flow via vasoconstriction, increased myocardial dysfunction post arrest, and decreased cerebral perfusion (Angelosa et al., 2008; Ristagno et al., 2009). It is also less effective in acidotic environments that can develop with prolonged arrest (>10 min). A higher incidence of cardiac arrhythmia in the post-resuscitation period has also been associated with epinephrine. The 'high dose' therapy (0.1 mg/kg versus 0.01 mg/kg) has not been associated with increased survival, may be detrimental, and is no longer recommended.

Vasopressin has been demonstrated to improve outcome in humans and animals with cardiac arrest, especially those with asystole (Wenzel et al., 2004; Grmec & Mally, 2006; Mally et al., 2007, Stroumpoulis et al., 2008). Also known as antidiuretic hormone (ADH), vasopressin is an endogenous peptide released by the neurohypophysis to regulate water balance that generally has no effect on blood pressure at physiological doses in healthy patients. However, at high doses, vasopressin produces intense vasoconstriction, acting on vasopressin 1 receptors of vascular smooth muscle. It has been shown to improve pulmonary blood flow and gas exchange (Loeckinger et al., 2002) and coronary and cerebral circulation (Prengel et al., 2005). It has no adrenergic effects, is still effective in acidotic states, and is not associated with arrhythmia in the post-resuscitation period.

There is no definitive work that has determined which vasopressor medication(s) to use, what dose to use, or when to give such therapy. Vasopressin was previously recommended to replace one dose of epinephrine in patients with PEA, VT, or VF; and as an alternative to epinephrine during CPCR in patients with asystole (ILCOR, 2005; AHA, 2005). Some authors have recommended using multiple doses of vasopressin, combining it with epinephrine, or alternating vasopressin with epinephrine (Krismer et al., 2004; Wenzel et al., 2004). Recent randomized trials in humans comparing epinephrine and vasopressin have not shown a difference between eventual outcome when either drug was used (Gueugniaud et al., 2008; ICCOR, 2010). Since no difference has been documented, the European Resuscitation Council has never recommended vasopressin over epinephrine for treatment of cardiac arrest. However, because of evidence for better short-term outcomes *and* this lack of a difference, the 2010 ICCOR group and the 2010 AHA guidelines take a different view and continue to suggest that one dose of vasopressin may replace epinephrine during the first or second resuscitation cycle in all patients with cardiac arrest.

Most of the research and clinical studies on CPCR has focused on healthy animals with induced VF or humans with VF or PVT at the onset of cardiac arrest. Asystole is the more common initial rhythm in animals, and there are no prospective controlled trials of techniques or medical therapy used for CPCR in clinical veterinary patients for comparison, so it is difficult to extrapolate findings of the human literature to our patients. One recent retrospective analysis of factors associated with survival in dogs and cats with cardiac arrest did find a positive association with the use of vasopressin (Hofmeister et al., 2009), and successful ROSC in an anaesthetized dog using multiple doses of vasopressin during CPCR has been reported (Schmittinger et al., 2005). The laboratory studies in animals with induced cardiac arrest have consistently shown better outcomes with vasopressin, even after long durations of arrest (>10 min) (Wenzel et al., 2000; Stadlbauer et al., 2003; Stroumpoulis et al., 2008), and vasopression has been associated with better outcome in patients with asystole (Mally et al., 2007; Wenzel et al., 2004). Vasopressin may therefore be a reasonable alternative or adjunct to the use of epinephrine in animals (Plunkett & McMichael, 2008; Scroggin & Quandt, 2009).

Anti-arrhythmic medication

Atropine

Atropine is a muscarinic receptor (M2) antagonist that increases heart rate by blocking parasympathetic input to cardiac muscle, resulting in increased automaticity of the sinus node and improved conduction at the atrioventricular node. Atropine was previously recommended for use in the management of asystole, PEA, or PEA with bradycardia (ILCOR, 2005), however, it is no longer recommended for routine use in humans with cardiac arrest. Glycopyrrolate or atropine is still recommended for patients with symptomatic bradycardia (AHA, 2010). Since vagal tone can be increased by anaesthetic drugs and surgery, it is still recommended in CPCR for anaesthetized patients (Plunkett & McMichael, 2008). When atropine has been given, pupillary response may not be a reliable clinical sign in dogs for monitoring in the post-arrest period since it causes mydriasis.

Amiodarone

Amiodarone is currently recommended when ventricular fibrillation or ventricular tachycardia are refractory to repeated electrical conversion (ILCOR, 2005; Plunkett & McMichael, 2008; ICCOR, 2010). Outcome was improved when amiodarone administration was compared with lidocaine or placebo (Dorian et al., 2002). It is a mixed class anti-arrhythmic drug, with actions at sodium, potassium, and calcium channels as well as α- and β-adrenergic effects. Amiodarone must be diluted and should be given slowly IV whenever possible. It can be given as continuous infusion post resuscitation as well if ventricular arrhythmias persist or recur. Significant hypotension can develop with intravenous use, thought to be associated with the solvent vehicle used and the speed of administration. Reversible hepatic dysfunction is reported in dogs, associated with chronic oral therapy (Jacobs et al., 2000). Severe skin reactions with erythema, urticaria, and pruritus were seen in five dogs when IV amiodarone was given for ventricular arrhythmias. Clinical signs resolved when the infusion was stopped, and corticosteroids were also administered to some of the dogs (Cober et al., 2009). An aqueous preparation of amiodarone (Amio-Aqueous®) is now approved in the USA that has fewer side effects (Somberg et al., 2004; ICCOR, 2010).

Lidocaine

Lidocaine is a local anaesthetic and anti-arrhythmic drug that prevents the influx of sodium into cells, inhibiting depolarization of the cell membrane, thereby blocking the generation or conduction of an action potential. It has minimal effects on normal cardiac pacemaker cells, but is active in the Purkinje fibres of the ventricles, especially in damaged or ischaemic tissue. Lidocaine is not useful for ventricular fibrillation and, in fact, increases the defibrillation threshold, and should be avoided if defibrillation is possible. It may be useful to control ventricular arrhythmias post ROSC when amiodarone is unavailable. Preparations without preservative are best for intravenous use rather than those used for local anaesthesia. Overdose is characterized by central nervous system side effects such as excitement, tremors, and collapse. If this occurs, the infusion should be slowed or stopped temporarily and restarted at a lower rate.

Other medication or therapy

Fluid therapy

Fluid therapy is an important adjunct to the medical therapy of CPCR, however, it is primarily effective when patients are hypovolaemic, especially when this is the primary cause of the arrest. More commonly, too much fluid is given to patients in cardiac arrest rather than inadequate amounts. This can be harmful as excessive fluid volume increases right atrial pressure (RAP). Increased RAP without an increase of systolic pressure will decrease coronary perfusion since coronary blood flow is proportional to the difference between aortic pressure and RAP. Crystalloid solutions decrease osmotic pressure and dilute plasma proteins and coagulation factors, which may cause tissue oedema and hypocoagulability. To avoid hypervolaemia in normovolaemic patients, infusions of balanced electrolyte solution in normovolaemic patients should be on the order of 20 ml/kg in dogs, 10 ml/kg in cats (Plunkett & McMichael, 2008), and 20 ml/kg in horses (Muir & Hubbell, 2009). Improved circulation is obtained when crystalloid and colloid solutions are used together. Many combinations of dosages have been reported, and Table 22.4 lists the more common doses. Recently, use of a low dose of a combination product with 6% hydroxyethylstarch (colloid) and 7.2% hypertonic saline (HSS) at 2 ml/kg/10 minutes was reported to improve cerebral microcirculation and neurological scores in swine and cerebral perfusion pressures in swine and humans (Noppens et al., 2006; Bender et al., 2007). Hypertonic saline improves cardiac function during and after ROSC and is used to treat or prevent cerebral oedema. It increases serum sodium levels and osmolarity, creating an osmotic gradient between the blood and the tissues that promotes the passive movement of fluid into the vascular system. This increases plasma volume, producing greater cardiac output and higher mean arterial pressure, and decreases oedema and intracranial pressure (ICP). The combination of increased MAP and decreased ICP results in improved cerebral perfusion pressure (CPP). It may also improve perfusion by decreasing resistance in injured tissues by reducing oedema in vascular endothelium and by improving viscosity. Hypertonic saline should be used very carefully in patients with hyponatraemia to avoid cellular swelling and hypomyelinosis. Hypertonic saline also effectively increases blood volume in patients with trauma, haemorrhage, sepsis, and endotoxaemia.

Sodium bicarbonate

Sodium bicarbonate ($NaHCO_3$) therapy is still debated. Earlier guidelines suggested that $NaHCO_3$ be given at 0.5–1 mEq/kg IV at 10 minute intervals during CPCR. However, both the 2005 and 2010 guidelines do not recommend it for routine use during CPCR in humans. This is based on the premise that the acidosis seen during CPCR is a lactic acidosis secondary to the lack of perfusion and the subsequent increase in anaerobic metabolism in tissues, and is best treated by restoration of blood flow. Potential side effects of $NaHCO_3$ therapy that are frequently identified are hypernatraemia, intracellular acidosis, and decreased tissue oxygenation due to a left shift of the oxyhaemoglobin dissociation curve. However, it is not clear how often these effects occur in levels significant enough to be detrimental. Acidosis and hyperkalaemia often develop after 10 minutes of CPCR, and these abnormalities could be countered with bicarbonate therapy. Some studies have shown better outcomes with the use of sodium bicarbonate in CPCR (Bar-Joseph et al., 1998; Leong et al., 2001). These authors believe that the decision of the ILCOR group in regard to the use of bicarbonate is not based on thorough controlled and randomized clinical trials of its use in CPCR. Bicarbonate therapy is recommended when metabolic acidosis was present prior to arrest, in cases with extreme hyperkalaemia, for calcium channel blocker overdose, and in patients where loss of bicarbonate via the kidney or gastrointestinal tract is significant. The dose utilized and the osmolality of the solution given may be factors to consider. Acid–base status should therefore be evaluated using mixed venous or jugular venous blood samples when $NaHCO_3$ is utilized. The amount of bicarbonate needed can be calculated as follows:

$$\text{mEq of bicarbonate} = \text{BW (kg)} \times [\text{base deficit or} \\ (24 - HCO3)] \times 0.3 \text{ (or 0.5 for neonates)}.$$

This calculation is an estimate of the total extracellular fluid (ECF) deficit of bicarbonate, however, this amount is rarely necessary and no more than ⅓–½ of the deficit should be given at a time over 15 minutes. When ROSC occurs, acid–base status should then be re-evaluated after an hour to allow equilibration between the tissues and the ECF. Blood volume status and blood pressure deficits should also be addressed. Sodium bicarbonate decreases serum potassium and ionized calcium levels, therefore, administration should be postponed until after correction of ionized hypocalcaemia or hypokalaemia.

Mannitol

A potent osmotic diuretic, mannitol has been the mainstay of therapy to treat or prevent cerebral oedema and increased ICP, and improve CPP in patients with cerebral disease or injury. Mannitol stimulates a reflex vasoconstriction in the cerebral vessels and improves blood viscosity in the first few minutes after administration. The osmotic effect of pulling fluid out of the tissues into the vasculature is seen after approximately 15–20 minutes. Cerebral oedema is not common in the immediate post-resuscitation period but may develop later when significant neuronal cell damage has occurred. Mannitol is used in the post-resuscitation phase in patients with neurological deficits and administered at 0.5–1.5 g/kg IV over 20 minutes, up to three times a day. Mannitol is administered intermittently rather than as an infusion to avoid increased permeability of the blood–brain barrier by continuous exposure. The diuretic effect of mannitol precludes its use in hypovolaemic patients until after fluid volume is replaced, especially since a rebound hypotension may occur following its use. Acute renal failure has developed in people when serum osmolality exceeded 320 mOsm/L, therefore, monitoring of serum osmolality is recommended when either mannitol or HSS is used. Results of recent investigations indicate that HSS may be preferred for ICP control as it has a longer duration, can be given more often, has fewer adverse side effects, has positive effects on the myocardium, cardiac output, and peripheral circulation, and may be associated with better outcomes (Krieter et al., 2002; Noppens et al., 2006; Bender et al., 2007). Rebound hypotension following therapy is less likely with HSS since the sodium is reabsorbed by the kidneys.

Glucose

Glucose is required only when the patient is hypoglycaemic and is not given routinely for CPCR. Both hypoglycaemia and hyperglycaemia have been associated with poorer outcomes in critically ill patients. Therapy should be guided by periodic assessment of blood glucose levels.

Treatment for severe hyperglycaemia is recommended but hypoglycaemia must be avoided (ICCOR, 2010). Neonates, toy breeds, birds, small mammals, and patients with insulinoma, liver failure, portosystemic shunt, diabetes, and sepsis may require IV dextrose to maintain normal glucose levels during anaesthesia.

Electrolyte abnormalities

Electrolyte abnormalities secondary to a primary disease can cause cardiac arrest and interfere with therapy. Calcium, potassium, and magnesium are most often involved and will be briefly discussed here.

Calcium

Calcium is not recommended during CPCR except in cases of pre-existing hypocalcaemia. Poorer outcome has been seen when patients are given calcium, presumably because cell death is associated with increased release of intracellular calcium. Therapy should be conservative and guided by ionized calcium measurements whenever possible. Ionized calcium levels are decreased by general anaesthesia and alkalosis, and can be seen with endotoxaemia and gastrointestinal disease, especially in horses. Heavily pregnant or lactating females may also become hypocalcaemic when ill or anaesthetized. Overdose of calcium channel blockers may produce decreased myocardial contractility that may respond to calcium administration. The effects of hyperkalaemia may be temporarily ameliorated by calcium infusion as it is thought to readjust the change in resting membrane potential back to normal (Hyperkalemic Periodic Paralysis in horses, uroperitoneum), allowing more time for other treatments given to decrease potassium to be effective.

Hyperkalaemia

Hyperkalaemia is a cause of life-threatening cardiac arrhythmia. It is seen in cases with urinary tract obstruction, uroperitoneum, severe dehydration, Addison's disease, acute renal failure, and acidosis. It develops quickly during CPR, doubling in magnitude by 10 minutes, and can be associated with post-arrest arrhythmias. Bradycardias, tachycardia, and normal heart rates can be seen, although slower heart rates and heart block may be more common since sinus node activity is sensitive to potassium concentrations. Treatments to decrease serum potassium concentration depend somewhat on the severity of hyperkalaemia. Serum levels ≤6.5 mEq/L may respond to dilution and diuresis with intravenous administration of isotonic electrolyte solution that is potassium free (0.9% saline) or potassium deficient (Normosol R®, lactated Ringer's solution). Higher blood potassium concentrations may require infusion of dextrose with or without insulin to facilitate movement of K^+ into cells by activation of the Na^+K^+ ATPase pump. Five percent dextrose solution, 4.4–6.6 ml/kg IV, can be given to large animals, and

0.7–1 g/kg of 25% dextrose IV administered over 3–5 minutes in small animals will decrease potassium levels in less than 1 hour. Insulin is not always necessary but 0.5 U/kg of regular insulin can be given to small animals. Glucose concentrations should be monitored closely. Sodium bicarbonate can be given to produce alkalinization that encourages the shift of H^+ out of cells and K^+ into cells to maintain electroneutrality. For example, 1–2 mEq/kg or ½–⅓ of the ECF deficit of bicarbonate (see above) can be given slowly IV in both small and large animals. Calcium can be given as a more immediate palliative treatment for severe hyperkalaemia to antagonize its effects on the myocardium by restoration of the resting membrane potential that decreases hyperexitability of myocytes. Ten percent calcium gluconate, 0.5–1.5 ml/kg IV, can be administered over 5–10 minutes to small animals and 23% calcium gluconate, 0.2–0.4 ml/kg, in 1–2 L of 5% dextrose administered to large animals. The ECG should be monitored during administration of calcium (Burns, 2008; Riordan & Schaer, 2009). Abdominal drainage or cystocentesis may be necessary to remove the source of potassium in cases of uroperitoneum or urinary tract obstruction, respectively.

Hypokalaemia

Hypokalaemia occurs less commonly but may be associated with alkalosis, diarrhoea and diuretic therapy. Hypokalaemia can lead to muscular weakness and cardiac arrhythmia, and may cause the myocardium to become refractory to the effects of some anti-arrhythmic drugs. Animals with significant hypokalaemia should receive IV fluids that contain up to 40 mEq/L of potassium. Saline should be used in patients with alkalaemia, whereas an alkalinizing fluid such as acetated or lactated electrolyte solution should be used in acidaemic patients. A separate infusion of potassium chloride (KCl) can be given to patients that require rapid fluid resuscitation. The usual guideline is to avoid administration rates for potassium greater than 0.5 mEq/kg/min. In severely hypokalaemic (<2.0 mg/dl), non-oliguric small animals, the infusion rate for potassium may be increased to 1–1.5 mEq/kg/min. The rate should be tailored to the individual patient's need, and the electrocardiogram should be monitored continuously (Riordan & Schaer, 2009). It may be difficult to improve serum potassium concentrations intravenously in large animal patients and oral supplementation via nasogastric tube is often necessary.

Magnesium

Magnesium is not recommended for routine use. However, it is an important emergency treatment for torsades des pointes in dogs and horses to prevent ventricular fibrillation, and may help with refractory ventricular tachycardias. It may also be necessary to affect a response to calcium administration when hypocalcaemia is present. Hypomagnesaemia is likely more common than is currently realized. It has recently been associated with general anaesthesia in dogs and cats (Brainard et al., 2007) and is associated with critical illness in horses (Johansson et al., 2003) and dogs (Khanna et al., 1998).

Therapeutic hypothermia

Therapeutic hypothermia is recommended by the 2010 ICCOR guidelines for all patients that achieve ROSC but remain comatose. Both increased survival and better neurological outcome have been associated with its use in many species (Alzagaa et al., 2006; Polderman, 2008). Mild to moderate hypothermia is considered one of the more useful treatments for cerebral protection since it is directed at multiple pathways of neuronal death. It is thought to prevent tissue damage by several mechanisms, including decreasing the metabolic requirements of tissues, especially the brain, by reducing the cellular inflammatory response to ischaemia. Its use is not common in clinical veterinary medicine, however, it has been used successfully in a dog with refractory seizures following a traumatic brain injury (Hayes, 2009). It is probably not practical and is potentially dangerous in large animal species that must stand following general anaesthesia. Since patients often become hypothermic under anaesthesia and temperature may continue to decrease with cardiac arrest, avoidance of rewarming may be appropriate. Maintenance of a temperature a few degrees below the normal range may be helpful. However, severe hypothermia should be avoided as it is a risk factor for cardiac arrest itself, especially in cats.

POST RESUSCITATION

Patients that suffer cardiac arrest and are quickly resuscitated may require little supportive therapy. However, those who do not recover quickly may develop numerous problems post ROSC. Re-arrest following ROSC is common, especially when pre-existing conditions are severe or the primary cause has not been identified. Unfortunately, many more patients are successfully resuscitated than are actually discharged from the hospital. Therefore, treatment during the post-arrest period is essential to survival as well as to ensure an outcome with a good quality of life. Immediate, good quality post-arrest care is re-emphasized in the 2010 ICCOR guidelines. The following information is a summary of the most important aspects of care in the post-ROSC period. See the suggested readings for more details on this topic.

The whole body ischaemia that occurs during arrest is followed by poor perfusion during CPCR, and then further tissue damage occurs with reperfusion injury. The pathophysiological changes that occur in the post-arrest period are considered to be a separate syndrome. The most important areas of concern are brain injury, myocardial dysfunction, ischaemia and reperfusion injury, and persistence of pre-existing problems. Therapy is therefore directed to all these areas, initially to stabilize the patient and then therapy to treat or prevent complications. If the initial damage is severe or not adequately reversed in the immediate post-ROSC period, the patient may develop a condition similar to that of septic shock with evidence of a systemic inflammatory response, and may succumb to infection or multiorgan failure.

Following ROSC, a short period of hyperperfusion occurs that is followed by a longer period of poor perfusion due to myocardial dysfunction, vasodilation, and cardiac arrhythmias. During this latter period, the brain is especially susceptible to further injury as autoregulation of CBF is usually dysfunctional, and CPP is dependent on systemic MAP. Hypovolaemia may be present following cardiac arrest and should be treated, avoiding hypervolaemia or inappropriate increases in right atrial pressure. Blood pressure should be monitored frequently and, if possible, continuously with placement of an arterial catheter. A mean arterial pressure of >65 mmHg or a systolic pressure >80–90 mmHg should be maintained. If available, echocardiography is recommended to identify myocardial dysfunction and to determine the need for inotrope therapy. Administration of one or more inotropes is indicated when impaired contractility is identified, or in patients that are hypotensive but not vasodilated or hypovolaemic. Dobutamine is usually preferred for post-resuscitation management. Vasopressor therapy is needed if vasodilation is a significant cause of hypotension. Vasopressin, norepinephrine, epinephrine, or dopamine can be used as continuous infusions to support blood pressure. Treatment should be titrated to the lowest possible effective dose to avoid excessive vasoconstriction of peripheral and splanchnic vasculature. Hypertension (MAP >100 mmHg) should also be avoided as this may exacerbate reperfusion injury. The ECG should be monitored and significant dysrhythmias treated accordingly. Persistent ventricular tachycardia is not uncommon. Infusion of lidocaine or amiodarone may be necessary to maintain sinus rhythm (see Table 22.4).

Respiratory depression is common following cardiac arrest. Hypoxaemia and hyperoxia are both detrimental. Oxygen supplementation is almost always necessary and should be titrated to achieve arterial oxygen levels between 80 and 100 mmHg. Flow-by oxygen or nasal insufflation therapy can be utilized, however, some patients may have to remain connected to the anaesthesia machine and artificially ventilated to maintain carbon dioxide tension within the normal range ($PaCO_2$ 35–45, $ETCO_2$ 30–40 mmHg). Hyperoxia can be avoided by using a mixture of oxygen and air. Some anaesthesia machines will mix these gases automatically and others require manual adjustment of the flow meters. Hypocarbia should be avoided as this greatly decreases CBF. Pulse oximetry can be used to identify hypoxaemia, however, it does not recognize hyperoxia that can exacerbate reperfusion injury. When available, blood gas analysis should be performed periodically because hypotension and inconsistent perfusion can affect capnography and pulse oximetry measurements. Sedation of the patient may be necessary to facilitate ventilation. Analgesic agents should be utilized as pain can impair cardiopulmonary function through mechanisms such as tachycardia, vasoconstriction, and laboured breathing.

Temperature should be monitored closely. Inability to maintain a normal temperature may be seen in some patients, especially when blood pressure is variable. Patients can be allowed to remain mildly hypothermic by avoidance of rewarming but, some species such as birds, small mammals, and cats, may be more prone to complications with hypothermia. Hyperthermia should be avoided since it increases metabolic oxygen requirements. Metabolic status should be monitored regularly with serial measurement of glucose and electrolytes, and organ function should be evaluated as needed with laboratory tests of kidney and liver function, and coagulation. Urine output should be monitored as part of the assessment of renal function and efficacy of fluid therapy. In dogs, placement of a urinary catheter with a closed urine collection system facilitates accurate evaluation.

Neurological status is a major component of post-ROSC care and eventual outcome. The brain is very susceptible to continued injury in the post-arrest period because of cardiovascular dysfunction, reperfusion injury, lack of CBF autoregulation, and regional damage or dysfunction of the cerebral microcirculation. Optimization of neurological recovery first involves appropriate cardiovascular and respiratory interventions as previously discussed. In addition, therapy for intracranial hypertension and cerebral oedema may be necessary. As previously mentioned, these are not always seen post ROSC but may be more likely if pre-existing cerebral disease was present, when asphyxia is a cause of the arrest, or if arrest or resuscitation was prolonged. A test dose of mannitol or HSS may be helpful in diagnosis if improvement is observed following administration. If dysregulation of CBF is suspected, MAP should maintained at a higher value (100 mmHg) than that usually needed to ensure adequate CPP. Hyperventilation can be used to treat sudden increases in ICP, and to allow time for the onset of intravenous therapy. However, hyperventilation will eventually be ineffective as the brain 'resets' to the lower CO_2 level and intracranial hypertension will return. Elevation of the head to approximately 30° from horizontal with the head and neck straight and the jugular veins unobstructed (e.g. loose neck wraps) can help to decrease ICP. Great care should be taken when performing procedures that could decrease PaO_2 or stimulate coughing or sneezing, such as endotracheal tube exchange or suctioning and changing nasal oxygen tubing. Sedation may be necessary in some patients to avoid

increases in ICP during such procedures. Seizure activity should be immediately treated with diazepam or midazolam. If needed, longer-acting anticonvulsant therapy should be instituted.

Although neurological outcome of cardiac arrest survivors has not been evaluated in clinical veterinary medicine as thoroughly as in people, one retrospective study of 18 survivors to discharge of cardiac arrest at a veterinary teaching hospital over a 5-year period found that two of the 18 had neurological deficits at discharge. Both were dogs and one was normal at a 2-month follow-up examination (Waldrop et al., 2004). Clinical investigations in humans and research studies using animal species have looked at neurological outcome. Most authors recommend observation for 24–48 hours to determine a prognosis. A poor outcome is expected when corneal reflexes, pupillary responses, withdrawal response to pain, and motor responses remain absent at 24 hours following ROSC.

Supportive care, similar to basic care of anaesthetized or critical care patients, is important to ensure a good outcome in the post-ROSC period. Nutrition should be provided as soon as possible depending on the particular patient's abilities. Catheter sites and bandaged areas should be examined regularly. The eyes should be examined for corneal damage and lubricated often. Comfortable padding for pressure points and painful areas should be provided. Patients should be examined regularly for passage of faeces or urine to prevent scalding of skin or soiling of bandages, catheters, and drains. Positioning in sternal recumbency is usually better for gas exchange and may help avoid regurgitation and aspiration of gastric contents in depressed or comatose individuals.

SUMMARY AND FUTURE THERAPIES

In spite of much research in animals and humans, clinical trials in humans, and years of debate by those directly involved, there are very few definitive conclusions in regard to recommendations for treatments that will ensure an excellent long-term outcome following CPCR. The best therapies to date are the application of early and excellent quality basic life support, defibrillation as soon as a shockable rhythm is identified, and thorough post-resuscitation care. Outcome is much better in those patients who require only BLS; when medical therapy is required, the likelihood of survival decreases greatly and only becomes worse with time. Specific guidelines for veterinary anaesthesia patients will not be known until controlled and randomized trials of clinical veterinary patients are conducted.

Therapies that may be included in the future could be some of the following: intravenous erythropoietin, which improves myocardial haemodynamics during CPCR

(Grmec et al., 2009); treatments aimed at preventing mitochondrial dysfunction (Ayoub et al., 2008); injection of mesenchymal stem cells from bone marrow to replace myocardial cells damaged by ischaemia/reperfusion (Wang et al., 2008); and combination medical therapy using corticosteroids (Mentzelopoulos et al., 2009) and/or beta-blockers and/or cerebral vasodilators (Xanthos et al., 2009) in addition to vasopressors during ACLS.

REFERENCES

Abeysekera, A., Bergman, I.J., Kluger, M.T., et al., 2005. Drug error in anaesthetic practice: a review of 896 reports from the Australian Incident Monitoring Study database. Anaesthesia 60, 220–227.

Alzagaa, A.G., Cerdanb, M., Varonc, J., 2006. Therapeutic hypothermia. Resuscitation 70, 369–380.

American Heart Association (AHA), 2010. Guidelines for Cardiopulmonary Resuscitation and Emergency Cardiovascular Care. Circulation 122 (18, suppl 3), S640–S933.

Angelosa, M.G., Butkea, R.L., Panchala, A.R., et al., 2008. Cardiovascular response to epinephrine varies with increasing duration of cardiac arrest. Resuscitation 77, 101–110.

Arbous, M.S., Brobbee, D.E., Van Kleef, J.W., et al., 2001. Mortality associated with anaesthesia: a qualitative analysis to identify risk factors. Anaesthesia 56, 1141–1153.

Arbous, M.S., Meursing, A.E., Van Kleef, J.W., et al., 2005. Impact of anesthesia management characteristics on severe morbidity and mortality. Anesthesiology 102, 257–268.

Aufderheide, T.P., Sigurdsson, G., Pirrallo, R.G., et al., 2004. Hyperventilation-induced hypotension during cardiopulmonary resuscitation. Circulation 109, 1960–1965.

Ayoub, I.M., Radhakrishnan, J., Gazmuri, R.J., 2008. Targeting mitochondria for resuscitation from cardiac arrest. Crit Care Med 36, S440–S446.

Bar-Joseph, G., Weinberger, T., Castel, T., et al., 1998. Comparison of sodium bicarbonate, Carbicarb, and THAM during CPR in dogs. Crit Care Med 26, 1397–1408.

Bidwell, L.A., Bramlage, L.R., Rood, W.A., 2007. Equine perioperative fatalities associated with general anaesthesia at a private practice-a retrospective case series. Vet Anaesth Analg 34, 23–30.

Beecher, H.K., Todd, D.P., 1954. Ann Surg 140, 2–34.

Bender, R., Breil, M., Heistera, U., et al., 2007. Hypertonic saline during CPR: Feasibility and safety of a new protocol of fluid management during resuscitation. Resuscitation 72, 74–81.

Brainard, B.M., Campbell, V.L., Drobatz, K.J., et al., 2007. The effects of surgery and anesthesia on blood magnesium and calcium concentrations in canine and feline patients. Vet Anaesth Analg 34, 89–98.

Brodbelt, D.C., 2009. Perioperative mortality in small animal anaesthesia. Vet J 182, 152–161.

Brodbelt, D.C., Blisset, K.J., Hammond, R.A., et al., 2008. The risk of death: the Confidential Enquiry into Perioperative Small Animal Fatalities. Vet Anaesth Analg 35, 365–373.

Burns, T.A., 2008. Potassium, hyperkalemia. In: Lavoie, J.P., Hinchcliff, K.W. (Eds.), Blackwell's Five Minute Veterinary Consult: Equine, second ed. Wiley-Blackwell, Ames, p. 618.

Cole, S., 2009. Cardiopulmonary resuscitation. In: Silverstein, D.C., Hopper, K. (Eds.), Small Animal Critical Care Medicine. Saunders Elsevier, St Louis, pp. 14–21.

Cooper, J.A., Cooper, J.D., Cooper, J.M., 2006. Cardiopulmonary resuscitation: history, current practice, and future direction. Circulation 114, 2839–2849.

Cober, R.E., Schober, K.E., Hildebrandt, N., et al., 2009. Adverse effects of intravenous amiodarone in 5 dogs. J Vet Int Med 23, 657–661.

Domino, K.B., Bowdle, T.A., Posner, K.L., et al., 2004. Injuries and liability related to central vascular catheters, a closed claims analysis. Anesthesiology 100, 1411–1418.

Dorian, P., Cass, D., Schwartz, B., et al., 2002. Amiodarone as compared with lidocaine for shock-resistant ventricular fibrillation N Engl J Med 346, 884–890.

Eichhorn, J.H., 1989. Prevention of intraoperative anesthesia accidents and related severe injury through safety monitoring. Anesthesiology 70, 572–577.

Fecho, K., Jackson, F., Smith, F., et al., 2009. In-hospital resuscitation: opioids and other factors influencing survival. Ther Clin Risk Manag 5, 961–968.

Frauenfelder, H.C., Fessler, J.F., Latshaw, H.S., et al., 1981. External cardiovascular resuscitation of the anesthetized pony. J Am Vet Med Assoc 179, 673–676.

Gaynor, J.S., Dunlop, C.I., Wagner, A.E., et al., 1999. Complications and mortality associated with anesthesia in dogs and cats. J Am Anim Hosp Assoc 35, 13–17.

Geddes, L.A., Tacker, N.A., Rosborouci, J.P., et al., 1974. Electrical dose for ventricular defibrillation of large and small animals using precordial electrodes. J Clin Invest 53, 310–319.

Greene, S.A., Marks, S.L., 2007. Gastrointestinal disease. In: Tranquilli, W.J., Thurmon, J.C., Grimm, K.A. (Eds.), Lumb & Jones Veterinary Anesthesia and Analgesia, fourth ed. Blackwell Publishing, Ames, pp. 927–932.

Gross, M.E., Giuliano, E.A., 2007. Ocular patients. In: Tranquilli, W.J., Thurmon, J.C., Grimm, K.A. (Eds.), Lumb & Jones Veterinary Anesthesia and Analgesia, fourth ed. Blackwell Publishing, Ames, pp. 943–954.

Grmec, S., Mally, S., 2006. Vasopressin improves outcome in out-of-hospital cardiopulmonary resuscitation of ventricular fibrillation and pulseless ventricular tachycardia: a observational cohort study. Critical Care 10 (1), R13.

Grmec, S., Strnad, M., Kupnik, D., et al., 2009. Erythropoietin facilitates the return of spontaneous circulation and survival in victims of out-of-hospital cardiac arrest. Resuscitation 80, 631–637.

Gueugniaud, P.-Y., David, J.-S., Chanzy, E., et al., 2008. Vasopressin and epinephrine vs. epinephrine alone in cardiopulmonary resuscitation. N Engl J Med 359, 21–30.

Gunew, M., Marshall, R., Lui, M., et al., 2008. Fatal venous air embolism in a cat undergoing dental extractions. J Small Anim Pract 49, 601–604.

Harvey, R.C., Schaer, M., 2007. Endocrine disease. In: Tranquilli, W.J., Thurmon, J.C., Grimm, K.A. (Eds.), Lumb & Jones Veterinary Anesthesia and Analgesia, fourth ed. Blackwell Publishing, Ames, pp. 933–936.

Haskin, S.C., 1992. Internal cardiac compressions. J Am Vet Med Assoc 200, 1945–1946.

Hayes, G.M., 2009. Severe seizures associated with traumatic brain injury managed by controlled hypothermia, pharmacologic coma, and mechanical ventilation in a dog. J Vet Emerg Crit Care 19, 29–34.

Hofmeister, E.H., Brainard, B.M., Egger, C.M., et al., 2009. Prognostic indicators for dogs and cats with cardiopulmonary arrest treated by cardiopulmonary cerebral resuscitation at a university teaching hospital. J Am Vet Med Assoc 235, 50–57.

Hwang, S.O., Kim, S.H., Kim, H., et al., 2008. Comparison of 15:1, 15:2, and 30:2 compression-to-ventilation ratios for cardiopulmonary resuscitation in a canine model of a simulated, witnessed cardiac arrest. Acad Emerg Med 2, 183–189.

Hubbell, J.A.E., Muir, W.W., Gaynor, J.S., 1993. Cardiovascular effects of thoracic compression in horses subjected to euthanasia. Equine Vet J 25, 282–284.

ICCOR, 2010. International Consensus on Cardiopulmonary Resuscitation and Emergency Cardiovascular Care Science With Treatment Recommendations 2010 Circulation 122 (16, suppl 2), S298–S421.

Iff, I., Moens, Y., 2008. Two cases of bradyarrhythmia and hypotension after extradural injections in dogs. Vet Anaesth Analg 35, 265–269.

International Liaison Committee on Resuscitation (ILCOR), 2005. American Heart Association, and European Resuscitation Council. Circulation 112, III-1-III-4.

Jacobs, G., Calvert, C., Kraus, M., 2000. Hepatopathy in 4 dogs treated with amiodarone. J Vet Int Med 14, 96–99.

Janssens, L., Altman, S., Rogers, P.A., 1979. Respiratory and cardiac arrest under general anaesthesia: treatment by acupuncture of the nasal philtrum. Vet Rec 105, 273–276.

Johansson, A.M., Gardner, S.Y., Jones, S.L., et al., 2003. Hypomagnesemia in hospitalized horses. J Vet Int Med 17, 860–867.

Johnston, G.M., Eastman, J.K., Taylor, P.M., et al., 2002. Confidential enquiry of perioperative equine fatalities (CEPEF): mortality results of Phases 1 and 2. Vet Anaesth Analg 29, 159–170.

Kass, P.H., Haskins, S.C., 1992. Survival following cardiopulmonary resuscitation in dogs and cats. Vet Emerg Crit Care 2, 57–65.

Kellagher, R.E.B., Watney, G.C.G., 1986. Cardiac arrest during anaesthesia in two horses. Vet Rec 119, 347–349.

Khanna, C., Lund, E.M., Raffe, M., et al., 1998. Hypomagnesemia in 188 dogs: a hospital population-based prevalence study. J Vet Int Med 2, 304–309.

Kilgannon, J.H., Jones, A.E., Shapiro, N.I., et al., 2010. Association between arterial hyperoxia following resuscitation from cardiac arrest and in-hospital mortality. J Am Med Assoc 303, 2165–2171.

Krieter, H., Denz, C., Janke, C., et al., 2002. Hypertonic-hyperoncotic solutions reduce the release of cardiac troponin i and s-100 after successful cardiopulmonary resuscitation in pigs. Anesth Analg 95, 1031–1036.

Krismer, A.C., Wenzel, V.,Karl, H., et al., 2004. Vasopressin during cardiopulmonary resuscitation: A progress report. Crit Care Med 32 (9, Suppl), S432–S435.

Lagasse, R.S., 2002. Anesthesia safety: model or myth? A review of the published literature and analysis of current original data. Anesthesiology 97, 1609–1617.

Lienhart, A., Auroy, Y., Péquignot, F., et al., 2006. Survey of anesthesia-related mortality in France. Anesthesiology 105 (6), 1087–1097.

Loeckinger, A., Kleinsasser, A., Wenzel, V., et al., 2002. Pulmonary gas exchange after cardiopulmonary resuscitation with either vasopressin or epinephrine. Crit Care Med 30, 2059–2062.

Leong, E.C.M., Bendall, J.C., Boyd, A.C., et al., 2001. Sodium bicarbonate improves the chance of resuscitation after 10 minutes of cardiac arrest in dogs. Resuscitation 51, 309–315.

Lottes, A.E., Rundell, A.E., Geddes, L.A., et al., 2007. Sustained abdominal compression during CPR raises coronary perfusion pressures as much as vasopressor drugs. Resuscitation 75, 515–524.

Mally, S., Jelatancev, A., Grmec, S., 2007. Effects of epinephrine and vasopressin on end-tidal carbon dioxide tension and mean arterial blood pressure in out-of-hospital cardiopulmonary resuscitation: an observational study. Critical Care 11 (2), R39.

McGoldrick, T.M.E., Bowen, I.M., Clarke, K.W., 1998. Sudden cardiac arrest in an anaesthetized horse associated with low venous oxygen tensions. Vet Rec 142, 610–611.

Mentzelopoulos, S.D., Zakynthinos, S.G., Tzoufi, M., et al., 2009. Vasopressin, epinephrine, and corticosteroids for in-hospital cardiac arrest. Arch Intern Med 169, 15–24.

Mitchell, S.J., McCarthy, R., Rudloff, K., et al., 2000. Tracheal rupture associated with intubation in cats: 20 cases (1996–1998). J Am Vet Med Assoc 216, 1592–1595.

Mosing, M., Iff, I.K., Nemetz, W., 2008. Cardiopulmonary arrest and resuscitation following an extradural injection in a normovolemic dog. J Vet Emerg Crit Care 18, 532–536.

Muir, W.W., Hubbell, J.A.E., 2009. Cardiopulmonary resuscitation. In: Muir, W.W., Hubbell, J.A.E. (Eds.), Equine Anesthesia, Monitoring and Emergency Therapy, second ed. Saunders/Elsevier, St Louis, pp. 418–429.

Nagao, K., 2009. Chest compression-only cardiocerebral resuscitation. Curr Opin Crit Care 15, 189–197.

Noppens, R.R., Christ, M., Brambrink, A.M., 2006. An early bolus of hypertonic saline hydroxyethyl starch improves long-term outcome after global cerebral ischemia. Crit Care Med 34, 2194–2200.

Ober, C.P., Spotswood, T.C., Hancock, R., 2006. Fatal venous air embolism in a cat with a retropharyngeal diverticulum. Vet Radiol Ultrasound 47, 153–158.

Pargett, M., Geddes, L.A., Otlewski, M.P., et al., 2008.

Rhythmic abdominal compression CPR ventilates without supplemental breaths and provides effective blood circulation. Resuscitation 79, 460–467.

Pilchera, J., Weatherall, M., Shirtcliffe, P., et al., 2012. The effect of hyperoxia following cardiac arrest - A systematic review and meta-analysis of animal trials. Resuscitation 83, 417–422.

Plunkett, S.J., McMichael, M., 2008. Cardiopulmonary resuscitation in small animal medicine: an update. J Vet Int Med 22, 9–25.

Polderman, K.H., 2008. Hypothermia and neurological outcome after cardiac arrest: state of the art. Eur J Anaesth 25 (S42), 23–30.

Prengel, A.W., Linstedt, U., Zenz, M., et al., 2005. Effects of combined administration of vasopressin, epinephrine, and norepinephrine during cardiopulmonary resuscitation in pigs. Crit Care Med 33, 2587–2591.

Raptopoulos, D., Karatzias, C., 1981. Successful resuscitation after cardiac arrest in a cow. Veterinary Record 109, 17.

Rieser, T.M., 2000. Cardiopulmonary resuscitation. Clin Tech Small Anim Pract 15, 76–81.

Riordan, L.L., Schaer, M., 2009. Potassium disorders. In: Silverstein, D.C., Hopper, K. (Eds.), Small Animal Critical Care Medicine. Saunders Elsevier, St Louis, pp. 229–233.

Ristagno, G., Tang, W., Chang, Y.T., et al., 2007. The quality of chest compressions during CPR overrides importance of timing of defibrillation. Chest 132, 70–75.

Ristagno, G., Tang, W., Huang, L., et al., 2009. Epinephrine reduces cerebral perfusion during cardiopulmonary resuscitation. Crit Care Med 37, 1408–1415.

Rush, J.E., Wingfield, W.E., 1992. Recognition and frequency of dysrhythmias during cardiopulmonary arrest. J Am Vet Med Assoc 200, 1932–1937.

Sanehi, O., Calder, I., 1999. Capnography and the differentiation between tracheal and oesophageal intubation. Anaesthesia 54, 604–605.

Schmittinger, C.A., Astner, S., Astner, L., et al., 2005. Cardiopulmonary resuscitation with vasopressin in a dog. Vet Anaesth Analg 32, 112–114.

Schneider, A., Bottiger, B.W., Popp, E., 2009. Cerebral resuscitation after cardiocirculatory arrest. Anesth Analg 108, 971–979.

Scofield, D.B., Alexander, D.L., Franklin, R.P., et al., 2010. Review of fatalities and adverse reactions after administration of α-2 adrenergic agonist reversal agents in the horse. Proc Am Assoc Eq Pract 56, 44–49.

Scroggin, R.D., Quandt, J., 2009. The use of vasopressin for treating vasodilatory shock and cardiopulmonary arrest. J Vet Emerg Crit Care 19, 135–137.

Somberg, J.C., Timar, S., Bailin, S.J., 2004. Lack of a hypotensive effect with rapid administration of a new aqueous formulation of intravenous Amiodarone. Am J Card 93, 576–581.

Stadlbauer, K.H., MD, Wagner-Berger, H.G., Wenzel, V., et al., 2003. Survival with full neurologic recovery after prolonged cardiopulmonary resuscitation with a combination of vasopressin and epinephrine in pigs. Anesth Analg 96, 1743–1749.

Sternbach, G.L., Varon, J., Fromm Jr, R., et al., 2005. The Resuscitation Greats: The humane societies. Resuscitation 45, 71–75.

Stroumpoulis, K., Xanthos, T., Rokas, G., et al., 2008. Vasopressin and epinephrine in the treatment of cardiac arrest: an experimental study. Crit Care 12, R40.

Tacker, W.A., Geddes, L.A., Rosborough, J.P., et al., 1973. Ventricular defibrillation of a 341 kg horse using precordial electrodes. Can J Comp Med 37, 382–390.

Tiret, L., Desmonts, J.M., Hatton, F., et al., 1986. Complications associated with anaesthesia – a prospective survey in France. Can Anaesth Soc J 33, 336–344.

Waldrop, J.E., Rozanski, E.A., Swank, E.D., et al., 2004. Causes of cardiopulmonary arrest, resuscitation management, and functional outcome in dogs and cats surviving cardiopulmonary arrest. J Vet Emerg Crit Care 14, 22–29.

Wang, T., Tang, W., Sun, S., et al., 2008. Intravenous infusion of bone marrow mesenchymal stem cells improves brain function after resuscitation from cardiac arrest. Crit Care Med 36, S486–S491.

Wenzel, V., Krismer, A.C., Arntz, R., et al., 2004. A comparison of vasopressin and epinephrine for out-of-hospital cardiopulmonary resuscitation. N Engl J Med 350, 105–113.

Wenzel, V., Lindner, K.H., Krismer, A.C., et al., 2000. Survival with full neurologic recovery and no cerebral pathology after prolonged cardiopulmonary resuscitation with vasopressin in pigs. J Am Coll Cardiol 35, 527–533.

Wess, G., Thomas, W.P., Berger, D.M., et al., 2006. Applications, complications, and outcomes of transvenous pacemaker implantation in 105 dogs (1997–2002). J Vet Intern Med 20, 877–884.

Wingfield, W.E., Van Pelt, D.R., 1992. Respiratory and cardiopulmonary arrest in dogs and cats: 265 cases (1986–1991). J Am Vet Med Assoc 200, 1993–1996.

Xanthos, T., Bassiakou, E., Koudouna, E., et al., 2009. Combination pharmacotherapy in the treatment of experimental cardiac arrest. Am J Emerg Med 27, 651–659.

Yu, T., Weil, M.H., Tang, W., et al., 2002. Adverse outcomes of interrupted precordial compression during automated defibrillation. Circulation 106, 368–372.

SUGGESTED READING

As previously mentioned, the most recent ILCOR review of the guidelines for CPCR in humans was published in the October and November 2010 issues of *Resuscitation* (ERC) and *Circulation* (ICCOR and AHA). Further updates to the 2010 guidelines will appear soon thereafter and can be found at www.erc.edu/index.php/ilcor/en/ or www.ilcor.org/en/home/.

American Heart Association (AHA), 2010. Guidelines for Cardiopulmonary Resuscitation and Emergency Cardiovascular Care. 2010 Circulation 122 (18, suppl 3), S640–S933.

Cooper, J.A., Cooper, J.D., Cooper, J.M., 2006. Cardiopulmonary resuscitation: history, current practice, and future direction. Circulation 114, 2839–2849.

Hofmeister, E.H., Brainard, B.M., Egger, C.M., et al., 2009. Prognostic indicators for dogs and cats with cardiopulmonary arrest treated by cardiopulmonary cerebral resuscitation at a university teaching hospital. J Am Vet Med Assoc 235, 50–57.

International Liaison Committee on Resuscitation (ILCOR), 2005. American Heart Association, and European Resuscitation Council, Circulation 112, III-1–III-4.

International Consensus on Cardiopulmonary Resuscitation (ICCOR) and Emergency Cardiovascular Care Science With Treatment Recommendations, 2010.

Circulation 122 (16 suppl 2), S249–S638.

Muir, W.W., Hubbell, J.A.E., 2009. Cardiopulmonary resuscitation. In: Muir, W.W., Hubbell, J.A.E. (Eds.), Equine Anesthesia, Monitoring and Emergency Therapy, second ed. Saunders/Elsevier, St Louis, pp. 418–429.

Neumar, R.W., Nolan, J.P., Adrie, C., et al., 2008. Post-cardiac arrest syndrome epidemiology, pathophysiology, treatment, and prognostication, a consensus statement from ILCOR. Circulation 118, 2452–2483.

Plunkett, S.J., McMichael, M., 2008. Cardiopulmonary resuscitation in small animal medicine: an update. J Vet Intern Med 22, 9–25.

Reassessment Campaign on Veterinary Resuscitation (RECOVER) Initiative, 2012. RECOVER evidence and knowledge gap analysis on veterinary CPR. Parts 1–7. J Vet Emerg Crit Care 22 (S1), S4–S131.

Rush, J.E., Wingfield, W.E., 1992. Recognition and frequency of dysrhythmias during cardiopulmonary arrest. J Am Vet Med Assoc 200, 1932–1937.

Schneider, A., Böttiger, B.W., et al., 2009. Cerebral resuscitation after cardiocirculatory arrest. Anesth Analg 108, 971–979.

Scroggin, R.D., Quandt, J., 2009. The use of vasopressin for treating vasodilatory shock and cardiopulmonary arrest. J Vet Emerg Crit Care 19, 135–137.

Wang, T., Tang, W., Sun, S., et al., 2008. Intravenous infusion of bone marrow mesenchymal stem cells improves brain function after resuscitation from cardiac arrest. Crit Care Med 36, S486–S491.

Wenzel, V., Lindner, K.H., Krismer, A.C., et al., 2000. Survival with full neurologic recovery and no cerebral pathology after prolonged cardiopulmonary resuscitation with vasopressin in pigs. J Am Coll Cardiol 35, 527–533.

Wenzel, V., Krismer, A.C., Arntz, R., et al., 2004. A comparison of vasopressin and epinephrine for out-of-hospital cardiopulmonary resuscitation. N Engl J Med 350, 105–113.

Wess, G., Thomas, W.P., Berger, D.M., et al., 2006. Applications, complications, and outcomes of transvenous pacemaker implantation in 105 dogs (1997–2002). J Vet Intern Med 20, 877–884.

Wingfield, W.E., Van Pelt, D.R., 1992. Respiratory and cardiopulmonary arrest in dogs and cats: 265 cases (1986–1991). J Am Vet Med Assoc 200, 1993–1996.

Xanthos, T., Bassiakou, E., Koudouna, E., et al., 2009. Combination pharmacotherapy in the treatment of experimental cardiac arrest. Am J Emerg Med 27, 651–659.

Yu, T., Weil, M.H., Tang, W., et al., 2002. Adverse outcomes of interrupted precordial compression during automated defibrillation. Circulation 106, 368–372.

Appendix

ABBREVIATIONS

ABG	arterial blood gas
ABP	arterial blood pressure
AC	alternating current
ADH	antidiuretic hormone
AFib	atrial fibrillation
AV	atrioventricular
BAR	standard atmospheric pressure
BMR	basal metabolic rate
BP	blood pressure
Ca^{++} or Ca^{2+}	calcium, calcium ion
CI	cardiac index
CNS	central nervous system
CO	cardiac output
COPD	chronic obstructive airways disease
CPAP	continuous positive airway pressure
CPCR	cardiopulmonary cerebral resuscitation
CSF	cerebrospinal fluid
CVC	caudal vena cava
CVP	central venous pressure
DAP	diastolic arterial pressure
DC	direct current
ECG	electrocardiogram, electrocardiograph
$ETCO_2$	end-tidal carbon dioxide tension or concentration
FiO_2	fractional inspired oxygen percent
FRC	functional residual capacity
g	gramme, gram
Hb	haemoglobin
HCO_3^-	bicarbonate, bicarbonate ion
Hct	haematocrit, packed cell volume
HR	heart rate
IM	intramuscular, intramuscularly
IO	intraosseous, intraosseously
IP	intraperitoneal, intraperitoneally
IPPV	intermittent positive pressure ventilation
IT	intratracheal
IV	intravenous, intravenously
kPa	kilopascal (1 kPa = approximately 7.5 mmHg)
L	litre
MAP	mean arterial pressure
mg	milligramme, milligram
Mg^{++} or Mg^{2+}	magnesium, magnesium ion
mg/kg	milligrammes per kilogramme body weight
mL	millilitre
mL/kg	millilitres per kilogramme body weight
mmH_2O	millimetres of water
mmHg	millimetres of mercury
N_2	nitrogen
N_2O	nitrous oxide
NO	nitric oxide
O_2	oxygen
°C	degree Celsius
°F	degree Fahrenheit
PAWP	pulmonary artery wedge pressure
$PACO_2$	alveolar carbon dioxide tension
$PaCO_2$	arterial carbon dioxide tension
PAO_2	alveolar oxygen tension
PaO_2	arterial oxygen tension
PCO_2	carbon dioxide tension
PEEP	positive end-expiratory pressure
PiO_2	inspired oxygen tension
PO_2	oxygen tension
psi	pounds per square inch
PVC	premature ventricular complex
$P\bar{v}CO_2$	mixed venous carbon dioxide tension
$P\bar{v}O_2$	mixed venous oxygen tension
PVR	(1) pulmonary vascular resistance, (2) peripheral vascular resistance
SAP	systolic arterial pressure
SC	subcutaneous, subcutaneously
SVR	systemic vascular resistance
swg	standard wire gauge
TLC	total lung capacity
UK	United Kingdom
USA	United States of America

Appendix

V_D	respiratory dead space volume
VIC	vaporizer in the (breathing) circuit
VOC	vaporizer outside the (breathing) circuit
V/Q	ventilation: perfusion ratio
µg	microgramme, microgram
µg/kg	microgrammes per kilogramme body weight
µL	microlitre

WEIGHTS

1 gram (g) = weight of 1 mL water at 4°C
1 kilogram (kg) = 1000 g (grams)
1 gram (g) = 1000 mg (milligrams)
1 milligram (mg) = 1000 µg (micrograms)

CONVERSIONS

Measurement	SI unit	Old unit	Conversion factors	
			Old to SI (exact)	SI to old (approx.)
PCO_2	kPa	mmHg	0.133	7.5
PO_2	kPa	mmHg	0.133	7.5
Standard bicarbonate	mmol/L	mEq/L	Equivalent	
Base excess	mmol/L	mEq/L	Equivalent	
Haematocrit (packed cell volume)	Decimal fraction	%	0.01	100
Total protein	g/L	g/100 mL	10.0	0.1
Glucose	mmol/L	mg/100 mL	0.0555	18
Creatinine	µmol/L	mg/100 mL	88.4	0.01
Urea	mmol/L	mg/100 mL	0.166	6.0
Pressure	mmHg	cmH_2O	0.73554	1.36
Weight	kg	lb	0.4545	2.2

Endotracheal tube sizes: The French number is divided by four for conversion to approximate internal diameter in millimetres

UNITS OF PRESSURE

Atmospheric pressure is important in relation to uptake of gases (oxygen and anaesthetic gases). Many different units are used in weather forecasts. Cylinder pressures may be given in psi or BAR. Relevant conversions of the most common are as follows:

The 'Standard Atmosphere' at sea level = 760 mmHg = 29.92 inchesHg = 101.3 kPa = 1013.25 millibar (hectapascals).

1 BAR = 100 kPa = (approx) 14.5038 psi

Index

Page numbers followed by 'f' indicate figures, 't' indicate tables, and 'b' indicate boxes.

Index